CAMPBELL-WALSH

UROLOGY

ELEVENTH EDITION REVIEW

CAMPBELL-WALSH
UROLOGY
ELEVENTH EDITION REVIEW

EDITION 2

Editors

W. SCOTT MCDOUGAL, MD, MA (HON)
Walter S. Kerr, Jr. Distinguished Professor of
Urology
Harvard Medical School
Chief Emeritus, Massachusetts General
Hospital
Boston, Massachusetts

ALAN J. WEIN, MD, PhD (HON), FACS
Founders Professor of Urology
Division of Urology
Penn Medicine, Perelman School of Medicine
Chief of Urology
Division of Urology
Penn Medicine, Hospital of the University of
Pennsylvania
Program Director, Residency in Urology
Division of Urology
Penn Medicine, University of Pennsylvania
Health System
Philadelphia, Pennsylvania

LOUIS R. KAVOUSSI, MD, MBA
Waldbaum-Gardner Distinguished Professor
of Urology
Department of Urology
Hofstra North Shore-LIJ School of Medicine
Hampstead, New York
Chairman of Urology
The Arthur Smith Institute for Urology
Lake Success, New York

ALAN W. PARTIN, MD, PhD
Professor and Director of Urology
Department of Urology
The Johns Hopkins School of Medicine
Baltimore, Maryland

CRAIG A. PETERS, MD
Chief, Surgical Innovation
Principal Investigator
Sheikh Zayed Institute for Pediatric
Surgical Innovation
Children's National Medical Center
Washington, DC

ELSEVIER

ELSEVIER

1600 John F. Kennedy Blvd.
Ste 1800
Philadelphia, PA 19103–2899

CAMPBELL-WALSH UROLOGY ELEVENTH EDITION REVIEW, SECOND EDITION   ISBN: 978-0-323-32830-2

Notices

Knowledge and best practice in this field are constantly changing. As new research and experience broaden our understanding, changes in research methods, professional practices, or medical treatment may become necessary.

Practitioners and researchers must always rely on their own experience and knowledge in evaluating and using any information, methods, compounds, or experiments described herein. In using such information or methods they should be mindful of their own safety and the safety of others, including parties for whom they have a professional responsibility.

With respect to any drug or pharmaceutical products identified, readers are advised to check the most current information provided (i) on procedures featured or (ii) by the manufacturer of each product to be administered, to verify the recommended dose or formula, the method and duration of administration, and contraindications. It is the responsibility of practitioners, relying on their own experience and knowledge of their patients, to make diagnoses, to determine dosages and the best treatment for each individual patient, and to take all appropriate safety precautions.

To the fullest extent of the law, neither the Publisher nor the authors, contributors, or editors, assume any liability for any injury and/or damage to persons or property as a matter of products liability, negligence or otherwise, or from any use or operation of any methods, products, instructions, or ideas contained in the material herein.

Previous edition copyrighted 2012.

Library of Congress Cataloging-in-Publication Data

Campbell-Walsh urology review.
  Campbell-Walsh urology eleventh edition review / editors, W. Scott McDougal, Alan J. Wein, Louis R. Kavoussi, Alan W. Partin, Craig A. Peters. – Second edition.
       p. ; cm.
  Urology eleventh edition review
  A companion to the 11th edition of Campbell-Walsh Urology. This text includes review questions and answers and chapter review points for each chapter of Campbell-Walsh Urology, 11 ed.
  Revised edition of Campbell-Walsh urology tenth edition review / editors, W. Scott McDougal ... [et al.]. c2012.
  ISBN 978-0-323-32830-2 (pbk. : alk. paper)
  I. McDougal, W. Scott (William Scott), 1942- , editor. II. Wein, Alan J., editor. III. Kavoussi, Louis R., editor. IV. Partin, Alan W., editor. V. Peters, Craig (Craig Andrew), editor. VI. Title. VII. Title: Urology eleventh edition review.
  [DNLM: 1. Female Urogenital Diseases–Problems and Exercises. 2. Male Urogenital Diseases–Problems and Exercises. 3. Urology–methods–Problems and Exercises. WJ 18.2]
  RC871
  616.60076–dc23
                                                                        2015025014

Senior Content Strategist: Charlotta Kryhl
Content Development Manager: Katie DeFrancesco
Publishing Services Manager: Patricia Tannian
Project Manager: Amanda Mincher
Senior Book Designer: Amy Buxton

Printed in the United States of America

Last digit is the print number: 9 8 7 6 5 4

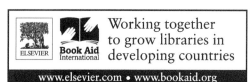

CONTRIBUTORS

Paul Abrams, MD, FRCS
Professor of Urology
Bristol Urological Institute
Southmead Hospital
Bristol, United Kingdom

Mark C. Adams, MD, FAAP
Professor of Urologic Surgery
Department of Urology
Division of Pediatric Urology
Monroe Carell Jr. Children's Hospital at Vanderbilt
Nashville, Tennessee

Mohamad E. Allaf, MD
Associate Professor of Urology, Oncology, and Biomedical
    Engineering
Director of Minimally Invasive and Robotic Surgery
Department of Urology
Brady Urological Institute
Johns Hopkins University School of Medicine
Baltimore, Maryland

Sero Andonian, MD, MSc, FRCS(C), FACS
Assistant Professor
Department of Urology
McGill University
Montreal, Quebec, Canada

Jennifer Tash Anger, MD, MPH
Associate Professor
Department of Surgery
Cedars-Sinai Medical Center;
Adjunct Assistant Professor
Urology
University of California, Los Angeles
Los Angeles, California

Kenneth W. Angermeier, MD
Associate Professor
Glickman Urological and Kidney Institute
Cleveland Clinic
Cleveland, Ohio

Emmanuel S. Antonarakis, MD
Associate Professor of Oncology
Sidney Kimmel Comprehensive Cancer Center
Johns Hopkins University
Baltimore, Maryland

Jodi A. Antonelli, MD
Assistant Professor
Department of Urology
University of Texas Southwestern Medical Center
Dallas, Texas

Anthony Atala, MD
Director, Wake Forest Institute for Regenerative Medicine
William H. Boyce Professor and Chair
Department of Urology
Wake Forest School of Medicine
Winston-Salem, North Carolina

Paul F. Austin, MD
Professor
Division of Urologic Surgery
Washington University School of Medicine in St. Louis
St. Louis, Missouri

Darius J. Bägli, MDCM, FRCSC, FAAP, FACS
Professor of Surgery and Physiology
Division of Urology, Departments of Surgery and
    Physiology
University of Toronto;
Senior Attending Urologist, Associate Surgeon-in-Chief, Senior
    Associate Scientist
Division of Urology, Department of Surgery, Division of
    Developmental and Stem Cell Biology
Sick Kids Hospital and Research Institute
Toronto, Ontario, Canada

Daniel A. Barocas, MD, MPH, FACS
Assistant Professor
Urologic Surgery
Vanderbilt University Medical Center
Nashville, Tennessee

Julia Spencer Barthold, MD
Associate Chief
Surgery/Urology
Nemours/Alfred I. duPont Hospital for Children
Wilmington, Delaware;
Professor
Departments of Urology and Pediatrics
Sidney Kimmel Medical College of Thomas Jefferson University
Philadelphia, Pennsylvania

Stuart B. Bauer, MD
Professor of Surgery (Urology)
Harvard Medical School;
Senior Associate in Urology
Department of Urology
Boston Children's Hospital
Boston, Massachusetts

Arie S. Belldegrun, MD
Roy and Carol Doumani Chair in Urologic Oncology
Professor and Chief, Urologic Oncology
Director, Institute of Urologic Oncology
David Geffen School of Medicine at UCLA
Department of Urology
Ronald Reagan UCLA Medical Center
Los Angeles, California

Mitchell C. Benson, MD
Herbert and Florence Irving Professor and Chairman Emeritus
Department of Urology
Columbia University
Attending Physician
Department of Urology
New York-Presbyterian Hospital/Columbia University Medical Center
New York, New York
Attending Physician
Department of Urology
Mount Sinai Medical Center
Miami Beach, Florida

Brian M. Benway, MD
Director, Comprehensive Kidney Stone Program
Urology Academic Practice
Cedars-Sinai Medical Center
Los Angeles, California

Jonathan Bergman, MD, MPH
Assistant Professor
Departments of Urology and Family Medicine
David Geffen School of Medicine at UCLA
Los Angeles, California

Sara L. Best, MD
Assistant Professor
Department of Urology
University of Wisconsin School of Medicine and
    Public Health
Madison, Wisconsin

Sam B. Bhayani, MD, MS
Professor of Surgery
Urology
Department of Surgery
Washington University School of Medicine in St. Louis;
Vice President, Chief Medical Officer
Barnes West Hospital
St. Louis, Missouri

Lori A. Birder, PhD
Associate Professor of Medicine and Pharmacology
Medicine-Renal Electrolyte Division
University of Pittsburgh School of Medicine
Pittsburgh, Pennsylvania

Jay T. Bishoff, MD, FACS
Director, Intermountain Urological Institute
Intermountain Health Care
Salt Lake City, Utah

Brian G. Blackburn, MD
Clinical Associate Professor
Department of Internal Medicine/Infectious Diseases and
    Geographic Medicine
Stanford University School of Medicine
Stanford, California

Jeremy Matthew Blumberg, MD
Chief of Urology
Harbor-UCLA Medical Center
Assistant Professor of Urology
David Geffen School of Medicine at UCLA
Los Angeles, California

Michael L. Blute, Sr., MD
Chief, Department of Urology
Walter S. Kerr, Jr., Professor of Urology
Massachusetts General Hospital/Harvard Medical School
Boston, Massachusetts

Timothy B. Boone, MD, PhD
Professor and Chair
Department of Urology
Houston Methodist Hospital and Research Institute
Houston, Texas
Professor
Department of Urology
Weill Medical College of Cornell University
New York, New York

Stephen A. Boorjian, MD
Professor of Urology
Department of Urology
Mayo Clinic
Rochester, Minnesota

Joseph G. Borer, MD
Associate Professor of Surgery (Urology)
Harvard Medical School
Reconstructive Urologic Surgery Chair
Director, Neurourology and Urodynamics
Director, Bladder Exstrophy Program
Department of Urology
Boston Children's Hospital
Boston, Massachusetts

Charles B. Brendler, MD
Co-Director, John and Carol Walter Center for Urological
    Health
Department of Surgery
Division of Urology
NorthShore University HealthSystem
Evanston, Illinois
Senior Clinician Educator
Department of Surgery
Division of Urology
University of Chicago Pritzker School of Medicine
Chicago, Illinois

Gregory A. Broderick, MD
Professor of Urology
Mayo Clinic College of Medicine
Program Director, Urology Residency Program
Mayo Clinic
Jacksonville, Florida

James D. Brooks, MD
Keith and Jan Hurlbut Professor
Chief of Urologic Oncology
Department of Urology
Stanford University
Stanford, California

Benjamin M. Brucker, MD
Assistant Professor
Urology and Obstetrics and Gynecology
NYU Langone Medical Center
New York, New York

Kathryn L. Burgio, PhD
Professor of Medicine
Department of Medicine
Division of Gerontology, Geriatrics, and Palliative Care
University of Alabama at Birmingham;
Associate Director for Research
Birmingham/Atlanta Geriatric Research, Education
    and Clinical Center
Birmingham VA Medical Center
Birmingham, Alabama

Arthur L. Burnett II, MD, MBA, FACS
Patrick C. Walsh Distinguished Professor of Urology
Department of Urology
Johns Hopkins University School of Medicine
Baltimore, Maryland

Nicol Corbin Bush, MD, MSCS
Co-Director, PARC Urology
Dallas, Texas

Jeffrey A. Cadeddu, MD
Professor of Urology and Radiology
Department of Urology
University of Texas Southwestern Medical Center
Dallas, Texas

Anthony A. Caldamone, MD, MMS, FAAP, FACS
Professor of Surgery (Urology)
Division of Urology
Section of Pediatric Urology
Warren Alpert Medical School of Brown University;
Chief of Pediatric Urology
Division of Pediatric Urology
Hasbro Children's Hospital
Providence, Rhode Island

Steven C. Campbell, MD, PhD
Professor of Surgery
Department of Urology
Glickman Urological and Kidney Institute
Cleveland Clinic
Cleveland, Ohio

Douglas A. Canning, MD
Professor of Urology (Surgery)
Perelman School of Medicine
University of Pennsylvania
Chief, Division of Urology
The Children's Hospital of Philadelphia
Philadelphia, Pennsylvania

Michael A. Carducci, MD
AEGON Professor in Prostate Cancer Research
Sidney Kimmel Comprehensive Cancer Center
Johns Hopkins University
Baltimore, Maryland

Peter R. Carroll, MD, MPH
Professor and Chair
Ken and Donna Derr–Chevron Distinguished Professor
Department of Urology
University of California, San Francisco
San Francisco, California

Herbert Ballentine Carter, MD
Professor of Urology and Oncology
Department of Urology
Johns Hopkins School of Medicine and James Buchanan Brady
    Urological Institute
Baltimore, Maryland

Clint Cary, MD, MPH
Assistant Professor
Department of Urology
Indiana University
Indianapolis, Indiana

Pasquale Casale, MD
Professor
Department of Urology
Columbia University Medical Center;
Chief, Pediatric Urology
Morgan Stanley Children's Hospital of New York-Presbyterian
New York, New York

William J. Catalona, MD
Professor
Department of Urology
Northwestern University Feinberg School of Medicine
Chicago, Illinois

Frank A. Celigoj, MD
Male Infertility/Andrology Fellow
Department of Urology
University of Virginia
Charlottesville, Virginia

Toby C. Chai, MD
Vice Chair of Research
Department of Urology
Yale School of Medicine
Co-Director of Female Pelvic Medicine and Reconstructive Surgery
    Program
Department of Urology
Yale New Haven Hospital
New Haven, Connecticut

Alicia H. Chang, MD, MS
Instructor
Department of Internal Medicine/Infectious Diseases and
    Geographic Medicine
Stanford University School of Medicine
Stanford, California
Medical Consultant
Los Angeles County Tuberculosis Control Program
Los Angeles County Department of Public Health
Los Angeles, California

Christopher R. Chapple, MD, FRCS (Urol)
Professor and Consultant Urologist
Department of Urology
The Royal Hallamshire Hospital
Sheffield Teaching Hospitals
Sheffield, South Yorkshire, United Kingdom

Mang L. Chen, MD
Assistant Professor
Department of Urology
University of Pittsburgh
Pittsburgh, Pennsylvania

Ronald C. Chen, MD, MPH
Associate Professor
Department of Radiation Oncology
University of North Carolina at Chapel Hill
Chapel Hill, North Carolina

Benjamin I. Chung, MD
Assistant Professor
Department of Urology
Stanford University School of Medicine
Stanford, California

Michael J. Conlin, MD, MCR
Associate Professor of Urology
Portland VA Medical Center
Portland, Oregon

Christopher S. Cooper, MD, FAAP, FACS
Professor
Department of Urology
University of Iowa
Associate Dean, Student Affairs and Curriculum
University of Iowa Carver College of Medicine
Iowa City, Iowa

Raymond A. Costabile, MD
Jay Y. Gillenwater Professor of Urology
Department of Urology
University of Virginia
Charlottesville, Virginia

Paul L. Crispen, MD
Assistant Professor
Department of Urology
University of Florida
Gainesville, Florida

Juanita M. Crook, MD, FRCPC
Professor
Division of Radiation Oncology
University of British Columbia, Okanagan
Radiation Oncologist
Center for the Southern Interior
British Columbia Cancer Agency
Kelowna, British Columbia, Canada

Douglas M. Dahl, MD, FACS
Associate Professor of Surgery
Harvard Medical School
Chief, Division of Urologic Oncology
Department of Urology
Massachusetts General Hospital
Boston, Massachusetts

Marc Arnaldo Dall-Era, MD
Assistant Professor
Department of Urology
University of California, Davis
Sacramento, California

Anthony V. D'Amico, MD, PhD
Eleanor Theresa Walters Distinguished Professor and Chief of
    Genitourinary Radiation Oncology
Department of Radiation Oncology
Brigham and Women's Hospital and Dana-Farber Cancer Institute
Boston, Massachusetts

Siamak Daneshmand, MD
Professor of Urology (Clinical Scholar)
Institute of Urology
University of Southern California
Los Angeles, California

John W. Davis, MD, FACS
Associate Professor
Division of Surgery
Director, Urosurgical Prostate Program
Department of Urology
The University of Texas MD Anderson Cancer Center
Houston, Texas

Shubha De, MD, FRCPC
Assistant Professor
University of Alberta
Edmonton, Alberta, Canada

G. Joel DeCastro, MD, MPH
Assistant Professor of Urology
Department of Urology
New York-Presbyterian Hospital/Columbia University
    Medical Center
New York, New York

Michael C. Degen, MD, MA
Clinical Assistant
Department of Urology
Hackensack University Medical Center
Hackensack, New Jersey

Sevag Demirjian, MD
Assistant Professor
Cleveland Clinic Lerner College of Medicine
Department of Nephrology and Hypertension
Cleveland Clinic
Cleveland, Ohio

Francisco Tibor Dénes, MD, PhD
Associate Professor
Division of Urology
Chief, Pediatric Urology
University of São Paulo Medical School
Hospital das Clínicas
São Paulo, Brazil

John D. Denstedt, MD, FRCSC, FACS
Professor of Urology
Chairman of the Department of Surgery
Western University
London, Ontario, Canada

Theodore L. DeWeese, MD, MPH
Professor and Chair
Radiation Oncology and Molecular Radiation Sciences
Johns Hopkins University School of Medicine
Baltimore, Maryland

David Andrew Diamond, MD
Urologist-in-Chief
Department of Urology
Boston Children's Hospital
Professor of Surgery (Urology)
Department of Surgery
Harvard Medical School
Boston, Massachusetts

Colin P.N. Dinney, MD
Chairman and Professor
Department of Urology
The University of Texas MD Anderson Cancer Center
Houston, Texas

Roger R. Dmochowski, MD, MMHC, FACS
Professor of Urology and Gynecology
Vanderbilt University Medical School
Nashville, Tennessee

Charles G. Drake, MD, PhD
Associate Professor of Oncology, Immunology, and Urology
James Buchanan Brady Urological Institute
Johns Hopkins University
Attending Physician
Department of Oncology
Johns Hopkins Kimmel Cancer Center
Baltimore, Maryland

Marcus John Drake, DM, MA, FRCS (Urol)
Senior Lecturer in Urology
School of Clinical Sciences
University of Bristol
Consultant Urologist
Bristol Urological Institute
Southmead Hospital
Bristol, United Kingdom

Brian D. Duty, MD
Assistant Professor of Urology
Oregon Health & Science University
Portland, Oregon

James A. Eastham, MD
Chief, Urology Service
Surgery
Memorial Sloan Kettering Cancer Center
Professor
Department of Urology
Weill Cornell Medical Center
New York, New York

Louis Eichel, MD
Chief, Division of Urology
Rochester General Hospital
Director, Minimally Invasive Surgery
Center for Urology
Rochester, New York

J. Francois Eid, MD
Attending Physician
Department of Urology
Lenox Hill Hospital
North Shore-LIJ Health System
New York, New York

Mario A. Eisenberger, MD
R. Dale Hughes Professor of Oncology and Urology
Sidney Kimmel Comprehensive Cancer Center
Johns Hopkins University
Baltimore, Maryland

Mohamed Aly Elkoushy, MD, MSc, PhD
Associate Professor
Department of Urology
Faculty of Medicine
Suez Canal University
Ismailia, Egypt

Jonathan I. Epstein, MD
Professor of Pathology, Urology, and Oncology
Reinhard Professor of Urological Pathology
Director of Surgical Pathology
The Johns Hopkins Medical Institutions
Baltimore, Maryland

Carlos R. Estrada, Jr., MD
Associate Professor of Surgery
Harvard Medical School
Director, Center for Spina Bifida and Spinal Cord Conditions
Co-Director, Urodynamics and Neurourology
Boston Children's Hospital
Boston, Massachusetts

Michael N. Ferrandino, MD
Assistant Professor
Division of Urologic Surgery
Duke University Medical Center
Durham, North Carolina

Lynne R. Ferrari, MD
Associate Professor of Anesthesiology
Department of Anaesthesia
Harvard Medical School
Medical Director, Perioperative Services and
    Operating Rooms
Chief, Division of Perioperative Anesthesia
Robert M. Smith Chair in Pediatric Anesthesia
Department of Anesthesiology, Perioperative and
    Pain Medicine
Boston Children's Hospital
Boston, Massachusetts

Fernando A. Ferrer, MD
Peter J. Deckers, MD, Endowed Chair of Pediatric Surgery
Surgeon-in-Chief
Director, Division of Urology
Connecticut Children's Medical Center
Hartford, Connecticut
Vice Chair
Department of Surgery
Professor of Surgery, Pediatrics, and Cell Biology
University of Connecticut School of Medicine
Farmington, Connecticut

Richard S. Foster, MD
Professor
Department of Urology
Indiana University
Indianapolis, Indiana

Dominic Frimberger, MD
Professor of Urology
Department of Urology
University of Oklahoma
Oklahoma City, Oklahoma

Pat F. Fulgham, MD
Director of Surgical Oncology
Texas Health Presbyterian Dallas
Dallas, Texas

John P. Gearhart, MD
Professor of Pediatric Urology
Department of Urology
Johns Hopkins University School of Medicine
Baltimore, Maryland

Glenn S. Gerber, MD
Professor
Department of Surgery
University of Chicago Pritzker School of Medicine
Chicago, Illinois

Bruce R. Gilbert, MD, PhD
Professor of Urology
Hofstra North Shore-LIJ School of Medicine
New Hyde Park, New York

Scott M. Gilbert, MD
Associate Member
Department of Genitourinary Oncology
H. Lee Moffitt Cancer Center and Research Institute
Tampa, Florida

Timothy D. Gilligan, MD, MS
Associate Professor of Medicine
Department of Solid Tumor Oncology
Cleveland Clinic Lerner College of Medicine
Co-Director, Center for Excellence in Healthcare
    Communication
Program Director, Hematology/Oncology Fellowship
Medical Director, Inpatient Solid Tumor Oncology
Taussig Cancer Institute
Cleveland Clinic
Cleveland, Ohio

David A. Goldfarb, MD
Professor of Surgery
Cleveland Clinic Lerner College of Medicine
Surgical Director, Renal Transplant Program
Glickman Urological and Kidney Institute
Cleveland Clinic
Cleveland, Ohio

Irwin Goldstein, MD
Director of Sexual Medicine
Alvarado Hospital
Clinical Professor of Surgery
University of California, San Diego
Director, San Diego Sexual Medicine
San Diego, California

Marc Goldstein, MD, DSc (Hon), FACS
Matthew P. Hardy Distinguished Professor of Urology and Male
    Reproductive Medicine
Department of Urology and Institute for Reproductive
    Medicine
Weill Medical College of Cornell University
Surgeon-In-Chief, Male Reproductive
    Medicine and Surgery
New York-Presbyterian Hospital/Weill Cornell Medical
    Center
Adjunct Senior Scientist
Population Council
Center for Biomedical Research at Rockefeller University
New York, New York

Leonard G. Gomella, MD, FACS
Bernard Godwin Professor of Prostate Cancer and Chair
Department of Urology
Associate Director, Sidney Kimmel Cancer Center
Thomas Jefferson University
Philadelphia, Pennsylvania

Mark L. Gonzalgo, MD, PhD
Professor of Urology
University of Miami Miller School of Medicine
Miami, Florida

Hans Albin Gritsch, MD
Surgical Director, Kidney Transplant
Department of Urology
University of California, Los Angeles
Los Angeles, California

Frederick A. Gulmi, MD
Chairman and Residency Program Director
Chief, Division of Minimally Invasive and
    Robotic Surgery
Department of Urology
Brookdale University Hospital and Medical Center
Brooklyn, New York
Clinical Associate Professor of Urology
New York Medical College
Valhalla, New York

Khurshid A. Guru, MD
Robert P. Huben Endowed Professor of Urologic Oncology
Director, Robotic Surgery
Department of Urology
Roswell Park Cancer Institute
Buffalo, New York

Thomas J. Guzzo, MD, MPH
Associate Professor of Urology
Penn Medicine, Perelman School of Medicine
Division of Urology
Hospital of the University of Pennsylvania
University of Pennsylvania Health System
Philadelphia, Pennsylvania

Jennifer A. Hagerty, DO
Attending Physician
Surgery/Urology
Nemours/Alfred I. duPont Hospital for Children
Wilmington, Delaware
Assistant Professor
Departments of Urology and Pediatrics
Sidney Kimmel Medical College of Thomas
    Jefferson University
Philadelphia, Pennsylvania

Ethan J. Halpern, MD, MSCE
Professor of Radiology and Urology
Department of Radiology
Thomas Jefferson University
Philadelphia, Pennsylvania

Misop Han, MD, MS
David Hall McConnell Associate Professor
    in Urology and Oncology
Johns Hopkins University School of Medicine
Baltimore, Maryland

Philip M. Hanno, MD, MPH
Professor of Urology
Department of Surgery
University of Pennsylvania
Philadelphia, Pennsylvania

Hashim Hashim, MBBS, MRCS (Eng), MD, FEBU,
FRCS (Urol)
Consultant Urological Surgeon and Director of the
    Urodynamics Unit
Continence and Urodynamics Unit
Bristol Urological Institute
Bristol, United Kingdom

Sender Herschorn, MD, FRCSC
Professor
Division of Urology
University of Toronto
Urologist
Division of Urology
Sunnybrook Health Sciences Centre
Toronto, Ontario, Canada

Piet Hoebeke, MD, PhD
Full Professor
Ghent University
Chief of Department of Urology and Pediatric Urology
Ghent University Hospital
Ghent, Belgium

Michael H. Hsieh, MD, PhD
Associate Professor
Departments of Urology (primary), Pediatrics
    (secondary)
and Microbiology, Immunology, and Tropical Medicine
    (secondary)
The George Washington University
Washington, DC
Attending Physician
Division of Urology
Children's National Health System
Washington, DC
Stirewalt Endowed Director
Biomedical Research Institute
Rockville, Maryland

Tung-Chin Hsieh, MD
Assistant Professor of Surgery
Department of Urology
University of California, San Diego
La Jolla, California

Douglas A. Husmann, MD
Professor
Department of Urology
Mayo Clinic
Rochester, Minnesota

Thomas W. Jarrett, MD
Professor and Chairman
Department of Urology
George Washington University
Washington, DC

J. Stephen Jones, MD, MBA, FACS
President, Regional Hospitals and Family Health Centers
Cleveland Clinic
Cleveland, Ohio

Gerald H. Jordan, MD, FACS, FAAP (Hon), FRCS (Hon)
Professor
Department of Urology

Eastern Virginia Medical School
Norfolk, Virginia

David B. Joseph, MD, FACS, FAAP
Chief of Pediatric Urology
Children's Hospital at Alabama
Professor of Urology
Department of Urology
University of Alabama at Birmingham
Birmingham, Alabama

Martin Kaefer, MD
Professor
Department of Urology
Indiana University School of Medicine
Indianapolis, Indiana

Jose A. Karam, MD
Assistant Professor
Department of Urology
The University of Texas MD Anderson Cancer Center
Houston, Texas

Louis R. Kavoussi, MD, MBA
Waldbaum-Gardner Distinguished Professor of Urology
Department of Urology
Hofstra North Shore-LIJ School of Medicine
Hampstead, New York
Chairman of Urology
The Arthur Smith Institute for Urology
Lake Success, New York

Parviz K. Kavoussi, MD
Reproductive Urologist
Austin Fertility & Reproductive Medicine
Adjunct Assistant Professor
Neuroendocrinology and Motivation Laboratory
Department of Psychology
The University of Texas at Austin
Austin, Texas

Antoine E. Khoury, MD, FRCSC, FAAP
Walter R. Schmid Professor of Urology
University of California, Irvine
Head of Pediatric Urology
CHOC Children's Urology Center
Children's Hospital of Orange County
Orange, California

Roger S. Kirby, MD, FRCS
Medical Director
The Prostate Center
London, United Kingdom

Eric A. Klein, MD
Chairman
Glickman Urological and Kidney Institute
Cleveland Clinic
Professor of Surgery
Cleveland Clinic Lerner College of Medicine
Cleveland, Ohio

David James Klumpp, PhD
Associate Professor
Department of Urology
Northwestern University
    Feinberg School of Medicine
Chicago, Illinois

Bodo E. Knudsen, MD, FRCSC
Associate Professor and Interim Chair, Clinical Operations
Department of Urology
Wexner Medical Center
The Ohio State University
Columbus, Ohio

Kathleen C. Kobashi, MD, FACS
Section Head
Urology and Renal Transplantation
Virginia Mason Medical Center
Seattle, Washington

Thomas F. Kolon, MD, MS
Associate Professor of Urology (Surgery)
Perelman School of Medicine
University of Pennsylvania
Director, Pediatric Urology Fellowship Program
The Children's Hospital of Philadelphia
Philadelphia, Pennsylvania

Bridget F. Koontz, MD
Butler-Harris Assistant Professor
Department of Radiation Oncology
Duke University Medical Center
Durham, North Carolina

Martin Allan Koyle, MD, FAAP, FACS, FRCSC, FRCS (Eng)
Division Head
Pediatric Urology
Women's Auxiliary Chair in Urology and Regenerative
    Medicine
Hospital for Sick Children
Professor
Department of Surgery
Division of Urology
Institute of Health Policy, Management, and Evaluation
University of Toronto
Toronto, Ontario, Canada

Amy E. Krambeck, MD
Associate Professor
Department of Urology
Mayo Clinic
Rochester, Minnesota

Ryan M. Krlin, MD
Assistant Professor of Urology
Department of Urology
Louisiana State University Health Science Center
New Orleans, Louisiana

Bradley P. Kropp, MD, FAAP, FACS
Professor of Pediatric Urology
Department of Urology
University of Oklahoma Health Sciences Center
Oklahoma City, Oklahoma

Alexander Kutikov, MD, FACS
Associate Professor of Urologic Oncology
Department of Surgery
Fox Chase Cancer Center
Philadelphia, Pennsylvania

Raymond S. Lance, MD
The Paul F. Schellhammer Professor of Cancer Research
Associate Professor
Departments of Urology and Microbiology and
    Cancer Biology
Eastern Virginia Medical School
Sentara Norfolk General Hospital
Sentara Medical Group–Urology of Virginia
Norfolk, Virginia

Jaime Landman, MD
Professor of Urology and Radiology
Chairman, Department of Urology
University of California, Irvine
Orange, California

Brian R. Lane, MD, PhD
Betz Family Endowed Chair for Cancer Research
Spectrum Health Regional Cancer Center
Chief of Urology
Spectrum Health Medical Group
Associate Professor of Surgery
Michigan State University
Grand Rapids, Michigan

Stephen Larsen, MD
Chief Resident
Department of Urology
Rush University Medical Center
Chicago, Illinois

Eugene Kang Lee, MD
Assistant Professor
Department of Urology
University of Kansas Medical Center
Kansas City, Kansas

Richard S. Lee, MD
Assistant Professor of Surgery (Urology)
Harvard Medical School
Department of Urology
Boston Children's Hospital
Boston, Massachusetts

W. Robert Lee, MD, MEd, MS
Professor
Department of Radiation Oncology
Duke University School of Medicine
Durham, North Carolina

Dan Leibovici, MD
Chairman of Urology
Kaplan Hospital
Rehovot, Israel

Gary E. Lemack, MD
Professor of Urology and Neurology
Department of Urology
University of Texas Southwestern Medical Center
Dallas, Texas

Herbert Lepor, MD
Professor and Martin Spatz Chairman
Department of Urology
NYU Langone Medical Center
New York, New York

Laurence A. Levine, MD, FACS
Professor
Department of Urology
Rush University Medical Center
Chicago, Illinois

Sey Kiat Lim, MBBS, MRCS (Edinburgh), MMed (Surgery),
    FAMS (Urology)
Consultant
Department of Urology
Changi General Hospital
Singapore

W. Marston Linehan, MD
Chief, Urologic Oncology Branch
Physician-in-Chief, Urologic Surgery
National Cancer Institute
National Institutes of Health Clinical Center
Bethesda, Maryland

James E. Lingeman, MD
Professor
Department of Urology
Indiana University School of Medicine
Indianapolis, Indiana

Richard Edward Link, MD, PhD
Associate Professor of Urology
Director, Division of Endourology and Minimally Invasive
    Surgery
Scott Department of Urology
Baylor College of Medicine
Houston, Texas

Michael E. Lipkin, MD
Associate Professor
Division of Urologic Surgery
Duke University Medical Center
Durham, North Carolina

Mark S. Litwin, MD, MPH
The Fran and Ray Stark Foundation Chair in Urology
Professor of Urology and
    Health Policy & Management
David Geffen School of Medicine at UCLA
UCLA Fielding School of Public Health
Los Angeles, California

Stacy Loeb, MD, MSc
Assistant Professor
Urology, Population Health, and Laura and Isaac Perlmutter
    Cancer Center
New York University and
    Manhattan Veterans Affairs
New York, New York

Armando J. Lorenzo, MD, MSc, FRCSC, FAAP, FACS
Staff Paediatric Urologist
Hospital for Sick Children
Associate Scientist
Research Institute, Child Health Evaluative Sciences
Associate Professor
Department of Surgery
Division of Urology
University of Toronto
Toronto, Ontario, Canada

Yair Lotan, MD
Professor
Department of Urology
University of Texas Southwestern
    Medical Center
Dallas, Texas

Tom F. Lue, MD, ScD (Hon), FACS
Professor
Department of Urology
University of California, San Francisco
San Francisco, California

Dawn Lee MacLellan, MD, FRCSC
Associate Professor
Departments of Urology and Pathology
Dalhousie University
Halifax, Nova Scotia, Canada

Vitaly Margulis, MD
Assistant Professor
Department of Urology
University of Texas Southwestern
    Medical Center
Dallas, Texas

Stephen David Marshall, MD
Chief Resident
Department of Urology
SUNY Downstate College of Medicine
Brooklyn, New York

Aaron D. Martin, MD, MPH
Assistant Professor
Department of Urology
Louisiana State University Health Sciences Center
Pediatric Urology
Children's Hospital New Orleans
New Orleans, Louisiana

Darryl T. Martin, PhD
Associate Research Scientist
Department of Urology
Yale University School of Medicine
New Haven, Connecticut

Neil Martin, MD, MPH
Assistant Professor
Department of Radiation Oncology
Brigham and Women's Hospital and Dana-Farber
    Cancer Institute
Boston, Massachusetts

Timothy A. Masterson, MD
Associate Professor
Department of Urology
Indiana University Medical Center
Indianapolis, Indiana

Ranjiv Mathews, MD
Professor of Urology and Pediatrics
Director of Pediatric Urology
Southern Illinois University School of Medicine
Springfield, Illinois

Surena F. Matin, MD
Professor
Department of Urology
Medical Director
Minimally Invasive New Technology in Oncologic
    Surgery (MINTOS)
The University of Texas MD Anderson Cancer Center
Houston, Texas

Brian R. Matlaga, MD, MPH
Professor
James Buchanan Brady Urological Institute
Johns Hopkins Medical Institutions
Baltimore, Maryland

Richard S. Matulewicz, MS, MD
Department of Urology
Northwestern University Feinberg School of Medicine
Chicago, Illinois

Kurt A. McCammon, MD, FACS
Devine Chair in Genitourinary Reconstructive Surgery
Chairman and Program Director
Professor
Department of Urology
Eastern Virginia Medical School
Sentara Norfolk General Hospital
Urology
Norfolk, Virginia
Devine-Jordan Center for Reconstructive Surgery and
    Pelvic Health
Urology of Virginia, PLLC
Virginia Beach, Virginia

James M. McKiernan, MD
Chairman
Department of Urology
New York-Presbyterian Hospital/Columbia University
    Medical Center
New York, New York

Alan W. McMahon, MD
Associate Professor
Department of Medicine
University of Alberta
Edmonton, Alberta, Canada

Chris G. McMahon, MBBS, FAChSHM
Director, Australian Centre for Sexual Health
Sydney, New South Wales, Australia

Thomas Anthony McNicholas, MB, BS, FRCS, FEBU
Consultant Urologist and Visiting Professor
Department of Urology
Lister Hospital and University of Hertfordshire
Stevenage, United Kingdom

Kevin T. McVary, MD, FACS
Professor and Chairman, Division of Urology
Department of Surgery
Southern Illinois University School of Medicine
Springfield, Illinois

Alan K. Meeker, PhD
Assistant Professor of Pathology
Assistant Professor of Urology
Assistant Professor of Oncology
Johns Hopkins University School of Medicine
Baltimore, Maryland

Kirstan K. Meldrum, MD
Chief, Division of Pediatric Urology
Professor of Surgery
Michigan State University
Helen DeVos Children's Hospital
Grand Rapids, Michigan

Cathy Mendelsohn, PhD
Professor
Departments of Urology, Pathology, and Genetics &
    Development
Columbia University College of Physicians and
    Surgeons
New York, New York

Maxwell V. Meng, MD
Professor
Chief, Urologic Oncology
Department of Urology
University of California
San Francisco
San Francisco, California

David C. Miller, MD, MPH
Assistant Professor
Department of Urology
University of Michigan Medical School
Ann Arbor, Michigan

Alireza Moinzadeh, MD
Director of Robotic Surgery
Institute of Urology
Lahey Hospital & Medical Center
Burlington, Massachusetts
Assistant Professor
Department of Urology
Tufts University School of Medicine
Boston, Massachusetts

Manoj Monga, MD, FACS
Director, Stevan B. Streem Center for Endourology and
    Stone Disease
Glickman Urological and Kidney Institute
Cleveland Clinic
Cleveland, Ohio

Allen F. Morey, MD, FACS
Professor
Department of Urology
University of Texas Southwestern Medical Center
Dallas, Texas

Todd M. Morgan, MD
Assistant Professor
Department of Urology
University of Michigan
Ann Arbor, Michigan

Ravi Munver, MD, FACS
Vice Chairman
Chief of Minimally Invasive and Robotic
    Urologic Surgery
Department of Urology
Hackensack University Medical Center
Hackensack, New Jersey
Associate Professor of Surgery (Urology)
Department of Surgery

Division of Urology
Rutgers New Jersey Medical School
Newark, New Jersey

Stephen Y. Nakada, MD, FACS
Professor and Chairman
The David T. Uehling Chair of Urology
Department of Urology
University of Wisconsin School of Medicine and
    Public Health
Chief of Service
Department of Urology
University of Wisconsin Hospital and Clinics
Madison, Wisconsin

Leah Yukie Nakamura, MD
Associate in Urology
Orange County Urology Associates
Laguna Niguel, California

Neema Navai, MD
Assistant Professor
Department of Urology
The University of Texas MD Anderson Cancer Center
Houston, Texas

Joel B. Nelson, MD
Frederic N. Schwentker Professor and Chairman
Department of Urology
University of Pittsburgh School of Medicine
Pittsburgh, Pennsylvania

Diane K. Newman, DNP, ANP-BC, FAAN
Adjunct Associate Professor of Urology in Surgery
Division of Urology
Research Investigator Senior
Perelman School of Medicine
University of Pennsylvania
Co-Director, Penn Center for
    Continence and Pelvic Health
Division of Urology
Penn Medicine
Philadelphia, Pennsylvania

Paul L. Nguyen, MD
Associate Professor
Department of Radiation Oncology
Harvard Medical School
Director of Prostate Brachytherapy
Department of Radiation Oncology
Brigham and Women's Hospital and Dana-Farber
    Cancer Institute
Boston, Massachusetts

J. Curtis Nickel, MD, FRCSC
Professor and Canada Research Chair
Department of Urology
Queen's University
Kingston, Ontario, Canada

Craig Stuart Niederberger, MD, FACS
Clarence C. Saelhof Professor and Head
Department of Urology
University of Illinois at Chicago College of Medicine
Professor of Bioengineering
University of Illinois at
    Chicago College of Engineering
Chicago, Illinois

Victor W. Nitti, MD
Professor
Urology and Obstetrics and Gynecology
NYU Langone Medical Center
New York, New York

Victoria F. Norwood, MD
Robert J. Roberts Professor of Pediatrics
Chief of Pediatric Nephrology
Department of Pediatrics
University of Virginia
Charlottesville, Virginia

L. Henning Olsen, MD, DMSc, FEAPU, FEBU
Professor
Department of Urology & Institute of Clinical Medicine
Section of Pediatric Urology
Aarhus University Hospital & Aarhus University
Aarhus, Denmark

Aria F. Olumi, MD
Associated Professor of Surgery/Urology
Department of Urology
Massachusetts General Hospital/Harvard Medical
    School
Boston, Massachusetts

Michael Ordon, MD, MSc, FRCSC
Assistant Professor
Division of Urology
University of Toronto
Toronto, Ontario, Canada

David James Osborn, MD
Assistant Professor
Division of Urology
Walter Reed National Military
    Medical Center
Uniformed Services University
Bethesda, Maryland

Nadir I. Osman, MBChB (Hons), PhD, MRCS
Department of Urology
The Royal Hallmashire Hospital Sheffield Teaching
    Hospitals
Sheffield, South Yorkshire, United Kingdom

Ganesh S. Palapattu, MD
Chief of Urologic Oncology
Associate Professor
Department of Urology
University of Michigan
Ann Arbor, Michigan

Drew A. Palmer, MD
Institute of Urology
Lahey Hospital & Medical Center
Burlington, Massachusetts
Clinical Associate
Tufts University School of Medicine
Boston, Massachusetts

Jeffrey S. Palmer, MD, FACS, FAAP
Director
Pediatric and Adolescent Urology Institute
Cleveland, Ohio

Lane S. Palmer, MD, FACS, FAAP
Professor and Chief
Pediatric Urology
Cohen Children's Medical Center of New York/Hofstra North
    Shore-LIJ School of Medicine
Long Island, New York

John M. Park, MD
Cheng Yang Chang Professor of Pediatric Urology
Department of Urology
University of Michigan Medical School
Ann Arbor, Michigan

J. Kellogg Parsons, MD, MHS, FACS
Associate Professor
Department of Urology
Moores Comprehensive Cancer Center
University of California, San Diego
La Jolla, California

Alan W. Partin, MD, PhD
Professor and Director of Urology
Department of Urology
Johns Hopkins School of Medicine
Baltimore, Maryland

Margaret S. Pearle, MD, PhD
Professor
Departments of Urology and Internal Medicine
University of Texas Southwestern Medical Center
Dallas, Texas

Craig A. Peters, MD
Chief, Surgical Innovation
Principal Investigator
Sheikh Zayed Institute for Pediatric Surgical Innovation
Children's National Medical Center
Washington, DC

Andrew Peterson, MD, FACS
Associate Professor
Urology Residency Program Director
Surgery
Duke University
Durham, North Carolina

Curtis A. Pettaway, MD
Professor
Department of Urology
The University of Texas MD Anderson Cancer Center
Houston, Texas

Louis L. Pisters, MD
Professor
Department of Urology
The University of Texas MD Anderson Cancer Center
Houston, Texas

Emilio D. Poggio, MD
Associate Professor of Medicine
Cleveland Clinic Learner College of Medicine
Medical Director, Kidney and Pancreas Transplant Program
Department of Nephrology and Hypertension

Cleveland Clinic
Cleveland, Ohio

Hans G. Pohl, MD, FAAP
Associate Professor of Urology and Pediatrics
Children's National Medical Center
Washington, DC

Michel Arthur Pontari, MD
Professor
Department of Urology
Temple University School of Medicine
Philadelphia, Pennsylvania

John C. Pope IV, MD
Professor
Departments of Urologic
    Surgery and Pediatrics
Vanderbilt University Medical Center
Nashville, Tennessee

Glenn M. Preminger, MD
Professor and Chief
Division of Urology
Duke University Medical Center
Durham, North Carolina

Mark A. Preston, MD, MPH
Instructor in Surgery
Division of Urology
Brigham and Women's Hospital/Harvard Medical School
Boston, Massachusetts

Raymond R. Rackley, MD
Professor of Surgery
Glickman Urological Institute
Cleveland Clinic
Cleveland, Ohio

Soroush Rais-Bahrami, MD
Assistant Professor of Urology and Radiology
Department of Urology
University of Alabama at Birmingham
Birmingham, Alabama

Jay D. Raman, MD
Associate Professor
Surgery (Urology)
Penn State Milton S. Hershey Medical Center
Hershey, Pennsylvania

Art R. Rastinehad, DO
Director of Interventional Urologic Oncology
Assistant Professor of Radiology and Urology
The Arthur Smith Institute for Urology and Interventional
    Radiology
Hofstra North Shore-LIJ School of Medicine
New York, New York

Yazan F.H. Rawashdeh, MD, PhD, FEAPU
Consultant Pediatric Urologist
Section of Pediatric Urology

Aarhus University Hospital
Aarhus, Denmark

Shlomo Raz, MD
Professor of Urology
Department of Urology
Division of Pelvic Medicine and Reconstructive Surgery
UCLA School of Medicine
Los Angeles, California

Ira W. Reiser, MD
Associate Professor of Clinical Medicine
State University of New York Health Science Center at Brooklyn
Attending Physician and Chairman Emeritus
Department of Medicine
Division of Nephrology and Hypertension
Brookdale University Hospital and Medical Center
Brooklyn, New York

Neil M. Resnick, MD
Thomas Detre Endowed Professor of Medicine
University of Pittsburgh School of Medicine
Chief, Division of Geriatric Medicine and Gerontology
Department of Medicine
Associate Director, Institute on Aging
University of Pittsburgh Medical Center
Pittsburgh, Pennsylvania

W. Stuart Reynolds, MD, MPH
Assistant Professor
Department of Urologic Surgery
Vanderbilt University
Nashville, Tennessee

Koon Ho Rha, MD, PhD, FACS
Professor
Department of Urology
Urological Science Institute
Yonsei University College of Medicine
Seoul, South Korea

Kevin R. Rice, MD
Urologic Oncologist
Urology Service, Department of Surgery
Walter Reed National Military Medical Center
Bethesda, Maryland

Lee Richstone, MD
System Vice Chairman
Department of Urology
Associate Professor
Hofstra North Shore-LIJ School of Medicine
Lake Success, New York
Chief
Urology
The North Shore University Hospital
Manhasset, New York

Richard C. Rink, MD, FAAP, FACS
Robert A. Garret Professor
Pediatric Urology
Riley Hospital for Children

Indiana University School of Medicine
Faculty
Pediatric Urology
Peyton Manning Children's Hospital at St. Vincent
Indianapolis, Indiana

Michael L. Ritchey, MD
Professor
Department of Urology
Mayo Clinic College of Medicine
Phoenix, Arizona

Larissa V. Rodriguez, MD
Professor
Vice Chair, Academics
Director, Female Pelvic Medicine and Reconstructive Surgery (FPMRS)
Director, FPMRS Fellowship
University of Southern California Institute of Urology
Beverly Hills, California

Ronald Rodriguez, MD, PhD
Professor and Chairman
Department of Urology
University of Texas Health Science Center at San Antonio
San Antonio, Texas
Adjunct Professor
Department of Urology
Johns Hopkins University School of Medicine
Baltimore, Maryland

Claus G. Roehrborn, MD
Professor and Chairman
Department of Urology
University of Texas Southwestern Medical Center
Dallas, Texas

Lisa Rogo-Gupta, MD
Assistant Professor
Urogynecology and Pelvic Reconstructive Surgery
Urology
Stanford University
Palo Alto, California

Ashley Evan Ross, MD, PhD
Assistant Professor of Urology, Oncology, and Pathology
James Buchanan Brady Urological Institute
Johns Hopkins Medicine
Baltimore, Maryland

Eric S. Rovner, MD
Professor of Urology
Department of Urology
Medical University of South Carolina
Charleston, South Carolina

Richard A. Santucci, MD, FACS
Specialist-in-Chief
Department of Urology
Detroit Medical Center
Clinical Professor
Department of Osteopathic Surgical Specialties
Michigan State College of Osteopathic Medicine
Detroit, Michigan

Anthony J. Schaeffer, MD
Herman L. Kretschmer Professor of Urology
Department of Urology
Northwestern University Feinberg School of
   Medicine
Chicago, Illinois

Edward M. Schaeffer, MD, PhD
Associate Professor of Urology and Oncology
Johns Hopkins University School of Medicine
Baltimore, Maryland

Douglas S. Scherr, MD
Associate Professor of Urology
Clinical Director of Urologic Oncology
Department of Urology
Weill Medical College of Cornell University
New York, New York

Francis X. Schneck, MD
Associate Professor of Urology
Division of Pediatric Urology
Children's Hospital of Pittsburgh at the University of Pittsburgh
   Medical Center
Pittsburgh, Pennsylvania

Michael J. Schwartz, MD, FACS
Assistant Professor of Urology
Hofstra North Shore-LIJ School of Medicine
New Hyde Park, New York

Karen S. Sfanos, PhD
Assistant Professor of Pathology
Assistant Professor of Oncology
Johns Hopkins University
   School of Medicine
Baltimore, Maryland

Robert C. Shamberger, MD
Chief of Surgery
Department of Surgery
Boston Children's Hospital
Robert E. Gross Professor of Surgery
Department of Surgery
Harvard Medical School
Boston, Massachusetts

Ellen Shapiro, MD
Professor of Urology
Director, Pediatric Urology
Department of Urology
New York University School of Medicine
New York, New York

David S. Sharp, MD
Assistant Professor
Department of Urology
Ohio State University
   Wexner Medical Center
Columbus, Ohio

Alan W. Shindel, MD, MAS
Assistant Professor
Department of Urology
University of California, Davis
Sacramento, California

Daniel A. Shoskes, MD, MSc, FRCSC
Professor of Surgery (Urology)
Glickman Urological and Kidney Institute
Department of Urology
Cleveland Clinic
Cleveland, Ohio

Aseem Ravindra Shukla, MD
Director of Minimally Invasive Surgery
Pediatric Urology
Children's Hospital of Philadelphia
Philadelphia, Pennsylvania

Eila C. Skinner, MD
Professor and Chair
Department of Urology
Stanford University
Stanford, California

Ariana L. Smith, MD
Associate Professor of Urology
Penn Medicine, Perelman School of Medicine
Division of Urology
Hospital of the University of Pennsylvania
University of Pennsylvania Health System
Philadelphia, Pennsylvania

Armine K. Smith, MD
Assistant Professor of Urology and Director of Urologic Oncology
   at Sibley Hospital
James Buchanan Brady Urological Institute
Johns Hopkins University
Assistant Professor of Urology
Department of Urology
George Washington University
Washington, DC

Joseph A. Smith, Jr., MD
William L. Bray Professor of Urology
Department of Urologic Surgery
Vanderbilt University School of Medicine
Nashville, Tennessee

Warren T. Snodgrass, MD
Co-Director
PARC Urology
Dallas, Texas

Rene Sotelo, MD
Chairman, Department of Urology
Minimally Invasive and Robotic Surgery Center
Instituto Médico La Floresta
Caracas, Miranda, Venezuela

Mark J. Speakman, MBBS, MS, FRCS
Consultant Urological Surgeon
Department of Urology
Musgrove Park Hospital
Consultant Urologist
Nuffield Hospital
Taunton, Somerset, United Kingdom

Philippe E. Spiess, MD, MS, FACS, FRCS(C)
Associate Member
Department of Genitourinary Oncology
Moffitt Cancer Center
Associate Professor
Department of Urology

University of South Florida
Tampa, Florida

Samuel Spitalewitz, MD
Associate Professor of Clinical Medicine
State University of New York Health Science Center
    at Brooklyn
Attending Physician
Division of Nephrology and Hypertension
Supervising Physician of Nephrology and Hypertension,
    Outpatient Services
Brookdale University Hospital and Medical Center
Brooklyn, New York

Ramaprasad Srinivasan, MD, PhD
Head, Molecular Cancer Section
Urologic Oncology Branch
Center for Cancer Research
National Cancer Institute
National Institutes of Health
Bethesda, Maryland

Andrew J. Stephenson, MD, MBA, FACS, FRCS(C)
Associate Professor of Surgery
Department of Urology
Cleveland Clinic Lerner College of Medicine
Case Western Reserve University
Director, Urologic Oncology
Glickman Urological and Kidney Institute
Cleveland Clinic
Cleveland, Ohio

Julie N. Stewart, MD
Assistant Professor
Department of Urology
Houston Methodist Hospital
Houston, Texas

Douglas W. Storm, MD, FAAP
Assistant Professor
Department of Urology
University of Iowa Hospitals and Clinics
Iowa City, Iowa

Li-Ming Su, MD
David A. Cofrin Professor of Urology
Chief, Division of Robotic and Minimally Invasive
    Urologic Surgery
Department of Urology
University of Florida College of Medicine
Gainesville, Florida

Stasa D. Tadic, MD, MS
Assistant Professor
Department of Medicine
Division of Geriatric Medicine and Gerontology
University of Pittsburgh School of Medicine
Attending Physician, Department of Medicine
Division of Geriatric Medicine and Gerontology
University of Pittsburgh Medical Center
Pittsburgh, Pennsylvania

Thomas Tailly, MD, MSc
Fellow in Endourology
Department of Surgery
Division of Urology
Schulich School of Medicine and Dentistry
Western University
London, Ontario, Canada

Shpetim Telegrafi, MD
Associate Professor (Research) of Urology
Senior Research Scientist
Director, Diagnostic Ultrasound
Department of Urology
New York University School of Medicine
New York, New York

John C. Thomas, MD, FAAP, FACS
Associate Professor of Urologic Surgery
Department of Urology
Division of Pediatric Urology
Monroe Carell Jr. Children's
    Hospital at Vanderbilt
Nashville, Tennessee

J. Brantley Thrasher, MD
Professor and William L. Valk Chair of Urology
Department of Urology
University of Kansas Medical Center
Kansas City, Kansas

Edouard J. Trabulsi, MD, FACS
Associate Professor
Department of Urology
Kimmel Cancer Center
Thomas Jefferson University
Philadelphia, Pennsylvania

Chad R. Tracy, MD
Assistant Professor
Department of Urology
University of Iowa
Iowa City, Iowa

Paul J. Turek, MD, FACS, FRSM
Director, the Turek Clinic
Beverly Hills and San Francisco, California

Robert G. Uzzo, MD, FACS
Chairman
G. Willing "Wing" Pepper
    Professor of Cancer Research
Department of Surgery
Deputy Chief Clinical Officer
Fox Chase Cancer Center
Philadelphia, Pennsylvania

Sandip P. Vasavada, MD
Professor of Surgery (Urology)
Glickman Urological Institute
Cleveland Clinic
Cleveland, Ohio

David J. Vaughn, MD
Professor of Medicine
Division of Hematology/Oncology
Department of Medicine
Abramson Cancer Center at the University of
    Pennsylvania
Philadelphia, Pennsylvania

Manish A. Vira, MD
Assistant Professor of Urology
Vice Chair for Urologic Research
The Arthur Smith Institute for Urology
Hofstra North Shore-LIJ School of Medicine
New Hyde Park, New York

Gino J. Vricella, MD
Assistant Professor of Urologic Surgery
Urology Division
Washington University School of Medicine in St. Louis
St. Louis, Missouri

John T. Wei, MD, MS
Professor
Department of Urology
University of Michigan
Ann Arbor, Michigan

Alan J. Wein, MD, PhD (Hon), FACS
Founders Professor of Urology
Division of Urology
Penn Medicine, Perelman School of Medicine
Chief of Urology
Division of Urology
Penn Medicine, Hospital of the University of Pennsylvania
Program Director, Residency in Urology
Division of Urology
Penn Medicine, University of Pennsylvania Health System
Philadelphia, Pennsylvania

Jeffrey Paul Weiss, MD
Professor and Chair
Department of Urology
SUNY Downstate College of Medicine
Brooklyn, New York

Robert M. Weiss, MD
Donald Guthrie Professor of Surgery/Urology
Department of Urology
Yale University School of Medicine
New Haven, Connecticut

Charles Welliver, MD
Assistant Professor of Surgery
Division of Urology
Albany Medical College
Albany, New York

Hunter Wessells, MD, FACS
Professor and Nelson Chair
Department of Urology
University of Washington
Seattle, Washington

J. Christian Winters, MD, FACS
Professor and Chairman
Department of Urology
Louisiana State University Health Sciences Center
New Orleans, Louisiana

J. Stuart Wolf, Jr., MD, FACS
David A. Bloom Professor of Urology
Associate Chair for Clinical Operations
Department of Urology
University of Michigan
Ann Arbor, Michigan

Christopher G. Wood, MD
Professor and Deputy Chairman
Douglas E. Johnson, M.D. Endowed Professorship
    in Urology
Department of Urology
The University of Texas MD Anderson Cancer Center
Houston, Texas

David P. Wood, Jr., MD
Chief Medical Officer
Beaumont Health
Professor of Urology
Department of Urology
William Beaumont School of Medicine
Royal Oak, Michigan

Christopher R.J. Woodhouse, MB, FRCS, FEBU
Emeritus Professor
Adolescent Urology
University College
London, United Kingdom

Subbarao V. Yalla, MD
Professor of Surgery (Urology)
Harvard Medical School
Urologist, Surgical Service
Brigham and Women's Hospital
VA Boston Healthcare System
Boston, Massachusetts
Urologist, Surgical Service
Togus VA Medical Center
Augusta, Maine

Stephen Shei-Dei Yang, MD, PhD
Professor
Department of Urology
Buddhist Tzu Chi University
Hualien, Taiwan
Chief of Surgery
Taipei Tzu Chi Hospital
New Taipei, Taiwan

Jennifer K. Yates, MD
Assistant Professor
Department of Urology
University of Massachusetts Medical School
Worcester, Massachusetts

Chung Kwong Yeung, MBBS, MD, PhD, FRCS, FRACS, FACS
Honorary Clinical Professor in Pediatric Surgery and Pediatric
    Urology
Department of Surgery
University of Hong Kong
Chief of Pediatric Surgery and Pediatric Urology
Union Hospital
Hong Kong, China

Richard Nithiphaisal Yu, MD, PhD
Instructor in Surgery
Harvard Medical School
Associate in Urology
Department of Urology
Boston Children's Hospital
Boston, Massachusetts

Lee C. Zhao, MD, MS
Assistant Professor
Department of Urology
New York University
New York, New York

Jack M. Zuckerman, MD
Fellow in Reconstructive Surgery
Department of Urology
Eastern Virginia Medical School
Norfolk, Virginia

HOW TO USE THIS STUDY GUIDE

This study guide is designed to provide the reader with a comprehensive review of urology based on the text *Campbell-Walsh Urology*, eleventh edition. Each chapter includes a series of questions and possible answers, explanations for each answer, and a collection of chapter review points. Within the answer explanations, text of particular importance has been highlighted in blue. If the reader knows the blue highlighted text and the chapter review points, he or she will know the majority of important points for that particular chapter. Moreover, if the questions are understood and the emphasized points are remembered, then the reader will have a thorough understanding of the important aspects of each chapter.

It is important to note that some of the questions are not of the format used in standardized tests such as the Qualifying Examination of the American Board of Urology. The proper format for examination questions is a question that asks for the one best possible answer out of five. While many questions in this review guide are in the proper format, some additional formats are used for teaching purposes. For example, "all of the following are true except" allows the author to provide the reader with four true statements regarding the question, and "more than one answer may be correct" also allows the author to make several points. Both formats serve to broaden the reader's knowledge.

Both the Pathology and the Imaging questions have been updated from the previous edition. The Pathology questions have been updated to be consistent with the new format proposed by the American Board of Urology. New Imaging questions have been included where new modalities have been introduced. Both sets of questions provide valuable additional information for review.

The authors of the 156 chapters and I hope that this study guide will be helpful to both the student in training and the practicing clinician in refreshing knowledge as well as in preparing for a Urology examination.

W. Scott McDougal, MD, MA (Hon)
Walter S. Kerr, Jr. Distinguished Professor of Urology
Harvard Medical School
Chief Emeritus, Massachusetts General Hospital
Boston, Massachusetts
2015

CONTENTS

1

Evaluation of the Urologic Patient: History, Physical Examination, and Urinalysis

Glenn S. Gerber and Charles B. Brendler

QUESTIONS

1. Pain associated with a stone in the ureter is the result of:
   a. obstruction of urine flow with distention of the renal capsule.
   b. irritation of the ureteral mucosa by the stone.
   c. excessive ureteral peristalsis in response to the obstructing stone.
   d. irritation of the intramural ureter.
   e. urinary extravasation from a ruptured calyceal fornix.

2. The most common cause of gross hematuria in a patient older than 50 years is:
   a. renal calculi.
   b. infection.
   c. bladder cancer.
   d. benign prostatic hyperplasia.
   e. trauma.

3. The most common cause of pain associated with gross hematuria is:
   a. simultaneous passage of a kidney stone.
   b. ureteral obstruction due to blood clots.
   c. urinary tract malignancy.
   d. prostatic inflammation.
   e. prostatic enlargement.

4. All of the following are typical lower urinary tract symptoms associated with benign prostatic hyperplasia EXCEPT:
   a. urgency.
   b. frequency.
   c. nocturia.
   d. dysuria.
   e. weak urinary stream.

5. The most likely cause of continuous incontinence (loss of urine at all times and in all positions) is:
   a. enterovesical fistula.
   b. noncompliant bladder.
   c. detrusor hyperreflexia.
   d. vesicovaginal fistula.
   e. sphincteric incompetence.

6. All of the following are potential causes of anejaculation EXCEPT:
   a. sympathetic denervation.
   b. pharmacologic agents.
   c. bladder neck and prostatic surgery.

   d. androgen deficiency.
   e. cerebrovascular accidents.

7. What percentage of patients with multiple sclerosis will present with urinary symptoms as the first manifestation of the disease?
   a. 1%
   b. 5%
   c. 10%
   d. 15%
   e. 20%

8. What important information is gained from pelvic bimanual examination that cannot be obtained from radiologic evaluation?
   a. Presence of bladder mass
   b. Invasion of bladder cancer into perivesical fat
   c. Presence of bladder calculi
   d. Presence of associated pathologic lesion in female adnexal structures
   e. Mobility/fixation of pelvic organs

9. With which of the following diseases is priapism most commonly associated?
   a. Peyronie disease
   b. Sickle cell anemia
   c. Parkinson disease
   d. Organic depression
   e. Leukemia

10. What is the most common cause of cloudy urine?
    a. Bacterial cystitis
    b. Urine overgrowth with yeast
    c. Phosphaturia
    d. Alkaline urine
    e. Significant proteinuria

11. Conditions that decrease urine specific gravity include all of the following EXCEPT:
    a. increased fluid intake.
    b. use of diuretics.
    c. decreased renal concentrating ability.
    d. dehydration.
    e. diabetes insipidus.

12. Urine osmolality usually varies between:
    a. 10 and 200 mOsm/L.
    b. 50 and 500 mOsm/L.
    c. 50 and 1200 mOsm/L.
    d. 100 and 1000 mOsm/L.
    e. 100 and 1500 mOsm/L.

13. Elevated ascorbic acid levels in the urine may lead to false-negative results on a urine dipstick test for:
    a. glucose.
    b. hemoglobin.
    c. myoglobin.
    d. red blood cells.
    e. leukocytes.

14. Hematuria is distinguished from hemoglobinuria or myoglobinuria by:
    a. dipstick testing.
    b. the simultaneous presence of significant leukocytes.
    c. microscopic presence of erythrocytes.
    d. examination of serum.
    e. evaluation of hematocrit.

15. The presence of one positive dipstick reading for hematuria is associated with significant urologic pathologic findings on subsequent testing in what percentage of patients?
    a. 2%
    b. 10%
    c. 25%
    d. 50%
    e. 75%

16. The most common cause of glomerular hematuria is:
    a. transitional cell carcinoma.
    b. nephritic syndrome.
    c. Berger disease (immunoglobulin A nephropathy).
    d. poststreptococcal glomerulonephritis.
    e. Goodpasture syndrome.

17. The most common cause of proteinuria is:
    a. Fanconi syndrome.
    b. excessive glomerular permeability due to primary glomerular disease.
    c. failure of adequate tubular reabsorption.
    d. overflow proteinuria due to increased plasma concentration of immunoglobulins.
    e. diabetes.

18. Transient proteinuria may be due to all of the following EXCEPT:
    a. exercise.
    b. fever.
    c. emotional stress.
    d. congestive heart failure.
    e. ureteroscopy.

19. Glucose will be detected in the urine when the serum level is above:
    a. 75 mg/dL.
    b. 100 mg/dL.
    c. 150 mg/dL.
    d. 180 mg/dL.
    e. 225 mg/dL.

20. The specificity of dipstick nitrite testing for bacteriuria is:
    a. 20%.
    b. 40%.
    c. 60%.
    d. 80%.
    e. >90%.

21. All of the following are microscopic features of squamous epithelial cells EXCEPT:
    a. large size.
    b. small central nucleus.
    c. irregular cytoplasm.
    d. presence in clumps.
    e. fine granularity in the cytoplasm.

22. The number of bacteria per high-power microscopic field that corresponds to colony counts of 100,000/mL is:
    a. 1.
    b. 3.
    c. 5.
    d. 10.
    e. 20.

23. Pain in the flaccid penis is usually due to:
    a. Peyronie disease.
    b. bladder or urethral inflammation.
    c. priapism.
    d. calculi impacted in the distal ureter.
    e. hydrocele.

24. Chronic scrotal pain is most often due to:
    a. testicular torsion.
    b. trauma.
    c. cryptorchidism.
    d. hydrocele.
    e. orchitis.

25. Terminal hematuria (at the end of the urinary stream) is usually due to:
    a. bladder neck or prostatic inflammation.
    b. bladder cancer.
    c. kidney stones.
    d. bladder calculi.
    e. urethral stricture disease.

26. Enuresis is present in what percentage of children at age 5 years?
    a. 5%
    b. 15%
    c. 25%
    d. 50%
    e. 75%

27. All of the following in the medical history suggest that erectile dysfunction is more likely due to organic rather than psychogenic causes EXCEPT:
    a. sudden onset.
    b. peripheral vascular disease.
    c. absence of nocturnal erections.
    d. diabetes mellitus.
    e. inability to achieve adequate erections in a variety of circumstances.

28. All of the following should be routinely performed in men with hematospermia EXCEPT:

    a. cystoscopy.

    b. digital rectal examination.

    c. serum prostate-specific antigen (PSA) level.

    d. genital examination.

    e. urinalysis.

29. Pneumaturia may be due to all of the following EXCEPT:

    a. diverticulitis.

    b. colon cancer.

    c. recent urinary tract instrumentation.

    d. inflammatory bowel disease.

    e. ectopic ureter.

30. Which of the following disorders may commonly lead to irritative voiding symptoms?

    a. Parkinson disease

    b. Renal cell carcinoma

    c. Bladder diverticula

    d. Prostate cancer

    e. Testicular torsion

ANSWERS

1. **a. Obstruction of urine flow with distention of the renal capsule.** Pain is usually caused by acute distention of the renal capsule, usually from inflammation or obstruction.

2. **c. Bladder cancer.** The most common cause of gross hematuria in a patient older than age 50 is bladder cancer.

3. **b. Ureteral obstruction due to blood clots.** Pain in association with hematuria usually results from upper urinary tract hematuria with obstruction of the ureters with clots.

4. **d. Dysuria.** Dysuria is painful urination that is usually caused by inflammation.

5. **d. Vesicovaginal fistula.** Continuous incontinence is most commonly due to a urinary tract fistula that bypasses the urethral sphincter or an ectopic ureter.

6. **e. Cerebrovascular accidents.** Anejaculation may result from several causes: (1) androgen deficiency, (2) sympathetic denervation, (3) pharmacologic agents, and (4) bladder neck and prostatic surgery.

7. **b. 5%.** In fact, 5% of patients with previously undiagnosed multiple sclerosis present with urinary symptoms as the first manifestation of the disease.

8. **e. Mobility/fixation of pelvic organs.** In addition to defining areas of induration, the bimanual examination allows the examiner to assess the mobility of the bladder; such information cannot be obtained by radiologic techniques such as computed tomography (CT) and magnetic resonance imaging (MRI), which convey static images.

9. **b. Sickle cell anemia.** Priapism occurs most commonly in patients with sickle cell disease but can also occur in those with advanced malignancy, coagulation disorders, and pulmonary disease, as well as in many patients without an obvious cause.

10. **c. Phosphaturia.** Cloudy urine is most commonly caused by phosphates in the urine.

11. **d. Dehydration.** Conditions that decrease specific gravity include (1) increased fluid intake, (2) diuretics, (3) decreased renal concentrating ability, and (4) diabetes insipidus.

12. **c. 50 and 1200 mOsm/L.** Osmolality is a measure of the amount of solutes dissolved in the urine and usually varies between 50 and 1200 mOsm/L.

13. **a. Glucose.** False-negative results for glucose and bilirubin may be seen in the presence of elevated ascorbic acid concentrations in the urine.

14. **c. Microscopic presence of erythrocytes.** Hematuria can be distinguished from hemoglobinuria and myoglobinuria by microscopic examination of the centrifuged urine; the presence of a large number of erythrocytes establishes the diagnosis of hematuria.

15. **c. 25%.** Investigators at the University of Wisconsin found that 26% of adults who had at least one positive dipstick reading for hematuria were subsequently found to have significant urologic pathologic findings.

16. **c. Berger disease (immunoglobulin A [IgA] nephropathy).** IgA nephropathy, or Berger disease, is the most common cause of glomerular hematuria, accounting for about 30% of cases.

17. **b. Excessive glomerular permeability due to primary glomerular disease.** Glomerular proteinuria is the most common type of proteinuria and results from increased glomerular capillary permeability to protein, especially albumin. Glomerular proteinuria occurs in any of the primary glomerular diseases such as IgA nephropathy or in glomerulopathy associated with systemic illness such as diabetes mellitus.

18. **e. Ureteroscopy.** Transient proteinuria occurs commonly, especially in the pediatric population, and usually resolves spontaneously within a few days. It may result from fever, exercise, or emotional stress. In older patients, transient proteinuria may be due to congestive heart failure.

19. **d. 180 mg/dL.** This so-called renal threshold corresponds to a serum glucose level of about 180 mg/dL; above this level, glucose will be detected in the urine.

20. **e. >90%.** The specificity of the nitrite dipstick test for detecting bacteriuria is greater than 90%.

21. **d. Presence in clumps.** Squamous epithelial cells are large, have a central small nucleus about the size of an erythrocyte, and have an irregular cytoplasm with fine granularity.

22. **c. 5.** Therefore 5 bacteria per high-power field in a spun specimen reflect colony counts of about 100,000/mL.

23. **b. Bladder or urethral inflammation.** Pain in the flaccid penis is usually secondary to inflammation in the bladder or urethra, with referred pain that is experienced maximally at the urethral meatus.

24. **d. Hydrocele.** Chronic scrotal pain is usually related to noninflammatory conditions such as a hydrocele or varicocele, and the pain is usually characterized as a dull, heavy sensation that does not radiate.

25. **a. Bladder neck or prostatic inflammation.** Terminal hematuria occurs at the end of micturition and is usually secondary to inflammation in the area of the bladder neck or prostatic urethra.

26. **b. 15%.** Enuresis refers to urinary incontinence that occurs during sleep. It occurs normally in children as old as 3 years but persists in about 15% of children at age 5 and about 1% of children at age 15.

27. **a. Sudden onset.** A careful history will often determine whether the problem is primarily psychogenic or organic. In men with psychogenic impotence, the condition frequently develops rather quickly, secondary to a precipitating event such as marital stress or change or loss of a sexual partner.

28. **a. Cystoscopy.** A genital and rectal examination should be done to exclude the presence of tuberculosis, a PSA assessment and digital rectal examination should be done to exclude prostatic carcinoma, and a urinary cytologic assessment should be done to exclude the possibility of transitional cell carcinoma of the prostate.

29. **e. Ectopic ureter.** Pneumaturia is the passage of gas in the urine. In patients who have not recently had urinary tract instrumentation or a urethral catheter placed, this is almost always due to a fistula between the intestine and bladder. Common causes include diverticulitis, carcinoma of the sigmoid colon, and regional enteritis (Crohn disease).

30. **a. Parkinson disease.** The second important example of nonspecific lower urinary tract symptoms that may occur secondary to a variety of neurologic conditions is irritative symptoms resulting from neurologic disease such as cerebrovascular accident, diabetes mellitus, or Parkinson disease.

CHAPTER REVIEW

1. See Table 1-1 in *Campbell-Walsh Urology, 11th edition* for the International Prostate Symptom Score (IPSS).
2. IPSS score: 0 to 7 mild symptoms, 8 to 19 moderate symptoms, 20 to 35 severe symptoms.
3. Renal pain radiates from the flank anteriorly to the respective lower quadrant and may be referred to the testis, labium, or medial aspect of the thigh. The pain is colicky (fluctuates). It may be associated with gastrointestinal symptoms due to reflex stimulation of the celiac ganglion.
4. Patients with slowly progressive urinary obstruction with bladder distention often have no pain, despite residual volumes in excess of a liter.
5. Pain of prostatic origin is poorly localized.
6. Scrotal pain may be primary or referred. Pain referred to the testicle originates in the retroperitoneum, ureter, or kidney.
7. Hematuria, particularly in adults, should be regarded as a symptom of malignancy until proven otherwise.
8. Adults normally arise no more than twice a night to void. Urine production increases at night (recumbent position) in older patients and those with cardiac disease, particularly congestive heart failure (CHF).
9. Postvoid dribbling: Urine escapes into the bulbar urethra and then leaks at the end of micturition. This may be alleviated by perineal pressure following voiding.
10. Those who present with microscopic hematuria and irritative voiding symptoms should be suspected of having carcinoma in situ of the bladder until proven otherwise.
11. Continuous incontinence is most commonly due to ectopic ureter, urinary tract fistula, or totally incompetent sphincter.
12. Hematospermia almost always resolves spontaneously and is rarely associated with any significant urologic pathology.
13. When urinary obstruction is associated with fever and chills, it should be regarded as a urologic emergency.
14. It is always worthwhile to obtain the previous operative report in patients who are to be operated on.
15. If the patient is uncircumcised, the foreskin must be retracted for inspection of the glans.
16. The testes are normally 6 cm in length and 4 cm in width.
17. If one obtains a stool guaiac test (hemoccult) as a screen for colon cancer, two subsequent stool specimens must be obtained for an adequate test. If the hemoccult is positive, the patient should be on a red meat–free diet for 3 days before collection of three specimens.
18. A male urologist should always perform a female pelvic examination with a female nurse in attendance.
19. The bulbocavernosus reflex tests the integrity of this spinal cord reflex involving S2 to S4.
20. A positive dipstick for blood in the urine indicates hematuria, hemoglobinuria, or myoglobinuria. Hematuria is distinguished from hemoglobinuria and myoglobinuria by microscopic examination of the centrifuged urine and identification of red blood cells (more than three red blood cells per high-power field is abnormal).
21. Hematuria of nephrologic origin is frequently associated with proteinuria and dysmorphic erythrocytes.
22. Anticoagulation at normal therapeutic levels does not predispose patients to hematuria.
23. The most accurate method to diagnosis urinary tract infection is by microscopic examination of the urine and identifying pyuria and bacteria. This is confirmed by urine culture.
24. The chief complaint is the focus of the visit and is the reason the patient seeks consultation. It should be the lead sentence in the History and Physical (H&P).
25. A family history should always include questions about renal and prostate cancer, renal cysts, and stone disease.
26. Priapism occurs most commonly in patients with sickle cell disease but can also occur in those with advanced malignancy, coagulation disorders, or pulmonary disease, as well as in many patients without an obvious cause.
27. On urine dipstick, false-negative results for glucose and bilirubin may be seen in the presence of elevated ascorbic acid concentrations in the urine.
28. Glomerular proteinuria is the most common type of proteinuria and results from increased glomerular capillary permeability to protein, especially albumin. Glomerular proteinuria occurs in any of the primary glomerular diseases such as IgA nephropathy or in glomerulopathy associated with systemic illness such as diabetes mellitus.
29. Five bacteria per high-power field in a spun specimen reflect colony counts of about 100,000/mL.
30. An important example of nonspecific lower urinary tract symptoms that may occur secondary to a variety of neurologic conditions is irritative symptoms resulting from neurologic disease such as cerebrovascular accident, diabetes mellitus, and Parkinson disease.
31. The renal threshold for glucose corresponds to a serum glucose level of about 180 mg/dL; above this level, glucose will be detected in the urine.

2 Urinary Tract Imaging: Basic Principles of CT, MRI, and Plain Film

Jay T. Bishoff and Art R. Rastinehad

QUESTIONS

1. The measure of the potential adverse health effects of ionizing radiation in sieverts (Sv) is known as:
   a. radiation exposure.
   b. absorbed dose.
   c. equivalent dose.
   d. effective dose.
   e. relative radiation levels.

2. The relative radiation level associated with abdominal computed tomography (CT) without and with contrast is:
   a. none.
   b. minimal, <0.1 mSv.
   c. low, 0.1-1.0 mSv.
   d. moderate, 1-10 mSv.
   e. high, 10-100 mSv.

3. Bladder filling may precipitate autonomic dysreflexia in patients with a spinal cord injury above:
   a. S2.
   b. L4.
   c. T10.
   d. T12.
   e. T6.

4. Radiation exposure diminishes as the square of the distance from the radiation source. An exposure of 9 mSv at 1 foot from the source would be how much at 3 feet from the source?
   a. 0.09 mSv
   b. 1 mSv
   c. 3 mSv
   d. 9 mSv
   e. 27 mSv

5. Type 2 diabetics on oral metformin biguanide hyperglycemic therapy are at risk for biguanide lactic acidosis after exposure to intravascular radiological contrast media if they:
   a. discontinue metformin 48 hours before the study.
   b. have severe renal insufficiency and take metformin the day of the study.
   c. are given a saline injection while taking metformin.
   d. have normal kidney function and fail to stop metformin 48 hours before the study.
   e. decrease metformin dose and increase other antihyperglycemic agents on the day of the study.

6. All of the following are true EXCEPT:
   a. Patients with a history of asthma are at greater risk of having an adverse reaction to contrast media.
   b. Severe allergic reactions are not dose dependent.
   c. Hyperosmolar contrast media are more likely to cause contrast reactions than are iso-osmolar agents.
   d. The mechanism of action associated with severe idiosyncratic anaphylactoid (IA) reactions is an immunoglobulin E (IgE) antibody reaction to the contrast media.
   e. Severe cardiac disease is a risk factor for an adverse reaction to contrast media.

7. After rapidly assessing airway, breathing, and circulation, the medical treatment of choice for a severe, life-threatening adverse drug reaction following exposure to contrast media is:
   a. subcutaneous injection of epinephrine 0.5 mg of 1 : 10,000 epinephrine.
   b. intravenous injection of 100 mg of methylprednisone.
   c. 0.01 mg/kg of epinephrine (1 : 10,000 concentration), given intramuscularly in the lateral thigh.
   d. intravenous diphenhydramine, 50 mg.
   e. 0.01 mg/kg of epinephrine (1 : 1000 concentration), given intramuscularly in the lateral thigh.

8. Which of the following is NOT a risk factor for developing contrast-induced nephropathy (CIN)?
   a. Type 2 diabetes mellitus
   b. Dehydration
   c. Hypertension
   d. Ventricular ejection fraction < 50%
   e. Chronic kidney disease (glomerular filtration rate [GFR] <60 mL/min)

9. Nephrogenic systemic fibrosis (NSF) is:
   a. a rare genetic condition exacerbated by the use of gadolinium-based contrast medium (GBCM).
   b. immediately evident after exposure to gadolinium in 10% of exposed patients.
   c. fibrosis of the skin, subcutaneous tissue, and skeletal muscle seen in patients with chronic hypertension exposed to gadolinium contrast medium.
   d. not seen in patients with GFR > 60 mL/min/1.73 m^2.
   e. mainly seen in dialysis patients exposed to gadolinium contrast medium.

10. During a diuretic renal scintigraphy:
    a. the diuretic is administered approximately 2 minutes after peak activity is seen in the collecting system.
    b. a $T_{1/2}$ of greater than 14 minutes is consistent with obstruction.
    c. ^{99m}Tc-DMSA is the most sensitive for obstruction and determination of glomerular filtration rate.
    d. intestinal or gallbladder activity should never be seen with ^{99m}Tc-MAG3.
    e. a $T_{1/2}$ of less than 10 minutes is consistent with a nonobstructed system.

11. Positron emission tomography (PET):
    a. has a higher diagnostic accuracy than CT for seminoma and nonseminoma testis cancer following chemotherapy.
    b. is sensitive and specific for detection of postchemotherapy teratoma.
    c. Can be used with high positive predictive value within 2 weeks of completion of chemotherapy for bulky lymph adenopathy.
    d. Has greater predictive value of primary disease in metastatic urothelial carcinoma than magnetic resonance imaging (MRI).
    e. Is able to detect local or systemic recurrence of prostate cancer in 74% of patients with prostate-specific antigen recurrence.

12. What is the minimum estimated GFR for use of gadolinium-based contrast agents?
    a. Less than 30 mL/min/1.73 m^2
    b. Greater than 50 mL/min/1.73 m^2
    c. Greater than 35 mL/min/1.73 m^2
    d. Greater than 30 mL/min/1.73 m^2
    e. There are no restrictions with patients with renal insufficiency.

13. In magnetic resonance (MR) images using T2-weighted sequences, fluid appears as:
    a. dark.
    b. bright.
    c. low signal.
    d. signal void.
    e. indeterminate.

14. What lesions may have a high signal (bright) on T2-weighted MRI of the adrenal gland?
    a. Pheochromocytoma
    b. Metastasis
    c. Adrenal cortical carcinoma (ACC)
    d. None of the above
    e. All of the above

15. MR chemical shift imaging for adrenal adenoma takes advantage of which of the following phenomena to aid in the diagnosis?
    a. Water and fat within the same voxels signals are canceled out in opposed-phase imaging.
    b. Opposed-phase imaging will exhibit a high signal (bright).
    c. Intracellular lipid content within an adenoma is low.
    d. Intravenous contrast is required.
    e. All of the above.

16. Oncocytoma typically has been characterized by a central scar. Which other renal lesion may also exhibit a central scar on T2-weighted images?
    a. Clear cell carcinoma
    b. Angiomyolipoma
    c. Chromophobe carcinoma
    d. Transitional cell carcinoma
    e. No other renal masses exhibit a central scar.

17. Which renal mass exhibits signal drop on opposed phase imaging?
    a. Papillary renal cell
    b. Chromophobe carcinoma
    c. Angiomyolipoma
    d. Clear cell carcinoma
    e. Transitional cell carcinoma

18. What signal characteristics do kidney stones exhibit on MR urography?
    a. High signal on T2-weighted images
    b. Low signal on T2-weighted images
    c. Signal void
    d. High signal on T1-weighted images
    e. Low signal on T1-weighted images

19. Multiparametric imaging of the prostate consists of anatomic and functional sequences. Match the correct pair.
    a. Anatomic : Diffusion-weighted imaging
    b. Functional : T1- and T2-weighted images
    c. Anatomic : Dynamic contrast enhanced sequences
    d. Functional : Apparent diffusion coefficient maps
    e. All of the above

ANSWERS

1. **d. Effective dose.** The distribution of energy absorption in the human body will be different based on the body part being imaged and a variety of other factors. The most important risk of radiation exposure from diagnostic imaging is the development of cancer. The effective dose is a quantity used to denote the radiation risk (expressed in sieverts) to a population of patients from an imaging study.

2. **e. High, 10-100 mSv.** The average person living in the United States is exposed to 6.2 mSv of radiation per year from ambient sources, such as radon, cosmic rays, and medical procedures, which account for 36% of the annual radiation exposure (NCRP, 2012). The recommended occupational exposure limit to medical personnel is 50 mSv per year (NCRP, 2012). The effective dose from a three-phase CT of the abdomen and pelvis without and with contrast may be as high as 25 to 40 mSv.

3. **e. T6.** Autonomic dysreflexia, also known as hyperreflexia, means an overactivity of the autonomic nervous system that can result in an abrupt onset of excessively high blood pressure. Persons at risk for this problem generally have injury levels above T5. Autonomic dysreflexia can develop suddenly, is potentially life threatening, and is considered a medical emergency. If not treated promptly and correctly, it may lead to seizures, stroke, and even death.

4. **b. 1 mSv.** Maintaining the maximum practical distance from an active radiation source significantly decreases exposure to medical personnel.

5. **b. Have severe renal insufficiency and take metformin the day of the study.** Patients with type 2 diabetes mellitus on metformin may have an accumulation of the drug after administering intravascular radiologic contrast medium (IRCM), resulting in biguanide lactic acidosis presenting with vomiting, diarrhea and somnolence. This condition is fatal in approximately 50% of cases (Wiholm, 1993).* Biguanide lactic acidosis is rare in patients with normal renal function. Consequently in patients with normal renal function and no known comorbidities, there is no need to discontinue metformin before IRCM use, nor is there a need to check creatinine following the imaging study.

6. **d. The mechanism of action associated with severe idiosyncratic anaphylactoid (IA) reactions is an IgE antibody reaction to the contrast media.** The IA reactions are most concerning, because they are potentially fatal and can occur without any predictable or predisposing factors. Approximately 85% of IA reactions occur during or immediately after injection of IRCM and are more common in patients with a prior adverse drug reaction to contrast media; patients with asthma, diabetes,

---

*Sources referenced can be found in *Campbell-Walsh Urology, 11th Edition,* on the Expert Consult website.

impaired renal function, or diminished cardiac function; and patients on beta-adrenergic blockers (Spring et al, 1997).

7. e. **0.01 mg/kg of epinephrine (1:1,000 concentration) intramuscularly in the lateral thigh.** Rapid administration of epinephrine is the treatment of choice for severe contrast reactions. Epinephrine can be administered intravenously (IV) 0.01 mg/kg body weight of 1 : 10,000 dilution or 0.1 mL/kg slowly into a running IV infusion of saline and can be repeated every 5 to 15 minutes as needed. If no IV access is available, the recommended intramuscular dose of epinephrine is 0.01 mg/kg of 1 : 1000 dilution (or 0.01 mL/kg to a maximum of 0.15 mg of 1 : 1000 if body weight is <30 kg; 0.3 mg if weight is >30 kg) injected intramuscularly in the lateral thigh.

8. d. **Ventricular ejection fraction <50%.** The most common patient-related risk factors for CIN are chronic kidney disease (CKD) (creatinine clearance< 60 mL/min), diabetes mellitus, dehydration, diuretic use, advanced age, congestive heart failure, age, hypertension, low hematocrit, and ventricular ejection fraction< 40%. The patients at highest risk for developing CIN are those with both diabetes *and* preexisting renal insufficiency.

9. d. **Not seen in patients with GFR >60 mL/min/1.73 m^2.** Patients with CKD but GRF >30 mL/min/1.73 m^2 are considered to be at extremely low or no risk for developing NSF if a dose of GBCM of 0.1 mmol/kg or less is used. Patients with GFR >60 mL/min/1.73 m^2 do not appear to be at increased risk of developing NSF, and the current consensus is that all GBCM can be administered safely to these patients.

10. a **T$_{1/2}$ of less than 10 minutes is consistent with a nonobstructed system.** Transit time throughout the collecting system in less than 10 minutes is consistent with a normal, nonobstructed collecting system. A T$_{1/2}$ of 10-20 minutes shows mild to moderate delay and may be a mechanical obstruction. The patient's perception of pain after diuretic administration can be helpful for the treating urologist to consider when planning surgery in the patient with middle to moderate obstruction. A T$_{1/2}$ of greater than 20 minutes is consistent with a high-grade obstruction.

11. a. **Has a higher diagnostic accuracy than CT for seminoma and nonseminoma testis cancer following chemotherapy.** There are

data on the use of PET/CT in testis cancer, where PET/CT was found to have a higher diagnostic accuracy than CT for staging and restaging in the assessment of a CT-visualized residual mass following chemotherapy for seminoma and nonseminomatous germ-cell tumors (Hain et al, 2000; Albers et al, 1999).

12. d. **Greater than 30 mL/min/1.73 m^2.** NSF occurs in patients with acute or chronic renal insufficiency with a GFR < 30 mL/min/1.73 m^2.

13. b. **Bright.** High signal on T2-weighted images. Fluid exhibits a low signal on T1-weighted images.

14. e. **All of the above.** Traditional teaching reported the lightbulb sign to be consistent with pheochromocytoma. However, metastasis and ACC also have a high signal on T2-weighted images. Furthermore, Varghese and colleagues reported that 35% of pheochromocytomas demonstrated low T2 signal, contrary to conventional teaching. Therefore the conventional teaching of the "lightbulb sign" is incorrect.

15. a. **Water and fat within the same voxels signals are canceled out in opposed-phase imaging.** MR chemical shift imaging (CSI) is performed on T1-weighted images. Opposed-phase imaging will demonstrate a low signal (dark) if fat and water occupy the same voxel. Adrenal adenomas have high intracytoplasmic fat. CSI is performed without the use of intravenous contrast.

16. c. **Chromophobe carcinoma.** Chromophobe carcinoma exhibits a high signal on T2-weighted images.

17. d. **Clear cell carcinoma.** Microscopic intracytoplasmic lipids have been found in 59% of clear cell carcinomas, which allows it to be differentiated from other renal cell carcinoma cell types.

18. c. **Signal void.** Nephrolithiasis/calcification on MR imaging has no signal characteristics; therefore it appears as a void on imaging.

19. d. **Functional : Apparent diffusion coefficient maps.** Multiparametric MRI refers to the use of anatomic sequences (T1-weighted images, T2 triplanar [axial, sagittal, and coronal] images) and functional sequences (diffusion-weighted imaging/apparent diffusion coefficient maps, dynamic contrast-enhanced MRI, spectroscopy). The combined approach has reported negative and positive predictive values to be greater than 90% in detecting prostate cancer.

CHAPTER REVIEW

1. Absorbed dose for therapy is measured in units called gray (Gy); 1 rad=0.01 Gy, or 1 centigray (cGy)=1 rad.
2. The amount of energy absorbed by a tissue for diagnostic purposes is referred to as the equivalent dose and is measured in sieverts (Sv). Exposure of the eyes and gonads to radiation has a more significant biologic impact than exposure of other parts of the body. The occupational safety limit is 50 mSv. Exposure time during fluoroscopy should be minimized by the use of short bursts of fluoroscopy; positioning the image intensifier as close to the patient as feasible substantially reduces scatter radiation.
3. There are four basic types of iodinated contrast media: (1) ionic monomer, (2) nonionic monomer, (3) ionic dimer, (4) nonionic dimer.
4. Idiosyncratic anaphylactoid reactions are potentially fatal, are not dose dependent, and are more common in patients with a history of adverse reactions to contrast media, those with asthma or diabetes, those with impaired renal and cardiac function, and those on β-adrenergic blockers.
5. It is common to have nausea, flushing, pruritus, urticaria, headache, and occasionally emesis after administration of contrast media.
6. Patients at high risk for adverse allergic reactions should be medicated with steroids, given 12 to 24 hours

before the injection of contrast media, as well as antihistamines.
7. For retrograde pyelography, it is useful to dilute contrast media by half with sterile saline, which facilitates identifying filling defects in the collecting system. There is a low risk of contrast reactions in patients in whom a retrograde or loopogram is performed.
8. Metformin does not need to be held before contrast administration in a patient with normal renal function and no comorbidities.
9. The risk of developing contrast induced nephropathy is increased in patients with decreased renal function (GFR <60 mL/min), diabetes mellitus, dehydration, advanced age, congestive heart failure, liver disease, and cardiac ejection fraction less than 40%.
10. TcDTPA is primarily filtered by the glomerulus. It is a good agent to assess renal function.
11. Because TcDMSA is both filtered by the glomerulus and secreted by the proximal tubule, it localizes in the renal cortex and is a good agent for assessing cortical scarring and ectopic renal tissue.
12. TcMAG3 is cleared mainly by tubular secretion; it has a limited ability to access renal function.
13. A T$_{1/2}$ less than 10 minutes suggests an unobstructed system. A T$_{1/2}$ greater than 20 minutes is consistent with renal obstruction.

14. A positive bone scan is not specific for cancer. Moreover, the volume of cancer cannot be quantitated on bone scan. Patients with widely metastatic disease may have diffuse uptake (hyper scan) and no discrete lesions.

15. Glucose, choline, and amino acids have been used as imaging agents for PET scans.

16. ^{18}F-fluorodeoxyglucose (FDG) is used as an imaging agent in PET scanning and takes advantage of the fact that tumors have increased glycolysis and decreased dephosphorylation. This scan is useful in testicular germ cell tumors, particularly seminomas, in determining residual viable tumor following chemotherapy.

17. The Hounsfield units scale assigns a value of −1000 Hounsfield units for air. Dense bone is assigned a value of +1000 Hounsfield units, and water is assigned 0 Hounsfield units.

18. With the exception of some indinavir stones, all renal and ureteral calculi may be detected by helical CT.

19. The advantage of MRI is high-contrast resolution of soft tissue on T1-weighted images. Fluid has a low signal and appears dark on T1-weighted images; on T2-weighted images, fluid has a high signal and appears bright. Gadolinium increases the brightness of T1-weighted images. Hemorrhage within a cyst results in a high signal on T1-weighted images. MRI is the imaging modality of choice for patients with iodine contrast allergies.

20. The risk of developing nephrogenic systemic fibrosis after gadolinium administration is increased in patients with GFRs below 30 mL/min.

21. Adrenal adenomas have high lipid content and may be differentiated from adrenal cancers or metastatic disease by specialized CT or MRI scans.

22. Thirty-five percent of pheochromocytomas do not enhance on T2-weighted images.

23. MRI and CT are excellent imaging studies to determine the presence and extent of renal vein and vena cava tumor thrombus. Uptake of gadolinium by the thrombus on MRI differentiates tumor from bland (blood clot) thrombus.

24. Prostate MRI coupled with an assessment of dynamic contrast uptake and washout increases the diagnostic accuracy for detecting cancer.

25. MR spectroscopy for prostate cancer is based on decreased citrate levels and increased creatine and choline levels.

26. Bladder filling in patients with spinal cord injuries higher than T6 may precipitate autonomic dysreflexia.

27. Radiation exposure diminishes as the square of the distance from the radiation source.

3   Urinary Tract Imaging: Basic Principles of Urologic Ultrasound

Bruce R. Gilbert and Pat F. Fulgham

QUESTIONS

1. The maximum excursion of a wave above and below the baseline is known as its:
   a. wavelength.
   b. frequency.
   c. period.
   d. cycle.
   e. amplitude.

2. The artifact that occurs when an ultrasound wave strikes an interface at a critical angle and is refracted with limited reflection is:
   a. a reverberation artifact.
   b. an increased through-transmission artifact.
   c. an edging artifact.
   d. a comet-tail artifact.
   e. an aliasing artifact.

3. Which ultrasound mode allows for detection and characterization of the velocity and direction of motion?
   a. Harmonic scanning
   b. Color Doppler
   c. Power Doppler
   d. Spatial compounding
   e. Gray-scale ultrasonography

4. If the kidney is less echogenic than the liver, it is described as:
   a. hyperechoic.
   b. hypoechoic.
   c. isoechoic.
   d. anechoic.
   e. echogenic.

5. The sonographic hallmark of testicular torsion is:
   a. the "blue dot" sign.
   b. epididymal edema.
   c. paratesticular fluid.
   d. increased epididymal blood flow.
   e. absence of intratesticular blood flow.

6. Ultrasound waves are examples of:
   a. radio waves.
   b. mechanical waves.
   c. electromagnetic waves.
   d. ionizing radiation.
   e. light waves.

7. The most important determinant of axial resolution is:
   a. impedance.
   b. speed of propagation.
   c. acoustic power.
   d. frequency.
   e. number of foci.

8. Increasing frequency results in a loss of:
   a. absorption.
   b. axial resolution.
   c. lateral resolution.
   d. depth of penetration.
   e. mechanical index.

9. When sound waves encounter the interface between two tissues with large differences in impedance, the waves are:
   a. increased in frequency.
   b. decreased in frequency.
   c. reflected.
   d. refracted.
   e. reverberated.

10. When a tissue appears darker than the surrounding tissue on ultrasound, it is said to be relatively:
    a. hypoechoic.
    b. hyperechoic.
    c. hypodense.
    d. isoechoic.
    e. anechoic.

11. The focal zone represents the area of best:
    a. lateral resolution.
    b. axial resolution.
    c. echogenicity.
    d. blood flow.
    e. tissue penetration.

12. Increasing the gain has the effect of:
    a. increasing amplitude of the sound waves.
    b. increasing acoustic power.
    c. increasing thermal index.
    d. increasing mechanical index.
    e. increasing transducer sensitivity.

13. One way to improve the visualization of deep structures is to:
    a. increase the frequency.
    b. decrease the frequency.
    c. increase the wave velocity.
    d. decrease the gain.
    e. use Doppler flow.

14. The best frequency for performing external renal ultrasound in most adults is:
    a. 3.5 to 5 MHz.
    b. 6 to 10 MHz.
    c. 7.5 MHz.
    d. 10 to 12 MHz.
    e. none of the above.

15. A simple cyst of the kidney would NOT display which of the following characteristics?

    a. Bright back wall

    b. Increased through transmission

    c. Anechoic interior

    d. Edging artifact

    e. Hyperechoic internal nodule

16. Which of the following is correct?

    a. Measuring bladder volume requires three-dimensional scanning.

    b. A nearly empty bladder is desirable for bladder scanning.

    c. A curved array transducer is preferred for bladder ultrasound in most patients.

    d. Ureteroceles are usually poorly visualized because the membrane is thin.

    e. Bladder ultrasound is a sensitive screening exam for suspected bladder tumors.

17. Which of the following are evaluable by transabdominal bladder ultrasound?

    a. Urine volume

    b. Bladder wall characteristics

    c. Stones or diverticulum

    d. Dilated ureters

    e. All of the above

18. Scrotal ultrasound for the evaluation of possible testicular torsion may include all of the following but must include:

    a. B-mode ultrasound.

    b. multiple scrotal views.

    c. Doppler flow studies.

    d. simultaneous bilateral views.

    e. harmonic scanning.

19. The most important limitation of ultrasound in attempting to characterize complex renal cysts as benign or malignant is:

    a. refraction.

    b. inability to evaluate enhancement.

    c. lack of axial resolution.

    d. increased through transmission with artifact.

    e. reverberation artifact.

20. A complete transrectal ultrasound of the prostate should include an evaluation of:

    a. the rectal wall.

    b. the seminal vesicles and ejaculatory ducts.

    c. the bladder.

    d. prostate.

    e. all of the above.

21. Which of the following would NOT typically be visible in a sagittal midline prostate ultrasound?

    a. Middle lobe of the prostate

    b. Central zone

    c. Ejaculatory duct

    d. Tip of the right seminal vesicle

    e. Apex of the prostate

22. Characteristics of prostate cancer as demonstrated on transrectal ultrasound of the prostate may include:

    a. hypoechogenicity.

    b. hyperechogenicity.

    c. prostate asymmetry.

    d. increased vascularity.

    e. all of the above.

23. The single most important determinant of patient safety in ultrasound use is:

    a. multifrequency probes.

    b. good documentation.

    c. an informed operator.

    d. periodic equipment inspection.

    e. Doppler capability.

24. The disinfection level protocol required for transrectal ultrasound probes following needle biopsy is:

    a. low.

    b. moderate.

    c. high.

    d. critical.

    e. none of the above.

25. For patient safety it is preferable to maximize _____ and limit _____:

    a. acoustic power, exam duration

    b. acoustic power, gain

    c. gain, acoustic power

    d. gain, use of cine function

    e. images, description

ANSWERS

1. **e. Amplitude.** In ultrasound physics it is crucial to understand the concept of amplitude. The amplitude of an ultrasound wave represents its relative energy state, and it is the amplitude of the returning sound wave that determines the pixel brightness to be displayed on a monitor during real-time gray-scale imaging.

2. **c. An edging artifact.** Echo reflection is the primary mechanism whereby sound waves are returned to a transducer. It is important to understand how the angle of insonation affects the reflection and refraction of sound waves. There is a critical angle at which waves will travel along an interface rather than being returned to the probe. When this angle is encountered, it provides a dark or hypoechoic "shadow" called an edging artifact. A reverberation artifact is caused by multiple transits of a sound wave between the transducer and the reflecting object. Increased through-transmission artifact is caused by decreased attenuation of sound waves as they travel through a fluid-filled structure. Comet tail artifact is a special form of reverberation artifact and occurs when highly refractive objects, such as calcific or crystalline objects, are interrogated. Aliasing artifact is seen with Doppler ultrasonography.

3. **b. Color Doppler.** Doppler ultrasonography is important for evaluating motion and flow. The critical difference between color Doppler and power Doppler is that color Doppler is able to evaluate both flow velocity and direction. Power Doppler evaluates integrated amplitude of the returning sound waves. Although gray-scale ultrasonography does permit the evaluation of motion, it does not permit the characterization of velocity or direction. Harmonic scanning and spatial compounding are modes that allow the selective evaluation of, or combination of, reflected frequencies in ways that improve image quality.

4. **b. Hypoechoic.** In describing ultrasound images, it is important to use correct terminology. Descriptive terms involving echogenicity are relative terms. A hyperechoic or hypoechoic structure is being described in relation to the echogenicity of a reference standard. In most cases, the reference standard is the liver. In the adult, the normal kidney is hypoechoic relative to the normal liver in approximately 75% of patients.

5. **e. Absence of intratesticular blood flow.** The absence of intratesticular blood flow is the classic sonographic finding in testicular torsion. However, there are many documented cases of some preserved intratesticular blood flow even in cases with significant torsion. Therefore testicular torsion remains a clinical diagnosis. Epididymal edema, paratesticular fluid, and increased epididymal blood flow may be seen with testicular torsion but may also be seen with other clinical conditions. The blue dot sign is a classic physical finding in torsion of the appendix testis.

6. **b. Mechanical waves.** Mechanical waves are represented graphically as a sine wave alternating between a positive and negative direction from the baseline.

7. **d. Frequency.** Axial resolution is directly dependent on the frequency of sound waves. The higher the sound wave's frequency, the better the axial resolution.

8. **d. Depth of penetration.** The optimal ultrasound image requires trade-offs between resolution and depth of penetration. High-frequency transducers of 6 to 10 MHz may be used to image structures near the surface of the body (e.g., testis, pediatric kidney) with excellent resolution. However, deeper structures (e.g., right kidney, bladder) require lower frequencies of 3.5 to 5 MHz to penetrate. Such images will have poorer axial resolution.

9. **c. Reflected.** The shape and size of the object and the angle at which the advancing wave strikes the object are critical determinants of the amount of energy reflected. The amount of energy reflected from an interface is also influenced by the impedance of the two tissues at the interface. Impedance is a property that is influenced by tissue stiffness and density. The difference in impedance allows an appreciation of interfaces between different types of tissue.

10. **a. Hypoechoic.** The liver is usually used as a benchmark for echogenicity. A hypoechoic area is described as darker and black on B-mode ultrasound.

11. **a. Lateral resolution.** Lateral resolution refers to the ability to identify separately objects that are equidistant from the transducer. Lateral resolution is a function of the focused width of the ultrasound beam and is a characteristic of the transducer. The location of the narrowest beam width can be adjusted by the user. The more focused the beam, the better the lateral resolution at that location. Thus image quality can be enhanced by locating the narrowest beam width (focus or focal zone) at the depth of the object or tissue of interest

12. **e. Increasing transducer sensitivity.** Gain is a control mechanism for varying the sensitivity of the transducer to returning ultrasound waves.

13. **b. Decrease the frequency.** The optimal ultrasound image requires trade-offs between resolution and depth of penetration. High-frequency transducers of 6 to 10 MHz may be used to image structures near the surface of the body (e.g., testis, pediatric kidney) with excellent resolution. However, deeper structures (e.g., right kidney, bladder) require lower frequencies of 3.5 to 5 MHz to penetrate. Such images will have poorer axial resolution.

14. **a. 3.5 to 5 MHz.** Deeper structures (e.g., right kidney, bladder) require lower frequencies of 3.5 to 5 MHz to penetrate.

15. **e. Hyperechoic internal nodule.** A simple cyst is an example of a structure that is well circumscribed, with an anechoic interior and through transmission.

16. **c. A curved array transducer is preferred for bladder ultrasound in most patients.** A curved array transducer is of lower frequency (3.5 to 6 MHz) and provides greater depth of penetration however with less axial resolution. It is most often the transducer of choice for imaging the kidney and urinary bladder.

17. **e. All of the above.** Urine volume, bladder wall characteristics, the presence of calculi or diverticulum, and the presence of dilated ureters just outside the bladder are all evaluable by transabdominal bladder ultrasound.

18. **c. Doppler flow studies.** Caution should be used when interpreting Doppler flow studies in the evaluation of suspected testicular torsion. The hallmark of testicular torsion is the absence of intratesticular blood flow. Paratesticular flow in epididymal collaterals may appear within hours of torsion. Comparison with the contralateral testis should be performed to ensure that the technical attributes of the study are adequate to demonstrate intratesticular blood flow.

19. **b. Inability to evaluate enhancement.** Unlike CT, presently ultrasound cannot evaluate enhancement. However, use of Doppler and elastography might aid in evaluation.

20. **e. All of the above.** When evaluating the prostate, surrounding structures need to be accessed. Rectal lesions, including cancer, dilated seminal vesicles, and/or ejaculatory ducts as well as bladder pathology should all be evaluated for a complete examination.

21. **d. Tip of the right seminal vesicle.** In a midline sagittal view, the tips of the seminal vesicles are not normally visualized on ultrasound. A lateral projection, however, must be obtained to allow measurement of the length of each seminal vesicle.

22. **e. All of the above.** Although excellent resolution and tissue characteristics are possible with transrectal ultrasound, a diagnosis of prostate cancer often cannot be made with ultrasound alone.

23. **c. An informed operator.** The ALARA principle ("as low as reasonably achievable") is intended to limit the total energy imparted to the patient during an examination. This can be accomplished by (1) keeping power outputs low, (2) using appropriate scanning modes, (3) limiting examination times, (4) adjusting focus and frequency, and (5) using the cine function during documentation. All of these are dependent on an informed sonographer.

24. **d. Critical.** Any time body fluids or tissues come in contact with an ultrasound transducer, critical or high-level disinfection protocols must be strictly adhered to.

25. **c. Gain, acoustic power.** Unlike gain, which refers to amplification of the acoustic signal returning to the transducer, acoustic power is the amount of acoustic energy applied to the tissue. The biologic effects of ultrasound in terms of power are in the milliwatt range. High levels generate heat and cavitation, which might result in tissue damage.

CHAPTER REVIEW

1. One cycle per second is known as 1 hertz (Hz). High-frequency ultrasonic transducers of 6 to 10 MHz are used to image structures near the surface. Deeper structures require lower frequencies of 3.5 to 5 MHz. Axial resolution improves with increasing frequency, and depth of penetration decreases with increasing frequency.

2. Resistive index is the peak velocity minus the end-diastolic velocity over the peak systolic velocity. This is measured using the color flow Doppler with spectral display and is used to characterize renal artery stenosis, ureteral obstruction, and penile arterial insufficiency.

3. By convention, the liver is used as a benchmark for echogenicity. Tissues with a high water content are generally hypoechoic; tissues with a high fat content appear hyperechoic.

4. By convention, the cephalad aspect of the structure is to the left of the image.

5. Ultrasonography may produce injury due to mechanical effects caused by cavitation or by heat generation.

6. Color Doppler evaluates velocity and direction of motion. Blue usually indicates motion away from the transducer, red indicates motion toward the transducer—the colors DO NOT signify arterial and venous flow.

7. Sonoelastography evaluates tissue elasticity. Less elastic tissues within a soft tissue organ, such as the prostate, are thought to be pathologic.

8. Contrast agents used in ultrasound are generally compounds containing microbubbles that create strong echoes.

9. The central band of echoes in the kidney is hyperechoic and represents renal hilar fat, blood vessels, and the collecting system.

10. Ultrasound measurements of bladder volume have an error of 10% to 20%.

11. Ultrasound is very helpful in defining the extent of corporal fibrosis in urethral stricture disease.

12. Doppler ultrasound is useful in quantization of penile blood flow. It is also useful in helping to diagnose testicular torsion by evaluating testicular blood flow. It is not diagnostic of vasculogenic impotence in the former case or testicular torsion in the latter.

4 Outcomes Research

Mark S. Litwin and Jonathan Bergman

QUESTIONS

1. Barriers to health care access may include which of the following?
   a. Lack of health insurance.
   b. Lack of transportation.
   c. Beliefs about the health care system.
   d. Culture.
   e. All of the above.

2. Costs of hospital care are best approximated by measuring:
   a. charges.
   b. collections.
   c. resources used.
   d. severity of illness.
   e. all of the above.

3. A true assessment of health care costs must include the amount of money spent on:
   a. facilities.
   b. disposable supplies.
   c. personnel.
   d. equipment.
   e. all of the above.

4. The introduction of diagnosis-related groups (DRGs) in the 1980s led to:
   a. longer hospital stays for most patients.
   b. shorter hospital stays for most patients.
   c. higher reimbursements for hospitals.
   d. higher reimbursements for physicians.
   e. increased costs.

5. Quality-adjusted life years (QALYs) are a metric used in:
   a. basic quality-of-life analysis in individual patients.
   b. cost-effectiveness analysis for populations of patients.
   c. patient satisfaction analysis for individual patients.
   d. cost-benefit analysis for individual patients.
   e. determining the number of years an individual is free of the condition.

6. Case mix is a metric that may be used in the study of medical outcomes to adjust for:
   a. comorbidity of a population cared for by a given provider.
   b. severity of illness in a population cared for by a given provider.
   c. both.
   d. neither.

7. In the Donabedian model of quality of care, measures of structure include:
   a. interpersonal skill with which a physician interacts with patients.
   b. perioperative mortality rates.
   c. patient satisfaction.
   d. board certification of physicians in a provider group.
   e. complication rates.

8. In the Donabedian model of quality of care, measures of outcome include:
   a. patient satisfaction.
   b. health-related quality of life.
   c. survival.
   d. all of the above.

9. Health-related quality of life is best assessed by:
   a. patients themselves.
   b. spouses or immediate family members of patients.
   c. primary care physicians caring for patients.
   d. specialists caring for patients.
   e. specially trained examiners.

10. Dysfunction and its related distress (also called "bother") are generally:
    a. perfectly correlated.
    b. completely independent.
    c. related but imperfectly correlated.
    d. measures of the same phenomenon.
    e. meaningful when the correlation coefficient is 0.1.

11. Disease-specific health-related quality of life domains in patients with urologic cancer include:
    a. physical function.
    b. emotional well-being.
    c. social function.
    d. sexual dysfunction.
    e. cardiac function.

12. In psychometric terms, reliability refers to how free an instrument is of:
    a. missing data.
    b. measurement error.
    c. grammatical or typographic errors.
    d. invalid data.
    e. selection bias.

13. When a scale has a coefficient alpha of 0.90, the scale has a high degree of:
    a. alternate form reliability.
    b. test-retest reliability.
    c. internal consistency reliability.
    d. concurrent validity.
    e. construct validity.

ANSWERS

1. **e. All of the above.** Barriers to access may be financial or nonfinancial and include any factor that decreases the likelihood that an individual in need will receive medical services.
2. **c. Resources used.** Charges are notoriously poor proxies for actual medical costs because of the way in which hospital budgets are calculated; actual collections do not account for deductibles, copayments, and opportunity costs.
3. **d. All of the above.** Each of the factors mentioned contributes to the total cost of health care.
4. **b. Shorter hospital stays for most patients.** DRGs allow for the calculation of prospective payments to hospitals and thus have led to shorter lengths of stay; they have also led to decreased reimbursements to hospitals.
5. **b. Cost-effectiveness analysis for populations of patients.** QALYs are used in population analysis and not for individual patients.
6. **c. Both.** Measuring case mix allows for outcomes to be controlled for both the underlying medical diseases and the severity of the disease of interest among groups of patients under the care of a provider.
7. **d. Board certification of physicians in a provider group.** Structural attributes of health care include clinician characteristics such as board certification, but not measures of process such as interpersonal style or outcome measures such as mortality and patient satisfaction.
8. **d. All of the above.** Each of these factors may be considered a valid measure of medical outcomes.
9. **a. Patients themselves.** It is axiomatic that health-related quality-of-life outcomes must be reported by patients themselves, as they perceive them.
10. **c. Related but imperfectly correlated.** In the various domains of disease-specific health-related quality of life, function and bother are loosely associated with each other but measure discrete phenomena.
11. **d. Sexual dysfunction.** Disease-specific, health-related, quality-of-life instruments focus on domains that are directly relevant to the specific disease or treatment.
12. **b. Measurement error.** Reliability refers to what proportion of a test score is true and what proportion is due to chance variation (or measurement error).
13. **c. Internal consistency reliability.** The Cronbach coefficient alpha is a well-established measure of internal consistency reliability.

CHAPTER REVIEW

1. Costs—what the provider spends to supply the service.
2. Charges—what the provider bills for the service, not necessarily what the provider collects for the service.
3. Resource utilization takes into account the duration, frequency, and intensity of the service.
4. Length of stay may be used to quantify resource utilization.
5. Cost-effectiveness is calculated by developing a probability model of possible medical outcomes for different interventions. The different interventions may then be compared taking into account costs.
6. Life years—the number of years lived for a population, not an individual patient.
7. Quality-adjusted life years—adjustment of the life years to account for the impact of various treatments on the health status of an individual.
8. Cost-benefit analysis takes into account not only cost but other factors that may not have a monetary value such as extra years of life.
9. Case mix refers to the severity of illness and the degree of comorbidity in a group of patients.
10. The most financially burdensome urologic conditions include stones, urinary tract infections, incontinence, and benign prostatic hyperplasia.
11. Proxy measures may be used to measure outcomes when actual measurement of the outcome is impossible or impractical; they are surrogate end points thought to be predictive of the actual true outcome.
12. Reliability refers to what proportion of a test score is true and what proportion is due to chance variation (or measurement error).

5 Core Principles of Perioperative Care

Manish A. Vira and Louis R. Kavoussi

QUESTIONS

1. A 64-year-old male is found to have an 8-cm left renal mass and presents to the office for evaluation regarding laparoscopic radical nephrectomy. He has a history of hypertension, non–insulin-dependent diabetes, and 30-pack-year tobacco use, which he quit 10 years ago. He has a strong family history of heart disease in that his father died at the age of 55 years from a myocardial infarction. Further questioning reveals that he does not regularly exercise but is able to walk up three flights of stairs without shortness of breath. Before surgery, to minimize the risk of complications, the patient should:

   a. undergo routine preoperative testing with complete blood count, basic metabolic panel, electrocardiogram, and chest radiograph.

   b. be referred to cardiology consultation to determine if further testing is necessary.

   c. undergo noninvasive cardiac stress testing.

   d. undergo pulmonary function testing to determine the need for preoperative bronchodilators.

   e. be started on a perioperative β blocker to reduce the risk of perioperative myocardial ischemia.

2. With regard to unique patient populations, which of the following statements is TRUE?

   a. Although elderly patients have an increased perioperative risk, recent larger trials have not found age to be an independent risk factor for perioperative morbidity and mortality.

   b. Morbidly obese patients should undergo open rather than laparoscopic surgery because of increased risk of pulmonary complications.

   c. In a pregnant patient presenting with urolithiasis operative intervention should be delayed, if possible, until the second trimester.

   d. A patient who presents with a 30-pound weight loss over the previous 3 months should be started on parenteral feedings immediately postoperatively after elective surgery.

   e. In patients with liver disease, the primary determinant of postoperative risk is degree of liver function enzyme abnormality.

3. A 74-year-old male with muscle-invasive bladder cancer is scheduled for radical cystectomy and ileal conduit urinary diversion. Preoperative urine culture shows no growth at 72 hours. The most important factor in the prevention of surgical site infection in this patient is:

   a. preoperative bowel preparation with oral antibiotics (Nichols prep) and sodium phosphate solution (Fleet).

   b. administration of 2 g cefoxitin 1 hour before incision.

   c. continuation of perioperative antibiotics for 48 hours following surgery.

   d. preoperative hair removal with mechanical clippers and proper sterile preparation of the operative field.

   e. optimization of comorbid illness and nutritional status.

4. According to current guidelines in the prevention of thromboembolic complications, a 78-year-old male with a recent history of colon cancer, medical history of hypertension, coronary artery disease (postoperative angioplasty with two coronary stents), and chronic renal insufficiency (creatinine, 2.9 mg/dL) undergoing laparoscopic transabdominal surgery should have pneumatic compression stockings and:

   a. early ambulation.

   b. aspirin and early ambulation.

   c. low-molecular-weight heparin.

   d. low-molecular-weight heparin and aspirin.

   e. unfractionated heparin and aspirin.

5. A 72-year-old female with a history of asthma, mild congestive heart failure, and breast cancer is to undergo cystoscopy and placement of a midurethral sling. Of the following agents, the best choice for anesthesia induction would be:

   a. inhaled halothane.

   b. intravenous thiopental.

   c. inhaled desflurane.

   d. inhaled sevoflurane.

   e. intravenous succinylcholine.

6. The most appropriate indication for blood product transfusion is:

   a. packed red blood cells for an 82-year-old male with coronary artery disease and hematocrit of 31%.

   b. fresh frozen plasma for a 69-year-old patient with an international normalized ratio (INR) of 1.6 scheduled to undergo laparotomy for a small bowel obstruction.

   c. platelet transfusion for a 78-year-old male with chronic renal insufficiency who was scheduled to undergo partial nephrectomy and found to have a platelet count of 55,000 on preoperative testing.

   d. packed red blood cells for a healthy 22-year-old male with a stable large retroperitoneal hematoma after motor vehicle accident and hematocrit of 21%.

   e. Fresh frozen plasma for a 64-year-old female during resection of a large renal mass with inferior vena cava thrombus who experiences significant blood loss requiring 4 U of packed red blood cell transfusion.

7. To reduce the risk of iatrogenic injury to a patient in the operating room, the patient should:

    a. be maintained with core body temperature between 36° C and 38° C throughout the perioperative period.

    b. be instructed to bathe with an antiseptic solution the night before surgery.

    c. be secured to the operating room table with fixed shoulder braces for procedures in steep Trendelenburg.

    d. be positioned in the lithotomy position one leg at a time to ensure safe flexion of the hips.

    e. be positioned and draped by the operating room staff before arrival of the surgeon.

8. In a patient undergoing an exploratory laparotomy for pelvic abscess following radical cystectomy, the best method of abdominal fascial closure is with:

    a. polyglycolic acid (Dexon) suture with continuous closure.

    b. silk suture with continuous closure.

    c. polypropylene (Prolene) suture with interrupted closure.

    d. polyglactin (Vicryl) suture with interrupted closure.

    e. polydioxanone suture (PDS) with continuous closure.

ANSWERS

1. **e. Be started on preoperative β blocker to reduce the risk of myocardial ischemia during the perioperative period.** This choice is best given the patient's multiple risk factors. Although cardiac stress testing may be considered, the patient's ability to climb three flights of stairs indicates a capacity of greater than 4 METS and therefore a low risk of significant coronary artery disease. Although routine preoperative testing is performed widely, there is no evidence that routine testing reduces the risk of perioperative complications.

2. **c. In a pregnant patient presenting with urolithiasis operative intervention should be delayed, if possible, until the second trimester.** The second trimester represents the least anesthetic risk to the mother and fetus with regard to spontaneous abortion and teratogenicity. Although controversy exists as to the exact etiology, several recent trials have found age to be an independent predictor of morbidity on multivariate analyses. Laparoscopic surgery is the preferred approach in morbidly obese patients secondary to the reduced risk of pulmonary and wound complications. Literature suggests that severely malnourished patients (>20 pounds weight loss in 3 months) significantly benefit from 7 to 10 days of enteral (not parenteral) feedings before elective surgery. The primary determinants of the degree of severity in patients with cirrhosis are hepatic function and severity of clinical manifestations.

3. **b. Administration of 2 g cefoxitin 1 hour before incision.** Administration of appropriate antibiotics within 60 minutes of incision has been shown to significantly decrease the incidence of surgical site infections. Recent meta-analyses from the colorectal literature indicate that mechanical bowel preparation does not decrease the risk of postoperative infections. Unless in the presence of active infection, perioperative antibiotics should be stopped 24 hours after incision to decrease the risk of *Clostridium difficile* colitis. Although preoperative hair removal and optimization of nutritional status and comorbid illness improve surgical outcomes, there is no specific evidence that this reduces surgical site infections.

4. **e. Unfractionated heparin and aspirin.** The clinical scenario describes a patient with high to highest risk of venous thromboembolism. Such a patient would require both mechanical and pharmacologic prophylaxis. In a patient with renal insufficiency, unfractionated heparin is a better choice than low-molecular-weight heparin. There is no evidence that aspirin is effective in the prevention of venous thromboembolism, but in a patient with coronary stents, aspirin is important in the prevention of stent thrombosis in the perioperative period.

5. **d. Inhaled sevoflurane.** This is an excellent choice for rapid induction in this patient secondary to its odorless and bronchodilation properties. Halothane can adversely affect left ventricular function and should be used with caution in patients with congestive heart failure. Desflurane has a pungent odor and is more suitable for maintenance of anesthesia during prolonged procedures. Intravenous thiopental can increase airway reactivity and is not appropriate in patients with asthma. Succinylcholine is appropriate for neuromuscular blockade and not commonly used for induction.

6. **c. Platelet transfusion for a 78-year-old male with chronic renal insufficiency who was scheduled to undergo partial nephrectomy and found to have a platelet count of 55,000 on preoperative testing.** This patient has moderate thrombocytopenia with likely platelet dysfunction secondary to uremia undergoing a high-bleeding-risk procedure; therefore platelet transfusion is indicated. Current indications for packed red blood cell transfusion are maintenance of hematocrit of greater than 30% in patients with high risk of myocardial ischemia or in patients with hematocrit 21% to 30% with signs of inadequate oxygen carrying capacity. Fresh frozen plasma transfusion is indicated only in the presence of active bleeding rather than isolated INR elevation or large-volume transfusion.

7. **a. Be maintained with core body temperature between 36° C and 38° C throughout the perioperative period.** Hypothermia by as little as 1° C has been shown to increase surgical site infection and postoperative complications. There is no evidence that showering with an antiseptic solution the night before surgery decreases the incidence of wound infection. Fixed shoulder braces have been associated with an increased risk of brachial plexus injury and should not be used in the operating room. Both legs should be positioned simultaneously when placing patients in the dorsal lithotomy position. Everyone in the operating room is responsible for patient safety, and therefore the surgeon should always be present for patient positioning.

8. **e. Polydioxanone suture with continuous closure.** Continuous closure with PDS (slowly absorbable) suture has been shown to have the lowest wound failure rates. In the presence of infection, braided sutures (silk and Vicryl) should be avoided to prevent secondary wound infection and failure. Although nonabsorbable sutures may be used, these have been associated with increased postoperative patient discomfort. Fast-absorbing sutures (such as Dexon) should not be used in continuous fascial closure because of increased wound failure risks.

CHAPTER REVIEW

1. One must always determine whether a woman in the childbearing years is pregnant before a surgical procedure. A urine pregnancy test is a simple method to do this.
2. The American Society of Anesthesiologists' classification is a significant predictor of operative mortality.
3. Preoperative cardiac evaluation is meant to identify serious coronary artery disease, heart failure, symptomatic arrhythmias, and the presence of a pacemaker or defibrillator. Major clinical predictors of cardiovascular risk are a recent myocardial infarction (within 1 month), unstable angina, evidence of an ischemic burden, decompensated heart failure, significant arrhythmias, and severe valvular disease.
4. A patient's ability to climb two flights of stairs is a good assessment of adequate functional capacity.
5. Patients with an FEV1 of less than 30% predicted are at high risk for complications.
6. Smoking must be discontinued at least 8 weeks before surgery to be effective in reducing risk.
7. Perioperative β blockade is associated with a reduced risk of death among high-risk patients undergoing major noncardiac surgical procedures. However, more recent data bring this into question.
8. Patients who have a depressed hypothalamic pituitary adrenal axis due to exogenous steroids should receive 50 to 100 mg of intravenous hydrocortisone before the induction of anesthesia and 25 to 50 mg every 8 hours thereafter until the patient's medication is resumed.
9. In the elderly, delirium can be the first clinical sign of hypoxia or of metabolic or infectious complications.
10. In the pregnant patient, postoperative pain is best managed with narcotic analgesics.
11. A preoperative electrocardiogram should be obtained in all patients older than 40 years and in those with a significant cardiac history.
12. It is important to remember that for prophylaxis of venous thromboembolic disease and the use of antibiotic and mechanical bowel preps before intestinal surgery, the studies are often based on data obtained from nonurologic patients. The urologist must consider this when the procedure being performed is significantly different from the standard general surgical operation on which the data are based. This is particularly true for bowel preparation, as urologic reconstructive procedures often require opening the isolated intestinal segment to be used in the procedure, exposing the entire contents to the operative field.
13. Parenteral antibiotics should be given before intestinal surgery.
14. Nitrous oxide inhalation anesthesia results in bowel distention.
15. The half-life of warfarin is 36 to 42 hours, and it is recommended that warfarin be stopped 5 days before the surgical event. Immediate reversal may be accomplished by giving fresh frozen plasma.
16. Aspirin and clopidogrel are irreversible inhibitors of platelet function and should be discontinued 7 to 10 days before surgery if bleeding risk is to be minimized.
17. For moderate- to high-risk groups on anticoagulation therapy, a therapeutic bridge is performed using low-molecular-weight heparin. This may be stopped 12 hours before the procedure and instituted shortly after its completion.
18. The indications for fresh frozen plasma are immediate reversal of warfarin and replacement of specific clotting factors.
19. The most common cause of transfusion-related fatality is transfusion-related acute lung injury.
20. Hypothermia results in increased blood loss and an increased incidence of wound infection.
21. If hair is to be removed, it should preferably be removed immediately before the surgical event with clippers.
22. The surgical scar regains 3% of strength at 1 week, 20% at 3 weeks, and 80% at 3 months.
23. Rapidly absorbable sutures used for continuous fascia closure are associated with an increased incidence of incisional hernias.
24. Fascia dehiscence generally occurs 7 to 10 days postoperatively. The use of retention sutures does not prevent dehiscence; it prevents evisceration.
25. The need for postoperative parenteral nutrition should be anticipated in patients undergoing major urologic procedures involving the use of bowel. If it is likely the patient will not be able to take an adequate caloric intake orally by 7 to 10 days, postoperative parenteral nutrition should be instituted.
26. The second trimester represents the least anesthetic risk to the mother and fetus with regard to spontaneous abortion and teratogenicity.
27. Severely malnourished patients (>20 pounds weight loss in 3 months) significantly benefit from 7 to 10 days of enteral (not parenteral) feedings *before* elective surgery.
28. In a patient with renal insufficiency, unfractionated heparin is a better choice than low-molecular-weight heparin.
29. Current indications for packed red blood cell transfusion are maintenance of hematocrit of greater than 30% in patients with high risk of myocardial ischemia, or in patients with hematocrit 21% to 30% with signs of inadequate oxygen carrying capacity.
30. In the presence of infection, braided sutures (silk and Vicryl) should be avoided.

6 Fundamentals of Urinary Tract Drainage

John D. Denstedt and Thomas Tailly

QUESTIONS

1. A 24-French (Fr) Foley balloon catheter:
   a. measures 24 cm long.
   b. measures 8 mm in outer diameter.
   c. measures 8 mm in inner diameter.
   d. measures 1 cm in outer diameter.
   e. can hold 24 mL of fluid in the retainment balloon.

2. Which of the following statements about the healthy adult male urethra is TRUE?
   a. The external meatus is the narrowest and should allow a 24-Fr catheter to pass.
   b. The bladder neck is the narrowest and should allow for a 24-Fr catheter to pass.
   c. The prostatic urethra is the narrowest and should allow for a 24-Fr catheter to pass.
   d. The prostatic urethra is the widest and should allow for a 24-Fr catheter to pass.
   e. The external meatus is the widest and should allow for a 32-Fr catheter to pass.

3. Which measures can be taken to maximize anesthetic lubrication effect?
   a. Lubricant at body temperature, 11 mL of fluid, fast instillation, 3 minutes indwelling time
   b. Lubricant cooled to 4° C, 20 mL of fluid, slow instillation, >15 minutes indwelling time
   c. Lubricant at body temperature, 30 mL of fluid, slow instillation, >25 minutes indwelling time
   d. Lubricant cooled to 4° C, 11 mL of fluid, fast instillation, 3 minutes indwelling time
   e. Lubricant cooled to 4° C, 11 mL of fluid, fast instillation, >15 minutes indwelling time

4. Asymptomatic bacteriuria:
   a. in the presence of a urinary catheter or ureter stent constitutes a catheter-associated urinary tract infection (CAUTI).
   b. should be screened for in patients with a bladder catheter or indwelling ureteral stent.
   c. should be treated as a urinary tract infection.
   d. should not be screened for in nonpregnant patients with a bladder catheter or indwelling ureteral stent.
   e. never evolves into a urinary tract infection.

5. What is the reported incidence of adjacent organ perforation during suprapubic catheter placement?
   a. 0% to 0.5%
   b. <0.1% to 2.7%
   c. 2.7% to 5%
   d. 5% to 10%
   e. 10% to 15%

6. Which of the following is NOT considered an indication for ureteral stent placement?
   a. Ureteric obstruction in a patient with a solitary functional kidney
   b. After a failed initial attempt at ureteroscopic treatment of a 12-mm ureteral stone
   c. Persistent urinary extravasation after blunt renal trauma
   d. After an uncomplicated ureteroscopy with no residual fragments
   e. After a laparoscopic pyeloplasty for ureteropelvic obstruction

7. What is the most important contributing factor resulting in stent failure?
   a. Small stent caliber
   b. Too soft stent material
   c. Ureteric obstruction by malignant external compression
   d. Female gender
   e. Biofilm-producing bacteria

ANSWERS

1. **b. Measures 8 mm in outer diameter.** The French or Charrière scale was introduced by Joseph E. B. Charrière as a measurement unit for the circumference of a catheter. One unit on the scale equals 0.33 mm in external diameter. A 24-Fr catheter is therefore 8 mm in outer diameter.

2. **a. The external meatus is the narrowest and should allow a 24-Fr catheter to pass.** The caliber of the urethra varies throughout its course. The normal healthy external meatus should allow for a 24-Fr catheter to pass. Subsequent portions of the adult urethra have a larger caliber, the largest being the prostatic urethra with a caliber of approximately 32 Fr. The bladder neck should be large enough to allow for passage of a 28-Fr catheter.

3. **b. Lubricant cooled to 4° C, 20 mL of fluid, slow instillation, >15 minutes indwelling time.** If anesthetic lubricant is to be used, the evidence available suggests instilling a minimum amount of 20 mL of cooled lubricant to be instilled slowly (>3 to 10 seconds) and to allow for a minimum of 15 minutes of exposure to maximize benefit to the patient.

4. **d. Should not be screened for in nonpregnant patients with a bladder catheter or indwelling ureteral stent.** As of January 2009, the definition for CAUTI was modified to exclude asymptomatic bacteriuria. In current guidelines, a CAUTI is defined as significant bacteriuria in a patient with symptoms or signs indicating a urinary tract infection. As there is no evidence supporting that treatment of asymptomatic bacteriuria provides any benefit in reducing morbidity or mortality, EAU and IDSA guidelines specifically recommend against screening and treatment of asymptomatic bacteriuria.

5. **b. <0.1% to 2.7%.** Surrounding organ injury is the most severe complication of suprapubic catheter placement and has been reported to occur in <0.1% to 2.7% of procedures. Ultrasound-guided suprapubic catheter placement is the safest method to avoid this complication.

6. **d. After an uncomplicated ureteroscopy with no residual fragments.** Indications for stent placement have changed in the past decade, with evidence-based medicine calling for stent placement only when specific conditions apply. Relieving obstruction in an obstructed solitary kidney is an absolute indication for stent placement. Current literature suggests that stenting after failed attempt at ureteroscopy may be beneficial. Meta-analysis has demonstrated that stent placement after uncomplicated ureteroscopy is not beneficial.

7. **e. Biofilm-producing bacteria.** The most common cause of stent failure is biofilm-producing bacteria. Together with a prolonged indwelling time, this is the most important factor inducing encrustation, which can lead to stent blockage.

CHAPTER REVIEW

1. The average length of the adult male urethra is 20 cm; the average length of the female urethra is 4 cm. The average caliber of the female urethra is 22 Fr.
2. The use of feeding tubes as urethral catheters is to be discouraged.
3. The use of silicone catheters is associated with a lower incidence of urinary tract infections when compared with those made with latex.
4. Many studies have shown that topical anesthesia is not helpful in reducing pain in routine catheterization.
5. Routine use of catheter coatings is currently not supported by the available literature. Silicone catheters induce less inflammation and are preferred over latex for long-term catheterization.
6. For selected patients, a suprapubic catheter results in less discomfort than a urethral catheter.
7. More than 80% of patients experience ureteral stent-related pain affecting daily activities, and 58% report reduced work capacity.
8. The use of an α_1-adrenergic blocker has been demonstrated to be beneficial in reducing stent symptoms and pain.
9. Indwelling stent time should be limited to 4 months; after that it should be changed or removed. For pregnant patients, the time limit is 4 to 6 weeks.
10. A biofilm is the microorganism's attempt to control its immediate environment by limiting exposure to harmful factors while enhancing exposure to tropic factors. It usually consists of three layers: (1) innermost or linking film that is attached to the surface, (2) a base film that contains exopolysaccharides and the microorganisms, and (3) an outer layer, which is the point of egress or access for organisms.
11. Patients who are catheterized for urinary retention should be decompressed efficiently and completely—there is no role for prolonged slow decompression.
12. Long-term antibiotic prophylaxis for patients with uncomplicated chronic indwelling urethral catheters or ureteral stents has not been shown to be beneficial.
13. Absolute indications for emergent upper track decompression include: (1) bilateral obstruction (unilateral in the case of a solitary kidney) and (2) an obstructed kidney that is infected.
14. One unit on the French scale equals 0.33 mm in external diameter.
15. The normal healthy external meatus should allow for a 24-Fr catheter to pass. Subsequent portions of the adult urethra have a larger caliber.
16. A catheter-associated urinary tract infection is defined as significant bacteriuria in a patient with symptoms or signs indicating a urinary tract infection. There is no evidence that treatment of asymptomatic bacteriuria provides any benefit in reducing morbidity or mortality.

7 Principles of Urologic Endoscopy

Brian D. Duty and Michael J. Conlin

QUESTIONS

1. Patients undergoing diagnostic cystoscopy should receive prophylactic antibiotics if they have any of the following risk factors EXCEPT:
   a. poor nutritional status.
   b. anatomical anomalies.
   c. hypertension.
   d. corticosteroid use.
   e. smoking history.

2. Compared to digital cystourethroscopes, fiberoptic scopes have improved:
   a. illumination.
   b. contrast evaluation.
   c. resolution.
   d. depth of field.
   e. color representation.

3. Techniques that have been shown to improve flexible cystourethroscopy tolerance in men include all of the following EXCEPT:
   a. allowing the patient to observe the procedure.
   b. having the patient empty his bladder before the procedure.
   c. playing classical music during the procedure.
   d. using lidocaine lubricating gel.
   e. increasing the hydrostatic pressure of the irrigant during scope passage.

4. Indications for ureteroscopy include all of the following EXCEPT:
   a. obstructing ureteral calculus.
   b. filling defect of the renal pelvis.
   c. 1.2-cm renal calculus in the lower pole.
   d. ureteropelvic junction obstruction with a large crossing vessel present.
   e. 1.5-cm midureteral stricture.

5. Which of the following statements about ureteroscopy are TRUE?
   a. Ureteral access sheaths decrease intrarenal pressure during ureteroscopy.
   b. Flexible ureteroscopes accept working instruments 3.6 Fr in diameter.
   c. Normal saline should be used for irrigation during ureteroscopy.
   d. A preoperative antibiotic is needed only in high-risk patients.
   e. a and c.

6. Compared to white light endoscopy, narrow band imaging has been shown to:
   a. predict favorable response to bacille Calmette-Guérin intravesical therapy.
   b. accurately differentiate between low- and high-grade lesions.
   c. obviate the need for re-resection in high-grade pT1 patients.
   d. significantly improve detection accuracy of muscle-invasive lesions.
   e. improve detection of noninvasive lesions, including carcinoma in situ.

7. Which of the following statements is TRUE?
   a. The holmium laser is absorbed in 3 cm of water.
   b. Water is the preferred irrigant for ureteroscopy because of improved visibility.
   c. Baskets made of nitinol are more "kink resistant" compared to stainless steel.
   d. Balloon dilation of the intramural ureter is usually necessary before flexible ureteroscopy.
   e. Compared to fiberoptic flexible ureteroscopes, digital flexible ureteroscopes less frequently require the use of ureteral access sheaths.

8. Techniques to minimize staff radiation exposure include all of the following EXCEPT:
   a. using "last image hold" setting.
   b. using fixed fluoroscopy units.
   c. surgeon control of the foot pedal.
   d. using image collimation.
   e. using pulse fluoroscopy mode.

ANSWERS

1. **c. Hypertension.** The American Urological Association's Best Practice Policy Statement on Antimicrobial Prophylaxis did not recommend routine antibiotic administration for diagnostic cystourethroscopy. This recommendation was based on the recognition that some randomized studies have shown antibiotic prophylaxis reduces bacteriuria and symptomatic infection rates, whereas others have not. However, antibiotic administration was advocated by the panel for patients with host factors increasing their risk of infection. These include advanced age, anatomic anomalies, poor nutritional status, smoking, chronic corticosteroid use, immunodeficiency, chronic indwelling hardware infected with endogenous or exogenous material, distant coinfection, and prolonged hospitalization.

2. **a. Illumination.** An in vitro study from the University of California at Irvine compared the resolution, contrast evaluation, depth of field, color representation, and illumination of fiberoptic, standard-definition, and high-definition digital flexible cystoscopes (Lusch et al, 2013).* All three scopes were by the same manufacturer (Olympus, Center Valley, PA). The high-definition digital cystourethroscope was found to have a significantly higher resolution and depth of field compared to the standard-definition digital and fiberoptic models. Color representation was also slightly improved. There was no difference in contrast evaluation among the three models. The only parameter that was found to be superior in the fiberoptic model was illumination.

3. **b. Having the patient empty his bladder before the procedure.** A variety of prospective studies have been performed with the aim of improving patient tolerance during office-based diagnostic flexible cystourethroscopy. A meta-analysis of four randomized trials involving 411 patients found that patients receiving lidocaine gel were 1.7 times less likely to experience moderate to severe pain during the procedure (Aaronson et al, 2009). Results

---

*Sources referenced can be found in *Campbell-Walsh Urology, 11th Edition,* on the Expert Consult website.

of a randomized trial involving 151 men indicated that increasing the hydrostatic pressure of the irrigation solution during passage of the scope through the membranous urethra was associated with significantly less discomfort on an analog pain scale (Gunendran et al, 2008). In another study, men who were allowed to watch the procedure had significantly less pain on a 100-mm visual analog scale (Patel et al, 2007). Last, 70 men were randomly assigned to hear either no music or classical music during cystourethroscopy (Yeo et al, 2013). Patients listening to classical music had significantly less pain, greater satisfaction, lower postprocedure pulse rates, and lower systolic blood pressures.

4. **d. Ureteropelvic junction obstruction with a large crossing vessel present.** All of the options are common indications for ureteroscopy except ureteropelvic junction obstruction due to a large crossing vessel. Although ureteropelvic junction obstruction can be managed with ureteroscopic endopyelotomy, patients with a large crossing vessel are better treated by laparoscopic pyeloplasty.

5. **e. a and c.** Auge and colleagues measured the pressure within the renal pelvis, proximal, mid and distal ureter before and after ureteral access sheath placement in five patients who had previously undergone nephrostomy tube placement (Auge et al, 2004). The pressure within the collecting system was found to be significantly lower at each location following access sheath placement.

6. **e. Improve detection of noninvasive lesions, including carcinoma in situ.** Narrow-band imaging uses only blue (415 nm) and green (540 nm) wavelengths to image the urothelium compared to white light endoscopy, which uses the entire visible light spectrum. Blue and green wavelengths are strongly absorbed by hemoglobin, improving visibility of urothelial capillaries, small papillary lesions, and carcinoma in situ. A meta-analysis of eight studies including 1022 patients found that narrow-band imaging improves detection accuracy of noninvasive lesions, including carcinoma in situ (Zheng et al, 2012).

7. **c. Baskets made of nitinol are more "kink resistant" compared to stainless steel.** Nitinol has a variety of advantageous properties compared to stainless steel. Nitinol is more biocompatible, has greater torqueability and improved "memory," and is more resistant to kinking. These properties make it ideal for stone basket construction. Holmium laser energy is absorbed by 3 mm of water. Saline is the preferred irrigation solution because of the decreased risk of "transurethral resection syndrome" compared to hypotonic solutions. The need for ureteral dilation has decreased over time with the advent of smaller diameter ureteroscopes. However, digital models have larger tip and shaft diameters, making them more likely to need ureteral dilation or access sheath placement compared to their fiberoptic counterparts.

8. **b. Using fixed fluoroscopy units.** All endourologic procedures using fluoroscopy should operate on the ALARA principle (as low as reasonably achievable). Techniques that have been shown to minimize radiation exposure include surgeon control of the foot pedal, using "last image hold," image collimation, and pulsed fluoroscopy mode. Compared to fixed units, mobile C-arm fluoroscopy machines are able to position the image intensifier closer to the patient, thereby reducing exposure while improving image quality.

CHAPTER REVIEW

1. Simple cystoscopy does not require prophylactic antibiotics unless there are risk factors.
2. If electrocautery is used, an electrolyte-free solution should be employed.
3. Narrow-band imaging filters light into two separate bands, blue and green wavelengths, which are absorbed by hemoglobin, aiding in identifying hypervascular lesions. Narrow-band imaging improves detection accuracy of noninvasive lesions, including carcinoma in situ.
5. The designation of the size of an instrument in French (Fr) is approximately the circumference of the instrument. To determine the diameter of the instrument, the French size is divided by 3. Thus a 21-Fr cystoscope is 7 mm in diameter. For ureteroscopy, the irrigants are typically physiologic solutions, such as normal saline. However, with a ureteral access sheath in place, low-osmolarity irrigant fluids may be used.
6. Complications of basketing include ureteral avulsion, intussusception, abrasion, perforation, postoperative stricture formation, and basket entrapment and retention.
7. When introducing an instrument into the bladder through the male urethra, the most uncomfortable area is the membranous urethra.
8. One should not step on the pedal when using the holmium laser if the tip of the fiber cannot be seen in contact with the stone; otherwise the ureter or the ureteroscope may be damaged.
9. Hydrophilic-coated guidewires should not be used as safety wires.

8 Percutaneous Approaches to the Upper Urinary Tract Collecting System

J. Stuart Wolf, Jr.

QUESTIONS

1. Percutaneous nephrostomy is not indicated for:
   a. instillation of intracavitary topical therapy for urothelial carcinoma.
   b. Whitaker test.
   c. management of fungal bezoars.
   d. urinary retention.
   e. ureteral injury.

2. Relative to retrograde ureteral stent placement, percutaneous nephrostomy:
   a. has a lower success rate.
   b. requires less anesthesia.
   c. is preferred in cases of ureteral obstruction owing to malignancy.
   d. is less commonly complicated by bacteriuria after indwelling for 1 week.
   e. is associated with worse health-related quality-of-life scores.

3. Which of the following is correct regarding the orientation of the kidney?
   a. The right kidney is slightly cephalad to the left kidney.
   b. The longitudinal axis is 45 degrees from vertical, with the lower pole lateral to the upper pole.
   c. The longitudinal axis is 45 degrees from vertical, with the lower pole anterior to the upper pole.
   d. The apposition of the colon to the kidney is greatest on the left side at the upper pole.
   e. Immediately posterior to the kidneys are the quadratus lumborum muscle, the psoas muscle, and the diaphragm.

4. Which of the following is correct regarding the intrarenal collecting system?
   a. Paired anterior and posterior calyces enter the infundibula about 90 degrees from each other.
   b. Compound calyces are most common in the lower pole
   c. Most kidneys have three distinct infundibula: the upper, middle, and lower.
   d. There are 8 to 16 minor calyces
   e. There is a consistent relationship between anterior and posterior calyces and their medial-lateral position on anterior-posterior radiography.

5. The correct order of the division of the intrarenal branches of the renal artery is:
   a. segmental, arcuate, interlobar (infundibular), interlobular.
   b. segmental, arcuate, interlobular, interlobar (infundibular).
   c. segmental, interlobar (infundibular), arcuate, interlobular
   d. interlobular, segmental, interlobar (infundibular), arcuate.
   e. segmental, interlobular, interlobar (infundibular), arcuate.

6. To reduce the risk of infectious complications from percutaneous renal surgery:
   a. all patients should receive prophylactic antimicrobials.
   b. urine cultures should be obtained on all patients.
   c. urine must be sterile before the procedure.
   d. gentamicin is an acceptable single agent for antimicrobial prophylaxis.
   e. ampicillin/sulbactam is not an acceptable single agent for antimicrobial prophylaxis.

7. To reduce the risk of hemorrhagic complications associated with percutaneous renal access, the minimum recommended preoperative cessation period for:
   a. herbal medications is 2 weeks.
   b. clopidogrel is 10 days.
   c. aspirin is 5 days.
   d. warfarin is 5 days.
   e. nonsteroidal inflammatory agents is 1 day.

8. Which of the following have NOT been demonstrated in randomized controlled clinical trials to reduce pain associated with percutaneous renal access?
   a. Tract infiltration with local anesthetic
   b. Intercostal nerve block
   c. Thoracic paravertebral block
   d. Balloon dilation compared to semirigid plastic dilation of the access tract
   e. Smaller compared to larger caliber postprocedure nephrostomy tubes

9. An advantage of the supine versus prone position for percutaneous renal surgery is:
   a. improved pulmonary mechanics.
   b. a large horizontal working surface.
   c. easier entry into upper pole calyces.
   d. easier entry into posterior calyces.
   e. reduced pressure in the collecting system.

10. Access into which site provides the optimal versatility and safety for percutaneous renal surgery in the prone position?
    a. Upper pole posterior calyx
    b. Upper pole infundibulum
    c. Renal pelvis
    d. Middle calyx
    e. Lower pole anterior calyx

11. Techniques for retrograde assistance for percutaneous renal access include all but which of the following?
    a. Straight ureteral catheter to inject air
    b. Ureteral access sheath to facilitate drainage
    c. Ureteroscopy to retrieve guidewire

d. Retrograde approach to percutaneous access

e. Retrograde placement of externalized (single pigtail) ureteral stent for drainage

12. Compared to an 18-gauge needle, the 21-gauge needle for percutaneous renal access:

a. should not be used by inexperienced operators.

b. requires a 0.025-inch guidewire.

c. cannot be directed as easily.

d. entails less risk of loss of access.

e. is more traumatic.

13. Compared to ultrasonography, fluoroscopy for percutaneous renal access:

a. is less suited in the morbidly obese.

b. provides more rapid evaluation of the entire kidney.

c. cannot be used to monitor tract dilation.

d. visualizes the access needle better.

e. is preferred in transplant kidneys.

14. The "triangulation" technique for fluoroscopic percutaneous renal access:

a. increases radiation exposure to the operator's hands compared to the "eye-of-the-needle" technique.

b. cannot be performed in malrotated kidneys.

c. is not as dependent on retrograde assistance as the "eye-of-the-needle" technique.

d. is less suitable than the "eye-of-the-needle" technique in morbidly obese patients.

e. continuously monitors depth of needle penetration.

15. Dilation of the tract for percutaneous renal surgery is:

a. not effective with a balloon dilator in hypermobile kidneys.

b. most effective with semirigid dilator.

c. least expensive with metal dilators.

d. most rapid with metal dilators.

e. easiest with a one-shot semirigid dilator.

16. When considering percutaneous renal surgery in horseshoe kidneys:

a. upper pole access is dangerous.

b. lower pole access is preferred in most cases.

c. computed tomography can be misleading.

d. the puncture site is more lateral than in normal kidneys.

e. lower hemorrhage rates than in normal kidneys can be expected.

17. When considering percutaneous renal surgery in transplant kidneys:

a. retrograde assistance is difficult.

b. fluoroscopy is more useful than ultrasonography for initial access.

c. the typical hypermobility renders tract dilation difficult.

d. semirigid plastic dilators should not be used.

e. secondary procedures are usually required.

18. Foley catheters for postprocedure nephrostomy drainage:

a. do not need to be secured at the skin.

b. can have a ureteral catheter passed through the end.

c. should have the balloon filled with dilute contrast material.

d. stay more securely in the kidney than Malecot catheters.

e. are less likely to become infected than Malecot catheters.

19. The Cope retention mechanism:

a. is used in nephro-ureteral stents.

b. is used in internal ureteral stents.

c. is more secure than a balloon catheter.

d. requires cutting the tube to disengage.

e. should not be used in more than one access site.

20. Alternatives to a nephrostomy tube after percutaneous renal surgery include all EXCEPT:

a. maintenance of the working sheath.

b. an internal ureteral stent that is removed cystoscopically.

c. an internal ureteral stent with an attached string that exits out the flank.

d. a ureteral stent externalized out the urethra.

e. no drainage tube at all.

21. A postoperative nephrostomy tube:

a. offers greater assurance of upper urinary tract drainage than an internal ureteral stent.

b. should be placed in the dilated access site.

c. does not maintain the percutaneous access tract unless > 18 Fr.

d. reduces postoperative bleeding.

e. is associated with pain unrelated to tube diameter.

22. A small-caliber (8 to 18 Fr) compared to a large-caliber (20 to 24 Fr) nephrostomy tube after percutaneous renal surgery is associated with:

a. equivalent pain.

b. more urinary leakage.

c. less postprocedure blood loss.

d. less need for removal in the radiology suite.

e. earlier hospital discharge.

23. Adjuncts intended to enhance hemostasis of the percutaneous tract include all EXCEPT:

a. direct cauterization of the tract.

b. microwave treatment of the tract.

c. cryotreatment of the tract.

d. insertion of oxidized cellulose.

e. instillation of fibrin glue.

24. Compared to internal ureteral stents after percutaneous renal surgery, nephrostomy tubes are associated with:

a. reduced need for a second procedure for removal.

b. greater technical success rate.

c. greater narcotic use.

d. fewer complications.

e. less urinary leakage from skin entry site.

25. Following an unremarkable percutaneous nephrolithotomy, there is nonpulsatile bleeding from the tract when the sheath is removed around a 12-Fr nephrostomy tube. The next step is:

a. replace the nephrostomy tube with an 18-Fr Malecot catheter.

b. replace the nephrostomy tube with a ureteral stent and suture the skin.

c. irrigate the nephrostomy tube.

d. occlude the nephrostomy tube and apply pressure to the incision.

e. replace the nephrostomy tube with a Kaye nephrostomy tamponade balloon.

26. During a percutaneous resection of a 2-cm upper pole urothelial neoplasm, there is sudden hemorrhage from the resection site. The next step is:
    a. continue with the procedure if vision is adequate.
    b. insert a percutaneous nephro-ureteral stent.
    c. instill gelatin granules plus thrombin into the collecting system.
    d. place an 18-Fr Councill catheter with the balloon inflated at the injury site.
    e. prepare the patient for selective angioembolization.

27. A 65-year-old man calls the office 1 week after percutaneous nephrolithotomy complaining of bright red blood in the urine on his last two urinations. He is otherwise feeling well. He should next:
    a. check the percutaneous access site and come to the hospital if there is external bleeding.
    b. force fluids and call back if bleeding persists.
    c. take aminocaproic acid (Amicar).
    d. apply pressure to the percutaneous access site.
    e. come to the hospital.

28. Which of the following has NOT been reported to cause renal pelvic perforation in association with percutaneous renal surgery?
    a. Wire passage
    b. Tract dilation
    c. Massive hemorrhage
    d. Use of resectoscope
    e. Ultrasonic lithotripsy

29. Two days after percutaneous endopyelotomy in a 65-year-old woman, nephrostography reveals contrast entering the colon. The next step is to:
    a. perform exploratory laparotomy.
    b. maintain the nephrostomy tube in place and insert a ureteral stent.
    c. maintain the nephrostomy tube in place and insert a colostomy tube.
    d. back out the nephrostomy tube into the colon and insert a new nephrostomy tube.
    e. start parenteral feeding, after appropriate tube insertions.

30. Injury to which organ during percutaneous renal surgery can often be managed with little additional interventions?
    a. Liver
    b. Spleen
    c. Duodenum
    d. Jejunum
    e. Gallbladder

31. Regarding pleural injuries in association with percutaneous renal surgery:
    a. access below the 12th rib results in hydropneumothorax in 1% to 2% of cases.
    b. supra-12th rib punctures (the 11th intercostal space) result in hydropneumothorax in 20% to 40% of cases.
    c. supra-11th rib punctures (the 10th intercostal space) result in hydropneumothorax in 50% to 75% of cases.
    d. combined with distal ureteral obstruction, a nephropleural fistula can occur.
    e. thoracostomy to water seal drainage and suction is recommended.

32. Irrigation fluid during percutaneous renal surgery:
    a. is not absorbed systemically unless there is significant venous injury.
    b. should be normal saline except during percutaneous nephrolithotomy.
    c. can have fatal consequences.
    d. should not be glycine.
    e. will not create a defined extrarenal collection.

33. A 55-year-old woman has an oral temperature of 38.5° C on the first night after an uncomplicated percutaneous nephrolithotomy for a partial staghorn renal calculus. A nephrostomy tube is in place. She is hemodynamically stable. The preoperative urine culture had grown a pansensitive *Proteus* sp., and she had received oral trimethoprim sulfamethoxazole for 2 weeks preoperatively. One g of cefazolin had been administered on call to the operating room. The next step is:
    a. observation.
    b. culture aspirate from nephrostomy tube and irrigate nephrostomy tube.
    c. Doppler ultrasonography of lower extremities and/or pulmonary embolus-protocol computed tomography scan.
    d. administer broad-spectrum antibiotics.
    e. culture urine and blood, obtain chest radiograph, and administer broad-spectrum antibiotics.

34. Following percutaneous renal surgery, loss of renal function is:
    a. approximately 5% of ipsilateral function per access site.
    b. minimal in the absence of vascular injury.
    c. greater than after shock wave lithotripsy.
    d. less in pelvic compared to orthotopic kidneys.
    e. greater in solitary compared to nonsolitary kidneys.

ANSWERS

1. **d. Urinary retention.** Obstruction of the lower urinary tract is best treated by drainage of the bladder rather than the kidney, unless secondary obstruction of the upper tract has developed that is refractory to vesical drainage. The other indications are appropriate ones for percutaneous nephrostomy.
2. **b. Requires less anesthesia.** Percutaneous nephrostomy can be done under local anesthesia, as opposed to retrograde ureteral stent placement, which usually requires at least intravenous sedation, and commonly general or regional anesthesia. Percutaneous nephrostomy has a greater initial success rate than retrograde ureteral stent placement, at least when the collecting system is dilated. Percutaneous nephrostomy is commonly associated with bacteriuria and has health-related quality-of-life scores that are equivalent to those associated with retrograde ureteral stent placement. Ureteral stents provide satisfactory drainage in most cases of ureteral obstruction owing to malignancy.
3. **e. Immediately posterior to the kidneys are the quadratus lumborum muscle, the psoas muscle, and the diaphragm.** The upper poles are anterior to attachments of the diaphragm. It is the left kidney that is slightly cephalad to the right one. The second two statements are correct, except that the angulation is 30 degrees rather than 45 degrees. The apposition of the colon to the kidney varies with location; it is greatest on the left side, but at the lower rather than upper pole.
4. **a. Paired anterior and posterior calyces enter the infundibula about 90 degrees from each other.** The paired anterior and posterior calyces enter about 90 degrees from each other. Although compound calyces are common in the lower pole, they are almost always present in the upper pole. In about two thirds of kidneys, there are only two major calyceal systems (upper

and lower). There are 5 to 14 minor calyces in each kidney. Because variation is considerable, the lateral-medial orientation of the calyces on anteroposterior radiography cannot be used to reliably determine which calyces are posterior.

5. **c. Segmental, interlobar (infundibular), arcuate, interlobular.**

6. **a. All patients should receive prophylactic antimicrobials.** The American Urological Association recommends periprocedural antimicrobial prophylaxis for all cases of percutaneous renal surgery. Urine cultures are considered standard only in patients where bacteriuria is likely; in other cases a screening urinalysis likely is adequate, with urine culture when the urinalysis is suspicious. The urine cannot be sterilized in some patients, especially in the presence of an externalized urinary catheter or an infected calculus, and the goal in these situations is only to suppress the bacterial count before intervention. Aminoglycosides (e.g., gentamicin) are acceptable for antimicrobial prophylaxis when combined with another agent. Ampicillin/sulbactam, first- and second-generation cephalosporins, and fluoroquinolones are acceptable single agents for antimicrobial prophylaxis.

7. **d. Warfarin is 5 days.** The recommended preoperative cessation periods are as follows: herbal medicines, 1 week; clopidogrel, 5 days; aspirin, 1 week; warfarin, 5 days; nonsteroidal inflammatory agents, 3 to 7 days.

8. **d. Balloon dilation compared to semirigid plastic dilation of the access tract.** There is no evidence that balloon dilation is associated with less pain compared to semirigid plastic dilation of the access tract. All of the other maneuvers have been demonstrated in randomized controlled clinical trials to reduce pain associated with percutaneous renal access.

9. **e. Reduced pressure in the collecting system.** The angle of the sheath is more horizontal in the supine compared to the prone position for percutaneous renal surgery, which reduces pressure in the collecting system (the volume also is reduced, which is a disadvantage). When padding is appropriate, pulmonary mechanics are better in the prone position. The prone position also provides a large horizontal working surface and easier entry into posterior and upper pole calyces compared to the supine position.

10. **a. Upper pole posterior calyx.** This offers the most versatile access to the intrarenal collecting system, and as long as the entry is below the 11th rib, the advantages generally outweigh the risks. Percutaneous access into an infundibulum or the renal pelvis poses a greater risk of vascular injury than calyceal entry. Middle calyceal access provides good access to the ureter, but usually does not provide good access to the upper and lower calyces. In the prone position an anterior calyx offers little access to the rest of the kidney.

11. **e. Retrograde placement of externalized (single pigtail) ureteral stent for drainage.** This can be performed at the conclusion of the procedure for drainage as an alternative to a nephrostomy tube, but it is not useful before access because the pigtail might interfere with the procedure and it would not have any advantage over a straight ureteral catheter or an occlusion balloon catheter. The other choices are all well-described techniques of retrograde assistance for percutaneous renal access.

12. **e. Is more traumatic.** A 21-gauge needle is not as easy to direct as an 18 gauge needle because it is more flexible. A 21 gauge needle requires a 0.018-inch guidewire, and because of this extra step (exchanging the 0.018-inch guidewire for a 0.035-inch guidewire) there is a greater risk of loss of access. Compared to an 18-gauge needle, the 21-gauge needle is less traumatic; this is its primary advantage, and it is for this reason that the 21-gauge needle should be used when the operator is less experienced or if minimizing trauma is paramount.

13. **d. Visualizes the access needle better.** It is easier to see a needle and monitor tract dilation with fluoroscopy than with ultrasonography. Percutaneous access is always more difficult in the morbidly obese, and ultrasonography is no better than fluoroscopy in this situation. Ultrasonography is more portable, can more rapidly evaluate different views of the kidney, and is preferred in settings in which retrograde access cannot be attained or is difficult to attain (kidneys above urinary diversions, transplanted kidneys, kidneys above a completely obstructed ureter, etc.).

14. **e. Continuously monitors depth of needle penetration.** The "triangulation" technique monitors depth of needle placement in all fluoroscopic views, whereas the "eye-of-the-needle" technique assesses depth only at the final step. If the fluoroscopy field is collimated down and the needle is held with a hemostat, sponge forceps, or purpose-built needle holder, then radiation exposure to the operator's hands can be avoided with both techniques. Retrograde assistance is useful with any fluoroscopic percutaneous renal access, and both techniques are more difficult in morbidly obese patients.

15. **c. Least expensive with metal dilators.** Metal dilators are least expensive on a per-case basis because they are reusable. The metal dilators are also the most effective dilators. It is uncertain which are the safest dilators, at least in terms of association with hemorrhage. The balloon dilators are more effective in hypermobile kidneys than other techniques, and also more rapid than sequential passage of metal or semirigid dilators. The one-shot semirigid dilator technique requires considerable manual force to create the tract.

16. **e. Lower hemorrhage rates than in normal kidneys can be expected.** The rate of major hemorrhagic complications during percutaneous renal surgery in horseshoe kidneys (4.3%) is less than in normal kidneys (6% to 20%). Upper pole access is useful, and direct lower pole access is usually not possible. Cross-sectional imaging is useful in assessing the anatomy of horseshoe kidneys. The initial entry into a horseshoe kidney usually is more medial than in normal kidneys.

17. **a. Retrograde assistance is difficult.** Because of the site of ureteral implantation in the bladder, retrograde assistance for percutaneous renal surgery in transplant kidneys is difficult. Given this, ultrasonography is more useful than fluoroscopy for guiding initial access. Semirigid plastic and metal dilators are often more useful than balloon dilators because of the perinephric scarring, which makes the transplant kidney quite fixed in place rather than hypermobile. Despite the challenges, percutaneous renal surgery in transplant kidneys has a high success rate, and secondary procedures are usually not required.

18. **d. Stay more securely in the kidney than Malecot catheters.** Malecot tubes are the easiest to pull out, and circle nephrostomy tubes are the hardest. All tubes should be secured at the skin to reduce the risk of at least one mechanism of tube removal. A ureteral catheter can be passed through the end hole of a Councill catheter; a Foley catheter does not have this end hole. Saline or water should be used to inflate the balloon, as the more viscous contrast material might hinder emptying of the balloon when removal is attempted. All nephrostomy tubes, even ones with robust internal retention devices, should be fixed to the skin externally with a suture or other mechanism. There is no evidence that Foley and Malecot catheters differ in propensity for infection.

19. **a. Is used in nephro-ureteral stents.** The Cope retention mechanism is used in the renal pelvic portion of nephro-ureteral stents. According to one study, the Cope retention mechanism is more secure than Malecot wings, but does not retain as well as a balloon. It is more secure than a passive pigtail retention mechanism owing to the string that holds the coil in place. There is no evidence that more than one Cope-type nephrostomy tube should not be used.

20. **a. Maintenance of the working sheath.** The stiff working access sheath would be a poor choice for postprocedure collecting system drainage. All of the other options have been described.

21. **a. Offers greater assurance of upper urinary tract drainage than an internal ureteral stent.** Drainage of upper urinary tract after percutaneous renal surgery is adequate with an internal ureteral stent in most cases (or with no tube at all in selected cases), but when hemorrhage occurs, the larger caliber of a nephrostomy tube provides better drainage of the upper urinary tract collecting system than an internal ureteral stent. The nephrostomy tube does not have to be placed in the dilated access site (i.e., it can be placed at a new site), although that is common practice. Although redilation may be required, any external nephrostomy

tube maintains the percutaneous access tract. There is actually less hemorrhage when a postoperative nephrostomy tube is omitted. Most studies suggest that the pain associated with nephrostomy tubes is related to tube diameter, with smaller-caliber tubes causing less pain.

22. **d. Less need for removal in the radiology suite.** The removal of larger tubes occasionally can be followed by immediate hemorrhage; this is rare with smaller tubes. Therefore large-caliber nephrostomy tubes should be removed in a radiology suite where there is the opportunity for immediate replacement of the tube. Small-caliber tubes can be removed safely at the bedside after a period of clamping to assess clinically for distal ureteral obstruction. A number of studies have compared the impact of nephrostomy tube diameter after percutaneous renal surgery. Only one study found no benefit to the smaller tube. Otherwise consistent advantages of the small-caliber tubes are less pain, less urinary leakage, and no change in postprocedure blood loss. There is no consistent evidence that small-caliber tubes are associated with shorter duration of hospitalization compared to large-caliber tubes.

23. **b. Microwave treatment of the tract.** Microwave treatment of the tract would be difficult with current instruments. The other options have all been described. Other hemostatic agents that have been inserted/instilled into the tract include gelatin sponge and gelatin granules plus thrombin.

24. **c. Greater narcotic use.** Most randomized controlled trials comparing internal ureteral stents to large-caliber nephrostomy tubes after percutaneous renal surgery have shown reduced narcotic use in the stented patients. The difference is less significant when a small-caliber nephrostomy tube is used. Depending on physician preference, both internal ureteral stents (if attached to a string that exits via the flank) and small-caliber nephrostomy tubes can be removed at the bedside. Randomized controlled trials comparing internal ureteral stents to nephrostomy tubes have not revealed any difference in technical success rates, complication rates, or incidence of urinary leakage from the skin entry site.

25. **d. Occlude the nephrostomy tube and apply pressure to the incision.** The first step in this situation is to occlude the nephrostomy tube and apply pressure to the incision. Let the collecting system clot off, and do not irrigate until the following morning. This management is successful in the majority of cases. If bleeding persists, then insert a Kaye nephrostomy tamponade balloon. An 18-Fr Malecot catheter will be no more effective than the 12-Fr Cope nephrostomy tube. Irrigation is not useful, and removing the nephrostomy tube altogether is ill-advised.

26. **a. Continue with the procedure if vision is adequate.** If the procedure can be continued with acceptable vision, then the blood loss cannot be great. If vision is lost, however, then the procedure must be aborted. If so, then inserting and occluding a nephrostomy tube, as well as applying pressure to the incision so that the collecting system clots off, will suffice in most cases. If this is not successful, then place a Councill catheter and attempt to inflate the balloon at the injury site. Instillation of gelatin granules plus thrombin into the collecting system can create a clot that is difficult to manage. Selective angioembolization is required only when an arterial injury does not respond to less intensive management, or if the injury is obviously a significant one that will not respond to these maneuvers.

27. **e. Come to the hospital.** Any report of bright red blood in the urine after percutaneous renal surgery should prompt hospital admission. This man likely has an arteriovenous fistula or arterial pseudoaneurysm. The conservative measures are not likely to be helpful, and aminocaproic acid (Amicar) is contraindicated in the setting of upper tract hemorrhage.

28. **c. Massive hemorrhage.** The renal pelvis will clot off before the pressure from hemorrhage would rupture it. Any manipulation during percutaneous renal surgery can cause renal pelvic perforation.

29. **d. Back out the nephrostomy tube into the colon and insert a new nephrostomy tube.** The main principle of care of a colon injury associated with percutaneous renal surgery is prompt and separate drainage of the colon and urinary collecting system. If detected postoperatively, the simplest management is to back the nephrostomy tube out of the kidney and into the colon to serve as a colostomy, and then obtain separate access to the upper urinary tract, with either a new percutaneous access that does not traverse the colon or a retrograde-placed ureteral stent. Parenteral feeding is usually not required, and for the typical extraperitoneal injury, open surgical repair usually is needed only if the patient develops peritonitis or sepsis.

30. **a. Liver.** Although splenic injuries have been managed conservatively, the need for surgical intervention is more likely than with liver injuries. Injuries to small bowel or the biliary system require prompt treatment.

31. **d. Combined with distal ureteral obstruction, a nephropleural fistula can occur.** Nephropleural fistula (urinothorax) is a direct and persistent communication between the intrarenal collecting system and the intrathoracic cavity, which can follow percutaneous renal access of the upper urinary tract in the setting of pleural transgression. Some degree of distal ureteral obstruction usually contributes to the problem. The rates of pleural injures for infra-12th rib, supra-12th rib, and supra-11th rib punctures are approximately less than 0.5%, 5%, and 25%, respectively. Thoracostomy is not necessary for all patients with hydrothorax. If one is needed, then a small-caliber tube with a Heimlich valve is all that is required in the absence of lung injury.

32. **c. Can have fatal consequences.** Intravascular hemolysis from the extravasated water irrigant can be fatal. The irrigant for percutaneous renal surgery should be saline, with the exception of glycine or similar nonelectrolytic isotonic fluids when monopolar electrocautery is used. Intravascular or extravascular extravasation of fluid from continued irrigation in the setting of a large venous injury or collecting system perforation can lead to clinically significant sequelae including volume overload and extrarenal fluid collections that require drainage.

33. **a. Observation.** Preoperative and perioperative management of this patient has been appropriate. In this setting, most patients with fever after percutaneous nephrolithotomy do not have infection. If the fever is an isolated postoperative one, then standard postoperative care (early ambulation, use of incentive spirometry, etc.) is all that is needed. If the fever does not resolve promptly, then appropriate diagnostic evaluation and initiation of antimicrobial therapy and other supportive care are indicated.

34. **b. Minimal in the absence of vascular injury.** The kidney suffers little permanent damage after uncomplicated percutaneous renal surgery. If there is significant loss of function, it is usually owing to disastrous vascular injury or the angioembolization used to treat hemorrhage. Loss of renal function associated with percutaneous renal surgery is less than or equal to the loss associated with shock wave lithotripsy. There is no evidence that damage to the kidney is any more or less in pelvic, orthotopic, solitary, or nonsolitary kidneys.

CHAPTER REVIEW

1. Percutaneous nephrostomy and retrograde ureteral stents are generally equivalent in their capacity to resolve fever in patients with upper urinary tract obstruction. However, obstruction complicated by infection is an emergency, and in the unstable patient, percutaneous drainage may be more efficacious.

2. The colon can be lateral or posterior to the right and left kidney.

3. A guidewire that enters the kidney percutaneously and exits the urethra via the meatus (through and through access) may be the only guidewire used when operating on the upper urinary tract. However, in all other situations, two guidewires—a safety and a working guidewire—are required. No matter what the access, it is always prudent to have a safety guidewire in addition to the working guidewire.

4. It is imperative that the dilators do not pass too far into the collecting system because this results in renal pelvic injury.

5. Percutaneous nephrostomy is generally the preferred approach for endoscopy of the obstructed collecting system in the transplanted kidney.

6. Approximately 1% of percutaneous procedures are complicated by delayed hemorrhage. Delayed hemorrhage is usually due to arteriovenous fistulas or arterial pseudoaneurysms. The preferred management is selective angioembolization.

7. Renal arteries are end arteries and result in loss of the segment of renal parenchyma they supply when occluded. Renal veins communicate with each other.

8. Complications of percutaneous nephrostomy include hemorrhage, collecting system injury, colon injury, pleural injury, neuromuscular injuries, air embolism, and infundibular stenosis.

9. Although compound calyces are common in the lower pole, they are almost always present in the upper pole.

10. The recommended preoperative cessation periods are as follows: herbal medicines, 1 week; clopidogrel, 5 days; aspirin, 1 week; warfarin, 5 days; nonsteroidal inflammatory agents, 3 to 7 days.

11. The main principle of care of a colon injury associated with percutaneous renal surgery is prompt and separate drainage of the colon and urinary collecting system. The simplest management is to back the nephrostomy tube out of the kidney and into the colon to serve as a colostomy, and then obtain separate access to the upper urinary tract, either with a new percutaneous access that does not traverse the colon or with a retrograde-placed ureteral stent.

12. Intravascular hemolysis from the extravasated water irrigant can be fatal. The irrigant for percutaneous renal surgery should be saline, with the exception of glycine or similar nonelectrolytic isotonic fluids when monopolar electrocautery is used.

9

Evaluation and Management of Hematuria

Stephen A. Boorjian, Jay D. Raman, and Daniel A. Barocas

QUESTIONS

1. Microhematuria sufficient to trigger a diagnostic evaluation is defined as:
   a. a positive chemical test (urine dipstick) showing small, moderate, or large blood on one properly collected specimen.
   b. a positive chemical test (urine dipstick) showing small, moderate, or large blood on at least two of three properly collected specimens.
   c. a positive chemical test (urine dipstick) showing large blood on one properly collected specimen.
   d. urine microscopy showing three or more red blood cells per high-powered field (RBCs/HPF) on one properly collected urine specimen.
   e. urine microscopy showing three or more RBCs/HPF on at least two of three properly collected urine specimens.

2. The likelihood of finding a malignancy in a patient with microhematuria is influenced by all of the following, EXCEPT:
   a. age.
   b. gender.
   c. use of anticoagulants.
   d. tobacco use.
   e. degree of hematuria.

3. According to American Urological Association guidelines, the proper initial assessment of a 50-year-old patient with asymptomatic microhematuria includes:
   a. blood pressure measurement, serum creatinine level, cystoscopy, and computed tomographic (CT) urogram.
   b. urine cytology, cystoscopy, and CT urogram.
   c. urine cytology, blue-light cystoscopy, and any upper tract imaging.
   d. urine cytology and renal/bladder ultrasound.
   e. no evaluation unless microhematuria is persistent/recurrent or hematuria is visible.

4. In the evaluation of patients with microhematuria, cystoscopy may be safely avoided if:
   a. there are no associated symptoms in a patient of any age.
   b. the patient is younger than 35 years and without symptoms or risk factors for malignancy.
   c. the patient is taking aspirin or warfarin.
   d. the cytology is negative.
   e. the patient has a history of urinary tract infection, and hematuria is still present after treatment.

5. Patients presenting with gross hematuria in the absence of recent trauma or concurrent infection who are on anticoagulation medications should be evaluated with:
   a. urinalysis, urine cytology, and cystoscopy only.
   b. CT urogram, with cystoscopy only if symptomatic.
   c. no evaluation is necessary.

   d. assessment of anticoagulation status, and evaluation only if supratherapeutic.
   e. urine cytology, cystoscopy, and CT urogram.

6. The metabolite of oxazaphosphorine chemotherapeutic agents that is responsible for hemorrhagic cystitis is:
   a. mesna.
   b. acrolein.
   c. formalin.
   d. gemcitabine.
   e. methotrexate.

7. Use of intravesical alum for hemorrhagic cystitis should be avoided in patients with:
   a. a history of malignancy.
   b. a history of detrusor instability.
   c. active gross hematuria.
   d. renal insufficiency.
   e. vesicoureteral reflux.

8. The molecular pathophysiology linking benign prostatic hyperplasia (BPH) and hematuria is exemplified by the identification of which of the following in the prostate tissue from men with BPH?
   a. Decreased microvessel density
   b. Androgen-independent angiogenesis
   c. Elevated expression of vascular endothelial growth factor (VEGF)
   d. Reduced cell proliferation
   e. Diminished blood flow

9. A 65-year-old man with a history of BPH has recurrent gross hematuria. The patient is clinically stable, with no transfusion requirement, no clots in urine, and no difficulty with bladder emptying. A hematuria evaluation with CT urogram, cystoscopy, and urine cytology is unremarkable. The best next step in management is:
   a. five-alpha reductase inhibitor.
   b. alpha-blocker therapy.
   c. angioembolization of internal iliac artery.
   d. channel transurethral resection of the prostate (TURP).
   e. trial of antibiotic therapy.

10. A 35-year-old man presents with the complaint of penile pain and immediate detumescence during intercourse. Physical examination notes blood at the urethral meatus. The next step should be:
    a. immediate operative exploration.
    b. CT scan of the pelvis.
    c. retrograde urethrography.
    d. to obtain serum coagulation parameters.
    e. conservative management with serial examinations.

11. A 55-year-old woman presents with intermittent gross hematuria 2 weeks after undergoing a right partial nephrectomy for a 4-cm solid enhancing renal mass. She is afebrile with stable vital signs. She is able to void to completion, and her urine is red without clots. Her creatinine is 1.1 mg/dL. The next step should be:

    a. surgical exploration.
    b. renal angiography.
    c. continuous bladder irrigation.
    d. observation.
    e. noncontrast CT scan of the abdomen/pelvis.

ANSWERS

1. **d. Urine microscopy showing three or more red blood cells per high-powered field (RBCs/HPF) on one properly collected urine specimen.** The presence of three or more RBCs/HPF on a single urine microscopy is associated with malignancy in 2.3% to 5.5% of patients. Chemical tests for hematuria detect the peroxidase activity of erythrocytes by using benzidine and can render false results in the presence of dehydration, myoglobinuria, high doses of vitamin C, improper technique, and other factors. Although higher levels of microhematuria (>25 RBCs/HPF) are known to be associated with higher rates of malignancy on evaluation, setting the threshold higher than 3 RBCs/HPF or requiring more than one positive urinalysis would lead to an unknown number of missed opportunities for diagnosis.

2. **c. Use of anticoagulants.** Increasing age, male gender, and tobacco use are risk factors for urologic cancers and specifically for urothelial carcinoma. In addition, although there are few data to distinguish among thresholds of 2, 3, 4, or 5 RBCs/HPF, it is clear that a high level of microhematuria (>25 RBCs/HPF) is associated with a greater likelihood of malignancy. By contrast, patients using anticoagulant medications or antiplatelet medications have a risk of malignancy similar to that of those who do not use these medications. Therefore, such patients should be evaluated comparably to those who do not use anticoagulants or antiplatelet agents.

3. **a. Blood pressure measurement, serum creatinine level, cystoscopy, and computed tomographic (CT) urogram.** The AUA suggests that adult patients presenting with asymptomatic microhematuria should undergo evaluation to determine the cause. Blood pressure measurement and serum creatinine level may help identify patients who require concurrent nephrologic workup, and creatinine level also helps determine patient eligibility for contrast imaging. The evaluation of asymptomatic microhematuria includes imaging (preferably with CT urogram) and cystoscopy in patients 35 and older and those under 35 with risk factors for malignancy.

4. **b. The patient is younger than 35 years and without symptoms or risk factors for malignancy.** The AUA guidelines call for use of cystoscopy for evaluation of hematuria in all patients 35 years and older (Recommendation). The risk of malignancy is very low in persons younger than 35 years, such that the potential benefits of cystoscopy may be outweighed by the very small risks associated with the procedure. Therefore, it is an option to omit cystoscopy in patients younger than the age of 35, provided that the patient does not have risk factors for a urologic malignancy.

5. **e. Urine cytology, cystoscopy, CT urogram.** Given the increased frequency with which clinically significant findings are associated with gross hematuria, the recommended evaluation in this setting is relatively uniform. That is, patients presenting with gross hematuria in the absence of antecedent trauma or culture-documented urinary tract infection should be evaluated with a urine cytology, cystoscopy, and upper tract imaging, preferably CT urogram. Importantly, patients who develop hematuria and are on anticoagulation medications should undergo a complete evaluation in the same manner as patients not taking such medications, because the prevalence of hematuria, as well as the likelihood of finding genitourinary cancers, among patients with hematuria on anticoagulation has been reported to be no different from that for patients not taking such medications.

6. **b. Acrolein.** Bladder toxicity with oxazaphosphorine chemotherapeutic agents results from renal excretion of the metabolite acrolein, which is produced by the liver and which stimulates bladder mucosal sloughing and subsequent tissue edema/fibrosis. Mesna (2-mercaptoethane sulfonate), which binds to acrolein and renders it inert, has been suggested for prophylaxis against cyclophosphamide-induced hemorrhagic cystitis.

7. **d. Renal insufficiency.** Alum may be considered for first-line intravesical therapy among patients with hemorrhagic cystitis failing initial supportive measures. However, although cell penetration and therefore overall toxicity of this agent is low, systemic absorption may nevertheless occur and may result in aluminum toxicity, with consequent mental status changes, particularly among patients with renal insufficiency. Meanwhile, before intravesical administration of silver nitrate or formalin, a cystogram should be obtained to evaluate for the presence of vesicoureteral reflux.

8. **c. Elevated expression of vascular endothelial growth factor (VEGF).** The etiology for BPH-related hematuria has been thought to be increased prostatic vascularity due to higher microvessel density in hyperplastic prostate tissue. This noted increase in microvessel density has in turn been linked to higher levels of VEGF. Moreover, because the pathophysiology of BPH-related bleeding has been postulated as increased cell proliferation stimulating increased vascularity, efforts to suppress prostate growth via androgen ablation have been explored. Indeed, both estrogens and antiandrogens have, in small case reports, been associated with decreased prostate bleeding, presumably through the repression of androgen-stimulated angiogenesis and the induction of programmed cell death within the prostate.

9. **a. Five-alpha reductase inhibitor.** Treatment with finasteride is associated with decreased VEGF expression, prostate microvessel density, and prostatic blood flow. Clinically, multiple series have demonstrated the efficacy of finasteride for BPH-related hematuria, with symptom improvement or resolution consistently noted in approximately 90% of patients. Therefore, in otherwise stable patients, finasteride represents a reasonable first-line therapy for BPH-related gross hematuria after the completion of an initial diagnostic evaluation. Channel TURP has typically been used in the setting of prostate cancer, whereas a "standard" TURP or an alternative form of such endoscopic prostate tissue removal/destruction may be used for patients with persistent bleeding from BPH despite conservative therapies and/or endoscopic fulguration, particularly when additional indications for BPH surgery coexist. In cases with persistent bleeding despite TURP, selective angioembolization should be considered.

10. **c. Retrograde urethrography.** The clinical scenario is consistent with an acute penile fracture. Blood at the meatus raises suspicion for concomitant urethral injury, which requires investigation by retrograde urethrography before planned operative repair. Conservative management poses the risk of untreated urethral and corporal injury, which can result in urethral stricture disease and erectile dysfunction.

11. **b. Renal angiography.** The clinical scenario is consistent with a renal arteriovenous malformation (AVM). Renal angiography is both diagnostic and therapeutic in this scenario, with the ability to coil or embolize this abnormal vascular communication. Observation and bladder irrigation do not address the underlying causative factor, and noncontrast CT imaging fails to delineate the vascular anatomy. Surgical exploration has a high likelihood of renal loss and is reserved for cases refractory to angiographic modalities.

CHAPTER REVIEW

1. Initial hematuria most commonly originates from the urethra; terminal hematuria is usually from the trigone, bladder neck, or prostate.

2. Substances that may make the urine appear to contain blood include bilirubin, myoglobin, porphyrins, ingested foods such as beets and rhubarb, and phenazopyridine.

3. Malignancy is found in 2% to 4% of patients evaluated for microhematuria.

4. Vigorous exercise may cause hematuria.

5. Patients who are on anticoagulants and have hematuria, microscopic or gross, should be fully evaluated.

6. None of the urinary biomarkers, including cytology, are sufficiently sensitive to eliminate cystoscopy in the evaluation.

7. Alum concentration should not exceed 1%; aluminum toxicity may be a complication. It should not be used in patients with renal insufficiency.

8. Silver nitrate concentration should not exceed 1%; formalin concentration should not exceed preferably 1% or 2% at most (it is normally supplied in a 10% concentration). Higher concentrations of silver nitrate and formalin markedly increase serious complications such as bladder wall slough, bladder contracture, and perforation. Before intravesical administration of silver nitrate or of formalin, a cystogram should be obtained to evaluate for the presence of vesicoureteral reflux.

9. Bilateral nephrostomy tubes may be helpful in patients with persistent hemorrhagic cystitis when all other conservative methods fail.

10. Laser fulguration has shown promise in controlling bleeding in patients with persistent hemorrhagic cystitis.

11. Signs that the bleeding is glomerular in origin include red blood cell casts, dysmorphic red cells, and significant proteinuria.

12. BPH is the most common cause of prostate bleeding; when the bleeding is due to untreated prostate cancer, one should think of more advanced disease, such as invasion into the bladder neck.

13. Microhematuria is defined as urine microscopy showing three or more red blood cells per high-powered field on one properly collected urine specimen.

14. The evaluation of asymptomatic hematuria includes imaging (preferably with CT urogram), cytology, and cystoscopy in patients 35 and older and those younger than 35 years with risk factors for malignancy.

15. Mesna (2-mercaptoethane sulfonate), which binds to acrolein and renders it inert, has been suggested for prophylaxis against cyclophosphamide-induced hemorrhagic cystitis.

16. The etiology for BPH-related hematuria has been thought to be increased prostatic vascularity due to higher microvessel density in hyperplastic prostate tissue. Treatment with finasteride is associated with decreased VEGF expression, prostate microvessel density, and prostatic blood flow

17. In cases with persistent prostatic bleeding despite TURP, selective angioembolization should be considered.

10 Fundamentals of Laparoscopic and Robotic Urologic Surgery

Michael Ordon, Jaime Landman, and Louis Eichel

QUESTIONS

1. Absolute contraindications to laparoscopic surgery include all of the following EXCEPT:
   a. uncorrectable coagulopathy.
   b. hemodynamic instability.
   c. significant abdominal wall infection.
   d. suspected malignant ascites.
   e. extensive prior abdominal or pelvic surgery.

2. Of the following, which is considered a relative contraindication to laparoscopic surgery?
   a. Generalized peritonitis
   b. Massive hemoperitoneum
   c. Intestinal obstruction with intention to treat
   d. Extensive prior abdominal or pelvic surgery
   e. Abdominal wall infection

3. The best method of preoperative preparation for patients undergoing laparoscopic renal surgery is:
   a. a 3-day mechanical bowel preparation if an extraperitoneal or retroperitoneoscopic approach is anticipated.
   b. a mechanical bowel preparation and antibiotic preparation with neomycin and metronidazole.
   c. for most uncomplicated patients, a clear liquid diet and a light mechanical bowel preparation the day before surgery.
   d. both an antibiotic and 3-day mechanical bowel preparation in patients who have had previous abdominal surgery if one anticipates encountering dense intra-abdominal adhesions.
   e. intravenous antibiotics 1 hour before surgery.

4. Which of the statements regarding pneumoperitoneum is TRUE?
   a. CO_2 as an insufflant can be dangerous because it can support combustion.
   b. CO_2 is most commonly used because it is insoluble in the blood.
   c. In patients with chronic respiratory disease, CO_2 is advantageous because it does not accumulate in the bloodstream.
   d. Argon gas would be an ideal insufflant because of its low cost and poor solubility in blood.
   e. Nitrous oxide has previously been used for insufflation; however, it is no longer routinely used because of the potential for intra-abdominal explosion.

5. When a patient has had multiple prior abdominal surgeries and extensive adhesions are anticipated, which of the following access techniques is recommended for obtaining a pneumoperitoneum and access to the abdomen for laparoscopy?
   a. Closed technique with Veress needle
   b. Closed technique with blind trocar insertion
   c. Open-access technique
   d. Hand-port access
   e. EndoTip entry

6. Which of the following port sites most often requires formal closure with a fascial and peritoneal suture?
   a. 5-mm nonbladed ports
   b. 5-mm bladed ports
   c. 10- to 12-mm bladed ports placed on the midclavicular line
   d. 10- to 12-mm nonbladed ports placed on the midclavicular line
   e. 10- to 12-mm nonbladed ports placed on the anterior axillary line

7. Which of the following pneumoperitoneum pressures is associated with the least perturbation in cardiac parameters, that is, change in stroke volume?
   a. 12 mm Hg
   b. 15 mm Hg
   c. 18 mm Hg
   d. 21 mm Hg
   e. 24 mm Hg

8. Which of the following physiologic effects has been noted with establishment of pneumoperitoneum?
   a. Increase in diaphragmatic motion
   b. Increase in disturbances of gastrointestinal motility
   c. Alkalosis
   d. Decrease in urinary output
   e. Increase in mesenteric vessel blood flow

9. What is the most common intra-abdominal site of injury associated with laparoscopic surgery?
   a. Bowel injury
   b. Vascular injury
   c. Liver injury
   d. Splenic laceration
   e. Bladder injury

10. What is a characteristic of a blunt trocar, compared with a bladed trocar?
    a. The blunt trocar requires formal closure of the port site regardless of its size.
    b. The blunt trocar takes less force to insert than the bladed trocar.
    c. The blunt trocar decreases the chance of injury to the epigastric vessels.
    d. The blunt trocar should only be placed in the midline.
    e. The blunt trocar eliminates possible trocar injury to the bowel.

11. All of the following options for treatment of a gas embolism during laparoscopy are true EXCEPT:
    a. Hyperventilate the patient with 100% oxygen.
    b. Immediately cease insufflation.
    c. Place the patient in a head-down position.
    d. Advance a central venous line into the right side of the heart.
    e. Place the patient in a right lateral decubitus position with the left side up.

12. Pneumomediastinum, pneumothorax, and pneumopericardium associated with laparoscopy are a result of:
    a. gas leaking along major blood vessels through congenital defects in the diaphragm.
    b. gas passing through secondary enlargement of openings in the diaphragm.
    c. diffusion of gas across the peritoneum and diaphragm.
    d. a and b.
    e. a and c.

13. If during insufflation of the abdomen the Veress needle is determined to have been placed into the iliac artery, which of the following is the best course of action?
    a. Remove the Veress needle and proceed to open the abdomen.
    b. Remove the Veress needle and then proceed with insufflating at a different location.
    c. Leave the Veress needle in place and open the abdomen.
    d. Leave the Veress needle in place and proceed with insufflation of the abdomen at a different location.
    e. Call for a vascular surgery consult.

14. What is the best management option if trocar injury to the iliac artery should occur during the placement of the first trocar?
    a. Remove the trocar and open the abdomen immediately.
    b. Remove the trocar immediately and proceed with re-insufflation of the abdomen and placement of the trocar at an alternate site.
    c. Leave the trocar in place, consult a vascular surgeon, and convert to open laparotomy.
    d. Leave the trocar in place and proceed with insufflation of the abdomen and placement of another port at an alternate site.
    e. Remove the obturator and immediately flush the port with fibrin glue.

15. Thermal bowel injury during laparoscopy can occur as a result of all of the following EXCEPT:
    a. capacitive coupling.
    b. insulation failure.
    c. inappropriate direct activation.
    d. electrode resistance.
    e. coupling to another instrument.

16. When a bladder injury is diagnosed postoperatively after a laparoscopic procedure, what is the best treatment?
    a. Transurethral indwelling Foley catheter if it is an intraperitoneal injury of the bladder
    b. Open repair if it is an extraperitoneal injury of the bladder
    c. Laparoscopic or open repair if it is an intraperitoneal injury to the bladder
    d. Laparoscopic repair if it is an extraperitoneal injury to the bladder
    e. Transurethral injection of fibrin glue into the bladder injury site if it is an extraperitoneal injury to the bladder

17. Hypercarbia during laparoscopy may be related to all of the following EXCEPT:
    a. severe chronic respiratory disease.
    b. subcutaneous emphysema.
    c. increased insufflation pressures.
    d. prolonged operative time.
    e. radical nephrectomy.

18. Possible advantages of retroperitoneal laparoscopy include all of the following EXCEPT:
    a. less need for lysis of adhesions.
    b. decreased risk of paralytic ileus.
    c. decreased risk of port-site hernias.
    d. direct rapid access to the renal hilum.
    e. technically easier to learn.

19. After extraperitoneal pelvic lymph node dissection, the incidence of which one of the following is higher than with transperitoneal pelvic node dissection?
    a. Urinoma
    b. Lymphocele
    c. Bowel injury
    d. Laparoscopic repair if it is an extraperitoneal injury to the bladder
    e. Shoulder/hip pain

20. All of the following instruments might be part of a hemorrhage control tray EXCEPT:
    a. laparoscopic needle drivers.
    b. laparoscopic Satinsky clamp and accompanying trocar.
    c. Lapra-Ty clip applier and 6-inch length of 3-0 absorbable suture.
    d. hemostatic agents (fibrin glue, gelatin matrix thrombin, etc.) plus laparoscopic applicators.
    e. laparoscopic renal biopsy forceps.

21. Which of the following hemostatic agents requires a 20-minute setup time before use?
    a. Tisseel
    b. FloSeal
    c. CrossSeal
    d. BioGlue
    e. CoSeal

22. Which of the following relationships is true for port placement for laparoscopic suturing?
    a. The angle produced by the horizontal plane and the instruments should be greater than 55 degrees and the angle between the needle drivers should be less than 25 degrees.
    b. The angle produced by the horizontal plane and the instruments should be less than 55 degrees and the angle between the needle drivers should be between 25 and 45 degrees.
    c. The angle produced by the horizontal plane and the instruments should be greater than 55 degrees and the angle between the needle drivers should be greater than 45 degrees.
    d. The angle produced by the horizontal plane and the instruments should be less than 55 degrees and the angle between the needle drivers should be less than 25 degrees.
    e. The angle produced by the horizontal plane and the instruments should be greater than 55 degrees and the angle between the needle drivers should be between 25 and 45 degrees.

23. During a procedure using the Da Vinci Robotic System, the robot malfunctions and one of the grasping forceps is closed on a vital structure. The system is completely unresponsive. The appropriate action to safely disengage the instrument from the vital structure is to:
    a. use the surgeon's console to override the system and robotically disengage the grasper.
    b. remove the robotic instrument from the robotic arm.

c. use the sterile Allen wrench provided by the company to manually disengage the instrument and then remove it from the robotic arm.

d. use a handheld laparoscopic instrument to pry open the jaws of the robotic instrument.

e. unplug the surgeon's console and robotic tower, plug them back in, and restart the system.

24. After placement of the Veress needle, insufflation should never be initiated unless all of the following signs for proper peritoneal entry are confirmed EXCEPT?
    a. Negative aspiration
    b. Easy irrigation of saline
    c. Negative pressure test
    d. Positive drop test
    e. Normal advancement test

25. Carbon dioxide is the most commonly used insufflant because it is:
    a. noncombustible.
    b. rapidly absorbed.
    c. inexpensive.
    d. colorless.
    e. all of the above.

26. Helium is a useful insufflant in patients with:
    a. coronary artery disease.
    b. peripheral vascular disease.
    c. pulmonary disease.
    d. inflammatory bowel disease.
    e. chronic kidney disease.

27. Which of the following are signs of bowel insufflation with the Veress needle?
    a. Asymmetrical abdominal distention
    b. Flatus
    c. High pressures reached after a large amount of CO_2 is insufflated
    d. a and c
    e. a and b

28. The diagnosis of air embolism is usually made by the anesthesiologist based on an initial abrupt:
    a. increase in end-tidal CO2.
    b. decrease in end-tidal CO_2.
    c. increase in oxygen saturation.
    d. increase in mean arterial pressure.
    e. decrease in airway pressures.

29. Laparoscopic virtual reality trainers have been shown to:
    a. increase the operating time and improve the operative performance of surgical trainees with limited laparoscopic experience when compared with no training or with box-trainer training.
    b. decrease the operating time and improve the operative performance of surgical trainees with limited laparoscopic experience when compared with no training or with box-trainer training.
    c. decrease the operating time and improve the operative performance of surgical trainees with extensive laparoscopic experience when compared with no training or with box-trainer training.

d. a and b.

e. a and c.

30. All of the following increase the risk of developing rhabdomyolysis from flank pressure when the patient is positioned in the modified flank position EXCEPT:
    a. BMI $\geq$ 25.
    b. elevation of the kidney rest.
    c. age < 45 years.
    d. male gender.
    e. full table flexion.

31. When using a laparoscopic stapling device, the 2.0-mm or 2.5-mm staple cartridges are preferred for:
    a. bowel.
    b. bladder.
    c. ureter.
    d. vascular (renal artery or vein).
    e. a and d.

32. All of the following represent options for port site fascial closure EXCEPT:
    a. retractors and direct vision.
    b. Endo Stitch.
    c. Carter-Thomason needlepoint suture passer.
    d. disposable Endo Close suture carrier.
    e. angiocatheter technique.

33. The basic principles of Hem-o-Lok clip placement include all of the following EXCEPT:
    a. incomplete circumferential dissection of the vessel.
    b. visualization of the curved tip of the clip around and beyond the vessel.
    c. confirmation of the tactile snap when the clip engages.
    d. during transaction of vessels, only a partial division is performed initially to confirm hemostasis before complete transaction.
    e. no cross clipping.

34. Balloon trocars are advantageous because they can help reduce the risk of:
    a. air embolism.
    b. alkalosis.
    c. subcutaneous emphysema.
    d. hypothermia.
    e. all of the above.

35. Certain precautions must be followed during monopolar electrosurgery to avoid local or distant transmitted thermal injury, including:
    a. checking the insulation of the electrosurgical instrument carefully for damage.
    b. not activating the electrosurgical probe unless the metal part is in complete view.
    c. not activating the probe unless it is in direct contact with the tissue to be incised.
    d. never using a metal trocar in conjunction with an outer plastic retaining ring.
    e. all of the above.

ANSWERS

1. **e. Extensive prior abdominal or pelvic surgery.** Absolute contraindications for laparoscopic surgery include uncorrectable coagulopathy, intestinal obstruction, abdominal wall infection, massive hemoperitoneum or hemoretroperitoneum, generalized peritonitis or retroperitoneal abscess, and suspected malignant ascites.

2. **d. Extensive prior abdominal or pelvic surgery.** When extensive intra-abdominal or pelvic adhesions are suspected, close attention must be given to access into the abdomen whether this is by Veress needle (Ethicon Endo-Surgery, Blue Ash, OH) or some open-access technique. Alternatively, in these patients, a retroperitoneal approach may be preferable to a transperitoneal approach, but this is only a relative contraindication to performing laparoscopic surgery. All of the other options listed are absolute contraindications to laparoscopic surgery.

3. **e. Intravenous antibiotics 1 hour before surgery.** For extraperitoneoscopy and retroperitoneoscopy, no bowel preparation is necessary. Similarly, for transperitoneal laparoscopic/robotic procedures *not* involving the use of bowel segments for urinary tract reconstruction, a mechanical bowel preparation is not necessary. A recent large-scale propensity score-matched analysis demonstrated no benefit for mechanical bowel preparation in operative time, postoperative stay, or overall complications for patients undergoing laparoscopic nephrectomy (Sugihara et al, 2013).*

4. **e. Nitrous oxide has previously been used for insufflation; however, it is no longer routinely used because of the potential for intra-abdominal explosion.** Most commonly, CO_2 is used as the insufflant because it does not support combustion and is very soluble in blood. However, in patients with chronic respiratory disease CO_2 may accumulate in the bloodstream to dangerous levels. In these patients, helium may be used for insufflation once the initial pneumoperitoneum has been established with CO_2. The drawback of helium is that, like air, it is much less soluble in the blood than CO_2. However, its use averts problems with hypercarbia. Other gases that were once used for insufflation, including room air, oxygen, and nitrous oxide, are no longer routinely used because of their potential side effects, such as air embolus or intra-abdominal explosion and potential to support combustion.

5. **c. Open-access technique.** A pneumoperitoneum can be more easily and, in one's early experience, more safely established using an open technique, especially in patients with multiple prior surgeries, who are at high risk for intra-abdominal adhesions. However, its use involves making a larger incision and increases the chances of port-site gas leakage during the procedure. Studies in general surgery have shown the open technique to be as efficient as a closed approach.

6. **c. 10- to 12-mm bladed ports placed on the midclavicular line.** All bladed port sites that are greater than 5 mm should be formally closed, independent of location.

7. **a. 12 mm Hg.** Recent studies support a pneumoperitoneum pressure of 12 mm Hg, because this results in no perturbation in cardiac parameters, that is, no change in stroke volume, versus a pressure of 15 mm Hg. Working at lower pneumoperitoneum pressures has also been found to reduce postoperative pain. Also, a marked reduction in oliguria has been associated with working at 10 mm Hg pressure.

8. **d. Decrease in urinary output.** Because of increased intra-abdominal pressure from the pneumoperitoneum, diaphragmatic motion is limited. Laparoscopic surgery causes less significant disturbances of the gastrointestinal motility pattern compared with open surgery. Insufflation with CO_2 results in variable amounts of gas absorption, thereby raising the Pco_2 in the blood and creating an acidosis. Increased intra-abdominal pressure was found to be associated with a significant decrease in urinary output secondary to decreased blood flow to the renal cortex with an associated decrease in renal vein blood flow of up to 90% at 15 mm Hg.

9. **b. Vascular injury.** The most common site of injury during laparoscopic surgery, in reports in the literature, is vascular in origin, occurring in 2.8% of patients, followed by bowel injury at 1.1%. The most often injured intra-abdominal organ was the bowel, at an incidence of 1.2%.

10. **c. The blunt trocar decreases the chance of injury to the epigastric vessels.** The use of only blunt trocars decreases the chance of injury to the epigastric vessels by fivefold.

11. **e. Place the patient in a right lateral decubitus position with the left side up.** The treatment for a suspected gas embolism is immediate cessation of insufflation and prompt desufflation of the peritoneal cavity. The patient is turned into a left lateral decubitus head-down position (i.e., right side up) to minimize right ventricular outflow problems. The patient is hyperventilated with 100% oxygen. Advancement of a central venous line into the right side of the heart with subsequent attempts to aspirate the gas may rarely be helpful. Use of hyperbaric oxygen and cardiopulmonary bypass have also been reported.

12. **d. a and b.** Gas leaking along major blood vessels through congenital defects or secondary enlargement of openings in the diaphragm may lead to pneumomediastinum, pneumopericardium, and pneumothorax.

13. **d. Leave the Veress needle in place and proceed with insufflation of the abdomen at a different location.** If vascular injury should occur with the Veress needle, the needle should be left in place to identify the area of injury, and insufflation of the abdomen can be re-performed at an alternate site and then the laparoscope inserted to identify the area of injury and to observe this as the Veress needle is removed to control any hemorrhage that may occur from the site.

14. **c. Leave the trocar in place, consult a vascular surgeon, and convert to open laparotomy.** A trocar injury to a major arterial vessel is a potentially life-threatening complication. The trocar should remain in place to tamponade the bleeding and also identify the area of injury once the abdomen is opened. The patient's blood should be typed and crossmatched, and immediate laparotomy should be performed and the site of vascular injury identified. A vascular surgery consult may be needed.

15. **d. Electrode resistance.** Electrosurgically induced thermal injury may occur through of one of four mechanisms: inappropriate direct activation; coupling to another instrument; capacitive coupling; and insulation failure.

16. **c. Laparoscopic or open repair if it is an intraperitoneal injury to the bladder.** When bladder injury is diagnosed postoperatively, the surgeon must determine whether the perforation is extraperitoneal or intraperitoneal. Extraperitoneal injury, without any complicating additional problems, may be treated by simple placement of a transurethral indwelling Foley catheter. Intraperitoneal injury is an indication for subsequent laparoscopic or open repair.

17. **e. Radical nephrectomy.** The potential for developing hypercarbia exists during both transperitoneal and preperitoneal laparoscopic procedures. Conceivably, this assumes greater importance in patients with preexisting airway and cardiovascular compliance. Vigilant perioperative anesthetic management is essential to prevent the development of potential complications related to CO_2 buildup. A rise in end-tidal CO_2 should prompt the anesthesiologist to adjust the respiratory rate and tidal volume to enhance CO_2 elimination. Simultaneously, the insufflation pressure of CO_2 should be decreased by the surgeon or, if need be, the operation should be halted and the abdomen desufflated until the end-tidal CO_2 returns to an acceptable level.

18. **e. Technically easier to learn.** Retroperitoneoscopy is associated with unique anatomic orientation and a relatively restricted initial working area compared with transperitoneal laparoscopy. This results in a steeper learning curve.

---

*Sources referenced can be found in *Campbell-Walsh Urology, 11th Edition*, on the Expert Consult website.

19. **b. Lymphocele.** Absence of the peritoneal absorptive surface after extraperitoneoscopic lymphadenectomy may increase the risk of development of postoperative lymphocele

20. **e. laparoscopic renal biopsy forceps.** The contents of a hemorrhage tray for laparoscopic surgery include the following:
    - Laparoscopic Satinsky clamp (Medline Industries Inc., Mundelein, IL)
    - 10-mm suction/irrigation tip
    - Endo Stitch device with a 4-0 absorbable suture
    - Lapra-Ty clip (Ethicon US, LLC, CA) applier and a packet of Lapra-Ty clips
    - 6-inch length of 4-0 vascular suture on an SH needle with a Lapra-Ty clip preplaced on the end
    - Two laparoscopic needle drivers
    - Topical hemostatic agent of choice

21. **a. Tisseel.** Tisseel (Baxter, Glendale, CA) is a form of fibrin glue containing fibrinogen, calcium chloride, aprotinin, and thrombin. It is useful as a topical hemostatic agent as well as a tissue glue, but it has a 20-minute setup time and thus must be prepared well in advance of potential use.

22. **b. The angle produced by the horizontal plane and the instruments should be less than 55 degrees and the angle between the needle drivers should be between 25 and 45 degrees.** Frede and colleagues performed an in vitro experiment performing laparoscopic suturing while varying trocar relationship to the horizontal plane and the distance between the two instrument trocars. They found that suturing was easiest when the angle between the horizontal plane and the instruments was less than 55 degrees and the angle between the two instruments was between 25 and 45 degrees (Frede et al, 1999).*

23. **c. Use the sterile Allen wrench provided by the company to manually disengage the instrument and then remove it from the robotic arm.** In the event of a system failure of the da Vinci Robotic System (Intuitive Surgical, Sunnyvale, CA) during which the robotic arms are rendered nonfunctional, instrument jaws can be manually opened using a sterile Allen wrench provided by the company for this purpose.

24. **c. Negative pressure test.** Several tests can be performed in an attempt to confirm proper placement of the Veress needle within the peritoneal cavity before insufflation to reduce the risk of insufflation related complications. These tests include: the aspiration/irrigation/aspiration test, the advancement test, and the drop test. Insufflation should never be initiated unless *all* of the signs for proper peritoneal entry (negative aspiration, easy irrigation of saline, negative aspiration of saline, positive drop test, and normal advancement test) have been confirmed.

25. **e. All of the above.** CO_2 is the most commonly used insufflant for laparoscopic surgery and is favored by most laparoscopists thanks to its properties (colorless, noncombustible, very soluble in blood, and inexpensive).

26. **c. Pulmonary disease.** Helium is an inert and noncombustible insufflant. Initial studies performed in various animal models showed favorable effects on arterial partial pressure of CO_2 and pH with no evidence of hypercarbia (Fitzgerald et al, 1992; Leighton et al, 1993; Rademaker et al, 1995). These results were corroborated by clinical studies (Bongard et al, 1991; Fitzgerald et al, 1992; Leighton et al, 1993; Neuberger et al, 1994; Rademaker et al, 1995; Jacobi et al, 1997). Therefore, helium is particularly useful for the patient with pulmonary disease in whom hypercarbia would be poorly tolerated.

27. **e, a, and b.** If entry into the bowel is not recognized at the time of irrigation and aspiration through the Veress needle, then the surgeon may insufflate the small or large bowel. The first sign of this problem is asymmetrical abdominal distention followed by

flatus and insufflation of only a small amount of CO_2 (<2 L) before high pressures are reached.

28. **a. Increase in end-tidal CO_2.** The diagnosis of CO_2 gas embolism is usually made by the anesthesiologist based on an abrupt increase of end-tidal CO_2 accompanied by a sudden decline in oxygen saturation and then a marked decrease in end-tidal CO_2. Sometimes, a "millwheel" precordial murmur can be auscultated. In addition, the anesthesiologist may notice foaming of a blood sample, if drawn, owing to the presence of insufflated CO_2.

29. **b. Decrease the operating time and improve the operative performance of surgical trainees with limited laparoscopic experience when compared with no training or with box-trainer training.** Virtual reality (VR) trainers are computer-based simulators that offer the opportunity to practice laparoscopic and robotic skills through specific tasks, as well as whole procedures. VR trainers have been shown to improve the skills of trainees helping to prepare them for better performance during live surgery (Seymour et al, 2002; Lucas et al, 2008). A recent systematic review demonstrated that VR training appears to decrease the operating time and improve the operative performance of surgical trainees with limited laparoscopic experience when compared with no training or with box-trainer training (Nagendran et al, 2013).

30. **c. Age <45 years.** Male patients with a BMI ≥ 25 undergoing laparoscopic surgery in the lateral position with the kidney rest elevated and the table completely flexed are at highest risk of developing rhabdomyolysis due to flank pressure.

31. **d. Vascular (renal artery or vein).** Various stapling devices are available for tissue occlusion and division. Each staple load cartridge is color-coded depending on the size of the staples: 2.0-mm staples (gray) or 2.5-mm staples (white) are preferred for vascular (renal vein or renal artery) stapling, whereas 3.8-mm (blue) and 4.8-mm (green) staples are used in thicker tissues (ureter, bowel, bladder).

32. **b. Endo Stitch.** The Endo Stitch (Covidien, Mansfield, MA) device is an innovative, disposable, 10-mm instrument that facilitates laparoscopic suture placement and knot tying, not port site closure.

33. **a. Incomplete circumferential dissection of the vessel.** The basic principles of Hem-o-Lok (Teleflex, Morrisville, NC) placement include the following:
    - Complete circumferential dissection of the vessel
    - Visualization of the curved tip of the clip around and beyond the vessel, often with curved end of the clip placed between artery and vein
    - Confirmation of the tactile snap when the clip engages
    - No cross clipping
    - Not squeezing clip handles too hard (compared with the application of metal clips)
    - Careful removal of the applier after application given; the tips are sharp and can cause a laceration of nearby vessels (e.g., renal vein)
    - During transection of vessels only a partial division is performed initially to confirm hemostasis before complete transection
    - Minimum of two clips placed on the patient side of the renal hilar vessel

34. **c. Subcutaneous emphysema.** Once the balloon cannula is positioned in the abdominal cavity, the balloon is inflated; the cannula is pulled upward until the balloon is snug on the underside of the abdominal wall. Next, the soft foam or rubber collar on the outside surface of the cannula is slid down until it is snug on the skin and locked in place. This process creates an excellent seal, precluding gas leakage and subcutaneous emphysema.

35. **e. All of the above.** Several actions can be taken by the surgeon to lessen the risks of a thermal complication. First, electrosurgical instruments must be carefully inspected before use for any "breaks" in the insulation; if these are found, the instrument must be sent for recoating. Second, electrosurgical instruments should never be left untended within the abdomen; when not

---

*Sources referenced can be found in *Campbell-Walsh Urology, 11th Edition,* on the Expert Consult website.

in use they must be removed from the abdomen. Third, *only* the primary surgeon should control electrode activation. Fourth, isolation of the area to be cauterized from the surrounding tissues, as well as use of bipolar electrocautery, reduces the risk of thermal spread and injury to other tissues. Fifth, the electrosurgical device should never be activated unless the entire extent of the metal portion of the instrument is in view. Sixth, problems of capacitive coupling can be precluded by not creating a situation in which a mixture of conducting and nonconducting elements are used by the surgeon (e.g., metal trocars combined with plastic retainers). Last, an active electrode monitoring system (Encision, Boulder, CO) is extremely helpful, as any sudden break in the insulation of the electrosurgical instrument results in immediate shutdown of the electrosurgical current, thereby precluding an electrosurgical injury.

CHAPTER REVIEW

1. Patients with massive ascites have an increased incidence of bowel injury when trocars are placed because of the closer proximity of the bowel loops to the anterior abdominal wall.
2. The Veress needle is commonly placed at the superior border of the umbilicus; there is a potential risk of injury to the left common iliac vessels, aorta, and vena cava.
3. The signs of proper peritoneal entry using the Veress needle include negative aspiration, easy irrigation of saline, negative aspiration of saline, positive drop test, and normal advancement test.
4. When using a stapler, the tissue must be properly situated between the markers before the cartridge is fired. Otherwise, a portion of the tissue will not be encompassed by the stapler. A stapler should not be fired across any previously placed clips.
5. Before port removal is initiated, the operative site and the intra-abdominal entry sites of each cannula should be carefully inspected for bleeding with the intra-abdominal pressure lowered to 5 mm Hg.
6. Patients with chronic obstructive pulmonary disease (COPD) may not be able to compensate for the absorbed CO_2 by increased ventilation and are at increased risk for hypercarbia as long as 2 to 3 hours after the procedure.
7. Nitrous oxide insufflation reduces cardiac output and increases mean arterial pressure, heart rate, and central venous pressure. It also supports combustion.
8. In patients with severe COPD, one should consider using helium as an alternative for insufflation.
9. A drawback of helium for insufflation is that it is much less soluble in blood than CO_2. Helium may be associated with a higher risk of gas embolism because of its lower blood solubility, and thus the initial pneumoperitoneum should be established with CO_2 and then the insufflation should be maintained with helium.
10. Intra-abdominal pressures during laparoscopy should not be allowed to exceed 20 mm Hg over extended periods of time, and a working pressure of 10 to 12 mm Hg is recommended.
11. Increased intra-abdominal pressures may artificially elevate central venous pressure readings; thus if it is critical to know right atrial filling pressures, a Swan-Ganz catheter (Edwards Lifesciences, Irvine, CA) should be placed.
12. During laparoscopy, diaphragmatic motion is limited and functional reserve capacity is decreased. There is a significant decrease in urinary output and decreased blood flow to mesenteric vessels as well as other abdominal organs, including liver, pancreas, stomach, spleen, and small and large bowel.
13. Excessive intra-abdominal pressure usually presents as an increase in ventilation pressure noted by the anesthesiologist.
14. During removal of laparoscopic ports and desufflation, bowel and omentum may be entrapped at one of the port sites.
15. Absolute contraindications for laparoscopic surgery include uncorrectable coagulopathy, intestinal obstruction, abdominal wall infection, massive hemoperitoneum or hemoretroperitoneum, generalized peritonitis or retroperitoneal abscess, and suspected malignant ascites.
16. Increased intra-abdominal pressure is associated with a significant decrease in urinary output secondary to decreased blood flow to the renal cortex with an associated decrease in renal vein blood flow of as high as 90% at 15 mm Hg.

11 Basic Energy Modalities in Urologic Surgery

Manoj Monga, Shubha De, and Bodo E. Knudsen

QUESTIONS

1. What is the mechanism electrosurgery uses to affect tissues?
   a. Current is delivered to the tip of the instrument, causing it to heat and affect the tissue.
   b. Current is delivered to the tissue directly, causing it to heat.
   c. Current is conducted through a fluid medium to affect the tissue.
   d. Electrons are excited, creating increased light energy, which directly affects the tissue.

2. What is the mechanism electrocautery uses to affect tissues?.
   a. Current is delivered to the tip of the instrument, causing it to heat and affect the tissue.
   b. Current is delivered to the tissue directly, causing it to heat.
   c. Current is conducted through a fluid medium to affect the tissue.
   d. Electrons are excited, creating increased light energy, which directly affects the tissue.

3. When cautery is set to "pure cut," the current is:
   a. interrupted, but mainly on.
   b. interrupted, but mainly off.
   c. continuous.
   d. continuous, but oscillates between high and low voltage.
   e. variable in both intermittency and voltage.

4. An argon beam coagulator:
   a. works by igniting a column of argon gas.
   b. uses an argon laser to diffusely coagulate tissues.
   c. should be used in direct contact with the tissue's surface.
   d. should be used in a dry environment.
   e. uses a column of argon gas that passes over an electrode.

5. Bipolar and monopolar cautery differ in that:
   a. monopolar does not require a dispersive electrode.
   b. monopolar can be used at much higher voltages.
   c. bipolar does not require a dispersive electrode.
   d. bipolar can be used at much higher voltages.
   e. there are no differences.

6. The LigaSure and Gyrus PK both show benefits over the Thunderbeat and Ultrashears in that they:
   a. are able to produce less smoke and keep a clear visual field.
   b. seal vessels faster, and with higher burst pressures.
   c. function more reliably in wet environments.
   d. are cheaper and reusable.
   e. show no benefits and are inferior products.

7. The wavelength for the holmium:YAG (Ho:YAG) laser is:
   a. 488 nm—blue; 514 nm—green.
   b. 1064 nm.
   c. 1318 nm.
   d. 2140 nm.
   e. 2640 nm.

8. Stone fragmentation via Ho:YAG lasers occurs by:
   a. cavitation bubble collapse and resulting shock waves.
   b. fluid jets created by rapid heating of the surrounding fluid.
   c. pneumatic activity of the laser tip against the stone.
   d. direct energy absorption.
   e. ultrasonic thermal ablation of the stone surface.

9. The major downside of pneumatic lithotripsy in the ureter is:
   a. cost.
   b. ureteral injury.
   c. poor visualization.
   d. stone retropulsion.
   e. all of the above.

10. Which instruments can be used through flexible ureteroscopy?
    a. Electrohydraulic lithotripsy (EHL), pneumatic, ultrasonic
    b. Laser, ultrasonic, combination (pneumatic and ultrasonic)
    c. Ultrasonic, laser, EHL
    d. Combination (pneumatic and ultrasound), laser, EHL
    e. All modalities

ANSWERS

1. **b. Current is delivered to the tissue directly, causing it to heat.** Electrosurgery uses radiofrequency current in the range of 400,000 to 600,000 Hz to pass through tissue and create the desired effects. The generators deliver more than 100 W of power to the tissue at voltages ranging from 100 to 5000 V. While the current is delivered to the tissue, the tissue is heated and the effect occurs. This is in contrast to electrocautery, in which the instrument itself is heated and then applied to the tissue.

2. **a. Current is delivered to the tip of the instrument, causing it to heat and affect the tissue.** In contrast to electrosurgery, where radiofrequency current in the range of 400,000 to 600,000 Hz passes through tissue and create the desired effects, with electrocautery the tip of the instrument is heated and then applied to the tissue to create the desired effect.

3. **c. Continuous.** Pure cut uses continuous delivery, whereas coagulation uses interrupted delivery. Generators will also usually provided "blended" modes that modify the degree of interruption to gain the desired effect.

4. **e. Uses a column of argon gas that passes over an electrode.** The argon beam coagulator works by adding a column of argon gas that passes over the electrode; electrosurgical energy ionizes the argon gas and helps to displace the blood in the surgical field. Because argon is a noble gas, the current from the electrode is effectively transmitted to the underlying tissue.

5. **c. Bipolar does not require a dispersive electrode.** Unlike monopolar systems in which a circuit is created by delivering the energy via an electrode and then removed from the patient using a dispersive electrode (grounding pad), bipolar delivery does not require a dispersive electrode. Rather, the active and return electrodes are integrated in the delivery hand piece. The tissue contained between the electrodes is the target tissue.

6. **b. Seal vessels faster, and with higher burst pressures.** A comparison study comparing the vessel sealing times and thermal spread of two bipolar vessel sealing systems (LigaSure and Gyrus PK) as well as an ultrasonic devise (Ethicon Harmonic Scalpel) was performed. This demonstrated that the two bipolar systems had faster vessel sealing times with higher burst pressures compared to the ultrasonic device. However, the ultrasonic device had less thermal spread and smoke production (Lamberton et al, 2008).*

7. **d. 2140 nm.** Ho:YAG laser is a 2140-nm pulsed laser that is used for both soft tissue and lithotripsy applications in urology. The 2140-nm wavelength is strongly absorbed in water, traveling only approximately 0.5 mm in the fluid medium, making it ideal for the urologic environment. Both the argon (488 nm—blue; 514 nm—green) and Nd:YAG (1064 nm, 1318 nm) lasers use two different wavelengths.

8. **d. Direct energy absorption.** Previous laser technologies (Ruby, Nd:YAG) used photoacoustic or photomechanical processes, where light energy created shock waves that fragmented stones. In contrast, the Ho:YAG laser uses photothermal lithotripsy, which involves direct light energy absorption ("photo") by stone surfaces, causing rapid temperature ("thermal") increases, before significant heat diffusion can occur. A "Moses effect" occurs by the rapid vaporization of fluid creating a vapor channel between the fiber tip and stone's surface, allowing for more direct energy transfer. Interstitial water may also become vaporized, leading to fragment ejection; however, these forces are not great enough to directly lead to stone fracture.

9. **d. Stone retropulsion.** Pneumatic lithotripsy uses ballistic forces to transfer kinetic energy from a handheld probe to the stone surface. Repetitive strikes (12 Hz LithoClast, 15 to 30 Hz Electrokinetic lithotripter) from the probe tip act as a jackhammer, fragmenting stones at the point of contact. Stone migration is a significant disadvantage when treating ureteric stones because the probe's ballistic effect can propel stones in capacious ureters into the kidney. Retropulsion has been reported in as much as 10% of distal and 40% of proximal stones treated with pneumatic lithotripsy. In a four-way comparison of intracorporeal lithotripters on iatrogenic urothelial trauma, pneumatic probes were found to be the least traumatic (compared to laser, ultrasonic, and electrohydraulic lithotripsy). Pneumatic lithotripters are currently one of the most cost effective because of their durability and use of reusable probes.

10. **c. Ultrasonic, laser, EHL.** Because of their mechanisms of action, EHL probes and laser fibers can fragment stones while being flexed. 200-μm laser fibers can be readily flexed 270 degrees in flexible ureteroscopes, whereas thin EHL probes (1.9 Fr) are flexible enough to reach the lower pole while conducting electrical pulses for spark discharge. Thin ultrasonic probes can be moderately deflected using flexible scopes; however, these wire-like probes lack a lumen for suction and suffer from significant dampening and reduced efficiency with flexion. Any amount of torque applied to pneumatic lithotrites significantly reduces the jackhammer-like movements and reduces fragmentation potential. Similarly, combination lithotrites cannot be flexed, nor are they available in sizes compatible with ureteroscopy.

CHAPTER REVIEW

1. When alternating current is employed, the term for resistance is impedance; impedance increases when charring occurs.
2. Lasers with shorter wavelengths have a much greater amount of scatter than those with longer wavelengths.
3. The depth of tissue penetration for Nd:YAG is 10 mm, KTP 1 to 2 mm, Ho:YAG 0.4 mm, and CO_2 no significant penetration.
4. The electrohydraulic probe produces a spark that creates a shock wave; one should place the probe 1 mm away from the stone.
5. Stone composition and surface characteristics affect the efficiency of EHL, with uric acid stones taking the most time to fragment.
6. The pneumatic device is the only modality that does not cut through wire, such as a safety guidewire or stone basket.
7. The ultrasonic probe results in vibration at the end of the probe that is transferred to the stone, causing it to fracture.
8. Ho:YAG laser stone fragmentation is primarily due to a photothermal effect.
9. Laser lithotripsy produces the smallest fragments and is useful for all stone compositions.
10. The argon beam coagulator works by adding a column of argon gas that passes over the electrode, and then electrosurgical energy ionizes the argon gas and helps to displace the blood in the surgical field. Because argon is a noble gas, the current from the electrode is effectively transmitted to the underlying tissue.
11. Bipolar delivery does not require a dispersive electrode (grounding pad). The active and return electrodes are integrated in the delivery hand piece.
12. The bipolar systems for sealing tissue have faster vessel sealing times with higher burst pressures compared to the ultrasonic device. However, the ultrasonic device has less thermal spread and smoke production.
13. Pneumatic probes are the least traumatic to ureteral tissue compared to laser, ultrasonic, and electrohydraulic lithotripsy.

---

*Sources referenced can be found in *Campbell-Walsh Urology, 11th Edition,* on the Expert Consult website.

12   Infections of the Urinary Tract

Anthony J. Schaeffer, Richard S. Matulewicz, and David James Klumpp

QUESTIONS

1. Acute pyelonephritis is the most likely diagnosis in a patient with:
   a. chills, fever, and flank pain.
   b. bacteria and pyuria.
   c. focal scar in renal cortex.
   d. delayed renal function.
   e. vesicoureteral reflux.

2. Bacteriuria without pyuria is indicative of:
   a. infection.
   b. colonization.
   c. tuberculosis.
   d. contamination.
   e. stones.

3. Nosocomial urinary tract infections (UTIs):
   a. occur in patients who are hospitalized or institutionalized.
   b. are caused by common bowel bacteria.
   c. can be suppressed by low-dose antimicrobial therapy.
   d. are due to reinfection.
   e. are due to bacterial persistence.

4. Most recurrent infections in female patients are:
   a. complicated.
   b. reinfections.
   c. due to bacterial resistance.
   d. due to hereditary susceptibility factors.
   e. composed of multiple organisms.

5. Rates of reinfection (i.e., time to recurrence) are influenced by:
   a. bladder dysfunction.
   b. renal scarring.
   c. vesicoureteral reflux.
   d. antimicrobial treatment.
   e. age.

6. The long-term effect of uncomplicated recurrent UTIs is:
   a. renal scarring.
   b. hypertension.
   c. azotemia.
   d. ureteral vesical reflux.
   e. minimal.

7. The ascending route of infection is least enhanced by:
   a. catheterization.
   b. spermicidal agents.
   c. indwelling catheter.
   d. fecal soilage of perineum.
   e. frequent voiding.

8. Approximately 10% of symptomatic lower UTIs in young, sexually active female patients are caused by:
   a. *Escherichia coli.*
   b. *Staphylococcus saprophyticus.*
   c. *Pseudomonas.*
   d. *Proteus mirabilis.*
   e. *Staphylococcus epidermidis.*

9. The virulence factor that is most important for adherence is:
   a. hemolysin.
   b. K antigen.
   c. pili.
   d. colicin production.
   e. O serogroup.

10. Phase variation of bacterial pili:
    a. occurs only in vitro.
    b. affects bacterial virulence.
    c. is characteristic of pyelonephritic *E. coli.*
    d. is irreversible.
    e. refers to change in pilus length.

11. The finding that first suggested a biologic difference in women susceptible to UTIs is:
    a. increased adherence of bacteria to vaginal cells.
    b. decreased estrogen concentration in vaginal cells.
    c. elevated vaginal pH.
    d. nonsecretor status.
    e. postmenopausal status.

12. Increased bacterial adherence resulting in increased susceptibility of women to recurrent UTIs has not been demonstrated in:
    a. introital mucosa.
    b. urethral mucosa.
    c. buccal mucosa.
    d. vaginal fluid.
    e. bladder mucosa.

13. The primary bladder defense is:
    a. low urine pH.
    b. low urine osmolarity.
    c. voiding.
    d. Tamm-Horsfall protein (uromucoid).
    e. vaginal mucus.

14. The most significant sequela of renal papillary necrosis is renal:
    a. failure.
    b. abscess.
    c. obstruction.
    d. stone.
    e. cancer.

15. Severity and morbidity of bacteriuria is most morbid in patients with:
    a. spinal cord injuries.
    b. pregnancy.
    c. reflux.
    d. diabetes mellitus.
    e. human immunodeficiency virus (HIV) infection.

16. The most reliable urine specimen is obtained by:
    a. urethral catheterization.
    b. catheter aspiration.
    c. midstream voiding.
    d. suprapubic aspiration.
    e. antiseptic periurethral preparation.

17. The validity of a midstream urine specimen should be questioned if microscopy reveals:
    a. squamous epithelial cells.
    b. red blood cells.
    c. bacteria.
    d. white blood cells.
    e. casts.

18. Rapid screening methods for detecting UTIs should be used primarily for:
    a. low-risk asymptomatic patients.
    b. pregnant women.
    c. children.
    d. catheterized patients.
    e. elderly patients.

19. The most accurate test for evaluation of infection in the kidney is:
    a. the Fairley bladder washout test.
    b. ureteral catheterization.
    c. gallium scanning.
    d. computed tomography (CT).
    e. the antibody-coated bacteria test.

20. Urinary tract imaging is NOT usually indicated for recurrent UTIs in:
    a. women.
    b. girls.
    c. men.
    d. boys.
    e. spinal cord-injured patients.

21. The most sensitive imaging modality for diagnosing renal abscess is:
    a. ultrasonography.
    b. indium scanning.
    c. gallium scanning.
    d. excretory urography.
    e. CT.

22. Cure of UTIs depends most on an antimicrobial agent's:
    a. serum half-life.
    b. serum level.
    c. urine level.
    d. duration of therapy.
    e. frequency of therapy.

23. During the past 5 years, the least development of antimicrobial resistance has been observed for:
    a. ampicillin.
    b. cephalosporins.
    c. nitrofurantoin.
    d. fluoroquinolones.
    e. trimethoprim-sulfamethoxazole (TMP-SMX).

24. The ideal class of drugs for empirical treatment of uncomplicated UTIs is:
    a. aminopenicillins.
    b. aminoglycosides.
    c. fluoroquinolones.
    d. cephalosporins.
    e. nitrofurantoins.

25. Antimicrobial prophylaxis is characterized as:
    a. administration of an antimicrobial agent within 4 to 6 hours of the procedure.
    b. administration of an antimicrobial agent for a period of time covering the first 48 hours after the procedure.
    c. administration of an antimicrobial agent within 30 minutes of the initiation of a procedure and for a period of time covering the first 48 hours after the procedure.
    d. administration of an antimicrobial agent within 30 minutes of the initiation of a procedure and for a period of time that covers the duration of the procedure.
    e. administration of an antimicrobial agent the night before the initiation of a procedure and for a period of time that covers the duration of the procedure.

26. Antimicrobial prophylaxis for transurethral resection of the prostate is not indicated for patients with:
    a. valvular heart disease.
    b. prosthetic valves.
    c. unknown urine culture.
    d. sterile urine.
    e. indwelling catheter.

27. Prophylaxis for endocarditis should not be administered in patients with:
    a. a history of childhood heart murmurs.
    b. heart valves inserted more than 5 years ago.
    c. calcified heart valves associated with a murmur.
    d. all synthetic heart valves.
    e. cadaveric heart valves.

28. The host factor least likely to be associated with an increased risk of infection is:
    a. advanced age.
    b. a history of previous infection in the site/organ of interest.
    c. residence in a chronic care facility.
    d. indwelling orthopedic pins.
    e. coexistent infection.

29. Urine culture is not routinely recommended for the clinical diagnosis of acute cystitis in:
    a. young women.
    b. elderly women.
    c. children.
    d. men.
    e. patients with hematuria.

30. The drug of choice for uncomplicated cystitis in most young women is:
    a. TMP-SMX.
    b. fluoroquinolone.
    c. penicillin.
    d. cephalosporin.
    e. nitrofurantoin.

31. The optimal duration of antimicrobial therapy for symptomatic acute uncomplicated cystitis in women is:
    a. 1 day.
    b. 3 days.
    c. 7 days.
    d. 14 days.
    e. 21 days.

32. Treatment of asymptomatic bacteriuria is most indicated in patients who are:
    a. elderly.
    b. catheterized.
    c. pregnant.
    d. confused.
    e. incontinent.

33. Screening for bacteriuria is beneficial in:
    a. pregnant women.
    b. elderly patients.
    c. men.
    d. children.
    e. spinal cord-injured patients.

34. The most common cause of unresolved bacteriuria during antimicrobial therapy is:
    a. development of bacterial resistance.
    b. rapid reinfections.
    c. azotemia.
    d. staghorn calculi.
    e. initial bacterial resistance.

35. Nitrofurantoin prophylaxis is effective because of the concentration of the drug in the:
    a. urine.
    b. vaginal mucus.
    c. bowel.
    d. serum.
    e. bladder.

36. The ideal antimicrobial agent for self-start therapy for a UTI is:
    a. a fluoroquinolone.
    b. a cephalosporin.
    c. nitrofurantoin.
    d. TMP-SMX.
    e. tetracycline.

37. The most common cause of acute pyelonephritis in young women is:
    a. vesicoureteral reflux.
    b. P-piliated bacteria.
    c. type 1 piliated bacteria.
    d. recurrent UTIs.
    e. bacterial endotoxin.

38. The optimal antimicrobial agent for treatment of acute uncomplicated pyelonephritis in women is:
    a. TMP-SMX.
    b. a cephalosporin.
    c. an aminoglycoside.
    d. a fluoroquinolone.
    e. nitrofurantoin.

39. A patient with acute pyelonephritis, persistent fever, and flank pain for 24 hours warrants:
    a. observation.
    b. CT.
    c. change in antimicrobial therapy.
    d. ultrasonography.
    e. blood cultures.

40. The overall mortality rate in emphysematous pyelonephritis is approximately:
    a. 5%.
    b. 10%.
    c. 20%.
    d. 40%.
    e. 60%.

41. In chronic renal abscess the predominant urographic abnormality is:
    a. calyceal distortion.
    b. renal mass.
    c. calculi.
    d. hydronephrosis.
    e. calyceal amputation.

42. The high mortality rate associated with perinephric abscess is primarily attributed to:
    a. bacterial hemolysis.
    b. diabetes mellitus.
    c. delay in diagnosis.
    d. inappropriate antimicrobial therapy.
    e. inadequate drainage.

43. The primary treatment for a small perirenal abscess in a functioning kidney is:
    a. nephrectomy.
    b. partial nephrectomy.
    c. open surgical drainage.
    d. percutaneous drainage.
    e. retrograde ureteral drainage.

44. Most patients with chronic pyelonephritis present with:
    a. hypertension.
    b. renal failure.
    c. chronic infection.
    d. flank pain.
    e. no symptoms.

45. The most common bacterial cause of xanthogranulomatous pyelonephritis is:
    a. *Escherichia coli.*
    b. *Pseudomonas.*
    c. *Klebsiella.*
    d. *Proteus mirabilis.*
    e. *Staphylococcus.*

46. It is hypothesized that the nidus for the Michaelis-Gutmann body is:
    a. renal papillae.
    b. bacterial fragments.
    c. calcium crystals.
    d. macrophages.
    e. uric acid stones.

47. Echinococcosis is rare in/among:
    a. the former Soviet Union.
    b. Eskimos.
    c. Native Americans.
    d. the United States.
    e. Eastern Europe.

48. The most reliable early clinical indicator of septicemia is:
    a. chills.
    b. fever.
    c. hyperventilation.
    d. lethargy.
    e. change in mental status.

49. Compared with nonpregnant women, pregnant women have a higher prevalence of:
    a. asymptomatic bacteriuria.
    b. acute cystitis.
    c. acute pyelonephritis.
    d. recurrent cystitis.
    e. bacterial persistence.

50. Clinical pyelonephritis during pregnancy is most commonly linked to:
    a. maternal sepsis.
    b. maternal anemia.
    c. maternal hypertension.
    d. eclampsia.
    e. congenital malformations.

51. The drug thought to be safe in any phase of pregnancy is:
    a. a fluoroquinolone.
    b. nitrofurantoin.
    c. a sulfonamide.
    d. penicillin.
    e. tetracycline.

52. The majority of elderly patients with bacteriuria are:
    a. asymptomatic.
    b. febrile.
    c. incontinent.
    d. confused.
    e. dysuric.

53. In the absence of obstruction, treatment of asymptomatic bacteriuria in the elderly:
    a. is cost effective.
    b. prevents renal failure.
    c. reduces mortality.
    d. reduces morbidity.
    e. is unnecessary.

54. The most common predisposing factor for hospital-acquired UTIs is:
    a. surgery.
    b. antimicrobial therapy.
    c. age.
    d. catheterization.
    e. diabetes mellitus.

55. The most effective measure for reducing catheter-associated UTI is:
    a. closed drainage.
    b. antimicrobial prophylaxis.
    c. catheter irrigation.
    d. intermittent catheterization.
    e. daily meatal care.

56. In spinal cord-injured patients the bladder drainage technique with the lowest complication rate is:
    a. clean intermittent catheterization (CIC).
    b. suprapubic drainage.
    c. indwelling catheter.
    d. condom catheter.
    e. suprapubic pressure.

57. Fournier gangrene in the early stage is least likely to be associated with scrotal:
    a. pain.
    b. discharge.
    c. crepitation.
    d. erythema.
    e. swelling.

Pathology

1. See Figure 12-1.
   A 65-year-old woman has the acute onset of right flank pain, fever, and an enlarged kidney on imaging. Blood cultures and urine cultures are obtained and broad-spectrum antibiotics administered. The patient improves, but the kidney on imaging remains enlarged. A needle biopsy of the kidney is obtained. The pathology report is acute pyelonephritis with numerous neutrophils within the interstitium and the renal tubules. The biopsy:
   a. provides information as to the length of time antibiotics should be administered.
   b. suggests that the antibiotics should be changed.
   c. is unnecessary.
   d. suggests the need for a percutaneous drain.
   e. suggests that an abscess is likely to develop.

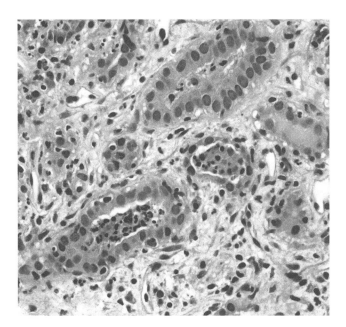

Figure 12-1. (From Bostwick DG, Qian J, Hossain D. Non-neoplastic diseases of the prostate. In: Bostwick DG, Cheng L, editors. Urologic surgical pathology. 2nd ed. Edinburgh: Mosby; 2008.)

2. A 65-year-old man has fever and malaise. A CT scan reveals an 8-cm solid mass in his left kidney with marked thickening of the retroperitoneum around the kidney and pancreas. The kidney is poorly functioning and there is a 1 cm stone in the renal pelvis. A biopsy is done and reveals xanthogranulomatous pyelonephritis, which is depicted in Figure 12-2. The next step in management is:

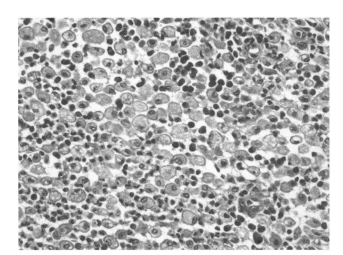

Figure 12-2. (From Bostwick DG, Cheng L, editors. Urologic surgical pathology. 2nd ed. Edinburgh: Mosby; 2008.)

a. extracorporeal shockwave lithotripsy.
b. biopsy of the retroperitoneum.
c. left nephrectomy.
d. urine culture and treatment according to sensitivities.
e. partial left nephrectomy

3. A 45-year-old woman is found to have a raised bladder lesion on cystoscopy. The biopsy shown in Figure 12-3 reveals malakoplakia. The nest step in management is:

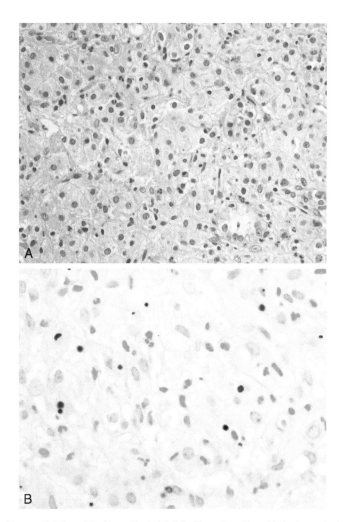

Figure 12-3A and B. (From Bostwick DG, Cheng L, editors. Urologic surgical pathology. 2nd ed. Edinburgh: Mosby; 2008.)

a. intravesical bacille Calmette-Guérin.
b. fulguration of the lesions.
c. intravesical mitomycin C.
d. treat with a sulfonamide for several months.
e. a 3-day course of ciprofloxacin.

Imaging

1. A 72-year-old man presents with right flank pain and fever. A contrast-enhanced CT scan is shown in Figure 12-4. The most likely diagnosis is:

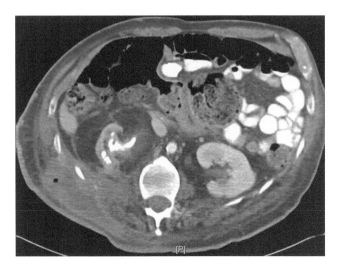

Figure 12-4.

a. acute right renal obstruction.
b. delayed excretion in left kidney.
c. cellulitis in right flank.
d. right perinephric abscess.
e. xanthogranulomatous pyelonephritis.

2. A 40-year-old woman presents with pelvic pain and fever. A contrast-enhanced CT scan is shown in Figure 12-5. The most likely diagnosis is:

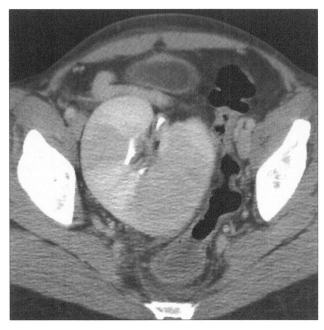

Figure 12-5.

a. renal infarct.
b. renal artery occlusion.
c. chronic pyelonephritis.
d. acute urinary obstruction.
e. acute pyelonephritis.

3. A 22-year-old woman presents with shaking chills and fever. An enhanced CT image is shown in Figure 12-6. The next step in management is:

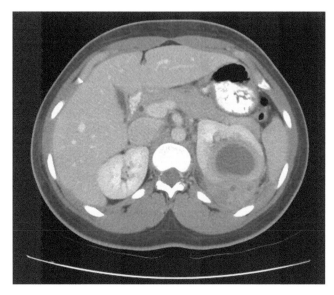

Figure 12-6.

a. percutaneous drainage.
b. nephrectomy.
c. partial nephrectomy.
d. open surgical drainage.
e. cystoscopy and retrograde urography.

ANSWERS

1. **a. Chills, fever, and flank pain.** Acute pyelonephritis is a clinical syndrome of chills, fever, and flank pain that is accompanied by bacteriuria and pyuria, a combination that is reasonably specific for an acute bacterial infection of the kidney.
2. **b. Colonization.** Bacteriuria without pyuria is generally indicative of bacterial colonization without infection of the urinary tract.
3. **a. Occur in patients who are hospitalized or institutionalized.** Nosocomial or health care–associated UTIs occur in patients who are hospitalized or institutionalized and may be caused by *Pseudomonas* and other more antimicrobial-resistant strains.
4. **b. Reinfections.** Of these recurrent infections, 71% to 73% are caused by reinfection with different organisms, rather than recurrence with the same organism.
5. **d. Antimicrobial treatment.** Whether a patient receives no treatment or short-term, long-term, or prophylactic antimicrobial treatment, the risk of recurrent bacteriuria remains the same; antimicrobial treatment appears to alter only the time until recurrence.
6. **e. Minimal.** The long-term effects of uncomplicated recurrent UTIs are not completely known, but, so far, no association between recurrent infections and renal scarring, hypertension, or progressive renal azotemia has been established.
7. **e. Frequent voiding.** This route is further enhanced in individuals with significant soilage of the perineum with feces, women using spermicidal agents, and patients with intermittent or indwelling catheters.
8. **b. *Staphylococcus saprophyticus*.** *S. saprophyticus* is now recognized as causing approximately 10% of symptomatic lower UTIs in young, sexually active females, whereas it rarely causes infection in males and elderly individuals.

9. **c. Pili.** Studies have demonstrated that interactions between FimH and receptors expressed on the luminal surface of the bladder epithelium are critical to the ability of many uropathogenic *E. coli* strains to colonize the bladder and cause disease.

10. **b. Affects bacterial virulence.** This process is called phase variation and has obvious biologic and clinical implications. For example, the presence of type 1 pili may be advantageous to the bacteria for adhering to and colonizing the bladder mucosa but disadvantageous because the pili enhance phagocytosis and killing by neutrophils.

11. **a. Increased adherence of bacteria to vaginal cells.** These studies established increased adherence of pathogenic bacteria to vaginal epithelial cells as the first demonstrable biologic difference that could be shown in women susceptible to UTI.

12. **e. Bladder mucosa.** These studies individually and collectively support the concept that there is an increased epithelial receptivity for *E. coli* on the introital, urethral, and buccal mucosa that is characteristic of women susceptible to recurrent UTIs and may be a genotypic trait. Thus the vaginal fluid appears to influence adherence to cells and presumably vaginal mucosal colonization.

13. **c. Voiding.** Bacteria presumably make their way into the bladder fairly often. Whether small inocula of bacteria persist, multiply, and infect the host depends in part on the ability of the bladder to empty.

14. **c. Obstruction.** A patient who suffers from an acute ureteral obstruction caused by a sloughed papilla and who has a concomitant UTI should have the condition treated as a urologic emergency.

15. **a. Spinal cord injuries.** Of all patients with bacteriuria, no group compares in severity and morbidity with those who have spinal cord injury.

16. **d. Suprapubic aspiration.** A single aspirated specimen reveals the bacteriologic status of the bladder urine without introducing urethral bacteria, which can start a new infection.

17. **a. Squamous epithelial cells.** The validation of the midstream urine specimen can be questioned if numerous squamous epithelial cells (indicative of preputial, vaginal, or urethral contaminants) are present.

18. **a. Low-risk asymptomatic patients.** The main role of rapid screening methods for UTIs is in screening asymptomatic patients.

19. **b. Ureteral catheterization.** Ureteral catheterization allows not only separation of bacterial persistence into upper and lower urinary tracts but also separation of the infection between one kidney and the other.

20. **a. Women.** Several reports of women patients with recurrent UTIs show that excretory urograms are unnecessary for routine evaluation in women. Those who have special risk factors are excluded.

21. **e. CT.** CT and magnetic resonance imaging are more sensitive than excretory urography or ultrasonography in the diagnosis of acute focal bacterial nephritis, renal and perirenal abscesses, and radiolucent calculi.

22. **c. Urine level.** Efficacy of the antimicrobial therapy is critically dependent on the antimicrobial levels in the urine and the length of time that this level remains above the minimum inhibitory concentration of the infecting organism. Thus resolution of infection is closely associated with the susceptibility of the bacteria to the concentration of the antimicrobial agent achieved in the urine.

23. **c. Nitrofurantoin.** Over a 5-year period the prevalence of resistance to trimethoprim-sulfamethoxazole, ampicillin, and cephalothin increased significantly, whereas resistance to nitrofurantoin and ciprofloxacin remained uncommon.

24. **c. Fluoroquinolones.** The fluoroquinolones have a broad spectrum of activity that makes them ideal for the empirical treatment of UTIs.

25. **d. Administration of an antimicrobial agent within 30 minutes of the initiation of a procedure and for a period of time that covers the duration of the procedure.** Surgical antimicrobial prophylaxis entails treatment with an antimicrobial agent before and for a limited time after a procedure to prevent local or systemic postprocedural infections.

26. **d. Sterile urine.** Prolonged use of an indwelling urethral catheter is common in hospitalized patients and is associated with an increased risk of bacterial colonization, with a 3% to 10% incidence of bacteriuria per catheter day in one study and 100% incidence of bacteriuria with long-term catheterization (>30 days). Prophylactic antimicrobial therapy during catheterization is not generally recommended because bacterial resistance can develop rapidly. Chronically catheterized patients have bacteriuria and should be treated therapeutically, not with prophylaxis.

27. **a. A history of childhood heart murmurs.** The American Heart Association's recommendations on the prevention of bacterial endocarditis are based on the patient's risk of developing endocarditis and the likelihood that a procedure will cause bacteremia with an organism that can cause endocarditis. Prophylaxis is recommended for both high- and moderate-risk patients. High-risk patients include individuals with prosthetic heart valves, previous bacterial endocarditis, cyanotic congenital heart disease, and systemic-pulmonary shunts or conduits. Moderate-risk patients include other congenital malformations (excluding isolated secundum atrial septal defects, surgically repaired atrial septal defect, ventricular septal defects, or patent ductus arteriosus), acquired valvular dysfunction, hypertrophic cardiomyopathy, and mitral valve prolapse with valvular regurgitation and/or thickened leaflets. Antimicrobial prophylaxis is not recommended for patients with congenital malformations including isolated secundum atrial septal defects, surgically repaired atrial septal defect, ventricular septal defects, or patent ductus arteriosus; previous coronary artery bypass graft surgery; benign heart murmurs; previous Kawasaki disease or rheumatic fever without valvular dysfunction; or implanted pacemakers or defibrillators.

28. **d. Indwelling orthopedic pins.** Bacterial seeding of implanted orthopedic hardware is a rare but morbid event. A joint commission of the American Urological Association, the American Academy of Orthopaedic Surgeons, and infectious disease specialists convened in 2003 and released an advisory statement on antibiotic prophylaxis for urologic patients with total joint replacement. In general, antimicrobial prophylaxis for urologic patients with total joint replacements, pins, plates, or screws is not indicated. Prophylaxis is advised for individuals at higher risk of seeding a prosthetic joint and include those with recently inserted implants (within 2 years).

29. **a. Young women.** In women with recent onset of symptoms and signs suggesting acute cystitis and in whom factors associated with upper tract or complicated infection are absent, a urinalysis that is positive for pyuria, hematuria, or bacteriuria or a combination should provide sufficient documentation of UTI and a urine culture may be omitted.

30. **a. TMP-SMX.** TMP and TMP-SMX are recommended in areas where the prevalence of resistance to these drugs among *E. coli* strains causing cystitis is less than 20%.

31. **b. 3 days.** Three-day therapy is the preferred regimen for uncomplicated cystitis in women.

32. **c. Pregnant.** In populations other than those for whom treatment has been documented to be beneficial (e.g., pregnant women and patients undergoing urologic interventions), screening for or treatment of asymptomatic bacteriuria is not appropriate and should be discouraged.

33. **a. Pregnant women.** In populations other than those for whom treatment has been documented to be beneficial (e.g., pregnant women and patients undergoing urologic interventions), screening for or treatment of asymptomatic bacteriuria is not appropriate and should be discouraged.

34. **e. Initial bacterial resistance.** Most commonly, the bacteria are resistant to the antimicrobial agent selected to treat the infection.

35. **a. Urine.** Nitrofurantoin, which does not alter the bowel flora, is present for brief periods at high concentrations in the urine and leads to repeated elimination of bacteria from the urine, presumably by interfering with bacterial initiation of infection.

36. **a. A fluoroquinolone.** Fluoroquinolones are ideal for self-start therapy because they have a spectrum of activity broader than that of any of the other oral agents and are superior to many parenteral antimicrobial agents, including aminoglycosides.

37. **b. P-piliated bacteria.** If vesicourethral reflux is absent, a patient bearing the P blood group phenotype may have special susceptibility to recurrent pyelonephritis caused by *E. coli* that have P pili and bind to the P blood group antigen receptors.

38. **d. A fluoroquinolone.** For patients who will be managed as outpatients, single-drug oral therapy with a fluoroquinolone is more effective than TMP-SMX for patients with domiciliary infections.

39. **a. Observation.** Even though the urine usually becomes sterile within a few hours of starting antimicrobial therapy, patients with acute uncomplicated pyelonephritis may continue to have fever, chills, and flank pain for several more days after initiation of successful antimicrobial therapy. They should be observed.

40. **d. 40%.** Emphysematous pyelonephritis should be considered a complication of severe pyelonephritis rather than a distinct entity. The overall mortality rate is 43%.

41. **b. Renal mass.** In a more chronic abscess, the predominant urographic abnormalities are those of a renal mass lesion.

42. **c. Delay in diagnosis.** Although 71% of all the patients had eventual surgical treatment of their perinephric abscesses, the diagnostic delay of those patients admitted to medical services postponed definitive treatment and consequently caused higher mortality.

43. **d. Percutaneous drainage.** Although surgical drainage, or nephrectomy if the kidney is nonfunctioning or severely infected, is the classic treatment for perinephric abscesses, renal ultrasonography and CT make percutaneous aspiration and drainage of small perirenal collections possible.

44. **e. No symptoms.** There are no symptoms of chronic pyelonephritis until it produces renal insufficiency, and then the symptoms are similar to those of any other form of chronic renal failure.

45. **d. Proteus mirabilis.** Although review of the literature shows *Proteus* to be the most common organism involved with xanthogranulomatous pyelonephritis, *E. coli* is also common.

46. **b. Bacterial fragments.** It is hypothesized that bacteria or bacterial fragments form the nidus for the calcium phosphate crystals that laminate the Michaelis-Gutmann bodies.

47. **d. The United States.** In the United States the disease is rare, but it is found in immigrants from Eastern Europe or other foreign endemic areas or as an indigenous infection among Native Americans in the Southwest United States and in Eskimos.

48. **c. Hyperventilation.** Even before temperature extremes and the onset of chills, bacteremic patients often begin to hyperventilate. Thus the earliest metabolic change in septicemia is a resultant respiratory alkalosis.

49. **c. Acute pyelonephritis.** Pyelonephritis develops in 1% to 4% of all pregnant women and in 20% to 40% of pregnant women with untreated bacteriuria.

50. **a. Maternal sepsis.** Pregnant women with asymptomatic bacteriuria are at higher risk for developing a symptomatic UTI that results in adverse fetal sequelae, complications associated with bacteriuria during pregnancy, and pyelonephritis and its possible sequelae, such as sepsis in the mother. Therefore all women with asymptomatic bacteriuria should be treated.

51. **d. Penicillin.** The aminopenicillins and cephalosporins are considered safe and generally effective throughout pregnancy. In patients with penicillin allergy, nitrofurantoin is a reasonable alternative.

52. **a. Asymptomatic.** Most elderly patients with bacteriuria are asymptomatic; estimates among women living in nursing homes range from 17% to 55%, as compared with 15% to 31% for their male cohorts.

53. **e. Is unnecessary.** Prospective randomized comparative trials of antimicrobial or no therapy in elderly male and female nursing home residents with asymptomatic bacteriuria consistently document no benefit of antimicrobial therapy. There

was no decrease in symptomatic episodes and no improvement in survival. In fact, treatment with antimicrobial therapy increases the occurrence of adverse drug effects and reinfection with resistant organisms and increases the cost of treatment. Therefore asymptomatic bacteriuria in elderly residents of long-term care facilities should not be treated with antimicrobial agents.

54. **d. Catheterization.** Catheter-associated bacteriuria is the most common hospital-acquired infection, accounting for up to 40% of such infections.

55. **a. Closed drainage.** Careful aseptic insertion of the catheter and maintenance of a closed dependent drainage system are essential to minimize development of bacteriuria.

56. **a. Clean intermittent catheterization.** Although never rigorously compared with indwelling urethral catheterization, CIC has been shown to decrease lower urinary tract complications by maintaining low intravesical pressure and reducing the incidence of stones.

57. **b. Discharge.** Early on, the involved area is swollen, erythematous, and tender as the infection begins to involve the deep subcutaneous tissue. Pain is prominent, and fever and systemic toxicity are marked. The swelling and crepitus of the scrotum quickly increase, and dark purple areas develop and progress to extensive gangrene.

Pathology

1. **c. Is unnecessary.** The figure shows numerous neutrophils within the interstitium and the renal tubules. The neutrophils in the tubules become white blood cell casts. The pathologic findings including an enlarged kidney may persist for several weeks despite appropriate treatment. There is no indication for a biopsy in this patient.

2. **c. Left nephrectomy.** The figure shows the foamy macrophages with neutrophils and cellular debris characteristic of xanthogranulomatous pyelonephritis. It may be associated with renal calculi and *Proteus* infection. *E. coli* is also a common organism found in this disease. Although partial nephrectomy has been performed for a small localized mass in a functioning kidney, a left nephrectomy in this situation is likely required and is necessary to rid the patient of the infection. An associated retroperitoneal inflammatory process with thickening is not uncommon.

3. **d. Treat with a sulfonamide for several months.** Figure 12-3A shows von Hansemann histiocytes, and Figure 12-3B demonstrates the Michaelis-Gutmann bodies, both of which are characteristic of malakoplakia. It is thought to be infectious in origin, and therefore the treatment is an extended course of an antibiotic that achieves a high intracellular concentration.

Imaging

1. **d. Right perinephric abscess.** The CT scan is obtained in the late arterial to nephrographic phase of the examination (the aorta is still opacified with contrast agent), before the excretion of the contrast agent. Thus option b is incorrect. There are multiple calculi in the right kidney, which is small and atrophic, indicating a chronic process (thus option a is incorrect). There is thickening of the perinephric fascia, and gas bubbles are seen in the posterior paranephric space, extending to the right flank. In addition, there are fluid collections in the posterior paranephric space and in the soft tissues of the right flank, making option d the most likely diagnosis. Xanthogranulomatous pyelonephritis is a chronic inflammatory condition associated with staghorn calculi. The affected kidney is usually enlarged rather than shrunken, as is the case here (making option e unlikely).

2. **e. Acute pyelonephritis.** The image demonstrates a pelvic kidney with wedge-shaped area of decreased enhancement, characteristic of acute pyelonephritis. Renal infarcts cause areas of poor perfusion that are more sharply defined and more poorly enhancing than in the present case (making option a unlikely). The clinical history of fever also supports an infection. With renal artery

occlusion (option b) the kidney would demonstrate no enhancement. Chronic pyelonephritis causes scarring in the kidney, and the nephrogram is usually normal. The renal contour in the present case is smooth, making option c unlikely. Acute urinary obstruction (option d) is ruled out because the visualized collecting system does not appear dilated.

3. **a. Percutaneous drainage.** The image demonstrates a low-attenuation area in the posterior interpolar region of the left kidney, with perinephric fascial thickening, consistent with a renal abscess. Intravenous antimicrobial therapy with percutaneous drainage of renal abscesses is highly effective and is the treatment of choice. Antimicrobial therapy alone is unlikely to be effective, given the size of the abscess. Nephrectomy, partial nephrectomy, and surgical drainage are rarely indicated in young patients with normally functioning kidneys. Cystoscopy is not warranted.

CHAPTER REVIEW

1. UTIs cause significant morbidity; they do not cause progressive renal failure unless significant comorbidities are present.
2. Increased receptors for uropathogenic *E. coli* on vaginal epithelial cells and buccal mucosal cells in women with recurrent UTIs imply a genetic etiology; moreover, hormonal changes may alter adherence of bacteria to the receptors in the vaginal epithelial cells, explaining the cyclic nature of UTIs in women.
3. If appropriate antimicrobial therapy fails to eradicate bacteria and there is a rapid recurrence, imaging is indicated to determine abnormalities that may cause persistence.
4. When a patient has a symptomatic UTI and gram-negative rods are seen on the urine analysis but the routine culture is negative, an anaerobic infection should be suspected.
5. 10^2 cfu/mL in a symptomatic patient confirms a UTI.
6. Patients with indwelling catheters should be treated only when symptomatic.
7. Whether a patient receives no treatment or short-term, long-term, or prophylactic antimicrobial treatment, the risk of recurrent bacteriuria remains the same; antimicrobial treatment appears to alter only the time until recurrence.
8. There is no association between recurrent infections and renal scarring, hypertension, or progressive renal azotemia
9. *Staphylococcus saprophyticus* is now recognized as causing approximately 10% of symptomatic lower UTIs in young, sexually active females, whereas it rarely causes infection in males and elderly individuals.
10. The validation of the midstream urine specimen can be questioned if numerous squamous epithelial cells (indicative of preputial, vaginal, or urethral contaminants) are present.
11. The fluoroquinolones have a broad spectrum of activity that makes them ideal for the empirical treatment of UTIs.
12. Prophylaxis is recommended for both high- and moderate-risk patients. High-risk patients include individuals with prosthetic heart valves, previous bacterial endocarditis, cyanotic congenital heart disease, and systemic-pulmonary shunts or conduits. Moderate-risk patients include other congenital malformations (excluding isolated secundum atrial septal defects, surgically repaired atrial septal defect, ventricular septal defects, or patent ductus arteriosus), acquired valvular dysfunction, hypertrophic cardiomyopathy, and mitral valve prolapse with valvular regurgitation and/or thickened leaflets. Antimicrobial prophylaxis is not recommended for patients with congenital malformations including isolated secundum atrial septal defects, surgically repaired atrial septal defect, ventricular

septal defects, or patent ductus arteriosus; previous coronary artery bypass graft surgery; benign heart murmurs; previous Kawasaki disease or rheumatic fever without valvular dysfunction; or implanted pacemakers or defibrillators.
13. In general, antimicrobial prophylaxis for urologic patients with total joint replacements, pins, plates, or screws is not indicated. Prophylaxis is advised for individuals at higher risk of seeding a prosthetic joint and include those with recently inserted implants (within 2 years).
14. Three-day therapy is the preferred regimen for uncomplicated cystitis in women.
15. If vesicourethral reflux is absent, a patient bearing the P blood group phenotype may have special susceptibility to recurrent pyelonephritis caused by *E. coli* that have P pili and bind to the P blood group antigen receptors.
16. Emphysematous pyelonephritis should be considered a complication of severe pyelonephritis rather than a distinct entity. The overall mortality rate is 43%.
17. Although surgical drainage, or nephrectomy if the kidney is nonfunctioning or severely infected, is the classic treatment for perinephric abscesses, renal ultrasonography and CT make percutaneous aspiration and drainage of small perirenal collections possible.
18. *Proteus* is the most common organism involved with xanthogranulomatous pyelonephritis; *E. coli* is also common.
19. Even before temperature extremes and the onset of chills, bacteremic patients often begin to hyperventilate. Thus the earliest metabolic change in septicemia is a resultant respiratory alkalosis.
20. Pregnant women with asymptomatic bacteriuria are at higher risk for developing a symptomatic UTI that results in adverse fetal sequelae, complications associated with bacteriuria during pregnancy, and pyelonephritis and its possible sequelae, such as sepsis in the mother. Therefore all pregnant women with asymptomatic bacteriuria should be treated.
21. The aminopenicillins and cephalosporins are considered safe and generally effective throughout pregnancy.
22. In elderly male and female nursing home residents with asymptomatic bacteriuria there is no benefit to administering antimicrobial therapy.
23. In the early stages of Fournier gangrene, the involved area is swollen, erythematous, and tender as the infection begins to involve the deep subcutaneous tissue. Pain is prominent, and fever and systemic toxicity are marked. The swelling and crepitus of the scrotum quickly increase, and dark purple areas develop and progress to extensive gangrene.

Inflammatory and Pain Conditions of the Male Genitourinary Tract: Prostatitis and Related Pain Conditions, Orchitis, and Epididymitis

J. Curtis Nickel

QUESTIONS

1. The most likely candidate for cryptic infection in category III prostatitis is:
   a. *Chlamydia*.
   b. *Ureaplasma*.
   c. nanobacteria.
   d. *Corynebacteria*.
   e. unknown.

2. The presence of white blood cells (WBCs) in the expressed prostatic secretion (EPS) of patients with category III chronic prostatitis/chronic pelvic pain syndrome (CP/CPPS):
   a. confirms significant prostatic inflammation.
   b. correlates with severity of symptoms.
   c. differentiates CP/CPPS patients from control patients.
   d. differentiates CP/CPPS category IIIA patients from category IIIB patients.
   e. differentiates CP category II patients from CP/CPPS category III patients.

3. The National Institutes of Health Chronic Prostatitis Symptom Index is:
   a. a research tool that is useful only in clinical trials.
   b. a research tool that is useful in clinical practice.
   c. another invalidated and unreliable clinical symptom index.
   d. an index that has been validated only in English.
   e. a simple pain questionnaire that can be applied to prostatitis patients.

4. An obese 26-year-old man has an 8-hour history of severe dysuria, stranguria, and suprapubic and perineal pain with fever. On examination, he has suprapubic tenderness, and his prostate is enlarged, boggy, and exquisitely tender. Urinalysis shows pyuria. He continues to complain of symptoms despite insertion of a Foley catheter and has persistent fever following 30 hours of intravenous gentamicin and ampicillin. Culture grew *Escherichia coli*. What is the best next step?
   a. Change antibiotic to a third-generation cephalosporin.
   b. Perform a transrectal ultrasonographic examination.
   c. Perform a cystoscopic examination.
   d. Perform a bladder scan ultrasonographic examination.
   e. Perform a computed tomography scan.

5. A 36-year-old man has a 4-month history of dull perineal and suprapubic discomfort, postejaculatory pain, and moderate obstructive voiding symptoms. A preprostatic massage urine sample was sterile, and microscopic evaluation of the sediment showed 2 white blood cells (WBCs) per high power field (HPF). No EPS was obtained during an uncomfortable digital rectal examination. A postprostatic massage urine sample grew 10^2

Staphylococcus epidermidis organisms per mL, and microscopy of the sediment showed 10 to 12 WBCs/HPF. What is the National Institutes of Health (NIH) chronic prostatitis classification?
   a. Category I
   b. Category II
   c. Category IIIA
   d. Category IIIB
   e. Category IV

6. A 24-year-old man has an 8-month history of obstructive voiding symptoms and perineal and ejaculatory discomfort. A preprostatic massage urine sample was sterile, and microscopic evaluation of sediment showed 1 WBC/HPF. Microscopy of a minute amount of EPS showed 3 WBCs/HPF. A post-prostatic massage urine sample was sterile, and microscopy of the sediment showed 2 WBCs/HPF. The CP/CPPS classification is:
   a. Category I.
   b. Category II.
   c. Category IIIA.
   d. Category IIIB.
   e. Category IV.

7. A 42-year-old man was treated for cystitis but continued to have dysuria, ejaculatory pain, and perineal/testicular discomfort after 7 days of antibiotics. The prostate examination was unremarkable. A midstream urine sample was sterile, but culture of a drop of EPS produced moderate growth of *Enterococcus faecalis*. A post-prostatic massage urine sample grew 10^2 *E. faecalis* organisms, and microscopic examination of the sediment showed 12 WBCs/HPF. What is the NIH classification?
   a. Category I
   b. Category II
   c. Category IIIA
   d. Category IIIB
   e. Category IV

8. A 32-year-old man had been successfully treated for an *E. coli* cystitis with trimethoprim-sulfamethoxazole (7-day course) 4 months previously. A recurrence of similar symptoms was again successfully treated with ciprofloxacin (3 days), but no culture was done at this time. The patient presents 3 days after antibiotics were discontinued with continued perineal discomfort, ejaculatory pain, and mild dysuria. Pre- and post-prostatic massage urine and EPS samples were sterile. Evaluation of the EPS showed 20 WBCs/HPF. The prostate felt normal. The best next step is:
   a. treat with anti-inflammatory agents.
   b. do a standard Meares-Stamey 4-glass test.
   c. wait for 3 days and do standard Meares-Stamey 4-glass test.
   d. restart trimethoprim-sulfamethoxazole.
   e. restart fluoroquinolone antibiotics.

9. A 47-year-old man has a 5-year history of perineal and suprapubic pain/discomfort and obstructive voiding symptoms that has not responded to multiple courses of antibiotics, α-blockers, anti-inflammatory agents, repetitive prostatic massage, or phytotherapy. The prostate is tender, and the post-prostatic massage urine sample was sterile and showed 20 WBCs/HPF. The PSA value was 1.2 mg/mL. What is the best next step?

   a. Incision of bladder neck

   b. Flow rate and bladder scan for residual urine

   c. Video-urodynamics

   d. CT scan of pelvis

   e. Cystoscopy and transrectal ultrasound

10. A 28-year-old man has been successfully treated for three episodes of cystitis (cultures not performed). He now presents with a 3-day history of frequency, urgency, dysuria, and suprapubic discomfort. The prostate feels normal and is nontender. An abdominal and pelvic ultrasonographic study had normal results. A midstream culture done 24 hours earlier by his family physician grew 10^5 E. coli organisms per mL. What is the best next step?

    a. A lower urinary tract localization test (2- or 4-glass test)

    b. Several days of nitrofurantoin therapy followed by lower urinary tract localization test

    c. Four weeks of fluoroquinolone antibiotics therapy

    d. Cystoscopy

    e. Transrectal ultrasonography

11. A 37-year-old man has a 3-month history of urinary frequency and urgency and discomfort localized to the perineum, suprapubic area, testicles, and penis. A sterile post-prostatic massage urine sample showed 15 WBCs/HPF on microscopy. A year earlier, the patient had been successfully treated for moderately severe symptoms with an unspecified antibiotic. He is allergic to many medications, including ciprofloxacin. The symptoms are now a significant bother and affecting his quality of life. The best initial treatment is a trial of:

    a. anti-inflammatory agents.

    b. tetracycline.

    c. trimethoprim-sulfamethoxazole.

    d. trimethoprim.

    e. carbenicillin.

12. A 58-year-old man with a 2-year history of symptomatic recurrent urinary tract infections with *Pseudomonas* (6 to 8 per year) is asymptomatic between treated episodes. *Pseudomonas aeruginosa* is localized to the EPS and postprostatic massage (voided bladder 3, VB3) samples (but not the midstream urine sample, or VB2) during a period when he was asymptomatic. The EPS shows severe pyuria with WBC plugs or aggregates on microscopy. Transrectal ultrasonography shows extensive prostatic calcifications. Cystoscopy results are normal, residual urine is negligible, and the PSA value is 1.0 mg/mL. What is the best treatment?

    a. Low-dose prophylactic antibiotics

    b. Intraprostatic antibiotic injection

    c. Radical TURP

    d. Radical prostatectomy

    e. Transurethral microwave thermotherapy

13. A 24-year-old man with a 6-year history of severe perineal pain with irritative and obstructive voiding symptoms has no significant benefits with 4 weeks of therapy with trimethoprim-sulfamethoxazole, anti-inflammatory agents, α-blockers, or phytotherapy respectively. Prostate-specific specimens were sterile, and no WBCs were noted on microscopy. The physical examination had normal findings except for anal sphincter spasm and a tender but normal-feeling prostate gland. Video-urodynamics showed adequate funneling of the bladder neck with seemingly poor opening of the striated sphincter area and abnormal striated sphincter EMG activity during the emptying phase of micturition. What is the best next step?

    a. Four weeks of fluoroquinolone therapy

    b. Muscle relaxant therapy

    c. Bladder neck incision

    d. Biofeedback

    e. Transurethral microwave thermotherapy

14. A 52-year-old man continues to have high, spiking fever despite suprapubic catheterization and 36 hours of treatment with wide-spectrum intravenous antibiotics. Transrectal ultrasonography confirms a large prostatic abscess. What is the best next step?

    a. Transperineal drainage

    b. Transrectal aspiration

    c. Transurethral drainage

    d. Open drainage

    e. Suprapubic aspiration

15. Alpha blocker therapy for CP/CPPS:

    a. is of proven value for Category I.

    b. is of proven value for Category II.

    c. is of proven value for Category III.

    d. is of proven value for Category II and III.

    e. May have value in some patients with Category III.

16. Mandatory evaluation of a patient with CP/CPPS includes history, physical examination, and:

    a. urine analysis, urine culture.

    b. urine analysis, urine culture, Chronic Prostatitis Symptom Index (CPSI).

    c. urine analysis, urine culture, CPSI, urine cytology.

    d. urine analysis, urine culture, CPSI, urine cytology, postvoid residual.

    e. urine analysis, urine culture, CPSI, urine cytology, postvoid residual, sexual function questionnaire.

17. An asymptomatic 65-year-old man undergoes a prostate biopsy because of an indistinct prostate asymmetry on digital rectal examination. The PSA value is 2.2 ng/mL. Pathology reveals extensive glandular and periglandular infiltration with acute and chronic inflammatory cells. What is the best next step?

    a. Observation

    b. Four weeks of antibiotics and then reassess

    c. Four weeks of antibiotics and anti-inflammatories and then reassess

    d. Repeat biopsy

    e. Cystoscopy

18. UPOINT is:

    a. a painful urological trigger point.

    b. an inflammatory biomarker.

    c. a phenotype categorization.

    d. a chronic prostatitis diagnosis.

    e. a microscopic technique.

19. Acupuncture as a treatment for CP/CPPS:

    a. cannot be tested because of difficulty in developing a validated sham procedure.

    b. is characterized by the increased effectiveness of electro-acupuncture over traditional acupuncture.

c. has been proved ineffective in randomized controlled trials.

d. is a reasonable choice for selected patients.

e. has been shown to compare favorably to alpha blockers in comparative clinical trials.

20. The following conservative therapy is associated with increased pain and disability in CP/CPPS patients:

a. rest.

b. diet modification.

c. exercise.

d. heat therapy.

e. physiotherapy.

21. The following minimally invasive procedure does not provide any proven efficacy to ameliorate symptoms in men with CP/CPPS:

a. extracorporeal shock wave therapy.

b. electrical neuromodulation.

c. microwave thermotherapy.

d. botulinum toxin.

e. balloon dilation.

22. Alpha blocker monotherapy for CP/CPPS category III is:

a. not recommended.

b. recommended for patients with obstructive voiding symptoms.

c. recommended for patients who are alpha blocker naïve.

e. recommended for patients who are alpha blocker naïve and have obstructive voiding symptoms.

f. recommended for patients who are newly diagnosed, alpha blocker naïve, and have obstructive voiding symptoms.

23. Epididymectomy for chronic epididymalgia provides the best results when performed:

a. in recently diagnosed patients.

b. in postinfection cases.

c. when the etiology is traumatic.

d. postvasectomy.

e. when associated with Behçet disease.

Pathology

1. A 65-year-old man undergoes a transurethral resection of the prostate. The pathology is depicted in Figure 13-1, and the report states that there is amyloid that fills several benign prostatic acini. The next step in management is to:

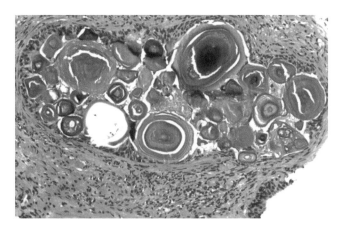

Figure 13-1. (From Bostwick DG, Cheng L. Urologic surgical pathology. 2nd ed. Edinburgh: Mosby; 2008.)

a. perform a transrectal biopsy.

b. refer to medicine for evaluation of systemic amyloidosis.

c. inquire as to whether the patient has been on estrogens.

d. ask the pathologist to perform immune stains for basal cells.

e. ask the pathologist if the diagnosis could be corpora amylacea.

2. A 70-year-old man had a transurethral resection of the prostate 10 years previously. A repeat procedure is performed, and the pathology depicted in Figure 13-2 is reported as showing granulomatous prostatitis. The next step in management is to:

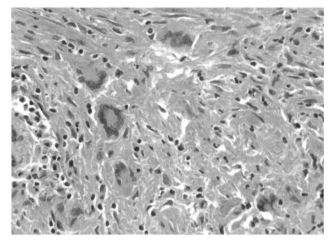

Figure 13-2. (From Bostwick DG, Cheng L. Urologic surgical pathology. 2nd ed. Edinburgh: Mosby; 2008.)

a. have the patient obtain a PPD.

b. refer to Infectious Disease for treatment.

c. inquire as to whether the patient received BCG.

d. observe the patient.

e. ask the pathologist to stain the slide for tuberculosis.

Imaging

1. A 40-year-old man with right scrotal pain is seen in the emergency department. Scrotal ultrasonography is performed (Figure 13-3). The most likely diagnosis is:

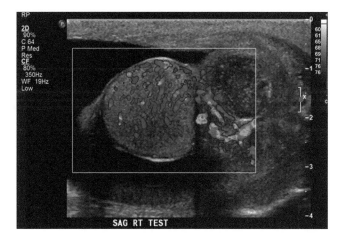

Figure 13-3.

a. adenomatoid tumor of epididymis.

b. testicular torsion.

c. primary testicular neoplasm.

d. epididymo-orchitis.

e. orchitis.

2. A 60-year-old man presents with pelvic and perineal discomfort, fever, and chills. A CT image is shown in Figure 13-4. The next step in management is:

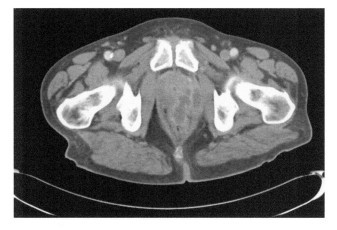

Figure 13-4.

a. magnetic resonance imagine (MRI) for staging.

b. antimicrobial therapy.

c. drainage.

d. retrograde urethrography.

e. transrectal prostate biopsy.

ANSWERS

1. **e. unknown.** A careful review of the evidence for and against the role of microorganisms—culturable, fastidious, or nonculturable—leaves the reviewer undecided, and etiologic mechanisms other than microorganisms must be considered.

2. **d. differentiates CP/CPPS category IIIA patients from category IIIB patients.** The differentiation of the two subtypes of category III CPPS is dependent on cytologic examination of the urine and/or EPS.

3. **b. a research tool that is useful in clinical practice.** The National Institutes of Health Chronic Prostatitis Collaborative Research Network developed a reproducible and valid instrument to measure the symptoms and quality of life/impact of chronic prostatitis for use in research protocols as well as in clinical practice. The symptom index has also proved its usefulness in the evaluation and follow-up of patients in general clinical urologic practice.

4. **b. Perform a transrectal ultrasonographic examination.** Development of a prostate abscess is best detected with transrectal ultrasonography. Patients with acute bacterial prostatitis are easily diagnosed and successfully treated with appropriate antibiotic therapy, as long as the clinician keeps a high index of suspicion for prostate abscess in patients who fail to respond quickly to the antibiotics.

5. **c. Category IIIA.** Diagnosis of category IIIA CP/CPPS, or inflammatory CPPS, is based on the presence of excessive leukocytes in EPS, a postprostatic massage urine sample, or semen.

6. **d. Category IIIB.** Diagnosis of category IIIB CP/CPPS, or noninflammatory CPPS, rests on no significant leukocytes being found in similar specimens.

7. **b. Category II.** Category I is identical to the acute bacterial prostatitis category of the traditional classification system. Category II is identical to the traditional chronic bacterial prostatitis classification.

8. **e. restart fluoroquinolone antibiotics.** The most important clue in the diagnosis of category II, chronic bacterial prostatitis is a history of documented recurrent urinary tract infections. The fluoroquinolone should be continued for a minimum of 4 weeks.

9. **c. Video-urodynamics.** A wide constellation of irritative and obstructive voiding symptoms is associated with CP/CPPS. Proposed etiologies to account for the persistent irritative and obstructive voiding symptoms include detrusor vesical neck or external sphincter dyssynergia, proximal or distal urethral obstruction, and fibrosis or hypertrophy of the vesical neck. Although flow rate and bladder scan can be done to further delineate these conditions, these abnormalities can be clarified and diagnosed best by urodynamics, particularly video-urodynamics.

10. **b. Several days of nitrofurantoin therapy followed by a lower urinary tract localization test.** In a patient who has acute cystitis, the localization of bacteria in the EPS or VB3 specimen (postprostatic massage sample) is impossible, and, in this case, the patient can be treated with a short course (1 to 3 days) of antibiotics such as nitrofurantoin, which penetrates the prostate poorly but eradicates the bladder bacteriuria. Subsequent localization of bacteria in the postprostatic massage urine sample or EPS sample is then diagnostic of category II prostatitis.

11. **d. trimethoprim.** Studies of animals with and without infection showed that trimethoprim concentrated in prostatic secretion and prostatic interstitial fluid (exceeding plasma levels), whereas sulfamethoxazole and ampicillin did not. It would be appropriate therefore to not prescribe the combination trimethoprim-sulfamethoxazole in a patient with multiple allergies.

12. **a. Low-dose prophylactic antibiotics.** Prolonged therapy with low-dose prophylactic or suppressive antimicrobials can be considered for recurrent or refractory prostatitis, respectively.

13. **d. Biofeedback.** On the basis of the possibility that the voiding and pain symptoms associated with CPPS may be secondary to some form of pseudodyssynergia during voiding or repetitive perineal muscle spasm, biofeedback has the potential to improve this process. Bladder neck incision in a young man should be avoided until after he has his family because of the possibility of retrograde ejaculation.

14. **c. Transurethral drainage.** In patients who fail to respond quickly to antibiotics, a prostatic abscess is optimally drained

by the transurethral incision route, although ultrasound-guided percutaneous aspiration (via any route) could be attempted first.

15. **e. May have value in some patients with Category III.** Six randomized placebo-controlled trials have shown efficacy for terazosin, alfuzosin, and tamsulosin in patients with CPPS. However, two recent NIH-sponsored large randomized placebo controlled trials have not confirmed its efficacy in heavily pretreated chronic patients, or in recently diagnosed α-blocker naive patients. A number of meta-analyses have confirmed a modest treatment effect, but it appears that the best results are obtained when α-blockers are used as part of a multimodal treatment strategy.

16. **a. urine analysis, urine culture.** Mandatory evaluation of a typical man presenting with CP/CPPS includes history-taking, physical examination, urinalysis, and urine culture.

17. **a. Observation.** Asymptomatic inflammatory prostatitis (Category IV) by definition does not require symptomatic therapy.

18. **c. a phenotype categorization.** UPOINT is a classification system that categorizes CP/CPPS patients into one or more of six distinct clinical phenotypes.

19. **d. is a reasonable choice for selected patients.** In a number of sham-controlled trials, acupuncture was shown to be effective in some patients.

20. **a. rest.** Studies show that the maladaptive pain coping technique of using "pain contingent resting" (the use of rest rather than more active behaviors to control pain) is not beneficial.

21. **e. balloon dilation.** Some minimally invasive surgical procedures (electrical neuromodulation, extracorporeal shock wave therapy, electroacupuncture, and perhaps transurethral microwave therapy and botulinum toxin injection) may be beneficial for treatment for CP/CPPS in selected patients, however, large, well designed sham controlled trials are required before they can be considered recommended therapy. Balloon dilation is ineffective.

22. **a. not recommended.** Alpha-blocker monotherapy is not recommended. Alpha-blocker therapy may be considered as part of multimodal treatment strategy for newly diagnosed, alpha-blocker naïve patients who have voiding symptoms (Table 13-1).

23. **d. postvasectomy.** Better surgical results (up to 70%) have been reported for epididymectomy for postvasectomy pain.

TABLE 13-1 Suggested Therapies for Chronic Prostatitis/Chronic Pelvic Pain Syndrome (NIH Category III)

RECOMMENDED

1. Alpha-blocker therapy as part of multimodal treatment strategy for newly diagnosed, alpha-blocker naïve patients who have voiding symptoms
2. Antimicrobial therapy trial for selected newly diagnosed, antimicrobial naïve patients
3. Selected phytotherapies: cernilton and quercetin
4. Multimodal therapy directed by clinical phenotype
5. Directed physiotherapy—although level 1 evidence is not available, evidence from multiple weak trials and vast clinical experience strongly suggests benefit for selected patients

NOT RECOMMENDED

1. Alpha-blocker monotherapy, particularly in patients previously treated with α-blockers
2. Anti-inflammatory monotherapy
3. Antimicrobial therapy as primary therapy, particular in patients who have previously failed treated with antibiotics
4. Five alpha-reductase inhibitor monotherapy; can be considered in older patients with co-existing benign prostatic hyperplasia
5. Most minimally invasive therapies such as transurethral needle ablation, laser therapies
6. Invasive surgical therapies such as transurethral resection of the prostate and radical prostatectomy

REQUIRING FURTHER EVALUATION

1. Low-intensity shock wave treatment
2. Acupuncture
3. Biofeedback
4. Invasive neuromodulation (e.g., pudendal nerve modulation)
5. Electromagnetic stimulation
6. Botulinum toxin A injection
7. Medical therapies including mepartricin, muscle relaxants, neuromodulators, immunomodulators

Modified from evidence based consensus, International Consultation of Urologic Disease, Fukuoko, Japan, 2012. (Nickel JC, Shoskes DA, Wagenlehner FM. Management of chronic prostatitis/chronic pelvic pain syndrome [CP/CPPS]: the studies, the evidence and the impact. World J Urol 2013;31:747-53.)

Pathology

1. **e. Ask the pathologist if the diagnosis could be corpora amylacea.** Corpora amylacea are most often associated with BPH. Amyloid of the prostate does not look like this; moreover, if there is concern for amyloid, a Congo Red stain should be obtained. Asking the pathologist to clarify the diagnosis, which would be unusual given the circumstances, is most appropriate.

2. **d. observe the patient.** The pathology shows multinucleated giant cells, which are not uncommonly seen after chronic irritation. There is no evidence of caseating necrosis and, in this patient with a cause for the giant cells, observation is the correct course.

Imaging

1. **d. epididymo-orchitis.** The image demonstrates skin thickening in the scrotum, hydrocele, and a complex hypoechoic mass in the enlarged epididymis that has no flow; color flow Doppler images demonstrate increased flow in the testis and in the remainder of the epididymis, consistent with epididymo-orchitis complicated by an epididymal abscess. These composite findings make the other listed possibilities less likely.

2. **c. drainage.** The CT image demonstrates low-attenuation areas in the prostate, primarily the left posterolateral aspect, with extension into the left periprostatic region. The appearance is most compatible with an abscess. This could be confirmed with transrectal ultrasonography. These findings on CT along with the clinical history and a rectal examination, which would reveal extreme tenderness, are sufficient to suggest a prostate abscess. Urgent drainage is prudent in such patients. Although urethral strictures and upper tract abnormalities may be the cause of recurrent urinary tract infections in a male, neither study is required urgently in a patient with a prostatic abscess. Antimicrobial therapy alone is not sufficient treatment at this stage of the infection. MRI may help in delineating the extent of involvement in equivocal cases but is unlikely to add more useful information when the results of CT and the physical examination are flagrantly abnormal. The appearance of the prostate on the CT image is not consistent with prostate cancer.

CHAPTER REVIEW

1. Granulomatous prostatic inflammation is a common occurrence following surgery or BCG treatment.
2. The most common cause of acute bacterial prostatitis is the Enterobacteriaceae family of gram-negative bacteria.
3. Bacteria reside deep in the ducts of the prostate gland and form aggregates called biofilms that allow the bacteria to persist in the presence of antibiotics.
4. Factors that increase the risk of bacterial colonization of the prostate include (1) intraprostatic ductal reflux, (2) phimosis, (3) specific blood groups, (4) unprotected anal intercourse, (5) urinary tract infections, (6) acute epididymitis, (7) indwelling urethral catheters, (8) condom catheter drainage, and (9) transurethral surgery.
5. Prostate-specific antigen levels can be markedly elevated during an episode of prostatitis.
6. Cytokines appear to play an important role in the development of prostatitis.
7. There is no validated level of WBCs in prostatic fluid that differentiates noninflammatory from inflammatory conditions; however, a finding of 5 to 10 WBCs/HPF is considered by many to be the upper limit of normal for prostatic fluid.
8. Patients with prostatitis-like symptoms who have no evidence of infection and complain of irritative voiding symptoms should have urine cytology performed.
9. It may not be the specific type of bacteria that causes CPPS but rather the individual's response to the infection being greater in those prone to get CPPS. The symptoms may continue chronically because of persistent immunologic mechanisms long after the bacterial infection has been eradicated.
10. Dysfunctional voiding may be a cause of CPPS.
11. Altered autonomic function may be responsible for the pain.
12. The NIH Chronic Prostatitis Symptom Index has three domains: pain, urinary function, and quality of life.
13. UPOINT is a 6-point clinical classification that includes the following categories: urinary, psychosocial, organ specific, infection, neurologic/systemic, and tenderness.
14. Orchitis is rare and usually viral in origin; most cases of bacterial orchitis are secondary to local spread from the epididymis.
15. Epididymitis usually results from spread of infection from bladder, urethra, or prostate via the vas deferens.
16. Development of a prostate abscess is best detected with transrectal ultrasonography. A prostatic abscess is optimally drained by the transurethral incision route,
17. The classification of prostatitis is as follows: Category I is identical to the acute bacterial prostatitis category of the traditional classification system. Category II is identical to the traditional chronic bacterial prostatitis classification. Category IIIA CP/CPPS, or inflammatory CPPS, is based on the presence of excessive leukocytes in EPS, a postprostatic massage urine sample, or semen. Category IIIB CP/CPPS, or noninflammatory CPPS, rests on no significant leukocytes being found in similar specimens.

14   Bladder Pain Syndrome (Interstitial Cystitis) and Related Disorders

Philip M. Hanno

QUESTIONS

1. Essential for the diagnosis of bladder pain syndrome/interstitial cystitis (BPS/IC) is the presence of:
   a. urinary urgency.
   b. pain or discomfort related to the bladder.
   c. glomerulations on cystoscopy.
   d. Hunner lesion.
   e. urinary frequency.

2. The definition of interstitial cystitis proposed by the National Institute of Arthritis, Diabetes, Digestive and Kidney Diseases (NIDDK) is best considered a:
   a. de facto definition of the disease.
   b. diagnostic pathway.
   c. definition applicable mainly to clinical research studies.
   d. historic document of no current value.
   e. purely symptom-based description of BPS/IC.

3. The best clinical evidence for a urine abnormality in BPS comes from:
   a. the absence of pain when a Foley catheter is left indwelling.
   b. relief of symptoms as a result of using narcotic analgesics.
   c. failure of conduit diversion to relieve symptoms.
   d. late occurrence of pain and bowel segment contraction after substitution cystoplasty and continent diversion.
   e. symptom relief associated with urinary alkalinization.

4. BPS/IC symptom and problem indices have been validated to:
   a. monitor disease progression or regression with or without treatment.
   b. correctly choose who should undergo cystectomy and diversion.
   c. determine on whom to perform diagnostic testing.
   d. accurately diagnose BPS/IC.
   e. determine appropriate candidates for clinical research.

5. Which of the following statements best categorizes the natural history of BPS/IC?
   a. The onset is generally insidious, occurring gradually over many years.
   b. Major deterioration in symptom severity is the rule.
   c. Symptoms follow a culture-documented urinary tract infection.
   d. Symptom resolution regardless of treatment after 1 to 2 years.
   e. Subacute onset with full development of the symptom complex over a relatively short time span.

6. Which statement best describes the relationship of BPS/IC to bladder cancer?
   a. BPS/IC is a premalignant lesion.
   b. BPS/IC is often associated with bladder cancer.
   c. A positive urine cytology can safely be ignored in patients with BPS/IC.
   d. The vast majority of reports fail to document an association of BPS/IC with subsequent development of bladder cancer.
   e. Dysplasia is a typical pathologic finding on bladder biopsy in BPS/IC patients.

7. The only animal that appears to spontaneously develop a syndrome similar to BPS/IC is the:
   a. cat.
   b. rabbit.
   c. dog.
   d. goat.
   e. rat.

8. The antibiotic of choice for diagnosed BPS/ IC is:
   a. doxycycline.
   b. none.
   c. gentamicin.
   d. ciprofloxacin.
   e. amoxicillin.

9. The cell most likely to play a central role in the pathogenesis of BPS is the:
   a. granulocyte.
   b. lymphocyte.
   c. mast cell.
   d. platelet.
   e. eosinophil.

10. Which statement best categorizes the potassium chloride test?
    a. It is soothing and calming to the painful bladder.
    b. It has high sensitivity and specificity for diagnosing BPS/IC.
    c. It is an important element in choosing effective therapy.
    d. It provides proof of abnormal mucosal permeability.
    e. None of the above.

11. A circumscribed inflammatory bladder lesion:
    a. is required to make a diagnosis of BPS/IC.
    b. is generally found in less than 30% of BPS patients.
    c. was not considered a part of the syndrome when it was initially described by Hunner.
    d. is synonymous with glomerulation.
    e. is pathognomonic of BPS/IC even in the absence of symptoms.

12. Exclusive use of the NIDDK criteria to diagnose BPS/IC would result in:
    a. an accurate depiction of the true prevalence of the condition.
    b. an improved treatment algorithm.
    c. increased diagnostic specificity.
    d. increased diagnostic sensitivity.
    e. a minimum of diagnostic testing and significant cost savings.

13. All but which of the following disorders have a much higher prevalence in the BPS population than in the general population?
    a. Irritable bowel syndrome
    b. Diabetes
    c. Fibromyalgia
    d. Allergy
    e. Chronic fatigue syndrome

14. Where is the antiproliferative factor (APF) produced?
    a. Bladder urothelial cells
    b. Glomeruli
    c. Transitional urothelial cells in the upper tracts
    d. Mast cells
    e. Neutrophils

15. The postulated direct effect of antiproliferative factor is to:
    a. increase afferent neuron sensitivity.
    b. increase potassium efflux into urothelial cells.
    c. protect the surface glycosaminoglycan layer.
    d. elevate leukotriene levels.
    e. regulate growth factor production by bladder cells.

16. The central role of histopathology in BPS is to:
    a. determine whether the patient has ulcerative or nonulcerative disease (Hunner lesion).
    b. help determine the most efficacious treatment modality.
    c. predict prognosis.
    d. rule out other disorders that might be responsible for the symptoms.
    e. confirm the diagnosis with pathologic criteria.

17. Which of the following has the least in common with BPS?
    a. Vulvodynia
    b. Chronic bacterial prostatitis
    c. Orchalgia
    d. Penile pain
    e. Perineal and scrotal pain

18. Urodynamic findings typical of BPS include:
    a. uninhibited detrusor contractions.
    b. obstructed flow patterns.
    c. abnormal bladder compliance.
    d. decreased capacity and hypersensitivity.
    e. increased volume at first urge to void.

19. The finding of glomerulations:
    a. is significant only when cystoscopy is performed with the patient under anesthesia.
    b. is of no significance in an asymptomatic patient.
    c. indicates a likelihood of response to laser fulguration of the bladder.
    d. is present only in patients with BPS.
    e. is sufficient to make a diagnosis of BPS.

20. The incidence of short-term spontaneous remission in BPS approaches:
    a. 50%.
    b. 100%.
    c. 30%.
    d. 10%.
    e. 75%.

21. Which test is potentially most helpful for diagnosis, prognosis, and therapy?
    a. Potassium chloride test
    b. Intravesical heparin trial
    c. Cystoscopy and low-pressure bladder hydrodistention
    d. Bladder biopsy
    e. Urodynamics

22. Which of the following treatments is targeted to the glycosaminoglycan layer of the bladder?
    a. Sodium pentosan polysulfate
    b. Amitriptyline
    c. Hydroxyzine
    d. L-Arginine
    e. None of the above

23. Which of the following intravesical treatments has shown proven efficacy for BPS in pivotal U.S. Food and Drug Administration trials?
    a. BCG (bacille Calmette-Guérin)
    b. Hyaluronic acid
    c. Botulinum toxin
    d. Heparin
    e. None of the above

24. Which of the following statements is true of narcotic analgesics?
    a. They have no place in the treatment of a chronic, nonmalignant condition such as BPS.
    b. They can make patients physically dependent on them.
    c. They generally result in drug addiction when used for chronic pain.
    d. They tend to cause diarrhea and sleeplessness.
    e. All of the above.

25. Which of the following is a reasonable surgical procedure to relieve the pain of BPS?
    a. Transurethral fulguration of Hunner lesion
    b. Reduction cystoplasty
    c. Sympathectomy and intraspinal alcohol injections
    d. Cystolysis
    e. Transvesical infiltration of the pelvic plexuses with phenol

26. The most important early step in the management of BPS is:
    a. initiating intravesical treatment.
    b. patient education.
    c. starting oral pentosan polysulfate therapy.
    d. physical therapy.
    e. strict adherence to "IC" diet.

27. A finding of detrusor overactivity on urodynamics in a patient with bladder pain in the absence of urinary urgency indicates:
    a. the patient needs treatment with antimuscarinic medication.
    b. the patient does not have BPS.
    c. a urinary tract infection is likely.
    d. neuromodulation would be the most effective treatment.
    e. none of the above.

28. Men with irritative voiding symptoms and pelvic pain should be evaluated for:
    a. chronic pelvic pain syndrome.
    b. bacterial prostatitis.
    c. bladder pain syndrome.

d. bladder carcinoma in situ.

e. all of the above.

29. The NIDDK Multidisciplinary Approach to the Study of Pelvic Pain (MAPP) is a 10-year multicenter program designed to:

a. test new treatments for BPS.

b. compile a long-term national database registration to follow BPS patients into the future.

c. gather data to justify officially changing the designation of "interstitial cystitis" to "bladder pain syndrome."

d. develop a rational treatment algorithm for BPS.

e. examine the chronic pelvic pain syndrome in men and BPS along with associated syndromes to better characterize the relationship among these disorders and enhance future diagnosis and treatment efforts.

30. Emotional, sexual, or physical abuse can be categorized as:

a. risk factors for bladder pain syndrome.

b. behaviors often attributed to patients with BPS.

c. unequivocally unrelated to BPS.

d. rare adverse events caused by medications used to treat BPS.

e. conditions for which there are no data to allow any tentative conclusions with regard to the relationship to BPS.

31. The only phenotype of IC/BPS currently shown to have a unique response to therapy and different natural history is

a. nocturia.

b. daytime frequency.

c. absence of bladder pain.

d. glomerulation.

e. Hunner lesion.

32. Epidemiologic information gathered by the Rand Corporation suggests which of the following?

a. BPS is never familial.

b. BPS may be as common in men as it is in women.

c. A male with BPS should be given a diagnosis of prostatitis.

d. BPS is a rare disease that should qualify for orphan drug classification by the Food and Drug administration.

e. BPS is common in children with urinary frequency.

ANSWERS

1. **b. Pain or discomfort related to the bladder.** Pain, pressure, or discomfort related to the bladder is necessary to make a diagnosis of bladder pain syndrome. Urgency, frequency, and the presence of glomerulations or Hunner ulcer on endoscopy are often associated with BPS, but the presence of pain or discomfort is the primary component. IC may form a subgroup of the painful bladder group, but the criteria are not clear, and at this point the terms can be used interchangeably.

2. **c. Definition applicable mainly to clinical research studies.** The definition of IC proposed by the NIDDK is best considered a definition applicable for use in research studies. It was never meant to define the disease but rather was developed to ensure that patients included in basic and clinical research studies were homogeneous enough that experts could agree on the diagnosis.

3. **d. Late occurrence of pain and bowel segment contraction after substitution cystoplasty and continent diversion.** Substitution cystoplasty and continent diversion both fail in some BPS patients because of the development of pain in the bowel segment used or contraction of the bowel segment. Some studies have shown histologic changes in bowel segments used in BPS patients similar to those that occur in the IC bladder. Both of these findings provide circumstantial clinical evidence that the urine of BPS patients may have toxicity associated with the symptomatic expression of the disorder. However, data with regard to antiproliferative factor make this evidence suspect.

4. **a. Monitor disease progression or regression with or without treatment.** Symptom and problem indices like the one developed by O'Leary and Sant are not intended to diagnose BPS/IC. Like the American Urologic Association Symptom Score for benign prostatic hypertrophy, these indices are designed to evaluate the severity of symptoms and to monitor disease progression or regression and response to treatment.

5. **e. Subacute onset with full development of the symptom complex over a relatively short time span.** Several epidemiologic studies have concluded that the onset of BPS is commonly subacute rather than insidious. It presents more as one would expect an infectious disorder to present, rather than a chronic disease process. Full development of the classic symptom complex takes place over a relatively short period of time. In the majority of cases, it does not progress continuously but reaches its final stage rapidly and then continues without significant change in overall symptoms.

6. **d. The vast majority of reports fail to document an association of BPS/IC with subsequent development of bladder cancer.** Until recently, no relationship has ever been shown between BPS and the subsequent development of bladder carcinoma. In the 1970s, the Mayo Clinic documented bladder cancer in 12 of 53 men who had been treated for IC, but the association was the result of incorrect diagnosis rather than progression. Peters and others have noted that patients with bladder cancer can be misdiagnosed with BPS/IC. A recent study from Taiwan reported a 2.95 relative risk compared with controls.

7. **a. Cat.** The feline urologic syndrome may represent the animal equivalent of BPS/IC. Approximately two thirds of cats with lower urinary tract disease have sterile urine and no evidence of other urinary tract disorders. Some of these cats experience frequency and urgency of urination, pain, and bladder inflammation. Glomerulations have been found in some of these cat bladders. Other findings similar to BPS include bladder mastocytosis, increased histamine excretion, and increased bladder permeability.

8. **b. None.** Antibiotics are not indicated for the treatment of BPS/IC, nor have they been implicated as a causative factor. An empiric trial of doxycycline is reasonable in patients who have never had an antibiotic trial to treat the symptoms. Numerous studies have concluded that it is unlikely that active infection is involved in the ongoing pathologic process or that antibiotics have a role to play in treatment.

9. **c. Mast cell.** Mast cells are strategically localized in the urinary bladder close to blood vessels, lymphatics, nerves, and detrusor smooth muscle. BPS appears to be a syndrome with neural, immune, and endocrine components in which activated mast cells play a central, although not primary, role in many patients.

10. **e. None of the above.** As many as 25% of patients who meet the NIDDK criteria for BPS/IC will have a negative KCl test. It is positive in the majority of patients with radiation cystitis, urinary tract infection, or nonbacterial prostatitis and in women with pelvic pain. It is neither sensitive nor specific for BPS/IC, is uncomfortable for patients, and does not help to guide therapeutic decisions.

11. **b. Is generally found in less than 30% of BPS patients.** Bladder ulceration (so-called Hunner ulcer) is more appropriately referred to as Hunner lesion and is found in a minority of patients with symptoms of BPS/IC. It is not a true ulcer, but a "vulnus" or weakness or vulnerable area of the mucosa. A circumscribed red patch that cracks and bleeds with distention is best appreciated with the patient under anesthesia.

12. **c. Increased diagnostic specificity.** Exclusive use of the NIDDK criteria to diagnose BPS would result in increased specificity and decreased sensitivity. Ninety percent of expert clinicians in the NIDDK database study agreed that patients diagnosed with IC by those criteria had IC. However, 60% of patients diagnosed

by these clinicians as having BPS/IC did not fulfill the NIDDK criteria. Using the criteria as a basis for diagnosis would probably exclude the majority of patients with this symptom complex from the correct diagnosis.

13. **b. Diabetes.** Fibromyalgia, irritable bowel syndrome, chronic fatigue syndrome, and atopic allergic reactions are overrepresented in the BPS population. Studies are ongoing to find out the reason for such relationships in the NIDDK MAPP (Multidisciplinary Approach to the Study of Chronic Pelvic Pain) 5-year study. Diabetes has never been associated with an increased prevalence in patients with BPS.

14. **a. Bladder urothelial cells.** APF can be obtained from cultured uroepithelial cells and is not present in renal pelvic urine. It is associated with decreased production of heparin binding epidermal growth factor–like growth factor.

15. **e. Regulate growth factor production by bladder cells.** APF regulates growth factor production by bladder epithelial cells. It has been postulated that any of a variety of injuries to the bladder (infection, trauma, overdistention) in a susceptible individual may result in BPS if APF is present and suppresses production of heparin binding epidermal growth factor–like growth factor.

16. **d. Rule out other disorders that might be responsible for the symptoms.** The primary value of histopathology in BPS is to rule out other diseases that may account for the symptoms. The differentiation between ulcerative and nonulcerative disease is based on endoscopic features. There is no pathognomonic histologic finding for the disorder, nor can histology predict prognosis. Even a severely abnormal microscopic picture does not necessarily indicate a poor prognosis. At this time, no data suggest that the treatment algorithm can be rationally predicated on the basis of the histologic findings alone.

17. **b. Chronic bacterial prostatitis.** BPS can be considered one of the pain syndromes of the urogenital and rectal area, all of which are well described but poorly understood. These include vulvodynia, orchialgia, perineal pain, penile pain, and rectal pain. Bacterial prostatitis is a well-understood entity with a known etiology and generally responds to treatment directed at the offending organism. NIH type 1 includes acute bacterial prostatitis and NIH type 2 denotes chronic bacterial prostatitis. Unlike NIH type 3 chronic pelvic pain syndrome/nonbacterial prostatitis, types 1 and 2 have no relationship to BPS.

18. **d. Decreased capacity and hypersensitivity.** Cystometry in conscious BPS patients generally demonstrates normal function, the exception being decreased bladder capacity and hypersensitivity, perhaps exaggerated by the use of carbon dioxide as a medium. Pain on bladder filling, which reproduces the patient's symptoms, is very suggestive of IC. Bladder compliance in patients with IC is normal, as hypersensitivity would prevent the bladder from filling to the point of noncompliance.

19. **b. Is of no significance in an asymptomatic patient.** Glomerulations are not specific for BPS, and only when seen in conjunction with the clinical criteria of pain and frequency can the presence of glomerulations be viewed as potentially significant. Glomerulations can be seen after radiation therapy, in patients with bladder carcinoma, after exposure to toxic chemicals or chemotherapeutic agents, and in patients undergoing dialysis or after urinary diversion when the bladder has not filled for extended periods. They have also been reported in the majority of men with prostate pain syndromes. In the United States and Europe they are not longer viewed as important for diagnosis or to guide management.

20. **a. 50%.** There is a 50% incidence of temporary remission unrelated to therapy, with a mean duration of 8 months. The clinical course of BPS is extremely variable, and it can be difficult to differentiate the effects of treatment from the natural history of the disease.

21. **c. Cystoscopy and low-pressure bladder hydrodistention.** Bladder hydrodistention with the patient under anesthesia is a common therapeutic modality used for BPS, frequently as part of the diagnostic evaluation. Its primary value is in diagnosis of a Hunner lesion. Between 30% and 50% of patients experience

some short-term relief in symptoms after the procedure. If a Hunner lesion is present, therapeutic response to resection or fulguration is excellent in many patients. About 30% of patients will note a brief exacerbation in their symptoms following hydrodistention. A bladder capacity under anesthesia of less than 200 mL is a sign of poor prognosis.

22. **a. Sodium pentosan polysulfate.** The target of sodium pentosan polysulfate therapy is the glycosaminoglycan (GAG) layer of the urothelium. This agent is an oral analogue of heparin. About 6% of an ingested dose is excreted in the urine. The proposed mechanism of action is the correction of a GAG dysfunction, thus presumably reversing the abnormal epithelial permeability. It is marginally effective in about 30% of patients in placebo-controlled trials.

23. **e. None of the above.** None of these treatments has been proven efficacious for BPS in double-blind placebo-controlled trials. Hyaluronic acid in both high and low concentrations and BCG have recently failed to show significant efficacy in large, multicenter American trials.

24. **b. They can make patients physically dependent on them.** Narcotic analgesics can be very useful in a subset of BPS patients with severe disease. Unlike other classes of analgesics, they have no therapeutic ceiling, dosing being limited by tolerance of side effects. They tend to cause constipation and can cause some sedation. Physical dependence is unavoidable, but physical addiction, a chronic disorder characterized by the compulsive use of a substance resulting in physical, psychological, or social harm to the user and the continued use despite that harm, is rare.

25. **a. Transurethral fulguration of Hunner lesion.** Transurethral fulguration or laser irradiation of a Hunner lesion can provide symptomatic relief. None of the other procedures listed have any place in the treatment of BPS.

26. **b. Patient education.** Patient education is the most important step in the initial treatment of BPS. This condition is chronic, the symptoms wax and wane, and remissions are not uncommon. It lends itself to practitioner abuse, and the uninformed, desperate patient is easy prey. Treatment is symptom-driven, and an informed patient makes the best decisions.

27. **e. None of the above.** Clinically insignificant detrusor overactivity may be seen in 15% of patients with BPS, a rate of involuntary contractions that has been reported in normal patients undergoing ambulatory urodynamics. The finding does not rule out the diagnosis of BPS, and treatment of this finding would be unlikely to result in improvement of the patient's bladder pain.

28. **e. All of the above.** BPS should be considered in the differential diagnosis of voiding disorders in men accompanied by irritative symptoms and pelvic pain. A rigorous BPS evaluation can be useful in differentiating BPS from bladder carcinoma in situ, functional or anatomic bladder outlet obstruction, and bacterial prostatitis. Many men with BPS have undergone what has proved to be unnecessary and ill-founded bladder neck surgery.

29. **e. Examine the chronic pelvic pain syndrome in men and BPS along with associated syndromes to better characterize the relationship among these disorders and enhance future diagnosis and treatment efforts.** The question as to whether chronic pelvic pain syndrome in men (CPPS III), previously referred to as "nonbacterial prostatitis," and BPS are two different disorders or manifestations of one pathologic process forms part of the goal of the MAPP. Other goals are to outline the relationship of the urologic chronic pelvic pain syndromes with other chronic pain syndromes and learn why such syndromes tend to be associated clinically in the same patients. (*http://www.mappnetwork.org/*)

30. **a. Risk factors for bladder pain syndrome.** Emotional, sexual, and physical abuse was shown to be a risk factor in the Boston Area Community Health Survey, and this has been borne out in other studies. A Michigan study compared a control group of 464 women with 215 BPS/IC patients and found that 22% of the control group had experienced abuse versus 37% of the patient group. Those with a history of sexual abuse may present with more pain and fewer voiding symptoms. How reliable

these data are is not clear, and it would be wrong to jump to any conclusions about abuse in an individual patient. However, practitioners need to have sensitivity for the possibility of an abusive relationship history in all pain patients, and BPS patients in particular. When patients are found to have multiple diagnoses, the rate of previous abuse also increases, and these patients may need referral for further counseling at a traumatic stress center.

31. **e. Hunner lesion.** Patients with Hunner lesions form a distinct subset of those with bladder pain syndrome. They have identifiable endoscopic and pathologic findings, are less likely to have comorbid conditions, tend to be older, and respond clinically to bladder fulguration and local steroid injection into the lesions.

32. **b. BPS may be as common in men as it is in women.** The Rand Corporation high specificity criteria data show a male prevalence of BPS of 1.9% compared with a 1.8% prevalence of nonbacterial prostatitis/chronic pelvic pain syndrome. Thus, the prevalence of BPS in men approaches that in women, suggesting that many men previously diagnosed with "prostatitis" actually have BPS as it is currently defined. The overlap of BPS and chronic pelvic pain syndrome was 17%.

CHAPTER REVIEW

1. Bladder pain syndrome/interstitial cystitis (BPS/IC) is a condition that is diagnosed on a clinical basis and consists of chronic pelvic pain often exacerbated by bladder filling and associated with urinary frequency. This is a diagnosis of exclusion because there is no specific test or marker that is diagnostic. Interstitial cystitis may be a subgroup of this population that has typical histologic and cystoscopic features; however, those specific features are still subject to debate.

2. Patients with bladder pain syndrome have a 10-fold higher incidence of childhood voiding problems than do patients without the syndrome.

3. A childhood presentation is extremely rare. The average age of onset is 40 years.

4. Antiproliferative factor (APF) is secreted by bladder epithelial cells, inhibits bladder epithelial cell proliferation, and is used as a marker of the disease. It may be the primary cause of syndrome in some patients. Urine APF appears to have the highest sensitivity and specificity of the markers studied for this disease.

5. Numerous studies indicate a role for increased sympathetic activity in interstitial cystitis. Whether this is a cause or effect is unknown.

6. Cross-sensitization among pelvic structures may contribute to chronic pain syndromes because this may result in alteration in function of adjacent pelvic organs.

7. Bladder compliance in patients with interstitial cystitis is normal.

8. Many patients find their symptoms adversely affected by certain food groups.

9. Amitriptyline, a tricyclic antidepressant, is the staple of oral treatment. Histamine-2 blockers such as cimetidine have shown some efficacy.

10. Intravesical agents such as silver nitrate, oxychlorosene (Clorpactin), dimethyl sulfoxide (DMSO), and sodium pentosan polysulfate (repairs the glycosaminoglycan layer) have all been used with limited success.

11. Long-term appropriate use of pain medication is an integral part of treatment of this disease.

12. Surgical treatment of this disease other than fulguration of a Hunner ulcer or hydrodistention should be an absolute last resort. Removal of the bladder or portions of the bladder has met with extremely limited success and is only rarely appropriate in highly selected circumstances. If frequency is a major symptom, it may be helped; however, relief of pain is unlikely to occur. Moreover, if intermittent catheterization is required, it may be very poorly tolerated.

13. Patient education, dietary manipulation, nonprescription analgesics, and pelvic floor relaxation sensation techniques constitute the initial treatment of BPS.

14. Sexual dysfunction is not uncommon in these patients.

15. A subpopulation of patients may have increased bladder mucosal permeability.

16. Pain memory in the spinal cord may be what causes the patient to become refractory to different therapies.

17. There may be a genetic component to the disease.

18. Urgency, frequency, and the presence of glomerulations or Hunner ulcer on endoscopy are often associated with BPS, but the presence of pain or discomfort is the primary component.

19. Substitution cystoplasty and continent diversion both fail in some BPS patients because of the development of pain in the bowel segment used or contraction of the bowel segment.

20. BPS appears to be a syndrome with neural, immune, and endocrine components in which activated mast cells play a central, although not primary, role in many patients.

21. Fibromyalgia, irritable bowel syndrome, chronic fatigue syndrome, and atopic allergic reactions are overrepresented in the BPS population.

22. Pain syndromes of the urogenital and rectal area include vulvodynia, orchialgia, perineal pain, penile pain, and rectal pain.

23. Cystometry in conscious BPS patients generally demonstrates normal function, the exception being decreased bladder capacity and hypersensitivity.

24. Glomerulations are not specific for BPS.

25. BPS is chronic, the symptoms wax and wane, and remissions are not uncommon.

26. The prevalence of BPS in men approaches that in women, suggesting that many men previously diagnosed with "prostatitis" actually have BPS as it is currently defined.

15 Sexually Transmitted Diseases

Michel Arthur Pontari

QUESTIONS

1. The most commonly diagnosed bacterial sexually transmitted infection (STI) in the United States is:
   a. gonorrhea.
   b. ureaplasma.
   c. syphilis.
   d. chlamydia.
   e. chancroid.

2. The major health risk to untreated *Chlamydia* infection in men is:
   a. epididymitis.
   b. Reiter syndrome.
   c. orchitis.
   d. chronic prostatitis/chronic pelvic pain syndrome.
   e. transmission to a female partner resulting in pelvic inflammatory disease.

3. In addition to treatment for chlamydia, what other medication is recommended as a first-line treatment for gonorrhea?
   a. Ciprofloxacin
   b. Levofloxacin
   c. Ceftriaxone
   d. Cefixime
   e. Penicillin VK

4. Which subtypes of human papillomavirus (HPV) are responsible for development of malignancies including cervical, penile, and anal?
   a. 16 and 18
   b. 13 and 14
   c. 6 and 11
   d. 31 and 33
   e. 26 and 28

5. HPV vaccines are indicated for which groups?
   a. All sexually active women
   b. All sexually active men who have sex with men (MSMs)
   c. Men and women up to age 26 years
   d. Only women up to age 26 years
   e. Only women with a family history of cervical cancer

6. Which STI often has no visible genital lesion because it has usually resolved by the time of presentation and is associated with tender, often suppurative adenopathy?
   a. Chancroid
   b. Herpes simplex virus type 2 (HSV-2)
   c. Herpes simplex virus type 1 (HSV-1)
   d. Donavanosis
   e. Lymphogranuloma venereum

7. Which of the following is not a reportable STI in every state?
   a. HSV
   b. Syphilis
   c. Chancroid
   d. Chlamydia
   e. Human immunodeficiency virus (HIV)

8. Which of the following tests should be used to monitor the clinical response to treatment in patients with syphilis?
   a. *Treponema pallidum* particle agglutination (TP-PA)
   b. Rapid plasma reagin (RPR)
   c. Fluorescent treponemal antibody absorption (FTA-ABS)
   d. Darkfield microscopy
   e. Tzanck test

9. What is the treatment of choice for primary, secondary, and early latent syphilis?
   a. Azithromycin
   b. Benzathine penicillin
   c. Probenecid penicillin
   d. Ceftriaxone
   e. Procaine penicillin

10. Which statement is true regarding the likelihood of recurrent genital lesions in patients with HSV-1 and HSV-2?
    a. No difference except in HIV patients in whom HSV-1 recurs more often
    b. No difference except in HIV patients in whom HSV-2 recurs more often
    c. HSV-1 recurs more often
    d. HSV-2 recurs more often
    e. No difference

11. What is the causative organism for lymphogranuloma venereum?
    a. *Calymmatobacterium*
    b. *Klebsiella*
    c. *Chlamydia*
    d. *Haemophilus ducreyi*
    e. *Trichomonas*

12. Gardasil in males is recommended:
    a. to prevent transmission of HPV to their partners.
    b. only for persons with documented HPV.
    c. to prevent anal cancer and genital warts.
    d. to prevent genital warts only.
    e. only in men older than 26 years.

13. Donovan bodies are seen on:
    a. Thayer-Martin medium in gonorrhea.
    b. ulcer scraping in primary syphilis.
    c. biopsy of condyloma acuminata.
    d. lymph node aspiration in lymphogranuloma venereum.
    e. biopsy of ulcer in granuloma inguinale.

14. Clue cells are diagnostic of:
    a. Bacterial vaginosis (BV).
    b. *Trichomonas*.
    c. Scabies.
    d. *Candida* vulvovaginitis.
    e. *Torulopsis glabrata* vulvovaginitis.

15. HIV is what type of virus?
    a. Single-stranded RNA
    b. Double-stranded RNA
    c. Single-stranded messenger RNA (mRNA)
    d. Single-stranded DNA
    e. Double-stranded DNA

16. The HIV envelope precursor protein gp160 is cleaved into what two envelope proteins?
    a. gp 123 and gp33
    b. gp 124 and gp40
    c. gp 141 and gp 20
    d. gp 120 and gp41
    e. gp 120 and gp6

17. HIV infects which immune cells?
    a. Macrophages
    b. B cells
    c. CD4 T cells
    d. CD8 T cells
    e. Natural killer (NK) cells

18. The initial screening test for HIV is:
    a. Western blot.
    b. indirect immunofluorescence assay.
    c. nucleoside amplification assay.
    d. rapid enzyme immunoassay (EIA).
    e. viral culture.

19. Antiretroviral therapy is recommended for:
    a. patients with CD4 count of <200 only.
    b. patients with CD4 count of <350 only.
    c. patients with CD4 count of <500 only.
    d. patients with CD4 count of <500 and symptoms.
    e. all patients with HIV.

20. What factor is not associated with increased risk of seroconversion with HIV after a needle stick?
    a. Recent infection by patient
    b. Deep exposure of needle
    c. Visible blood on injuring device
    d. Prior placement of injuring device in artery or vein
    e. Patient dying within 2 months of exposure

21. Polymorphisms of which gene are associated with development of HIV-associated nephropathy (HIVAN) in African-American patients?
    a. Tyrosine kinase
    b. Antichymotrypsin-1
    c. Apolipoprotein-1
    d. Tumor necrosis alpha
    e. Interleukin-10

22. Which type of antiretroviral medications are associated with formation of urinary tract stones?
    a. Integrase inhibitors
    b. Fusion inhibitors
    c. Protease inhibitors
    d. Non-nucleoside reverse-transcriptase inhibitors (NNRTIs)
    e. CCR5 blockers

23. What is the best diagnostic test to detect HIV in the acute phase of infection?
    a. Indirect immunofluorescence assay
    b. Viral load assay
    c. Western blot
    d. HIV-1/HIV-2 serology assay
    e. Rapid enzyme immunoassay

24. What class of medication can have a prolonged half-life when used in association with protease inhibitors and NNRTI's for treatment of HIV?
    a. Alpha-blockers
    b. 5-alpha reductase inhibitors
    c. Beta-3 agonists
    d. PDE5 inhibitors
    e. Fluoroquinolones

25. What type of genitourinary (GU) cancer is not increased in frequency in patients with HIV?
    a. Prostate cancer
    b. Kidney cancer
    c. Penile cancer
    d. Testis cancer
    e. Kaposi sarcoma

Pathology

1. A 32-year-old sexually active woman has the lesion in Figure 15-1A and B excised from her vulva. The diagnosis is condyloma acuminata. The most appropriate next step is:

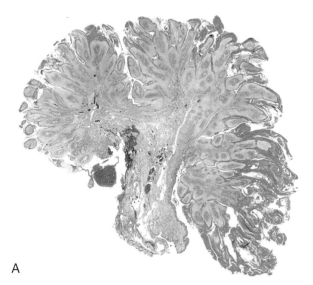

A

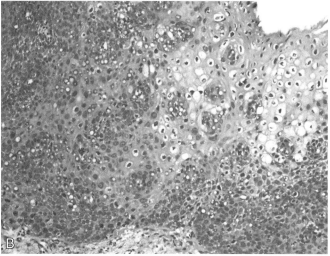

B

Figure 15-1A and B. (From Bostwick DG, Cheng L. Urologic surgical pathology. 3rd ed. St. Louis: Saunders; 2014.)

a. acetic acid test.

b. podophyllin to the base of the lesion.

c. HPV vaccine.

d. vaginoscopy.

e. cystoscopy.

2. A 22-year-old sexually active man has a 2-mm raised red lesion in the suprapubic area. A biopsy is performed (depicted in Figure 15-2) and read as molluscum contagiosum. The patient is concerned and desires treatment. The most appropriate treatment is:

a. wide local excision.

b. 5-Fluorouracil cream.

c. Ciprofloxacin for 2 weeks.

d. Bactrim for 4 weeks.

e. Liquid nitrogen application.

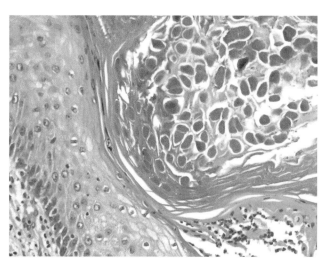

Figure 15-2. (From Bostwick DG, Cheng L. Urologic surgical pathology. 3rd ed. St. Louis: Saunders; 2014.)

ANSWERS

1. **d. *Chlamydia*.** *Chlamydia* is the most common bacterial STI in the United States. The 1,422,976 cases of *Chlamydia trachomatis* infection reported to the Centers for Disease Control and Prevention (CDC) in 2012 was the largest number ever reported to the CDC for any condition. The second most common bacterial STI is gonorrhea.

2. **e. Transmission to a female partner resulting in pelvic inflammatory disease.** Up to 75% of women with chlamydial infection can be asymptomatic. Ascending chlamydial infection can result in scarring of the fallopian tubes, pelvic inflammatory disease, risk for ectopic pregnancy, pelvic pain, and infertility. The risk of untreated chlamydial infection producing pelvic inflammatory disease is estimated to be between 9.5% and 27% of cases.

3. **c. Ceftriaxone.** As of 2007, quinolones are no longer recommended in the United States for treatment of gonorrhea and associated conditions such as pelvic inflammatory disease. As of August 2012, because of high resistance, cefixime is no longer recommended as first-line therapy to treat gonorrhea. Current treatment of uncomplicated gonococcal infections of the cervix, urethra, and rectum are ceftriaxone, 250 mg IM, single dose PLUS azithromycin, 1 g orally in single dose, or doxycycline, 100 mg orally twice per day for 7 days.

4. **a. 16 and 18.** Types 6 and 11 are nononcogenic and are responsible for about 90% of anogenital warts. Other subtypes including 16 and 18 account for cervical cancer, and other types of anogenital cancer including vulvar, vaginal, anal, and penile.

5. **c. Men and women up to age 26 years.** In June 2006, a quadrivalent HPV vaccine (Gardasil; Merck, Sharpe, and Dohme Corporation) was licensed for use in the United States in females aged 9 to 26 years. In October 2009, this vaccine also was licensed for use in males aged 9 to 26 years. This vaccine provides protection against HPV types 6, 11, 16, and 18. In October 2009, a bivalent HPV vaccine (Cervarix; Glaxo SmithKline Biologicals, Research Triangle Park, NC) that provides protection against types 16 and 18 was licensed for use in females aged 10 to 25 years.

6. **e. Lymphogranuloma venereum.** A self-limited genital ulcer or papule sometimes is present at the site of infection but usually has disappeared by the time of presentation. The secondary stage is the most common presentation in heterosexuals and is marked by tender inguinal and/or femoral lymphadenopathy, typically unilateral.

7. **a. HSV.** Diseases that must be reported to local health authorities: Syphilis, gonorrhea, chlamydia, chancroid, HIV infection, and acquired immunodeficiency syndrome (AIDS) are reportable diseases in every state.

8. **b. RPR.** Nontreponemal tests (RPR or VDRL) are used to monitor disease activity. A fourfold change in titer equivalent to a change of 2 dilutions (e.g., from 1:16 to 1:4) is considered necessary to demonstrate a clinically significant difference.

9. **b. Benzathine penicillin.** Benzathine penicillin is the treatment of choice for all of the stages of syphilis. Treatment varies by dose and duration of therapy. Not considered appropriate treatments are combinations of benzathine and procaine penicillin (Bicillin C-R), or oral penicillin.

10. **d. HSV-2 recurs more often.** Genital HSV-1 recurs much less frequently (0.02 per month) than genital HSV-2 infections (0.23 per month), on the order of 10-fold less.

11. **c. *Chlamydia*.** Lymphogranuloma venereum (LGV) is an infection by *Chlamydia*, specifically serovars L1, L2, or L3.

12. **c. To prevent anal cancer and genital warts.** The quadrivalent vaccine is used in males to prevent genital warts and in both genders to prevent anal cancer. MSMs are particularly at risk for developing anal intraepithelial neoplasia and anal cancer. As in women, it is best started in males before the onset of sexual activity.

13. **e. Biopsy of ulcer in granuloma inguinale.** Granuloma inguinale (GI) is an infection by the intracellular gram-negative bacterium *Klebsiella granulomatis* (formerly called *Calymmatobacterium granulomatis*) that produces genital ulcers. The bacterium is a strict human pathogen, which makes culture difficult. Diagnosis requires visualization of dark-staining Donovan bodies on crush preparation or biopsy, described by Donovan in 1905. These are intracellular inclusions of the bacteria within the cytoplasm of macrophages and appear deep purple when stained with a Wright, Giemsa, or Leishman stain.

14. **a. Bacterial vaginosis (BV).** Characteristic findings for BV on microscopic exam are clue cells, which are vaginal epithelial cells covered with bacteria.

15. **a. Single-stranded RNA.** The genetic material in HIV is single-stranded RNA. After entry into the targeted cell, the RNA is reverse transcribed by a reverse transcriptase into a double-stranded DNA. This new DNA is assembled into complexes, which then associate with the target cell chromatin and integrate via the action of viral integrase. The cell then translates and transcribes the viral genes to produce proteins that will assemble new copies of the virus. Copies of the virus are called virions.

16. **d. gp 120 and gp41.** The virus is shaped like a sphere. It is covered by an outer envelope that is a lipid bilayer derived from the host cell when it buds out of the cell. Embedded in the envelope is a complex of proteins known as Env. There is initially a precursor gp160 that is cleaved by a protease in the trans-Golgi network. It is cleaved into an outer subunit glycoprotein 120 (gp120) and a transmembrane subunit glycoprotein 41 (gp41). After proteolysis, the gp120 and gp41 remain coupled as noncovalent heterodimers.

17. **c. CD4 T cells.** Glycoprotein gp120 has a high-affinity binding site for the T lymphocyte receptor CD4.

18. **d. Rapid enzyme immunoassay (EIA).** Diagnosis of HIV includes the use of serologic tests that detect antibodies against HIV-1 (and HIV-2) and by virologic tests that detect HIV antigens RNA. The initial test is a screening test for antibodies, the conventional or rapid EIA. The initial result can be obtained in 30 minutes. Positive or reactive screening tests must be confirmed by a supplemental antibody test, Western blot, and indirect immunofluorescence assay (IFA) or by a virologic test, the HIV-1 RNA assay.

19. **e. All patients with HIV.** The benefit of treatment may depend on the starting CD4 count, but treatment guidelines recommend treatment for all patients regardless of CD4 count.

20. **a. Recent infection by patient.** A review of factors for increased risk of infection done by the CDC identified four that increased risk: deep as opposed to superficial exposure (odds ratio [OR] 15, 95% confidence index [CI] 6-41), visible blood on the injuring device (OR 6.2, 95% CI 2.2-21), prior placement of the injuring device in an artery or vein (OR 4.3, 95% CI 1.7-12), and patient dying within 2 months of the exposure (preterminal disease) (OR 5.6, 95% CI 2-16). Recent infection by the patient was not associated with an increased risk of seroconversion.

21. **c. Apolipoprotein-1.** African-Americans carrying two variants of the APOL-1 gene are at very high risk for HIVAN. These genes encode a secreted lipid binding protein called apolipoprotein-1 (apoL1). The variants G1 and G2 are common in African chromosomes but absent in European chromosomes; these variants lyse trypanosomes, including *Trypanosoma brucei rhodesiense*, which causes African sleeping sickness. Thus, these loci are thought to be selected out in this population. The presence of these two genes together increases the risk 29-fold, resulting in a 50% risk of developing HIVAN in untreated individuals as compared with a 12% baseline risk. Focal segmental glomerulosclerosis (FSGS) found in individuals with the two risk genes also occurs at an earlier age and progresses much more rapidly.

22. **c. Protease inhibitors.** The protease inhibitors specifically have the possibility of stone formation. Indinavir can form crystals in the urine. Indinavir stones are typically radiolucent on both plain film and computed tomography scan but can also be mixed with calcium and appear radio-opaque. Newer inhibitors including lopinavir, atazanavir, amprenavir, and nelfinavir have also been associated with the development of stones, but with less frequency than reported for indinavir.

23. **b. Viral load assay.** During this initial 3-month period, the "window" period, antibody screening tests may be negative but the person still infected. Virologic tests for HIV-1 RNA can be used to detect an acute infection in persons negative for HIV antibodies.

24. **d. PDE5 inhibitors.** PDE5 inhibitors depend on CYP3A for clearance, and all protease inhibitors and NNRTIs are inhibitors of CYP3A to some extent. This can lead to a significant increase in the serum dose of PDE5 inhibitors, and therefore they should be started at the lowest dose possible in patients on these antiretroviral medications.

25. **a. Prostate cancer.** The relative risk of prostate cancer in men with HIV compared to uninfected individuals has been reported as either no different or even less at 0.70.

Pathology

1. **d. Vaginoscopy.** The figure shows marked papillomatosis with koilocytic atypia. The patient should have a thorough genital examination, including vaginoscopy for other lesions.

2. **e. Liquid nitrogen application.** The biopsy shows an epidermal crater filled with molluscum bodies. This is usually a self-limited disease and requires no treatment. If treatment is desired, a local therapy is appropriate, such as curettage or liquid nitrogen application.

CHAPTER REVIEW

1. When exposed to STIs, women are more likely to become infected and less likely to be symptomatic.
2. Chlamydia is the most common sexually transmitted disease in the United States.
3. Herpes simplex virus type 2 accounts for 90% of the genital herpes infections. Herpes simplex virus type 1 accounts for the remainder and is the common cause of cold sores; silent infection is common in this disease. The diagnosis is made by viral culture and subtyping. HSV enters the nerve and remains latent in the nerve cell body. It may cause aseptic meningitis and autonomic dysfunction, which may lead to urinary retention.
4. Chancroid is caused by *Haemophilus ducreyi* and results in a painful, nonindurated ulcer covered by an exudate. Inguinal adenopathy occurs and may become suppurative.
5. Chancre of syphilis is single, painless, indurated, and clean. It is associated with nontender inguinal lymphadenopathy.
6. Latent syphilis is seropositive with no evidence of disease. Early latent syphilis occurs in less than 1 year. Late latent syphilis occurs beyond 1 year.
7. Primary syphilis is the acute infection. Secondary syphilis is manifested by mucocutaneous and constitutional signs and symptoms that are often associated with a maculopapular rash. Tertiary syphilis is a systemic disease involving the cardiovascular, skeletal, and central nervous system.
8. Treponemal tests for syphilis are generally positive for life and do not indicate treatment response. RPR, Venereal Disease Research Laboratory (VDRL), and the toluidine red unheated serum test (TRUST) are nontreponemal tests and correlate with disease activity. They usually become negative after treatment. Nontreponemal tests (RPR or VDRL) are used to monitor disease activity.
9. The Jarisch-Herxheimer reaction occurs when patients with syphilis are treated with penicillin, resulting in the release of toxic products when the treponemes are killed. The symptoms include headache, myalgia, fever, tachycardia, and increased respiratory rate.
10. Lymphogranuloma venereum presents as a single painless ulcer and painful inguinal adenopathy. Lymphogranuloma venereum is marked by tender inguinal and/or femoral lymphadenopathy, typically unilateral.
11. Polymerase chain reaction (PCR) assays are used for diagnosing chlamydial infection.
12. A strawberry rash on the vulva or strawberry cervix is seen in trichomoniasis.
13. More than 99% of cervical cancers and 84% of anal cancers are associated with HPV 16 or 18. The most common serotype associated with squamous cell carcinoma of the penis is HPV 16.
14. Biopsies of genital warts are not routinely indicated but should be performed when the wart is atypical, pigmented, indurated, or fixed and ulcerated.
15. HPV vaccine is recommended for females age 9 to 26 years and may also be given to males of the same age range.
16. The presence of sexually transmitted infections increases the risk for concurrent HIV.
17. Ulcerative sexually transmitted infections including herpes, syphilis, and chancroid enhance the susceptibility to HIV per sexual contact.
18. Antiviral therapy for HIV does not necessarily make the patient noninfectious.
19. Men who are circumcised are at lower risk for HIV infection.
20. There are two types of HIV viruses: HIV-1 and HIV-2. There are very few cases of HIV-2 in the developed world, and it is less easily transmitted and less virulent than HIV-1.
21. HIV is a retrovirus that infects T cells and dendritic cells.
22. Antiretroviral combination therapy delays the rate of progression of the disease and prolongs survival.
23. Overt AIDS is marked by a low CD4+ T-cell count.
24. Plasma HIV RNA load is the most accurate predictor of disease progression.
25. The diagnosis of HIV is made by screening for anti-HIV-1 and anti-HIV-2 antibodies. If this is positive, confirmation is made by using Western blot analysis. After treatment, the nadir of plasma HIV RNA predicts long-term outcome.
26. HIV testing is recommended for anyone diagnosed with a sexually transmitted infection or at risk for sexually transmitted infections.
27. Herpes simplex virus increases HIV replication in persons infected with both viruses.
28. Human papillomavirus infection increases the risk for carcinoma, especially in HIV-infected hosts.
29. The most common intrascrotal pathologic process in AIDS patients is testicular atrophy.
30. Voiding dysfunction is common in patients with advanced HIV infection.
31. Urinary calculi have been associated with, most notably, protease inhibitors such as indinavir. These stones are soluble at an acidic pH.
32. HIV-associated nephropathy is a glomerular disease that often presents as proteinuria.
33. Patients with HIV are at particular increased risk for Kaposi sarcoma and non-Hodgkin lymphoma. Kaposi sarcoma presents as a raised, firm, indurated purplish plaque, reflecting the presence of abundant blood vessels, extravasated erythrocytes, and siderophages.
34. Human herpesvirus 8 is essential for all forms of Kaposi sarcoma.
35. HIV protease inhibitors are also potent antiangiogenic molecules and are useful in treating Kaposi sarcoma. However, localized lesions may be treated by irradiation, laser, cryotherapy, or intralesional injections of antineoplastic drugs. Corticosteroids should not be used to treat the lesions.
36. There is an increased incidence of Kaposi sarcoma, non-Hodgkin lymphoma, and cervical cancer in patients with HIV infection. There also appears to be an increased incidence of the following GU tumors: testicular, renal, and penile.
37. The risk of untreated chlamydial infection producing pelvic inflammatory disease is estimated to be between 9.5% and 27% of cases.
38. Current treatment of uncomplicated gonococcal infections of the cervix, urethra, and rectum are ceftriaxone 250 mg IM single dose PLUS azithromycin, 1 g orally in single dose or doxycycline, 100 mg orally twice per day for 7 days.
39. Donovan bodies noted in granuloma inguinale are intracellular inclusions of the bacteria within the cytoplasm of macrophages and appear deep purple when stained with a Wright, Giemsa, or Leishman stain.
40. Characteristic findings for bacterial vaginosis on microscopic exam are clue cells, which are vaginal epithelial cells covered with bacteria.
41. Factors that increase the risk for transmitting HIV include deep as opposed to superficial exposure (OR 15, 95% CI 6-41), visible blood on the injuring device (OR 6.2, 95% CI 2.2-21), prior placement of the injuring device in an artery or vein (OR 4.3, 95% CI 1.7-12), and patient dying within 2 months of the exposure (preterminal disease) (OR 5.6, 95% CI 2-16).
42. PDE5 inhibitors depend on CYP3A for clearance, and all protease inhibitors and NNRTIs are inhibitors of CYP3A to some extent. This can lead to a significant increase in the serum dose of PDE5 inhibitors, and therefore they should be started at the lowest possible dose in patients on these antiretroviral medications.

16 Cutaneous Diseases of the External Genitalia

Richard Edward Link

QUESTIONS

1. The periodic acid–Schiff stain is used to identify what organism in scraped or touched skin preparations?
   a. *Pseudomonas* sp.
   b. *Candida*
   c. *Corynebacterium minutissimum*
   d. Herpes simplex
   e. Molluscum contagiosum

2. Oral glucocorticosteroids are often used to treat dermatologic conditions and have a duration of effect lasting:
   a. 2 to 3 weeks.
   b. 30 to 90 minutes.
   c. 1 to 5 hours.
   d. 8 to 48 hours.
   e. 5 to 7 days.

3. The preferred dosage schedule for a short course of oral glucocorticosteroids used to treat a cutaneous disorder is:
   a. a single morning dose.
   b. a single evening dose.
   c. doses in the morning and evening.
   d. a dose every other day in the morning.
   e. redosing every 8 hours.

4. A 12-year-old boy has a long-standing history of asthma and occasional outbreaks of erythematous, pruritic papules on his scrotum and lower extremities. Which of the following options represents a rational approach to treating this condition?
   a. Long-term suppressive topical corticosteroids
   b. Frequent soaking in warm water to prevent the development of lesions
   c. Low-dose systemic corticosteroids
   d. The frequent application of emollients
   e. Application of a topical calcineurin inhibitor

5. Patch testing is a useful diagnostic test to identify:
   a. psoriasis.
   b. contact dermatitis.
   c. erythema gangrenosum.
   d. atopic dermatitis.
   e. Behçet disease.

6. The North American Contact Dermatitis Group identified a series of common allergens that were associated with contact dermatitis. Which allergen was the most common offending agent in contact dermatitis cases?
   a. Silver
   b. Textile dyes
   c. Ragweed
   d. Nickel sulfate
   e. Pet dander

7. A 35-year-old textile worker spills a small amount of green dye onto her left thigh. By the end of the workday, she is complaining of pain and burning over a 5-cm irregular patch of skin on her left thigh. What is the most likely diagnosis?
   a. Erysipelas
   b. Allergic contact dermatitis
   c. Hailey-Hailey disease
   d. Irritant contact dermatitis
   e. Koebner phenomenon

8. Following a recent exacerbation of genital herpes, a 22-year-old man notes the development of erythematous papules and targetoid lesions on his thighs, scrotum, and oral mucosa. The best next course of action is:
   a. oral antihistamines.
   b. systemic corticosteroids.
   c. observation.
   d. oral acyclovir.
   e. topical corticosteroids.

9. A 19-year-old woman is 2 days into a course of sulfonamides for an *Escherichia coli* urinary tract infection. She develops painful labial erosions that progress to a generalized rash with the formation of blisters. The most likely diagnosis is:
   a. erythema multiforme minor.
   b. Reiter syndrome.
   c. Stevens-Johnson syndrome.
   d. pyoderma gangrenosum.
   e. Sézary syndrome.

10. A 42-year-old circumcised man has a history of widely distributed erythematous plaques—most severe on his knees, elbows, inguinal folds, and glans penis. The condition has waxed and waned since he was in his early twenties. What is an appropriate therapy during an exacerbation?
    a. Topical 3% liquor carbonis detergens in 1% hydrocortisone cream
    b. Oral psoralen combined with ultraviolet radiation (PUVA)
    c. Systemic corticosteroids
    d. Topical 5-fluorouracil cream
    e. Oral azathioprine

11. A 21-year-old man presents with dysuria, blurred vision, oral ulcers, and erythematous plaques in his genitalia. He has mild soreness in his knees and ankles. He is negative for human immunodeficiency virus (HIV) and has no history of sexually transmitted disease. What is a likely risk factor for development of this disorder?
    a. Genital herpes simplex
    b. The human leukocyte antigen [HLA]-B27 haplotype
    c. A history of atopic dermatitis
    d. Exposure to benzene-containing chemicals
    e. Family history of psoriasis

12. Which of the following statements is true about the treatment of symptomatic genital lichen planus?
    a. Systemic corticosteroids can prevent the development of lesions.
    b. In clinical trials, the most effective agent for treating lichen planus is systemic acitretin.
    c. Systemic corticosteroids can shorten the time to clearance of existing lesions from 29 to 18 weeks.
    d. Phytotherapy is the therapeutic modality of choice for treating lichen planus.
    e. Metronidazole is an effective and well-established, first-line agent in the treatment of lichen planus.

13. The late stage of lichen sclerosus involving the glans penis is termed:
    a. keratinizing balanoposthitis.
    b. pseudoepitheliomatous, keratotic, and micaceous balanitis.
    c. bowenoid papulosis.
    d. balanitis xerotica obliterans.
    e. Hailey-Hailey disease.

14. Which of the following cutaneous conditions has been associated with an increased risk of squamous cell carcinoma?
    a. Lichen sclerosus et atrophicus
    b. Lichen planus
    c. Psoriasis
    d. Bullous pemphigoid
    e. Lichen nitidus

15. An 18-year-old man has a history of seizures following an automobile accident 2 weeks ago. He was sexually active before the accident. Today, he presents with a solitary, painful erosion on the penis. What course of action is appropriate at this time?
    a. Perform a urethral swab for gonorrhea and chlamydia
    b. Consult with neurology to alter his antiseizure medication regimen
    c. Start oral acyclovir
    d. Perform a punch biopsy of the lesion
    e. Start oral doxycycline

16. A 35-year-old, previously healthy woman has noted the rapid development of sharply demarcated, pruritic, red-brown plaques over a large extent of her skin surface. The plaques are particularly dense in her nasolabial folds and perianal area, and the nails are spared. What is the next step?
    a. Systemic corticosteroids
    b. HIV test
    c. Skin culture for *Malassezia furfur*
    d. Examination of the lesions under ultraviolet (UV) light
    e. Biopsy of the lesions

17. In patients with pemphigus vulgaris, the characteristic clinical sign showing loss of epidermal cohesion is:
    a. the dimple sign.
    b. the Asboe-Hansen sign.
    c. the Leser-Trélat sign.
    d. the dimple sign.
    e. the bullous blanching sign.

18. Which of the following statements is FALSE concerning pemphigus vulgaris?
    a. The majority of pemphigus patients have painful oral mucosal erosions.
    b. Pemphigus appears to have an autoimmune pathogenesis.
    c. Blisters appear to form due to loss of keratinocyte cell-cell adhesion.

    d. Treatment of pemphigus relies on systemic corticosteroids.
    e. Given enough time, even advanced cases of pemphigus generally resolve spontaneously without sequelae.

19. Which of the following dermatoses has an association with celiac disease?
    a. Dermatitis herpetiformis
    b. Hailey-Hailey disease
    c. Behçet disease
    d. Bullous pemphigoid
    e. Psoriasis

20. Which of the following is not a vesicobullous dermatosis?
    a. Hailey-Hailey disease
    b. Pyoderma gangrenosum
    c. Pemphigus vulgaris
    d. Zoon balanitis
    e. Linear IgA bullous dermatoses

21. Which agent has been shown to be effective in treating linear IgA bullous dermatoses?
    a. Azathioprine
    b. Cyclosporine
    c. Dapsone
    d. Metronidazole
    e. Sulfonylurea

22. A 45-year-old woman has pruritic, foul-smelling blistering in the inframammary folds and groin. The skin findings are confluent areas of vesicles with fragile blisters. Which of the following statements is FALSE concerning this condition?
    a. The condition is usually worse during the summer months.
    b. Intralesional corticosteroids may be effective for treatment.
    c. Involvement of the vulva is common in women.
    d. Wide local excision may be necessary in refractory cases.
    e. Laser vaporization has been applied successfully to this condition.

23. A 35-year-old man presents with painful ulcerations in his mouth and on his penis, as well as blurred vision and a history of recurrent epididymitis. What is the likely diagnosis?
    a. Behçet disease
    b. Oculocutaneous aphthous ulcer syndrome
    c. Epidermolysis bullosa
    d. Fabry disease
    e. Pyoderma gangrenosum

24. Which of the following statements is FALSE concerning pyoderma gangrenosum?
    a. Pyoderma gangrenosum most likely has an autoimmune mechanism of pathogenesis.
    b. There is an association with collagen vascular disease.
    c. Corticosteroids may play a role in management.
    d. The presence of vacuolated keratinocytes in an inflammatory background is pathognomonic for this condition.

25. Which of the following cutaneous conditions has an association with borderline personality disorder?
    a. Factitial dermatitis
    b. "Innocent" traumatic dermatitis
    c. Sézary syndrome
    d. Munchausen syndrome by proxy
    e. Behçet disease

26. The most common organisms causing erysipelas are:
    a. dermatophytes.
    b. *S. aureus.*
    c. *S. pyogenes.*
    d. *Escherichia coli.*
    e. *Pseudomonas* sp.

27. Which of the following statements is FALSE concerning Fournier gangrene?
    a. The mortality rate even with modern treatment may be greater than 15%.
    b. Most cases of Fournier gangrene are caused by *S. pyogenes.*
    c. Alcoholism is a significant risk factor for development of Fournier gangrene.
    d. In severe cases, debridement may need to extend into the chest wall.
    e. Fournier gangrene can be caused by a cutaneous, urethral, or perirectal source of infection.

28. An 18-year-old woman develops a pruritic rash over her thighs and buttocks after using a whirlpool spa. Her face and upper extremities are spared. What is the likely diagnosis?
    a. Candidal intertrigo
    b. Pseudomonal folliculitis
    c. Contact dermatitis
    d. Scabies infestation
    e. Herpes simplex

29. Which of the following conditions has an association with hyperhidrosis?
    a. Atopic dermatitis
    b. Trichomycosis axillaris
    c. Hidradenitis suppurativa
    d. Psoriasis
    e. Genital lichen planus

30. A patient being treated for tinea cruris has significant scrotal involvement. What alternative diagnosis does this suggest?
    a. Seborrheic dermatitis
    b. Erythrasma
    c. Cutaneous candidiasis
    d. Hidradenitis suppurativa
    e. Contact dermatitis

31. Which of the following is a treatment for scabies that is contraindicated in pediatric patients?
    a. Lindane
    b. Dapsone
    c. Permethrin
    d. Ivermectin
    e. Doxycycline

32. Which of the following statements concerning Bowen disease is FALSE?
    a. Bowen disease and squamous cell carcinoma in situ are the same condition.
    b. Bowen disease involving the glans penis is termed *erythroplasia of Queyrat.*
    c. Bowen disease may be treated with topical imiquimod.
    d. Bowen disease is associated with human papillomavirus (HPV) types 6 and 11.
    e. Mohs microsurgery may play a role when tissue preservation is critical.

33. Which of the following statements concerning verrucous carcinoma is TRUE?
    a. Verrucous carcinoma has a high propensity to metastasize.
    b. Verrucous carcinoma should not be treated with primary radiotherapy because of the risk of anaplastic transformation.
    c. Verrucous carcinoma is an exceedingly rare malignancy of the genitalia.
    d. Verrucous carcinoma is associated with HPV types 16 and 18.
    e. Verrucous carcinoma may grow very rapidly and destroy local tissue.

34. What is the most common site of presentation for Kaposi sarcoma in immunocompetent individuals?
    a. Chest
    b. Face
    c. Lower extremities
    d. Genitalia
    e. Palms

35. The following malignancy has been found concurrently in lesions of pseudoepitheliomatous, keratotic, and micaceous balanitis:
    a. Basal cell carcinoma
    b. Cutaneous T-cell lymphoma
    c. Squamous cell carcinoma
    d. Verrucous carcinoma
    e. Kaposi sarcoma

36. Which of the following statements about extramammary Paget disease (EPD) is FALSE?
    a. EPD is an adenocarcinoma.
    b. EPD is associated with another underlying malignancy in more than 60% of cases.
    c. EPD has been associated with malignancies of the urethra and bladder.
    d. EPD lesions show vacuolated Paget cells on histopathologic exam.
    e. The vulva is the most common genital site involved in women.

37. Patients with cutaneous T-cell lymphoma who develop hematologic involvement are given the diagnosis of:
    a. lymphoid papulosis.
    b. mycosis fungoides.
    c. pagetoid reticulosis.
    d. Sézary syndrome.
    e. Fabry disease.

38. Which of the following conditions has the most in common histologically with pearly penile papules?
    a. Psoriasis
    b. Tuberous sclerosis
    c. *Molluscum contagiosum*
    d. Herpes simplex

39. The most effective treatment for Zoon balanitis is:
    a. topical 5-fluorouracil.
    b. topical corticosteroids.
    c. circumcision.
    d. laser therapy.
    e. topical calcineurin inhibitors.

40. Skin tags are also termed:

    a. fibrofolliculomas.

    b. angiokeratomas.

    c. hamartomas.

    d. acrochordons.

    e. dermatofibromas.

41. The Leser-Trélat syndrome refers to:

    a. the rapid progression of lichen planus associated with the HLA-B27 haplotype.

    b. an abrupt increase in the size and number of seborrheic keratoses, suggesting internal malignancy.

    c. the combination of hand, foot, and genital psoriasis.

    d. the development of brown macules on the genitalia, unrelated to sun exposure.

    e. the combination of oral and genital ulcers often seen in Behçet disease.

Pathology

1. A 70-year-old uncircumcised man has noted an erythematous macular lesion on his glans at the corona. The pathology report of the biopsy (depicted in Figures 16-1A and B) reads plasma cell infiltrate consistent with Zoon balanitis. The next step in management is:

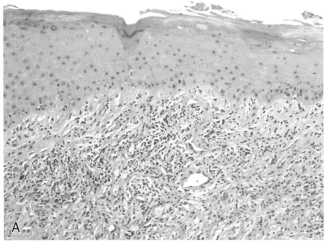

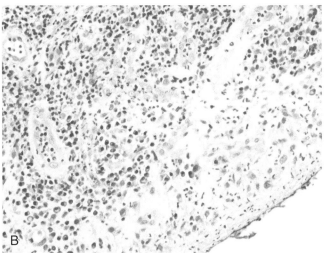

Figure 16-1. (From Bostwick DG, Cheng L. Urologic surgical pathology. 3rd ed. St. Louis: Saunders; 2014.)

    a. ask the pathologist if these are CD4 cells consistent with exposure to HIV.

    b. laser fulguration.

    c. ask the pathologist if he or she looked for an associated squamous cell carcinoma.

    d. circumcision.

    e. observation.

ANSWERS

1. **b. *Candida*.** To identify cutaneous fungi, such as dermatophytes and *Candida* species, PAS staining may be applied to scraped or touched skin specimens.

2. **d. 8 to 48 hours.** Oral glucocorticosteroids (GCS) are absorbed in the jejunum with peak plasma concentrations occurring in 30 to 90 minutes. Despite short plasma half-lives of 1 to 5 hours, the duration of effect of GCS is between 8 and 48 hours, depending on the agent.

3. **a. A single morning dose.** For short-term (≤3 weeks) treatment of dermatologic conditions such as allergic contact dermatitis, a single morning dose of oral glucocorticosteroids is given to minimize suppression of the hypothalamic-pituitary-adrenal axis.

4. **d. The frequent application of emollients.** The condition described is atopic dermatitis (AD or eczema), which is associated with susceptibility to irritants and proteins, as well as the tendency to develop asthma and allergic rhinitis. Intense pruritus is the hallmark of AD, and controlling the patient's urge to scratch is critical for successful treatment. Removal of various "trigger factors" from the environment (such as chemicals, detergents, and household dust mites) may be beneficial in some cases. The mainstay of treatment for AD includes gentle cleaning with nonalkali soaps and the frequent use of emollients.

5. **b. Contact dermatitis.** Patch testing is a simple technique of exposing an area of skin to a variety of potential allergens in a grid template. Generally performed by dermatologists, patch testing can help to confirm the diagnosis of allergic contact dermatitis and the allergen involved.

6. **d. Nickel sulfate.** In 2003, the North American Contact Dermatitis Group (NACDG) reported a long list of common allergens implicated in allergic contact dermatitis based on patch testing results. The most common sensitizing allergen identified was nickel sulfate, which is a common component of costume jewelry and belt buckles.

7. **d. Irritant contact dermatitis.** Irritant contact dermatitis results from a direct cytotoxic effect of an irritant chemical touching the skin and is responsible for approximately 80% of contact dermatitis cases. Occupational exposure is also common. Examples of offending agents include soaps, metal salts, acid- or alkali-containing compounds, and industrial solvents.

8. **c. Observation.** Erythema multiforme (EM) minor is an acute, self-limited skin disease characterized by the abrupt onset of symmetrical fixed red papules that may evolve into target lesions. The majority of cases are precipitated by herpesvirus type I and II, with herpetic lesions usually preceding the development of target lesions by 10 to 14 days. Although continuous suppressive acyclovir may prevent EM episodes in patients with herpes infection, administration of the drug after development of target lesions is of no benefit. With observation alone, the natural history of EM minor is spontaneous resolution after several weeks without sequelae, although recurrences are common.

9. **c. Stevens-Johnson syndrome.** Stevens-Johnson syndrome (SJS) is a life-threatening severe allergic reaction with features similar to extensive skin burns. A vast array of inciting factors has been implicated in the development of SJS, with drug exposures being the most commonly identified. Nonsteroidal

anti-inflammatory agents are the most frequent offending agents, followed by sulfonamides, tetracycline, penicillin, doxycycline, and anticonvulsants.

10. **a. Topical 3% liquor carbonis detergens in 1% hydrocortisone cream.** Psoriasis is a papulosquamous disorder affecting up to 2% of the population with a relapsing and remitting course. For genital psoriasis, the mainstay of therapy is the use of low-potency topical corticosteroid creams for short courses. Photochemotherapy combining an ingested psoralen with ultraviolet radiation (PUVA) has been used extensively to treat psoriasis. However, a dose-dependent increase in the risk of genital squamous cell carcinoma has been associated with high-dose PUVA therapy for psoriasis elsewhere on the body. Genital shielding during PUVA therapy is strongly recommended; therefore this modality is contraindicated for treating psoriatic lesions localized to genital skin.

11. **b. The HLA-B27 haplotype.** Reiter syndrome is a syndrome composed of urethritis, arthritis, ocular findings, oral ulcers and skin lesions. It is generally preceded by an episode of either urethritis (*Chlamydia, Gonococcus*) or gastrointestinal infection (*Yersinia, Salmonella, Shigella, Campylobacter, Neisseria,* or *Ureaplasma* species) and is more common in HIV- positive patients. There is a strong genetic association with the HLA-B27 haplotype.

12. **c. Systemic corticosteroids can shorten the time to clearance of existing lesions from 29 to 18 weeks.** Although bothersome pruritus is common with lichen planus (LP), asymptomatic lesions on the genitalia do not require treatment. The primary modality of treatment for symptomatic lesions is topical corticosteroids, although for severe cases, systemic corticosteroids have been shown to shorten the time course to clearance of LP lesions from 29 to 18 weeks.

13. **d. Balanitis xerotica obliterans.** Lichen sclerosis (LS) is a scarring disorder, with a predilection for the external genitalia of both sexes, characterized by tissue pallor, loss of architecture, and hyperkeratosis. The late stage of this disease is called *balanitis xerotica obliterans*, which can involve the penile urethra and result in troublesome urethral stricture disease.

14. **a. Lichen sclerosus et atrophicus.** Despite the similarities in name, LS shares little in common with lichen planus and lichen nitidus other than pruritus and a predilection for the genital region. Another critical distinction is that LS has been associated with squamous cell carcinoma of the penis, particularly those variants not associated with human papillomavirus, and may represent a premalignant condition. Biopsy is worthwhile both to confirm the diagnosis and to exclude malignant change.

15. **b. Consult with neurology to alter his antiseizure medication regimen.** The association of epileptic seizures and a solitary painful genital lesion is suspicious for a diagnosis of Behçet disease (BD). Other causes for genital ulceration, however, including aphthous ulcers, syphilis, herpes simplex, and chancroid, must be considered before a diagnosis of BD is made. In this case, the patient's neurologic issues should take priority over treatment for his genital ulcer.

16. **b. HIV test.** Seborrheic dermatitis (SD) is a common skin disease characterized by the presence of sharply demarcated, pink-yellow to red-brown plaques with a flaky scale. Particularly in immunosuppressed individuals, SD may involve a significant proportion of the body surface area. Extensive and/or severe SD should raise concerns for possible underlying HIV infection.

17. **b. The Asboe-Hansen sign.** The loss of epidermal cohesion seen in pemphigus vulgaris leads to the characteristic Asboe-Hansen sign: spreading of fluid under the adjacent normal-appearing skin away from the direction of pressure on a blister.

18. **e. Given enough time, even advanced cases of pemphigus generally resolve spontaneously without sequelae.** Severe cases of pemphigus vulgaris without appropriate treatment may be fatal because of the loss of the epidermal barrier function of large areas of affected skin. Treatment usually depends on systemic corticosteroids, although minimization of steroid dose is an important goal to limit side effects. The addition of immunosuppressive agents, such as azathioprine and cyclophosphamide, may be beneficial because of their corticosteroid-sparing effect.

19. **a. Dermatitis herpetiformis.** Dermatitis herpetiformis (DH) is a cutaneous manifestation of celiac disease and is generally associated with gluten sensitivity. Diagnosis can be confirmed by biopsy and direct immunofluorescence, which shows a granular pattern of IgA deposition at the basement membrane. Treatment includes the use of dapsone and a strict gluten-restricted diet.

20. **b. Pyoderma gangrenosum.** Pyoderma gangrenosum (PG) is an ulcerative skin disease associated with systemic illnesses, including inflammatory bowel disease, arthritis, collagen vascular disease, and myeloproliferative disorders. The classic morphologic presentation of PG is painful cutaneous and mucous membrane ulceration, often with extensive loss of tissue and a purulent base.

21. **c. Dapsone.** Characteristic clinical features of linear IgA bullous dermatosis (LABD) include vesicles and bullae arranged in a combination of circumferential and linear orientations. Treatment with either sulfapyridine or dapsone is usually effective in controlling LABD, and long-term spontaneous remission rates of 30% to 60% have been described.

22. **c. Involvement of the vulva is common in women.** Hailey-Hailey disease (HH) is an autosomal dominant blistering dermatosis that has a predilection for the intertriginous areas, including the groin and perianal region. Symptoms include an unfortunate combination of pruritus, pain, and a foul odor. Because heat and sweating exacerbate the condition, HH tends to worsen during the summer months. In women, disease in the inframammary folds is common, although vulvar disease is unusual. For disease resistant to medical therapy, wide excision and skin grafting have been effective, as have local ablative techniques such as dermabrasion and laser vaporization.

23. **a. Behçet disease.** When oral and genital aphthous ulcers are coexistent, the clinician should consider the diagnosis of BD. BD is a generalized relapsing and remitting ulcerative mucocutaneous disease that likely involves a genetic predisposition and an autoimmune mode of pathogenesis. Affected individuals may also suffer from epididymitis, thrombophlebitis, aneurysms, and gastrointestinal, neurologic, and arthritic problems.

24. **d. The presence of vacuolated keratinocytes in an inflammatory background is pathognomonic for this condition.** Pyoderma gangrenosum (PG) is an ulcerative skin disease associated with systemic illnesses, including inflammatory bowel disease, arthritis, collagen vascular disease, and myeloproliferative disorders. It most commonly affects women between the second and fifth decade of life and likely has an autoimmune pathogenesis, given its association with other autoimmune diseases. As is the case in Behçet disease, no specific diagnostic laboratory test or histopathologic feature is pathognomonic for PG, although a history of underlying systemic disease may raise suspicion.

25. **a. Factitial dermatitis.** Factitial dermatitis is a psychocutaneous disorder in which the individual self-inflicts cutaneous lesions, usually for an unconscious motive. An association between factitial dermatitis and borderline personality disorder appears to exist.

26. **c. *S. pyogenes*.** Erysipelas is a superficial bacterial skin infection limited to the dermis with lymphatic involvement. In contrast to the cutaneous lesion of cellulitis, erysipelas generally has a raised and distinct border at the interface with normal skin. The causative organism is usually *S. pyogenes*.

27. **b. Most cases of Fournier gangrene are caused by *S. pyogenes*.** Fournier gangrene (FG) is a potentially life-threatening progressive infection of the perineum and genitalia. In the genital

region, most cases of FG are caused by mixed bacterial flora, which include gram-positive, gram-negative, and anaerobic bacteria.

28. **b. Pseudomonal folliculitis.** Folliculitis is a common disorder characterized by perifollicular pustules on an erythematous base. It occurs most frequently in heavily hair-bearing areas such as the scalp, beard, axilla, groin, and buttocks and can be exacerbated by local trauma from shaving, rubbing, or clothing irritation. Folliculitis has also been associated with the use of contaminated hot tubs and swimming pools, with the offending organism usually *Pseudomonas aeruginosa*.

29. **b. Trichomycosis axillaris.** Trichomycosis axillaris (TA) is a superficial bacterial infection of axillary and pubic hair caused by *Corynebacterium*, which is associated with hyperhidrosis. Shaving can provide immediate improvement, and antibacterial soaps may prevent further infection. For pubic TA, clindamycin gel, bacitracin, and oral erythromycin have also proven effective.

30. **c. Cutaneous candidiasis.** Tinea cruris is the term given to dermatophyte infection of the groin and genital area and is commonly known as "jock itch." The inner thighs and inguinal region are the most commonly affected areas, and the scrotum and penis are usually spared in men. Significant scrotal involvement should raise suspicion for cutaneous candidiasis as an alternative diagnosis.

31. **a. Lindane.** As in the case of pediculosis pubis, the treatment of choice for scabies is 5% permethrin cream applied to the entire body overnight, with a second application 1 week later. An alternative scabicide, lindane, is not favored because of both central nervous system (CNS) toxicity in children and a rising rate of resistance among mites.

32. **d. Bowen disease is associated with human papillomavirus (HPV) types 6 and 11.** Bowen disease occurring on the mucosal surfaces of the male genitalia is referred to as erythroplasia of Queyrat. In that location, coinfection with HPV type 8, 16, 39, and 51 has been identified. In contrast, the variant of squamous cell carcinoma termed "verrucous carcinoma" has been associated with HPV type 6 and 11 infection but not with the more classically oncogenic type 16 and 18.

33. **b. Verrucous carcinoma should not be treated with primary radiotherapy because of the risk of anaplastic transformation.** Verrucous carcinoma (VC) is a slow-growing, locally aggressive, exophytic, low-grade variant of squamous cell carcinoma that has little metastatic potential. It most commonly occurs in uncircumcised men on the glans or prepuce, although similar lesions can be found on the vulva, vagina cervix, or anus. Treatment is preferably by local excision. Primary radiotherapy is relatively contraindicated because of the potential for anaplastic transformation with a subsequent increase in metastatic potential.

34. **c. Lower extremities.** Kaposi sarcoma (KS) in immunocompetent individuals presents as slowly growing, blue-red pigmented macules on the lower extremities. Although oral and gastrointestinal lesions may occur, the genitalia are seldom involved. This is in contrast to the case with acquired immunodeficiency syndrome (AIDS), in which a solitary genital lesion may be the first manifestation of KS. The clinical features of KS in AIDS patients are diverse, ranging from a single lesion to disseminated cutaneous and visceral disease.

35. **d. Verrucous carcinoma.** Pseudoepitheliomatous, keratotic, and micaceous balanitis (PEKMB) is a rare entity characterized by the development of a thick, hyperkeratotic plaque on the glans penis of older men. There remains controversy as to whether PEKMB is a premalignant condition. PEKMB was originally thought to be a purely benign process, although several case reports have documented the presence of concurrent verrucous carcinoma associated with this lesion.

36. **b. EPD is associated with another underlying malignancy in more than 60% of cases.** Extramammary Paget disease (EPD) is an uncommon intraepithelial adenocarcinoma of sites bearing apocrine glands. There is an important association between EPD and another underlying malignancy in 10% to 30% of cases. In the male, associations of urethral, bladder, rectal, and apocrine malignancies with EPD have been described.

37. **d. Sézary syndrome.** Cutaneous T-cell lymphoma (CTCL) represents a group of related neoplasms derived from T cells that home to the skin. CTCL generally presents with pruritus, which must be differentiated from a variety of benign dermatoses, including psoriasis, eczema, superficial fungal infections, and drug reactions. Patients may subsequently develop hematologic involvement (termed Sézary syndrome) and cutaneous plaques, erosions, ulcers, or frank skin tumors.

38. **b. Tuberous sclerosis.** Pearly penile papules (PPP) are white, dome-shaped, closely spaced, small papules located on the glans penis. Histologically, these lesions are angiofibromas similar to the lesions seen on the face in tuberous sclerosis.

39. **c. Circumcision.** Zoon balanitis, also called plasma cell balanitis, occurs in uncircumcised men from the third decade onward. Squamous cell carcinoma and extramammary Paget disease should be excluded, often by biopsy. Circumcision appears to be proof against development of the disease and can be performed to cure the majority of cases. For patients averse to circumcision, topical corticosteroids may provide symptomatic relief, and laser therapy may also have a role.

40. **d. Acrochordons.** Skin tags (acrochordons, fibroepithelial polyps) are soft, skin-colored, pedunculated lesions that can be present anywhere on the body. It is important to distinguish these lesions from the hamartomatous skin lesions (multiple fibrofolliculomas) associated with Birt-Hogg-Dube syndrome, which are histologically distinct from common skin tags.

41. **b. An abrupt increase in the size and number of seborrheic keratoses, suggesting internal malignancy.** The presence of brown macules unrelated to sun exposure suggests a diagnosis of seborrheic keratoses (SK). This condition may commonly involve the genitalia but generally spares the mucous membranes, palms, and soles of the feet. An abrupt increase in the size and number of multiple seborrheic keratoses (SK) has been termed Leser-Trélat syndrome and has been implicated as a cutaneous marker of internal malignancy. The HLA-B27 haplotype is associated with Reiter syndrome, not rapidly progressive lichen planus.

Pathology

1. **d. Circumcision.** The patient has Zoon balanitis. The biopsy shows reactive epithelial changes with a plasma cell infiltrate into the dermis. Although the disease can be treated with immune modulators, these patients respond best to circumcision.

CHAPTER REVIEW

1. Topical application of steroids may result in systemic absorption resulting in significant side effects.
2. The majority of cases of erythema multiforme are precipitated by herpesvirus type I and II, with the herpetic lesions usually preceding the development of the target lesions by 2 weeks.
3. The major form of erythema multiforme is called Stevens-Johnson syndrome, which has a protracted course of 4 to 6 weeks and may have a mortality approaching 30%. Nonsteroidal anti-inflammatory agents, sulfonamides, tetracyclines, penicillin, doxycycline, and anticonvulsants are the most common offending agents.
4. Reiter syndrome comprises urethritis, arthritis, ocular findings (conjunctivitis), oral ulcers, and skin lesions. It is generally preceded by an episode of urethritis or a gastrointestinal infection. It is more common in HIV-positive patients. It is associated with HLA-B27 haplotype.
5. The triad of clinical features in Behçet syndrome consists of mucocutaneous lesions of the oral cavity, genitalia, and uveitis. The ulcers are painful.
6. Hidradenitis suppurativa is an epithelial disorder of hair follicles that occurs in the apocrine gland–bearing skin, which results in a marked inflammatory response with formation of abscesses and sinus tracks. Bacterial infection does not appear to be the primary initiator. Rupture of the follicular contents—bacteria and keratin—into the dermis causes a marked inflammatory response.
7. Ecthyma gangrenosum is a result of pseudomonal septicemia and may result in gangrenous ulcers.
8. Dermatophytes are fungi of three genera: *Trichophyton, Microsporum,* and *Epidermophyton.* Tinea cruris, an infection of the groin and genital skin, may be caused by one of these fungi. Postinflammatory hyperpigmentation occurs with this disease and may not indicate an active infection.
9. Bowenoid papulosis consists of multiple small erythematous papules and is associated with HPV type 16.
10. Angiokeratomas of Fordyce are vascular ectasias of dermal blood vessels. They are 1- to 2-mm red or purple papules and may be the source of troublesome scrotal bleeding.
11. CIS of the penis rarely progresses to invasive disease.
12. Whether Kaposi sarcoma is a neoplastic or hyperplastic process is debated. When it is associated with organ transplantation, alteration of the immunosuppressive regimen may result in resolution.
13. Epidermoid cysts are commonly found in the scrotum.
14. Extensive and/or severe seborrheic dermatitis should raise concerns for possible underlying HIV infection.
15. Pyoderma gangrenosum is an ulcerative skin disease associated with systemic illnesses, including inflammatory bowel disease, arthritis, collagen vascular disease, and myeloproliferative disorders.
16. In tinea cruris, the inner thighs and inguinal region are the most commonly affected areas, and the scrotum and penis are usually spared in men.
17. Extramammary Paget disease (EPD) is an uncommon intraepithelial adenocarcinoma of sites bearing apocrine glands. There is an important association between EPD and another underlying malignancy in 10% to 30% of cases.

17 Tuberculosis and Parasitic Infections of the Genitourinary Tract

Alicia H. Chang, Brian G. Blackburn, and Michael H. Hsieh

QUESTIONS

Tuberculosis

1. Which of the following mycobacteria does NOT cause tuberculosis (TB)?
   a. *Mycobacterium bovis*
   b. *Mycobacterium avium-intracellulare*
   c. *Mycobacterium africanum*
   d. *Mycobacterium microti*
   e. Bacille Calmette-Guérin (BCG)

2. Which of the following statements about the epidemiology of tuberculosis is FALSE?
   a. TB incidence and mortality have been decreasing worldwide since the year 2000.
   b. Tuberculosis incidence is higher in those who are foreign-born than in those born in the United States.
   c. Prevalence of multidrug-resistant (MDR) tuberculosis cases is now approaching 12% in the United States.
   d. The lifetime risk of reactivation of TB is 5% to 10% in most people.
   e. Worldwide, tuberculosis is the cause of death in 25% of persons who test positive for human immunodeficiency virus (HIV).

3. Which of the following routes of infection is the most common in genitourinary tuberculosis?
   a. Hematogenous seeding
   b. Lymphatic spread
   c. Direct inoculation
   d. Sexual transmission
   e. Ascending or retrograde infection

4. Which of the following is a not a late complication of genitourinary tuberculosis?
   a. Infertility
   b. Scrotal fistula
   c. Autonephrectomy
   d. Thimble bladder
   e. Papulonecrotic tuberculid

5. Which of the following persons is LEAST likely to have tuberculosis infection?
   a. A patient with fibrosis on chest radiograph and a tuberculin skin test (TST) of 5 mm
   b. A patient with HIV infection and a TST of 3 mm
   c. A recent immigrant from Vietnam with a TST of 11 mm
   d. A BCG-vaccinated patient with a TST of 14 mm
   e. A healthy U.S.-born teacher with a TST of 11 mm

6. Which of the following results most specifically diagnoses genitourinary tuberculosis?
   a. A positive interferon gamma release assay
   b. A positive urine polymerase chain reaction (PCR) for *Mycobacterium tuberculosis* complex
   c. A TST reaction of 25 mm
   d. A positive urine acid-fast bacilli (AFB) culture
   e. A renal biopsy showing AFB

7. Which of the following first-line antituberculosis agents does not cause hepatic toxicity?
   a. Isoniazid
   b. Rifampin
   c. Pyrazinamide
   d. Ethambutol
   e. Streptomycin

8. Which of the following drugs might have efficacy against extensively drug-resistant (XDR) tuberculosis?
   a. Isoniazid (INH)
   b. Rifampin
   c. Pyrazinamide
   d. Moxifloxacin
   e. Amikacin

9. Which of the urological interventions is emergently indicated?
   a. Nephrectomy of nonfunctional kidney in medically resistant hypertension
   b. Bladder augmentation of a contracted bladder in a patient with severe dysuria
   c. Percutaneous nephrostomy of obstructive hydronephrosis in acute renal failure
   d. Balloon dilatation and ureteral stenting of a proximal ureteral stricture
   e. Boari flap for a lower ureteral stricture that requires excision

10. Which of the following statements is FALSE about genitourinary (GU) TB patients?
    a. Magnetic resonance imaging (MRI) is often used to help diagnose patients with GU TB.
    b. Computed tomography (CT) is most useful in extensive TB disease when other organ systems might be involved.
    c. The most common finding of GU TB on plain film is calcification.
    d. Intravenous urography (IVU) is the best test to detect early renal changes due to TB.
    e. The most common finding on IVU is obstructive uropathy from scarring.

Schistosomiasis

1. Of the following drugs, the most effective to treat schistosomiasis is:
   a. albendazole.
   b. praziquantel.
   c. mebendazole.
   d. diethylcarbamazine.
   e. ivermectin.

2. The life cycle stage of *Schistosoma haematobium* that infects humans transdermally is:
   a. the worm.
   b. the schistosomule.
   c. the cercariae.
   d. the egg.
   e. the sporocyst.

3. *S. haematobium* infections are estimated to affect the following number of people:
   a. 1.1 billion
   b. 1.1 million
   c. 900,000
   d. 112 million
   e. 11 million

4. The life cycle stage of *S. haematobium* that induces the majority of human tissue pathology is:
   a. the worm.
   b. the schistosomule.
   c. the cercaria.
   d. the egg.
   e. the sporocyst.

5. The eponym for acute schistosomiasis is:
   a. Katayama fever.
   b. Bilharz syndrome.
   c. Barlow fever.
   d. Toshiro syndrome.
   e. Tan's triad.

6. The diagnostic, first-line gold standard for urogenital schistosomiasis is:
   a. polymerase chain reaction (PCR).
   b. serology.
   c. cystourethroscopy with bladder biopsy.
   d. rectal biopsy.
   e. urine egg counts.

7. Without treatment, *Schistosoma* worms can live in human hosts for an average of:
   a. 3 months.
   b. 9 months.
   c. 3 to 5 years.
   d. 5 decades.
   e. 5 weeks.

8. Surgical options for reconstruction of irreversible ureteral lesions caused by urogenital schistosomiasis include all of the following EXCEPT:
   a. renal autotransplantation.
   b. Boari flaps.
   c. ureteroureterostomies.
   d. ileal ureter.
   e. suprapubic intravesical ureterostomy.

9. Intermediate snail hosts for *S. haematobium* are members of the following genus:
   a. *Biomphalaria*.
   b. *Oncomelania*.
   c. *Bulinus*.
   d. *Helix*.
   e. *Achatina*.

Other Parasitic Infections

1. The rickettsia-like organism that is an endosymbiont of the parasites which cause lymphatic filariasis (LF) and onchocerciasis is:
   a. *Rickettsia rickettsii*
   b. *Wuchereria bancrofti*
   c. *Wolbachia* spp.
   d. *Brugia malayi*
   e. *Brugia timori*

2. The chronic manifestations of LF are mostly seen in:
   a. short-term missionaries to endemic areas.
   b. short-term aid workers to endemic areas.
   c. long-term (current) residents of endemic areas.
   d. short-term tourists to endemic areas.
   e. short-term visiting friends and relatives travelers (VFRs) to endemic areas.

3. Most patients infected with *Onchocerca volvulus* live in:
   a. Latin America.
   b. Oceania.
   c. Asia.
   d. Sub-Saharan Africa.
   e. the Middle East.

4. The majority of patients infected with *Wuchereria bancrofti* have:
   a. lymphedema.
   b. hydrocele.
   c. no clinical manifestations.
   d. acute adenolymphangitis (ADL).
   e. elephantiasis.

5. Which drug should not be given to patients infected with *O. volvulus* or to those infected with high-grade *Loa loa* microfilaremia?
   a. Diethylcarbamazine (DEC)
   b. Albendazole
   c. Doxycycline
   d. Azithromycin
   e. Amoxicillin

ANSWERS

Tuberculosis

1. **b. *Mycobacterium avium-intracellulare*.** M. bovis, M. africanum, and M. microti are members of the M. tuberculosis complex (MTBC) and can cause TB disease. BCG is derived from M. bovis and can cause TB in certain individuals. Of the mycobacteria listed, M. avium-intracellulare is one of the many nontuberculous mycobacteria.
2. **c. Prevalence of multidrug-resistant tuberculosis cases is now approaching 12% in the United States.** Although MDR TB is concerning because of the difficulty of treatment, in 2012, the proportion of TB cases caused by MDR TB was only 1.2% in the United States.
3. **a. Hematogenous seeding.** Each of the answers is a known route of infection for the development of GU TB. However, hematogenous seeding is by far the most common one.
4. **e. Papulonecrotic tuberculid.** Papulonecrotic tuberculid is the only manifestation listed that can present early in the course of TB disease. The tuberculids are hypersensitivity reactions to MTBC antigens that were disseminated to the skin from other infectious foci, and as such, they are culture negative and typically PCR negative.
5. **e. A healthy U.S.-born teacher with a TST of 11 mm.** Refer to Table 17-1 for the Centers for Disease Control and Prevention guidelines on TST interpretation. Patients (a), (b), and (c) are likely TB infected. A BCG-vaccinated person is likely from a country with high enough incidence of TB to warrant vaccination; hence a cutoff of 10 mm is likely to apply for this person. Patient (e) has no clear risk factors for TB; hence a cutoff of 15 mm would apply for this person.
6. **d. A positive urine AFB culture.**
7. **d. Ethambutol.** Ethambutol is rarely hepatotoxic. Its main toxicity is ocular, such as decreased visual acuity or red-green color blindness. Streptomycin is not considered hepatotoxic either, but it is also not considered a first-line agent in the United States.
8. **c. Pyrazinamide.** By definition, MDR TB is resistant to INH, rifampin, any quinolone, and at least an additional injectable aminoglycoside. Hence, of the choices, pyrazinamide is the most likely to have efficacy against XDR TB.
9. **c. Percutaneous nephrostomy of obstructive hydronephrosis in acute renal failure.** All of the choices are appropriate indications for urological intervention. However, only (c) is emergently indicated. For the other interventions, waiting at least 4 to 6 weeks after initiation of medical therapy is preferred.
10. **a. Magnetic resonance imaging (MRI) is often used to help diagnose patients with GU TB.** Although MRI has potential uses in the diagnosis of GU TB, it is not sufficiently superior to CT or IVU to warrant its frequent use.

Schistosomiasis

1. **b. Praziquantel.** Although all of the drugs listed are antiparasitic agents, only praziquantel is used to treat schistosomiasis. In fact, praziquantel is the only drug approved for schistosomiasis by the World Health Organization (WHO).
2. **c. The cercaria.** The worm and egg stages are found in chronically infected humans but are intravascular or deposited in tissues such as the bladder, respectively. Cercariae infect humans by burrowing through the skin, whereupon they transform into schistosomules.
3. **d. 112 million.** Although an estimated 1 billion people are at risk of contracting schistosomiasis because they live in endemic areas, only 112 million are actively infected with S. haematobium.
4. **d. The egg.** The majority of human tissue pathology caused by urogenital schistosomiasis is induced by the host immune response against S. haematobium eggs. In comparison to eggs, worms, schistosomules, and cercariae are much less immunogenic and are thought to correspondingly cause much less chronic tissue pathology.
5. **a. Katayama fever.** The syndrome associated with acute schistosomiasis is named after the Katayama valley in Japan, a formerly endemic region for Schistosoma japonicum.
6. **e. Urine egg counts.** Although PCR and serology are highly sensitive for detecting infection, they are not considered first-line diagnostic modalities. Cystourethroscopy with bladder biopsy and rectal biopsy are highly invasive and reserved for difficult-to-diagnose cases or suspected cancer. Microscopic enumeration of S. haematobium eggs shed in urine are the diagnostic, first-line gold standard (albeit slow and impractical in many field settings).
7. **c. 3 to 5 years.** Although there have been reports that some schistosome worms can live for several decades, on average they are believed to only live for 3 to 5 years.
8. **a. Renal autotransplantation.** Renal autotransplantation is reserved for reconstruction of the urinary tract in the setting of multiple and/or large renal tumors. There are much less morbid surgical options for reconstruction of schistosomiasis-associated ureteral lesions.
9. **c. Bulinus.** Biomphalaria and Oncomelania are host snails for Schistosoma mansoni and S. japonicum, respectively, but not

TABLE 17-1 Guidelines for Determining a Positive Tuberculin Skin Test Reaction

INDURATION ≥5 mm	INDURATION ≥10 mm	INDURATION ≥15 mm
• HIV-positive persons • Recent contacts of TB case • Fibrotic changes on chest radiograph consistent with old TB • Patients with organ transplants and other immunosuppressed patients (receiving the equivalent of >15 mg/day prednisone for >1 mo, or tumor necrosis factor α [TNF-α] antagonists)	• Recent arrivals (<5 yr) from high-prevalence countries • Injection drug users • Residents and employees* of high-risk congregate settings: prisons and jails, nursing homes and other health care facilities, residential facilities for patients with acquired immunodeficiency syndrome (AIDS), and homeless shelters • Mycobacteriology laboratory personnel • Persons with clinical conditions that make them high-risk: silicosis diabetes mellitus, chronic renal failure, some hematologic disorders (e.g., leukemias and lymphomas), other specific malignancies (e.g., carcinoma of the head or neck and lung), weight loss of >10% of ideal body weight, gastrectomy, jejunoileal bypass • Children <4 yr of age or infants, children, and adolescents exposed to adults in high-risk categories	• Persons with no risk factors for TB

From American Thoracic Society and Centers for Disease Control and Prevention. Diagnostic standards and classification of tuberculosis in adults and children. Am J Respir Crit Care Med 2000;161(4 Pt. 1): 1376–95.
*For persons who are otherwise at low risk and are tested at entry into employment, a reaction of 15 mm induration is considered positive.

S. haematobium. Helix and *Achatina* snails are terrestrial and not considered hosts for human-specific schistosomes.

Other Parasitic Infections

1. c. *Wolbachia* spp. *Wolbachia* endosymbionts infect *W. bancrofti, Brugia* spp., and *O. volvulus*. They appear to be involved in embryogenesis and, when killed with antimicrobial therapy (e.g., doxycycline), result in decreased microfilaria release and suppressed larval molting.
2. c. **Long-term (current) residents of endemic areas.** Because transmission is inefficient, long-term exposure to multiple infective bites appears to be necessary for transmission of LF and the development of chronic disease due to LF. Therefore, short-term visitors to endemic areas rarely develop LF, which is mostly seen in long-term residents of endemic areas.
3. d. **Sub-Saharan Africa.** Although endemic to Latin America and the Middle East as well, 99% of persons who have onchocerciasis live in sub-Saharan Africa.
4. c. **No clinical manifestations.** Although *W. bancrofti* infection can lead to all of these clinical manifestations, most infected persons remain asymptomatic.
5. a. **Diethylcarbamazine (DEC).** DEC can cause blindness in patients with onchocerciasis (due to the inflammatory response to parasites in the anterior chamber of the eye) and encephalopathy in patients with high-grade *L. loa* microfilaremia.

CHAPTER REVIEW

1. Hematogenous spread of tuberculosis occurs to the kidney, epididymis, and fallopian tubes.
2. The likelihood of reactivation of dormant TB increases with diabetes and immunosuppression, such as with HIV infection and malignancies.
3. Healing tubercles result in extensive fibrosis, which may cause infundibular stenosis and ureteral pelvic junction stricture.
4. Tuberculosis usually affects the lower ureter. Tuberculosis of the bladder is secondary to infection from the kidney.
5. Lower urinary tract symptoms are the commonest presentation of genitourinary tuberculosis; up to 25% of patients will present with sterile pyuria.
6. When culturing for tuberculosis, the first morning void specimen is most appropriate.
7. Pipestem ureter and bladder contracture may be sequelae of tuberculosis.
8. The dome of the bladder is most often affected in tuberculosis; the ureteral orifice may have the appearance of a "golf hole."
9. Surgical treatment is reserved for a nonfunctional kidney and to correct obstructive effects of fibrosis rather than to remove infected tissues.
10. First-line drugs for treating tuberculosis are rifampicin, INH, pyrazinamide, and ethambutol.
11. Pyridoxine must be given with INH to prevent a peripheral neuropathy.
12. Patients must have a minimum of 3 to 6 weeks of medical treatment before surgical therapy is undertaken in those with active tuberculous infection.
13. Strictures of the ureter usually occur in the distal third; however, they may occur throughout the ureter, resulting in a beaded corkscrew appearance when infected with TB.
14. Rifampin resistance serves a s surrogate marker for multidrug-resistant TB.
15. *S. haematobium* has a terminal spine and dwells principally in the perivesical venous plexuses.
16. Schistosomiasis may cause inflammatory polyps of the bladder, sandy spots in the bladder (which represent submucosal egg deposition), calcification of the entire outline of the bladder, and strictures of the ureter (usually in the distal portion) with hydronephrosis. It may be associated with bladder cancer.
17. Squamous cell carcinoma of the bladder is the most common histologic variant occurring as a result of schistosomiasis. These cancers are usually well differentiated or verrucous and therefore carry an overall good prognosis.
18. *W. bancrofti* accounts for 90% of human lymphatic filariasis.
19. Obstructive lymphatic disease typically occurs in people who have multiple reinfections following the initial infection with filaria.
20. *W. bancrofti* results in chyluria and filarial hydrocele and occasional extensive scrotal and penile lymphedema.
21. Echinococcosis may result in cysts in the kidney; cyst rupture or spillage during surgical removal can cause anaphylaxis.

18 Basic Principles of Immunology and Immunotherapy in Urologic Oncology

Charles G. Drake

QUESTIONS

1. Antigen presentation involves both uptake of foreign proteins and processing to form peptide/major histocompatibility complex (MHC) complexes. Each of the following immune-responsive cell types can carry out this function EXCEPT:
   a. granulocytes.
   b. vascular endothelial cells.
   c. monocytes.
   d. macrophages.
   e. dendritic cells.

2. Transplants between two siblings who are histocompatibility leukocyte antigen (HLA) identical (perfect class I and II match) can be rejected. This is primarily a consequence of:
   a. direct antigen presentation.
   b. differences in complement proteins.
   c. indirect antigen presentation.
   d. differences in childhood antimicrobial vaccination.
   e. differences in numbers of circulating platelets.

3. Lymphocyte activation depends on complex interactions among many intracellular enzymes, transcription factors, and electrolytes. The influx of which electrolyte is most important for T-cell activation?
   a. Sodium
   b. Magnesium
   c. Potassium
   d. Phosphorus
   e. Calcium

4. Anergy describes a state of immune nonresponsiveness to antigenic stimulation. The most effective way to induce a state of anergy is by:
   a. splenic irradiation.
   b. delivery of signal 1 and signal 2.
   c. depletion of complement proteins.
   d. delivery of signal 1 without signal 2.
   e. depletion of helper CD4+ T cells.

5. Each of the following characteristics describes the utility and adaptability of the immune system EXCEPT:
   a. memory.
   b. rapid amplification.
   c. identification of self.

   d. antigen restriction.
   e. nonspecific defense mechanisms.

6. Innate immune responses are nonspecific and include all of the following EXCEPT:
   a. natural killer cells.
   b. antibody-dependent cell-mediated cellular cytotoxicity.
   c. complement.
   d. acute-phase proteins.
   e. physical and mucosal barriers.

7. Which cell surface glycoprotein is commonly referred to as the "pan-T-cell marker" because of its presence on all T lymphocytes?
   a. CD3
   b. CD4
   c. CD8
   d. CD28
   e. CD45

8. The part of an Immunoglobulin (Ig)G antibody molecule that interacts with cell surface receptors on other immune reactive cells such as natural killer (NK) cells is the:
   a. hypervariable region.
   b. disulfide bonds.
   c. amino-terminal end of the antibody.
   d. Fc fragment.
   e. Fab fragment.

9. The family of transcription factors termed nuclear factor of activated T cells (NFAT) are essential for T-cell activation and clonal expansion through the expression of the gene for:
   a. interferon-γ (IF-γ).
   b. transferrin.
   c. tumor necrosis factor.
   d. interleukin-2 (IL-2).
   e. IL-10.

10. The receptor on B cells that recognizes antigen and transmits signals to the nucleus for gene expression is:
   a. the T-cell receptor.
   b. the surface IgD molecule.
   c. the surface IgM molecule.
   d. CD40.
   e. CD28.

11. The JAK/STAT signaling pathways are critical in regulating cytokine expression. Inborn deficiencies in these pathways may lead to diseases such as:
    a. Burkitt lymphoma.
    b. Wilms tumor.
    c. neuroblastoma.
    d. retinoblastoma.
    e. severe combined immunodeficiency.

12. The initial contact of host immunoresponsive cells with foreign antigen or transplanted donor tissue takes place in the:
    a. peripheral lymph nodes.
    b. thymus gland.
    c. spleen.
    d. bursa of Fabricius.
    e. bone marrow.

13. Programmed cell death, apoptosis, is a mechanism responsible for the elimination of aged, damaged, autoimmune, or redundant cells. Caspase proteins are responsible for executing the suicide program by:
    a. release of granzyme B.
    b. activating the alternative complement pathway.
    c. activating natural killer cells.
    d. mediating DNA fragmentation and condensation.
    e. release of perforin.

14. Tolerance describes the absence of lymphocyte reactivity to specific antigens that have been previously encountered by the immune system. Known mechanisms of tolerance include each of the following EXCEPT:
    a. deletion of reactive T cells.
    b. deletion of reactive B cells.
    c. blocking by antigen-antibody complexes.
    d. clonal anergy by delivery of signal 1 without costimulation.
    e. suppression of immune responses by regulatory cells.

15. Chemokines are chemoattractant cytokines that localize various cell populations to tissue sites of inflammation. Each of the following cell types respond to chemokines EXCEPT:
    a. erythrocytes.
    b. granulocytes.
    c. natural killer cells.
    d. dendritic cells.
    e. monocytes.

16. Although most human tumors are antigenic, the immune system is often not a significant barrier to tumor growth and metastasis. A major reason for the relative weakness of the immune system to eradicate tumors is:
    a. absence of costimulation by tumors leading to anergy.
    b. tumor-induced alterations of immune function.
    c. impaired function of tumor neovasculature.
    d. rapid tumor cell proliferation.
    e. lack of tumor cell Fc receptors.

17. Tumor cell destruction by the immune system often is weak because of tumor cell escape mechanisms, which include all of the following EXCEPT:
    a. tumor cell release of IL-2.
    b. reduced expression of MHC class I and II molecules on tumor cells.
    c. tumor cell and local release of IL-10.

    d. ligation of tumor cell FAS by the FAS ligand (FASL) to induce apoptosis of host T cells.
    e. tumor cell and local release of transforming growth factor-β (TGF-β).

18. Immunotherapy for metastatic renal cell carcinoma in humans has included the use of cytokines such as IFN-γ and IL-2. The objective response rate (both complete and partial responses) has been demonstrated in what percentage of patients?
    a. 95%
    b. 75%
    c. 55%
    d. 35%
    e. 15%

19. Extracellular bacteria are susceptible to killing by phagocytosis and complement, but some have developed capsules to block these mechanisms. The most effective immune countermeasure for bacterial encapsulation is the:
    a. classical complement pathway.
    b. alternative complement pathway.
    c. opsonization of bacteria by circulating antibodies.
    d. increased secretion of TGF-β in tears.
    e. increased beating of bronchial cilia.

20. Clearance of intracellular bacteria is most dependent on which immune cell population?
    a. Macrophages.
    b. Plasma cells.
    c. Natural killer cells.
    d. Dendritic cells.
    e. Primed T lymphocytes.

21. Passive immune therapy may be particularly useful for patients with immunodeficiency. Passive therapy is delivered by:
    a. attenuated viral organisms.
    b. lyophilized vaccines.
    c. heterologous serum.
    d. live viral organisms.
    e. cow's milk.

22. Toll-like receptors can be engaged by all of the following EXCEPT:
    a. bacterial flagellin.
    b. bacterial lipopolysaccharides.
    c. calcium.
    d. double-stranded viral RNA.
    e. paclitaxel.

23. Recognition of Toll-like receptors by microbial products can activate all of the following immune mechanisms EXCEPT:
    a. adaptive immunity.
    b. intracellular microbial killing.
    c. innate immunity.
    d. IgE antibody formation.
    e. expression of costimulatory molecules.

24. DNA microarrays depend on the ability of target nucleic acid sequences to:
    a. bind to the surface of activated lymphocytes.
    b. hybridize to complementary oligonucleotides or polymerase chain reaction (PCR) products.
    c. engage the T-cell receptor (TCR).

d. bind to antibody fixed to a glass slide.

e. fix complement.

25. Gene expression profiling using DNA microarrays can be used to distinguish the following characteristics of urologic cancers EXCEPT:

a. pathologic stage of the malignancy.

b. diagnosis and classification of the malignancy.

c. monitoring the host response to the malignancy.

d. discovery of targets for treatment of the malignancy.

e. definition of the clinical prognosis of the malignancy.

26. Which of the following events do not play a role in the initiation of TCR signaling after engagement with antigen and MHC class II molecules?

a. TCR interaction with CD4 coreceptor

b. TCR interaction with CD8 coreceptor

c. Phosphorylation of TCR and CD3 immunoreceptor tyrosine-based activation motifs (ITAMs) by LCK and FYN kinases

d. Recruitment of ZAP-70 to TCR and its activation

e. Activation of the adaptor molecule, linker of activation in T cells (LAT)

27. Which of the following is a FALSE statement regarding the JANUS family of kinases?

a. The four JAK kinases are not constitutively associated with various cytokine receptors.

b. The JAK kinases regulate different cytokine receptors.

c. The cytokine-receptor binding causes dimerization of receptor chains resulting in JAK activation and phosphorylation of receptors.

d. The STATs are recruited to receptors and phosphorylated by JAK kinases.

e. Mutation in JAK3 results in severe combined immunodeficiency.

28. Which of the following statements is TRUE regarding programmed cell death (apoptosis)?

a. It is a mechanism for the elimination of aged, damaged, and autoimmune cells or cells no longer needed for differentiation.

b. It is a mechanism for inducing a primary immune response.

c. The proteins responsible for executing apoptosis, caspases, are JAK kinases.

d. Caspase-8 is the initiator caspase for apoptosis initiated by FAS and the T-cell receptor.

e. BCL-2 and BCL-XL are antiapoptotic proteins that protect the nucleus from damage.

29. The development of an effective immune response to cancer cells is dependent on appropriate antigen presentation by dendritic cells and the subsequent activation of CD4+ and CD8+ T cells. Which of the statements listed below are TRUE?

a. Many human tumors express antigenic epitopes that can be recognized by either CD4+ T cells or by CD8+ T cells.

b. T cells can destroy tumor cells by several mechanisms, which include the elaboration of granules containing pore-forming proteins, the upregulation of FASL that can bind FAS receptors, and the activation of macrophages.

c. IFN-γ production by lymphocytes is necessary but not sufficient for promoting antitumor immune response.

d. Tumors may evade T-cell detection because of a loss of MHC class I/II molecules or because of a decrease in expression of transporter proteins associated with antigen processing.

e. All of the statements are true.

ANSWERS

1. **a. Granulocytes.** Macrophages, monocytes, some B cells, Langerhans cells of the skin, dendritic reticulum cells, and vascular endothelial cells can process and present antigen.

2. **c. Indirect antigen presentation.** The evidence for an indirect recognition pathway for alloantigens comes from observations that rejection can take place even if donor and recipient share most, if not all, MHC antigens.

3. **e. Calcium.** This event also leads to the opening of the calcium channels in the plasma membrane, which further increases Ca^{2+} levels. Elevated intracellular Ca^{2+} results in the activation of the enzyme calcineurin, which is a cytosolic serine/threonine protein phosphatase that regulates the activation of a family of transcription factors termed nuclear factor of activated T cells (NFAT).

4. **d. Delivery of signal 1 without signal 2.** In fact, stimulation by signal 1 alone leads to a state of anergy, whereby the T cell becomes unresponsive to further stimulation by antigen.

5. **d. Antigen restriction.** Unique characteristics that help explain the utility and adaptability of the immune system against many different foreign invaders include (1) the ability to identify self from nonself, (2) specificity, (3) memory, and (4) rapid amplification.

6. **b. Antibody-dependent cell-mediated cellular cytotoxicity.** Innate defense mechanisms represent nonspecific barriers to invaders, which rely primarily on physical barriers, phagocytic cells, natural killer cells, complement, acute phase proteins, lysozyme, and the interferons.

7. **a. CD3.** Each T-cell precursor retains the pan-T-cell CD3 marker, which is the signal-transducing complex closely linked to the T-cell receptor.

8. **d. Fc fragment.** The Fc fragment does not bind antibody but is responsible for fixation to complement and attachment of the molecule to the cell surface.

9. **d. Interleukin-2.** NFAT along with other transcription factors plays a critical role in T-cell activation and clonal expansion through activation of the IL-2 gene.

10. **b. The surface IgD molecule.** The receptor on B cells that recognizes antigen and transmits signals to the nucleus for gene expression is composed of a cell surface immunoglobulin containing heavy and light chains with variable regions.

11. **e. Severe combined immunodeficiency.** The biologic importance of different JAKs and STATs has been revealed by deficiencies of these proteins both in human and animal models. Mutations in JAK3 have resulted in patients having severe combined immunodeficiency (SCID) that is similar to X-linked SCID, which occurs because of a mutation in the common cytokine receptor chain.

12. **a. Peripheral lymph nodes.** Activation of specific T cells and the generation of an immune response require transport of antigenic components to the lymphoid tissue. For the induction of most T-cell–mediated immune responses, the crucial antigen-presenting cell is the dendritic cell, which is interspersed throughout peripheral tissues.

13. **d. Mediating DNA fragmentation and condensation.** The proteins responsible for executing the suicide program, the caspases, are essentially common to all the stimuli and pathways and mediate the nuclear and cytoplasmic alterations characteristic of apoptotic cell death. The specific roles of each member of the caspase cascade are gradually becoming defined, whereby caspases 3, 6, and 7 have been identified as the terminal effectors mediating DNA fragmentation and chromatin condensation.

14. **c. Blocking by antigen-antibody complexes.** An important mechanism mediating tolerance to self-proteins is the deletion of self-reactive T cells and B cells during maturation. Clonal anergy of T cells is induced by T-cell receptor engagement of peptide/MHC complexes in the absence of costimulatory signals. An active mechanism of tolerance mediated by T cells with suppressive or downregulatory activities may also be induced to inhibit immune responses to self and exogenous antigens.

15. **a. Erythrocytes.** Cytokines with chemoattractant properties, chemokines, are also crucial in mediating localization and trafficking of leukocytes to tissue sites during physiologic processes, including inflammation and homeostasis.

16. **b. Tumor-induced alterations of immune function.** Tumor-induced alterations in the functional status of immune cells may be responsible for the poor development of antitumor immunity in many cancer patients.

17. **a. Tumor cell release of IL-2.** Natural killer cells can recognize and destroy some tumors, particularly those of lymphoid origin, without any exogenous activation. Reduction in or loss of MHC class I and class II expression by tumors, including renal cell carcinoma, has been well documented. In some tumors, there is also decreased expression of transporter proteins associated with antigen processing (TAP proteins). Among the best studied immunosuppressive molecules overexpressed in the tumor microenvironment is the Th2 cytokine IL-10. TGF-β is also thought to contribute to the suppression of tumor immunity. Evidence suggests that the downregulation of antitumor immunity may be due in part to the induction of the FAS apoptotic pathway in T cells.

18. **e. 15%.** It is clear from these and other studies that a subset of individuals with metastatic renal cancer does respond favorably to cytokine therapy; however, they represent a minority of patients (< 15% response rate).

19. **c. Opsonization of bacteria by circulating antibodies.** Many of these bacterial mechanisms can be overridden by host antibodies, which are soluble or secreted on external mucosal surfaces. Circulating antibodies can directly bind to bacterial exotoxins and "neutralize" them. They can also bind to the encapsulated bacteria, which will permit ingestion by polymorphs and macrophages.

20. **e. Primed T lymphocytes.** Clearance of these intracellular microbes depends directly on T cells, which in turn must activate the infected macrophages. Specifically primed T cells react with processed antigen derived from the intracellular bacteria in association with MHC class II molecules on the macrophage surface.

21. **c. Heterologous serum.** Protection against a specific infection can be passively transferred from one individual to another by serum containing preformed antibodies. This type of passive immunity is generally short-lived, because the half-life of immunoglobulins is 1 to 2 weeks. Patients with immunodeficiency diseases may actually be sustained by regular treatments with pooled nonspecific human immune globulin treatments.

22. **c. Calcium.** Toll-like receptors are cell surface glycoproteins that need physical contact with other macromolecules such as bacterial flagellins, lipopolysaccharides, phytins, or nucleic acids. Minerals such as calcium are too small.

23. **d. IgE antibody formation.** Engagement of Toll-like receptors activates various cellular immune responses. IgE antibody on the surface of mast cells promotes degranulation and allergy. IgE antibody is constitutively expressed on basophils/mast cells.

24. **b. Hybridize to complementary oligonucleotides or PCR products.** DNA microarrays or gene chips are tests performed in a laboratory. They depend on the natural ability of two complementary strands of nucleic acids to hybridize to each other. The others are in vivo biologic processes.

25. **a. Pathologic stage of the malignancy.** DNA microarrays can identify a unique molecular signature of a cancer, which represents the sum of genes upregulated or downregulated by the tumor. This can help classify the specific cancer, aid in identifying potential molecular targets for therapy, or possibly predict the outcome of therapy. The pathologic stage of the cancer is a description of its extent in the host. It is usually defined clinically, often aided by radiologic and histologic evaluation.

26. **b. TCR interaction with CD8 coreceptor.** The interaction of the TCR and class II HLA antigens requires the stabilization of CD4 on T cells. Class I antigen would be required to engage the CD8 molecules. The initiation of further downstream intracellular events is dependent on the cell surface engagement of class II antigen and CD4.

27. **a. The 4 JAK kinases are not constitutively associated with various cytokine receptors.** The JANUS family of kinases are constitutively expressed and are associated with various cell surface cytokine receptors. Once these receptors are engaged, the JAK kinases become activated and promote cytokine gene expression.

28. **a. It is a mechanism for the elimination of aged, damaged, and autoimmune cells or cells no longer needed for differentiation.** The proteins responsible for executing the suicide program are the caspases, and they can be triggered by a number of mechanisms such as FAS and TNFR but not the T-cell receptor or JAK kinases.

29. **e. All of the statements are true.**

CHAPTER REVIEW

1. The immune response is divided into innate immunity and adaptive immunity.
2. Innate immunity is nonspecific and involves polymorphonuclear leukocytes, macrophages, natural killer cells, complement, acute-phase proteins, interferons, and lysosomes, among others.
3. Adaptive immunity is specific and involves lymphocytes, antibodies, and cytokines.
4. Natural killer cells do not require prior contact with the antigen and are not MHC restricted.
5. Immune responses may be either humoral or cellular. The humoral response involves antibodies, whereas the cellular response involves macrophages, T cells, dendritic cells, etc.
6. The thymus is responsible for the selection and education of T cells; the bone marrow is responsible for the education of B cells, which produce antibody.
7. Dendritic cells process antigen and present it to the T cells. T cells present antigen to B cells. B cells make antibody.
8. The MHC markers (HLA) are divided into class I and class II.
9. All nucleated cells express HLA class I antigens, whereas class II antigens are primarily found on B cells, monocytes, macrophages, and antigen-presenting cells.
10. The major histocompatibility complex (MHC) is located on chromosome 6. Current tissue typing checks for three class I antigens—HLA-A, HLA-B, and HLA-C—and two class II antigens—HLA-DR and HLA-DQ. A six-antigen match refers to HLA-A, HLA-B, and HLA-DR.

11. The T-cell receptor, or TCR, is responsible for the initial step in T-cell activation on encounter with an antigen. During antigen priming, CD4 + T cells produce cytokines.
12. Chemokine production is primarily regulated by the cytokine environment. Chemokines attract leukocytes to the area in which they are located.
13. T lymphocytes are central to the generation of an effective tumor immune response.
14. Activation of CD8 + T cells that recognize tumor-associated antigens presented by MHC class I molecules and CD4 + T cells that respond to tumor-associated antigens presented by MHC class II molecules represents the most effective tumor immune response.
15. There are five classes of antibodies: IgA, IgG, IgM, IgD, and IgE. They are produced by plasma cells (B cells).
16. Immune responses to cancer are restrained by a specific set of molecules expressed on CD4 and CD8 tumor infiltrating lymphocytes. These "checkpoint" molecules are critically important in restraining the antitumor response.
17. Interferons render cells more sensitive to attack.
18. The major goal of cancer vaccines is to activate antigen-specific CD8 T cells.
19. Inflammation has a role in the development of bladder cancer and possibly prostate cancer.
20. DNA microarrays can identify a unique molecular signature of a cancer, which represents the sum of genes upregulated or downregulated by the tumor.

19 Molecular Genetics and Cancer Biology

Mark L. Gonzalgo, Karen S. Sfanos, and Alan K. Meeker

QUESTIONS

1. DNA is composed of all of the following elements EXCEPT:
   a. a base, either a purine or a pyrimidine.
   b. a sugar, called ribose.
   c. a phosphate.
   d. two complementary strands.
   e. hydrogen bonds.

2. The physical chemistry of DNA bases requires:
   a. uracil to form hydrogen bonds with guanine.
   b. a purine to form hydrogen bonds with another purine.
   c. a pyrimidine to form hydrogen bonds with a purine.
   d. adenine to form hydrogen bonds with cytosine.
   e. thymine to form hydrogen bonds with guanine.

3. Which of the following does DNA gene expression require?
   a. Linear DNA to be converted into linear RNA, a process called translation
   b. Conversion of linear RNA into a linear set of amino acids, a process called transcription
   c. Protein synthesis exclusively within the nucleus
   d. Mitosis
   e. A mechanism to bridge the gap between the genetic code and protein synthesis

4. Which of the following statements about transcriptional regulation is FALSE?
   a. The two general components involved in transcriptional regulation are specific sequences in the RNA and proteins that interact with those sequences.
   b. In addition to the genetic information carried within the nucleotide sequence of DNA, it provides specific docking sites for proteins that enhance the activity of the transcriptional machinery.
   c. Specific sequences within the promoter or enhancer region of a gene are called response elements.
   d. DNA sequences, often referred to as consensus sequences, are found in many genes and respond in a coordinated manner to a specific signal.
   e. It is an important mechanism to ensure coordinated gene expression.

5. What is alternative splicing?
   a. A form of protein modification occurring after a mature polypeptide is produced
   b. A modification to DNA during meiosis
   c. A process of including or excluding certain exons in an mRNA transcript
   d. A process in which novel RNA sequences are randomly inserted into a transcript
   e. A method of RNA degradation

6. Which of the following statements is TRUE regarding the nuclear matrix?
   a. It has the same protein composition in every tissue type.
   b. It is the site of mRNA transcription.
   c. It has the same protein composition whether a cell is proliferating or undergoing differentiation.
   d. It provides a mechanism to trace the cell type of origin for a cancer, because the nuclear matrix is identical within tissue types.
   e. It is a form of DNA.

7. What happens in the process of translation?
   a. The RNA message of four parts (the nucleotides A, U, C, G) is converted into 20 amino acids by using a functional group of three adjacent nucleotides called a codon.
   b. Each amino acid is encoded by only one codon.
   c. Shifts in the reading frame are of no consequence in the production of the polypeptide chain because of the fidelity of template DNA.
   d. Single-base substitutions always encode for the identical amino acid, known as a polymorphism.
   e. Transfer of genetic information from the DNA to the RNA occurs.

8. Which of the following statements about ubiquitination is NOT true?
   a. Ubiquitination is an important regulatory mechanism of a cell, used in the efficient disposal of proteins.
   b. A small protein called ubiquitin is linked to a protein, tagging it for destruction.
   c. The proteosome is the site of protein-ubiquitin complex degradation.
   d. The proteosome has a cylindrical shape.
   e. The targeted inhibition of proteosome function appears to enhance cancer progression.

9. Which of the following statements about oncogenes is TRUE?
   a. They are mutated forms of abnormal genes, known as proto-oncogenes.
   b. They can be produced by an inactivating mutation of a proto-oncogene, resulting in the silencing of the gene.
   c. They can be produced by gene amplification, resulting in many copies of the gene, or by chromosomal rearrangement.
   d. They are always due to retroviruses, capable of inducing malignant transformation of normal cells.
   e. They are endogenous cancer-fighting genes.

10. Which of the following statements about *hyper*methylation is TRUE?
    a. It is a direct change to the DNA sequence, similar to a mutation which alters the normal base-pairing.
    b. It occurs exclusively on cytosine nucleotides in the dinucleotide sequence CG.

c. Somatic methylation of CpG dinucleotides in the regulatory regions of genes is very often associated with increased transcriptional activity, leading to increased expression of that gene.

d. In cancer, hypermethylation is associated with enhanced activity of oncogenes, and demethylation may be an effective strategy for the treatment of cancer.

e. It marks cells for ubiquitination.

11. Von Hippel-Lindau disease predisposes patients to:
    a. epididymal carcinoma.
    b. clear cell renal carcinoma.
    c. papillary renal cell carcinoma.
    d. adrenocortical carcinoma.
    e. all of the above.

12. Hereditary prostate cancer genes that have been proven to cause prostate carcinoma include:
    a. *ELAC2*.
    b. *MSR1*.
    c. *RNASEL*.
    d. none of the above.
    e. all of the above.

13. Which of the following hereditary tumor syndromes are associated with genitourinary tumors?
    a. Von-Hippel-Lindau syndrome
    b. Birt-Hogg-Dube syndrome
    c. Beckwith-Wiedemann syndrome
    d. None of the above
    e. All of the above

14. Which of the following cancer-associated chromosomal abnormalities would be most likely to be associated with inactivation of a tumor suppressor gene?
    a. Inversion
    b. Tetraploidy
    c. Amplification
    d. Deletion
    e. Double minutes

15. The two main points of control in the cell cycle are:
    a. S and G_0.
    b. S and the G_2M boundary.
    c. M and the G_1S boundary.
    d. G_1S and G_2M boundaries.
    e. G_2 and M.

16. The TP53 tumor suppressor gene plays a critical role in which of the following processes?
    a. Apoptosis
    b. Angiogenesis
    c. DNA replication
    d. Signal transduction
    e. All of the above

17. INK4 family members inhibit the activity of:
    a. cyclin D/cdk4.
    b. cyclin E/cdk2.
    c. cyclin A/cdk2.
    d. cyclin B/cdc2.
    e. all of the above.

18. Cyclin-cdk complexes primarily function at the G_1S boundary by:
    a. dephosphorylation of RB1.
    b. phosphorylation of MDM2.
    c. dephosphorylation of E2F.
    d. phosphorylation of E2F.
    e. phosphorylation of RB1.

19. The regulatory proteins at the G_2M checkpoint primarily respond to:
    a. hypoxia.
    b. nutrient-poor environment.
    c. DNA damage.
    d. cytokines.
    e. all of the above.

20. Nucleotide excision repair primarily protects the cell from DNA damage caused by:
    a. reactive oxygen species.
    b. DNA polymerase errors.
    c. double-strand breaks.
    d. ultraviolet light.
    e. all of the above.

21. Which of the following repair pathways is responsible for repairing double-strand DNA breaks?
    a. MSH2/MSH6
    b. Homologous recombination
    c. Nucleotide excision repair
    d. Mismatch repair
    e. None of the above

22. Which of the following genes has been linked to double-strand break repair?
    a. *TP53*
    b. *VHL*
    c. *BRCA1*
    d. *RB1*
    e. *PTEN*

23. Procaspases are activated by which of the following?
    a. Phosphorylation
    b. Ubiquitination
    c. Dimerization
    d. Mitochondrial import
    e. Proteolytic cleavage

24. Ligand-dependent apoptosis is an attractive therapeutic target because activation is:
    a. independent of *TP53*.
    b. dependent on *TP53*.
    c. independent of caspases.
    d. dependent on caspases.
    e. dependent on RB1.

25. The *TP53*-induced apoptosis is mediated through:
    a. APAF-1/caspase 9.
    b. CD95 receptor.
    c. TRAIL.
    d. Bcl-2.
    e. CDKN1A (p21^{cip}).

26. Proapoptotic bcl-2 family members function by:
    a. digesting the mitochondria.
    b. increasing the cellular membrane permeability.
    c. increasing the mitochondrial membrane permeability.
    d. directly activating executioner caspases.
    e. increasing nuclear membrane permeability.

27. The enzyme telomerase immortalizes cells by:
    a. protecting the cells from DNA damage.
    b. stabilizing *TP53*.
    c. allowing the cell to grow in a nutrient-poor environment.
    d. inhibiting apoptosis.
    e. maintaining chromosomal length.

28. Telomere loss can lead to all of the following EXCEPT:
    a. irreversible cell cycle exit termed senescence.
    b. apoptosis.
    c. DNA hypomethylation.
    d. chromosomal instability.
    e. increased tumor initiation.

29. Which of the following chromosomal rearrangements is NOT typically associated with a genitourinary malignancy?
    a. Fusion of BCR to Abl via chromosome translocation
    b. Fusion of TMPRSS2 to ERG via intra-chromosomal deletion
    c. Fusion of *MiTF/TFE* gene family members via chromosome translocation
    d. Isochromosome 8q
    e. Loss of chromosome 9

30. An isochromosome of 12p has been identified in which genito-urinary carcinoma?
    a. Testis
    b. Prostate
    c. Renal
    d. Bladder
    e. Penile

31. Which of the following has been most consistently implicated in prostate cancer risk from GWAS studies?
    a. The 8q24 chromosomal region
    b. *MSR1*
    c. *RNASEL*
    d. *TMPRSS2-ERG* fusions
    e. None of the above

32. What type of genetic alteration in cancer could be identified using next-generation RNA sequencing (RNA-seq)?
    a. MicroRNAs associated with cancer
    b. Noncoding RNAs associated with cancer
    c. Gene fusions
    d. mRNA overexpression in cancer
    e. All of the above

ANSWERS

1. **b. A sugar, called ribose.** Ribose is an element of RNA, not DNA. In a rudimentary form, DNA is the fusion of three different elements: a base (either a pyrimidine or a purine), a sugar (in the case of DNA called 2-deoxyribose; for RNA called ribose), and a phosphate (which links individual nucleotides). The repeating connections between the phosphates and the sugars provide the backbone from which the information-carrying bases protrude. In its "resting" or nonreplicating form, this chain of elements forms a helix of two complementary strands; this double helix is held together by the hydrogen bonds.

2. **c. A pyrimidine to form hydrogen bonds with a purine.** The double helix is held together by the formation of hydrogen bonds between the pyrimidine on one strand and the purine base on the other. Uracil is in RNA, not DNA. Purines do not form bases with purines. The purine adenine (A) always forms two hydrogen bonds to the pyrimidine thymine (T), and the purine guanine (G) always forms three hydrogen bonds to the pyrimidine cytosine (C), one consequence being that A-T bonding is weaker than G-C bonding.

3. **e. A mechanism to bridge the gap between the genetic code and protein synthesis.** The physical locations of DNA and its genetic code and protein synthesis and the manifestation of that code are separate: DNA is in the nucleus, and protein synthesis is cytoplasmic. The DNA message must be converted into mRNA by a process called transcription in the nucleus. The mRNA is transferred into the cytoplasm where the mRNA is converted into a protein by a process called translation.

4. **a. The two general components involved in transcriptional regulation are specific sequences in the RNA and proteins that interact with those sequences.** Specific sequences in the DNA called response elements bind to the nuclear proteins that control transcription. Importantly, this provides a mechanism to coordinate gene expression by providing similar docking sites for genes that need to be expressed at specific time points. Although mRNA transcription, stability, transport, and translation are all highly regulated, they are not controlled by the transcriptional machinery binding to specific mRNA sequences.

5. **c. A process of including or excluding certain exons in an mRNA transcript.** A specific gene may have multiple similar (not identical) forms (isoforms). This is accomplished by having specific exons included or excluded from the final mRNA transcript. This allows one DNA sequence to produce several protein products that have different functions. It is not a random process but is very tightly regulated to ensure that the correct mRNA transcript is produced in the correct cell at the correct point in time.

6. **b. It is the site of mRNA transcription.**

7. **a. The RNA message of four parts (the nucleotides A, U, C, G) is converted into 20 amino acids by using a functional group of three adjacent nucleotides called a codon.** There is significant redundancy with several codons encoding for each amino acid. As a result, the RNA sequence between individuals can be different and yet still encode the same amino acid sequence (a polymorphism). However, some polymorphisms do result in amino acid changes. Shifts in reading frame are the most deleterious mutations because they result in a change in all the codons after the insertion/deletion and, as a result, a dramatic change in the amino acid sequence.

8. **e. The targeted inhibition of proteosome function appears to enhance cancer progression.** Degradation of proteins in the cell is an active, not passive, process. Ubiquitination is the process by which proteins are tagged for transport to the proteosome for destruction. Perturbation of this process is often found in cancer, and therefore inhibition of ubiquitination is a promising therapy for cancer.

9. **c. They can be produced by gene amplification, resulting in many copies of the gene, or by chromosomal rearrangement.** There are at least three ways a proto-oncogene can be converted into an oncogene. First, a mutation can occur within the coding sequence, producing a permanently activated form of the gene. A second mechanism converting a proto-oncogene into an oncogene is through gene amplification. A third mechanism of oncogene formation is through chromosomal rearrangement.

10. **b. It occurs exclusively on cytosine nucleotides in the dinucleotide sequence CG.** Hypermethylation is a normal process by which DNA is modified by the addition of a methyl group to

a cytosine nucleotide in a CpG DNA sequence. There is no change in DNA sequence. Methylation results in gene silencing, that is, decreased expression of the gene. As a result, hypermethylation in cancer is associated with decreased transcription and, therefore, reduces expression of tumor suppressor genes. Ubiquitination decreases levels of proteins but does so by increasing the degradation of the protein. Although alterations in ubiquitination occur in cancer, they are not directly related to methylation.

11. **b. Clear cell renal carcinoma.** VHL is a hereditary tumor syndrome that predisposes patients to clear cell renal carcinoma, retinal angiomas, pheochromocytomas, hemangiomas of the central nervous system, epididymal cystadenomas, and pancreatic islet cell tumors. It is not associated with epididymal, papillary renal cell, or adrenocortical carcinomas.

12. **d. None of the above.** All of the genes listed have been linked to prostate cancer by linkage studies examining families with a strong predisposition to prostate cancer and, in some cases, by case control studies examining polymorphisms within these genes. However, no data have conclusively demonstrated that these genes cause prostate cancer.

13. **e. All of the above.** Each of these syndromes includes increased risk of specific genitourinary malignancies among their spectra of pathologies.

14. **d. Deletion.** A common mechanism of tumor suppressor gene inactivation is through deletion of the gene or a chromosomal region containing the gene. The other abnormalities listed produce either no net loss of genetic material or lead to a gain of genetic material, a finding often associated with increased oncogene activity due to increased copy number of the oncogene.

15. **d. G_1S and G_2M boundaries.**

16. **a. Apoptosis.** Active TP53 binds to the promoter region of TP53-responsive genes and stimulates the transcription of genes responsible for cell cycle arrest, repair of DNA damage, and apoptosis. TP53 responds to DNA damage by inducing cell cycle arrest through CDKN1A (p21cip1) and then transcriptionally activating DNA repair enzymes. If the cell cannot arrest growth and/or repair the DNA, TP53 induces apoptosis. Although angiogenesis, DNA replication, and signal transduction are all critical cellular processes, TP53 does not directly influence any of them.

17. **a. Cyclin D/cdk4.** The INK4 family of cdk inhibitors directly inhibits the assembly of cyclin D with cdk4 and cdk6 by blocking the phosphorylation of the cyclin D-cdk4/6 complex. This phosphorylation is necessary for activation of the complex.

18. **e. Phosphorylation of RB1.** Phosphorylation is the attachment of a phosphate to a protein. It alters the conformation of the protein and therefore is an excellent method of regulating gene function. Cyclin-cdk complexes phosphorylate RB1 or its family members, p107 and p130. Phosphorylated RB1 can no longer bind to members of the E2F family of transcription factors. Free E2F heterodimerizes with DP1 or DP2 and transcriptionally activates genes important in DNA replication, such as DNA polymerase-A, and in the cell cycle, such as E2F-1. Dephosphorylation of RB has the opposite effect. E2F regulation does not occur directly though phosphorylation or dephosphorylation. MDM2 regulates TP53 and is not directly affected by cyclin-cdk complexes.

19. **c. DNA damage.** Hypoxia, nutrient-poor environment, and cytokines are all signals to the cell that it is not in an environment that is conducive to cellular division. These signals influence the cell *before* it invests its energy in replicating the DNA—that is, it is a G1S checkpoint. If DNA damage occurs, it is critical that the errors be repaired before cellular division. Therefore, DNA damage can lead to cell cycle arrest at both the G_1S and G_2M checkpoints.

20. **d. Ultraviolet light.** Nucleotide excision repair (NER) is a major defense against DNA damage caused by ultraviolet radiation and chemical exposure. NER acts on a wide range of alterations that result in large local distortions in DNA by recognizing distortions in the DNA helix, excising the damaged DNA, and replacing it with the correct sequence. Base excision repair is the primary mechanism for repairing damage caused by reactive

oxygen species. Mismatch repair is the primary mechanism for polymerase errors. Double-strand break repair is the primary mechanism for repairing double-strand breaks.

21. **b. Homologous recombination.** Homologous recombination (HR) is one of two mechanisms for repairing DNA double strand breaks, the other being nonhomologous end joining (NHEJ). In homologous recombination, the normal undamaged sister chromatid is used as a template to repair the damaged segment of DNA.

22. **c. *BRCA1*.** BRCA1 is associated with familial breast and ovarian cancer. It is believed that the breast cancer susceptibility gene *BRCA1* (as well as *BRCA2*) play an important role in homologous recombination as well as sensing DNA damage. Both *BRCA1* and *BRCA2* are part of an enzymatic complex with RAD51- and BRCA1-associated RING domain 1 (BARD1). This complex is recruited by proliferating cell nuclear antigen (PCNA) to regions that have undergone DNA damage to repair DNA breaks.

23. **e. Proteolytic cleavage.** Procaspases are the larger, inactive precursor forms of the caspase proteins. Specific proteolytic cleavage is required for their activation. The caspases themselves are proteases and, once activated, proceed to cleave and activate other caspases, thus facilitating a proteolytic cascade that serves to amplify the initial apoptotic signal.

24. **a. Independent of *TP53*.** The identification of ligand-dependent apoptosis receptors may have a profound impact on therapy. Most cancer therapies (e.g., chemotherapy and external beam radiotherapy) depend on TP53 to induce apoptosis in the cancer cell. Because TP53 is mutated in more than half of malignancies, TP53-independent pathways for apoptosis are of great clinical interest. Because ligand-dependent apoptosis is independent of TP53, these receptors and ligands are attractive and novel treatment targets.

25. **a. APAF-1/caspase 9.** The TP53-induced apoptosis is dependent on the APAF-1/caspase 9 activation pathway.

26. **c. Increasing the mitochondrial membrane permeability.** Although each proapoptotic bcl-2 family member responds to different stimuli, the principal mechanism by which these family members induce cell death is by increasing mitochondrial membrane permeability.

27. **e. Maintaining chromosomal length.** Telomerase immortalizes cells by maintaining the ends of the chromosomes, or telomeres, which normally shorten with each cell division.

28. **c. DNA hypomethylation.** Normal cells closely monitor their telomere lengths and, should they fall below a critical threshold length, will initiate either cell senescence or apoptosis. If key players in these responses (e.g., *TP53*) are mutated, then chromosomal instability may result, contributing to cancer initiation. To date, no strong connection is known for telomere loss and loss of DNA methylation.

29. **a. Fusion of BCR to Abl via chromosome translocation.** This particular chromosomal abnormality is typically found in chronic myelogenous leukemia patients, not in solid tumors. TMPRSS2-ERG gene fusions are found in approximately 50% of prostate cancer cases. MiTF/TFE gene family translocations have been associated with a subset of renal cell carcinomas. Isochromosome 8q is found in a subset of prostate cancers and is often associated with the loss of 8p. Loss of chromosome 9 is observed in a subset of urothelial cancers, and enumeration of this chromosome by FISH is one of the components of a molecular test used for detecting bladder cancer.

30. **a. Testis.** The urologic malignancy most closely linked to a karyotypic abnormality is a testis tumor. A 12p isochromosome was first identified in a testis tumor in the 1980s, and experimentally this cytogenetic hallmark of testicular tumors has diagnostic and prognostic value.

31. **a. The 8q24 chromosomal region.** Systematic review of GWAS studies in prostate cancer indicate that the 8q24 region continues to be the most implicated in prostate cancer risk and among different racial cohorts.

32. **e. All of the above.** RNA-seq technologies can sequence all RNA species in a sample in an unbiased manner, with an analysis that is not limited to "annotated" sequences.

CHAPTER REVIEW

1. Cancer cells have (1) genetic instability, (2) autonomous growth, (3) insensitivity to internal and external antiproliferative signals, (4) resistance to apoptosis, (5) unlimited cell division, (6) angiogenesis, (7) invasive behavior, and (8) the ability to evade the immune system.

2. RNA contains coding sequences (exons) and noncoding sequences (introns).

3. Loss of function of both alleles of a tumor suppressor gene is typically required for carcinogenesis.

4. Tumor suppressor genes normally negatively regulate and control cellular growth. Oncogenes promote cell growth. Oncogenes are mutated forms of normal genes (proto-oncogenes)

5. Oncogenes often exert their effects by interfering with cell cycle checkpoints and apoptotic pathways.

6. Certain tumor suppressor genes do not follow the two-hit hypothesis and may be inhibited by one alteration on one allele that inhibits the normal protein from the unaltered allele.

7. Cyclin-dependent kinases (CDK) are involved in synthetic activities of the cell cycle.

8. The regulatory portion of the CDK protein is called the *cyclin* and may also assist in substrate specificity.

9. The key point in the late G_1 cell phase at which the cell cycle becomes insensitive to extracellular signals is termed the restriction point. Loss of R-point control is typically due to inactivation of the RB1 pathway. Many cancer cells exhibit loss of R-point control.

10. If the cell cannot arrest growth or repair DNA damage, *TP53* often induces apoptosis.

11. Hypermethylation of CpG islands results in transcriptional downregulation, whereas hypomethylation of these regions increases the potential for gene activity.

12. Many prostate cancers are thought to harbor some form of a recurrent gene fusion such as TMPRSS2 and ERG.

13. Spontaneous mutation rate is insufficient to explain the number of mutations observed in cancers. Genetic instability is required.

14. Family history is one of the strongest predictors of prostate cancer risk.

15. The *VHL* gene is found to be mutated in over half of sporadic renal cell carcinoma cases. *VHL* targets HIF-1 (hypoxia-inducible factor).

16. Telomeres are structures composed of specialized repetitive DNA complexed with telomere-specific binding proteins located at the ends of every human chromosome and serve to stabilize and protect the end.

17. Progressive telomere shortening acts as a mitotic clock, signaling cell cycle exit (death) once telomeres reach a shortened threshold length. The majority of cancers have short telomeres but restabilize their telomeres through activation of the enzyme telomerase.

18. Apoptosis is an orderly process in which the contents of dying cells are degraded, packaged, and then engulfed by neighboring macrophages. This activity does not produce an inflammatory response.

19. Defects in the apoptotic cascade can profoundly influence tumor response to chemotherapy and radiotherapy.

20. Effective chemotherapy and radiation therapy in large part are dependent on apoptosis.

21. Apoptosis is mediated by the caspases.

22. Large variations in chromosome number and structure are the hallmarks of most solid tumors. The greater these variations, the more aggressive the tumor.

23. Free radical scavengers such as alpha-tocopherol, vitamin C, carotenoids, bilirubin and urate, and the enzymes superoxide dismutase, glutathione peroxidase, and glutathione transferase detoxify carcinogens.

24. A specific gene may have multiple similar (not identical) forms (isoforms). This is accomplished by having specific exons included or excluded from the final mRNA transcript. This allows one DNA sequence to produce several protein products that have different functions.

20 Principles of Tissue Engineering

Anthony Atala

QUESTIONS

1. Currently, possible tissue replacements for reconstruction include which of the following?
   a. Native nonurologic tissues
   b. Homologous tissues
   c. Heterologous tissues
   d. Artificial biomaterials
   e. All of the above

2. What does tissue engineering involve?
   a. The principles of cell transplantation
   b. The principles of materials science
   c. The use of matrices alone
   d. The use of matrices with cells
   e. All of the above

3. In regenerative medicine, when autologous cells are used:
   a. donor tissue is dissociated into individual cells.
   b. cells are either implanted directly into the host or expanded in culture.
   c. cells are attached to a support matrix.
   d. the cells and matrix are implanted in vivo.
   e. all of the above.

4. Which of the following statements is TRUE regarding biomaterials?
   a. They facilitate the localization and delivery of cells.
   b. They facilitate the localization and delivery of bioactive factors.
   c. They define a three-dimensional space for the formation of new tissues.
   d. They guide the development of new tissues with appropriate function.
   e. All of the above.

5. Types of biomaterials that have been utilized for engineering genitourinary tissues include which of the following?
   a. Naturally derived materials
   b. Acellular tissue matrices
   c. Synthetic polymers
   d. All of the above
   e. None of the above

6. Procedures and techniques that allow for the exclusion of nonurologic tissues during augmentation cystoplasty include which of the following?
   a. Autoaugmentation
   b. Ureterocystoplasty
   c. Tissue expansion

   d. Tissue engineering
   e. All of the above

7. Permanent synthetic materials, when used in continuity with the urinary tract, have been associated with:
   a. mechanical failure.
   b. emboli.
   c. calculus formation.
   d. a and c.
   e. none of the above.

8. Urothelium is associated with:
   a. a high reparative capacity.
   b. an inherent capacity for artificial extracellular matrix attachment.
   c. frequent malignant differentiation.
   d. poor growth parameters.
   e. none of the above.

9. Major limitations in phallic reconstructive surgery include which of the following?
   a. The availability of adequate growth factors
   b. The availability of sufficient autologous tissue
   c. The availability of adequate surgical techniques
   d. All of the above
   e. None of the above

10. What is the most prevalent form of renal replacement therapy?
    a. Organ transplantation
    b. Dialysis
    c. Bioartificial hemofilters
    d. Bioartificial renal tubules
    e. Engineered functional renal structures

11. The ideal bulking substance for the endoscopic treatment of reflux and incontinence should have what characteristic(s)?
    a. Easily injectable
    b. Nonantigenic
    c. Nonmigratory
    d. Volume stable
    e. All of the above

12. What are the most common cell sources for regenerative medicine today?
    a. Embryonic stem cells
    b. Induced pluripotent stem cells
    c. Autologous cells
    d. Stem cells derived from nuclear transfer techniques
    e. None of the above

ANSWERS

1. **e. All of the above.** Whenever there is a lack of native urologic tissue, reconstruction may be performed with native nonurologic tissues (skin, gastrointestinal segments, or mucosa from multiple body sites), homologous tissues (cadaver fascia, cadaver or donor kidney), heterologous tissues (bovine collagen), or artificial materials (silicone, polyurethane, Teflon [DuPont, Wilmington, DE]).

2. **e. All of the above.** Regenerative medicine follows the principles of cell transplantation, materials science, and engineering toward the development of biologic substitutes that would restore and maintain normal function. Tissue engineering may involve matrices alone, wherein the body's natural ability to regenerate is used to orient or direct new tissue growth, or the use of matrices with cells.

3. **e. All of the above.** When cells are used for regenerative medicine, donor tissue is dissociated into individual cells, which either are implanted directly into the host or are expanded in culture, attached to a support matrix, and reimplanted after expansion. The implanted tissue can be heterologous, allogeneic, or autologous.

4. **e. All of the above.** Biomaterials are used to facilitate the localization and delivery of cells and/or bioactive factors (e.g., cell adhesion peptides and growth factors) to desired sites in the body, define a three-dimensional space for the formation of new tissues with appropriate structure, and guide the development of new tissues with appropriate function.

5. **d. All of the above.** Generally, three classes of biomaterials have been used for engineering genitourinary tissues: naturally derived materials (e.g., collagen and alginate), acellular tissue matrices (e.g., bladder submucosa and small intestinal submucosa), and synthetic polymers (e.g., polyglycolic acid [PGA], polylactic acid [PLA], and poly(lactic-*co*-glycolic acid) [PLGA]).

6. **e. All of the above.** Because of the problems encountered with the use of gastrointestinal segments, numerous investigators have attempted alternative methods, materials, and tissues for bladder replacement or repair. These include autoaugmentation, ureterocystoplasty, methods for tissue expansion, seromuscular grafts, matrices for tissue regeneration, and tissue engineering using cell transplantation.

7. **d. a and c.** Usually, permanent synthetic materials used for bladder reconstruction succumb to mechanical failure and urinary stone formation, and degradable materials lead to fibroblast deposition, scarring, graft contracture, and a reduced reservoir volume over time.

8. **a. a high reparative capacity.** It has been well established for decades that the bladder is able to regenerate generously over free grafts. Urothelium is associated with a high reparative capacity. Bladder muscle tissue is less likely to regenerate in a normal manner.

9. **b. The availability of sufficient autologous tissue.** One of the major limitations of phallic reconstructive surgery is the availability of sufficient autologous tissue.

10. **b. Dialysis.** Although dialysis therapy is currently the most prevalent form of renal replacement therapy, the relatively high morbidity and mortality rates have prompted investigators to seek alternative solutions involving ex vivo systems.

11. **e. All of the above.** The ideal substance for the endoscopic treatment of reflux and incontinence should be injectable, nonantigenic, nonmigratory, volume stable, and safe for human use.

12. **c. Autologous cells.** Most current strategies for engineering urologic tissues involve harvesting of autologous cells from the host diseased organ or from donor cells from other sources from the patient, such as fat or bone marrow. However, in situations in which extensive end-stage organ failure is present, a tissue biopsy may not yield enough normal cells for expansion. Under these circumstances, the availability of pluripotent stem cells may be beneficial.

CHAPTER REVIEW

1. Stem cells may be either embryonic or adult. Embryonic stem cells may be harvested from (1) a blastocyst, (2) amniotic fluid, or (3) the placenta. Adult stem cells are usually isolated from a specific organ or bone marrow.

2. Stem cells have the ability to self-renew, to differentiate into a number of cell types, and to form clonal populations.

3. Altered nuclear transfer is a technique in which a genetically modified nucleus from a somatic cell is transferred into a human oocyte. The resulting embryo develops into a blastocyst but cannot implant into a uterus. The ethical advantage is that a fully developed organism is not created.

4. Adult stem cells have been discovered in many organs in the body and may serve as primary mechanisms of repair for injuries of these organs.

5. The ideal biomaterial provides regulation of cell behavior to promote development of functional new tissue. The cell behavior regulated includes but is not limited to cell adhesion, proliferation, migration, and differentiation. There are three types of biomaterials that are used: (1) naturally derived materials such as collagen or alginate (a polysaccharide isolated from seaweed), (2) acellular tissue matrices such as bladder submucosa or small intestine submucosa, and (3) synthetic polymers such as polyglycolic acid.

6. Formation of new blood vessels and capillaries occur by two mechanisms: vasculogenesis, in which new capillaries are formed from undifferentiated cells, and angiogenesis, in which new capillaries form by sprouting from preexisting capillaries.

7. In normal wound healing, epithelial cell ingrowth is initiated from the wound edges. This type of healing results in normal epithelium for no more than a distance of a few millimeters. Beyond that limit, fibrosis and scar formation occur in the rest of the wound. Matrices or matrices implanted with cells on the open wound allow greater wound coverage with the hope of less fibrosis. Cell-seeded matrices are superior to nonseeded matrices.

8. Most free grafts for bladder replacement show an adequate urothelial layer, but the muscular layer is not fully developed. SIS (small intestine submucosa), a biodegradable, acellular, xenogeneic collagen based tissue matrix graft, has been successfully employed in surgical correction of urethral strictures and Peyronie disease.

21 Surgical, Radiographic, and Endoscopic Anatomy of the Male Reproductive System

Parviz K. Kavoussi

QUESTIONS

1. The route that sperm travel through from the seminiferous tubules to the epididymis, in order, is:
   a. straight tubules, efferent ductules, rete testis.
   b. rete testis, straight tubules, efferent ductules.
   c. efferent ductules, rete testis, straight tubules.
   d. straight tubules, rete testis, efferent ductules.
   e. rete testis, efferent ductules, straight tubules.

2. The testis is enveloped by a tough capsule composed from external to internal, in order, of the:
   a. visceral tunica vaginalis, tunica albuginea, tunica vasculosa.
   b. tunica vasculosa, tunica albuginea, visceral tunica vaginalis.
   c. tunica albuginea, tunica vasculosa, visceral tunica vaginalis.
   d. visceral tunica vaginalis, tunica vasculosa, tunica albuginea.
   e. tunica albuginea, visceral tunica vaginalis, tunica vasculosa.

3. What percentage of testicular volume is made up by interstitium?
   a. 10% to 20%
   b. 20% to 30%
   c. 30% to 40%
   d. 40% to 50%
   e. 50% to 60%

4. Which of the following is the main arterial supply to the testis?
   a. Testicular artery
   b. Superficial dorsal artery
   c. The artery of the vas deferens
   d. Cremasteric artery
   e. Deep dorsal artery

5. The lymphatic drainage from the testis drains to:
   a. superficial and deep inguinal nodes.
   b. external and internal iliac nodes.
   c. para-aortic and interaortocaval nodes.
   d. internal iliac and obturator nodes.
   e. external iliac and obturator nodes.

6. The cremaster muscle is innervated by the:
   a. ilioinguinal nerve.
   b. genital branch of the genitofemoral nerve.
   c. femoral branch of the genitofemoral nerve.
   d. terminal branches of the subcostal nerve (T12).
   e. iliohypogastric nerve.

7. The nerves thought to be the main contributors to pain in men with chronic orchialgia include:
   a. perivasal complex.
   b. posterior periarterial/lipomatous complex.
   c. intracremasteric complex.
   d. femoral branch of the genitofemoral nerve.
   e. a, b, and c.

8. The anatomic component of the blood-testis barrier is the:
   a. tight junctions between Sertoli cells.
   b. myoendothelial junctions.
   c. tunica albuginea.
   d. basement membrane of seminiferous tubules.
   e. centrifugal arteries.

9. The seminal vesicle:
   a. is normally palpable on digital rectal examination.
   b. is a lateral outpouching of the prostate (central zone).
   c. contracts in response to excitatory efferents from the sacral parasympathetic nerves.
   d. is medial to the vas deferens.
   e. stores sperm.

10. The ducts of which of the following prostatic zones drain into the preprostatic urethra?
    a. Periurethral glands
    b. Central zone
    c. Transition zone
    d. Peripheral zone
    e. a and c

11. Benign prostatic hyperplasia (BPH) arises from the:
    a. periurethral glands.
    b. central zone.
    c. transition zone.
    d. peripheral zone.
    e. a and c.

12. Lymphatic drainage from the prostate drains to the:
    a. external iliac and common iliac nodes.
    b. internal iliac and obturator nodes.
    c. para-aortic nodes.
    d. internal iliac and inguinal nodes.
    e. perirectal and common iliac nodes.

13. The apex of the prostate is continuous with the:
    a. bladder neck.
    b. pubococcygeal portion of the of the levator ani.
    c. arcus tendineus fascia pelvis.
    d. bulbar urethra.
    e. striated urethral sphincter.

14. Lymphatic drainage from the bulbar urethra travels:
    a. through the perianal nodes to reach the pelvis.
    b. directly to the deep pelvic lymph nodes.
    c. through the superficial and deep inguinal lymph nodes.
    d. to the prepubic nodes.
    e. to para-aortic lymph nodes along with testicular drainage.

15. The only segment of the urethra that does not have transitional epithelium is the:
    a. prostatic urethra.
    b. membranous urethra.
    c. bulbar urethra.
    d. bulbomembranous urethra.
    e. fossa navicularis.

16. The glans penis is the most distal expansion of the:
    a. corpus cavernosum.
    b. corpus spongiosum.
    c. prepuce.
    d. urethra.
    e. Bucks fascia.

17. The dartos layer of smooth muscle and fascia in the scrotum is continuous with:
    a. the dartos layer of the penis.
    b. Colles fascia.
    c. Scarpa fascia.
    d. Buck fascia.
    e. a, b, and c.

ANSWERS

1. **d. Straight tubules, rete testis, efferent ductules.** Septa form 200 to 300 cone-shaped lobules, each containing one or more convoluted seminiferous tubules. Each tubule is U-shaped and has a stretched length of nearly 1 m. Interstitial (Leydig) cells lie in the loose tissue surrounding the tubules and are responsible for testosterone production. Toward the apices of the lobules, the seminiferous tubules become straight (tubuli recti) and enter the mediastinum testis to form an anastomosing network of tubules lined by flattened epithelium. This network, known as the *rete testis*, forms 12 to 20 efferent ductules and passes into the largest portion of epididymis, the caput.

2. **a. Visceral tunica vaginalis, tunica albuginea, tunica vasculosa.** The testis is enveloped by a tough capsule composed, from external to internal, of the visceral tunica vaginalis, the tunica albuginea, and the tunica vasculosa, before reaching the parenchyma of the testis. The tunica albuginea is composed of smooth muscle cells that pass through collagenous tissue.

3. **b. 20% to 30%.** The testicular interstitial tissue includes Leydig cells, mast cells, macrophages, nerves, blood vessels, and lymphatic vessels. This interstitial tissue makes up 20% to 30% of the testicular volume.

4. **a. Testicular artery.** There are three arterial supplies to the testis: the testicular (internal spermatic) artery, the artery of the vas deferens (deferential artery), and the cremasteric (external spermatic) artery. The testicular artery is the main blood supply to the testis, and its diameter is greater than the deferential and cremasteric arteries combined.

5. **c. Para-aortic and interaortocaval nodes.** Lymphatic channels from the testis drain into the para-aortic and interaortocaval lymph nodes. These lymphatic channels ascend within the spermatic cord after leaving the testis.

6. **b. Genital branch of the genitofemoral nerve.** The genital branch of the genitofemoral nerve follows the spermatic cord through the inguinal canal, supplies the cremaster muscle, and supplies sensation to the anterior scrotum.

7. **e. a, b, and c.** Three distinct anatomic distributions of nerves have been isolated within the spermatic cord and are thought to be the primary contributors in men with chronic orchialgia. These include a perivasal complex, posterior periarterial/lipomatous complex, and intracremasteric complex.

8. **a. Tight junctions between Sertoli cells.** There are extremely strong tight junctions between Sertoli cells, which provide an intracellular barrier that allows for spermatogenesis in an immune-privileged site. This is the barrier known as the *blood-testis barrier*.

9. **c. Contracts in response to excitatory efferents from the sacral parasympathetic nerves.** Innervation arises from the pelvic plexus, with major excitatory efferents contributed by the (sympathetic) hypogastric nerves.

10. **a. Periurethral glands.** At its midpoint, the urethra turns approximately 35 degrees anteriorly, but this angulation can vary from 0 to 90 degrees. This angle divides the prostatic urethra into proximal (preprostatic) and distal (prostatic) segments, which are functionally and anatomically discrete. Small periurethral glands, lacking periglandular smooth muscle, extend between the fibers of the longitudinal smooth muscle to be enclosed by the preprostatic sphincter.

11. **e. a and c.** The periurethral glands can contribute significantly to prostatic volume in older men as one of the sites of origin of BPH. The transition zone commonly gives rise to BPH.

12. **b. Internal iliac and obturator nodes.** Lymphatic drainage is primarily to the obturator and internal iliac nodes.

13. **e. Striated urethral sphincter.** The prostate is enveloped by a collagen, elastin, and smooth muscle capsule. The capsule measures 0.5 mm in thickness posteriorly and laterally on average. There is no true prostatic capsule at the apex of the prostate, where normal prostate glands are seen blending into the striated muscle of the urethral sphincter.

14. **c. Through the superficial and deep inguinal lymph nodes.** The penis, scrotum, and perineum drain into the inguinal lymph nodes. These nodes can be divided into superficial groups and deep groups.

15. **e. Fossa navicularis.** Unlike the transitional epithelium of the remainder of the urethra, the urethral mucosa that traverses the glans penis is squamous epithelium. These cells become keratinized near the meatus.

16. **b. Corpus spongiosum.** The glans penis is an expansion of the corpus spongiosum.

17. **e. a, b, and c.** The dartos layer of smooth muscle is anatomically continuous with Colles fascia, Scarpa fascia, and the dartos fascia of the penis.

CHAPTER REVIEW

1. The normal testicle measures $2.5 \times 3 \times 4$ cm and has a volume of 15 to 25 mL.
2. Both ends of the seminiferous tubules end in the rete testis.
3. Although there are three arteries that supply the testis, the testicular artery is the most important, and its ligation may result in testicular atrophy.
4. The testis, epididymis, vas, and seminal vesicles are innervated by the autonomic system, which is made up of afferent and efferent nerves.
5. The anatomic zones of the prostate include the transition zone, which is the site of BPH; the central zone, which contains the ejaculatory ducts (glands arising in this zone are thought to be derived from the wolffian duct, unlike the glands in the rest of the prostate); the peripheral zone, which contains 70% of the glandular epithelium and where 70% of prostate cancers occur; and the anterior zone, which is made up of fibromuscular stroma.
6. Seventy percent of the prostate is made up of glandular tissue, and 30% is fibromuscular tissue.
7. A permeable septum separates the corpora cavernosa, one from the other, and allows for free communication between the vascular spaces of the corpora bodies.
8. Scrotal lymphatics do not cross the midline and drain into the ipsilateral groin, unlike the penis, where the lymphatics cross over, allowing drainage to either groin irrespective of the side of the lesion.
9. The rete testis forms 12 to 20 efferent ductules and passes into the largest portion of epididymis, the caput.
10. The tunica albuginea is composed of smooth muscle cells that pass through collagenous tissue.
11. The genital branch of the genitofemoral nerve follows the spermatic cord through the inguinal canal, supplies the cremaster muscle, and supplies sensation to the anterior scrotum.
12. There are extremely strong tight junctions between Sertoli cells, which provide an intracellular barrier that allows for spermatogenesis in an immune-privileged site.
13. There is no true prostatic capsule at the apex of the prostate.
14. The penis, scrotum, and perineum drain into the inguinal lymph nodes.
15. The urethral mucosa that traverses the glans penis is squamous epithelium.

22   Male Reproductive Physiology

Paul J. Turek

QUESTIONS

1. Embryologically, the vas deferens is derived from what developmental structure?
   a. Müllerian ducts
   b. Wolffian ducts
   c. Urogenital ridge
   d. Gubernaculum testis
   e. Metanephros

2. The bulk of testicular volume in the adult human testicle is composed of:
   a. Leydig cells.
   b. Sertoli cells.
   c. spermatogenic cells.
   d. myoid cells.
   e. vascular endothelium.

3. Which of the following anterior pituitary hormones directly influences testicular function?
   a. Estradiol and adrenocorticotropic hormone (ACTH)
   b. Follicle-stimulating hormone (FSH) and estradiol
   c. Luteinizing hormone (LH) and FSH
   d. Testosterone and LH
   e. Thyroid-stimulating hormone (TSH) and testosterone

4. The bulk of the ejaculate volume is derived from:
   a. the epididymides.
   b. the Cowper gland.
   c. the seminal vesicles.
   d. the testes.
   e. the prostate.

5. Which of the following veins are responsible for varicoceles?
   a. The hypogastric veins
   b. The deferential veins
   c. The internal iliac veins
   d. The internal spermatic veins
   e. The cavernosal veins

6. A 25-year-old body builder eschews the merits of "natural" bodybuilding and uses injectable anabolic steroids regularly to maximize muscle bulk. His fertility potential would be expected to be:
   a. normal, because exogenous testosterone does not impair production of endogenous testosterone.
   b. low, because exogenous testosterone stimulates pituitary production of FSH and LH.
   c. low, because exogenous testosterone inhibits pituitary production of FSH and LH.
   d. low, because exogenous testosterone is not as potent as endogenous testosterone at nurturing spermatogenesis.
   e. normal, because intratestis testosterone concentrations are 50 times higher than serum levels, whether or not the blood contains exogenous testosterone.

7. Tight junctions between which testis cell types are structurally integral to the blood-testis barrier?
   a. Sertoli-Sertoli cells
   b. Myoid-Leydig cells
   c. Spermatids-Sertoli cells
   d. Leydig-Leydig cells
   e. Endothelial-endothelial cells

8. A 26-year-old man has a 1-year history of infertility and abnormal bulk semen parameters (low sperm concentration and motility). Hormonal testing reveals normal testosterone, FSH, and LH levels, but an elevated serum prolactin level (20 ng/dL, normal level, 2-18 ng/dL). The most likely cause of his elevated prolactin level is:
   a. pituitary microadenoma.
   b. pituitary macroadenoma.
   c. drug polypharmacy.
   d. stressful blood draw.
   e. timing of blood draw relative to sleep-wake cycle.

9. What is the normal developmental progression of spermatogenic cells?
   a. Sertoli, spermatogonia, spermatocyte
   b. Spermatocyte, spermatogonia, spermatid
   c. Spermatid, Sertoli, spermatocyte
   d. Spermatogonia, spermatid, spermatocyte
   e. Spermatogonia, spermatocyte, spermatid

10. Which hormone is the primary feedback inhibitor of pituitary LH secretion?
    a. Inhibin
    b. Testosterone
    c. Activin
    d. Prolactin
    e. Sertolin

11. Which of the following testicular volumes would be considered low for an adult human of any ethnicity?
    a. 12 mL
    b. 18 mL
    c. 22 mL
    d. 30 mL
    e. 40 mL

12. Major anatomic regions of the epididymis include:
    a. septa, efferent ductules, and corpus
    b. globus minor, ductus deferens, and cauda.
    c. rete testis, efferent ductules, and caput.
    d. efferent ductules, caput, and cauda.
    e. caput, corpus, and cauda

13. Which of the following is characteristic of meiosis?
    a. It is a process that occurs in all somatic cells.
    b. The chromosome number is maintained with cell division.

c. It is a process that occurs only in gametes.

d. There is no chromosomal crossing over.

e. Daughter cells are identical to parent cells.

14. When do testosterone peaks occur during a human male's life?

a. First trimester gestation, 2 months of age, puberty

b. 1 year of age, puberty, 50 years of age

c. Puberty, 30 years of age, 70 years of age

d. Puberty, 50 years of age

e. First trimester gestation, puberty, 70 years of age

15. With chronic obstruction, sperm motility is highest in what region of the epididymis?

a. Rete testis

b. Efferent ducts

c. Caput epididymis

d. Corpus epididymis

e. Cauda epididymis

16. What occurs during spermiogenesis?

a. Division of spermatogonia to form primary spermatocytes

b. Division of primary spermatocytes to form secondary spermatocytes

c. Cellular remodeling and nuclear compaction of spermatid DNA

d. Cytokinesis

e. Meiosis

17. Changes to sperm during epididymal transit include:

a. decreased motility.

b. sulfhydryl reduction.

c. decreased phospholipid content.

d. reduced membrane rigidity.

e. increased capacity for glycolysis.

18. Which of the following germ cell types is considered a true stem cell?

a. Elongating spermatids

b. Primary spermatocytes

c. Round spermatids

d. Secondary spermatocytes

e. Type A spermatogonia

19. During their development within the male reproductive tract before ejaculation, sperm spend the majority of time in which organ?

a. Epididymis

b. Ejaculatory ducts

c. Seminal vesicle

d. Testis

e. Urethra

20. The sperm region containing mitochondria is the:

a. tail.

b. head.

c. acrosome.

d. midpiece.

e. axoneme.

21. Which of the following statements about testosterone is the most accurate?

a. It is produced by the exocrine testis.

b. It exists mainly in the unbound or "free" form in the circulation.

c. It is regulated by follicle-stimulating hormone.

d. Its production is increased by excess prolactin.

e. One of its metabolites is dihydrotestosterone (DHT).

22. Processes that must occur for a sperm to normally fertilize an egg include all of the following EXCEPT:

a. development of motility.

b. acrosome reaction.

c. capacitation.

d. zona pellucida binding.

e. sexual intercourse.

23. After ejaculation the contents of the vas deferens are:

a. returned to the seminal vesicles.

b. maintained in the ampulla.

c. released into the ejaculatory ducts.

d. propelled back into the epididymis.

e. released into the bladder.

ANSWERS

1. **b. Wolffian ducts.** Müllerian ducts regress in the male. The indifferent gonad migrates to the urogenital ridge to become the testis. The gubernaculum testis is associated with the testis.

2. **c. Spermatogenic cells.** In humans, interstitial tissue takes up 20% to 30% of the total testicular volume, whereas germ line cells constitute the remainder (70%-80%).

3. **c. Luteinizing hormone (LH) and FSH.** Estradiol and testosterone are not anterior pituitary hormones, although they influence pituitary function. TSH and ACTH are derived from the anterior pituitary but do not act directly on the testicle.

4. **c. The seminal vesicles.** At least 65% to 70% of ejaculate volume is derived from the seminal vesicles, with the remainder from the vas deferens (sperm) and prostatic secretions. Periurethral Cowper glands also contribute a small amount of fluid to the ejaculate.

5. **d. The internal spermatic veins.** The pampiniform plexus of veins forms from the internal spermatic or gonadal veins. Deferential veins follow the vas deferens and empty into the hypogastric veins. These veins are spared during varicocele ligation surgery.

6. **c. Low, because exogenous testosterone inhibits pituitary production of FSH and LH.** Negative feedback inhibition maintains homeostatic balance in the pituitary-gonadal axis. Excess testosterone from any source acts on the anterior pituitary to reduce the production of LH and FSH. Without appropriate FSH production, azoospermia results in most men taking anabolic steroids, but the effect varies based on the dose, frequency, and duration of the drugs.

7. **a. Sertoli-Sertoli cells.** Sertoli-Sertoli tight junctions are the strongest cell-cell interactions in the body and give the blood-testis barrier its name. They form a high-resistance barrier that prevents the deep penetration of most drugs, molecules, and electron-opaque tracers into the seminiferous epithelium from the testicular interstitium. Sertoli cell tight junctions also segregate premeiotic germ cells (spermatogonia) from meiotic and postmeiotic germ cells.

8. **d. Stressful blood draw.** All of the choices can cause elevated serum prolactin levels. However, pathologically high prolactin levels are associated with low LH, FSH, and testosterone levels and reduced semen quality. Because anterior pituitary function is preserved, the elevated prolactin is likely spurious and due to a stressful blood draw. The measurement should be repeated with a blood draw at least 2 hours after awakening from sleep.

9. **e. Spermatogonia, spermatocyte, spermatid.** Proceeding from the least to the most differentiated, they are named dark type A spermatogonia (Ad); pale type A spermatogonia (Ap); type B spermatogonia (B); preleptotene primary spermatocytes (R);

leptotene primary spermatocytes (L); zygotene primary spermatocytes (z); pachytene primary spermatocytes (p); secondary spermatocytes (II); and Sa, Sb1, Sb2, Sc, Sd1, and Sd2 spermatids.

10. **b. Testosterone.** Inhibin and activin regulate FSH secretion. Prolactin, in excess, can downregulate LH but is not the primary regulator of LH secretion.

11. **a. 12 mL.** Although ethnic and racial differences do exist, a normal testis volume is generally above 16 mL and averages 20 mL.

12. **e. Caput, corpus, and cauda.** Anatomically, the epididymis is divided into three regions: the caput, the corpus, and the cauda epididymis. On the basis of histologic criteria, each of these regions can be subdivided into distinct zones separated by transition segments.

13. **c. It is a process that occurs only in gametes.** Crossing over of sister chromatids, exchange of genetic material, creation of unique daughter cells, and halving of chromosomal number are the hallmarks of meiosis. Meiosis occurs only in gametes whereas mitosis occurs in somatic cells.

14. **a. First trimester gestation, 2 months of age, puberty.** Testosterone peaks occur during early gestation and at approximately 2 months of age; a third spike occurs at puberty. Testosterone levels fall about 1%/year after age 30 and may fall more dramatically in the seventh and eighth decades of life.

15. **c. Caput epididymis.** Studies in men with congenital absence of the vas deferens or epididymal obstruction from vasectomy generally report better sperm motility in caput versus cauda epididymal sperm.

16. **c. Cellular remodeling and nuclear compaction of spermatid DNA.** In spermiogenesis, massive remodeling of postmeiotic germ cells (spermatids) occurs that involves nuclear compaction, tail and acrosome development, and cytoplasmic stripping of the mature germ cell. This is a postmeiotic process, and cell division, or cytokinesis, does not occur.

17. **e. Increased capacity for glycolysis.** Sperm undergo many metabolic changes during epididymal transit. Animal studies describe an increased capacity for glycolysis, changes in intracellular pH and calcium content, modification of adenylate cyclase activity, and alterations in cellular phospholipid and phospholipid-like fatty acid content. Sperm motility increases with epididymal transit.

18. **e. Type A spermatogonia.** Type A spermatogonia are the only true stem cell in the testis because they can either self-renew or differentiate to become sperm. All of the other cell types listed do not share this dual potential.

19. **d. Testis.** Sperm spend 45 to 60 days developing in the testis and 2 to 12 days in the epididymis. They are not routinely found in the seminal vesicle, and spend only seconds in the ejaculatory ducts and urethra during ejaculation.

20. **d. Midpiece.** The middle segment of sperm is highly organized, consisting of helically arranged mitochondria that surround a set of outer dense fibers and the 9 + 2 microtubular structure of the axoneme. The sperm head contains an acrosome and the nucleus, and the tail contains the axoneme.

21. **e. One of its metabolites is dihydrotestosterone (DHT).** Testosterone is produced by the endocrine testes, exists mainly in bound forms in plasma, and is regulated by LH, not FSH. Testosterone is converted to DHT in target tissue by 5-α reductase. It is also converted to estrogen by aromatase enzymes. Excess prolactin decreases testosterone production.

22. **e. Sexual intercourse.** For physiologic egg fertilization, all of the processes listed must occur. Intrauterine insemination (IUI) can replace sexual intercourse and improve the odds of natural conception. The process of in vitro fertilization (IVF)–intracytoplasmic sperm injection (ICSI) avoids many of these physiologic processes by simply injecting a sperm from any reproductive-tract source into a mature oocyte or egg.

23. **d. Propelled back into the epididymis.** Studies have shown that after sexual stimulation or ejaculation, the contents of the vas deferens are propelled back toward the cauda epididymis, because of differences in the amplitude, frequency, and duration of vas deferens contractility along its length.

CHAPTER REVIEW

1. The steroid hormones testosterone, dihydrotestosterone, and estradiol are translocated to nuclear DNA recognition sites and regulate the transcription of target genes.

2. The hypothalamus is anatomically linked to the pituitary gland by both a portal vascular system and neuronal pathway. The hypothalamic hormone GnRH (sometimes called LHRH) stimulates the secretion of luteinizing hormone and follicle-stimulating hormone.

3. GnRH output exhibits three types of rhythmicity: (1) seasonal, peaking in the spring; (2) circadian, peaking in the early morning; and (3) pulsatile, periodic peaks per 24 hours. The importance of pulsatile GnRH secretory pattern is demonstrated when a GnRH agonist is given; this eliminates the pulsatile activity and therefore suppresses GnRH output.

4. Both androgens and estrogens regulate LH secretion through negative feedback.

5. Increased levels of prolactin abolish gonadotropin pulsatility by interfering with the episodic GnRH release, thus causing a reduction in LH and FSH.

6. Testosterone is metabolized to dihydrotestosterone (5-α reductase) and estradiol (aromatase).

7. Sertoli cells produce inhibin, which inhibits FSH, and activin, which stimulates FSH. The presence of these hormones accounts for the relatively secondary independence of FSH from GnRH secretion. Sertoli cells produce androgen-binding protein, which maintains high levels of androgen in the seminiferous tubules and epididymis.

8. Negative feedback for testosterone occurs at the hypothalamus; for estrogens, it occurs at the pituitary.

9. The SRY (sex-determining region Y gene) on the short arm of the Y chromosome is a critical gene for sex determination.

10. Dihydrotestosterone masculinizes the external genitalia; müllerian-inhibiting substance prevents müllerian duct development, that is, the uterus, fallopian tubes, and proximal third of the vagina.

11. A slow but progressive decline in testosterone production occurs with age > 30 years.

12. Androgen production during the early male neonate's life is thought to hormonally imprint the hypothalamus, liver, and prostate.

13. The blood-testis barrier is more appropriately termed blood-seminiferous tubule barrier; it allows sperm development to occur in an immunologically privileged way.

14. An insult to the testes, such as biopsy, torsion, or trauma, will not induce anti-sperm antibodies if the event occurs before puberty.

15. The X chromosome appears to be important for spermatogenesis.

16. The azoospermic factor region (AZF) is located on the long arm of the Y chromosome. Deletions in this region are found in some patients with abnormal spermatogenesis. Microdeletions in the AZF region are subdivided into a, b, and c. Sperm may be found in AZFc microdeletions but not in AZFa and AZFb.

17. With paternal age, there are increases in structural chromosomal abnormalities in sperm and autosomal-dominant mutations leading to specific (sentinel) phenotypes in offspring.

18. Lymph from the caput and corpus epididymis travels the same route as that for the testes. Lymph from the cauda epididymis joins the vas deferens and terminates in the external iliac nodes. There is a blood-epididymis barrier that extends from caput to cauda epididymis.

19. The epididymis serves to transport sperm, store it, increase fertility, and promote motility maturation. Epididymal function is temperature and androgen (DHT) dependent. Sperm fertility maturation is achieved at the level of the late corpus or early cauda epididymis.

20. Semenogelin, a component of semen that results in semen coagulation, is produced in the seminal vesicle. Seminal vesicle secretions have an alkaline pH and contain antioxidant enzymes, fructose, vitamin C, flavins, and prostaglandins.

21. At least 65% to 70% of ejaculate volume is derived from the seminal vesicles,

22. Testosterone peaks occur during early gestation and at approximately 2 months of age, and a third spike occurs at puberty.

23. Sperm spend 45 to 60 days developing in the testis and 2 to 12 days in the epididymis.

23 Integrated Men's Health: Androgen Deficiency, Cardiovascular Risk, and Metabolic Syndrome

J. Kellogg Parsons and Tung-Chin Hsieh

QUESTIONS

Sections 1 and 2

1. Systemic illnesses associated with increased risk for androgen deficiency are:
   a. traumatic brain injury.
   b. sepsis.
   c. chronic obstructive pulmonary disease.
   d. rheumatoid arthritis.
   e. all of the above.

2. All of the following diseases are associated with primary hypogonadism, EXCEPT:
   a. cryptorchidism.
   b. Klinefelter syndrome.
   c. Pasqualini syndrome.
   d. orchitis.
   e. Noonan syndrome.

3. All of the following conditions are associated with abnormal sex hormone–binding globulin (SHBG), EXCEPT:
   a. diabetes mellitus.
   b. coronary heart disease.
   c. aging.
   d. hepatic cirrhosis.
   e. acromegaly.

4. Evaluation for suspected androgen deficiency should include all of the following, EXCEPT:
   a. complete history and physical exam.
   b. measurement of serum luteinizing hormone (LH) and follicle-stimulating hormone (FSH).
   c. confirmatory repeat testosterone (T) testing if initial T level is in the mildly hypogonadal range.
   d. digital rectal exam and prostate-specific antigen (PSA) testing.
   e. scrotal sonography.

5. Which of the following statements regarding the diagnosis of androgen deficiency in aging is TRUE?
   a. Screening questionnaires are highly specific.
   b. Serum T threshold for symptoms ranges narrowly among individuals.
   c. Recurrence of symptoms is highly reproducible for each individual with interruption of therapy.
   d. Signs and symptoms of hypogonadism are specific; biochemical support is desirable but not mandatory.
   e. Sarcopenia and osteoporosis are fundamental elements for the diagnosis of the condition.

6. For which of the following conditions is T supplemental therapy indicated?
   a. Male infertility

   b. Inability to concentrate
   c. Obesity
   d. Sleep disturbance
   e. None of the above

7. Which of the following is NOT a contraindication for T supplemental therapy?
   a. Polycythemia
   b. Congestive heart failure
   c. Breast cancer
   d. Angina pectoris
   e. Gynecomastia

8. T therapy preparations associated with the highest risk of polycythemia are:
   a. topical T gels.
   b. subcutaneous T implants.
   c. intramuscular injectable preparations.
   d. oral T undecanoate.
   e. T buccal formulation.

9. Recommended follow-up monitoring after initiation of T therapy includes all of the following, EXCEPT:
   a. yearly PSA testing.
   b. monitoring T level 3 to 6 months after initiation of T therapy.
   c. measuring bone mineral density of lumbar spine and/or femoral neck in men with osteoporosis and history of low-trauma fracture.
   d. checking baseline hematocrit and then annually.
   e. evaluating patients 3 to 6 months after initiation of T therapy, and then annually to assess symptomatic response and adverse effects.

10. Aspects of metabolic syndrome (MetS) are associated with the development of the following urologic diseases, EXCEPT:
    a. nephrolithiasis.
    b. prostate cancer.
    c. benign prostatic hypertrophy.
    d. erectile dysfunction.
    e. testicular cancer.

Section 3

11. According to the National Cholesterol Education Program guidelines, all of the following are components of the metabolic syndrome EXCEPT:
    a. elevated serum triglycerides.
    b. hypertension.
    c. decreased high-density lipoprotein (HDL) cholesterol.
    d. abdominal obesity.
    e. increased low-density lipoprotein (LDL) cholesterol.

12. Which of the following is TRUE of the MetS?
    a. It is associated with an increased risk of urinary stones.
    b. Definitive guidelines exist regarding the evaluation and treatment of MetS in the context of urologic diseases.
    c. It is associated with an increased risk of erectile dysfunction.
    d. a and c
    e. None of the above

13. Regarding obesity:
    a. Level 1 evidence indicates that weight loss may improve stress urinary incontinence in obese women.
    b. It is associated with a decreased risk of prostate enlargement.
    c. Weight loss will not improve erectile function in obese men.
    d. Weight loss will improve fertility in obese men.
    e. For the MetS, obesity is measured using body mass index (BMI).

14. Which of the following potentially contributes to infertility in the setting of the MetS?
    a. Ejaculatory dysfunction
    b. Azoospermia
    c. Hypogonadism
    d. Spermatic DNA damage
    e. All of the above

15. Which of the following is NOT true of erectile dysfunction (ED)?
    a. ED increases the risk of incident cardiovascular disease, including myocardial infarction.
    b. For obese men with ED, evidence-based guidelines recommend lifestyle modifications, including weight loss, before initiating pharmacotherapy.
    c. ED is as strong a risk factor for cardiovascular disease as smoking and family history.
    d. ED is associated with increased risks of insulin resistance and diabetes.
    e. Men with hypertension are more likely to develop ED than men without hypertension.

ANSWERS

Sections 1 and 2

1. **e. All of the above.** Many systemic diseases are associated with increased risk of androgen deficiency. Physicians need to be aware of these disorders when evaluating patients with suspected hypogonadism and offer appropriate screening for at-risk patients. T therapy has been shown to improve outcomes and quality of life in patients with systemic illnesses.
2. **c. Pasqualini syndrome.** Pasqualini syndrome is a condition characterized by isolated LH deficiency. It is important to differentiate between primary and secondary hypogonadism during the evaluation of suspected patients. In patients with secondary hypogonadism with possible central nervous system abnormalities, magnetic resonance imaging of the pituitary is indicated.
3. **b. Coronary heart disease.** Serum total T concentration represents the sum of unbound and protein-bound T in circulation. Most T is bound to SHBG and to albumin; only 0.5% to 3% of circulation T is unbound or "free." When interpreting biochemical measurements, clinicians need to be aware of conditions associated with alterations in SHBG concentration.
4. **e. Scrotal sonography.** Guidelines on the evaluation for suspected androgen deficiency are well established. History and physical examination with biochemical testing are required for the initial workup. Although genital and testicular examination is indicated, scrotal imaging is warranted only when an abnormality is found.
5. **c. Recurrence of symptoms is highly reproducible for each individual with interruption of therapy.** Validated questionnaires are ideal for screening with high sensitivity (~80%) but poor specificity (<50%). There is a wide interpersonal variability among T cutoff for clinical hypogonadal symptoms. However, after adequate response to treatment, discontinuation of T administrations triggers predictable symptom recurrence with reproducible T decline.
6. **e. None of the above.** T was studied as male contraception and is contraindicated in men desiring future fertility. Although T therapy has been shown to positively impact body composition, obesity alone is not an indication for therapy. Indications for T therapy include delayed puberty, symptomatic hypogonadism, and testicular dysgenesis. Many hypogonadal symptoms are nonspecific, and multiple signs and symptoms before initiating therapy are preferred.
7. **d. Angina pectoris.** Peripheral aromatization of T to estrogen can stimulate the growth of breast cancer and gynecomastia. Fluid retention is sometimes observed with T therapy and can exacerbate preexisting heart failure. Despite conflicting literature on the cardiovascular risks associated with T therapy, T has been shown to induce coronary vasodilation.
8. **c. Intramuscular injectable preparations.** Polycythemia is a known complication of T therapy (incidence 5%-30% with elderly men at highest risk). Although the exact mechanism is unknown, both androgen receptor and dihydrotestosterone were implicated. Erythrocytosis is often dose limiting and is the most common reason for treatment modification/cessation. Injectable formulations are associated with the highest rate of T therapy-related polycythemia.
9. **a. Yearly PSA testing.** Routine scheduled follow-up is important after initiation of T therapy. Monitoring should include assessment of symptomatic response, adverse events, and biochemical testing (Table 23-1). Although baseline PSA testing and digital rectal exam should be performed before initiation of therapy, prostate cancer screening for men undergoing T therapy is the same as for eugonadal men and should follow the current American Urological Association Guidelines.
10. **e. Testicular cancer.** Metabolic syndrome can be found in up to 40% of U.S. adults. Growing evidence suggests a link between aspects of metabolic syndrome and urologic diseases. An increased prevalence of nephrolithiasis is parallel with metabolic syndrome in countries with a Western lifestyle. Insulin appears to be the strongest promoter of both prostate growth and development of high-risk prostate cancer. Aspects of metabolic syndrome are known risk factors for ED.

Section 3

11. **e. Increased low-density lipoprotein (LDL) cholesterol.** Whereas decreased HDL cholesterol is a component of the metabolic syndrome (MetS), increased LDL cholesterol is not. The fifth component of the MetS is elevated blood glucose, defined as fasting plasma glucose ≥ 100 mg/dL or drug treatment for elevated blood glucose.
12. **d. a and c.** The MetS increases the risk of urinary stones, erectile dysfunction, and several other urologic diseases. However, there are currently no evidence-based guidelines for MetS and urologic diseases, and practical applications of these data to the urologic practice remain limited.
13. **a. Level 1 evidence indicates that weight loss may improve stress urinary incontinence in obese women.** The Program to Reduce Incontinence by Diet and Exercise (PRIDE) trial demonstrated that overweight or obese women with 10 or more incontinence episodes per week benefited from a behavioral intervention focused on weight loss. Obesity is associated with an increased risk of prostate enlargement. A randomized trial of 110 obese men observed that weight loss significantly improved erectile function, but weight loss trials have as yet not been performed in obese infertile men. For the obesity component of the MetS, abdominal adiposity is measured using waist circumference.
14. **e. All of the above.** Ejaculatory dysfunction, azoospermia, hypogonadism, and spermatic DNA damage are all putative causes of

TABLE 23-1   Monitoring after Initiation of Testosterone Therapy: Endocrine Guideline

1. Evaluate the patient every 3-6 months after treatment initiation and then annually to asses symptom response and assess adverse effects.
2. Monitor T level 3-6 months after treatment initiation with goal to raise serum T level into the mid-normal range.
   Injectable formulations: measure serum T level midway between injections.
   Transdermal patch: assess T level 3-12 hr after application.
   Transdermal gels: assess T level anytime after 1 wk of treatment.
   Buccal T: assess T level immediately before or after application.
   Oral agent: monitor T level 3-5 hr after ingestion.
   T pellets: measure T levels at the end of the dosing interval.
3. Check hematocrit at baseline, at 3-6 mo, and then annually.
   If Hct > 54%, stop therapy until Hct has decreased to a safe level.
4. Measure bone mineral density of lumbar spine and/or femoral neck after 1-2 yr of T therapy in men with osteoporosis or low-trauma fracture.
5. Perform digital rectal examination and check PSA before initiation of therapy, at 3-6 mo, and then in accordance with prostate cancer screening guidelines.
6. Additional urologic workup if there is abnormal digital rectal exam, elevation of PSA, worsening lower urinary tract symptom, International Prostate Symptom Score > 19
7. Evaluation formulation-specific adverse effects at each visit
   Buccal: alterations in taste and examination of gum and oral mucosa for irritation
   Injectable: fluctuations in symptom, fluid retention
   T patches: irritation at the application site
   T gels: advise patient to cover the application sites with clothing, local hygiene before skin-to-skin contact with women or children. Serum T levels are maintained when application site is washed 4-6 hr after application.
   T pellet: check for signs of infection, fibrosis, or pellet extrusion.

From Bhasin et al. *J Clin Endocrinol Metab* 2010;95(6):2536–59; Table 8.

infertility in men with the MetS. Other potential factors include low ejaculate volume and diminished sperm motility.

15. **b. For obese men with ED, evidence-based guidelines recommend lifestyle modifications, including weight loss, before initiating pharmacotherapy.** Although level 1 evidence supports the concept that weight loss improves erectile function in obese men, evidence-based guidelines for ED do not as yet formally address the topic of lifestyle interventions. Robust data indicate that ED substantially increases the risk of incident cardiovascular disease and is as strong an independent risk factor as current smoking or family history. Insulin resistance, diabetes, and hypertension are all strongly associated with ED.

CHAPTER REVIEW

1. With aging, there is a change in the gonadal hypothalamic pituitary axis.
2. The number of Leydig cells decrease with aging, and there is a reduction in the diurnal variation of T, suggesting desensitization of Leydig cells to LH with aging.
3. Circulating T is 98% bound to SHBG and albumin. T bound to albumin is more readily unbound than that bound to SHBG. Bioavailable T includes albumin bound and free T.
4. With aging, changes in enzyme receptor function and responsiveness of cells to the balance between T and dihydrotestosterone occur at different rates in individuals, which makes setting an absolute level of hormone deficiency difficult for a particular individual.
5. Metabolism of T takes place mainly in the liver, prostate, and skin; the catabolic products are excreted in the urine.
6. The CAG repeat sequence on the androgen receptor is maximal in humans (about 22 triplets) and is less in other species. There is an increased androgen response of the receptor in men with shorter CAG repeats. The androgen receptor may be activated not only by T but also by protein kinase C and other factors.
7. Hypogonadal men have increased levels of leptin and insulin. They are more likely to be obese. Hypogonadism correlates with elevated serum glucose and triglyceride levels. There is an increase in total body fat mass and fasting insulin resistance index.
8. Administration of T in older men is associated with decreased visceral fat, decreased glucose concentration, and increased sensitivity to insulin.
9. The diagnosis of T deficiency syndrome (TDS) cannot be based on absolute levels of serum T or symptoms and is a matter of judgment. However, among the most prominent symptoms of this syndrome are tiredness, decreased sexual desire, and dysphoria (mood of general dissatisfaction, depression).
10. It appears that bioavailable free T is better correlated with symptoms of TDS than is total T. Measurement of T should be restricted to the morning hours because that is the peak point of secretion. In younger men there is a normal circadian rhythm that is blunted as men age.
11. While men age, growth hormone decreases, which may result in changes in lean muscle mass, bone density, hair distribution, and the pattern of obesity. In addition, there is a reduction in dehydroepiandrosterone (DHEA), melatonin, and thyroxine. Serum leptin levels increase.
12. Hypogonadism is associated with increased mortality in males.
13. Serum T increases bone mineral density. Higher levels of circulating T correlate with a lower cardiovascular risk. Lower levels correlate with hypoactive sexual desire.
14. The presence of prostate or breast cancer is an absolute contraindication for T treatment. There is little evidence to indicate that in the normal male without prostate cancer, supplementation with T for periods of up to 3 years increases prostate growth.
15. Serum PSA thresholds for normal values are less in hypogonadal men.
16. T increases red cell mass (erythrocytosis).
17. Exogenous T suppresses spermatogenesis.
18. Peripheral aromatization of T to estrogen can stimulate the growth of breast cancer and gynecomastia.
19. ED substantially increases the risk of incident cardiovascular disease and is as strong an independent risk factor as current smoking or family history. Insulin resistance, diabetes, and hypertension are all strongly associated with ED.

24   Male Infertility

Craig Stuart Niederberger

QUESTIONS

1. For couples practicing optimal timing methods to conceive, the proportion who conceive after six cycles should be approximately:
   a. 1/2.
   b. 1/3.
   c. 1/5.
   d. 2/5.
   e. 4/5.

2. For couples desiring to conceive, around the time of ovulation, they should have intercourse:
   a. daily.
   b. twice daily.
   c. every other day.
   d. in the morning.
   e. near noon.

3. In the industrialized world, female fecundity typically declines most rapidly after:
   a. puberty.
   b. age 30 years.
   c. age 35 years.
   d. age 40 years.
   e. menopause.

4. All of the following medications are associated with male reproductive dysfunction EXCEPT:
   a. cimetidine.
   b. spironolactone.
   c. indinavir.
   d. prednisone.
   e. lisinopril.

5. A man with oligoasthenospermia has inflammatory bowel disease and is prescribed sulfasalazine. He should be counseled to:
   a. repeat a semen analysis.
   b. continue sulfasalazine.
   c. substitute sulfasalazine with colchicine.
   d. substitute sulfasalazine with mesalazine.
   e. discontinue all medications.

6. A 30-year-old man is attempting to conceive with his 28-year-old wife. She is diagnosed with premature ovarian failure, and hematoxylin and eosin microscopic staining of his sperm is consistent with the presence of *Escherichia coli*. His bulk seminal parameters are otherwise unremarkable. You recommend:
   a. swim up and intrauterine insemination.
   b. a 3-week course of ciprofloxacin, 500 mg twice daily.
   c. prostatic culture.
   d. seminal vesicle aspiration for culture.
   e. observation.

7. The effect of human immunodeficiency virus (HIV) infection on bulk seminal parameters is:
   a. none.
   b. decreased motility.
   c. increased number of morphologically abnormal forms.
   d. decreased concentration.
   e. decreased volume.

8. Direct exposure of the testis to ionizing radiation causes irreparable damage to spermatogenesis at doses at and above:
   a. 2.5 Gy.
   b. 5 Gy.
   c. 7.5 Gy.
   d. 10 Gy.
   e. 20 Gy.

9. The typical differential between core body and scrotal temperature is:
   a. 0.5° C.
   b. 0.5° F.
   c. 1° to 2° C.
   d. 2° to 4° C.
   e. 6° C.

10. An 18-year-old man has bilateral testes palpable at the external inguinal rings. He desires to father children in the future. Two centrifuged semen analyses reveal azoospermia. Serum testosterone is 410 ng/dL, and follicle-stimulating hormone is 22 IU/L. The best next step is:
    a. counsel that when he is ready, he and his partner should use donor sperm or adopt.
    b. clomiphene citrate, 50 mg every other day.
    c. testis biopsy.
    d. microsurgical testis sperm extraction with cryopreservation if sperm are found.
    e. bilateral orchidopexy.

11. The lubricant that does NOT affect sperm function or DNA integrity is:
    a. Astroglide.
    b. K-Y Jelly.
    c. Pre-Seed.
    d. Replens.
    e. saliva.

12. The serum hormonal pattern commonly observed in male obesity is:

	TESTOSTERONE	SHBG	ESTRADIOL
a.	↓	↓	↓
b.	↓	↓	↑
c.	↓	↑	↓
d.	↓	↑	↑
e.	↑	↑	↑

13. The finding most consistent with spermatogenic impairment is:
    a. a testis volume as measured by Prader orchidometer less than 30 mL.
    b. a testis volume as measured by scrotal ultrasonography less than 30 mL.
    c. a testis longitudinal axis as measured by caliper orchidometer less than 4.6 cm.
    d. an engorged epididymis.
    e. an absent vas deferens.

14. A man evaluated for azoospermia has absent vasa bilaterally. The next step is cystic fibrosis transmembrane conductance regulator (CFTR) gene sequence assay for him and his partner and:
    a. transrectal ultrasound.
    b. renal ultrasound.
    c. postejaculatory urinalysis.
    d. seminal vesicle aspiration.
    e. testis biopsy.

15. The following condition increases sex hormone–binding globulin (SHBG):
    a. aging.
    b. diabetes mellitus.
    c. hypothyroidism.
    d. obesity.
    e. testosterone therapy.

16. A man is found to be azoospermic. The following most strongly suggests spermatogenic dysfunction as a cause rather than obstruction:
    a. testis long axis on physical examination 4.2 cm, FSH assay 4 IU/L.
    b. testis long axis on physical examination 4.3 cm, FSH assay 10 IU/L.
    c. bioavailable testosterone, 166 ng/dL, FSH assay 6 IU/L.
    d. luteinizing hormone (LH), 2 IU/L, FSH 2 IU/L.
    e. testosterone, 160 ng/dL, LH 9 IU/L.

17. A reasonable threshold for sperm concentration above which a man can be considered fertile is:
    a. 15 million/mL.
    b. 20 million/mL.
    c. 48 million/mL.
    d. 80 million/mL.
    e. 200 million/mL.

18. Brown-hued semen is often associated with:
    a. ingested asparagus.
    b. ejaculatory ductal obstruction.
    c. sexual activity.
    d. spinal cord injury.
    e. urinary tract infection.

19. The optimal time in days of abstinence to wait after an ejaculate for a semen analysis is:
    a. 1.
    b. 2.
    c. 3.
    d. 5.
    e. 7.

20. A man who has been unsuccessful in impregnating his wife during the past year is identified to have azoospermia and semen volumes of 0.8 and 0.5 mL. The next step is:
    a. testis biopsy.
    b. scrotal ultrasound.
    c. postejaculatory urinalysis.
    d. clomiphene citrate, 50 mg every other day.
    e. transurethral resection of ejaculatory ducts.

21. A 32-year-old man presents for fertility evaluation. Physical exam and endocrine assessment are normal. Semen analysis demonstrates volume 2.5 mL, density 84 million/mL, motility 71%, and strict morphology 0% with a variety of abnormal forms. The next step is:
    a. vitamin E.
    b. reassurance.
    c. testis biopsy.
    d. scrotal ultrasound.
    e. antisperm antibody assay.

22. Two semen analyses from a man undergoing a reproductive evaluation include volumes of 2.5 and 1.8 mL, densities of 24 and 28 million/mL, and motility 0%. The next step is:
    a. vital stain.
    b. immunobead assay.
    c. repeat semen analysis.
    d. sperm chromatin structure assay (SCSA).
    e. computer-assisted semen analysis (CASA).

23. Semen observed under phase contrast light microscopy reveals abundant round cells similar in size and shape to leukocytes. The next step is:
    a. semen culture.
    b. Papanicolaou staining.
    c. transrectal ultrasound.
    d. ciprofloxacin, 1 g daily for 4 weeks.
    e. ibuprofen, 400 mg daily for 2 weeks.

24. A direct assay of sperm-head DNA fragmentation is the:
    a. terminal deoxynucleotidyl transferase dUTP nick end labeling (TUNEL) assay.
    b. acid comet assay.
    c. alkaline comet assay.
    d. sperm chromatin dispersion (SCD) assay.
    e. SCSA.

25. The assay that most closely models incubational in vitro fertilization is:
    a. reactive oxygen species-total antioxidant capacity (ROS-TAc).
    b. Penetrak assay.
    c. Tru-trax assay.
    d. sperm penetration assay.
    e. acrosomal assay.

26. A 26-year-old man presenting for fertility evaluation has two semen analyses, one with volume 2.1 mL and density 32 million/mL, and another with volume 2.3 mL and density 28 million/mL. No motile sperm are observed in either, and vital stain demonstrated greater than 80% metabolically active sperm in both. The next step is:
    a. immunobead assay.
    b. pyospermia stain.
    c. electron microscopy.

d. SCSA.

e. repeat semen analysis.

27. A 30-year-old man has azoospermia. Physical examination reveals absent vasa bilaterally. CFTR analysis reveals a ΔF508 mutation. The next step is:

   a. repeat CFTR analysis of the man with a 1600-mutation screen.

   b. repeat semen analysis.

   c. CFTR analysis of his wife.

   d. testicular sperm extraction.

   e. testis biopsy.

28. A 28-year-old man desires a biological child. Physical examination is normal. Two semen analyses reveals azoospermia with volumes of 0.8 and 0.7 mL, and no sperm is identified in a post-ejaculatory urinalysis. FSH is 3.2 IU/L. Transrectal ultrasound reveals seminal vesicles of 0.9 and 1.1 cm in largest diameter, and no midline cyst is visualized. The next step is:

   a. reassurance.

   b. testis biopsy.

   c. repeat semen analysis.

   d. transurethral resection of ejaculatory ducts.

   e. testis sperm extraction and cryopreservation.

29. A 33-year-old man desires a biological child and is found to have azoospermia with semen volumes 2.2 and 2.4 mL on two analyses. Longitudinal axis of the left testis is 3.3 cm, and the right is 3.5 cm. Serum FSH is 9.3 IU/L, and testosterone is 440 ng/dL. The next step is:

   a. testis biopsy.

   b. epididymovasostomy.

   c. repeat semen analysis.

   d. microsurgical testis sperm extraction.

   e. clomiphene citrate, 50 mg every other day.

30. A 30-year-old man desires a biological child with his 28-year-old wife. Her evaluation is normal. Semen analysis reveals density 84 million/mL and globozoospermia. The next step is:

   a. repeat semen analysis.

   b. clomiphene citrate, 50 mg every other day.

   c. in vitro fertilization after incubation of sperm with pentoxifylline.

   d. intracytoplasmic sperm injection with ejaculated sperm.

   e. microsurgical testis sperm extraction.

31. The most common genetic cause of male infertility is:

   a. r(Y).

   b. 45,X0.

   c. 47,XXY.

   d. 47,XYY.

   e. 46,XY/47,XXY.

32. The biological system responsible for protecting haploid male germ cells from the immune system is:

   a. IgG.

   b. PSA.

   c. natural killer cells.

   d. reactive oxygen species.

   e. Sertoli cell tight junctions.

33. A man presents with azoospermia. Testis longitudinal axis is 3.0 cm bilaterally, and the testes are soft. Laboratory evaluation reveals testosterone 140 ng/dL, LH less than 1.0 IU/L, and FSH less than 1.0 IU/L. The next step is:

   a. repeat semen analysis.

   b. transrectal ultrasound.

   c. microsurgical testis sperm extraction.

   d. smell test.

   e. Y-chromosomal microdeletion assay.

34. A man presents with erectile dysfunction and azoospermia. Testis longitudinal axis is 5 cm bilaterally, and the testes are firm. Laboratory evaluation reveals bioavailable testosterone 150 ng/dL and prolactin 42 μg/L. The next step is:

   a. repeat prolactin.

   b. bromocriptine, 2.5 mg orally per day.

   c. cabergoline, 0.25 mg orally twice a week.

   d. clomiphene citrate, 50 mg orally every other day.

   e. cranial magnetic resonance imaging.

35. Laboratory values associated with androgen receptor insensitivity include:

   a. significantly elevated testosterone, LH, and FSH.

   b. mildly elevated testosterone, LH, and FSH.

   c. significantly elevated testosterone, mildly elevated LH, and normal FSH.

   d. decreased testosterone, and elevated LH and FSH.

   e. decreased testosterone, LH, and FSH.

36. The most common mutation in the cystic fibrosis transmembrane conductance region, or CFTR, is:

   a. R117H.

   b. R334W.

   c. R347P.

   d. ΔF508.

   e. G542X.

37. A man presents with a palpable right-sided varicocele of 3 months onset and no varicocele palpable on the left side. Testis longitudinal axis is 5 cm bilaterally, and a semen analysis reveals volume 2.0 mL, density 33 million/mL, and motility 38%. The next step is:

   a. semen analysis with strict morphology.

   b. renal ultrasound.

   c. CFTR testing.

   d. right varicocelectomy.

   e. bilateral varicocelectomy.

38. Electroejaculation is planned for a man with anejaculation due to spinal cord injury at T5. Treatment should include monitoring and therapy before the procedure with oral:

   a. lisinopril.

   b. nifedipine.

   c. pseudoephedrine.

   d. captopril.

   e. ciprofloxacin.

39. A couple desires children. Semen analysis reveals volume 2.2 mL, density 58 million/mL, and motility 18%, and all sperm have enlarged heads with multiple tails. The next step is:

   a. testis biopsy.

   b. scrotal ultrasound.

   c. repeat semen analysis.

   d. intrauterine insemination with donor sperm.

   e. in vitro fertilization with intracytoplasmic sperm injection.

ANSWERS

1. **e. 4/5.** Cumulative pregnancy rates in a well-conducted study were 38% at one cycle, 68% at three cycles, 81% at six cycles, and 92% at 12 cycles (Gnoth et al., 2003).*

2. **a. Daily.** Although prior recommendations specified intercourse every other day to optimize the probability of conception, a recent study demonstrated that intercourse every day around the time of ovulation is likely the best strategy (Scarpa et al., 2007).

3. **c. Age 35 years.** Whereas women in developing nations may experience a rapid decline in fecundity at a younger age, in the industrialized world, female fecundity declines precipitously after age 35 years (Balasch and Gratacós, 2012).

4. **e. Lisinopril.** All agents listed are spermatotoxins except lisinopril, which may improve bulk seminal parameters (Mbah et al., 2012).

5. **d. Substitute sulfasalazine with mesalazine.** Sulfasalazine is associated with oligoasthenospermia (Stein and Hanauer, 2000). If sulfasalazine is substituted with mesalazine, adverse effects on sperm are generally reversible (Riley et al., 1987).

6. **e. Observation.** Limited seminal concentrations of the majority of bacteria including *E. coli* have minimal or no effects on sperm motility in vivo (Diemer et al., 2003; Lackner et al., 2006).

7. **a. None.** HIV does not appear to be correlated with a direct negative effect on sperm function (Garrido et al., 2005).

8. **c. 7.5 Gy.** The probability of future fatherhood is significantly decreased with radiation doses to the testes of 7.5 Gy and above (Green et al., 2010). The testis does not need to be directly exposed for adverse spermatogenic effects to occur.

9. **d. 2 to 4° C.** Unlike female gonads, the testes are extracorporeal and subject to thermal regulation by a vascular heat exchange mechanism and muscular activity controlling proximity to the body, resulting in a scrotal temperature maintained between 2° and 4° C. below body core temperature (Setchell, 1998; Thonneau et al., 1998).

10. **e. Bilateral orchidopexy.** The most significant feature affecting this man's reproductive potential is bilateral cryptorchidism. Although the likelihood of improving fertility is hampered by his advanced age, no value will be derived from waiting. Testis biopsy is unnecessary, and his total testosterone is adequate. In this patient with distal cryptorchidism who does not desire offspring presently, removing the spermatotoxic insult of cryptorchidism is the most prudent course.

11. **c. Pre-Seed.** Nearly all lubricants are spermatotoxic, including saliva. In a study of a variety of lubricants, Pre-Seed did not result in a significant decrease in sperm motility or chromatin integrity (Agarwal et al., 2008).

12. **Row b.** In obese males, serum testosterone is decreased (Hammoud et al., 2006). SHBG is typically reduced, likely because of increased circulating insulin (Hammoud et al., 2006; 2008; Pauli et al., 2008; Teerds et al., 2011). Estradiol is increased because of peripheral conversion from testosterone by an overabundance of adipose cells containing the enzyme aromatase (Aggerholm et al., 2008; Chavarro et al., 2010; Hammoud et al., 2006, 2010; Hofny et al., 2010).

13. **c. A testis longitudinal axis as measured by caliper orchidometer less than 4.6 cm.** A measurement of the long axis of the testis of 4.6 cm or less is associated with spermatogenic impairment (Schoor et al., 2001).

14. **b. Renal ultrasound.** Renal agenesis is noted in 11% of men with congenital bilateral absence of the vas deferens (Schlegel et al., 1996).

15. **a. Aging.** Concentration of SHBG increases with age, resulting in decreased bioavailable testosterone (Bhasin et al., 2010).

16. **b. Testis long axis on physical examination 4.3 cm, FSH assay, 10 IU/L.** If the FSH assay result is 7.6 IU/L or less and the testis long axis is greater than 4.6 cm, the probability of obstruction is 96%; conversely, if the FSH values is greater than 7.6 IU/L and the testis long axis 4.6 cm or less, the probability that azoospermia is due to spermatogenic dysfunction is 89% (Schoor et al., 2001).

17. **c. 48 million/mL.** By classification and regression tree analysis, or CART, one large study demonstrated that for sperm concentration, 13.5 million/mL was found to be the lower parameter below which intrauterine insemination (IUI) success would be unlikely, and 48.0 million/mL was identified as the upper parameter above which IUI outcomes were favorable (Guzick et al., 2001).

18. **d. Spinal cord injury.** The ejaculate is normally white or light gray. A brown hue is often observed in spinal cord–injured men (Centola, 2011; World Health Organization, 2010).

19. **a. 1.** A single day of abstinence is optimal for assessing bulk seminal parameters (Elzanaty, 2008; Levitas et al., 2005).

20. **c. Postejaculatory urinalysis.** The differential diagnosis of seminal hypovolemia includes retrograde ejaculation, ejaculatory ductal obstruction, and accessory sex gland hypoplasia. The simplest and least invasive test to exclude a diagnosis of retrograde ejaculation is postejaculatory urinalysis, and this should be performed first.

21. **b. Reassurance.** This man's bulk seminal parameters are adequate with the exception of morphology. The variety of abnormal forms excludes rare genetic conditions such as failure of formation of the acrosomal cap. The assessing technician likely overread abnormal forms, and the patient should be reassured.

22. **a. Vital stain.** In cases of complete asthenospermia, assessment of antisperm antibodies with the immunobead assay is not possible, as it requires some motile sperm. The first diagnosis to exclude is necrospermia, which may be investigated with a vital stain.

23. **b. Papanicolaou staining.** Leukocytes and immature germ cells are not differentiable with light microscopy. A simple stain such as Papanicolaou allows the two to be distinguished (World Health Organization, 2010).

24. **a. Terminal deoxynucleotidyl transferase dUTP nick end labeling (TUNEL) assay.** Direct measures of sperm DNA fragmentation include the TUNEL assay and the comet assay at neutral pH. The other assays listed include denatured DNA (Sakkas and Alvarez, 2010).

25. **d. Sperm penetration assay.** To simulate incubational in vitro fertilization, human sperm are incubated with denuded hamster ova in the sperm penetration assay, or SPA (Margalioth et al., 1986; Yanagimachi et al., 1976).

26. **c. Electron microscopy.** Vital stain excluded necrospermia in this patient with complete asthenospermia. Electron microscopy will identify ultrastructural tail defects if present in the immotile cilia syndrome (Zini and Sigman, 2009).

27. **c. CFTR analysis of his wife.** Should the wife of this azoospermic man with a severe CFTR mutation harbor a severe mutation as well, a child born from surgically extracted sperm and intracytoplasmic sperm injection may be homozygous for a severe mutation and have clinical cystic fibrosis. In order to counsel the couple regarding the probability of that result, CFTR analysis of the wife is indicated.

28. **e. Testis sperm extraction and cryopreservation.** This man's normal physical examination and relatively low FSH indicates a high likelihood of adequate spermatogenesis and obstructive azoospermia. The lack of seminal vesicle dilation suggests that the probability of ejaculatory ductal obstruction is low. The next step is surgical sperm retrieval.

29. **d. Microsurgical testis sperm extraction.** With the FSH assay result greater than 7.6 IU/L and the testes long axis measurements of 4.6 cm or less, the probability that azoospermia is due to spermatogenic dysfunction is 89% (Schoor et al., 2001). The next step is microsurgical testis sperm extraction.

30. **d. Intracytoplasmic sperm injection with ejaculated sperm.** In globozoospermia, the sperm lack acrosomal caps, and sperm heads are rendered spheric rather than ovoid. Without the

---

*Sources referenced can be found in *Campbell-Walsh Urology, 11th Edition*, on the Expert Consult website.

acrosome, fertilization with sperm in the natural setting or with incubational in vitro fertilization will not be successful. Intracytoplasmic sperm injection is required. Ejaculated sperm is available in this patient, and surgical sperm extraction is consequently unnecessary.

31. **c. 47,XXY.** The presence of a supernumerary X chromosome in 47,XXY, or Klinefelter syndrome, is the most common genetic cause of male infertility (Groth et al., 2013; Oates and Lamb, 2009; Sigman, 2012).

32. **e. Sertoli cell tight junctions.** The haploid male gamete expresses different surface antigens than other diploid cells and is protected from the immune system by tight junctions between Sertoli cells (Walsh and Turek, 2009).

33. **d. Smell test.** Anosmia associated with hypogonadotropic hypogonadism is known as Kallmann syndrome (Kallmann and Schoenfeld, 1944). In a patient with significantly low gonadotropin assay results, the presence of the syndrome is confirmed by a smell test.

34. **a. Repeat prolactin.** Prolactin is a labile assay. Before continuing with further diagnostic assessment or therapy, moderately elevated assay results should first be confirmed with a second test.

35. **c. Significantly elevated testosterone, mildly elevated LH, and normal FSH.** Male infertility associated with androgen receptor insensitivity is characterized by increased testosterone, increased estradiol, increased LH to variable degrees, and typical FSH levels (Sokol, 2009).

36. **d. ΔF508.** The most common CFTR mutation is ΔF508, which is severe (Hampton and Stanton, 2010).

37. **b. Renal ultrasound.** Solitary right varicoceles are rare. Should one be of abrupt onset, renal pathology such as tumor should be considered (Masson and Brannigan, 2014).

38. **b. Nifedipine.** Ejaculatory stimulation for men with spinal cord injuries at a level of T6 or above may result in autonomic dysreflexia, which can be addressed before stimulation by treatment with nifedipine and during the procedure with monitoring of cardiac activity and blood pressure (Brackett et al., 2009; Phillips et al., 2014).

39. **d. Intrauterine insemination with donor sperm.** Because of the high rate of aneuploidy in sperm associated with macrocephaly and multiple tails, intracytoplasmic sperm injection with biological gametes is not recommended (Machev et al., 2005; Perrin et al., 2012; Sun et al., 2006).

CHAPTER REVIEW

1. Human spermatogenesis requires 64 days to complete and 5 to 10 days of epididymal transit time.
2. 5-α reductase inhibitors have a limited effect on spermatogenesis.
3. Cannabis decreases plasma testosterone; heavy alcohol use increases the conversion of testosterone to estradiol.
4. DNA damage can be detected up to 2 years following chemotherapy.
5. Following torsion of the testis, 11% of men develop antisperm antibodies.
6. Testis size correlates well with sperm production.
7. Patients with bilateral absence of the vas should be evaluated for a cystic fibrosis gene mutation.
8. Varicoceles are present in 15% of the adult population but occur in 30% to 50% of men presenting with fertility problems.
9. Normal semen volume is between 1 and 5 mL.
10. Progressive motility should be between 32 and 63%.
11. Antisperm antibodies are associated with vasectomy, testes trauma, orchitis, cryptorchidism, testis cancer, and varicocele.
12. Genetic testing should be considered in those with spermatogenic dysfunction causing azoospermia and in those with sperm densities of less than 5 million/mL.
13. The AZF factor is found on the long arm of the Y chromosome; the DAZ genes are located in the AZFc region. A microdeletion of the AZFc region may result in spermatogenic impairment but not necessarily absence of spermatogenesis, but a microdeletion of the AZFa and AZFb regions generally result in absence of spermatogenesis.
14. Spermatogenesis may be highly focal in men with azoospermia so that a random biopsy may miss areas of sperm production.
15. Cumulative pregnancy rates in a well-conducted study were 38% at one cycle, 68% at three cycles, 81% at six cycles, and 92% at 12 cycles.
16. Female fecundity declines precipitously after age 35 years.
17. Limited seminal concentrations of the majority of bacteria, including *E. coli*, have minimal or no effects on sperm motility in vivo.
18. If the FSH assay result is 7.6 IU/L or less and the testis long axis is greater than 4.6 cm, the probability of obstruction is 96%. Conversely, if the FSH value is greater than 7.6 IU/L and the testis long axis 4.6 cm or less, the probability that azoospermia is due to spermatogenic dysfunction is 89%.
19. A sperm concentration of 13.5 million/mL has been found to be the lower parameter below which IUI success is unlikely, and 48.0 million/mL is identified as the upper parameter above which IUI outcomes are favorable.
20. A single day of abstinence is optimal for assessing bulk seminal parameters.
21. The differential diagnosis of seminal hypovolemia includes retrograde ejaculation, ejaculatory ductal obstruction, and accessory sex gland hypoplasia.
22. Leukocytes and immature germ cells are not differentiable with light microscopy. A simple stain such as Papanicolaou allows the two to be distinguished.
23. Direct measures of sperm DNA fragmentation include the terminal deoxynucleotidyl transferase dUTP nick end labeling, or TUNEL.
24. To simulate incubational in vitro fertilization, human sperm are incubated with denuded hamster ova in the sperm penetration assay, or SPA.
25. In globozoospermia, the sperm lack acrosomal caps, and sperm heads are rendered spheric rather than ovoid. Without the acrosome, fertilization with sperm in the natural setting or with incubational in vitro fertilization will not be successful.
26. Klinefelter syndrome is the most common genetic cause of male infertility.
27. Male infertility associated with androgen receptor insensitivity is characterized by increased testosterone, increased estradiol, increased LH to variable degrees, and typical FSH levels.
28. Solitary right varicoceles are rare. Should one be of abrupt onset, renal pathology such as tumor should be considered.

25 Surgical Management of Male Infertility

Marc Goldstein

QUESTIONS

1. Which of the following venous structures are intentionally preserved during varicocelectomy?
   a. External spermatic veins
   b. Internal spermatic veins
   c. Gubernacular veins
   d. Deferential (vasal) veins
   e. Cremasteric veins

2. In the evaluation for vasectomy reversal, which clinical finding is suggestive of epididymal obstruction?
   a. Varicocele
   b. Hydrocele
   c. Sperm granuloma
   d. Normal serum follicle-stimulating hormone (FSH) level
   e. Vasal gap larger than 2 cm

3. Which of the following is NOT an indication for crossed vasovasostomy?
   a. Right: inguinal vas obstruction and normal testis; left: patent vas and atrophic testis
   b. Right: epididymal obstruction, patent vas, and normal testis; left: ejaculatory duct obstruction and normal testis
   c. Right: inguinal vas obstruction and normal testis; left: epididymal obstruction, patent vas, and normal testis
   d. Right: epididymal obstruction and patent vas above vasectomy site; left: sperm in testicular end of vas and vasectomy site in convoluted vas
   e. Right: congenital absence of epididymis and normal patent vas; left: normal testis and partial absence of vas ending retroperitoneally

4. Compared with the other surgical options for varicocelectomy, the advantages of performing a subinguinal microsurgical varicocelectomy include all of the following EXCEPT:
   a. lower rate of arterial injury.
   b. lower rate of postoperative hydrocele.
   c. lower rate of varicocele recurrence.
   d. fewer veins ligated.
   e. lower overall complication rate.

5. Which maneuvers should be avoided when bridging a large vasal gap during vasovasostomy?
   a. Mobilization of the vas deferens toward the external inguinal ring
   b. Dissection of the sheath of the convoluted vas deferens off the epididymis and allowing the testis to drop upside-down
   c. Separation of the cauda and corpus epididymis from the testis
   d. Mobilization of the vas deferens toward the internal inguinal ring
   e. Unraveling of the convoluted vas deferens

6. In which of the following scenarios is a testis biopsy least helpful?
   a. Failure to retrieve motile sperm from the epididymis
   b. Sperm retrieval for nonobstructive azoospermia
   c. Diagnostic evaluation of men with congenital absence of vas and normal FSH levels
   d. Diagnostic evaluation in azoospermic men with normal findings on scrotal examination and normal serum testosterone and FSH levels
   e. Sperm retrieval for men diagnosed with Sertoli cell–only pattern in the testes

7. Which of the following scenarios has the lowest rate for sperm return to ejaculate after vasectomy reversal?
   a. Motile sperm in the vas and vasovasostomy
   b. Nonmotile sperm in the vas and vasovasostomy
   c. Motile sperm in the vas and unilateral crossed vasovasostomy
   d. Thick, white vasal fluid devoid of sperm and vasovasostomy
   e. Copious clear vasal fluid but no sperm and vasovasostomy

8. In the evaluation for azoospermia, all of the following tests should be considered to confirm a diagnosis of obstructive azoospermia EXCEPT:
   a. transrectal ultrasonography.
   b. testicular biopsy.
   c. serum antisperm antibody assay.
   d. epididymal biopsy.
   e. serum testosterone and FSH assay.

9. Which of the following is TRUE regarding varicocele?
   a. Treatment in infertile men rarely results in improved semen parameters.
   b. Severity of testicular insult is related to the size of the varicoceles.
   c. Severity of testicular insult from varicocele is duration independent.
   d. Because of the severity of testicular insult, repair of large varicoceles is not warranted.
   e. Surgical treatment of subclinical varicoceles results in greater improvement in semen quality than treatment of large varicoceles.

10. After a bilateral vasoepididymostomy, a patient remained azoospermic in two semen analyses until 6 months postoperative, when the analysis revealed 8 million sperm/mL with 60% motility. What is the next management step?
    a. A plan for intrauterine insemination with ejaculated sperm
    b. A plan for assisted reproduction with intracytoplasmic sperm injection (ICSI) and ejaculated sperm
    c. Cryopreservation of semen
    d. No follow-up necessary
    e. Scrotal ultrasound

11. Which of the following is a disadvantage of the intussusception vasoepididymostomy?

    a. Inability to assess epididymal fluid for sperm before setting up for anastomosis

    b. Lower patency rate than end-to-side techniques

    c. Difficult hemostasis

    d. Placement of sutures into a collapsed epididymal tubule

    e. Transection of the epididymis required before anastomosis

12. All of the following situations are appropriate for assisted reproduction with ICSI as a first line of treatment EXCEPT:

    a. obstruction with multiple failures of reconstruction.

    b. mild oligoasthenospermia with varicoceles and a female partner of 29 years of age.

    c. Klinefelter syndrome.

    d. only a few viable sperm found in the ejaculate.

    e. postchemotherapy azoospermia.

13. In which of the following settings are vasovasostomy and vasoepididymostomy contraindicated?

    a. Previous vasectomy more than 20 years ago

    b. Concomitant scrotal pain

    c. Concomitant hydrocele

    d. Concomitant varicoceles

    e. Nonobstructive azoospermia

14. In the presence of epididymal obstruction, which of the following statements is FALSE?

    a. The quality of sperm is better in caput than caudal tubules.

    b. Vasoepididymostomy to the caudal tubules has a better patency rate than to the caput tubules.

    c. Vasovasostomy can yield a satisfactory patency rate.

    d. A scrotal sonogram may demonstrate epididymal fullness and hydrocele.

    e. Intraoperative sperm cryopreservation is possible.

15. Which of the following statements is FALSE regarding microsurgical testicular sperm extraction?

    a. Sertoli cell–only pattern is a contraindication for the procedure.

    b. Large seminiferous tubules typically give a higher sperm yield.

    c. It is best performed percutaneously.

    d. It can better preserve the blood supply to testis parenchyma than a nonmicrosurgical wound.

    e. It should be used in men with nonobstructive azoospermia.

16. All of the following are expected outcomes of varicocele repair EXCEPT:

    a. improved sperm motility.

    b. increased risk of multiple gestation.

    c. improved sperm counts.

    d. elevated serum testosterone levels.

    e. return of sperm to the ejaculate in azoospermic men.

17. A 30-year-old man presenting with primary infertility was found to be azoospermic on two semen analyses. For which of the following findings is a diagnostic biopsy indicated?

    a. Ejaculate volume below 2 mL with negative fructose

    b. Semen pH less than 7.2

    c. Palpable vasa, normal serum FSH, normal testis volume, and negative antisperm antibodies

    d. Serum FSH of 25 IU/L and 12-mL soft testis

    e. Absence of vasa deferentia and normal serum FSH level

18. In which of the following scenarios is a vasogram indicated?

    a. Azoospermia, Sertoli cell only on testis biopsy

    b. Azoospermia, testicular volume of 10 mL, FSH value 25 IU/L

    c. Azoospermia, normal testicular volume, biopsy revealing active spermatogenesis

    d. Azoospermia, no palpable vasa deferential

    e. Sperm count 5 million/mL, 5% motility, grade 2 varicoceles bilaterally

19. All of the following diagnoses can be made from a radiocontrast vasogram EXCEPT:

    a. inguinal vasal obstruction.

    b. ejaculatory duct obstruction.

    c. seminal vesicle agenesis.

    d. spermatogenic failure.

    e. partial agenesis of vasa deferentia.

20. All of the following are potential complications of transurethral resection of the ejaculatory ducts EXCEPT:

    a. urinary incontinence.

    b. retrograde ejaculation.

    c. recurrent epididymitis.

    d. testicular atrophy.

    e. contamination of semen with urine.

21. What is the pathogenesis of postvaricocelectomy hydrocele?

    a. Increased testicular venous pressure

    b. Lymphatic obstruction

    c. Soft tissue fibrosis

    d. Arterial injury

    e. Catch-up growth of testes

22. Which of the following is TRUE regarding the ejaculatory duct?

    a. It is a single midline duct formed by the confluence of the seminal vesicle ducts.

    b. It enters into the middle of the verumontanum.

    c. It joins with the prostatic ducts.

    d. It is a paired duct formed by the confluence of each seminal vesicle duct and vasa deferentia.

    e. It enters directly into the vesicle trigone.

23. All of the following are potential complications of vasography EXCEPT:

    a. vasal obstruction at the site of vasography.

    b. perivasal hematoma.

    c. sperm granuloma at the site of vasography.

    d. injury to the vasal artery.

    e. retrograde ejaculation.

24. What is the estimated percentage of men who develop antisperm antibodies after vasectomy?

    a. 0% to 20%

    b. 20% to 40%

    c. 40% to 60%

    d. 60% to 80%

    e. 80% to 100%

25. Intraoperatively during a vasectomy reversal, a sperm granuloma is found on the left side. What does this indicate?

    a. Concomitant epididymal obstruction that requires a vasoepididymostomy

    b. Infection requiring postoperative antibiotics

c. The need for genetic counseling

d. That sperm will be found at the testicular end of the vas

e. That the procedure should be abandoned and the patient should undergo re-exploration in 3 months

26. When is the best time to perform vasography?

a. At the time of diagnostic testis biopsy

b. At the time of reconstruction, if a prior testis biopsy result was normal

c. At the time of scrotal ultrasonography with color flow Doppler

d. At the time of transrectal ultrasonography revealing normal seminal vesicles

e. At the time of electroejaculation

27. Twelve years after vasectomy, a man was found on routine examination to have asymptomatic sperm granulomas bilaterally. All of the following scenarios are true EXCEPT:

a. Microrecanalization is possible with the appearance of rare sperm in the ejaculate.

b. If vasectomy reversal is performed, only bilateral vasovasostomy is likely to be necessary.

c. The epididymides are unlikely to be indurated.

d. The epididymides are likely to be obstructed.

e. No treatment is necessary for asymptomatic sperm granuloma.

28. A midline cyst compressing the ejaculatory duct is found on a transrectal ultrasonographic scan. What does the presence of sperm in the cyst aspirate suggest?

a. Congenital absence of vas on at least one side

b. Nonobstructive azoospermia

c. Bilateral epididymal obstruction

d. The possibility of XXY karyotype

e. Patency of a vas deferens and epididymis on at least one side

29. After transurethral resection of the ejaculatory ducts, the patient develops retrograde ejaculation. What is the next step of management?

a. Watchful waiting

b. Intrauterine insemination

c. ICSI

d. A trial of pseudoephedrine

e. Electroejaculation

30. One year after vasovasostomy, a progressive decline in sperm motility and sperm counts is noted. What does this indicate?

a. Progressive spermatogenic failure

b. Infection

c. Arterial injury to the testis and epididymis

d. Ejaculatory duct obstruction

e. Stricture of the vasovasostomy

31. In which of the following scenarios would a diagnostic testicular biopsy provide valuable clinical information?

a. Men with azoospermia, atrophic testes, and an FSH level of 25 IU/L

b. Men with a 47,XXY karyotype

c. Men with a fecundity history who seek vasectomy reversal

d. Men with primary infertility, azoospermia, normal physical examination findings, and a normal serum FSH level

e. Men with anejaculation caused by high spinal cord injury

32. Which of the following is TRUE regarding retractile testes in adults?

a. As in the pediatric population, surgical repair is never indicated.

b. A dartos pouch operation is the treatment of choice.

c. Simple three-stitch orchiopexy of the tunica albuginea to the dartos, as for torsion prophylaxis, is effective in preventing retraction.

d. Bilateral orchiopexy is necessary for unilateral retractile testis.

e. Torsion of the testis is a common complication.

33. Which of the following is TRUE regarding vasoepididymostomy?

a. End-to-side anastomosis currently has the highest patency rate.

b. Microsurgical technique does not significantly improve the surgical outcome.

c. Assisted reproduction with ICSI is a more cost-effective option.

d. It should be reserved for azoospermia patients with spermatogenic arrest.

e. It should be performed only on an epididymal tubule containing sperm.

34. When a vasoepididymostomy is performed for fertility reasons, which of the following should be routinely done in the same setting?

a. Intraoperative epididymal sperm aspiration for sperm cryopreservation

b. Testicular biopsy for sperm cryopreservation

c. A touch preparation of testicular tissue

d. A squash preparation of testicular tissue

e. A radiocontrast vasogram

35. Which of the following is the most important factor in ensuring a high patency rate after a vasovasostomy?

a. Age of the patient

b. Time since vasectomy

c. Surgeon's technique and experience

d. Presence of motile sperm in the vasal fluid

e. Presence of a sperm granuloma at the vasectomy site

36. Which of the following surgical sperm retrieval techniques is inappropriate for the clinical situation indicated?

a. Percutaneous epididymal sperm aspiration (PESA) for congenital absence of vas

b. Percutaneous testicular sperm aspiration (TESA) after failed vasoepididymostomy

c. Electroejaculation in a man with postretroperitoneal lymph node dissection for left testicular embryonal carcinoma

d. Microsurgical epididymal sperm aspiration (MESA) for spermatogenic maturation arrest

e. Testicular sperm extraction (TESE) in a man with azoospermia from chemotherapy

ANSWERS

1. **d. Deferential (vasal) veins.** All veins within the cord, with the exception of the vasal veins, are doubly ligated. Scrotal or gubernacular collateral veins have been demonstrated radiographically to be the cause of 10% of recurrent varicoceles. All external spermatic veins are identified and doubly ligated with

hemoclips and divided. The gubernaculum is inspected for the presence of veins exiting from the tunica vaginalis. These are either cauterized or doubly ligated.

2. **b. Hydrocele.** The presence of a hydrocele in the presence of excurrent ductal system obstruction is often associated with secondary epididymal obstruction. Surgeons attempting reconstruction should be aware of the possibility of the need for a vasoepididymostomy.

3. **d. Right: epididymal obstruction, patent vas above vasectomy site, and normal testis; left: sperm in testicular end vas and vasectomy site in convoluted vas.** Crossover is indicated in the following circumstances: (1) unilateral inguinal obstruction of the vas deferens associated with an atrophic testis on the contralateral side. A crossover vasovasostomy should be performed to connect a healthy testicle to the contralateral unobstructed vas. (2) Obstruction or aplasia of the inguinal vas or ejaculatory duct on one side and epididymal obstruction on the contralateral side. It is preferable to perform one anastomosis with a high probability of success (vasovasostomy) than two operations with a much lower chance of success such as unilateral vasoepididymostomy and contralateral transurethral resection of the ejaculatory ducts.

4. **d. Fewer veins ligated.** At the subinguinal level, significantly more veins are encountered, the artery is more often surrounded by a network of tiny veins that must be ligated, and the testicular artery has often divided into two or three branches, making arterial identification and preservation more difficult without using a microscope for the procedure.

5. **e. Unraveling of the convoluted vas deferens.** When large vasal gaps are present, a gauze-wrapped index finger is used to bluntly separate the cord structures from the vas. Blunt finger dissection through the external ring will free the vas to the internal ring if additional abdominal side length is necessary. These maneuvers will leave all the vasal vessels intact. When the vasal gap is extremely large, additional length can be achieved by dissecting the entire convoluted vas free of its attachments to the epididymal tunica, allowing the testis to drop upside-down. If the amount of the vas removed is so large that even these measures fail to allow a tension-free anastomosis, the incision can be extended to the internal inguinal ring, the floor of the inguinal canal cut, and the vas rerouted under the floor, as in a difficult orchiopexy. An additional 4 to 6 cm of length can be obtained by dissecting the epididymis off of the testis from the vasoepididymal junction to the caput epididymis. The superior epididymal vessels are left intact and provide adequate blood supply to the testicular end of the vas. With this combination of maneuvers, gaps up to 10 cm wide can be bridged. The convoluted vas should not be unraveled. This disturbs the blood supply at the anastomotic line.

6. **c. Diagnostic evaluation of men with congenital absence of vas and normal FSH levels.** Testis biopsy is indicated in azoospermic men with testes of normal size and consistency, palpable vasa deferentia, and normal serum FSH levels. Under these circumstances, biopsy will distinguish obstructive azoospermia from primary seminiferous tubular failure. In the testes of men with congenital absence of vasa, biopsy always reveals normal or at least some spermatogenesis, and biopsy is not necessary before definitive sperm aspiration and in-vitro fertilization (IVF) with ICSI.

7. **d. Thick, white vasal fluid devoid of sperm and vasovasostomy.** If the fluid expressed from the vas is found to be thick, white, water insoluble, and like toothpaste in quality, microscopic examination rarely reveals sperm. Under these circumstances, the tunica vaginalis is opened and the epididymis inspected. If clear evidence of obstruction is found (e.g., an epididymal sperm granuloma with dilated tubules above and collapsed tubules below), vasoepididymostomy is performed. When the surgeon is in doubt or is not experienced with vasoepididymostomy, vasovasostomy should be performed. However, only 15% of men with bilateral absence of sperm in the vasal fluid after barbotage and intensive search will have sperm return to the ejaculate after vasovasostomy.

8. **d. Epididymal biopsy.** Before surgical reconstruction of the reproductive tract is attempted, spermatogenesis in the patient should be evident. A testicular biopsy may be indicated to confirm the presence of spermatogenesis. Men with a low semen volume should have a transrectal ultrasonographic scan to alert one to the possibility of an additional ejaculatory duct obstruction. For serum and antisperm antibody studies, the presence of serum antisperm antibodies corroborates the diagnosis of obstruction and the presence of active spermatogenesis. At present, this test is of unknown prognostic value and is optional. For serum FSH assay, men with small, soft testes should have serum FSH measured. An elevated FSH level suggests impaired spermatogenesis and potentially a poorer prognosis.

9. **b. Severity of testicular insult is related to the size of the varicoceles.** Larger varicoceles appear to cause more damage than small varicoceles; large varicoceles are associated with greater preoperative impairment in semen quality than are small varicoceles.

10. **c. Cryopreservation of semen.** With the older end-to-end or end-to-side vasoepididymostomy method, at 14 months after surgery 25% of initially patent anastomoses have shut down. For this reason, we recommend banking sperm both intraoperatively and as soon as sperm appear in the ejaculate postoperatively.

11. **a. Inability to assess epididymal fluid for sperm before setting up for anastomosis.** This method, also known as the *triangulation technique*, was introduced by Berger. There are several advantages of this method versus previous techniques. Two or three sutures placed in the epididymal tubule provide four and six points of fixation, and the anastomosis is virtually bloodless. However, one cannot assess tubular fluid for sperm before the anastomosis setup.

12. **b. Mild oligoasthenospermia with varicoceles and a female partner of 29 years of age.** Assisted reproduction can be offered to men with surgically unreconstructable obstruction such as congenital absence of the vas deferens; men with few viable sperm in the ejaculate; azoospermic men with varicoceles (half of these men will respond to varicocelectomy with return of enough sperm to ejaculate to achieve pregnancy using IVF with ICSI); and men with nonobstructive azoospermia.

13. **e. Nonobstructive azoospermia.** Before surgical reconstruction of the reproductive tract is attempted, spermatogenesis in the patient should be evident. A prior history of natural fertility prevasectomy is usually adequate. In other cases, a testicular biopsy may be indicated to confirm the presence of spermatogenesis.

14. **c. Vasovasostomy can yield a satisfactory patency rate.** If clear evidence of obstruction is found, vasoepididymostomy is performed. When there is doubt or the physician is not experienced with vasoepididymostomy, vasovasostomy should be performed. However, only 15% of men with bilateral absence of sperm in the vasal fluid after barbotage and an intensive search will have sperm return to the ejaculate after vasovasostomy.

15. **c. It is best performed percutaneously.** The use of an operating microscope for standard open diagnostic testes biopsy allows identification of an area in the tunica albuginea free of blood vessels, minimizing the risk of injury to the testicular blood supply and allowing a relatively blood-free biopsy specimen.

16. **b. Increased risk of multiple gestation.** Varicocelectomy results in significant improvement in the findings of semen analysis in 60% to 80% of men. Reported pregnancy rates after varicocelectomy vary from 20% to 60%. A randomized controlled trial of surgery versus no surgery in infertile men with varicoceles revealed a pregnancy rate of 44% at 1 year in the surgery group versus 10% in the control group. In our series of 1500 microsurgical operations, 43% of couples were pregnant at 1 year and 69% at 2 years when couples with female factors were excluded. Microsurgical varicocelectomy results in return of sperm to the ejaculate in 50% of azoospermic men with palpable varicoceles. Repair of large varicoceles results in a

significantly greater improvement in semen quality than repair of small varicoceles. In addition, large varicoceles are associated with greater preoperative impairment in semen quality than are small varicoceles, and consequently overall pregnancy rates are similar regardless of varicocele size. Some evidence suggests that the younger the patient is at the time of varicocele repair, the greater the improvement after repair and the more likely the testis is to recover from varicocele-induced injury. Varicocele recurrence, testicular artery ligation, and postvaricocelectomy hydrocele formation are often associated with poor postoperative results. In infertile men with low serum testosterone levels, microsurgical varicocelectomy alone results in substantial improvement in serum testosterone levels.

17. **c. Palpable vasa, normal serum FSH, normal testis volume, and negative antisperm antibodies.** Men with a positive antisperm antibody assay are always obstructed, and a biopsy is not necessary. Men with elevated FSH levels and small, soft testes always have nonobstructive azoospermia.

18. **c. Azoospermia, normal testicular volume, biopsy revealing active spermatogenesis.** The absolute indications for vasography are azoospermia, plus complete spermatogenesis with many mature spermatids on testis biopsy and at least one palpable vas. Relative indications for vasography are severe oligospermia with normal testis biopsy, a high level of sperm-bound antibodies that may be due to obstruction, low semen volume, and poor sperm motility (partial ejaculatory duct obstruction).

19. **d. Spermatogenic failure.** Vasography should answer the questions: Are there sperm in the vasal fluid? Is the vas obstructed? If the testis biopsy reveals many sperm, then the absence of sperm in vasal fluid indicates obstruction proximal to the vasal site examined, most likely an epididymal obstruction. Vasography is done in this case with saline or indigo carmine to confirm the patency of the seminal vesicle end of the vas before vasoepididymostomy. Copious vasal fluid containing many sperm indicates vasal or ejaculatory duct obstruction, and formal contrast vasography is performed to document the exact location of the obstruction. Copious thick, white fluid without sperm in a dilated vas indicates secondary epididymal obstruction in addition to potential vasal or ejaculatory duct obstruction.

20. **d. Testicular atrophy.** Reflux of urine into the ejaculatory ducts, vas, and seminal vesicles occurs after a majority of resections. This can be documented by voiding cystourethrography or by measuring semen creatinine levels. Reflux can lead to acute and chronic epididymitis. Recurrent epididymitis often results in epididymal obstruction. The incidence of epididymitis after transurethral resection is probably underestimated. Symptomatic chemical epididymitis may occur from refluxing urine. If epididymitis is chronic and recurrent, vasectomy or even epididymectomy may be necessary. Even when care has been taken to spare the bladder neck, retrograde ejaculation is common after transurethral resection. Transurethral instrumentation can increase the risk of urethral stricture.

21. **b. Lymphatic obstruction.** Analysis of the protein concentration of hydrocele fluid indicates that hydrocele formation after varicocelectomy is due to lymphatic obstruction.

22. **d. It is a paired duct formed by the confluence of each seminal vesicle duct and vasa deferentia.** The ejaculatory ducts course between the bladder neck and the verumontanum and exit at the level of and along the lateral aspect of the verumontanum.

23. **e. Retrograde ejaculation.** Complications of vasography include stricture, injury to the vasal blood supply, hematoma, and sperm granuloma. Multiple attempts at percutaneous vasography using sharp needles can result in stricture or obstruction at the vasography site. Careless or crude closure of a vasotomy can also result in stricture and obstruction. Non–water-soluble contrast agents may also result in stricture and should not be employed for vasography. If the vasal blood supply is injured at the site of vasography, vasovasostomy proximal to the vasography site may result in ischemia, necrosis, and obstruction of the intervening segment of vas. A bipolar cautery should be used for meticulous hemostasis at the time of vasostomy to

prevent hematoma in the perivasal sheath. Leaky closure of a vasography site may lead to the development of a sperm granuloma, which can result in stricture or obstruction of the vas.

24. **d. 60% to 80%.** Systemic effects of vasectomy have been postulated. Vasectomy disrupts the blood-testis barrier, resulting in detectable levels of serum antisperm antibodies in 60% to 80% of men. Some studies suggest that the antibody titers diminish 2 or more years after vasectomy. Others suggest that these antibody titers persist. However, neither circulating immune complexes nor deposits are increased after vasectomy.

25. **d. That sperm will be found at the testicular end of the vas.** A sperm granuloma at the testicular end of the vas suggests that sperm have been leaking at the vasectomy site. This vents the high pressures away from the epididymis and is associated with a better prognosis for restored fertility regardless of the time interval since vasectomy.

26. **b. At the time of reconstruction, if a prior testis biopsy result was normal.** There is no need to perform vasography at the time of testis biopsy for azoospermia unless immediate reconstruction is planned and the touch or wet-preparation biopsy reveals mature sperm with tails. If performed carelessly, vasography can cause stricture or even obstruction at the vasography site, which can complicate subsequent reconstruction.

27. **d. The epididymides are likely to be obstructed.** Sperm granulomas form when sperm leak from the testicular end of the vas. Sperm are highly antigenic, and an intense inflammatory reaction occurs when sperm escape outside the reproductive epithelium. Sperm granulomas are rarely symptomatic. The presence or absence of a sperm granuloma at the vasectomy site seems to be of importance in modulating the local effects of chronic obstruction on the male reproductive tract. The sperm granuloma's complex network of epithelialized channels provides an additional absorptive surface that helps vent the high intraluminal pressure in the obstructed excurrent ducts. Numerous animal studies have correlated the presence or absence of sperm granuloma at the vasectomy site with the degree of epididymal and testicular damage. Species that always develop granulomas after vasectomy have minimal damage to the seminiferous tubules. Some studies of men undergoing vasectomy reversal have revealed somewhat higher success rates in men who have a sperm granuloma at the vasectomy site, whereas another large study has not. Although sperm granulomas at the vasectomy site are present microscopically in 10% to 30% of men undergoing reversal, it is likely that, given enough time, virtually all men develop sperm granulomas at the vasectomy site, the epididymis, or the rete testis. When chronic postvasectomy pain is localized to the granuloma, excision and occlusion of the vasa with intraluminal cautery usually relieve the pain and prevent recurrence. Men with postvasectomy congestive epididymitis may be relieved of pain by open-ended vasectomy designed to purposefully produce pressure, relieving sperm granuloma.

28. **e. Patency of a vas deferens and epididymis on at least one side.** The fine-needle aspirate is examined for sperm. If sperm are present, it means at least one vas and epididymis are patent.

29. **d. A trial of pseudoephedrine.** Pseudoephedrine (Sudafed), 120 mg orally, 90 minutes before ejaculation, may prevent retrograde ejaculation. If this is not successful, sperm can be retrieved from alkalinized urine and used for either intrauterine insemination or IVF with ICSI.

30. **e. Stricture of the vasovasostomy.** Late stricture and obstruction are disappointingly common. Progressive loss of sperm motility followed by decreasing counts indicates stricture.

31. **d. Men with primary infertility, azoospermia, normal physical examination findings, and a normal serum FSH level.** Testis biopsy is indicated in azoospermic men with testis of normal size and consistency, palpable vasa deferentia, and normal serum FSH levels.

32. **b. A dartos pouch operation is the treatment of choice.** When scrotal orchiopexy is performed for retractile testis, a dartos pouch operation should be performed. Simple suture orchiopexy of the tunica albuginea of the testis to the dartos, such as

is performed sometimes to prevent torsion, will not prevent retraction of these testes into the groin. Creation of a dartos pouch will keep the testis well down into the scrotum and permanently prevent retraction. This is also the most reliable and safest technique for the prevention of testicular torsion.

33. **e. It should be performed only on an epididymal tubule containing sperm.** Specific treatments for male factor infertility such as microsurgical reconstruction for obstructive azoospermia and varicocelectomy for impaired testes remain the safest and most cost-effective ways of managing infertile men. Microsurgical approaches allow accurate approximation of the vasal mucosa to that of a single epididymal tubule, resulting in marked improvement in the patency and pregnancy rates. If the level of obstruction is not clearly delineated, after the buttonhole opening is made in the tunica, a 70-μm diameter tapered needle from the 10 to 0 nylon microsuture is used to puncture the epididymal tubule, beginning as distal as possible, and fluid is sampled from the puncture site. When sperm are found, the puncture sites are sealed with microbipolar forceps, a new buttonhole is made in the epididymal tunica just proximally, and

the tubule is prepared as described previously. Patency rates with the intussusception technique can exceed 80%. With the classic end-to-side or older end-to-end method, the patency rate is about 70%, and 43% of men with sperm will impregnate their wives after a minimum follow-up of 2 years.

34. **a. Intraoperative epididymal sperm aspiration for sperm cryopreservation.** Once sperm are identified, they are aspirated into glass capillary tubes and flushed into media for cryopreservation.

35. **c. Surgeon's technique and experience.** The responsibilities assumed by the surgeon demand the utmost in judgment and skill. Many of the procedures described in this chapter are among the most technically demanding in all of urology. Acquisition of the skills required to perform them demands intensive laboratory training in microsurgery and a thorough knowledge of the anatomy and physiology of the male reproductive system.

36. **d. Microsurgical epididymal sperm aspiration (MESA) for spermatogenic maturation arrest.** MESA is indicated for men with normal spermatogenesis and unreconstructable obstruction such as congenital bilateral absence of the vas deferens.

CHAPTER REVIEW

1. If the vas is transected at two different locations, the intervening segment will likely fibrose because of lack of blood supply.
2. In repairing a hydrocele, the epididymis is often splayed, and one should leave a generous border around the epididymis to avoid injuring it.
3. When sperm are retrieved before any repair, it is prudent to cryopreserve some for future use, if necessary.
4. Following vasoepididymotomy, 50% to 85% of men will have sperm in the ejaculate; about half of these men will foster a pregnancy.
5. The indications for testicular sperm extraction are failure to find sperm in the epididymis and nonobstructive azoospermia.
6. During microsurgical testicular sperm extraction, larger tubules are more likely to yield sperm.
7. About 85% of patients following vasovasostomy will have sperm in their ejaculate; a little more than half will foster a pregnancy.
8. During vasovasostomy repeated failure to identify sperm in the vasal fluid usually means epididymal obstruction; however, 15% of men with bilateral absence of sperm in the fluid will have sperm return in the ejaculate.
9. Testis biopsy is indicated in azoospermic men with testes of normal size and consistency, palpable vasa deferentia, and normal serum FSH level.
10. Varicocelectomy results in significant improvement in the findings of semen analysis in 60% to 80% of men. Reported pregnancy rates after varicocelectomy vary from 20% to 60%.
11. Men with a positive antisperm antibody assay are always obstructed, and a biopsy is not necessary.
12. A sperm granuloma at the testicular end of the vas suggests a better prognosis for fertility.
13. Progressive loss of sperm motility followed by decreasing counts indicates stricture.

26 Physiology of Penile Erection and Pathophysiology of Erectile Dysfunction

Tom F. Lue

QUESTIONS

1. Penile prosthesis tends to extrude more on the:
   a. lateral surface.
   b. ventral surface.
   c. crura.
   d. glans.
   e. dorsal surface.

2. Accessory pudendal artery is most likely to arise from:
   a. external iliac artery.
   b. femoral artery.
   c. obturator artery.
   d. superior vesical artery.
   e. bulbourethral artery.

3. During a rigid erection, all the following statements are true EXCEPT:
   a. dilation of the arterioles and arteries.
   b. sinusoidal relaxation.
   c. corporal pressure increase (to several hundred millimeters of mercury).
   d. subtunical venous compression reducing venous outflow.
   e. relaxation of the ischiocavernosus muscles.

4. All of the following are neurotransmitters that promote sexual function EXCEPT:
   a. dopamine.
   b. acetylcholine.
   c. oxytocin.
   d. serotonin (5-HT).
   e. nitric oxide (NO).

5. All of the following statements are true EXCEPT:
   a. NO stimulates the production of cyclic guanosine monophosphate (cGMP).
   b. NO released by endothelial nitric oxide synthase (eNOS) contained in the terminals of the cavernous nerve initiates the erection process, whereas nitric oxide released from neuronal nitric oxide synthase (nNOS) in the endothelium helps maintain erection.
   c. Cyclic GMP activates protein kinase G, which in turn opens the potassium channels and closes the calcium channels.
   d. Low cytosolic calcium favors smooth muscle relaxation.
   e. The smooth muscle regains its tone when cGMP is degraded by phosphodiesterase.

6. All the following statements about testosterone are true EXCEPT:
   a. It enhances sexual interest.
   b. It increases the frequency of sexual acts.
   c. It increases the frequency of nocturnal erection.
   d. It increases visually stimulated erections.
   e. It increases bone density and lean body mass.

7. All the following antihypertensives DO NOT negatively affect erection EXCEPT:
   a. hydrochlorothiazide.
   b. terazosin.
   c. losartan.
   d. amlodipine.
   e. captopril.

8. All of the following are possible causes of erectile dysfunction (ED) in end-stage renal disease (ESRD) patients EXCEPT:
   a. low NO.
   b. neuropathy.
   c. low prolactin.
   d. atherosclerosis.
   e. depression.

9. All of the following statements are true EXCEPT:
   a. NO is the principal neurotransmitter mediating penile erection.
   b. Oxytocin is a potent inducer of erection when injected into the central nervous system.
   c. Central norepinephrine transmission has a positive effect on sexual function.
   d. $GABA_B$ receptors are pro-erectile.
   e. Cannabinoid CB1 receptor activation inhibits sexual function.

10. All the following statements about smooth muscle contraction are true EXCEPT:
    a. Myosin light chain phosphatase (MLCP) is a holoenzyme consisting of a type 1 phosphatase (PP1c), a myosin-targeting subunit (MYPT1), and a 20-kDa subunit of unknown function.
    b. MLCP inhibition may lead to enhanced smooth muscle contraction.
    c. Phosphorylation of the regulatory subunit of MLCP by Rho kinase inhibits phosphatase activity and enhances the contractile response.
    d. One of the mechanisms of increased intracellular Ca^{2+} is by permitting entry of extracellular Ca^{2+} through receptor-operated channels without a change in membrane potential.
    e. Latch state refers to a period of smooth muscle relaxation after prolonged contraction.

11. All of the following are true statements about NO EXCEPT:
    a. Synthesis of NO is catalyzed by NOS, which converts L-arginine and oxygen to L-citrulline and NO.
    b. Upregulation of nNOS expression has been found in the corpus cavernosum of aging and diabetic rats.

c. NOS exists as three isoforms in mammals: nNOS, inducible nitric oxide synthase (iNOS), and eNOS.

d. Gene transfer of nNOS or eNOS to the penis has been shown to augment erectile responses in aging rats.

e. Gene transfer of iNOS has enhanced intracavernous pressure.

12. All the following statements are true EXCEPT:

a. C-type natriuretic peptide (CNP) is the most potent natriuretic peptide and it relaxes the isolated cavernous smooth muscle by binding to NPR-B.

b. Protein kinase G-I (PKGI) may induce relaxation via activation of the plasma membrane Ca^{2+}-ATPase pump, inhibition of IP3 generation, inhibition of Rho-kinase, stimulation of MLCP, and phosphorylation of heat shock proteins.

c. Reduced penile adenosine levels are associated with priapism.

d. Calcitonin gene-related peptide is a potent vasodilator released from perivascular nerve fibers.

e. The erectogenic effects of PGE1 as a pharmaceutic agent have been extensively documented.

13. All of the following statements about ED are true EXCEPT:

a. Psychogenic ED is the most common form of ED.

b. 10% to 19% of cases of ED are neurogenic.

c. In cases of pelvic fracture, ED can be a result of cavernous nerve injury or vascular insufficiency or both.

d. There is a decrease in penile tactile sensitivity with increasing age.

e. In diabetics, impairment of neurogenic and endothelium-dependent relaxation results in inadequate NO release.

14. All of the following statements about arteriogenic ED are true EXCEPT:

a. Atherosclerotic or traumatic arterial occlusive disease can decrease the perfusion pressure and arterial flow to the sinusoidal spaces.

b. Common risk factors associated with arterial insufficiency include hypertension, hyperlipidemia, cigarette smoking, diabetes mellitus, blunt perineal or pelvic trauma, and pelvic irradiation.

c. Long-distance cycling is also a risk factor for vasculogenic and neurogenic ED.

d. Lesions in the pudendal arteries are less common in men with ED than in the general population of similar age.

e. Among men with coronary arterial disease, the prevalence of ED increases while the severity of coronary arterial lesions increases.

15. All of the following statements are true EXCEPT:

a. Aging is the single most important contributing factor to ED.

b. The aging process can affect the central regulatory mechanism, hormonal and neural function, and penile structure.

c. Diabetes mellitus and metabolic syndrome may affect multiple organ systems and cause premature aging of both central and peripheral structures and molecules that regulate erectile process.

d. Primary ED may be due to psychogenic cause, inexperience, congenital arterial insufficiency or abnormal venous channels.

e. Primary ED refers to a recently developed ED of unknown etiology.

ANSWERS

1. **b. Ventral surface.** The strength and thickness of the tunica correlate in a statistically significant fashion with location. The most vulnerable area is located on the ventral groove (between the 5 and 7 o'clock positions), where the longitudinal outer layer is absent; most prostheses tend to extrude here (Hsu et al, 1994).*

2. **c. Obturator artery.** Nehra and colleagues (2008) studied 79 consecutive patients with a history of ED and noted that 35% had an accessory pudendal artery, typically arising from the obturator artery. In these men, the accessory pudendal was the dominant blood supply in 54% and the only corporal blood supply in 11%.

3. **e. Relaxation of the ischiocavernosus muscles.** Sexual stimulation triggers release of neurotransmitters from the cavernous nerve terminals. This results in relaxation of these smooth muscles and the following events: (1) dilation of the arterioles and arteries by increased blood flow in both the diastolic and systolic phases; (2) trapping of the incoming blood by the expanding sinusoids; (3) compression of the subtunical venous plexuses between the tunica albuginea and the peripheral sinusoids, reducing venous outflow; (4) stretching of the tunica to its capacity, which occludes the emissary veins between the inner circular and outer longitudinal layers and further decreases venous outflow; (5) an increase in Po_2 (to about 90 mm Hg) and intracavernous pressure (around 100 mm Hg), which raises the penis from the dependent position to the erect state (the full-erection phase); and (6) a further pressure increase (to several hundred millimeters of mercury) can occur with reflex contractions of the ischiocavernosus muscles (rigid-erection phase) during sexual stimulation.

4. **d. Serotonin (5-HT).** General pharmacologic data indicate that 5-HT pathways inhibit copulation, but 5-HT may have both facilitory and inhibitory effects on sexual function, depending on the receptor subtype, the receptor location, and the species investigated (de Groat and Booth, 1993).

5. **b. NO released by endothelial nitric oxide synthase (eNOS) contained in the terminals of the cavernous nerve initiates the erection process, whereas nitric oxide released from neuronal nitric oxide synthase (nNOS) in the endothelium helps maintain erection.** The consensus is that NO derived from nNOS in the nitrergic nerves is responsible for the initiation whereby NO from eNOS contributes to the maintenance of smooth muscle relaxation and erection (Hurt et al, 2002).

6. **d. It increases visually stimulated erections.** Mulligan and Schmitt (1993) concluded that testosterone (1) enhances sexual interest; (2) increases the frequency of sexual acts; and (3) increases the frequency of nocturnal erection, but has little or no effect on fantasy-induced or visually stimulated erections.

7. **a. Hydrochlorothiazide.** Data from a large U.K. trial showed that twice as many men taking thiazides for mild hypertension reported ED than those treated with propranolol or placebo.

8. **c. Low prolactin.** Many of the effects of uremia can potentially contribute to the development of ED, including disturbance of the hypothalamic-pituitary-testis sex hormone axis, hyperprolactinemia, accelerated atheromatous disease, and psychologic factors (Ayub and Fletcher, 2000).

9. **d. $GABA_B$ receptors are pro-erectile.** γ-Aminobutyric acid (GABA) activity in the paraventricular nucleus of the hypothalamus (PVN) provides a mechanism to balance (inhibit) proerectile signaling.

10. **e. Latch state refers to a period of smooth muscle relaxation after prolonged contraction.** Smooth muscle has the ability

---

*Sources referenced can be found in *Campbell-Walsh Urology, 11th Edition*, on the Expert Consult website.

to maintain tension for prolonged periods with minimal energy expenditure. This efficiency has been termed the *latch* state and is critical for sustaining the "basal" tone of the smooth muscle.

11. **b. Upregulation of nNOS expression has been found in the corpus cavernosum of aging and diabetic rats.** Downregulation of nNOS expression has been found in the corpus cavernosum of aging rats (Carrier et al, 1997), castrated rats (Penson et al, 1996), and diabetic rats (Rehman et al, 1997).

12. **c. Reduced penile adenosine levels are associated with priapism.** Excessive adenosine accumulation in the penis, coupled with increased A(2B)R signaling, contributes to priapism in two independent lines of mutant mice.

13. **a. Psychogenic ED is the most common form of ED.** Previously, psychogenic impotence was believed to be the most common, thought to affect 90% of impotent men (Masters and Johnson, 1965). This belief has given way to the realization that ED is usually a mixed condition that may be predominantly functional or physical.

14. **d. Lesions in the pudendal arteries are less common in ED men than in the general population of similar age.** Erectile dysfunction and cardiovascular disease share the same risk factors such as hypertension, diabetes mellitus, hypercholesterolemia, and smoking (Feldman et al, 1994; Martin-Morales et al, 2001). Lesions in the pudendal arteries are much more common in ED men than in the general population of similar age. Interestingly, natural remission and progression do occur in a substantial number of men with erectile dysfunction. The association of body mass index with remission and progression, as well as the association of smoking and health status with progression, offer potential avenues for facilitating remission and delaying progression using lifestyle intervention (Travison et al, 2007).

15. **e. Primary ED refers to a recently developed ED of unknown etiology.** Primary ED refers to a lifelong inability to initiate and/or maintain erections beginning with the first sexual encounter. Although most cases are caused by psychologic factors, a small number of afflicted men do have a physical cause resulting from maldevelopment of the penis or the blood and nerve supply. Primary psychologic dysfunction is usually related to anxiety about sexual performance stemming from adverse childhood events, traumatic early sexual experience, or misinformation.

CHAPTER REVIEW

1. Intracorporal smooth muscle is contracted in the flaccid state due to intrinsic myogenic activity, adrenergic neurotransmission, and endothelium-derived contracting factors.

2. Sexual stimulation triggers release of neurotransmitters from the cavernous nerve terminals. This results in relaxation of the smooth muscles and (a) dilation of arteries; (b) trapping of incoming blood by the expanding sinusoids; (c) compression of the subtunical venous plexuses between the tunica albuginea and the peripheral sinusoids reducing venous outflow; (d) stretching of the tunica to capacity, which occludes the emissary veins; (e) an increase in PO_2; and (f) further pressure increases with contraction of the ischiocavernosus muscles.

3. The sympathetic system causes detumescence (norepinephrine is the neural transmitter).

4. Thiazide diuretics may be responsible for impotence. Drugs most commonly associated with ED are antiandrogens, antidepressants, and antihypertensives.

5. Luteinizing hormone-releasing hormone agonists result in the reduction of sexual desire in 70% of patients.

6. Sexual dysfunction is a common event after the induction of antiretroviral therapy.

7. The prevalence of ED is three times higher in diabetic men, occurs at an earlier age, and increases with the duration of the disease.

8. The metabolic syndrome consisting of glucose intolerance, insulin resistance, obesity, dyslipidemia, and hypertension increases the risk of ED.

9. About half of people with chronic renal failure have significant sexual dysfunction. Moreover, following transplantation about half continue to have ED.

10. Primary ED is a lifelong inability to initiate or maintain an erection. In most cases it is psychogenic, but in a small number it is due to maldevelopment of the penis and/or blood and nerve supply.

11. Aging is the single most important contributing factory to ED.

12. Endothelial dysfunction is the final common pathway to ED in patients with hyperlipidemia, diabetes mellitus, hypertension, and chronic renal failure.

13. The strength and thickness of the tunica are correlated in a statistically significant fashion with location. The most vulnerable area is located on the ventral groove (between the 5 and 7 o'clock positions), where the longitudinal outer layer is absent; most prostheses tend to extrude here.

14. Testosterone (1) enhances sexual interest; (2) increases the frequency of sexual acts; and (3) increases the frequency of nocturnal erection, but has little or no effect on fantasy-induced or visually stimulated erections.

15. ED is usually a mixed condition that may be predominantly functional or physical.

27 Evaluation and Management of Erectile Dysfunction

Arthur L. Burnett II

QUESTIONS

1. The best predictor for the development of erectile dysfunction (ED) is:
   a. young age.
   b. higher education.
   c. underweight status.
   d. passive cigarette smoke exposure.
   e. prediabetes.

2. "Goal-directed management" is justified in the modern management of ED because of:
   a. availability of etiology-specific diagnostic testing.
   b. availability of increasingly invasive therapies.
   c. availability of irreversible therapies.
   d. central role of the clinician in directing proper treatment.
   e. acceptance of treatment preferences by patient and partner.

3. The risk association of ED with cardiovascular events:
   a. has not been established.
   b. is established unidirectionally to inform ED risk.
   c. is established unidirectionally to inform cardiovascular disease risk.
   d. is established bidirectionally to inform ED and cardiovascular disease risks.
   e. is established in conjunction with carcinogenesis risk.

4. Recommendations for lifestyle modification for the patient with ED requires:
   a. stratification of cardiovascular risk.
   b. determination of high and moderate cardiovascular disease risk.
   c. cardiologic workup with diagnostic stress testing standardly.
   d. cardiologic medical treatment.
   e. basic medical assessment and health monitoring.

5. The characteristic that is typically associated with "organic" ED, in contrast with "psychogenic" ED, is:
   a. sudden loss of erections.
   b. situational erectile difficulty.
   c. erection responses on awakening.
   d. gradual decline in erectile ability.
   e. existence of an interpersonal relationship factor.

6. Self-administered ED questionnaires serve to:
   a. document responsiveness to treatment of ED.
   b. define the etiology of ED.
   c. indicate the objective severity of ED.
   d. distinguish the systemic type of ED (e.g., vascular, neurologic, endocrinologic).
   e. evaluate ED in research settings alone.

7. The best rationale for using specialized diagnostic testing is:
   a. to assess complex ED clinical presentations.
   b. as a requirement to direct ED treatment decisions.
   c. to ascertain a specific diagnosis underlying the ED presentation.
   d. to determine ED causation.
   e. to apply Grade A level evidence-based ED diagnostic tools.

8. Duplex ultrasonography of the penis is a reliable diagnostic test when:
   a. combining pharmacostimulation.
   b. assessing intrapenile vascular communications.
   c. combining intracavernous pressure measurements.
   d. assessing penile and suprapubic penile flow velocities.
   e. indexing results to brachial systolic blood pressures.

9. A vascular test required for a patient under consideration for penile revascularization surgery is:
   a. combined intracavernosal injection and stimulation.
   b. duplex ultrasonography.
   c. dynamic infusion cavernosometry and cavernosography.
   d. penile angiography.
   e. radioisotopic penography.

10. Increased sex hormone–binding globulin (SHBG) is associated with:
    a. elevated bioavailable testosterone.
    b. lowered bioavailable testosterone.
    c. unaltered bioavailable testosterone.
    d. elevated total testosterone.
    e. lowered total testosterone.

11. The efficacy of testosterone therapy is best judged by:
    a. restored diurnal pattern of hormone levels.
    b. normal reference range serum testosterone level.
    c. midrange serum testosterone level.
    d. normal score using hypogonadism questionnaires.
    e. hypogonadism symptomatic improvement.

12. At the penile tissue level, a pharmacologic mechanism to promote penile erection is via the promoting actions of:
    a. cyclic nucleotides.
    b. phosphodiesterases.

c. α₁ adrenergic agonists.

d. dopaminergic D_2 receptor agonists.

e. serotonergic receptor antagonists.

13. Intracavernosal pharmacotherapy is contraindicated for a patient with a clinical history of:

a. neurological condition.

b. cardiovascular disease.

c. diabetes.

d. priapism.

e. anticoagulant use.

14. An advantage of alprostadil among pharmacologic agents for intracavernosal pharmacotherapy is:

a. lower incidence of prolonged erection.

b. lower incidence of painful erection.

c. lower cost.

d. long-term half-life once reconstituted.

e. role in combination therapy.

15. The vacuum erection device is most advantageous for ED associated with:

a. veno-occlusive dysfunction.

b. glanular insufficiency.

c. postpriapism.

d. postexplantation of a penile prosthesis.

e. Peyronie disease.

16. In patients with ED, the vascular lesion addressed by arterial revascularization surgery is:

a. internal pudendal artery stenosis.

b. penile dorsal artery stenosis.

c. cavernosal artery stenosis.

d. penile deep dorsal venous incompetence.

e. internal pudendal venous incompetence.

ANSWERS

1. **d. Passive cigarette smoke exposure.** Predictors for the development of ED include older age, lower education, diabetes, cardiovascular disease (such as hypertension and stroke), cigarette smoke exposure (active and passive), and overweight condition.

2. **e. Acceptance of treatment preferences by patient and partner.** Goal-directed management serves to allow the patient or couple to make an informed selection of the preferred therapy for sexual fulfillment on understanding all treatment options after completing a thorough discussion with the treating clinician.

3. **d. Is established bidirectionally to inform ED and cardiovascular disease risks.** Epidemiologic studies have documented a bidirectional risk relationship for ED and cardiovascular disease. This bidirectional paradigm carries ramifications with regard to overall male health status.

4. **e. Basic medical assessment and health monitoring.** All patients presenting for ED management carry some level of cardiovascular risk. Lifestyle modifications such as increased physical activity and improved weight control apply to all patients in accordance with a full medical assessment and regular health monitoring.

5. **d. Gradual decline in erectile ability.** "Organic" ED typically is characterized by a gradual onset of the problem, along with incremental progression, global dysfunction, and poor/absent erections on awakening.

6. **a. Document responsiveness to treatment of ED.** Self-administered ED questionnaires have served to document the presence, subjective severity, and responsiveness of treatment of ED in both clinical and research settings. They do not distinguish an etiologic basis for ED, differentiate among various causes of ED, or indicate an objective severity of ED.

7. **a. To assess complex ED clinical presentations.** Specialized diagnostic testing offers to improve diagnostic accuracy, but it is not a standard requirement to proceed therapeutically. Its best role at this time applies to the ED specialist who may elect certain tests to be done in settings of complex clinical presentations.

8. **a. Combining pharmacostimulation.** The combination of pharmacostimulation or combined intracavernosal injection and stimulation to duplex ultrasonography validates the imaging component of this test by establishing hemodynamic properties of a functionally relevant erection response. The quantification of blood flow in the penis applies to the main vascular tributaries and includes the entire penis from the crura in the perineum to the tip.

9. **d. Penile angiography.** Definition of the anatomy and radiographic appearance of the iliac, internal pudendal, and penile arteries by penile angiography is necessary in order to perform penile revascularization surgery.

10. **b. Lowered bioavailable testosterone.** Bioavailable testosterone can be affected to some extent by alterations in the SHBG fraction in serum associated with factors that increase SHBG, thereby accounting for a decrease in bioavailable testosterone.

11. **e. Hypogonadism symptomatic improvement.** The objective of testosterone therapy for hypogonadism is symptomatic improvement. The efficacy is not judged by a precise testosterone determination, although standard practice is to provide therapy at a normative serum testosterone level.

12. **a. Cyclic nucleotides.** Cyclic guanosine monophosphate and cyclic adenosine monophosphate act to promote proerectile molecular mechanisms resulting in corporal smooth muscle relaxation.

13. **d. Priapism.** Intracavernosal pharmacotherapy is contraindicated for men with psychological instability, a history or risk for priapism, histories of severe coagulopathy or unstable cardiovascular disease, reduced manual dexterity, and use of monoamine oxidase inhibitors.

14. **a. Lower incidence of prolonged erection.** Perceived advantages of alprostadil for intracavernosal pharmacotherapy relative to other agents are lower incidences of prolonged erection, systemic side effects, and penile fibrosis. Disadvantages include a higher incidence of painful erection, higher cost, and shortened half-life once reconstituted.

15. **b. Glanular insufficiency.** The effect of vacuum erection device therapy involves engorgement of the entire penis including the glans penis, such that it provides an advantage to patients experiencing glanular insufficiency. Special uses for this therapy such as preserving the elasticity of penile tissue after priapism or penile prosthesis explantation or after surgical correction of Peyronie disease have been suggested.

16. **a. Internal pudendal artery stenosis.** The penile arterial anatomic defect correctable by arterial revascularization commonly involves stenosis of the internal pudendal artery following perineal or pelvic trauma.

CHAPTER REVIEW

1. The prevalence of ED in the adult male is 20% and is correlated with age.
2. Men with ED are 45% more likely than men without ED to experience a cardiac event within 5 years of diagnosis.
3. The International Index of Erectile Function (IIEF) questionnaire has five domains: erectile function, orgasmic function, sexual desire, intercourse satisfaction, and overall satisfaction.
4. Erections observed with nocturnal penile tumescence monitoring do not necessarily equate with erections sufficient for sexual performance.
5. Cavernous arterial insufficiency is suggested when peak systolic velocity is less than 25 cm/sec. A peak systolic velocity greater than 35 cm/sec defines normal cavernous arterial inflow.
6. Testosterone circulates as free, bound to albumin, and bound to SHBG. Free testosterone and albumin-bound testosterone comprise the bioavailable testosterone.
7. Testosterone production is circadian, with the peak occurring in the morning. To evaluate testosterone status, blood should be drawn in the morning (between 7 AM and 11 AM).
8. Penile revascularization is reserved for patients in whom it is most likely to be successful: patients with a history of perineal trauma, age younger than 55 years, nondiabetic, nonsmoker, no venous leak, and a documented stenotic lesion in the internal pudendal artery on angiography.
9. Endocrine conditions that may be associated with erectile dysfunction include hypogonadism, hyperthyroidism, and diabetes.
10. Induction of a penile erection requires release of nitric oxide from penile nerve endings and vascular endothelium.
11. Nitrate use in any form is an absolute contraindication for the use of phosphodiesterase type 5 (PDE5) inhibitors.
12. Penile rehabilitation following radical prostatectomy using PDE5 inhibitors has not proved efficacious.
13. The vasoactive drugs commonly injected to produce an erection include prostaglandin E, papaverine, and phentolamine.
14. Predictors for the development of ED include older age, lower education, diabetes, cardiovascular disease (such as hypertension and stroke), cigarette smoke exposure (active and passive), and overweight condition.
15. Intracavernosal pharmacotherapy is contraindicated for men with psychological instability, a history or risk for priapism, histories of severe coagulopathy or unstable cardiovascular disease, reduced manual dexterity, and use of monoamine oxidase inhibitors.

28 Priapism

Gregory A. Broderick

QUESTIONS

1. Ischemic priapism is a persistent erection marked by each of the following clinical and pathophysiologic characteristics EXCEPT:
   a. rigidity of the corpora cavernosa.
   b. bright red corporal blood.
   c. hypoxic and acidotic corporal environment.
   d. painful rigidity.
   e. thrombus within the sinusoidal spaces.

2. Each of the following are etiologies typically associated with ischemic priapism EXCEPT:
   a. sickle cell disease (SCD).
   b. straddle injury.
   c. cocaine use.
   d. spider bite.
   e. pharmacologic erection therapy.

3. SCD is a risk factor for ischemic priapism; the pathophysiologic mechanisms include each of the following EXCEPT:
   a. decreased content of hemoglobin S (HgbS) in the plasma.
   b. the polymerization of HgbS when deoxygenated.
   c. scavenging of nitric oxide.
   d. arginine catabolism removing substrate for nitric oxide (NO) synthesis.
   e. adhesive interactions among sickle cells, endothelial cells, and leukocytes.

4. Prolonged erection in males 40 years of age and older is usually attributed to:
   a. SCD.
   b. hematologic malignancy.
   c. erectile dysfunction (ED) pharmacotherapy.
   d. prostate cancer.
   e. testosterone supplementation.

5. Case reports have documented prolonged erections and, rarely, priapism in men by using phosphodiesterase type 5 (PDE5) inhibitor therapies. Associated risks for prolonged erection/priapism include each of the following EXCEPT:
   a. daily dosing.
   b. combination with intracavernous injection.
   c. history of penile trauma.
   d. psychotropic medications.
   e. narcotic use.

6. The associations and pathophysiology of high-flow priapism include each of the following EXCEPT:
   a. straddle injury.
   b. coital trauma.
   c. birth canal injury to the newborn male.
   d. cold-knife urethrotomy.
   e. hemodialysis.

7. The critical pathologic change occurring in the cavernosal tissue at 4 hours after the onset of ischemic priapism is:
   a. irreversible cavernous damage and ED.
   b. the beginning of glucopenia.
   c. the beginning of hypercoagulable thrombotic conditions.
   d. the deterioration of cavernous smooth muscle contractile responses.
   e. cavernous fibrosis.

8. The nitric oxide/cyclic guanosine monophosphate (cGMP) signaling pathway is implicated in the pathogenesis of priapism on the basis of scientific work showing:
   a. guanylate cyclase activity upregulation.
   b. guanylate cyclase activity downregulation.
   c. nitric oxide synthase activity upregulation.
   d. PDE5 activity upregulation.
   e. PDE5 activity downregulation.

9. An adolescent with SCD presents with a 6-hour erection. Initial cavernous blood gas results show Po_2 30 mm Hg, Pco_2 60 mm Hg, and pH 7.25. The first therapeutic step should be:
   a. oral terbutaline.
   b. oral pseudoephedrine.
   c. intracavernous aspiration.
   d. exchange transfusion.
   e. distal surgical shunt.

10. The characteristic blood flow defect of ischemic priapism found on color duplex ultrasonography is:
    a. normal cavernosal artery inflow.
    b. increased cavernosal artery inflow.
    c. decreased or absent cavernosal artery inflow.
    d. arteriovenous blush.
    e. sinusoidal fistula.

11. After initial intracavernous treatment for ischemic priapism, blood gas sampling produces an equivocal mixed-venous blood result. Priapism resolution is best confirmed by:
    a. color duplex ultrasonography.
    b. penile scintigraphy.
    c. corpus cavernosography.
    d. penile arteriography.
    e. pelvic computed tomography scan.

12. After a second session of intracavernous treatment consisting of aspiration/irrigation with phenylephrine administration, the priapic penis remains turgid. Cavernosal blood gas results are Po_2 40 mm Hg, Pco_2 50 mm Hg, and pH 7.35. The next step should be:
    a. observation.
    b. oral sympathomimetic.
    c. repeat intracavernous treatment.
    d. distal surgical shunt.
    e. proximal surgical shunt.

13. Phenylephrine is the preferred sympathomimetic used in the treatment of ischemic priapism because of its:

    a. α_1-selective activity.

    b. α_1 and α_2 activity.

    c. β_1-selective activity.

    d. β_2-selective activity.

    e. combined α and β activities.

14. The best indication for arterial embolization in the management of high-flow priapism is:

    a. unlikely spontaneous resolution.

    b. failure of sympathomimetic therapy.

    c. reduction of recurrent priapism risk.

    d. reduction of subsequent ED risk.

    e. patient preference to intervene.

15. Persistent penile rigidity after a technically successful proximal surgical shunt procedure in a patient with a 72-hour episode of ischemic priapism is an indication for:

    a. observation.

    b. gonadotropin-releasing hormone agonist therapy.

    c. pudendal artery ligation.

    d. distal surgical shunt.

    e. penile prosthesis surgery.

16. The mother of a child with SCD complains that her son has recently been awakening with erections lasting 3 to 4 hours. She is concerned that similar occurrences have been a warning sign for a major priapism. All of the following are appropriate management options EXCEPT:

    a. trial of nightly oral sympathomimetic drug.

    b. trial of low-dosage, daily PDE5 inhibitor.

    c. a gonadotropin-releasing hormone agonist or antiandrogen.

    d. intracavernous injection of phenylephrine in the morning.

17. Evidence-based studies of priapism therapies and outcomes are rare. A recent investigation of adult SCD patients presenting with ischemic priapism subjected all men to a standard protocol of aspiration and phenylephrine injections. Long-term sexual health function outcomes revealed complete ED in men with duration of priapism:

    a. less than 12 hours.

    b. 12 to 24 hours.

    c. longer than 36 hours.

    d. longer than 48 hours.

    e. longer than 72 hours.

18. An adult male presents with ischemic priapism of 8 hours duration. He fails to respond to serial aspiration and intracavernous injection after 4 hours in the emergency department. The recommended intervention at this time should be:

    a. hydration, nasal oxygen, and keeping the patient NPO for 8 hours to avoid risks of emergent intubation.

    b. a percutaneous distal penile shunt.

    c. an open distal shunt.

    d. an open proximal shunt.

    e. a saphenous vein shunt.

19. Radiographic imaging may be helpful in the diagnosis and management of priapism. Each of the following is correct EXCEPT:

    a. color Doppler ultrasound (CDU) in the evaluation of a persistent erection following treatments for ischemic priapism.

    b. penile arteriography to differentiate high-flow from ischemic priapism.

    c. magnetic resonance imaging (MRI) to diagnose corporal thrombus in men with refractory priapism or when there has been a significant delay in presentation.

    d. MRI in the differential diagnosis of corporal metastasis.

20. A 36-year-old tech entrepreneur is referred for a diagnosis of priapism after he slipped while climbing aboard his yacht. He initially had a saddle bruise on his perineum and pain; the next morning he awoke with persistent erection. The patient has a board of directors meeting at the end of the week and wants immediate treatment. The correct management strategy is:

    a. penile aspiration and α-adrenergic injection in the office or emergency department.

    b. penile arteriography.

    c. angio-embolization after a thorough discussion of chances for spontaneous resolution and risks of treatment-related ED.

    d. CDU-guided corporal exploration to ligate fistula.

    e. distal penile shunt.

21. Priapism associated with SCD is ischemic. The current pathophysiology is believed to be:

    a. obstruction of venous outflow by sickled erythrocytes.

    b. hemolysis and reduced nitric oxide.

    c. increased blood viscosity.

    d. a blood dyscrasia associated with reduced reticulocyte counts.

    e. dysregulated cavernous arterial inflow.

22. Ischemic priapism in boys and men with SCD should focus on correcting the hemoglobinathy:

    a. with exchange transfusions.

    b. with hydration, alkalinization, and oxygen.

    c. with aspiration and pharmacologic detumescence.

    d. with hydroxyurea.

    e. with analgesia and expectant management.

23. A 27-year-old previously healthy white male is brought into the emergency department in the early morning hours by his girlfriend. She describes a night of partying with alcohol, energy drinks, and a small amount of cocaine. Her boyfriend has had a persistent erection for 6 to 8 hours. She says, "I've done all I can to help him—it won't go down!" The emergency department doctor calls the urologist to go over the case and initiate management. The best course of therapy would be:

    a. baclofen, 20 mg PO followed every 6 hours until erection subsides.

    b. pseudoephedrine, 60 mg PO.

    c. inhaled terbutaline, 4 mg.

    d. oral terbutaline, 4 mg.

    e. corporal aspiration and injection of phenylephrine, 200 μg.

24. Phosphodiesterase type 5 inhibitors are first-line therapy for ED, but like intracavernous therapy, PDE5inhibitors have been associated with prolonged erection and priapism. Which agent is most likely to cause priapism?

    a. Sildenafil, 100 mg PRN sex

    b. Avanafil, 200 mg PRN sex

    c. Levitra, 20 mg PRN sex

    d. Cialis, 5 mg daily

    e. None of these agents is more likely to result in priapism.

25. Early reviews concluded that the natural history of ischemic priapism is ED. Recent interventions have tracked sexual health function outcomes with evidence-based questionnaires such as the International Index of Erectile Function (IIEF-5). Improvements in medical and surgical management of ischemic priapism may preserve erectile function. Unfortunately, ED is likely to occur if reversal by medical or surgical means is not successful after how many hours?

    a. 8 hours
    b. 12 to 24 hours
    c. 36 hours
    d. 48 hours
    e. 72 hours

ANSWERS

1. **b. Bright red corporal blood.** Ischemic priapism is a persistent erection marked by rigidity of the corpora cavernosa and little or no cavernous arterial inflow. In ischemic priapism there are time-dependent changes in the corporal metabolic environment with progressive hypoxia, hypercarbia, and acidosis. The patient typically complains of penile pain after 6 to 8 hours, and examination reveals a rigid erection. After 48 hours, thrombus can be found in the sinusoidal spaces and smooth muscle necrosis with fibroblast-like cell transformation is evident.

2. **b. Straddle injury.** Nonischemic priapism is much rarer than ischemic priapism, and the etiology is largely attributed to trauma. Forces may be blunt or penetrating, resulting in laceration of the cavernous artery or one of its branches within the corpora. The etiology most commonly reported is a straddle injury to the crura.

3. **a. Decreased content of hemoglobin S (HgbS) in the plasma.** The clinical features are seen in homozygous SCD patients: chronic hemolysis, vascular occlusion, tissue ischemia, and end-organ damage. HgbS polymerizes when deoxygenated, injuring the sickle erythrocyte, activating a cascade of hemolysis and vaso-occlusion. Membrane damage results in dense sickling of red cells, causing adhesive interactions among sickle cells, endothelial cells, and leukocytes. Hemolysis releases hemoglobin into the plasma. Free Hgb reacts with nitric oxide (NO) to produce methemoglobin and nitrate. This is a scavenging reaction; the vasodilator NO is oxidized to inert nitrate. Sickled erythrocytes release arginase-I into blood plasma, which converts L-arginine into ornithine, effectively removing substrate for NO synthesis. Oxidant radicals further reduce NO bioavailability. The combined effects of NO scavenging and arginine catabolism result in a state of NO resistance and insufficiency termed *hemolysis-associated endothelial dysfunction.* Therapeutic interventions include transfusion to decrease the relative concentrations of HgbS in the plasma.

4. **c. Erectile dysfunction (ED) pharmacotherapy.** The introduction of intracavernous pharmacotherapy approximately 2 decades ago led to a pronounced increase in the incidence of prolonged erection and true priapism. Prolonged erection is more commonly reported than is priapism, following therapeutic or diagnostic injection of intracavernous vasoactive medications. In many communities patients receiving intracavernous medications for ED will outnumber patients with SCD. The majority of men requiring treatment for ED are middle-aged to older men. In worldwide clinical trials of the Alprostadil Study Group, prolonged erection (defined as 4–6 hours) was 5%, and priapism (>6 hours) was described in 1% of subjects. In papaverine/phentolamine/alprostadil intracavernous injection programs, prolonged erections have been reported in 5% to 35% of patients.

5. **a. Daily dosing.** Few cases reports have documented priapism following PDE5 inhibitor therapy. These reports suggest that men with the following conditions were at increased risk for priapism: SCD, spinal cord injury, men who used a PDE5 inhibitor recreationally, men who used a PDE5 inhibitor in combination with intracavernous injection, men with a history of penile trauma, men on psychotropic medications, and men abusing narcotics. Tadalafil, 5 mg daily dosing caused no priapism in a phase II clinical study of 281 men with history of lower urinary tract symptoms secondary to benign prostatic hyperplasia for 6 weeks, followed by dosage escalation to 20 mg once daily for 6 weeks.

6. **e. Hemodialysis.** Nonischemic priapism is much rarer than ischemic priapism, and the etiology is largely attributed to trauma. Forces may be blunt or penetrating, resulting in laceration of the cavernous artery or one of its branches within the corpora. The etiology most commonly reported is a straddle injury to the crura. Other mechanisms include coital trauma, kicks to the penis or perineum, pelvic fractures, birth canal trauma to the newborn male, needle lacerations, complications of penile diagnostics, and vascular erosions complicating metastatic infiltration of the corpora. Although accidental blunt trauma is the most common etiology, high-flow priapism has been described following iatrogenic injury: cold-knife urethrotomy, Nesbitt corporoplasty, and deep dorsal vein arterialization. Any mechanism that lacerates a cavernous artery or arteriole can produce unregulated pooling of blood in sinusoidal space with consequent erection.

7. **d. The deterioration of cavernous smooth muscle contractile responses.** In ischemic priapism there are time-dependent changes in the corporal metabolic environment with progressive hypoxia, hypercarbia, and acidosis. in vitro studies have demonstrated that when corporal smooth muscle strips are exposed to a hypoxic condition, α-adrenergic stimulation fails to induce corporal smooth muscle contraction. Histologically, by 12 hours corporal specimens show interstitial edema, progressing to destruction of the sinusoidal endothelium, exposure of the basement membrane, and thrombocyte adherence at 24 hours.

8. **e. PDE5 activity downregulation.** Recent scientific advances have shown that priapism is associated with decreased PDE5 functional regulation in the penis. The relative lack of this molecular factor needed for controlling chemical signaling of penile erection accounts for stuttering and ischemic priapism in sickle cell patients. Experimental models of corpus cavernosum smooth muscle cells suggest that the cyclic nucleotide cGMP is produced in low steady-state amounts under the influence of priapism-related destruction of the vascular endothelium and thus reduced endothelial nitric oxide activity. This situation downregulates the set point of PDE5 function, secondary to altered cGMP-dependent feedback control mechanisms. When nitric oxide is neuronally produced in response to erectogenic stimulus or during sleep-related erectile activity, cGMP production surges in a manner that leads to excessive erectile tissue relaxation because of basally insufficient functional PDE5 to degrade the cyclic nucleotide.

9. **c. Intracavernous aspiration.** The history and blood gases define an ischemic priapism event, which warrants immediate attempts at decompression/aspiration of the corpora cavernosa. In SCD, concurrent systemic treatments may be offered, but relief of the penile ischemia should be pursued aggressively. Aspiration should be repeated until no more dark blood can be seen coming out of the corpora and bright red blood is obtained. This process decreases the intracavernous pressure, relieves pain, and resuscitates the corporal environment, removing anoxic, acidotic, and hypercarbic blood.

10. **c. Decreased or absent cavernosal artery inflow.** In presentations of ischemic priapism, minimal or absent blood flow in the cavernosal arteries is found using color Doppler ultrasonography. CDU is an adjunct to the corporal aspirate in differentiating ischemic from nonischemic priapism. Patients with ischemic priapism will have no blood flow in the cavernous arteries; the return of the cavernous artery waveform will accompany successful detumescence. Patients with nonischemic

priapism have normal to high blood-flow velocities in the cavernous arteries; an effort should be made to localize the characteristic blush of color emanating from flow signal of the disrupted cavernous artery or arteriolar-sinusoidal fistula.

11. **a. Color duplex ultrasonography.** This tool is the most reliable and least invasive imaging technique to differentiate ischemic from nonischemic priapism. CDU should always be considered in the evaluation of a full or partial erection after treatments for ischemic priapism. The differential diagnosis includes resolved ischemia with persistent tenderness and penile edema, persistent ischemia, or conversion to a high-flow state.

12. **a. Observation.** These blood gas results are consistent with normal mixed venous blood. The turgid penis may be due to tissue edema. Observation is appropriate at this time.

13. **a. α_1-Selective activity.** According to American Urological Association Guidelines, aspiration followed by intracavernous injection of sympathomimetic drugs is the standard of care in the medical treatment of ischemic priapism. Sympathomimetic pharmacotherapies (phenylephrine, etilefrine, ephedrine, epinephrine, norepinephrine, metaraminol) cause smooth muscle contraction in the corpora. Phenylephrine is a selective α_1-adrenergic receptor agonist, with minimal β-mediated inotropic and chronotropic cardiac effects. There are no comparative trials of sympathomimetic injectables in the management of priapism.

14. **e. Patient preference to intervene.** Nonischemic priapism should generally be managed by observation. Arterial priapism is not an emergency. Spontaneous resolution or response to conservative therapy has been reported in up to 62% of published series. Persistent partial erection from high-flow priapism may continue from months to years. There are no comparative outcome studies of intervention versus conservative management, but there are sufficient case descriptions in children to recommend initial watchful waiting. Adult patients demanding immediate relief can be offered selective arterial embolization.

15. **e. Penile prosthesis surgery.** Unfortunately, the natural history of untreated ischemic priapism or priapism refractory to interventions is severe fibrosis, penile length loss, and complete ED. The exact time point when penile prosthesis becomes a reasonable option is unclear, but most series describe complete ED in men who have had ischemic priapism for 36 to 72 hours. The advantages of early penile implantation in the acute management of ischemic priapism are preservation of penile length and a technically easier implantation; delayed implantation is technically challenging due to corporal fibrosis.

16. **c. A gonadotropin-releasing hormone agonist or antiandrogen.** The goals of managing stuttering ischemic priapism are prevention of future episodes, preservation of erectile function, and reducing the trauma to the patient from priapism management. A trial of daily oral sympathomimetic therapy, a trial of oral PDE5 inhibitor therapy, or intracavernous injection of phenylephrine should be considered in the management of children and adults with stuttering ischemic priapism associated with hemoglobinopathies. GnRH agonists or antiandrogens may be used in adults but should not be used in patients who have not achieved full sexual maturation and adult stature.

17. **c. Longer than 36 hours.** In those patients in whom priapism was reversed, spontaneous erection (with or without sildenafil) was reported in 100% of men when priapism was reversed in less than 12 hours; 78% when reversed by 12 to 24 hours; and 44% when reversed by 24 to 36 hours. No patient reported spontaneous erection after priapism duration of more than 36 hours.

18. **b. A percutaneous distal penile shunt.** The objective of shunt surgery is reoxygenation of the corpus cavernosum. The shared principle of all shunting procedures is to reestablish corporal inflow by relieving venous outflow obstruction. A distal cavernoglanular shunt should be the first choice of shunting procedures because it is technically easier to perform than proximal shunting. Percutaneous distal shunting is less invasive than open distal shunting and can be attempted in the emergency department with local anesthetic. Anesthesiologists must be educated that ischemic priapism is an emergency and sexual function outcomes are time dependent; appropriate airway precautions should be taken for emergent intubation as needed in the surgical management of priapism.

19. **b. Penile arteriography to differentiate high-flow from ischemic priapism.** CDU is an adjunct to the corporal aspirate in differentiating ischemic from nonischemic priapism. CDU imaging should include corporal shaft and transperineal assessment of the crural bodies when there is a history of penile trauma or straddle injury. CDU should always be considered in the evaluation of a persistent or partial erection after treatments for ischemic priapism. Penile arteriography is too invasive as a diagnostic procedure to differentiate ischemic from nonischemic priapism. Penile arteriography should be reserved for the management of high-flow priapism, when embolization is planned. There are three possible roles for MRI: (1) imaging of a well-established arteriolar-sinusoidal fistula, (2) identifying corporal thrombus, and (3) identifying corporal metastasis.

20. **c. Angio-embolization after a thorough discussion of chances for spontaneous resolution and risks of treatment-related ED.** Arterial priapism is not an emergency and may be managed expectantly. Diagnosis of high-flow priapism is best made by penile/perineal color Doppler ultrasound. Penile aspiration and injection of α-adrenergic agents is not recommended for HFP. Angio-embolization should be preceded by a thorough discussion of chances for spontaneous resolution, risks of treatment-related ED, and lack of significant consequences expected from delaying interventions. Overall success rates with embolization are high, although a single treatment carries a recurrence rate of 30% to 40%. Where angio-embolization fails or is contraindicated, surgical ligation is reasonable. Formation of a pseudocapsule at the site of a sinusoidal fistula may take weeks to months following trauma. Color Doppler ultrasound guidance is recommended during exploration to locate the fistula.

21. **b. Hemolysis and reduced nitric oxide.** Contemporary science implicates hemolysis and reduced nitric oxide in the pathogenesis of pulmonary hypertension, leg ulcers, priapism, and stroke in SCD patients, whereas, increased blood viscosity is believed to be responsible for painful crises, osteonecrosis, and acute chest syndrome (Kato, 2006, 2010).* SCD patients with priapism have a fivefold greater risk of developing pulmonary hypertension. SCD priapism is also associated with reduced hemoglobin levels and increased hemolytic markers: reticulocyte count, bilirubin, lactate dehydrogenase, and aspartate aminotransferase.

22. **c. With aspiration and pharmacologic detumescence.** Classically, management of SCD-induced ischemic priapism involved analgesics, hydration, oxygen, bicarbonate, and exchange transfusion. It is very tempting, especially in boys, to defer management to pediatricians and hematologists. Hematologists have begun to question the emphasis on intravenous hydration, sodium bicarbonate for alkalinization, and exchange transfusion as first-line therapy for SCD-associated priapism (Kato, 2010). Unfortunately, acute neurologic complications may follow exchange transfusions. Hydroxycarbamide (hydroxyurea) is a hematologic agent used in the management of vaso-occlusive crises in SCD patients (Saad, 2004; Morrison, 2012). The proposed mechanisms of action are increase in production of hemoglobin F, lowering of leukocytes–platelets–reticulocytes, and promoting release of NO. In the best interest of the patient, the urologist should seek hematologic consultation in the management of boys and men with SCD priapism, but remain assertive that hematologic therapy alone is not effective management of SCD priapism (Rogers, 2005). One report suggested that blood transfusion may have no effective role in the treatment

---

*Sources referenced can be found in *Campbell-Walsh Urology, 11th Edition,* on the Expert Consult website.

of sickle cell-induced priapism (Merritt, 2006). Reports from hematology centers suggest high success rates using penile aspiration/injection/irrigation of intracavernous sympathomimetics for SCD priapism (Mantadakis, 2000).

23. **e. Corporal aspiration and injection of phenylephrine 200 μg.** Oral agents are not recommended in the management of acute ischemic priapism (>4 hours). Oral α-adrenergic agents may have a role in the management of stuttering priapism associated with prolonged nocturnal erections. The recommended initial treatment of ischemic priapism is the decompression of the corpora cavernosa by aspiration. Aspiration will immediately soften the erection and relieve pain. Aspiration alone may relieve priapism in 36% of cases. The AUA Guidelines Panel (2003) advised that there were not sufficient data to conclude that aspiration followed by saline intracorporal irrigation was any more effective than aspiration alone (Montague, 2003). Aspiration should be repeated until no more dark blood can be seen coming out from the corpora and fresh bright red blood is obtained. This process leads to a marked decrease in the intracavernous pressure, relieves pain, and resuscitates the corporal environment removing anoxic, acidotic, and hypercarbic blood. Corporal aspiration, if unsuccessful, should be followed by α-adrenergic injection.

24. **e. None of these agents is more likely to result in priapism.** The 2013 label for the most recently approved PDE5 inhibitor Stendra (avanafil 50 mg, 100 mg, 200 mg) contains precautionary wording virtually identical to that on prior labels for PRN oral dosing of sildenafil, vardenafil, and tadalafil: "There have been rare reports of prolonged erection greater than 4 hours and priapism (painful erections greater than 6 hours)." Once-daily tadalafil (2.5 mg and 5 mg) was approved for oral treatment of ED in 2008, and subsequently in 2011 tadalafil (2.5 mg and 5 mg) was approved for the signs and symptoms of benign prostatic hyperplasia (BPH) and treatment of ED and the signs and symptoms of BPH. Tadalafil 5 mg daily dosing caused no priapism in a phase II clinical study of 281 men with history of lower urinary tract symptoms secondary to benign prostatic hyperplasia for 6 weeks.

25. **d. 48 hours.** Bennett and Mulhall (2008) carefully documented 39 cases of SCD priapism presenting to their emergency department over 8 years; men were routinely interviewed for erectile function status within 4 weeks of priapism/interventions. Of the 39 African-American men followed, 73% acknowledged prior episodes of stuttering; 85% had previously been diagnosed with SCD; but only 5% had been counseled in SCD clinics or were aware that priapism was a complication of SCD. A standard protocol of aspiration and phenylephrine injection was performed; shunting for failure of medical management was performed in 28%. In those patients in whom priapism was reversed, spontaneous erections (with or without use of sildenafil) were reported in 100% of men when priapism was reversed by 12 hours; 78% when reversed by 12 to 24 hours; and 44% when reversed by 24 to 36 hours. In this contemporary series of SCD patients, no men reported the return of spontaneous erections after priapism lasting 36 hours or more. Ralph (2014) describes the efficacy and outcomes of combining the T-shunt (Brant and Lue, 2009) with the corporal "snake" maneuver in 45 patients. All were refractory to medical reversal of ischemic priapism. The combined distal surgical technique was successful in resolving the acute priapism if duration was less than 24 hours but had limited efficacy in cases of priapism greater than 48 hours. Corporal needle biopsies were performed in each case and documented smooth muscle necrosis, worsening as a function of time and uniform in all men with more than 48 hours of ischemia. At 6 months erectile function outcomes were assessed by the erectile function domain score from the IIEF-5. T-shunt with corporal snake tunneling successfully reversed ischemic priapism in all patients with less than 24 hours' duration, but at 6 months ED was complained of by 50% of men. The authors conclude that the cutoff for irreversible restoration of erectile tissue is 48 hours; aggressive combined distal shunting may resolve priapism in a small cohort (30%), but all will have severe ED. They advise that management of refractory ischemic priapism greater than 48 hours should include discussion of immediate insertion of penile implant.

CHAPTER REVIEW

1. Ischemic priapism is the result of little or no cavernous arterial inflow.
2. Interventions 48 hours beyond the onset of ischemic priapism may relieve pain but will have little benefit in preserving potency.
3. Stuttering priapism is recurrent, unwanted, painful erections in men, usually with sickle cell disease.
4. Nonischemic or high-flow arterial priapism is usually the result of trauma, and the corpora are tumescent but not rigid.
5. The etiology of the majority of ischemic priapism is idiopathic; however, it may be associated with psychotropic medications, alcohol or drug abuse, hematologic dyscrasias, metastatic disease, perineal trauma, intracavernous injection of vasoactive drugs, and sickle cell disease.
6. Priapism following a PDE5 inhibitor usually occurs in men with other risk factors.
7. On rare occasion, following reversal of ischemic priapism, high-flow priapism may occur. Doppler ultrasound is useful in making this diagnosis.
8. Ischemic priapism and stuttering priapism are the result of NO imbalance.
9. In ischemic priapism, aspiration alone will be curative in a third of the patients.
10. Phenylephrine, 200 μg/mL given in 0.5-mL aliquots, not to exceed a total dose of 1 mg, is used to treat ischemic priapism. Corporal aspiration, if unsuccessful, should be followed by α-adrenergic injection.
11. Aspiration has no role in high-flow priapism other than for diagnosis; it plays no role in treatment.
12. PDE5 inhibitor therapy has been used to treat stuttering priapism in men with sickle cell disease.
13. When surgical therapy is indicated, a cavernosal glanular shunt should be the first choice.
14. Spontaneous resolution of high-flow arterial priapism generally occurs in two thirds of patients.
15. If a distal shunt fails, a proximal shunt should be considered.
16. In sickle cell disease, concurrent systemic treatments may be offered, but relief of the penile ischemia should be pursued aggressively. Aspiration should be repeated until no more dark blood can be seen coming out of the corpora and bright red blood is obtained.
17. Increased risk for priapism occurs in sickle cell disease, spinal cord injury, men who used a PDE5 inhibitor recreationally, men who used a PDE5 inhibitor in combination with intracavernous injection, men with a history of penile trauma, men on psychotropic medications, and men abusing narcotics.

29 Disorders of Male Orgasm and Ejaculation

Chris G. McMahon

QUESTIONS

1. The most important inhibitory neurotransmitter in the central neurochemical control of ejaculation is:
   a. dopamine.
   b. serotonin.
   c. noradrenalin.
   d. oxytocin.
   e. γ-aminobutyric acid.

2. Which of the following is INCORRECT?
   a. The ejaculatory process comprises three phases: emission, ejection and orgasm.
   b. Emission is mediated by sympathetic nerves (T10 to L2).
   c. Ejection is mediated by somatic nerves (S2 to S4).
   d. Ejection also involves a parasympathetic spinal cord reflex on which there is limited voluntary control.
   e. Closure of bladder neck, rhythmic contraction of the bulbocavernosus, bulbospongiosus, and other pelvic floor muscles, and relaxation of the external urinary sphincter during emission prevents retrograde ejaculation.

3. The prevalence of intravaginal ejaculation latency times (IELT) of 1 minute or less in the general population is approximately:
   a. <1%.
   b. 2.5%.
   c. 5.5%.
   d. 11%.
   e. 20%.

4. Which of the following is INCORRECT?
   a. The Diagnostic and Statistical Manual (DSM) IV definition of premature ejaculation (PE) is an operationalized multivariate definition that captures the key dimensions of latency, control, and bother.
   b. Approximately 80% of heterosexual men seeking treatment for lifelong PE ejaculate within 1 minute after penetration.
   c. The consistent early ejaculations of lifelong PE suggest an underlying neurobiologic functional disturbance.
   d. Acquired PE is most often due to psychological factors or comorbid erectile dysfunction.
   e. Men with subjective PE complain of PE, often due to psychological and/or cultural factors, but have a normal or even extended IELT.

5. Which of the following is INCORRECT?
   a. The International Society for Sexual Medicine (ISSM) developed the first contemporary, evidence-based definition of lifelong and acquired PE.
   b. The main constructs in the ISSM definition of PE are time from penetration to ejaculation, inability to delay ejaculation, and the presence of negative personal consequences.
   c. Lifelong PE is, in part, defined by an IELT less than about 1 minute.

d. Acquired PE is, in part, defined by a clinically significant and bothersome reduction in latency time, often to about 3 minutes or less.
   e. This definition is applicable to all men regardless of their sexual orientation or type of sexual contact.

6. The rationale for the ISSM definition of lifelong and acquired PE includes which of the following?
   a. Men with acquired PE tend to have lower IELT than men with lifelong PE.
   b. Patient self-estimated IELT correlates poorly with stopwatch IELT.
   c. Most men do not use cognitive or behavioral techniques to prolong intercourse and delay ejaculation.
   d. Men with lifelong or acquired PE invariably experience a variety of negative psychological consequences such as bother, frustration, or the avoidance of sexual contact.
   e. Men with PE had similar overall health-related quality of life, self-esteem, and confidence compared with non-PE groups.

7. Which of the following is FALSE?
   a. There is a substantial disparity between the incidence of PE in epidemiologic studies that rely on patient self-reports of PE and/or inconsistent and poorly validated definitions of PE.
   b. Community-based stopwatch IELT studies demonstrate that the distribution of the IELT is positively skewed, with a median IELT of 5.4 minutes (range, 0.55-44.1 minutes).
   c. Community-based stopwatch IELT studies demonstrate that IELT decreases with age and varies among countries.
   d. Some men may have a neurobiologic and genetic predisposition toward early ejaculation.
   e. Hypothyroidism is a common cause of PE.

8. In men with acquired PE and comorbid erectile dysfunction (ED), which of the following is FALSE?
   a. Intentionally "rushing" intercourse to prevent early detumescence of a partial erection is common.
   b. PE is rarely compounded by the presence of high levels of performance anxiety related to their ED.
   c. Limitation of arousal during foreplay to prevent early ejaculation may result in an incomplete erection.
   d. The presence of vascular risk factors such as diabetes and hypertension is common.
   e. c and d

9. In the evaluation of men with acquired PE, which of the following is FALSE?
   a. A physical examination is mandatory in an effort to identify the etiology of the PE.
   b. The presence of comorbid ED can be evaluated using a validated instrument such as the International Index of Erectile Function (IIEF) or the IIEF-5 (SHIM).
   c. The Index of Premature Ejaculation (IPE) was developed specifically for use as a screening questionnaire.

d. Laboratory or imaging investigations are occasionally required based on the patient's medical history

e. A digital prostate examination, routine in an andrologic setting for all men older than 40 years, is useful in identifying possible evidence of prostatic inflammation or infection.

10. In the management of PE, which of the following is FALSE?

a. All men seeking treatment for PE should receive basic psychosexual education or coaching.

b. Present-day psychotherapy for PE is an integration of behavioral (e.g., the well known start-stop and pause-squeeze methods) and cognitive approaches within a short-term psychotherapy model.

c. Psychological-behavioral strategies for treating PE are moderately successful in the long term.

d. Drawbacks to the psychological-behavioral approach are that it is it is time-consuming, requires substantial resources of both time and money, lacks immediacy, and requires the partner's cooperation.

e. Combining PE pharmacotherapy and psychological approaches may be especially useful and potentially prevent symptom relapses.

11. In the pharmacotherapy management of PE, which of the following is FALSE?

a. Dapoxetine is a rapid acting and short half-life selective serotonin reuptake inhibitor (SSRI) taken 1 to 3 hours before sexual contact.

b. Daily dosing of SSRIs such as paroxetine, sertraline, fluoxetine, and citalopram are effective treatments for PE.

c. SSRIs inhibit the postsynaptic 5-HT transporter system in the serotonergic neuron synapse.

d. Dapoxetine can be combined with sildenafil as a treatment for PE in men with comorbid ED.

e. The use of on-demand clomipramine taken 4 to 6 hours before sexual contact is limited by the occurrence of nausea and dizziness.

12. Which of the following is/are TRUE?

a. The DSM-IV-TR definition of delayed ejaculation is evidence based on a small number of community-based IELT studies.

b. Men with IELT more than two standard deviations above the mean who report distress and/or cease sexual intercourse due to fatigue or irritation are regarded as suffering from delayed ejaculation.

c. An IELT of 40 to 45 minutes represents an IELT in excess of two standard deviations above the mean.

d. Many men with acquired DE can often masturbate to orgasm and may use idiosyncratic masturbation techniques that cannot be easily replicated during intercourse.

e. Both b and d

13. The causes of delayed ejaculation include which of the following?

a. Hypothyroidism

b. Hypogonadism

c. Multiple sclerosis

d. Antidepressants drugs such as SSRIs

e. All of the above

14. In men with a spinal cord injury (SCI), which of the following is FALSE?

a. The ability to ejaculate increases with descending levels of spinal injury.

b. Fewer than 5% of patients with complete upper motor neuron lesions retain the ability to ejaculate.

c. The ability to achieve an erection increases with descending levels of spinal injury.

d. Semen harvesting with electroejaculation or vibratory stimulation is associated with a significant risk of autonomic dysreflexia.

e. Both a and b

15. Which of the following is TRUE in men with retrograde ejaculation?

a. Retrograde ejaculation can be confirmed by the presence of spermatozoa in postmasturbation first-void urine.

b. Retrograde ejaculation is more common following a bladder neck incision than transurethral resection of the prostate (TURP).

c. Retrograde ejaculation may occur in men with diabetic autonomic neuropathy.

d. Retrograde ejaculation in men with diabetic autonomic neuropathy is usually associated with hypogonadism.

e. Both a and c

ANSWERS

1. **b. Serotonin.** Many neurotransmitters are involved in the control of ejaculation, including dopamine, norepinephrine, serotonin, acetylcholine, oxytocin, GABA, and nitric oxide (NO). Of the many studies conducted to investigate the role of the brain in the development and mediation of sexual functioning, dopamine and serotonin have emerged as essential neurochemical factors. Whereas dopamine promotes seminal emission/ejaculation via D2 receptors, serotonin is inhibitory.

2. **d. Ejection also involves a parasympathetic spinal cord reflex on which there is limited voluntary control.** Based on functional, central, and peripheral mediation, the ejaculatory process is typically subdivided into three phases: emission, ejection (or penile expulsion), and orgasm. Emission consists of contractions of seminal vesicles (SVs) and the prostate, with expulsion of sperm and seminal fluid into the posterior urethra, and is mediated by sympathetic nerves (T10 to L2). Ejection is mediated by somatic nerves (S2 to S4) and involves pulsatile contractions of the bulbocavernosus and pelvic floor muscles together with relaxation of the external urinary sphincter. Ejection also involves a sympathetic spinal cord reflex on which there is limited voluntary control. The bladder neck closes to prevent retrograde flow; the bulbocavernosus, bulbospongiosus, and other pelvic floor muscles contract rhythmically; and the external urinary sphincter relaxes. Intermittent contraction of the urethral sphincter prevents retrograde flow into the proximal urethra.

3. **b. 2.5%.** Community-based normative IELT research and observational studies of men with PE demonstrate that IELTs of less than 1 minute have a low prevalence of about 2.5% in the general population, although a substantially higher percentage of men with normal IELT complain of PE.

4. **a. The Diagnostic and Statistical Manual (DSM) IV definition of PE is an operationalized multivariate definition that captures the key dimensions of latency, control, and bother.** The medical literature contains several univariate and multivariate operational definitions of PE. Each of these definitions characterize men with PE by using all or most of the accepted dimensions of this condition: ejaculatory latency, perceived ability to control ejaculation, reduced sexual satisfaction, personal distress, partner distress, and interpersonal or relationship distress. The first official definition of PE was established in 1980 by the American Psychiatric Association (APA) in the DSM-III. The American Psychiatrist Association Diagnostic and Statistical Manual of Mental Disorders (DSM III/IV) definitions of PE were largely accepted with little discussion, despite having no evidence-based medical support.

Several observational studies in cohorts of heterosexual men with lifelong PE with prospective stopwatch IELT measurement showed that about 90% of men seeking treatment for lifelong PE ejaculated within 1 minute after penetration, and about 10% ejaculated between 1 and 2 minutes. These data support the proposal that lifelong PE is characterized by an IELT of less than or about 1 minute after vaginal penetration.

Recent studies have suggested that in some men neurobiologic and genetic variations could contribute to the pathophysiology of lifelong PE, as defined by the ISSM criteria, and that the condition may be maintained and heightened by psychological/environmental factors. Acquired PE is commonly due to sexual performance anxiety, psychological or relationship problems, ED, and occasionally prostatitis, hyperthyroidism, or during withdrawal/detoxification from prescribed or recreational drugs.

Four PE subtypes are distinguished on the basis of the duration of the IELT, frequency of complaints, and course in life. In addition to lifelong PE and acquired PE, this classification includes natural variable PE (or variable PE) and premature-like ejaculatory dysfunction (or subjective PE). Men with subjective PE complain of PE, while actually having a normal or even extended ejaculation time. The complaint of PE in these men is probably related to psychological and/or cultural factors.

5. **e. This definition is applicable to all men regardless of their sexual orientation or type of sexual contact.** In October 2007, the ISSM convened an initial meeting of the first Ad Hoc ISSM Committee for the Definition of Premature Ejaculation to develop the first contemporary, evidence-based definition of lifelong PE. Evidence-based definitions seek to limit errors of classification and thereby increase the likelihood that existing and newly developed therapeutic strategies are truly effective in carefully selected dysfunctional populations.

The committee unanimously agreed that the constructs that are necessary to define lifelong PE are time from penetration to ejaculation, inability to delay ejaculation, and negative personal consequences from PE, and they recommended the following definition. "Lifelong PE is a male sexual dysfunction characterized by the presence of all of these criteria: (1) ejaculation that always or nearly always occurs prior to or within about 1 minute of vaginal penetration; (2) the inability to delay ejaculation on all or nearly all vaginal penetrations; and (3) negative personal consequences such as distress, bother, frustration, and/or the avoidance of sexual intimacy."

In April 2013, a second Ad Hoc ISSM Committee for the Definition of Premature Ejaculation agreed that although lifelong and acquired PE are distinct and different demographic and etiologic populations, they can be jointly defined, in part, by the constructs of time from penetration to ejaculation, inability to delay ejaculation, and negative personal consequences from PE. The committee determined that the presence of a clinically significant and bothersome reduction in latency time, often to about 3 minutes or less, was an additional key defining dimension of acquired PE. This definition is limited to men engaging in vaginal intercourse, as there are few studies available on PE research in homosexual men or during other forms of sexual expression.

6. **d. Men with lifelong or acquired PE invariably experience a variety of negative psychological consequences such as bother, frustration, or the avoidance of sexual contact.** Waldinger et al. (1998)* reported IELTs <30 sec in 77% and <60 sec in 90% of 110 men with lifelong PE, with only 10% ejaculating between 1 and 2 minutes. These data are consistent with normative community IELT data, support the notion that IELTs of less than 1 minute are statistically abnormal, and confirm that an IELT cutoff of 1 minute will capture 80% to 90% of treatment-seeking men with lifelong PE. A post hoc analysis of the dapoxetine Phase III COUPLE trial data confirms a statistically significant higher IELT in men with acquired PE and comorbid ED

compared with men with lifelong PE with comorbid ED. Additional recent studies support this report and confirm that self-estimated IELT was lower in men with lifelong PE compared with acquired PE and highest in men with subjective PE. These data suggest 3 minutes as a valid cutoff for either self-estimated or stopwatch IELT for the diagnosis of acquired PE.

Several authors report that estimated and stopwatch IELT correlate reasonably well or are interchangeable in assigning PE status when estimated IELT is combined with PRO Inventory. Because patient self-report is the determining factor in treatment-seeking and satisfaction, it is recommended that self-estimation by the patient and partner of ejaculatory latency be accepted as the method for determining IELT in clinical practice.

The ability to prolong sexual intercourse by delaying ejaculation and the subjective feelings of ejaculatory control comprise the complex construct of ejaculatory control. Virtually all men report using at least one cognitive or behavioral technique to prolong intercourse and delay ejaculation, with varying degrees of success, and many young men reported using multiple different techniques (Grenier, 1997). Voluntary delay of ejaculation is most likely exerted either before or in the early stages of the emission phase of the reflex but progressively decreases until the point of ejaculatory inevitability.

Several authors have reported an association between lifelong or acquired PE and negative psychological outcomes in men with lifelong or acquired PE and their female partners. This personal distress has discriminative validity in diagnosing men with and without PE. The personal and/or interpersonal distress, bother, frustration and annoyance that results from PE may affect men's quality of life and partner relationships, their self-esteem, and their self-confidence and can act as an obstacle to single men forming new partner relationships.

7. **e. Hypothyroidism is a common cause of PE.** Reliable information on the prevalence of lifelong and acquired PE in the general male population is lacking. Premature ejaculation (PE) has been estimated to occur in 4% to 39% of men in the general community. Prevalence data derived from patient self-report are appreciably higher than prevalence estimates based on clinician diagnosis using the more conservative ISSM definition of PE. As a result, there is a substantial disparity between the incidence of PE in epidemiologic studies that rely on patient self-report of PE and/or inconsistent and poorly validated definitions of PE.

Community-based stopwatch studies of the IELT, the time interval between penetration and ejaculation, demonstrate that the distribution of the IELT is positively skewed with a median IELT of 5.4 minutes (range, 0.55-44.1 minutes), decreases with age, and varies between countries, and supports the notion that IELTs of less than 1 minute are statistically abnormal compared to men in the general Western population.

Early ejaculation in humans has been explained by either hyposensitivity of the 5-HT2C and/or hypersensitivity of the 5-HT1A receptor. Recent studies have suggested that in some men neurobiologic and genetic variations could contribute to the pathophysiology of lifelong PE, as defined by the ISSM criteria, and that the condition may be maintained and heightened by psychological/environmental factors.

The majority of patients with thyroid hormone disorders experience sexual dysfunction. Studies suggest a significant correlation between PE and suppressed TSH values in a selected population of andrologic and sexologic patients. One author reports that the 50% prevalence of PE in men with hyperthyroidism fell to 15% after treatment with thyroid hormone normalization. Although occult thyroid disease has been reported in the elderly hospitalized population, it is uncommon in the population who present for treatment of PE, and routine thyroid-stimulating hormone (TSH) screening is not indicated unless clinically indicated.

8. **b. PE is rarely compounded by the presence of high levels of performance anxiety related to their ED.** Recent data demonstrate that as many as half of subjects with ED also experience PE. Men with ED may either require higher levels of stimulation to achieve an erection or intentionally "rush" intercourse to

---

*Sources referenced can be found in *Campbell-Walsh Urology, 11th Edition,* on the Expert Consult website.

prevent early detumescence of a partial erection, resulting in ejaculation with a brief latency. This may be compounded by the presence of high levels of performance anxiety related to their ED, which serve only to worsen their prematurity.

ED is often associated with endothelial dysfunction and atherosclerosis of the internal pudendal and cavernous arteries due to the presence of vascular risk factors such as diabetes mellitus, hypertension, hyperlipidemia, and cigarette smoking.

Off-label on-demand or daily dosing of PDE5 inhibitors is not recommended for the treatment of lifelong PE in men with normal erectile function. However, ED pharmacotherapy alone or in combination with PE pharmacotherapy is recommended for the treatment of lifelong or acquired PE in men with comorbid ED. PDE5 inhibitors, sildenafil, tadalafil, and vardenafil, are effective treatments for ED. Several authors have reported experience with PDE5 inhibitors alone or in combination with SSRIs as a treatment for PE.

9. **c. The Index of Premature Ejaculation (IPE) was developed specifically for use as a screening questionnaire.** Men presenting with self-reported PE should be evaluated with a full medical/sexual history, a focused physical examination, inventory assessment of erectile function, and any investigations suggested by these findings. Current literature suggests that the diagnosis of lifelong PE is based purely on the medical history because there are no predictive physical findings or confirmatory investigations. However, in men with acquired PE, a physical examination is mandatory in an effort to identify the etiology of the PE and to alleviate its possible cause. Laboratory or imaging investigations are occasionally required based on the patient's medical history. A digital prostate examination, routine in an andrologic setting for all men older than 40 years, is useful in identifying possible evidence of prostatic inflammation or infection.

The presence of comorbid ED should be evaluated using a validated instrument such as the IIEF or the IIEF-5 (SHIM). The IIEF is not specifically validated in men with PE. Caution should be exercised in the IIEF diagnosis of comorbid ED in men with PE, because 33.3% of potent men with PE confuse the ability to maintain erections before ejaculation and after ejaculation; record contradictory responses to some or all questions of the SHIM, especially Q3 and Q4; and receive a false-positive IIEF/SHIM diagnosis of ED.

10. **c. Psychological-behavioral strategies for treating PE are moderately successful in the long term.** There are multiple psychosexual and pharmacologic treatments for PE. Graded levels of patient and couple counseling, guidance, and/or relationship therapy, either alone or ideally in combination with PE pharmacotherapy, should be offered as a treatment option for most men with PE. All men seeking treatment for PE should receive basic psychosexual education or coaching.

Although the new and often more expedient pharmacologic therapies are overshadowing traditional psychological-behavioral methods in the treatment of PE, the psychological-behavioral approach remains an attractive option but is time-consuming, requires substantial resources of both time and money, lacks immediacy, requires the partner's cooperation, and has mixed efficacy.

Psychological interventions are designed to achieve more than simply increasing the IELT. Targeted factors focus on the man, his partner, and their relationship. Psychotherapy and behavioral interventions improve ejaculatory control by helping men/couples to: (1) learn techniques to control and/or delay ejaculation, (2) gain confidence in their sexual performance, (3) lessen performance anxiety, (4) modify rigid sexual repertoires, (5) surmount barriers to intimacy, (6) resolve interpersonal issues that precipitate and maintain the dysfunction, and (7) increase communication.

Psychological-behavioral strategies for treating PE have been at least moderately successful in alleviating the dysfunction in the short term, but long-term outcome data are limited and suggest a significant relapse rate.

11. **c. SSRIs inhibit the postsynaptic 5-HT transporter system in the serotonergic neuron synapse.** Dapoxetine has received approval for the treatment of PE in more than 50 countries worldwide. Dapoxetine has not received marketing approval for the United States by the Food and Drug Administration (FDA). It is a rapid acting and short half-life SSRI with a pharmacokinetic profile supporting a role as an on-demand treatment for PE.

Several forms of pharmacotherapy have been used in the treatment of PE. These include the use of topical local anesthetics, SSRIs, tramadol, PDE5 inhibitors, and α-adrenergic blockers. The use of topical local anesthetics such as lidocaine, prilocaine, or benzocaine, alone or in association, to diminish the sensitivity of the glans penis is the oldest known pharmacologic treatment for PE. The introduction of the SSRIs paroxetine, sertraline, fluoxetine, and citalopram and the tricyclic antidepressant (TCA) clomipramine has revolutionized the treatment of PE. These drugs block presynaptic axonal reuptake of serotonin from the synaptic cleft of central serotonergic neurons by 5-HT transporters, resulting in enhanced 5-HT neurotransmission and stimulation of postsynaptic membrane 5-HT receptors.

On-demand administration of clomipramine, paroxetine, sertraline, or fluoxetine 3-6 hours before intercourse is modestly efficacious and well tolerated but is associated with substantially less ejaculatory delay than daily treatment in most studies.

12. **e. Both b and d.** The DSM-IV-TR definition of delayed ejaculation contains no clear criteria as to when a man actually meets the conditions for DE, because operationalized criteria do not exist. Most sexually functional men ejaculate within about 4 to 10 minutes following intromission, so a clinician might assume that men with latencies beyond 25 or 30 minutes (21-23 minutes represents about two standard deviations above the mean) who report distress or men who simply cease sexual activity due to exhaustion or irritation qualify for this diagnosis. Such symptoms, together with the fact that a man and/or his partner decide to seek help for the problem, are usually sufficient for a DE diagnosis.

Psychogenic DE, often described as inhibited ejaculation, is usually related to sexual performance anxiety that may draw the man's attention away from erotic cues that normally serve to enhance arousal. It is occasionally characterized by the use of idiosyncratic and vigorous masturbation styles that cannot be replicated during intercourse with a partner, or an "autosexual" orientation where men derive greater arousal and enjoyment from masturbation than from intercourse. These men precondition themselves to possible difficulty attaining orgasm with a partner and, as a result, experience acquired DE. These men appear able to achieve erections sufficient for intercourse despite a relative absence of subjective arousal, and their erections are taken as erroneous evidence by both the man and his partner that he was ready for sex and capable of achieving orgasm.

13. **e. All of the above.** Delayed ejaculation/anejaculation is associated with several differing pathophysiologies, including congenital disorders as well as ones caused by psychological factors, treatment of male pelvic cancers with surgery or radiotherapy, neurologic disease, endocrinopathy, infection, and treatment for other disorders. When a medical history or symptomatology so indicates, investigation of such possible etiologies may be necessary. The most common causes of DE seen in clinical practice are psychogenic inhibited ejaculation, degeneration of penile afferent nerves and pacinian corpuscles in the aging male, hypogonadism, diabetic autonomic neuropathy, treatment with SSRI antidepressants and major tranquilizers, radical prostatectomy, or other major pelvic surgery or radiotherapy.

14. **c. The ability to achieve an erection increases with descending levels of spinal injury.** The ability to ejaculate is severely impaired by spinal cord injury (SCI). The level and completeness of SCI determine the post-SCI erectile and ejaculatory capacity. Unlike erectile capacity, the ability to ejaculate increases with descending levels of spinal injury. Fewer than 5% of patients with complete upper motor neuron lesions retain the ability to ejaculate. Ejaculation rates are higher (15%) in patients with both lower motor

neuron lesions and an intact thoracolumbar sympathetic outflow. Approximately 22% of patients with an incomplete upper motor neuron lesion and almost all men with incomplete lower motor neuron lesions retain the ability to ejaculate. In those patients capable of successful ejaculation, the sensation of orgasm may be absent and retrograde ejaculation often occurs.

Several techniques for obtaining semen from spinal cord injured men with ejaculatory dysfunction have been reported. Vibratory stimulation is successful in obtaining semen in up to 70% of men with spinal cord injury. The use of electroejaculation to obtain semen by electrical stimulation of efferent sympathetic fibers of the hypogastric plexus is an effective and safe method of obtaining semen. Both vibratory stimulation and electroejaculation are associated with a significantly high risk of autonomic dysreflexia. Pretreatment with a fast-acting vasodilator such as nifedipine minimizes the risk of severe hypertension, should autonomic dysreflexia occur with either form of treatment (Steinberger, 1990).

15. **e. Both a and c.** Antegrade (normal) ejaculation requires a closed bladder neck (and proximal urethra). Surgical procedures that compromise the bladder neck closure mechanism may result in retrograde ejaculation. The occurrence of orgasm in the absence of prograde ejaculation suggests retrograde ejaculation and can be confirmed by the presence of spermatozoa in postmasturbation first-void urine.

Transurethral incision of the prostate (TUIP) results in retrograde ejaculation in 5% to 45% of patients and is probably related to whether one or two incisions are made and whether or not the incision includes primarily the bladder neck or extends to the level of the verumontanum. The importance of contraction of the urethral smooth muscle at the level of the verumontanum has been hypothesized to be important in preventing retrograde ejaculation. Transurethral resection of the prostate (TURP) carries a higher incidence of retrograde ejaculation than does TUIP. The reported incidence of retrograde ejaculation following TURP ranges from 42% to 100%.

Retrograde ejaculation is more common in men with diabetes mellitus (DM) than in age-matched controls ($p < 0.01$), has been reported in 30% of men with DM, and is not statistically associated with duration of DM, body mass index, waist circumference, or HgbA1c or total testosterone levels.

Several sympathomimetic amine agents have been described as useful with mixed results. These drugs include pseudoephedrine, ephedrine, midodrine, and phenylpropanolamine. These agents work by stimulating the release of noradrenaline from the nerve axon terminals but may also directly stimulate both alpha- and beta-adrenergic receptors. The tricyclic antidepressant imipramine, which blocks the reuptake of noradrenaline by the axon from the synaptic cleft, is also occasionally useful. The usual dose is 25 mg twice daily. The current feeling is that long-term treatment with imipramine is likely to be more effective. Although medical treatment may not always produce normal ejaculation, it may result in some improvement.

CHAPTER REVIEW

1. The ejaculatory process is divided into: (1) emission, mediated by the sympathetic nervous system, T10-L2; (2) ejection, a somatic S2-S4 response; and (3) orgasm, which involves a spinal cord reflex.
2. Premature ejaculation (PE) may be divided into lifelong and acquired.
3. PE is defined as ejaculation within approximately 1 minute following vaginal penetration and before the individual wishes it.
4. Acquired PE is situational and may be due to prostatitis, hyperthyroidism, or detoxification.
5. Erectile dysfunction is commonly associated with PE.
6. The majority of patients with thyroid hormone disorders experience sexual dysfunction.
7. Treatment of PE includes topical anesthetics, serotonin reuptake inhibitors, tramadol, PDE5 inhibitors, and α-adrenergic blockers.
8. The postorgasmic illness syndrome includes severe myalgias and fatigue associated with a flulike state that occurs within 30 minutes of orgasm.
9. Dopamine promotes seminal emission/ejaculation via D2 receptors; serotonin is inhibitory.
10. PE has been estimated to occur in 4% to 39% of men in the general community.
11. Most sexually functional men ejaculate within about 4 to 10 minutes following intromission.
12. In spinal cord injury patients, approximately 22% of patients with an incomplete upper motor neuron lesion and almost all men with incomplete lower motor neuron lesions retain the ability to ejaculate.
13. Retrograde ejaculation is more common in men with DM than in age-matched controls.

30 Surgery for Erectile Dysfunction

J. Francois Eid

QUESTIONS

1. The three treatments that have had the most impact on the history of erectile dysfunction management are:
   a. inflatable penile prostheses, penile arterial surgery, and phosphodiesterase-5 (PDE5) inhibitors.
   b. inflatable penile prostheses, penile venous ligation, and PDE5 inhibitors.
   c. inflatable penile prostheses, intracavernous injections, and PDE5 inhibitors.
   d. intracavernous injections, penile venous ligation, and PDE5 inhibitors.
   e. intracavernous injections, penile arterial surgery, and PDE5 inhibitors.

2. The most important difference between a prosthetic erection and a normal erection is that the prosthetic erection:
   a. is usually shorter.
   b. has less girth.
   c. has less sensitivity.
   d. has greater rigidity.
   e. is cooler.

3. The feature that differentiates the AMS 700 LGX prosthesis from others is:
   a. penile girth expansion.
   b. penile length expansion.
   c. that it has two pieces.
   d. that it is preconnected.
   e. that it is prefilled.

4. The three most commonly used surgical approaches for penile prosthesis implantation are:
   a. ventral penile, infrapubic, and inguinoscrotal.
   b. subcoronal, inguinoscrotal, and penoscrotal.
   c. ventral penile, infrapubic, and penoscrotal.
   d. inguinoscrotal, infrapubic, and penoscrotal.
   e. subcoronal, infrapubic, and penoscrotal.

5. Compared with the penoscrotal approach, the infrapubic approach has the following advantage:
   a. It avoids dorsal nerve injury.
   b. It allows scrotal pump anchoring.
   c. It provides better corporeal exposure.
   d. It allows reservoir placement under direct vision.
   e. There is less chance of infection.

6. The traditional method of sizing corpora for cylinders:
   a. sizes them correctly.
   b. undersizes them by 1 cm.
   c. undersizes them by 2 cm.
   d. oversizes them by 1 cm.
   e. oversizes them by 2 cm.

7. Cylinders that are too long for the corpora result in:
   a. an S-shaped deformity and premature failure.
   b. an S-shaped deformity and poor rigidity.
   c. premature failure and poor rigidity.
   d. premature failure and pain.
   e. an S-shaped deformity and pain.

8. For most patients, the ideal inflatable penile prosthesis reservoir location is:
   a. the inguinal canal.
   b. the scrotum.
   c. the retropubic space.
   d. between the rectus muscle and the peritoneum.
   e. extraperitoneal, lateral to the rectus muscle.

9. Wearing the penis up on the lower abdomen (anatomic position) postoperatively helps to:
   a. prevent upward penile curvature.
   b. prevent downward penile curvature.
   c. minimize pain.
   d. avoid infection.
   e. avoid autoinflation.

10. Following penile prosthesis implantation, failure to reach orgasm is best avoided by:
    a. supplemental testosterone.
    b. using a water-soluble lubricant.
    c. not inflating the device to high cylinder pressures.
    d. having adequate foreplay.
    e. using a rear-entry position.

11. Infected penile prostheses are best treated by:
    a. removal of the single infected component.
    b. removal of all prosthetic components.
    c. 12 weeks of broad-spectrum antibiotics.
    d. hyperbaric oxygen.
    e. 12 weeks of broad-spectrum antibiotics plus hyperbaric oxygen.

12. Five months following three-piece inflatable penile prosthesis implantation, the recipient complains of persistent scrotal pain. Physical examination is normal except for adherence of the scrotal skin to the pump. The most likely cause of this man's symptoms and physical findings is:
    a. allergy to silicone.
    b. mechanical irritation from too much pumping.
    c. overly tight undergarments.
    d. infection with gram-positive organisms.
    e. infection with gram-negative organisms.

13. The following coatings for penile prosthesis are being used in attempts to lower the infection rates:
    a. minocycline, rifampin, and polyvinylpyrrolidone.
    b. gentamicin, vancomycin, and polyvinylpyrrolidone.

c. gentamicin, vancomycin, and rifampin.

d. gentamicin, rifampin, and povidone-iodine (Betadine Purdue Products L.P., Stamford, CT).

e. minocycline, vancomycin, and povidone-iodine (Betadine).

14. Infection rates following penile prosthesis revision surgery have been shown to be equivalent to infection rates following first-time penile prosthesis implantation. This is most likely due to:

a. 6 weeks of postrevision, wide-spectrum, intravenous antibiotics.

b. irrigation with hydrogen peroxide, povidone-iodine (Betadine), and multiple antibiotic solutions.

c. hydrophilic-coated devices.

d. antibiotic-coated devices.

e. removal of all prosthetic components.

15. During three-piece inflatable penile prosthesis implantation, while the right corpus cavernosum is being dilated, the 8-mm dilator comes out the urethral meatus. Which approach should be used to manage this intraoperative complication?

a. Repair the urethra, continue using the implant, and leave the urethral catheter as a stent for 3 weeks.

b. Repair the urethra, continue using the implant, and insert a suprapubic tube.

c. Abandon the implant and leave the urethral catheter in for 10 days.

d. Abandon the implant, repair the urethra, and leave the urethral catheter as a stent for 3 weeks.

e. Abandon the implant, repair the urethra, and insert a suprapubic tube.

ANSWERS

1. **c. Inflatable penile prostheses, intracavernous injections, and PDE5 inhibitors.** In the 1970s and 1980s there was considerable enthusiasm regarding penile arterial revascularization and penile venous ligation surgery. However, long-term results with these two treatment modalities have generally been disappointing and consequently these procedures are no longer commonly performed.

2. **a. Is usually shorter.** In our experience shortness of the prosthetic erection is the most common cause for patient dissatisfaction. The other difference between a prosthetic erection and a normal erection is the absence of glans tumescence.

3. **b. Penile length expansion.** The middle fabric layer of the AMS 700 LGX cylinder (Endo International, Malvern, PA) provides both controlled girth and length expansion.

4. **e. Subcoronal, infrapubic, and penoscrotal.** The subcoronal incision should only be used to implant malleable or positionable devices.

5. **d. It allows reservoir placement under direct vision.** This is the only advantage of the infrapubic surgical approach.

6. **e. Oversizes them by 2 cm.** The correct cylinder size is one whose length is the same as the length of an imaginary line that runs lengthwise through the center of the corpus cavernosum. Traditional sizing techniques overestimate this length by approximately 2 cm.

7. **a. An S-shaped deformity and premature failure.** A malleable prosthesis that is too long may cause pain, but a cylinder that is too long does not. Rigidity is usually not affected.

8. **c. The retropubic space.** When the reservoir is in the retropubic space, autoinflation of the prosthesis is less likely.

9. **b. Prevent downward penile curvature.** While healing is taking place, a pseudocapsule forms around the prosthesis. If the cylinders are held down by an undergarment as this capsule is forming, they may develop downward curvature.

10. **d. Having adequate foreplay.** If a man inflates his prosthesis, he is able to have coitus. However, unless he is sexually aroused, he may be unable to reach orgasm.

11. **b. Removal of all prosthetic components.** Although only the scrotal pump may appear clinically to be infected, all components of the prosthesis are joined by tubing and the entire device should be considered infected.

12. **d. Infection with gram-positive organisms.** Organisms such as *Staphylococcus epidermidis* typically cause a low-grade infection manifested by these symptoms and clinical findings. Infections due to gram-negative organisms commonly occur earlier and are associated with erythema and often drainage of pus from the wound.

13. **a. Minocycline, rifampin, and polyvinylpyrrolidone.** Coloplast's three-piece inflatable penile prosthesis is coated with polyvinylpyrrolidone. American Medical Systems' three-piece inflatable penile prostheses are coated with minocycline and rifampin.

14. **e. Removal of all prosthetic components.** Infection rates following repeat penile prosthesis surgery approach the rates seen with first-time penile prosthesis implantation if the entire device is replaced.

15. **c. Abandon the implant and leave the urethral catheter in for 10 days.** If the implant is not abandoned, the urethra is unlikely to heal and the entire device is at risk of infection.

CHAPTER REVIEW

1. There are three types of penile prostheses in common use: (1) semirigid, (2) two-piece inflatable, and (3) three-piece inflatable. Normal penile flaccidity and erection is best achieved with a three-piece prosthesis.

2. Device removal is required when there is infection or erosion through the skin.

3. Safe insertion of the reservoir in the retropubic space requires an empty bladder.

4. Infections occurring within the first few weeks following an implant are more likely to be associated with gram-negative bacteria versus those occurring 6 months or later, which are associated with gram-positive bacteria. In the majority of circumstances, the source of infection is from the skin.

5. Late prosthetic infections can occur due to hematogenous spread.

6. Early penile prosthesis reimplantation after removal of an infection penile prosthesis following eradication of infection minimizes loss of penile length.

7. When one of the cylinders fails, many patients can have successful coitus with only one functional cylinder.

8. Sensation, orgasm, and ejaculatory function are not altered by the placement of a penile prosthesis.

9. The patient should understand preoperatively that implantation of a penile prosthesis causes irreversible changes.

10. Placement of the reservoir in the space of Retzius should be performed only in patients who have not had prior surgery in the area.

11. Peyronie disease compromises inflatable prosthetic device durability and increases malfunction rates.

12. Shortness of the prosthetic erection is the most common cause for patient dissatisfaction.

13. The subcoronal incision should only be used to implant malleable or positionable devices.

14. While healing is taking place, a pseudocapsule forms around the prosthesis. If the cylinders are held down by an undergarment as this capsule is forming, they may develop downward curvature.

31 Diagnosis and Management of Peyronie Disease

Laurence A. Levine and Stephen Larsen

QUESTIONS

1. Peyronie disease (PD):
   a. is a wound healing disorder.
   b. is an autoimmune disease.
   c. frequently spontaneously recovers (30% to 50% of the time).
   d. may degenerate into cancer.
   e. is associated with Dupuytren contracture in 40% of men.

2. The fibrous plaques in PD originate in:
   a. Buck fascia.
   b. the substance of the corpora cavernosa.
   c. the substance of the corpus spongiosum.
   d. the tunica albuginea surrounding the corpora cavernosa.
   e. the tunica albuginea surrounding the corpus spongiosum.

3. Based on recent natural history studies on PD, a 54-year-old man with a 60-degree dorsal curve 18 months after onset suggests:
   a. 40% chance of spontaneous improvement of deformity.
   b. 70% chance of getting worse.
   c. 10% chance of getting worse.
   d. 10% or less chance of spontaneous improvement of deformity.
   e. 80% chance of staying the same.

4. What is the prevalence of PD following radical prostatectomy?
   a. 4%
   b. 1% to 3%
   c. 11% to 16%
   d. >20%
   e. 0%

5. Plaque calcification:
   a. can be reliably identified on physical examination.
   b. can be found in 50% to 60% of men with PD.
   c. is not an indication of stable, mature disease.
   d. is associated with successful intralesional injection therapy.
   e. is a predictive factor for the need for surgical treatment.

6. Psychological distress in men with PD:
   a. is infrequent.
   b. is typically resolved by successful surgery.
   c. is frequently associated with penile shortening.
   d. correlates with degree of erect curvature.
   e. has no association with relationship issues with the patient's partner.

7. All of the following statements regarding the physical examination of a man presenting with PD are true EXCEPT that the examination:
   a. should include measurement of plaque size with calipers.
   b. should include direct assessment of curvature following injection of vasoactive agent.
   c. should include measurement of stretched penile length.
   d. can be supported with a picture of the erect penis by a smartphone.
   e. should include assessment of the patient's palms.

8. Penile duplex ultrasound is a valuable test for men with PD. Yet it does not provide information about:
   a. penile deformity when erect.
   b. erectile response to vasoactive penile injection.
   c. penile vascular flow parameters.
   d. penile sensory integrity.
   e. plaque calcification.

9. Pentoxifylline and the phosphodiesterase-5 (PDE5) inhibitors have been shown in an animal model of PD to reduce scarring by what proposed mechanism?
   a. Improved penile blood flow
   b. Anti-inflammatory
   c. Elevated local levels of nitric oxide (NO)
   d. Anti-transforming growth factor-β (TGF-β)
   e. Mechanotransduction

10. Penile injection therapy (i.e., prostaglandin E1, TriMix-gel, etc.) for ED is not directly responsible for:
    a. cavernosal fibrosis.
    b. Peyronie disease.
    c. penile pain.
    d. priapism.
    e. high success rate.

11. A 35-year-old man with Peyronie disease is able to achieve an erection adequate for intercourse with minimal discomfort and reported dorsal erect penile curvature of 20 degrees. The initial treatment should be:
    a. reassurance.
    b. oral vitamin E.
    c. intralesional steroids.
    d. oral tamoxifen.
    e. intralesional collagenase.

12. A 66-year-old man presents with a 2-year history of PD and a 55-degree dorsal curvature. He also notes that his average-grade erection with sexual stimulation at home is a grade 5/10, which would not be adequate for intromission even if the penis were straight. Duplex ultrasound analysis demonstrates arterial insufficiency and an inadequate erectile response to 90 mg of intracorporal papaverine. The most appropriate treatment option for this patient who wants to resume sexual activity would be:
    a. oral vitamin E or potassium para-aminobenzoate (Potaba).
    b. vacuum constriction device.
    c. penile prosthesis with penile straightening.
    d. intralesional verapamil injections.
    e. oral colchicine.

13. Tunica plication is preferred for mild to moderate curvature correction because of:
    a. less shortening compared with grafting.
    b. better sensory protection.
    c. diminished risk of postoperative ED.
    d. greater potential for loss of erect length.

14. Postoperative rehabilitation is designed to aid in postoperative healing and outcomes in the following ways, EXCEPT:
    a. to prevent shortening and possibly recover some lost length.
    b. to encourage straight healing.
    c. to enhance cicatrix contracture.
    d. to preserve vascular integrity.
    e. to encourage partner participation.

15. All of following are true regarding penile traction therapy after surgical penile straightening, EXCEPT:
    a. increases or preserves postoperative length.
    b. encourages tissue remodeling.
    c. should be used for 3 or more hours/day for optimum results.
    d. increases the risk of sensory change.
    e. results appear dose-related.

16. What is the most common adverse event occurring after manual modeling during placement of a penile prosthesis in a man with PD?
    a. Tunica tear proximal
    b. Urethral injury
    c. Sensory deficit
    d. Recurrent curvature
    e. Distal urethral perforation

17. Indications to perform a plaque incision or partial excision and grafting include all of the following, EXCEPT:
    a. severe curvature in excess of 70 degrees.
    b. indentation resulting in an unstable penis or hinge effect.
    c. a short penis (<9 cm) with severe curve and poor rigidity.
    d. a short penis with severe curvature and excellent rigidity.
    e. extensive plaque calcification associated with severe deformity.

18. The primary postoperative side effect occurring following a grafting procedure for PD is:
    a. erectile dysfunction.
    b. incomplete correction of hinge effect.
    c. shortening.
    d. diminished sexual sensation.
    e. infection.

19. The primary reason to consider a grafting procedure to correct penile deformity in a man with PD is:
    a. a severe ventral curve.
    b. suboptimal rigidity even with PDE5 inhibitors.
    c. severe curve greater than 60 to 70 degrees with or without hinge effect.
    d. a 90-degree lateral curve presenting 6 months after onset.
    e. to gain length as a result of surgery.

20. The ideal graft includes all of the following EXCEPT:
    a. thin, strong, and easy to suture.
    b. no rejection.
    c. resistant to infection.
    d. preserves erectile function.
    e. contracts during healing.

ANSWERS

1. **a. Is a wound healing disorder.** PD is currently recognized as a wound healing disorder of the tunica albuginea (Devine and Horton, 1988)* that results in the formation of an exuberant scar, occurring presumably after an injury to the penis, which activates an abnormal wound healing response (Ralph et al, 2010; Levine and Burnett 2013; Greenfield and Levine, 2005; Van De Water, 1997). PD is not a premalignant condition, spontaneous resolution is a rare event, and improvement likely does not take place in more than 13% of men over the first 12 to 18 months. Though an association with Dupuytren contracture has been described, studies vary widely on this association.

2. **d. The tunica albuginea surrounding the corpora cavernosa.** PD plaques originate in the tunica albuginea. Sixty percent to 70% of plaques are located on the dorsal aspect of the tunica albuginea and are usually associated with the septum (Pryor and Ralph, 2002). It is possible that pressures on the penis during intercourse result in a delamination between the two layers, activating the abnormal wound-healing process, which is trapped within the tunic, fostering the progressive scarring.

3. **d. 10% or less chance of spontaneous improvement of deformity.** Spontaneous regression has been looked at in several contemporary natural history studies, which have suggested that no more than 13% will experience improvement of deformity. Full spontaneous resolution is extremely rare. If no treatment is offered, up to 50% will experience worsening of their deformity (Mulhall et al, 2006).

4. **c. 11% to 16%.** Tal and associates (2010) demonstrated an incidence of PD of 15.9% with a mean time to development of disease of 13.9 months. Ciancio and Kim (2000) also examined the effects of prostatectomy on penile fibrosis and sexual dysfunction. Eleven percent of all patients undergoing prostatectomy developed fibrotic changes in the penis. This fibrosis led to penile curvature in 93%, "waistband" deformity in 24%, and palpable plaques in 69%.

5. **c. Is not an indication of stable, mature disease.** Only recently has it been recognized that calcification may occur early after the onset of the scarring process, and therefore, the previously held notion that calcification is an indication of chronic, severe, and/or mature disease appears untrue (Levine et al, 2013). Several investigators have indicated that intralesional injection therapy of verapamil and interferon is less likely to be successful in men with significant calcification (Levine et al, 2002b; Hellstrom et al, 2006). A "rock-hard" plaque may be an indicator of calcification but will need to be confirmed with some form of imaging, preferably ultrasound. A calcified plaque is readily identified by ultrasound because of the hyperdensity of the plaque with shadowing behind it. Calcification itself does not predict the need for surgery. Approximately 34% of PD patients will have some degree of plaque calcification.

---

*Sources referenced can be found in *Campbell-Walsh Urology, 11th Edition*, on the Expert Consult website.

6. **c. Is frequently associated with penile shortening.** Penile shortening and inability to have intercourse are the two most common and consistent risk factors for emotional distress and relationship problems associated with PD (Smith et al, 2008; Rosen et al, 2008). Psychosocial stress is common and is reported by 77% to 94% of men with PD (Gelbard et al, 1990; Tal et al, 2012; Nelson and Mulhall, 2013). PD also commonly affects the patient's sexual partner, causing feelings of helplessness, as well as feeling personally responsible for the PD due to trauma during intercourse and sadness over loss of intimacy (Rosen et al, 2008). For some patients even a lesser degree of curvature may be highly bothersome or provoke distress (Hellstrom et al, 2013). Despite "successful treatment" that may allow the patient to be sexually functional again, there is often persistent psychological distress, presumably due to the residual changes compared with that man's pre-PD penis (Jones, 1997; Gelbard et al, 1990).

7. **a. Should include measurement of plaque size with calipers.** Measurement of the size of the plaque with any modality has been found to be inaccurate, as the plaque is rarely a discrete lesion (Bacal et al, 2009; Levine and Burnett, 2013; Ralph et al, 2010; Hatzimouratidis et al, 2012). Deformity assessment via ultrasound after injection of vasoactive agent has been shown to be the best method of assessing curvature as well as erectile response. Pictures taken from multiple vantage points may give a better idea of deformity during initial consultation. Because of the association with other collagen vascular disorders, the patient's palms should be examined.

8. **d. Penile sensory integrity.** The benefits of a complete duplex ultrasound assessment include identification of calcification during initial surveillance in the flaccid state, assessment of penile vascular flow parameters following intracavernosal injection of vasoactive agent, observing the erectile response to the vasoactive injection compared to the patient's sexually induced erection at home, and finally providing the best opportunity to objectively assess deformity. These parameters are absolutely critical to the decision process for the patient who is considering surgery. Penile sensation is best evaluated with biothesiometry.

9. **c. Elevated local levels of nitric oxide (NO).** Pentoxifylline is a nonspecific phosphodiesterase inhibitor with combined antiinflammatory and antifibrogenic properties. NO synthesized by inducible nitric oxide synthase (iNOS) reacts with reactive oxygen species (ROS), thus reducing ROS levels and presumably inhibiting fibrosis. The antifibrotic effects of NO may be mediated at least in part by the reduction of myofibroblast abundance and lead to a reduction in collagen I synthesis (Vernet et al, 2002).

10. **b. Peyronie disease.** Injection therapy has no association with leading to PD. It may, however, lead to some degree of cavernosal fibrosis, pain, and priapism. When used in the appropriate population, intracavernosal injection therapy for ED does have a high success rate.

11. **a. Reassurance.** In this case, a young man presents with PD with a minimal curvature and minimal discomfort. Pursuing aggressive therapy is not indicated because the disease process may not worsen. Therefore, reassurance is the proper answer. This patient should also be counseled to follow up should he see any exacerbation of his symptoms. At this time, intralesional collagenase is not indicated for curvature less than 30 degrees, the two noted oral therapies are not noted to be beneficial, and intralesional steroids are not recommended because of lack of objective evidence of benefit.

12. **c. Penile prosthesis with penile straightening.** This man presents with stable PD, a borderline moderate to severe curvature, but a poor-quality erection at home and an inadequate erectile response during duplex ultrasound with a high dose of vasoactive intracorporal drug injection. Therefore, for the motivated patient who has both erectile dysfunction (ED) and PD, placement of a penile prosthesis with straightening maneuvers is the most likely treatment to address both problems. Use of oral therapy had not been proven to be beneficial in this circumstance. Intralesional injection of any sort may potentially benefit his deformity, but given that he has inadequate erectile response, intralesional injections would not result in ability to resume sexual activity.

13. **c. Diminished risk of postoperative ED.** A tunica plication procedure is the preferred approach because it has the least likelihood of causing injury to the underlying cavernosal tissue, which presumably is responsible for postsurgical ED seen most commonly with a grafting procedure. There is indeed a greater potential for loss of erect length with a plication and less likelihood of damaging the penile sensory nerves, but the diminished risk of postoperative ED is the strongest reason to pursue a plication rather than grafting procedure, particularly in patients with less than severe curvature.

14. **c. To enhance cicatrix contracture.** Postoperative rehabilitation with massage and stretch, nightly use of a PDE5 inhibitor, and traction therapy are designed to enhance postoperative healing in all listed ways except for c, which is the correct answer because enhancing cicatrix contracture would not enhance healing or postoperative outcomes.

15. **d. Increases the risk of sensory change.** Penile traction therapy has emerged as an effective treatment option for PD either preoperatively alone or in combination with other treatments, or postoperatively to aid in the rehabilitation of the penis. Traction therapy has been shown to increase or preserve postoperative length and encourage tissue modeling, and it does appear to be dose-related. In addition, one study suggested that the minimum average time for daily use following surgery would be 3 hours or more per day. There is no evidence that traction therapy causes injury to the sensory nerves, nor is there evidence to suggest that it increases the risk of sensory change.

16. **b. Urethral injury.** Manual modeling was introduced in the mid-1990s as a straightening maneuver to correct residual curvature after placement of a penile prosthesis. In performing this procedure, the primary reported risk is injury to the urethra at the meatus, where the prosthetic cylinder tips may extrude through the meatus as a result of pressure placed on the distal shaft during the modeling process. Although sensory deficit, recurring curvature, and tunica tear are possible complications, they have not been reported, nor has a proximal urethral perforation.

17. **c. A short penis (<9 cm) with severe curve and poor rigidity.** This is the only option noted that would not be appropriately treated by a grafting procedure for PD, primarily because of the poor rigidity. One of the primary indications to perform a grafting procedure would be the patient having a strong erection preoperatively with severe curvature in excess of 70 degrees, having indentation causing an unstable penis or hinge effect, or a short penis. The key here is the poor rigidity, which would be an absolute contraindication to performing a grafting procedure, as it is unlikely that the grafting will improve the quality of erection; it is more likely to cause further ED in this circumstance.

18. **a. Erectile dysfunction.** Although the other listed side effects have been reported, the primary concern with patients undergoing this procedure is postoperative ED. Therefore, proper patient selection preoperatively would include only those men who have excellent-quality rigidity with or without PDE5 inhibitor therapy and have a normal vascular response during duplex ultrasound assessment.

19. **c. Severe curve greater than 60 to 70 degrees with or without hinge effect.** Ventral curvatures when repaired with grafting have a much higher rate of complete ED. Those with suboptimal rigidity tend to also develop more erectile problems post-grafting. A 90-degree curve may be an indication, but it should be with at least 1 year from the time of onset with 6 months of stable disease, which would rule out option d, as this patient is still in the acute phase. Finally, it should be recognized that although a patient is more likely to recover some length after performing a grafting procedure, neither grafting nor plication operations should be expected to result in substantial gain of length; the primary goal is straightening.

20. **e. Contracts during healing.** Contraction during the healing process would not be included in the criteria for an ideal graft.

CHAPTER REVIEW

1. There are two phases in the natural history of Peyronie disease (PD): the acute phase, in which changes occur, and the stable chronic phase.

2. The incidence of PD is between 3% and 9% with a peak age of 50 years.

3. There is a high association (33%) of diabetes with PD.

4. Preoperative erectile function correlates strongly with postoperative results.

5. Combination therapy includes intralesional injection of verapamil, oral pentoxyfilline and L-arginine, and traction. Pentoxifylline is a nonspecific phosphodiesterase inhibitor with combined anti-inflammatory and antifibrogenic properties. Penile traction therapy has emerged as an effective treatment option for PD.

6. Patients with poor-quality erections preoperatively who have grafting procedures are likely to have significant problems postoperatively with erectile function.

7. PD is currently recognized as a wound healing disorder of the tunica albuginea.

8. Sixty percent to 70% of plaques are located on the dorsal aspect of the tunica albuginea and are usually associated with the septum.

9. The natural history of PD suggests that no more than 13% of patients will experience improvement of deformity.

10. Eleven percent of all patients undergoing prostatectomy developed fibrotic changes in their penis.

11. Penile shortening and inability to have intercourse are the two most common and consistent risk factors for emotional distress and relationship problems associated with PD.

12. Primary indications to perform a grafting procedure in a patient with a strong erection are severe curvature in excess of 70 degrees, an indentation causing an unstable penis or hinge effect, and a short penis. Poor rigidity is an absolute contraindication to performing a grafting procedure.

13. Ventral curvatures, when repaired with grafting, have a much higher rate of complete erectile dysfunction.

32 Sexual Function and Dysfunction in the Female

Alan W. Shindel and Irwin Goldstein

QUESTIONS

1. Sexual health encompasses which of the following concepts?
   a. Absence of sexual dysfunction/problem
   b. Mental well-being
   c. Human development and maturation
   d. All of the above
   e. a and c

2. Which of these molecules is thought to play only a minor role in female genital sexual response?
   a. Vasoactive intestinal polypeptide
   b. Nitric oxide
   c. Acetylcholine
   d. Norepinephrine
   e. Aquaporins

3. The Female Sexual Function Index (FSFI) assesses all but which of the following aspects of sexuality?
   a. Sexual distress
   b. Sexual desire
   c. Sexual arousal
   d. Sexual pain
   e. Orgasm

4. Which of the following is NOT an essential part of the physical examination in a woman with sexual concerns?
   a. Vital signs
   b. Assessment of vaginal pH
   c. Palpation of the levator ani musculature
   d. Careful inspection of the vulva
   e. Biothesiometry

5. Which of the following statements is TRUE?
   a. Assessment of the patient's intimate relationship(s) is a key aspect of treating sexual problems.
   b. Women with spinal cord injury cannot experience orgasm.
   c. A linear pattern for sexual response is typical for all women.
   d. Survey instruments may take the place of history in evaluation of sexual concerns.
   e. All women who have sex with women identify as lesbian or bisexual.

6. Which of the following statements is FALSE?
   a. Hysterectomy may improve or worsen sexual function in women depending on the indication.
   b. Low serum testosterone levels have been clearly linked to worse sexual function in all women.
   c. Phosphodiesterase type 5 inhibitors are not currently approved for the management of problems with sexual arousal response in women.
   d. Sexual activity during routine pregnancy is safe.
   e. Women may have genital arousal responses to erotic materials that they find mentally or emotionally unappealing.

7. Which of the following are potential adverse events associated with supplemental testosterone in women?
   a. Hirsutism
   b. Acne
   c. Decreased high-density lipoprotein
   d. Vaginal bleeding
   e. All of the above

8. Decreased sexual interest/desire has been associated with which of the following conditions in women?
   a. Use of antidepressants
   b. Life stressors
   c. Hypoestrogenism
   d. Relationship problems
   e. All of the above

9. Education on sexuality is always indicated; which of the following women is likely to also benefit from medical and/or psychological treatment?
   a. 24-year-old woman who does not climax with vaginal penetration but does climax with clitoral stimulation
   b. 56-year-old woman with vaginal dryness that is well managed with sexual lubricant
   c. 35-year-old woman with bothersome decline in sexual desire
   d. All of the above
   e. None of the above

10. Which of the following diagnoses are included in the *Diagnostic and Statistical Manual of Mental Illness Fifth Edition*?
    a. Female Orgasmic Disorder
    b. Hypoactive Sexual Desire Disorder
    c. Genitopelvic Pain/Penetration Disorder
    d. a and c above
    e. All of the above

11. Which of the following conditions has been associated with lower bioavailable androgen levels in women?
    a. Hormonal contraceptives
    b. Surgical menopause
    c. Elevated prolactin levels
    d. All of the above
    e. None of the above

12. Which of the following has NOT been shown to be useful in the management of problems with sexual arousal in women?
    a. Topical prostaglandins
    b. Muscle relaxants
    c. Vaginal lubricants

d. Hormonal supplementation with androgens and/or estrogens

e. Psychosocial counseling

13. Which of the following have been definitively linked to sexual dysfunction in women?

a. Postmenopausal estrogen replacement

b. Obesity

c. High educational achievement

d. Depression

e. Metabolic syndrome

14. Which of the following has the least evidence for efficacy in management of antidepressant-associated sexual dysfunction in women?

a. Use of an adjunctive antidepressant

b. Reassurance

c. Drug cessation

d. Drug holiday

e. Sildenafil

15. What is the most commonly purported etiology for the sexual problems that occur in some women using hormonal contraception?

a. Reduction of bioavailable testosterone

b. Reduction of bioavailable estrogen

c. Psychological distress

d. Partner dissatisfaction

e. Alteration of vascular response

ANSWERS

1. **d. All of the above**. Sexual wellness incorporates many aspects of human experience.
2. **c. Acetylcholine.** Acetylcholine is thought to play a relatively minor role in sexual response in women.
3. **a. Sexual distress.** The FSFI does not include a metric to quantify or measure sexuality-related distress.
4. **e. Biothesiometry.** Biothesiometry may be indicated in some cases of genital neuropathy but much of the same information can be gleaned from careful history and physical examination (with or without basic sensory testing).
5. **a. Assessment of the patient's intimate relationship(s) is a key aspect of treating sexual problems.** Women with spinal cord injury may experience orgasm, and women may endorse a circular or linear sexual response. A history is critical to evaluation of sexual wellness, and up to half of women who have had sex with another woman do not identify as lesbian or bisexual.
6. **b. Low serum testosterone levels have been clearly linked to worse sexual function in all women.** There are data to support a role for testosterone in sexual function in some women, but this is the least well supported of the statements in this question.
7. **e. All of the above**. These are well-established potential effects of testosterone. There are substantial concerns about the potential for cardiovascular disease or neoplasia, but robust data on risk are scant.
8. **e. All of the above.** There are numerous potential causes of low sexual desire.
9. **c. 35-year-old woman with bothersome decline in sexual desire**. Many sexually healthy women do not climax with vaginal penetration. Use of vaginal lubricant is an effective and safe management option for vaginal dryness.
10. **d. a and c above.** The DSM V combined Hypoactive Sexual Desire Disorder and Female Sexual Arousal Disorder into Female Sexual Interest/Arousal Disorder. Similarly, dyspareunia and vaginismus were combined into Genitopelvic Pain/Penetration Disorder. Female orgasmic disorder was carried over from DSM IV TR.
11. **d. All of the above.** Hormonal contraception, prolactin, and surgical menopause all tend to decrease bioavailable testosterone.
12. **b. Muscle relaxants.** Muscle relaxants have been used with good efficacy for issues of sexual pain but have not been shown to directly aid sexual arousal response in women.
13. **d. Depression.** Depression is unambiguously linked to sexual dysfunction in women; the other entities have been linked to sexual dysfunction in some but not all studies.
14. **b. Reassurance.** There are peer-reviewed, published data to support all but answer b. Reassurance may be indicated for some women but may be viewed by others as a dismissal of their concerns related to antidepressant treatment.
15. **a. Reduction of bioavailable testosterone.** Hormonal contraception has been clearly linked to lower bioavailable serum testosterone. Other etiologies may contribute.

CHAPTER REVIEW

1. The vagina is acidic, with a pH between 4 and 5, and is colonized by microorganisms that produce lactic acid.
2. Testosterone production in women comes directly from the ovaries and adrenal glands. Unlike estrogen and progesterone levels, which fall abruptly with menopause, testosterone levels diminish gradually throughout life.
3. Sexual neutrality or being receptive to rather than initiating sexual activity is considered a normal variation of female sexual functioning.
4. Women with incontinence are up to three times more likely to experience decreased arousal, infrequent orgasms, and increased dyspareunia.
5. Lack of estrogen may not directly impair female arousal and desire, but it impairs sexual function by resulting in a decreased vasocongestion and lubrication and increased vaginal epithelial atrophy. Estrogens maintain female genital tissue integrity and thickness.
6. Selective serotonin reuptake inhibitors have an inhibitory effect on sexual desire, arousal, and orgasm.
7. Optimal female sexual health requires physical, emotional, and mental well-being.
8. Hormonal contraception, prolactin, and elevated SHBG all tend to decrease bioavailable testosterone.

33 Surgical, Radiographic, and Endoscopic Anatomy of the Retroperitoneum

Drew A. Palmer and Alireza Moinzadeh

QUESTIONS

1. Which of the following structures is NOT in the retroperitoneum?
   a. Kidney
   b. Second portion of the duodenum
   c. Ascending colon
   d. Adrenal
   e. Transverse colon

2. Which muscle's function is most similar to psoas major?
   a. Iliacus
   b. Quadratus lumborum
   c. Transversus abdominis
   d. External oblique
   e. Vastus lateralis

3. Which fascial layer is immediately deep to the transversus abdominis muscle?
   a. Lumbodorsal fascia
   b. Lateroconal fascia
   c. Internal oblique fascia
   d. External oblique fascia
   e. Transversalis fascia

4. A 28-year-old urology resident is injured in a motorcycle accident and suffers Grade 2 renal trauma. The hematoma would most likely continue in which direction:
   a. Superior
   b. Lateral
   c. Medial
   d. Caudal
   e. Cephalad

5. The anterior and posterior laminae of Gerota fascia merge laterally to form:
   a. transversus abdominis.
   b. lumbodorsal fascia.
   c. lateral renal fascia.
   d. lateroconal fascia.
   e. perirenal fascia.

6. The blood supply to the adrenal gland may include branches from the:
   a. inferior phrenic artery.
   b. aorta.
   c. renal artery.
   d. a and b.
   e. a and c.
   f. a, b, and c.

7. Which of the following statements is TRUE?
   a. The superior mesenteric artery (SMA) may be sacrificed without causing bowel ischemia.
   b. Ligation of the inferior mesenteric artery (IMA) will cause ischemia to the large bowel but not the small bowel.
   c. The IMA may be sacrificed without colonic ischemia because of collateral circulation via the marginal artery and hemorrhoidal arteries.
   d. The IMA may be sacrificed without colonic ischemia because of collateral circulation via the ileocolic artery.
   e. Neither the superior nor the inferior mesenteric arteries may be sacrificed without causing bowel ischemia.

8. Which of the following statements is FALSE?
   a. The right testicular vein typically drains into the inferior vena cava (IVC).
   b. The left testicular vein typically drains into the left renal vein.
   c. Unilateral varicoceles are more common on the left side.
   d. A sudden onset unilateral right-sided varicocele should prompt retroperitoneal imaging.
   e. The left ovarian vein typically drains into the IVC.

9. What statement best describes the lymphatic drainage of the right testis?
   a. Superficial then deep right inguinal nodes
   b. Left para-aortic with some drainage to the interaortocaval nodes
   c. Only to the interaortocaval nodes
   d. Primarily to the interaortocaval nodes with some drainage to the right paracaval nodes
   e. Interaortocaval nodes primarily with some drainage to the right paracaval nodes and a small but appreciable amount of drainage to the left para-aortic nodes

10. What is the major function of the muscles innervated by the obturator nerve?
    a. Hip adduction
    b. Hip abduction
    c. Hip flexion
    d. Hip extension
    e. Knee flexion

ANSWERS

1. **e. Transverse colon.** The contents of the retroperitoneum include the kidneys, ureters, adrenals, pancreas, second and third portions of the duodenum, ascending colon, descending colon, arterial structures including the aorta and its branches, venous structures including the inferior vena cava and its tributaries, lymphatics, lymph nodes, sympathetic trunk, and lumbosacral plexus. The transverse colon is intraperitoneal.

2. **a. Iliacus.** Psoas major functions in flexion of the thigh at the hip joint and is innervated by the anterior rami of L1, L2, and L3. Iliacus is the only muscle listed that also functions in flexion of the thigh at the hip joint.

3. **e. Transversalis fascia.** The transversalis fascia lies deep to the transversus abdominis muscle and superficial to the preperitoneal fat and peritoneum.

4. **d. Caudal.** The perirenal space around the kidney is cone-shaped and is open at its inferior extent in the extraperitoneal pelvis. If a hematoma were to form within the Gerota fascia, it would be able to travel in a caudal direction.

5. **d. Lateroconal fascia.** The anterior and posterior laminae of Gerota fascia merge laterally to form the lateroconal fascia, which functions to separate the anterior and posterior pararenal spaces. It can be visualized radiographically on computed tomographic (CT) scan and continues anterolaterally deep to the transversalis fascia.

6. **f. a, b, and c.** The adrenal gland may receive branches from the superior adrenal artery off of the inferior phrenic artery, the middle adrenal artery off of the aorta, and the inferior adrenal artery off of the renal artery.

7. **c. The IMA may be sacrificed without colonic ischemia because of collateral circulation via the marginal artery and hemorrhoidal arteries.** The SMA supplies the pancreas (inferior pancreaticoduodenal artery), small intestine, and the majority of the large intestine (ileocolic, right colic, and middle colic). Ligation of the SMA will result in catastrophic bowel ischemia (without pancreatic ischemia because of collaterals from the celiac artery and the superior pancreaticoduodenal artery). The branches of the IMA are the left colic, sigmoid, and superior hemorrhoidal (rectal) arteries. The collateral circulation of the sigmoid artery via the marginal artery of Drummond and the inferior and middle hemorrhoidal arteries allows for the IMA to be sacrificed without colonic ischemia.

8. **e. The left ovarian vein typically drains into the IVC.** The venous drainage of the ovarian and testicular veins is similar. The right testicular and the right ovarian veins typically drain into the IVC while the left testicular and the left ovarian veins drain into the left renal vein. Unilateral varicoceles are more common on the left, which may be a result of the increased length and perpendicular entry of the left testicular vein into the left renal vein. Given the rarity of unilateral right-side varicocele, a sudden-onset right-side varicocele should increase suspicion for a renal or retroperitoneal malignancy leading to poor outflow and warrants retroperitoneal imaging.

9. **e. Interaortocaval nodes primarily with some drainage to the right paracaval nodes and a small but appreciable amount of drainage to the left para-aortic nodes.** The right testis drains primarily to the interaortocaval nodes with some drainage to the right paracaval nodes. The left para-aortic region does receive a small but appreciable amount of lymphatic drainage from the right testis. This drainage pattern is consistent with the global lymphatic flow from right to left.

10. **a. Hip adduction.** The obturator nerve innervates the muscles of the medial thigh compartment. These include the gracilis, adductor longus, adductor brevis, adductor magnus, and obturator externus muscles. The muscles function to adduct and rotate the thigh at the hip joint.

TABLE 33-1 Branches of the Abdominal Aorta

ARTERY	BRANCH	ORIGIN	SUPPLIES
Celiac trunk	Anterior	Immediately inferior to aortic hiatus of diaphragm	Abdominal foregut
Superior mesenteric artery	Anterior	Immediately inferior to celiac trunk	Abdominal midgut
Inferior mesenteric artery	Anterior	Inferior to renal arteries	Abdominal hindgut
Middle adrenal arteries	Lateral	Immediately superior to renal arteries	Adrenal glands
Renal arteries	Lateral	Immediately inferior to superior mesenteric artery	Kidneys
Testicular or ovarian arteries	Paired anterior	Inferior to renal arteries	Testes in male and ovaries in female
Inferior phrenic arteries	Paired lateral	Immediately inferior to aortic hiatus	Diaphragm
Lumbar arteries	Posterior	Usually four pairs	Posterior abdominal wall and spinal cord
Median sacral arteries	Posterior	Just superior to aortic bifurcation, pass inferiorly across lumbar vertebrae, sacrum, and coccyx	
Common iliac arteries	Terminal	Bifurcation usually occurs at the level of L4 vertebra	

Modified from Drake RL, Vogl W, Mitchell AWM. *Gray's anatomy for students*. Philadelphia: Elsevier; 2005. p. 331.

TABLE 33-2   Branches of the Lumbosacral Plexus

BRANCH	ORIGIN	SPINAL SEGMENTS	MOTOR FUNCTION	SENSORY FUNCTION
Subcostal	Anterior ramus T12	T12	Muscles of the abdominal wall	Skin over the hip
Iliohypogastric	Anterior ramus L1	L1	Internal oblique and transversus abdominis	Posterolateral gluteal skin and skin in pubic region
Ilioinguinal	Anterior ramus L1	L1	Internal oblique and transversus abdominis	Skin in the upper medial thigh, and either the skin over the root of the penis and anterior scrotum or the mons pubis and labium majus
Genitofemoral	Anterior rami L1 and L2	L1, L2	*Genital branch*: male cremasteric muscle	*Genital branch*: skin of anterior scrotum or skin of mons pubis and labium majus; *Femoral branch*: skin of upper anterior thigh
Lateral cutaneous nerve of the thigh	Anterior rami L2 and L3	L2, L3	None	Skin on anterior and lateral thigh to the knee
Obturator	Anterior rami L2 to L4	L2 to L4	Obturator externus, pectineus, and muscles in medial compartment of thigh	Skin on medial aspect of the thigh
Femoral	Anterior rami L2 to L4	L2 to L4	Iliacus, pectineus, and muscles in anterior compartment of thigh	Skin on anterior thigh and medial surface of leg

Modified from Drake RL, Vogl W, Mitchell AWM. *Gray's anatomy for students*. Philadelphia: Elsevier; 2005. p. 340.

CHAPTER REVIEW

1. The upper pole of the left kidney is located at the level of the 11th rib. The upper pole of the right kidney is located at the level of the 12th rib.
2. The tail of the pancreas lies in close proximity to the upper pole of the left kidney and left adrenal gland.
3. The superior arterial supply to the adrenal is from the phrenic artery and is constant; the middle and inferior arteries are variable.
4. The main renal vein courses ventral to the artery.
5. Lumbar veins often drain into the left renal vein and sometimes into the right renal vein and may be injured when dissecting the renal vein.
6. The general direction of lymph flow is from caudal to cephalad and right to left.
7. The perirenal space around the kidney is cone-shaped and is open at its inferior aspect in the extraperitoneal pelvis.

8. The IMA may be sacrificed without colonic ischemia because of collateral circulation via the marginal artery and hemorrhoidal arteries.
9. Ligation of the SMA will result in catastrophic bowel ischemia.
10. The venous drainage of the ovarian and testicular veins is similar. The right testicular and the right ovarian veins typically drain into the IVC, whereas the left testicular and the left ovarian veins drain into the left renal vein.
11. Unilateral varicoceles are more common on the left, which may be a result of the increased length and perpendicular entry of the left testicular vein into the left renal vein. Given the rarity of unilateral right-side varicocele, a sudden-onset right-side varicocele should increase suspicion for a renal or retroperitoneal malignancy.

34 Neoplasms of the Testis

Andrew J. Stephenson and Timothy D. Gilligan

QUESTIONS

1. The following adult male germ cell tumor (GCT) subtypes arise from intratubular germ cell neoplasia (ITGCN) EXCEPT:
   a. Embryonal tumor.
   b. Choriocarcinoma.
   c. Classic seminoma.
   d. Spermatocytic seminoma.
   e. Teratoma.

2. Which of the following statements is TRUE regarding spermatocytic seminoma?
   a. Cryptorchidism is a risk factor.
   b. It may occur as a mixed GCT with other histologic GCT subtypes.
   c. It may contain i(12p) mutations.
   d. Bilateral testicular involvement may occur in 2% to 3% of cases.
   e. Metastatic spermatocytic seminoma is rare.

3. Which of the following GCT subtypes is most likely to spread hematogenously?
   a. Choriocarcinoma
   b. Embryonal carcinoma
   c. Immature teratoma
   d. Teratoma with malignant transformation
   e. Seminoma

4. A 24-year-old man presents with a solid, painless, right intratesticular mass confirmed by scrotal ultrasonography. His left testis is normal. Serum tumor markers show a human chorionic gonadotropin (hCG) value of 96 mU/mL (upper limit: <5 mU/mL) and an α-fetoprotein (AFP) value of 58 ng/mL (upper limit: <11 ng/mL). The most likely histologic finding in the right testis is:
   a. Pure teratoma.
   b. Pure seminoma.
   c. Pure embryonal carcinoma.
   d. Pure yolk sac tumor.
   e. Choriocarcinoma.

5. Which of the following is an acceptable indication for testis-sparing surgery?
   a. 1.3-cm solid intratesticular mass with a normal contralateral testis
   b. Suspected benign testicular lesion
   c. 2.4-cm solid mass in a solitary testis
   d. Hypogonadal male with 1.2-cm solid intratesticular mass in a solitary testis
   e. Small (<1 cm) hyperechoic lesion suggestive of a "burned out" primary tumor in a patient with disseminated nonseminomatous GCT (NSGCT) with serum-elevated AFP and hCG

6. A 37-year-old man presents with a 5-cm left testicular mass. Computed tomography (CT) reveals a 6-cm para-aortic mass but no evidence of distant metastases. Serum tumor markers show an AFP level of 1100 ng/mL (upper limit: <11 ng/mL) and an hCG level of 80 mU/mL (upper limit: <5 mU/mL). Left inguinal orchiectomy reveals a mixed GCT with 60% embryonal carcinoma, 30% yolk sac tumor, 5% seminoma, and 5% teratoma. The next best management step is:
   a. Retroperitoneal lymph node dissection (RPLND).
   b. Induction chemotherapy with three cycles of bleomycin-etoposide-cisplatin.
   c. Induction chemotherapy with four cycles of bleomycin-etoposide-cisplatin.
   d. To obtain repeat serum tumor marker levels in 7 days.
   e. CT-guided biopsy of the para-aortic mass.

7. All of the following patients would be classified as "poor-risk" by International Germ Cell Cancer Collaborative Group (IGCCCG) classification criteria EXCEPT those with:
   a. Testicular seminoma with brain metastases.
   b. Primary mediastinal NSGCT.
   c. Testicular NSGCT with rising postorchiectomy AFP of 15,000 ng/mL (upper limit: <11 ng/mL).
   d. Primary retroperitoneal NSGCT with liver metastases.
   e. Testicular NSGCT with rising postorchiectomy hCG of 93,000 mU/mL (upper limit: <5 mU/mL).

8. A 34-year-old African-American man with a left testicular mass undergoes inguinal orchiectomy that reveals a 1.2-cm pure seminoma that is confined to the testis with no evidence of lymphovascular invasion or rete testis invasion. His postorchiectomy serum tumor markers are within the normal range. CT of the chest-abdomen-pelvis reveals no evidence of retroperitoneal lymphadenopathy and no evidence of pulmonary metastases. However, on the chest images, there is evidence of bulky hilar adenopathy bilaterally. The next best management step is:
   a. Induction chemotherapy with four cycles of bleomycin-etoposide-cisplatin.
   b. Induction chemotherapy with four cycles of etoposide-cisplatin.
   c. Mediastinoscopy and biopsy.
   d. Close observation.
   e. Bilateral thoracotomy and resection.

9. A 43-year-old man with clinical stage IIA left seminoma receives dog-leg radiation therapy to the retroperitoneum and ipsilateral pelvis with a boost to his solitary 2-cm para-aortic mass. Six months after completing treatment, surveillance CT reveals a persistent para-aortic mass that has now grown to 2.8 cm. The remainder of his metastatic evaluation is negative, and his serum tumor marker levels are all within normal limits. The next best management step is:
   a. RPLND.
   b. CT-guided biopsy of the retroperitoneal mass.
   c. Close observation until the mass regresses or the patient develops distant metastases.
   d. Induction chemotherapy with three cycles of bleomycin-etoposide-cisplatin.
   e. Salvage chemotherapy with four cycles of paclitaxel-ifosfamide-cisplatin.

10. A 41-year-old man has ITGCN discovered on biopsy of an atrophic right testis during investigations for infertility due to azoospermia. He has a history of left inguinal hernia repair. His left testis is normal in size and consistency, and there is evidence of normal spermatogenesis on testicular biopsy. His serum luteinizing hormone (LH), follicle-stimulating hormone (FSH), and testosterone levels are within the normal range. The most appropriate treatment for the ITGCN in the right testis at this time is:

    a. Inguinal orchiectomy.

    b. Low-dose radiation therapy.

    c. Carboplatin.

    d. Observation.

    e. Transscrotal orchiectomy.

11. Which of the following factors is NOT associated with the presence of occult metastases in clinical stage I NSGCT?

    a. Lymphovascular invasion

    b. Absence of yolk sac tumor in the primary tumor

    c. Percentage of embryonal carcinoma in the primary tumor

    d. Elevated preorchiectomy AFP level

    e. Advanced primary tumor stage

12. A 27-year-old convict at a correctional facility presents for management of clinical stage I left NSGCT. He has a history of enlarging left testicular mass for 12 months that was discovered incidentally during a routine physical examination by the prison physician. Pathologic examination of the orchiectomy specimen revealed a 1.2-cm mixed GCT (40% seminoma, 40% embryonal carcinoma, 20% yolk sac tumor) confined to the testis without evidence of lymphovascular invasion. His postorchiectomy serum tumor markers are within normal limits. He has a history of multiple incarcerations in the past, and his viral serology is positive for hepatitis C. The most appropriate treatment is:

    a. Adjuvant radiation therapy to the retroperitoneum and ipsilateral pelvis.

    b. Surveillance.

    c. Chemotherapy with two cycles of bleomycin-etoposide-cisplatin.

    d. Chemotherapy with two cycles of carboplatin.

    e. RPLND.

13. Which of the following factors is NOT associated with the presence of necrosis/fibrosis in residual masses after first-line chemotherapy?

    a. Absence of teratoma in the primary tumor

    b. Residual mass size

    c. Percentage shrinkage of mass after chemotherapy

    d. Prechemotherapy mass size

    e. Lymphovascular invasion

14. A 37-year-old man presents for treatment of a 1.2-cm left testicular mixed GCT (40% teratoma, 40% seminoma, 15% embryonal carcinoma, 5% yolk sac tumor) confined to the testis without evidence of lymphovascular invasion. His postorchiectomy serum tumor marker levels are within normal limits. Chest CT shows no evidence of metastatic disease. Abdominopelvic CT shows a 7-mm nodule in the paracaval location just inferior to the right renal hilum. The remainder of the CT study is unremarkable. His medical history is also unremarkable. The most appropriate management is:

    a. CT-guided biopsy of the paracaval lesion.

    b. RPLND.

    c. Two cycles of chemotherapy with bleomycin-etoposide-cisplatin.

    d. Observation.

    e. Three cycles of chemotherapy with bleomycin-etoposide-cisplatin.

15. The following factors are associated with the presence of occult distant metastases in patients with clinical stage IIA-B NSGCT EXCEPT:

    a. Elevated postorchiectomy hCG.

    b. Lymphovascular invasion.

    c. Retroperitoneal mass size.

    d. Large primary tumor with involvement of the scrotal skin.

    e. Retroperitoneal lymphadenopathy outside the primary landing zone.

16. The following are independent risk factors for relapse postchemotherapy RPLND EXCEPT:

    a. Evidence of viable malignancy in resected specimens.

    b. Incomplete resection.

    c. Rising pre-RPLND serum tumor markers.

    d. Poor-risk disease at diagnosis by IGCCCG criteria.

    e. Prior RPLND.

17. A 34-year-old man with right clinical stage III NSGCT (100% embryonal carcinoma) with good-risk features by IGCCCG criteria receives induction chemotherapy with three cycles of bleomycin-etoposide-cisplatin. At completion of chemotherapy his serum tumor markers are within normal limits. On postchemotherapy CT studies he has a 1.7-cm mass (4.8 cm at diagnosis) in the interaortocaval region and a 0.8-cm mass in the para-aortic region (2.3 cm at diagnosis). He also has bilateral pulmonary nodules in the right lower lobe (0.6 cm; 1.4 cm at diagnosis) and left upper lobe (0.8 cm; 1.6 cm at diagnosis). The most appropriate management is:

    a. Four cycles of vinblastine-ifosfamide-cisplatin second-line chemotherapy.

    b. Resection of the interaortocaval mass.

    c. Bilateral postchemotherapy RPLND.

    d. Bilateral thoracotomy and resection of residual pulmonary masses.

    e. CT-guided biopsy of the pulmonary mass(es).

18. Which of the following statements is FALSE concerning late relapse of NSGCT?

    a. Surgical resection is the primary treatment modality.

    b. Yolk sac tumor is the most common malignant histology.

    c. The incidence is increasing.

    d. The retroperitoneum is the most common site.

    e. The outcome is poor relative to those with early NSGCT relapse.

19. A 35-year-old man with clinical stage IIC left mixed GCT (50% embryonal, 40% teratoma, 10% yolk sac) with good-risk features by IGCCCG criteria receives three cycles of bleomycin-etoposide-cisplatin chemotherapy. At the start of chemotherapy his AFP was 380 ng/mL (upper limit: <11 ng/mL), and this has normalized at the end of chemotherapy. Restaging CT shows the solid para-aortic mass has increased from 5.3 cm to 8.9 cm with displacement of the aorta and left kidney as well as new lymphadenopathy in the left common iliac and left obturator region. The patient complains of recent onset of left-sided back pain. The most appropriate management is:

    a. RPLND and pelvic lymph node dissection.

    b. CT-guided biopsy of the para-aortic mass.

    c. Four cycles of paclitaxel-ifosfamide-cisplatin as second-line chemotherapy.

d. Two cycles of bleomycin-etoposide-cisplatin followed by carboplatin-etoposide high-dose chemotherapy and autologous stem cell rescue.

e. Bleomycin-etoposide-cisplatin plus radiation therapy.

20. The rationale for single-agent carboplatin as treatment for clinical stage I seminoma is based on all of the following factors EXCEPT:

a. Absence of teratoma.

b. Less neurotoxicity compared with cisplatin.

c. Less nephrotoxicity compared with cisplatin.

d. Less ototoxicity compared with cisplatin.

e. Similar efficacy to cisplatin.

21. Late complications of infradiaphragmatic dog-leg radiotherapy include all of the following EXCEPT:

a. Peptic ulcer disease.

b. Coronary artery disease.

c. Secondary malignancy.

d. Ejaculatory dysfunction.

e. Impaired spermatogenesis.

22. The rationale for surveillance in clinical stage I seminoma is based on all of the following factors EXCEPT:

a. Utility of serum tumor markers to identify relapse at an early and curable stage.

b. Relapses are cured in virtually all cases by deferred dog-leg radiotherapy.

c. Lack of validated histopathologic prognostic factors to identify a high-risk subset.

d. Improved short- and long-term toxicity compared with primary radiotherapy and carboplatin.

e. 15% to 20% of patients are cured by orchiectomy.

23. A 44-year-old man with clinical stage III left testicular seminoma with IGCCCG good-risk features has a discrete 2.4-cm residual para-aortic mass (3.8 cm at diagnosis) after receiving three cycles of bleomycin-etoposide-cisplatin chemotherapy. His pulmonary nodules have regressed completely. His serum tumor markers are within the normal range. The most appropriate management is:

a. Postchemotherapy radiation therapy to the residual mass.

b. Fluorodeoxyglucose-labeled positron emission tomography (FDG-PET) at least 4 weeks after completing chemotherapy.

c. Observation.

d. Postchemotherapy surgical resection of the residual mass.

e. Four cycles of paclitaxel-ifosfamide-cisplatin as second-line chemotherapy.

24. A 42-year-old asymptomatic man presents for management of right NSGCT (80% embryonal carcinoma, 10% teratoma, 10% choriocarcinoma). His preorchiectomy hCG value was 15,000 mU/mL (upper limit: <5 mU/mL), and this has risen to 50,800 mU/mL after orchiectomy. Chest CT shows numerous pulmonary nodules. There is evidence of multiple masses in the interaortocaval region (largest, 4.8 cm) and masses in the para-aortic region (largest, 2.6 cm). The most appropriate management is:

a. Three cycles of bleomycin-etoposide-cisplatin chemotherapy.

b. RPLND.

c. Four cycles of bleomycin-etoposide-cisplatin chemotherapy.

d. CT of the head.

e. Two cycles of bleomycin-etoposide-cisplatin followed by carboplatin-etoposide high-dose chemotherapy and autologous stem cell rescue.

25. Which of the following statements is FALSE regarding treatment-related toxicity?

a. Two cycles of platin-based chemotherapy does not increase one's risk of developing cardiovascular disease or secondary malignant neoplasm (SMN).

b. Frequent CT body imaging may increase the risk of SMN.

c. The risk of cardiovascular disease is highest among patients receiving mediastinal radiotherapy.

d. Exposure to cisplatin-based chemotherapy and history of cigarette smoking are associated with similar risks of cardiovascular disease and SMN.

e. Suprahilar dissection, vascular reconstruction, and hepatic resection are risk factors for chylous ascites after RPLND.

26. Which of the following are NOT similarities between Leydig cell tumors and GCT?

i. Both are associated with a history of cryptorchidism.

ii. Radical inguinal orchiectomy is the initial treatment of choice.

iii. Bilateral tumors occur in 2% to 3% of cases.

iv. Both may be associated with gynecomastia.

v. The retroperitoneum is the most common site of metastatic disease.
a. i, ii, and iii
b. i and iii
c. i, ii, iii, and iv
d. v only
e. All of the above

27. A 54-year-old man presents with an enlarging right inguinal mass. On examination, a palpable mass is noted in the right inguinal region that extends into the right hemiscrotum. The testis cannot be distinguished from this mass. Staging CT reveals a heterogeneous, infiltrative, area of low-intensity mass (−20 Hounsfield units), 6 × 9 cm, involving the right spermatic cord and extending from the inguinal canal into the scrotum with displacement of the right testis. There is no evidence of retroperitoneal lymphadenopathy or distant metastases. The most appropriate management is:

a. Inguinal orchiectomy followed by adjuvant radiotherapy.

b. Inguinal orchiectomy alone.

c. Transscrotal orchiectomy.

d. Inguinal orchiectomy followed by ifosfamide-based adjuvant chemotherapy.

e. Inguinal orchiectomy followed by RPLND.

Pathology

1. A 26-year-old man has a right radical orchiectomy for an embryonal carcinoma of the testis. At the time of surgery a contralateral biopsy is performed and reveals intratubular germ cell neoplasia (Fig. 34-1). The patient should be advised that he:

a. Should have a radical orchiectomy.

b. Has a significant chance of developing a germ cell tumor in the left testis.

c. Should not try to have a child.

d. Should immediately receive radiation to the testis.

e. Should receive salvage chemotherapy.

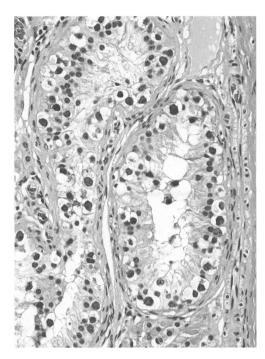

Figure 34-1. (From Bostwick DG, Cheng L. Urologic surgical pathology. 2nd ed. Edinburgh: Mosby; 2008.)

2. A 35-year-old man has an asymptomatic right scrotal mass. Testicular ultrasonography reveals a 3-cm heterogeneous intratesticular mass. A right radical orchiectomy is performed. The histology is depicted in Figure 34-2 and is reported as seminoma. Abdominal CT scan is normal. The patient should be advised to:

   a. Receive radiation to the contralateral testis.

   b. Receive at least four cycles of chemotherapy.

   c. Be advised that observation is not an option.

   d. Be advised to have radiation therapy to the retroperitoneum.

   e. Receive radiation to the abdomen and chest.

3. A 32-year-old man has a right radical orchiectomy for a testicular mass. Preoperatively his AFP value was normal and his hCG level was elevated at 5000 units. The histology is depicted in Figure 34-3 and is reported as seminoma with giant cells. The next step in management is:

   a. Follow markers and check half-life.

   b. Chemotherapy according to choriocarcinoma protocol.

   c. RPLND.

   d. Radiation therapy to retroperitoneum.

   e. Three cycles of chemotherapy.

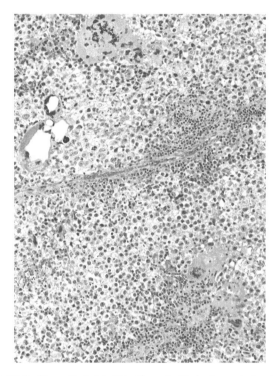

Figure 34-3. (From Bostwick DG, Cheng L. Urologic surgical pathology. 2nd ed. Edinburgh: Mosby; 2008.)

4. A 50-year-old man has a right radical orchiectomy for a testicular mass. The histology is depicted in Figure 34-4 and is a spermatocytic seminoma. Abdominal and chest CT are negative. Serum markers are normal. The patient should be advised to:

   a. Receive radiation to the retroperitoneum.

   b. Receive one cycle of chemotherapy.

   c. Have a biopsy of the contralateral testis.

   d. Not have any treatment.

   e. Have a PET-CT scan.

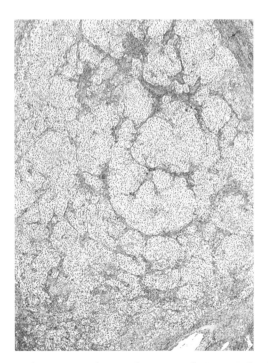

Figure 34-2. (From Bostwick DG, Cheng L. Urologic surgical pathology. 2nd ed. Edinburgh: Mosby; 2008.)

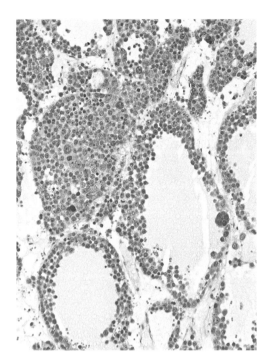

Figure 34-4. (From Bostwick DG, Cheng L. Urologic surgical pathology. 2nd ed. Edinburgh: Mosby; 2008.)

5. A 20-year-old man has a right radical orchiectomy. The pathology is depicted in Figure 34-5 and is read as embryonal carcinoma. His hCG and AFP values are elevated and a CT of abdomen and chest reveals no evidence of metastatic disease. Three weeks later repeat AFP and hCG testing show no change in either marker. The patient should be advised to:

a. Have induction chemotherapy.

b. Have an RPLND.

c. Have a PET-CT.

d. Receive radiotherapy below the diaphragm.

e. Repeat the hCG and AFP tests in another month.

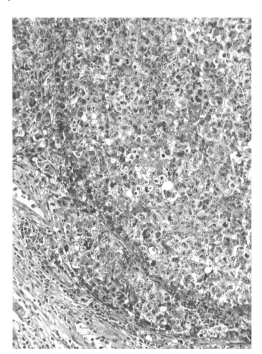

Figure 34-5. (From Bostwick DG, Cheng L. Urologic surgical pathology. 2nd ed. Edinburgh: Mosby; 2008.)

6. A 25-year-old man has a right radical orchiectomy. The histology is depicted in Figure 34-6 and is reported as a mature teratoma. The patient's AFP is slightly elevated, bHCG is negative; however, there is a 3-cm mass in the retroperitoneum on CT. He is given chemotherapy, and the mass shrinks to 1.8 cm. The patient should be advised to

a. Have a retroperitoneal lymphadenectomy (RPLND).

b. Have salvage chemotherapy.

c. Get an FDG-PET scan.

d. Receive radiation therapy.

e. Be observed.

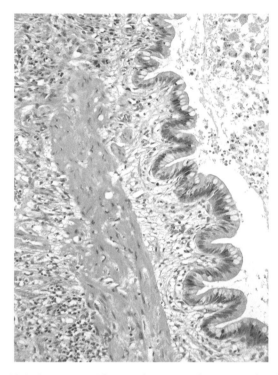

Figure 34-6. (From Bostwick DG, Cheng L. Urologic surgical pathology. 2nd ed. Edinburgh: Mosby; 2008.)

Imaging

1. A 36-year-old man noted a firm left scrotal mass. He was hit in the groin 1 month earlier with a tennis ball. Currently he has no pain, fever, or chills. The testicular ultrasound image is depicted in Figure 34-7. The most likely diagnosis is:

a. Ruptured testis with peritesticular hematoma.

b. Testicular neoplasm.

c. Epidermoid cyst.

d. Dilated rete testis.

e. Testicular abscess.

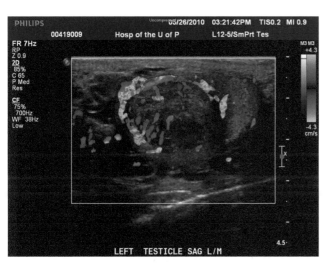

Figure 34-7.

2. A 32-year-old man had a left radical orchiectomy. Pathologic evaluation reveals a mixed GCT containing seminoma and embryonal cell carcinoma. Tumor markers are negative. The CT image depicted in Figure 34-8 was obtained 1 day postoperation. Chest CT is negative. The next step in management is:

  a. Biopsy.

  b. Radiation therapy.

  c. Chemotherapy.

  d. RPLND.

  e. Repeat CT in 1 week to confirm a postsurgical inflammatory response.

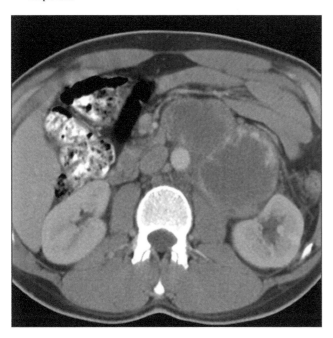

Figure 34-8.

ANSWERS

1. **d. Spermatocytic seminoma.** ITGCN is the common precursor lesion for all types of adult male GCT with the exception of spermatocytic seminoma. Pediatric GCTs do not typically arise from ITGCN.

2. **e. Metastatic spermatocytic seminoma is rare.** Spermatocytic seminoma differs from other GCT subtypes in that it does not arise from ITGCN, cryptorchidism is not a risk factor, bilaterality has not been reported, it does not express i(12p) or placental alkaline phosphatase, and it does not occur as a mixed GCT with other GCT subtypes. Only one documented case of metastasis has been reported, and these lesions are almost always cured by orchiectomy.

3. **a. Choriocarcinoma.** With the exception of choriocarcinoma, the most common route of disease dissemination is via lymphatic channels from the primary tumor to the retroperitoneal lymph nodes and subsequently to distant sites. Choriocarcinoma has a propensity for hematogenous dissemination. Yolk sac tumors in children are thought to spread hematogenously as well.

4. **c. Pure embryonal carcinoma.** Pure embryonal carcinoma may produce both AFP and hCG. Pure seminoma is associated with elevated serum hCG levels in 15% of cases but does not produce AFP. Pure teratoma typically is not associated with elevated serum tumor markers, although slightly elevated AFP levels may be observed. Choriocarcinoma is uniformly associated with elevated hCG levels but does not produce AFP. The vast majority of yolk sac tumors produce AFP, but they do not produce hCG.

5. **b. Suspected benign testicular lesion.** Testis-sparing surgery should be considered only in patients with suspected GCT who have normal testicular androgen production and who have a small (<2 cm) tumor either in a solitary testis or in the setting of bilateral synchronous testicular GCT. Testis-sparing surgery should not be performed in patients with suspected GCT who have a normal contralateral testis. Testis-sparing surgery may also be considered in patients with suspected benign testicular lesions such as an epidermoid cyst or adenomatoid tumor arising from the tunica albuginea.

6. **d. To obtain repeat serum tumor marker levels in 7 days.** Patients with elevated serum tumor markers before orchiectomy should have these levels measured after orchiectomy to assess whether the levels are declining, stable, or rising. Management decisions should not be made based on serum tumor marker levels before orchiectomy. Patients with rising postorchiectomy serum tumor marker levels should receive chemotherapy. The IGCCCG classification of metastatic NSGCT is based on the postorchiectomy serum tumor marker levels.

7. **a. Testicular seminoma with brain metastases.** According to IGCCCG classification criteria there is no "poor risk" category for metastatic seminoma. Patients with metastatic seminoma who have nonpulmonary visceral metastases (e.g., liver, bone, brain) are classified as at intermediate risk. Metastatic NSGCT patients with mediastinal primary tumor *or* nonpulmonary visceral metastases *or* postochiectomy AFP > 10,000 ng/mL, *or* postorchiectomy hCG of 50,000 mU/mL are classified as at poor risk.

8. **c. Mediastinoscopy and biopsy.** The presence of distant metastasis in the absence of retroperitoneal disease or elevated serum levels of tumor markers is uncommon, particularly for patients with testicular seminoma. Therefore, these patients should undergo biopsy and histologic confirmation of the suspected lesion before management decisions are made.

9. **b. CT-guided biopsy of the retroperitoneal mass.** The risk of teratoma at metastatic sites is less of a consideration for metastatic seminoma than for NSGCT. Although rare, seminoma may transform into NSGCT elements, and this should be considered in patients with metastatic seminoma who fail to respond to conventional therapy. These patients should undergo biopsy and histologic confirmation of the suspected lesion before management decisions are made. Either an open or a laparoscopic biopsy of the para-aortic mass is an acceptable approach if CT-guided biopsy is not feasible or the result is nondiagnostic. However, an RPLND should not be performed without histologic confirmation of NSGCT pathology.

10. **a. Inguinal orchiectomy.** Inguinal orchiectomy and low-dose radiation therapy are associated with the highest rates of local control of ITGCN. In a patient with a normal contralateral testis (particularly if future paternity is desired), inguinal orchiectomy is the preferred choice owing to the deleterious effects of radiation therapy on spermatogenesis within the contralateral testis.

11. **d. Elevated pre-orchiectomy AFP level.** Preorchiectomy serum tumor marker levels are not associated with the presence of occult metastases in clinical stage I NSGCT. The presence of postorchiectomy serum tumor marker levels in clinical stage I NSGCT indicates the presence of occult systemic disease.

12. **c. Chemotherapy with two cycles of bleomycin-etoposide-cisplatin.** Chemotherapy is associated with the lowest risk of recurrence and is thus preferred versus surveillance for patients who are anticipated to be noncompliant with surveillance imaging and testing (even for patients at low risk for occult metastases). Chemotherapy and RPLND are associated with similar rates of long-term cure, but the former may be preferable in patients with transmissible diseases. Adjuvant radiation therapy and carboplatin are standard treatment approaches for clinical stage I seminoma.

13. **e. Lymphovascular invasion.** Absence of teratoma in the primary tumor, prechemotherapy and postchemotherapy mass size, and percentage shrinkage of mass with chemotherapy are all associated with the presence of necrosis/fibrosis in residual masses after first-line chemotherapy. However, none of these factors (alone or together) is sufficiently accurate to exclude the presence of residual teratoma or viable malignancy in patients with residual masses greater than 1 cm. Lymphovascular invasion is associated with the presence of occult metastases in patients with clinical stage I NSGCT and has no impact on the histology of residual masses after chemotherapy.

14. **d. Observation.** Patients at low risk for metastatic disease with indeterminate CT findings should be closely observed because small (<1 cm) retroperitoneal lesions may represent false-positive findings, particularly if they are located outside the primary landing zone. A CT-guided biopsy would be technically difficult to perform given the lesion size and its proximity to the renal vessels.

15. **b. Lymphovascular invasion.** Lymphovascular invasion is associated with the presence of occult metastases in patients with clinical stage I NSGCT, but it has not been associated with an increased risk of distant metastases in patients with clinical or pathologic stage II disease. Elevated postorchiectomy serum tumor markers, bulky (>3 cm) retroperitoneal masses, or retroperitoneal lymphadenopathy outside the primary landing zone are associated with an increased risk of systemic relapse after RPLND. Thus clinical stage IIA-B patients with these features are recommended to receive induction chemotherapy. Scrotal invasion by the primary tumor is associated with an increased risk of metastasis to the inguinal lymph nodes, which are considered nonregional lymph nodes.

16. **d. Poor-risk disease at diagnosis by IGCCCG criteria.** Although patients with poor-risk GCT have diminished survival and are more likely to have viable malignancy or incomplete resection at postchemotherapy RPLND, IGCCCG risk category is not a predictor of relapse independent of the histology of resected masses or completeness of resection. "Desperation" postchemotherapy RPLND in the setting of rising serum tumor markers after second- or third-line chemotherapy and reoperative RPLND are other conditions associated with an increased risk of relapse.

17. **c. Bilateral postchemotherapy RPLND.** Approximately one third of patients will have residual masses at multiple anatomic sites, and these patients should undergo resection of all sites of measurable residual disease because discordant histology between anatomic sites is reported in 22% to 46% of cases. However, the presence of necrosis in postchemotherapy RPLND specimens is highly predictive of necrosis at other sites. Thus, postchemotherapy RPLND should be performed before resection of residual masses at other sites. Observation of small residual masses at other sites is a reasonable option if the histology of the RPLND specimen is necrosis. Patients with viable malignancy discovered at postchemotherapy resection should have all residual masses resected and are usually treated with an additional two cycles of chemotherapy. A full course of second-line chemotherapy is reserved for patients with either serologic or radiographic progression during or after first-line chemotherapy.

18. **e. The outcome is poor relative to those with early NSGCT relapse.** Until recently, late relapse has been associated with a worse prognosis than early relapse, although more recent data suggest these patient groups have a similar probability of cure. Disease-free rates of 50% to 60% are reported after treatment of early and late relapse.

19. **b. CT-guided biopsy of the para-aortic mass.** Patients with good-risk metastatic NSGCT who have dramatic progression of their disease with first-line chemotherapy despite normalization of serum tumor marker levels should be considered to have either growing teratoma syndrome or teratoma with malignant transformation. The presence of an enlarging solid mass and new sites of disease suggest a malignant process. An enlarging mass only with cystic appearance is more suggestive of growing teratoma syndrome. A CT-guided biopsy to identify the presence of malignant transformation is indicated because this finding may influence the choice of chemotherapy.

20. **e. Similar efficacy to cisplatin.** All of the randomized trials in advanced GCT in which a cisplatin-based regimen has been compared with a carboplatin-based regimen have reported superior outcomes with cisplatin. The rationale for single-agent carboplatin is based on reduced toxicity compared with cisplatin and 65% to 90% response rates reported in studies of carboplatin in advanced seminoma.

21. **d. Ejaculatory dysfunction.** Dog-leg radiotherapy for clinical stage I seminoma is associated with infertility due to the direct effects of radiation on the germinal epithelium with resultant impaired spermatogenesis. Infertility related to ejaculatory dysfunction is not associated with radiation therapy and is most commonly associated with RPLND.

22. **a. Utility of serum tumor markers to identify relapse at an early and curable stage.** Only 15% of seminomas produce elevations in serum hCG, and serum tumor marker levels are uncommonly elevated in the vast majority of patients with clinical stage I seminoma at diagnosis or at the time of relapse. This is in contrast to clinical stage I NGSCT, in which serum tumor markers are commonly the first (and only) manifestation of disease relapse.

23. **c. Observation.** In contrast to advanced NSGCT, only 10% of residual masses in advanced seminoma after first-line chemotherapy contain viable malignancy (90% contain fibrosis/necrosis only), and residual teratoma is less of a consideration. Spontaneous resolution of these masses will occur in the majority of cases. Approximately 30% of discrete residual masses greater than 3 cm will contain viable malignancy. FDG-PET is a useful adjunct to postchemotherapy staging CT to determine the need for postchemotherapy surgical resection. Residual masses larger than 3 cm that are PET negative and those less than 3 cm can be safely observed because of the high probability of necrosis/fibrosis. FDG-PET has no role in the characterization of residual masses less than 3 cm.

24. **d. CT of the head.** Choriocarcinoma spreads hematogenously and widely. Brain metastases should be suspected in any patient with a very high hCG level. Thus, patients with high hCG levels at diagnosis should have staging CT or magnetic resonance imaging (MRI) studies of the brain. Choriocarcinomas are highly vascular and tend to hemorrhage during chemotherapy, which may have catastrophic consequences in those patients with brain metastases. Brain metastases are also associated with a poor prognosis, and these patients should receive four cycles of bleomycin-etoposide-cisplatin as first-line chemotherapy, as should any patient with an hCG level over 5000 mU/mL at the time chemotherapy is initiated.

25. **a. Two cycles of platin-based chemotherapy does not increase one's risk of developing cardiovascular disease or SMN.** Although the risk of late complications of chemotherapy is dose dependent, there appears to be no safe lower limit. Thus even patients receiving one to two cycles of platin-based chemotherapy may have an increased risk of late toxicity.

26. **b. i and iii.** Unlike GCT, Leydig cell tumors are not associated with a history of cryptorchidism, and bilateral tumors have not been reported.

27. **a. Inguinal orchiectomy followed by adjuvant radiotherapy.** A large, infiltrative mass involving the spermatic cord in an adult man is a sarcoma until proved otherwise. The low-intensity signal on CT and patient age make liposarcoma the most common histology. Paratesticular liposarcoma rarely metastasize but tend to recur locally. Thus, adjuvant radiotherapy may be used to decrease the risk of local recurrence.

Pathology

1. **b. Has a significant chance of developing a germ cell tumor in the left testis.** The figure illustrates intratubular germ cell neoplasia as evidenced by enlarged hyperchromatic nuclei and a lack of a spermatogenesis. This carries a 50% risk of developing a germ cell tumor.
2. **d. Be advised to have radiation therapy to the retroperitoneum.** Notice in the figure the sheathlike pattern of small cells interspersed with fibrous septa that contain lymphocytes, the hallmarks of seminoma. Although observation is an option, most would recommend radiation to the retroperitoneum, because seminoma is very sensitive to radiation and the morbidity is low—although there is a risk for the development of secondary malignancies over the long term.
3. **a. Follow markers and check half-life.** The figure demonstrates seminoma with syncytiotrophoblasts. Approximately 15% of patients with seminoma have elevated hCG and will demonstrate syncytiotrophoblasts. Following orchiectomy, the hCG should

decline according to its 24-hour half-life. This should be determined first before any treatment decisions are made.
4. **d. Not have any treatment.** The figure shows a spermatocytic seminoma that has a very low malignant potential. Notice the small basophilic cells and the multinucleated tumor giant cell, which are characteristic for spermatocytic seminoma.
5. **a. Have induction chemotherapy.** This patient has an embryonal carcinoma: notice the primitive, anaplastic epithelial cells. With persistently elevated serum markers the patient should undergo induction chemotherapy. Surgery is not indicated, radiation therapy is inappropriate, and there is no reason to delay.
6. **a. Have an RPLND.** The tumor depicted is a teratoma: notice the mature enteric epithelium. Because the specimen is in the primary tumor, there is a high likelihood that there is residual teratoma in the retroperitoneal mass. This tumor is chemoinsensitive and should be resected.

Imaging

1. **b. Testicular neoplasm.** The ultrasound image shows an irregular, vascular mass in the left testis that also has microlithiasis. This is most consistent with a testicular neoplasm. It is not unusual for patients to have a history of groin trauma before presentation.
2. **c. Chemotherapy.** The CT image shows a large (>5 cm) para-aortic mass that represents metastatic adenopathy. Because this represents bulky retroperitoneal disease (stage IIC), chemotherapy is the best option.

CHAPTER REVIEW

1. Germ cell tumors (GCTs) occur bilaterally approximately 2% of the time. The risk factors for developing GCTs include cryptorchidism, a family history of testicular cancer, a previous history of testicular cancer, and intratubular germ cell neoplasia (ITGCN).
2. In men with a history of GCTs, the finding of testicular microlithiasis on ultrasonography in the contralateral testis is associated with an increased risk of intratubular germ cell neoplasia; the significance of microlithiasis in the general population, however, is unclear.
3. One percent to 5% of GCTs are extragonadal; they are generally less sensitive to chemotherapy and are more likely to contain yolk sac tumor elements than tumors arising in the testis.
4. On rare occasion teratomas may transform into somatic malignancies, such as rhabdomyosarcoma, adenocarcinoma, or neuroendocrine tumors.
5. Two thirds of patients with GCTs have diminished fertility.
6. Choriocarcinomas and seminomas do not produce AFP.
7. The half-life of AFP is 5 to 7 days, hCG is 24 to 36 hours, and LDH is 24 hours.
8. The primary landing zone in the retroperitoneum for right testicular tumors is the interaortocaval lymph nodes; for left testicular tumors it is the periaortic lymph nodes; the pattern of lymph drainage in the retroperitoneum is from right to left.
9. Patients with persistently elevated AFP and hCG after orchiectomy are given induction chemotherapy.
10. In clinical stage I disease approximately 25% of patients will have metastases.
11. Lymphovascular invasion and a prominent component of embryonal carcinoma are risk factors for metastases in NSGCTs.
12. In seminomas, risk factors for metastases are rete testis involvement and tumor size greater than 4 cm.
13. Patients with bulky retroperitoneal lymph node disease greater than 3 cm should receive induction chemotherapy.
14. After initial treatment, patients with enlargement of a retroperitoneal mass or an increase in markers should undergo salvage chemotherapy. Consideration may be given to a CT-guided biopsy under selected circumstances.
15. Patients with an NSGCT, undetectable markers, and a residual mass greater than 1 cm after chemotherapy should undergo surgical resection.
16. Approximately half of those patients who have surgical resection of a retroperitoneal mass following chemotherapy will harbor teratoma or a viable malignancy. The remainder will have fibrosis.
17. Patients with viable malignancy in residual masses after salvage chemotherapy have a poor prognosis.
18. Predictors of relapse in patients with stage I seminoma on surveillance include rete testis invasion and size of tumor greater than 4 cm. Lymphovascular invasion is not predictive as it is in NSGCT.
19. In patients with seminomas who are treated with chemotherapy, the size of the residual mass is highly predictive of viable tumor. Masses less than 3 cm rarely have viable tumor in them, whereas about a third of residual masses greater than 3 cm contain viable malignancy. FDG-PET is a useful adjunct to postchemotherapy staging CT to determine the need for postchemotherapy surgical resection. Residual masses larger than 3 cm that are PET negative and those less than 3 cm can be safely observed because of the high probability of necrosis/fibrosis.
20. Late toxicity of chemotherapy includes peripheral neuropathy, Raynaud phenomenon, hearing loss, hypogonadism and infertility, secondary malignant neoplasms, and cardiovascular disease.
21. There is an increased number of copies of genetic material from the short arm of chromosome 12 in germ cell tumors.
22. There is no clinical distinction between immature and mature teratoma. Teratomas are resistant to chemotherapy. They also tend to be infiltrative when large in size and can be extremely difficult to resect.
23. Of patients with testicular tumors, 52% are oligospermic and 10% are azoospermic at presentation.
24. Of patients who receive radiation as treatment for intratubular germ cell neoplasia, 40% require testosterone supplementation.

25. The risk for a secondary malignancy after radiation therapy for seminoma is 18% at 25 years.

26. Ninety percent of Leydig cell tumors and Sertoli cell tumors are benign and 10% are malignant.

27. The most common testicular neoplasm in men older than 50 years is lymphoma.

28. Cystadenoma of the epididymis is associated with von Hippel–Lindau syndrome; adenomatoid tumor of the epididymis is benign.

29. Liposarcoma is the most common paratesticular tumor in the adult. Rhabdomyosarcoma is the most common paratesticular tumor in the child.

30. ITGCN is the common precursor lesion for all types of adult male GCT, with the exception of spermatocytic seminoma.

31. Choriocarcinoma has a propensity for hematogenous dissemination. Yolk sac tumors in children are thought to spread hematogenously as well.

32. Pure embryonal carcinoma may produce both AFP and hCG. Pure seminoma is associated with elevated serum hCG levels in 15% of cases but does not produce AFP. Pure teratoma typically is not associated with elevated serum tumor markers, although slightly elevated AFP levels may be observed. Choriocarcinoma is uniformly associated with elevated hCG levels but does not produce AFP. The vast majority of yolk sac tumors produce AFP but they do not produce hCG.

33. Testis-sparing surgery should be considered only in patients with suspected GCT who have normal testicular androgen production and who have a small (<2 cm) tumor either in a solitary testis or in the setting of bilateral synchronous testicular GCT. Testis-sparing surgery should not be performed in patients with suspected GCT who have a normal contralateral testis. Testis-sparing surgery may also be considered in patients with suspected benign testicular lesions such as an epidermoid cyst or adenomatoid tumor arising from the tunica albuginea.

34. Absence of teratoma in the primary tumor, prechemotherapy and postchemotherapy mass size, and percentage shrinkage of mass with chemotherapy are all associated with the presence of necrosis/fibrosis in residual masses after first-line chemotherapy. However, none of these factors (alone or together) is sufficiently accurate to exclude the presence of residual teratoma or viable malignancy in patients with residual masses greater than 1 cm.

35. Approximately one third of patients who have residual masses following chemotherapy will have residual masses at multiple anatomic sites (sites outside the retroperitoneum), and these patients should undergo resection of all sites of measurable residual disease because discordant histology between anatomic sites is reported in 22% to 46% of cases. However, the presence of necrosis in postchemotherapy RPLND specimens is highly predictive of necrosis at other sites outside the retroperitoneum.

35 Surgery of Testicular Tumors

Kevin R. Rice, Clint Cary, Timothy A. Masterson, and Richard S. Foster

QUESTIONS

1. The following nerve is at risk for injury during radical orchiectomy:
   a. The genitofemoral nerve.
   b. The ilioinguinal nerve.
   c. The obturator nerve.
   d. The lateral femoral cutaneous nerve.
   e. The pudendal nerve.

2. Patients should NOT be considered for partial orchiectomy if they possess any of the following EXCEPT:
   a. A polar tumor >2 cm in greatest dimension.
   b. A normal contralateral testicle.
   c. Hypogonadism.
   d. Suspicion for benign tumor.
   e. Infertility.

3. All of the following are part of clinical staging for testicular cancer EXCEPT:
   a. Radical orchiectomy.
   b. Chest radiograph.
   c. Whole-body positron emission tomography (PET) scan.
   d. Serum alpha fetoprotein (AFP), human chorionic gonadotropin (hCG), and lactate dehydrogenase (LDH).
   e. Contrasted computed tomography (CT) scan of the abdomen and pelvis.

4. The incidence of perioperative acute respiratory distress syndrome (ARDS) in patients with prior receipt of bleomycin can be minimized by:
   a. Avoidance of the Trendelenburg position.
   b. Keeping the FiO_2 as low as possible.
   c. Short operating time.
   d. Minimization of intraoperative and perioperative fluid resuscitation.
   e. Both b and d.

5. Performing the aortic split-and-roll before that of the inferior vena cava (IVC):
   a. Allows prospective identification of right accessory lower pole renal arteries not identified on preoperative imaging.
   b. Facilitates identification of right-sided postganglionic sympathetic nerves as they cross over the aorta.
   c. Minimizes risk of left ureteral injury.
   d. Increases risk if injury to the inferior mesenteric artery.
   e. Should never be performed.

6. The ureter is typically located:
   a. Anterior to the ipsilateral renal artery.
   b. Anterior to the ipsilateral retroperitoneal nodal packet.
   c. Posterior to the ipsilateral gonadal vein adjacent to the lower pole of the ipsilateral kidney.
   d. Anterior to the ipsilateral gonadal vein adjacent to the lower pole of the ipsilateral kidney.
   e. Posterior to the ipsilateral common iliac artery.

7. Which of the following anatomic structures demonstrates the most predictable and constant anatomy?
   a. The postganglionic sympathetic nerve fibers
   b. The lumbar arteries
   c. The lumbar veins
   d. The number of nodes in each retroperitoneal packet
   e. The lymphatic vessels

8. The cisterna chylae is located:
   a. Immediately posterolateral to the IVC, just cephalad to the right renal artery.
   b. Immediately posterolateral to the IVC, just inferior to the right renal artery.
   c. Immediately posterolateral to the aorta, just cephalad to the left renal artery.
   d. Immediately posterolateral to the aorta, just inferior to the left renal artery.
   e. Immediately posteromedial to the aorta, just cephalad to the right renal artery.

9. The most common auxiliary procedure required to ensure complete resection of residual tumor at postchemotherapy (PC)-RPLND is:
   a. IVC resection.
   b. Retrocrural resection.
   c. Nephrectomy.
   d. Pelvic resection.
   e. Aortic resection.

10. All of the following are associated with an increased risk of nephrectomy EXCEPT:
    a. Left-sided primary testicular tumor.
    b. Prior receipt of salvage chemotherapy.
    c. Larger retroperitoneal mass size.
    d. Presence of ipsilateral accessory lower pole renal arteries.
    e. Elevated serum tumor markers at PC-RPLND.

11. The histology encountered most often at resection of residual hepatic lesions after chemotherapy is:
    a. Viable malignancy.
    b. Teratoma.
    c. Fibrosis/necrosis.
    d. Somatic-type malignancy.
    e. Hemangioma.

12. Which of the following are associated with an increased risk of pelvic germ cell tumor (GCT) metastases?
    a. Higher initial clinical stage
    b. Extragonadal primary GCT
    c. Prior pelvic surgery
    d. Congenital absence of the vasa deferentia
    e. a, b, c

13. Which of the following is TRUE?
    a. Patients with a PET-negative residual mass after induction chemotherapy for nonseminomatous GCT (NSGCT) can be safely observed.
    b. Performing PC-RPLND in patients with a clinical complete remission (no mass larger than 1 cm) of metastatic disease to induction chemotherapy has been shown to decrease recurrences.
    c. When PC-RPLND is performed in patients demonstrating complete clinical remission to induction chemotherapy, approximately 20% of specimens demonstrate residual microscopic teratoma or cancer.
    d. It is safe to observe patients experiencing a clinical complete remission if they have teratoma-negative primary tumors, but not if there is teratoma in the primary tumor.
    e. All International Germ Cell Cancer Collaborative Group (IGCCCG) intermediate- and poor-risk patients should undergo PC-RPLND, regardless of response to chemotherapy.

14. With regard to the use of postoperative adjuvant cisplatin-based chemotherapy in patients demonstrating pathologic stage IIA-B disease at primary RPLND, all of the following are true EXCEPT:
    a. It spares one to two cycles of chemotherapy for those patients destined to recur on postoperative observation.
    b. It nearly eliminates postoperative recurrences.
    c. It improves overall and cancer-specific survival.
    d. It results in overtreatment of 50% to 70% of patients if given to all patients.
    e. It is typically given in two cycles.

15. Which of the following characteristics has been associated with increased recurrence rate when teratoma is encountered at PC-RPLND?
    a. Large residual mass size
    b. Presence of somatic type malignancy
    c. Mediastinal primary GCT
    d. Presence of immature teratoma
    e. a, b, c

16. Which of the following factors have been associated with poorer prognosis when viable GCT is encountered at PC-RPLND?
    a. Incomplete resection
    b. >10% viable GCT in resection specimen
    c. IGCCCG intermediate or poor risk status
    d. Prior receipt of salvage chemotherapy
    e. All of the above

17. Which of the following patients is most likely to benefit from two cycles of adjuvant chemotherapy after PC-RPLND?
    a. 32-year-old male who received BEPx4 with persistently elevated AFP that normalized with salvage VelPx4, but has a 6-cm interaortocaval residual mass. PC-RPLND reveals viable yolk sac tumor in 50% of the resection specimen.
    b. 25-year-old male with a history of IGCCCG poor-risk NSGCT who after completing BEPx4 has a 15-cm para-aortic mass resected demonstrating teratoma and fibrosis.

    c. 28-year-old male with a 5-cm interaortocaval mass after completion of BEPx3 for IGCCCG good-risk disease. At PC-RPLND, viable embryonal cell carcinoma makes up 30% of his specimen, with the remainder being teratoma and a small amount of fibrosis.
    d. 31-year-old male with history of clinical stage IIC good-risk NSGCT who has a 5-cm residual mass after EPx4. PC-RPLND reveals teratoma with enteric-type adenocarcinoma.
    e. 27-year-old male who experienced a clinical CR of a 5 cm left para-aortic mass to BEPx3 approximately 5 years ago. He demonstrates an AFP of 150 on follow-up, and CT scan reveals a 7-cm left para-aortic recurrence. Resection reveals 100% viable yolk sac tumor. AFP normalizes postoperatively.

18. A patient has an isolated resectable residual retroperitoneal mass after induction chemotherapy without radiographic evidence of disease outside the retroperitoneum, but tumor markers have failed to normalize. Which of the following are reasonable indications for the consideration of desperation RPLND?
    a. Declining or plateauing AFP after induction chemotherapy
    b. Slowly rising AFP after a complete serologic response to induction chemotherapy
    c. All potentially curative chemotherapeutic options have been exhausted
    d. Persistently rising serum tumor markers (STMs) through induction chemotherapy
    e. a, b, c

19. Reoperative RPLND is thought to indicate a technical failure at prior RPLND. All of the following findings supportive of this hypothesis have been reported in the literature EXCEPT:
    a. The primary landing zone is the most common site of retroperitoneal recurrence.
    b. Ipsilateral pelvic recurrences are common.
    c. Incomplete ipsilateral lumbar vessel ligation encountered at reoperative RPLND has been associated with ipsilateral infield recurrence.
    d. Unresected ipsilateral gonadal vessels are frequently encountered at reoperative RPLND.
    e. The retroaortic and retrocaval regions are frequent sites of recurrence.

20. All of the following are true regarding late relapse of GCT EXCEPT:
    a. Yolk sac tumor is the most common viable histology encountered.
    b. First-line treatment is generally systemic chemotherapy followed by consolidative PC-RPLND.
    c. Patients who are chemotherapy-naïve demonstrate superior survival outcomes.
    d. GCT with somatic-type malignancy is seen with increased frequency in this population.
    e. The retroperitoneum is the most common site of late relapse.

21. What percentage of patients presenting with GCT have abnormal parameters on semen analysis?
    a. <10%
    b. 20% to 60%
    c. 70% to 80%
    d. >90%

22. Which processes are required to ensure antegrade ejaculation of sperm-containing semen?
    a. Seminal emission through vasa deferentia
    b. Closure of the bladder neck

c. Contraction of the bulbospongiosis muscles

d. Penile erection

e. a, b, c

23. All of the following interventions have demonstrated efficacy in managing chylous ascites EXCEPT:

    a. Medium-chain triglyceride (MCT) diet.

    b. Total parenteral nutrition.

    c. Subcutaneous octreotide.

    d. Limiting fat intake preoperatively.

    e. Placement of peritoneovenous shunt.

24. Which of the following patients is at the greatest risk for neurologic compromise due to spinal ischemia?

    a. 32-year-old male undergoing resection of left para-aortic mass with apparent aortic invasion who will most likely require resection of the infrahilar aorta and tube graft reconstruction.

    b. 29-year-old male with large-volume left para-aortic and interaortocaval masses that extend through the retrocrural region into the middle visceral mediastinum.

    c. 27-year-old male with a completed occluded IVC due to large interaortocaval, retrocaval, and right paracaval masses with a tumor thrombus up the inferior border of the right renal vein.

    d. 31-year-old male with a large infrarenal left para-aortic mass that is found to be invading the L2 vertebral foramina during resection.

ANSWERS

1. **b. The ilioinguinal nerve.** The ilioinguinal nerve will be encountered immediately on opening the external oblique fascia and entering the inguinal canal. It courses parallel to the spermatic cord along the cephalad aspect of its anterior surface. Care should be taken to preserve this structure in order to prevent postoperative numbness and paresthesia of the ipsilateral medial thigh and scrotum.

2. **d. Suspicion for benign tumor.** For obvious reasons, patients who are suspected to have a benign tumor are prime candidates for partial orchiectomy. Patients with larger tumors in the setting of normal contralateral testicle should be managed with radical orchiectomy as they will not likely suffer permanent postoperative infertility or hypogonadism. In addition, the benefits of partial orchiectomy with the goal of saving poorly functioning testicular parenchyma in a patient with baseline infertility and/or hypogonadism are most likely outweighed by the potential for incomplete resection of tumor and/or ipsilateral testicular recurrence.

3. **c. Whole-body positron emission tomography (PET) scan.** Testicular germ cell tumor patients are clinically staged with radical orchiectomy (T stage), chest imaging, a CT scan or magnetic resonance imaging (MRI) of the abdomen and pelvis (N and M stages), and postorchiectomy serum tumor markers (S stage). PET scans have no role in the clinical staging of seminomas or nonseminomas. PET scans do have a role in evaluating postchemotherapy residual masses in cases of pure seminoma.

4. **e. Both b and d.** Postoperative ARDS in patients with prior receipt of bleomycin is rare but most commonly encountered in patients having received four courses of bleomycin with significant pulmonary tumor burden. The two intraoperative factors that have been associated with an increased risk of developing postoperative ARDS have been (1) exposure to high FiO_2 and (2) high-volume administration of intravenous fluids and blood products. Anesthesiologists should be made aware of these risk factors.

5. **a. Allows prospective identification of right accessory lower pole renal arteries not identified on preoperative imaging.** The advantage of splitting of the aorta before the IVC is that it allows for the prospective identification of right accessory lower pole renal arteries not identified on preoperative imaging. Such vessels may be inadvertently divided if the IVC split is performed first. This can lead to significant blood loss and renal parenchymal loss. The disadvantage of splitting of the aorta first is inadvertent division of postganglionic sympathetic fibers involved in ejaculation. This can be minimized by stopping the aortic split at the inferior mesenteric artery and prospectively identifying the sympathetic efferents before continuing the split caudally.

6. **c. Posterior to the ipsilateral gonadal vein adjacent to the lower pole of the ipsilateral kidney.** The ureters provide the anatomic landmark for the lateral border of dissection for the para-aortic and paracaval lymph node packets. However, the ureters are vulnerable to injury if not prospectively identified. The ureter can be easily found at the inferior border of the ipsilateral kidney where it typically passes behind the ipsilateral gonadal vein. The ureter passes anterior to the ipsilateral common iliac artery as it descends into the pelvis.

7. **b. The lumbar arteries.** There are three paired lumbar arteries located between the renal hilum and the aortic bifurcation in nearly all patients. The only subtle anomaly commonly encountered with aortic lumbars is that the paired lumbars may exit the aorta through a short common trunk before bifurcating, a variant that can result in significant blood loss if not identified before these structures are ligated and divided. Lumbar vein anatomy is high variable, with these structures varying widely in location and caliber. While the number of postganglionic sympathetic roots in the field of retroperitoneal lymph node dissection (RPLND) tends to be relatively constant at four per side, the exact locations, paths, and patterns of fusion to adjacent roots is highly variable. Studies on lymph node counts have universally reported high standards of deviation and interquartile ranges.

8. **e. Immediately posteromedial to the aorta just cephalad to the right renal artery.** Failure to meticulously ligate large-caliber lymphatics in the region of the cisterna chylae can predispose patients to troublesome postoperative chylous ascites. Thus, use of clips and/or ties at the superior extent of the interaortocaval and para-aortic packets as well as during retrocrural dissections is advised.

9. **c. Nephrectomy.**

10. **d. Presence of ipsilateral accessory lower pole renal arteries.** Reported nephrectomy rates at PC-RPLND have ranged from 5% to 31%. Increased nephrectomy rates have been reported for patients undergoing salvage RPLND, desperation RPLND, reoperative RPLND, and resection of late relapse. In addition, large retroperitoneal mass size and left-sided primary tumors are associated with increased rates of nephrectomy.

11. **c. Fibrosis/necrosis.** Approximately three quarters of residual hepatic lesions after chemotherapy will demonstrate fibrosis/necrosis only at resection. There is a 94% concordance between retroperitoneal and hepatic fibrosis/necrosis. Thus, observation should be considered in patients with retroperitoneal necrosis and residual hepatic lesions that would require a potentially morbid resection.

12. **e. a, b, c.** Although the pelvis is the caudal extension of the retroperitoneum, it is not a common site of GCT metastases. Patients with high-volume retroperitoneal disease are thought to be at increased risk of pelvic metastases due to retrograde spread of tumor down the iliac lymphatic chains. A truly extragonadal primary GCT has less predictable lymphatic spread than testicular primaries; thus, pelvic spread seems to occur more often in these patients. Prior pelvic surgery likely leads to pelvic spread of disease by disrupting normal lymphatic drainage.

13. **c. When PC-RPLND is performed in patients demonstrating complete clinical remission to induction chemotherapy,**

approximately 20% of specimens demonstrate residual microscopic teratoma or cancer. Investigators at Memorial Sloan Kettering Cancer Center reported that approximately 20% of patients with postchemotherapy residual masses smaller than 1 cm demonstrated teratoma or viable GCT at resection, leading to a recommendation to perform PC-RPLND in all patients with history of retroperitoneal masses regardless of response to chemotherapy. To date, no study has demonstrated that this practice is associated with any improvement in recurrence-free or cancer-specific survival. Thus, observation is still considered a standard management, as this strategy has been associated with 97% to 100% cancer-specific survival. There is no role for PET scan in the assessment of postchemotherapy masses in nonseminomas.

14. **c. Improves overall and cancer-specific survival.** Adjuvant chemotherapy for pathologic stage IIA-B disease encountered at primary RPLND consists of two cycles of bleomycin, etoposide, and cisplatin (BEP) or two cycles of etoposide and cisplatin (EP). This nearly eliminates the risk of recurrence but has no effect on cancer-specific survival, which approaches 100% whether chemotherapy is administered in the adjuvant setting or reserved for patients who experience relapse. Patients who relapse will require full induction chemotherapy consisting of BEPx3 or EPx4. When pathologic stage IIA-B patients are observed after primary RPLND, approximately 30% to 50% of patients relapse.

15. **e. a, b, c.** Patients with high-volume teratoma, somatic-type malignancy, and mediastinal primary GCT disease have a higher risk of postoperative recurrence. Although once thought to be a marker of more aggressive behavior, immature teratoma has demonstrated no decrement in survival outcomes compared with mature teratoma.

16. **e. All of the above.** In a large multicenter review by Fizazi and colleagues, incomplete resection, proportion of viable GCT in resection specimen, and IGCCCG risk status were used to classify patients into three risk categories that predicted survival outcomes. When evaluating patients with viable GCT at PC-RPLND, prior receipt of salvage chemotherapy has consistently been associated with significantly poorer survival outcomes.

17. **c. 28-year-old male with a 5-cm interaortocaval mass after completion of BEPx3 for IGCCCG good-risk disease. At PC-RPLND viable embryonal cell carcinoma makes up 30% of his specimen, with the remainder being teratoma and a small amount of fibrosis.** Patients having received salvage chemotherapy who demonstrate viable GCT at PC-RPLND (option a), those demonstrating teratoma only at PC-RPLND (option b), and those demonstrating transformation to somatic-type malignancy (option d) have not been shown to benefit from adjuvant chemotherapy. In addition, patients with prior receipt of chemotherapy who experience late relapse do not often benefit from chemotherapy. The patient in option c would fall into the intermediate risk group for viable GCT encountered at PC-RPLND described by Fizazi and colleagues and, thus, would be a prime candidate for adjuvant cisplatin-based chemotherapy.

18. **e. a, b, c.** Investigators at Indiana University reported a 53.9% cancer-specific survival rate at a median follow-up of 6 years

when the criteria outlined in a-c were used to select patients to undergo desperation PC-RPLND. A patient with persistently rising STMs during chemotherapy should receive either standard or high-dose salvage chemotherapy.

19. **b. Ipsilateral pelvic recurrences are common.** Reoperative RPLND indicates a technical failure at prior RPLND in the majority of cases. Several reviews of reoperative experiences at high-volume centers have revealed that primary landing zone recurrence as well as signs of an inadequate prior resection (incomplete/absent lumbar vessel ligation, unresected ipsilateral gonadal vein, and recurrence posterior to the great vessels) are common in patients experiencing retroperitoneal recurrence after RPLND.

20. **b. First-line treatment is generally systemic chemotherapy followed by consolidative PC-RPLND.** Late relapse in patients with prior receipt of chemotherapy is often composed of yolk sac tumor and tends to be relatively chemorefractory regardless of histology. Thus, primary management of resectable disease at late relapse is surgical extirpation. Late relapse in chemotherapy-naïve patients has been associated with improved outcomes likely due to increased susceptibility to chemotherapy.

21. **b. 20% to 60%.** Infertility and subfertility are frequently present at GCT diagnosis. This can present challenges to pretreatment sperm banking. For unclear reasons, parameters occasionally improve after orchiectomy. However, this baseline infertility needs to be taken into account when evaluating fertility outcomes after treatment of GCT.

22. **e. a, b, c.** Seminal emission and bladder neck closure are both mediated by the L1-L4 postganglionic sympathetic nerve fibers vulnerable to resection during RPLND. Although contraction of the bulbospongiosis muscles is necessary for ejaculation, this phenomenon is not mediated by the sympathetic efferents. Penile erection is necessary for vaginal penetration, but not ejaculation. Notably, erection is a parasympathetic process.

23. **d. Limiting fat intake preoperatively.** Although it is a troublesome postoperative complication, chylous ascites tends to be transient, and management is usually directed at draining accumulated fluid and minimizing further production by instituting an MCT diet, progressing to total parenteral nutrition if the MCT diet fails, and possibly starting subcutaneous octreotide. A peritoneovenous shunt is an intervention of last resort. Limiting preoperative fat intake has not been shown to decrease the incidence of chylous ascites.

24. **b. 29-year-old male with large-volume left para-aortic and interaortocaval masses that extend through the retrocrural region into the middle visceral mediastinum.** Spinal ischemia leading to neurologic compromise is extremely rare. Patients at risk for this potentially devastating complication are those who will require resection of more than three sequential lumbar artery pairs. This tends to be in patients with high-volume para-aortic disease in the retroperitoneum, retrocrural region, and visceral mediastinum.

CHAPTER REVIEW

1. The proper performance of a radical inguinal orchiectomy includes mobilizing the cord 1 to 2 cm proximal to the internal inguinal ring and individually ligating the vas deferens and cord vessels with silk sutures so that the stump may be identified if an RPLND is performed.

2. When an orchiectomy has been performed through the scrotum in patients who have a low-stage seminoma, the radiation portals should be extended to include the ipsilateral groin and scrotum; for those with low-stage NSGCT, the scrotal scar should be excised along with the spermatic cord remnant; and for those who have received a full cycle of platinum-based chemotherapy, only the cord stump need be removed at the time of RPLND.

3. The right testicular lymphatics drain to the interaortocaval lymph nodes followed by paracaval and pericaval nodes. The left testicular lymphatics drain to the periaortic and preaortic lymph nodes.

4. Contralateral lymphatic flow is more commonly seen in right-sided tumors than left-sided tumors.

5. There is a 20% to 30% incidence of positive nodes in clinical stage I disease and approximately a 25% relapse rate in such patients who are placed on a surveillance protocol.

6. Suprahilar metastases are rare in low-stage NSGCT. Three percent to 23% of patients with positive nodes at RPLND will have extra-template disease. The most common site of residual suprahilar disease is in the retrocrural space.

7. It is extremely important, when performing a primary RPLND, to secure all lymphatic vessels with either clips or ties, particularly in the region of the right renal artery and diaphragmatic crus, to minimize injury to the cisterna chyli, which could result in chylous ascites.

8. In the presence of documented or suspected metastatic disease, a full bilateral dissection should be performed. In selected cases, preservation of individual nerve fibers may be performed.

9. The anterior split over the vena cava is not likely to damage nerve fibers; however, the anterior split over the aorta risks injury to these fibers.

10. The most important nerves to preserve antegrade ejaculation are those arising from the L1-L4 ganglia. To preserve nerve fibers, a dissection on the aorta should only be performed after the nerve fibers have been identified and isolated.

11. There is a sevenfold increase in cardiovascular complications in men treated with platinum-based chemotherapy.

12. All patients should be given the opportunity to bank sperm before RPLND.

13. In clinical stage I NSGCT lymphovascular invasion; higher T stage; tumor involvement of the cord, capsule, or scrotum; and a high percentage of embryonal carcinoma are associated with an increased incidence of retroperitoneal relapse. Most relapses occur within the first 2 years and are rare after 5 years. The absence of teratoma in the primary tumor does not preclude its presence in the retroperitoneum.

14. Persistently elevated tumor marker levels after orchiectomy require systemic chemotherapy as the next step is not RPLND.

15. Patients best suited for RPLND are those with clinical stage IIA and low-volume, less than 3-cm ipsilateral disease (stage IIB).

16. Sixty percent of patients with testicular cancer have subnormal pretreatment semen analyses. Sixty-five percent of men on surveillance can impregnate their partner after orchiectomy.

17. Bilateral RPLND is the standard template for patients with pathologic stage II NSGCT.

18. Bleomycin can cause restrictive pulmonary fibrosis with increased collagen deposition and makes the patient highly susceptible to fluid overload.

19. Increased serum concentration of AFP and hCG after primary platinum-based chemotherapy is usually characterized by unresectable viable tumor, and salvage chemotherapy rather than excision of the mass is recommended.

20. After chemotherapy, retroperitoneal masses are composed of necrosis/fibrosis in 40%, teratoma in 45%, and viable GCT in 15%. A residual mass after salvage chemotherapy is composed of viable GCT in 50%, teratoma in 40%, and fibrosis in 10%. The clinical behavior of a teratoma is unpredictable, and complete resection is required.

21. After chemotherapy, RPLND is indicated for NSGCT primary tumors in which the residual mass is larger than 1 cm. RPLND may be eliminated after chemotherapy if there was no evidence of the disease in the retroperitoneum before chemotherapy.

22. Late relapses occur in 2% to 4% of patients, and more than half of late relapses occur beyond 10 years, emphasizing the need for prolonged follow-up.

23. If the aortic wall is stripped of its adventitia, it should be replaced with a synthetic graft because delayed rupture may occur.

24. Tumor involvement of the superior mesenteric artery, celiac axis, or porta hepatis usually precludes resection. After chemotherapy, resection of residual masses should be accompanied by a complete RPLND. The standard bilateral dissection is the prudent approach.

25. Incidental appendectomy during RPLND increases the risk of infection and should not be performed.

26. After chemotherapy for seminoma, residual masses very rarely contain teratoma and are extremely difficult technically to remove. Thus a residual mass less than 3 cm should be observed, patients with masses larger than 3 cm should have PET, and if a viable seminoma is noted, then either additional chemotherapy or RPLND is indicated.

27. After chemotherapy, spermatogenesis may take 3 years to return to normal.

28. In the setting of complete or near complete occlusion, routine reconstruction of the vena cava following resection is not required.

29. RPLND histology is a strong predictor of histology at thoracotomy: if necrosis is all that is found in the retroperitoneum, 89% of the time the chest lesions will be necrotic.

30. The ureters provide the anatomic landmark for the lateral border of dissection for the para-aortic and paracaval lymph node packets.

31. There are three paired lumbar arteries located between the renal hilum and the aortic bifurcation in nearly all patients.

32. Patients having received salvage chemotherapy who demonstrate viable GCT at PC-RPLND, those demonstrating teratoma only at PC-RPLND, and those demonstrating transformation to somatic-type malignancy have not been shown to benefit from adjuvant chemotherapy.

33. Late relapse in patients with prior receipt of chemotherapy is often composed of yolk sac tumor and tends to be relatively chemorefractory regardless of histology. Thus, primary management of resectable disease at late relapse is surgical extirpation.

36

Laparoscopic and Robotic-Assisted Retroperitoneal Lymphadenectomy for Testicular Tumors

Mohamad E. Allaf and Louis R. Kavoussi

QUESTIONS

1. A 23-year old man presents after undergoing transscrotal orchiectomy for presumed hydrocele. Pathologic examination revealed embryonal carcinoma with vascular invasion. Serum levels of tumor markers and results of physical examination and computed tomography (CT) of the chest, abdomen, and pelvis were normal. Which of the following approaches is most appropriate?

   a. Observation

   b. Retroperitoneal lymph node dissection (RPLND)

   c. RPLND plus excision of scrotal scar and remnant cord

   d. RPLND plus scrotectomy and inguinal lymph node dissection

   e. RPLND plus scrotal and inguinal radiation

2. Late relapse is a feature most commonly associated with:

   a. seminoma.

   b. yolk sac tumor.

   c. embryonal carcinoma.

   d. choriocarcinoma.

   e. teratoma.

3. A 25-year-old man with a stage IIC nonseminomatous germ cell tumor (NSGCT) has completed primary platinum-based chemotherapy. Tumor marker levels have normalized according to appropriate half-life, and he has undergone bilateral postchemotherapy RPLND. Final pathologic analysis reveals a focus of yolk sac tumor. Appropriate therapy at this point is:

   a. careful observation.

   b. radiation therapy.

   c. two additional cycles of platinum-based chemotherapy.

   d. four additional cycles of platinum-based chemotherapy.

   e. re-exploration in 6 weeks.

4. A 20-year-old man with clinical stage I NSGCT undergoes laparoscopic RPLND. During surgery a 2-cm lymph node is encountered. Which of the following is the most appropriate next step?

   a. Abort the procedure and administer chemotherapy.

   b. Convert to an open procedure.

   c. Perform a unilateral template dissection and administer chemotherapy.

   d. Continue the procedure and perform a full bilateral dissection.

   e. None of the above.

5. The most common cause of open conversion during laparoscopic RPLND is:

   a. intraoperative discovery of bulky lymphadenopathy.

   b. failure to progress.

   c. bowel injury.

   d. hypercapnia.

   e. bleeding.

6. Two weeks after laparoscopic RPLND, a patient complains of abdominal distention and emesis. CT reveals ascites. Diagnostic paracentesis confirms the diagnosis of chylous ascites. The next best step is:

   a. reassurance and discharge.

   b. reoperation to identify and treat the source of lymphatic leak.

   c. placement of peritoneal drain and initiation of a low-fat diet.

   d. initiation of somatostatin.

   e. hydration and initiation of a low-fat diet.

7. A 20-year-old man undergoes laparoscopic RPLND after right radical orchiectomy for an NSGCT. All of the following regions should be dissected clear of all lymphatic tissue EXCEPT:

   a. right spermatic cord.

   b. paracaval region.

   c. interaortocaval region.

   d. retrocrural region.

   e. precaval region.

8. Potential advantages to laparoscopic compared with open RPLND include all of the following EXCEPT:

   a. improved cosmesis.

   b. shorter convalescence.

   c. improved disease-free survival.

   d. shorter interval to chemotherapy when necessary.

   e. faster return to normal activities.

ANSWERS

1. **c. RPLND plus excision of scrotal scar and remnant cord.** In the setting of scrotal contamination and clinical stage I disease, the patient is best managed with RPLND and wide excision of the scrotal scar. The remainder of the cord also should be removed. Observation is not optimal, because of the presence of vascular invasion and scrotal contamination.

2. **e. Teratoma.** Late relapse of germ cell tumor after definitive therapy is defined as recurrence more than 2 years after completion of therapy and occurring without evidence of disease. Teratoma is the most common histologic subtype involved in cases of late relapse. This is likely due to its combination of prolonged doubling time and chemotherapy resistance.

3. **c. Two additional cycles of platinum-based chemotherapy.** The patient's prognosis is related to serum tumor marker level at the time of RPLND, prior treatment burden, and the pathologic findings for the resected specimen. If viable germ cell tumor (GCT) is present at any site, but all disease is completely resected, two additional cycles provide survival benefit in this subset of patients. Einhorn reported only 2 long-term survivors of 22 patients (9%) with completely resected viable GCT after cisplatin, bleomycin, and vinblastine chemotherapy, if additional postoperative chemotherapy was not given. Fox and colleagues reported

that 70% of patients with completely resected viable GCT after primary chemotherapy followed by two cycles of postoperative chemotherapy remained disease free compared with none of seven patients without additional chemotherapy.

4. **d. Continue the procedure and perform a full bilateral dissection.** Whenever a suspicious lymph node is identified, a full bilateral dissection should be performed. Chemotherapy will not compensate for an inadequate retroperitoneal dissection.

5. **e. Bleeding.** The most common reason for conversion to an open procedure is uncontrollable bleeding, and vascular injury is cited as the most common intraoperative complication. This occurs less than 5% of the time in experienced hands.

6. **e. Hydration and initiation of a low-fat diet.** Chylous ascites is a devastating complication that occurs less than 2% of the time after primary laparoscopic (and open) RPLND. Initiation of a low-fat diet, hydration, and drainage of the fluid is usually the first step in management. Reoperation is considered only when all other options have been exhausted.

7. **d. Retrocrural region.** The superior boundary of dissection templates does not include lymph nodes superior to the renal hilum.

8. **c. Improved disease-free survival.** No study has demonstrated any difference in disease-free survival comparing open or laparoscopic approaches to node dissection.

CHAPTER REVIEW

1. Patients who have small volume retroperitoneal disease (pN1) are cured 70% of the time by a radical RPLND.

2. RPLND is the treatment of choice for patients with stage I NSGCTs with teratoma.

3. All patients undergoing RPLND should be offered preoperative sperm banking.

4. In nerve-sparing techniques for RPLND, great care should be taken around the lumbar veins because these are adjacent to the sympathetic chain.

37 Tumors of the Penis

Curtis A. Pettaway, Raymond S. Lance, and John W. Davis

QUESTIONS

1. Which of the following penile lesions does NOT have malignant potential?
   a. Balanitis xerotica obliterans
   b. Condylomata acuminatum
   c. Coronal papillae
   d. Bowen disease
   e. Leukoplakia

2. Which of the following infections is associated with cervical dysplasia?
   a. Human immunodeficiency virus (HIV) infection
   b. Herpesvirus infection
   c. Gonorrhea
   d. Human papillomavirus (HPV) infection
   e. Lymphogranuloma venereum

3. What is the major difference between Bowen disease and erythroplasia of Queyrat?
   a. Loss of rete pegs
   b. Keratin staining
   c. Viral etiologic agents
   d. Location
   e. Treatment options

4. Kaposi sarcoma of the acquired immunodeficiency syndrome (AIDS)-related (epidemic) type is associated with which of the following etiologic agents?
   a. HPV type 16
   b. Human herpesvirus (HHV) type 8
   c. HPV type 32
   d. *Haemophilus ducreyi* (chancroid [soft chancre])
   e. Coxsackievirus type 23

5. Where do penile cancers most commonly arise?
   a. Glans
   b. Shaft
   c. Frenulum
   d. Coronal sulcus
   e. Scrotum

6. Which of the following is not considered a risk factor for the development of squamous cell carcinoma of the penis?
   a. Cigarette smoke
   b. HPV infection
   c. Phimosis
   d. Gonorrhea
   e. Chewing tobacco

7. All of the following are preventive strategies to decrease the incidence of penile cancer EXCEPT:
   a. circumcision after 21 years of age.
   b. avoiding sexual promiscuity.
   c. daily genital hygiene.
   d. avoiding cigarette smoke.
   e. circumcision before puberty.

8. Which of the following statements regarding penile cancer is FALSE?
   a. Cancer may develop anywhere on the penis.
   b. Because of the associated discomfort, patients usually present to physicians within the first month of noting the lesion.
   c. Phimosis may obscure the nature of the lesion.
   d. Penetration of the Buck fascia and the tunica albuginea by the tumor permits invasion of the vascular corpora.
   e. Cancer cells reach the contralateral inguinal region because of lymphatic cross-communications at the base of the penis.

9. Before a treatment plan for penile cancer is initiated, which of the following is TRUE?
   a. Adequate biopsies to determine stage are unimportant because all patients should be treated with amputation.
   b. Radiologic studies play no role in decision making.
   c. DNA flow cytometry should be performed on virtually all specimens because it provides crucial information.
   d. Tumor stage, grade, and vascular invasion status all provide prognostically important information.
   e. No disfiguring therapy is indicated, because spontaneous remissions have been noted in approximately 10% of cases.

10. Which of the following statements is TRUE regarding the natural history of penile cancer?
    a. Metastases from the primary tumor often involve lung, liver, or bone as initial sites.
    b. Lymphatic drainage from the primary tumor is ipsilateral alone in most cases.
    c. Metastasis often initially involves spread from the corpora cavernosa to the pelvic lymph nodes.
    d. Metastasis initially involves inguinal lymph nodes beneath the fascia lata.
    e. Metastasis initially involves inguinal lymph nodes above the fascia lata.

11. Which of the following statements concerning hypercalcemia in patients with penile cancer is TRUE?
    a. It is more commonly due to massive bone metastases than bulky soft tissue metastases.
    b. It is often related to uremia due to ureteral obstruction.

c. It may be due to the action of parathyroid hormone-like substances released from the tumor.

d. It is related to the action of osteoblasts on bone formation.

e. It is managed with aggressive diuretic administration as first-line therapy.

12. The following statements are true regarding imaging tests in patients with penile cancer EXCEPT:

a. Both ultrasonography and magnetic resonance imaging (MRI) lack sensitivity for the detection of corpus cavernosum involvement.

b. Computed tomography (CT) is not an appropriate test for determining primary tumor stage.

c. CT may be beneficial in detecting enlarged inguinal nodes in obese patients or those who have had prior inguinal therapy.

d. Lymphangiography can detect abnormal architecture in normal-sized lymph nodes.

e. Inguinal palpation is preferred to CT and lymphangiography for determining inguinal nodal status.

13. According to the 2010 version of the International Union Against Cancer/TNM staging system for penile cancer, which of the following statements is TRUE?

a. Primary tumor stage is based on the size of the primary lesion.

b. Lymph node stage is based on the resectability of involved nodes.

c. Stage T2 tumors are based on biopsy and involve corpora cavernosa only.

d. Large verrucous carcinomas are considered stage Ta.

e. Stage T1 tumors may involve the urethra at the meatus.

14. What is the strongest prognostic factor for survival in penile cancer?

a. The presence of lymph node metastasis

b. The grade of the primary tumor

c. The stage of the primary tumor

d. Vascular invasion presence in the primary tumor

e. The extent of lymph node metastasis

15. Criteria for curative surgical resection (>70% 5-year survival) in patients treated for lymph node metastasis include all of the following EXCEPT:

a. no more than two positive inguinal lymph nodes.

b. no positive pelvic lymph nodes.

c. absence of extranodal extension of cancer.

d. unilateral metastasis.

e. a single metastasis of only 6 cm.

16. Surgical staging of the inguinal region is strongly considered under all of the following conditions EXCEPT:

a. palpable adenopathy.

b. stage T2 or greater primary tumor.

c. presence of vascular invasion in primary tumor.

d. presence of predominantly high-grade cancer in primary tumor.

e. stage Ta tumors.

17. A watchful waiting strategy toward the management of the inguinal region in patients with no palpable adenopathy is recommended for all of the following situations EXCEPT:

a. primary tumor stage Tis.

b. primary tumor stage Ta.

c. primary tumor stage T1, grade I.

d. primary tumor stage T1, grade II.

e. noncompliant patients.

18. Strategies to minimize the morbidity of inguinal staging in patients with no palpable adenopathy include all the following EXCEPT:

a. superficial inguinal lymph node dissection.

b. modified complete inguinal dissection.

c. standard ilioinguinal dissection.

d. sentinel lymph node biopsy.

e. dynamic sentinel node biopsy.

19. Which of the following inguinal staging procedures is considered the "gold standard" for detecting microscopic metastases while limiting both morbidity and false-negative findings?

a. Inguinal node biopsy

b. Superficial inguinal dissection

c. Sentinel lymph node dissection

d. Fine-needle aspiration cytology

e. Sentinel lymph node biopsy

20. For patients with proven unilateral metastasis involving 2 or more lymph nodes at presentation, all of the following surgical considerations are true EXCEPT:

a. Ipsilateral ilioinguinal lymphadenectomy should be performed.

b. A contralateral staging procedure is not indicated.

c. A contralateral staging procedure is indicated.

d. Both a superficial dissection and a deep ipsilateral dissection are performed.

e. Ipsilateral pelvic dissection provides useful prognostic information.

21. Adjuvant or neoadjuvant chemotherapy should be considered in addition to surgery for all of the following EXCEPT:

a. single pelvic nodal metastasis.

b. extranodal extension of cancer.

c. fixed inguinal masses.

d. two unilateral inguinal nodes with focal metastases.

e. single 6-cm inguinal lymph node.

22. The majority of penile cancers are histologically:

a. melanoma.

b. bowenoid papulosis.

c. squamous cell carcinoma.

d. epidemic Kaposi sarcoma.

e. verrucous carcinoma.

23. Which of the following chemotherapeutic agents used in combination therapy for penile cancer has been associated with significant pulmonary toxicity?

a. Bleomycin

b. Methotrexate

c. Cisplatin

d. 5-Fluorouracil (5-FU)

e. Paclitaxel

24. Indications for radiation therapy as primary treatment for penile cancer include which of the following?

a. Young, sexually active patient with a small lesion

b. Patient refuses surgery

c. Patient with inoperable tumor who needs local treatment but desires to retain the penis

d. None of the above

e. a, b, and c

25. Primary penile melanoma is thought to be rare for what reason?

a. Penile skin is protected from exposure to the sun

b. Keratin content in penile skin is decreased

c. Penile blood supply precludes such tumor development

d. Effective topical chemotherapy exists

e. None of the above

26. Lymphomatous infiltration of the penis is most likely secondary to which condition?

a. Autoimmune disorder

b. Diffuse disease

c. Metastasis from a distant primary tumor

d. Chronic infection

e. Previous venereal infection

27. What is the most frequently encountered sign of metastatic involvement of the penis?

a. Pain

b. Urethral discharge

c. Ecchymoses

d. Priapism

e. Preputial swelling

28. Which of the following features of Buschke-Löwenstein tumor characterizes it as different from condyloma acuminatum?

a. Propensity for early distant metastasis

b. Disruption of the rete pegs

c. Loss of pigmentation

d. Autoamputation

e. Invasion and destruction of adjacent tissues by compression

29. Which of the following statements about how verrucous carcinoma of the penis differs from classic Buschke-Löwenstein tumor is TRUE?

a. The terms describe the same disease.

b. Verrucous carcinoma sometimes exhibits spontaneous regression.

c. Proportion of melanin pigment in verrucous carcinoma is higher than in Buschke-Löwenstein tumor.

d. Simultaneous bilateral inguinal metastases occur commonly with Buschke-Löwenstein tumor.

e. Circumcision is not protective for verrucous carcinoma.

30. Small lesions of erythroplasia of Queyrat may be successfully treated with which of the following?

a. Topical 5% 5-FU

b. Neodymium:yttrium-aluminum-garnet (Nd:YAG) laser

c. Local excision

d. External-beam radiation therapy

e. All of the above

Pathology

1. A 65-year-old man has a cauliflower-type lesion on his foreskin involving a 3-mm area of the dorsal glans. He is sexually active. The lesion is biopsied and depicted in Figure 37-1. The pathology report is verrucous carcinoma, invasive. The most appropriate treatment is:

a. topical 5-FU cream.

b. laser photocoagulation.

c. circumcision and hemiglansectomy.

d. partial penectomy followed by bilateral groin dissection.

e. total penectomy.

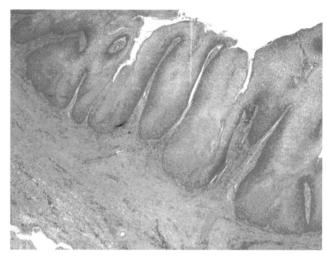

Figure 37-1. (From Bostwick D, Cheng L. Urologic surgical pathology. 2nd ed. Philadelphia, PA: Elsevier; 2008.)

2. A 55-year-old man has a red raised 2 × 3 mm lesion on his dorsal corona that has been present for the past 6 months. The lesion is biopsied and depicted in Figure 37-2. The diagnosis is well-differentiated squamous cell carcinoma with superficial invasion. The patient is sexually active and is very concerned about the appearance of his penis. The treatment most consistent with the patient's wishes and excellent cancer control is:

a. Hemiglansectomy.

b. External beam radiation therapy.

c. 5-FU cream application.

d. Laser photocoagulation.

e. Partial penectomy.

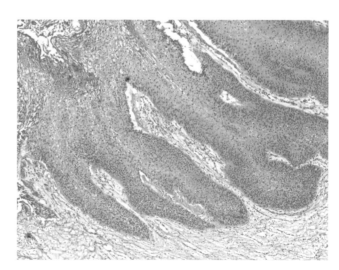

Figure 37-2. (From Bostwick D, Cheng L. Urologic surgical pathology. 3rd ed. Philadelphia, PA: Elsevier; 2014.)

ANSWERS

1. **c. Coronal papillae.** Coronal papillae present as linear, curved, or irregular rows of conical or globular excrescences, varying from white to yellow to red, arranged along the coronal sulcus. They are considered acral angiofibromas. These lesions have not been associated with malignancy.
2. **d. Human papillomavirus (HPV) infection.** HPV is recognized as the principal etiologic agent in cervical dysplasia and cervical cancer.
3. **d. Location.** Carcinoma in situ of the penis is referred to by urologists and dermatologists as erythroplasia of Queyrat if it involves the glans penis or prepuce and as Bowen disease if it involves the remainder of the penile shaft skin, genitalia, or perineal region.
4. **b. Human herpesvirus (HHV) type 8.** HHV type 8—also known as Kaposi sarcoma-associated herpesvirus—is strongly suspected to be the etiologic agent of epidemic (AIDS-related) Kaposi sarcoma.
5. **a. Glans.** Penile tumors may present anywhere on the penis but occur most commonly on the glans (48%) and prepuce (21%).
6. **d. Gonorrhea.** No convincing evidence has been found linking penile cancer to other factors such as occupation, other venereal diseases (gonorrhea, syphilis, herpes), marijuana use, or alcohol intake.
7. **a. Circumcision after 21 years of age.** Adult circumcision appears to offer little or no protection from subsequent development of the disease. These data suggest that the crucial period of exposure to certain etiologic agents may have already occurred at puberty and certainly by adult age, rendering later circumcision relatively ineffective as a prophylactic tool for penile cancer.
8. **b. Because of the associated discomfort, patients usually present to physicians within the first month of noting the lesion.** Patients with cancer of the penis, more than patients with other types of cancer, seem to delay seeking medical attention. In large series, from 15% to 50% of patients have been noted to delay medical care for more than a year.
9. **d. Tumor stage, grade, and vascular invasion status all provide prognostically important information.** Confirmation of the diagnosis of carcinoma of the penis, an assessment of the depth of invasion and tumor grade by the combination of an adequate biopsy, and complete clinical assessment are beneficial before the initiation of definitive therapy. Biopsy can be performed as a frozen section immediately before definitive therapy in some cases.
10. **e. Metastasis initially involves inguinal lymph nodes above the fascia lata.** The lymphatics of the prepuce form a connecting network that joins with the lymphatics from the skin of the shaft. These tributaries drain into the superficial inguinal nodes (the nodes external to the fascia lata).
11. **c. It may be due to the action of parathyroid hormone-like substances released from the tumor.** Parathyroid hormone and related substances may be produced by both tumor and metastases that activate osteoclastic bone resorption.
12. **a. Both ultrasonography and magnetic resonance imaging (MRI) lack sensitivity for the detection of corpus cavernosum involvement.** The sensitivity of ultrasonography for detecting cavernosum invasion was 100% in one study. This study confirmed the value of ultrasonography in assessing the primary tumor also reported by other investigators. For lesions suspected of invading the corpus cavernosum, both ultrasonography and contrast-enhanced MRI may provide unique information, especially when organ-sparing surgery is considered.
13. **d. Large verrucous carcinomas are considered stage Ta.** According to this staging system, designations for primary tumors are as follows: Tx indicates that the primary tumor cannot be assessed; T0 indicates no evidence of tumor; Tis indicates carcinoma in situ; Ta indicates noninvasive verrucous carcinoma; T1 indicates tumor invading subepithelial connective tissue; T2 indicates tumor invading corpus spongiosum or cavernosum; T3 indicates tumor invading urethra or prostate; and T4 indicates tumor invading other adjacent structures.
14. **e. The extent of lymph node metastasis.** The presence and extent of metastasis to the inguinal region are the most important prognostic factors for survival in patients with squamous penile cancer.
15. **e. A single metastasis of only 6 cm.** Pathologic criteria associated with long-term survival after attempted curative surgical resection of inguinal metastases (i.e., 80% 5-year survival) include (1) minimal nodal disease (up to two involved nodes in most series), (2) unilateral involvement, (3) no evidence of extranodal extension of cancer, and (4) the absence of pelvic nodal metastases. A lymph node larger than 4 cm is often associated with extranodal extension of cancer.
16. **e. stage Ta tumors.** Tumor histologic type associated with little or no risk for metastasis includes those patients with primary tumors exhibiting (1) carcinoma in situ or (2) verrucous carcinoma.
17. **e. noncompliant patients.** Noncompliant patients with any degree of invasion in the primary tumor specimen should have an inguinal staging procedure recommended.
18. **c. standard ilioinguinal dissection.** In patients with no evidence of palpable adenopathy who are selected to undergo inguinal procedures by virtue of adverse prognostic factors within the primary tumor, the goal is to define whether metastases exist with minimal morbidity for the patient. A variety of treatment options for this purpose have been reported and include (1) fine-needle aspiration cytology, (2) node biopsy, (3) sentinel lymph node biopsy, (4) extended sentinel lymph node dissection, (5) dynamic sentinel node biopsy, (6) superficial dissection, and (7) modified complete dissection.
19. **b. Superficial inguinal dissection.** One series found that the sensitivity of fine-needle aspiration cytology was approximately 71% in 18 patients with clinically negative lymph nodes. This finding and the technical difficulty with lymphangiography make aspiration less practical as a staging technique for patients with no palpable lymph nodes. Biopsies directed to a specific anatomic area can be unreliable in identifying microscopic metastasis and are no longer recommended.
20. **b. A contralateral staging procedure is not indicated.** Support for a bilateral procedure is based on the finding of bilateral lymphatic drainage from the primary site in the majority of cases and contralateral metastases in more than 50% of patients so treated in some series, even if the contralateral nodal region was negative to palpation.
21. **d. two unilateral inguinal nodes with focal metastases.** For patients requiring ilioinguinal lymphadenectomy because of the presence of metastases, adjuvant chemotherapy should be considered for those exhibiting more than two positive lymph nodes, extranodal extension of cancer, or pelvic nodal metastasis. Reports from one center further confirmed the value of adjuvant chemotherapy. Of 25 node-positive patients treated with adjuvant combination vincristine-bleomycin-methotrexate chemotherapy, 82% survived 5 years, compared with 37% of 31 patients treated with surgery alone.
22. **c. squamous cell carcinoma.** The majority of tumors of the penis are squamous cell carcinomas demonstrating keratinization, epithelial pearl formation, and various degrees of mitotic activity.
23. **a. Bleomycin.** Response rates of bleomycin, whether as a single agent or in combination with other agents, has not been shown to be superior to cisplatin alone, but has been associated with significant pulmonary toxicity and death in several series of patients treated for metastatic penile cancer.
24. **e. a, b, and c.** Radiation therapy may be considered in a select group of patients: (1) young individuals presenting with small (2 to 4 cm), superficial, exophytic, noninvasive lesions on the glans or coronal sulcus; (2) patients who refuse as an initial form of treatment; and (3) patients with inoperable tumor or distant metastases who require local therapy to the primary tumor but who express a desire to retain the penis.
25. **a. Penile skin is protected from exposure to the sun.** Melanoma and basal cell carcinoma rarely occur on the penis, presumably because the organ's skin is protected from exposure to the sun.

26. **b. Diffuse disease.** When lymphomatous infiltration of the penis is diagnosed, a thorough search for systemic disease is necessary.
27. **d. Priapism.** The most frequent sign of penile metastasis is priapism; penile swelling, nodularity, and ulceration have also been reported.
28. **e. Invasion and destruction of adjacent tissues by compression.** The Buschke-Löwenstein tumor differs from condyloma acuminatum in that condylomata, regardless of size, always remain superficial and never invade adjacent tissue. Buschke-Löwenstein tumor displaces, invades, and destroys adjacent structures by compression. Aside from this unrestrained local growth, it demonstrates no signs of malignant change on histologic examination and does not metastasize.
29. **a. The terms describe the same disease.** Buschke-Löwenstein tumor is synonymous with verrucous carcinoma and giant condyloma acuminatum.
30. **e. All of the above.** When lesions are small and noninvasive, local excision, which spares penile anatomy and function, is satisfactory. Circumcision will adequately treat preputial lesions. Fulguration may be successful but often results in recurrences. Radiation therapy has successfully eradicated these tumors, and well-planned, appropriately delivered radiation results in minimal morbidity. Topical 5-FU as the 5% base causes denudation of malignant and premalignant areas while preserving normal skin. There are also reports of successful treatment with Nd: YAG laser.

Pathology

1. **c. Circumcision and hemiglansectomy.** Verrucous carcinoma is locally invasive but normally does not metastasize. Note invasion at the base in the figure. Thus wide local excision is indicated.
2. **a. Hemiglansectomy.** Wide local excision of the well-differentiated superficially invasive (T1) squamous cell carcinoma will provide excellent cancer control while providing the best cosmetic result. Moreover, the permanent pathology will be very helpfuul in follow-up and prognosis.

CHAPTER REVIEW

1. Pearly penile papules or papillomas are normal and generally found on the glans penis or corona.
2. Zoon balanitis presents as an erythematous plaque that pathologically reveals a plasma cell infiltrate and is cured by circumcision. Grossly, it is difficult to distinguish from carcinoma in situ.
3. Lesions associated with the development of penile cancer include cutaneous horn, balanitis xerotica obliterans, and pseudoepitheliomatous micaceous and keratotic balanitis.
4. Bowenoid papulosis meets all the histologic criteria for carcinoma in situ; however, the course is invariably benign.
5. Kaposi sarcoma is classified as (1) not associated with immunodeficiency and with an indolent and rarely fatal course, (2) associated with immunosuppressive treatment that is often reversed by modification of the immunosuppressive medications, (3) African Kaposi sarcoma that may be either indolent or aggressive, and (4) HIV-related Kaposi sarcoma. If surgical treatment is required, localized excision is often successful.
6. Carcinoma in situ of the glans is called erythroplasia of Queyrat; if carcinoma in situ is on the shaft of the penis it is called Bowen disease.
7. On the penis there are multiple cross-connections of lymphatics so that drainage can occur to either inguinal region.
8. The overwhelming majority of penile squamous cell carcinomas occur on the glans, the prepuce, or corona.
9. Vascular invasion and perineural invasions are strong predictors of lymph node metastases. Distant metastases occur late in the course of the disease and are rare without recognized significant inguinal and pelvic lymphadenopathy.
10. Tis, TA, T1, grade 1 and grade 2 tumors are at low risk for metastases.
11. T2 or greater and grade 3 tumors have a greater than 50% incidence of metastases.
12. The criteria associated with long-term survival after inguinal lymphadenectomy include (1) minimal nodal disease, (2) unilateral involvement, (3) no evidence of extranodal extension, and (4) absence of pelvic node metastases.
13. Inguinal lymphadenectomy should be bilateral when performed on patients at initial presentation. If, on the other hand, the patient presents with unilateral adenopathy at a prolonged time after the initial presentation and treatment of the primary lesion, a unilateral inguinal node dissection may be considered.
14. HPV 16, 18, 31, and 33 are associated with carcinoma in situ and invasive squamous cell cancer.
15. Tumor grade correlates with microscopic contiguous spread: 5 mm for grade 1 and 2 and 10 mm for grade 3. Skip lesions generally do not occur.
16. There is an improved survival when lymphadenectomy is done early for nonpalpable microscopic disease as opposed to delaying it until the nodes become palpable. When the inguinal nodes are negative, the ipsilateral pelvic nodes are almost always negative as well.
17. Before radiation therapy, the patient should be circumcised.
18. Advanced disease may benefit from cisplatin-based combination chemotherapy.
19. Tx indicates that the primary tumor cannot be assessed; T0 indicates no evidence of tumor; Tis indicates carcinoma in situ; Ta indicates noninvasive verrucous carcinoma; T1 indicates tumor invading subepithelial connective tissue; T2 indicates tumor invading corpus spongiosum or cavernosum; T3 indicates tumor invading urethra or prostate; and T4 indicates tumor invading other adjacent structures.
20. The Buschke-Löwenstein tumor differs from condyloma acuminatum in that condylomata, regardless of size, always remain superficial and never invade adjacent tissue. Buschke-Löwenstein tumor displaces, invades, and destroys adjacent structures by compression. Aside from this unrestrained local growth, it demonstrates no signs of malignant change on histologic examination and does not metastasize.

38 Tumors of the Urethra

David S. Sharp and Kenneth W. Angermeier

QUESTIONS

1. What is the most frequent site of both stricture disease and urethral cancer in the male?
   a. Pendulous urethra
   b. Fossa navicularis
   c. Bulbomembranous urethra
   d. Prostatic urethra
   e. Urethral meatus

2. Which of the following is TRUE concerning distal urethral carcinoma in the male?
   a. Prognosis depends on histologic cell type.
   b. Penectomy is usually indicated for tumors infiltrating the corpus spongiosum.
   c. Prognosis is worse than for bulbomembranous urethral cancer.
   d. Conservative surgical therapy is not effective.
   e. Biopsy most commonly demonstrates transitional cell carcinoma.

3. When a delayed urethrectomy is performed in a male patient after radical cystectomy, which of the following is necessary to ensure a complete dissection and decrease the risk of a local recurrence?
   a. Removal of the fossa navicularis and urethral meatus
   b. Bilateral groin dissections
   c. Total penectomy
   d. Intraoperative ultrasound imaging
   e. Cauterization of the urethral bed

4. Which of the following statements regarding urethral tumor recurrence after cystectomy and orthotopic urinary diversion is FALSE?
   a. It seems to occur more frequently than after cutaneous diversion.
   b. Some patients with carcinoma in situ may be successfully treated with urethral infusion of bacillus Calmette-Guérin (BCG).
   c. Urethrectomy and cutaneous diversion can often be done using bowel tissue from the existing neobladder.
   d. Surveillance consists of urine cytology and symptom assessment.
   e. Urethrectomy with conversion to a continent cutaneous diversion may be possible in some patients.

5. Possible causes for female urethral carcinoma include all of the following EXCEPT:
   a. childhood urinary tract infections.
   b. leukoplakia.
   c. chronic irritation or urinary tract infections.
   d. proliferative lesions such as caruncles.
   e. human papillomavirus infection.

6. What is the most common histologic type of proximal urethral cancer in women?
   a. Adenocarcinoma
   b. Squamous cell carcinoma
   c. Melanoma
   d. Transitional cell carcinoma
   e. Lymphoma

7. What is the most significant prognostic factor for local control and survival in female urethral cancer?
   a. Anatomic location and extent of the tumor
   b. Age at presentation
   c. Histologic type of the tumor
   d. Hematuria
   e. Urinary retention

8. Radiation therapy for female urethral carcinoma is most successful:
   a. as a single modality for proximal invasive tumors.
   b. when used in conjunction with chemotherapy for low-stage distal urethral tumors.
   c. at controlling distant metastatic disease.
   d. at controlling small lesions in the distal urethra.
   e. as neoadjuvant therapy before excision of locally advanced proximal urethral cancer.

Pathology

1. A 64-year-old woman has had urethral pain for the past 6 months. A 0.5-cm mass is palpable in the distal urethra. A biopsy of the mass reveals adenocarcinoma and is depicted in the figure. The next step in management is:
   a. Imaging to rule out a primary gastrointestinal origin.
   b. Cystouretrectomy.
   c. Local excision.
   d. Radiation therapy.
   e. Pelvic magnetic resonance imaging (MRI).

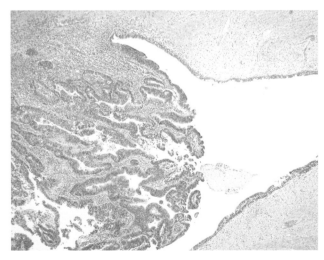

Figure 38-1. (From Bostwick D, Cheng L. *Urologic surgical pathology*. 3rd ed. Philadelphia: Elsevier; 2014.)

ANSWERS

1. **c. Bulbomembranous urethra.** The incidence of urethral stricture in men later developing a carcinoma of the urethra ranges from 24% to 76% and most frequently involves the bulbomembranous urethra, which is also the portion of the urethra most commonly involved by tumor.

2. **b. Penectomy is usually indicated for tumors infiltrating the corpus spongiosum.** In general, anterior urethral carcinoma is more amenable to surgical control, and the patient's prognosis is better than that for posterior urethral carcinoma, which is often associated with extensive local invasion and distant metastasis.

3. **a. Removal of the fossa navicularis and urethral meatus.** It is important that the fossa navicularis and meatus also be taken in the dissection, because of the high incidence of involvement of the squamous epithelium.

4. **a. It seems to occur more frequently than after cutaneous diversion.** Studies to date suggest that urethral tumor recurrence after orthotopic urinary diversion is less common than after cutaneous diversion. In the presence of an orthotopic neobladder, urethral surveillance consists of urine cytology and symptom assessment. Success has been reported in selected patients treated with urethral infusion of BCG for urethral carcinoma in situ after orthotopic diversion. After urethrectomy, cutaneous diversion can often be done using bowel tissue from the existing neobladder, eliminating the need to take additional small bowel tissue out of the circuit.

5. **a. Childhood urinary tract infections.** Causes associated with subsequent development of urethral malignancy in females include chronic irritation or urinary tract infections; proliferative lesions such as caruncles, papillomas, adenomas, and polyps; leukoplakia of the urethra; parturition; and human papillomavirus infection.

6. **b. Squamous cell carcinoma.** Carcinomas of the proximal or entire urethra tend to be high grade and locally advanced, with squamous cell carcinoma accounting for 60%; transitional cell carcinoma 20%; adenocarcinoma 10%; undifferentiated tumor and sarcomas 8%; and melanoma 2%.

7. **a. Anatomic location and extent of the tumor.** The most significant prognostic factor for local control and survival is the anatomic location and extent of the tumor, with low-stage distal urethral tumors having a better prognosis than high-stage proximal urethral tumors.

8. **d. At controlling small lesions in the distal urethra.** Radiation therapy alone, as with surgical excision, is often sufficient to control small lesions in the distal urethra.

Pathology

1. **e. Pelvic MRI.** An MRI may be very helpful in evaluating the extent of surgery required in this patient. If confined to the distal urethra, the adenocarcinoma may be removed by distal urethrectomy with inclusion of the anterior vaginal wall. In the female, adenocarcinoma accounts for about a third of the urethral tumors and is the most common tumor found in a urethral diverticulum.

CHAPTER REVIEW

1. The most common benign urethral tumors are leiomyoma, hemangioma, and fibroepithelial polyp.
2. In the male, the histology of cancer in the prostatic urethra is transitional cell in 90% and squamous cell carcinoma in 10%; in the penile urethra, 90% are squamous cell cancers and 10% are transitional cell tumors; and in the bulbomemebranous urethra 80% are squamous cell, 10% are transitional cell, and 10% are adenocarcinoma. In the female, squamous cell carcinoma accounts for one third, adenocarcinoma for one third, and transitional cell carcinoma for one third.
3. In the male, the anterior urethra lymphatics drain to the inguinal nodes, and the posterior urethra lymphatics drain to the pelvic nodes.
4. In the female, the anterior urethra (distal third) lymphatics drain to the inguinal nodes. The posterior urethra lymphatics (proximal two thirds) drain to the external and internal iliac and obturator lymph nodes.
5. Transitional cell carcinoma, which involves the prostatic urethral stroma, significantly increases the probability of urethral recurrence.
6. Adenocarcinoma is the most common type of tumor to occur in a urethral diverticulum.
7. Distal urethral cancers in both men and women have a more favorable prognosis than proximal urethral cancers.
8. The distal third of the female urethra may be excised with maintenance of continence.
9. Carcinomas of the proximal or entire urethra tend to be high grade and locally advanced, with squamous cell carcinoma accounting for 60%; transitional cell carcinoma 20%; adenocarcinoma 10%; undifferentiated tumor and sarcomas 8%; and melanoma 2%.
    Because of the poor prognosis of invasive proximal urethral cancers in both men and women, consideration should be given to multimodality therapy.
10. Survival in patients with invasive urethra cancer does not appear to be correlated with histologic type.
11. Causes associated with subsequent development of urethral malignancy in females include chronic irritation or urinary tract infections; proliferative lesions such as caruncles, papillomas, adenomas, and polyps; leukoplakia of the urethra; parturition; and human papillomavirus infection.
12. Radiation therapy alone, as with surgical excision, is often sufficient to control small lesions in the distal urethra.

39 Inguinal Node Dissection

Kenneth W. Angermeier, Rene Sotelo, and David S. Sharp

QUESTIONS

1. Efforts designed to improve the accuracy of dynamic sentinel lymph node biopsy include all of the following EXCEPT:
   a. use of an ultrasensitive gamma ray detection probe.
   b. routine inguinal exploration in the absence of radiotracer visualization.
   c. extended pathologic analysis of excised lymph nodes.
   d. intraoperative palpation of the wound for abnormal nodes.
   e. preoperative inguinal ultrasonography with fine-needle aspiration of any abnormal-appearing nodes.

2. When compared with the standard groin dissection, the modified groin dissection has all of the following features EXCEPT:
   a. The node dissection excludes regions lateral to the femoral artery and caudad to the fossa ovalis.
   b. The saphenous vein is preserved.
   c. The transposition of the sartorius muscle is eliminated.
   d. The required incision is longer.
   e. Decreased morbidity.

3. Which of the following statements regarding radical ilioinguinal lymphadenectomy is TRUE?
   a. The fascia lata remains intact.
   b. The saphenous vein may be preserved in the setting of low-volume disease.
   c. Rotation of the gracilis muscle is performed to cover the exposed femoral vessels.
   d. The femoral nerve is visualized superior to the iliacus fascia.
   e. A laparoscopic approach has not been reported.

4. A pelvic node dissection for male penile cancer should include all of the following areas EXCEPT:
   a. distal common iliac nodes.
   b. para-aortic and paracaval node dissection.
   c. external iliac nodes.
   d. obturator group of nodes.
   e. a and b

5. Which of the following measures may help prevent lymphedema after a radical ilioinguinal node dissection?
   a. Preservation of Colles fascia in the flap dissection
   b. Low-dose heparin in the perioperative period
   c. A 6-week delay between treatment of the primary tumor and the node dissection
   d. Postoperative bed rest and elastic stockings
   e. Obliteration of dead space during wound closure

ANSWERS

1. **a. Use of an ultrasensitive gamma ray detection probe.** Techniques reported to increase the accuracy of dynamic sentinel lymph node biopsy include preoperative inguinal ultrasonography with needle biopsy of any suspicious nodes, routine inguinal exploration even in the absence of radiotracer visualization, intraoperative palpation of the wound for abnormal nodes, and extended pathologic analysis of any excised lymph nodes.

2. **d. The required incision is longer.** The modified groin dissection differs from the standard dissection in that (1) the skin incision is shorter; (2) the node dissection is limited, excluding regions lateral to the femoral artery and caudad to the fossa ovalis; (3) the saphenous veins are preserved; and (4) the transposition of the sartorius muscles is eliminated.

3. **b. The saphenous vein may be preserved in the setting of low-volume disease.** In a radical inguinal lymphadenectomy, the fascia lata is divided longitudinally, and the sartorius muscle is rotated to cover the femoral vessels. The femoral nerve is usually not seen because it lies beneath the iliacus fascia lateral to the femoral artery. In the setting of low-volume nodal disease, it is acceptable to spare the saphenous vein, if feasible, to attempt decreasing the risk of lower-extremity complications.

4. **b. Para-aortic and paracaval node dissection.** The pelvic lymphadenectomy includes the distal common iliac, external iliac, and obturator groups of nodes. No further therapeutic benefit is gained from proximal iliac or para-aortic node dissection.

5. **d. Postoperative bed rest and elastic stockings.** Efforts to minimize lymphedema during the initial postoperative period include applying thigh-high elastic wraps or stockings and elevating the foot of the bed.

CHAPTER REVIEW

1. Penile cancer is not a unilateral disease and may metastasize to either groin regardless of location of the primary lesion.
2. Immediate resection of clinically occult lymph node metastases in patients with penile cancer results in improved survival when compared to waiting until metastatic lymph nodes become palpable before performing a groin dissection.
3. A radical groin dissection may be therapeutic and on occasion is used for palliation.
4. Penile cancer does not metastasize to the pelvic nodes without involvement of the inguinal nodes.
5. Twenty percent of patients with nonpalpable inguinal nodes harbor occult metastases.
6. Dynamic sentinel node biopsy has a false-negative rate of 5% to 15%. With the use of stage and grade, the false-negative rate is 20%.
7. The lymphatics drain to the groin beneath Camper fascia. When this fascia is included in the skin flaps, the dissection is less likely to compromise the overlying skin.
8. A transverse incision is least likely to compromise blood flow to the skin flaps.
9. The modified groin dissection differs from the standard dissection in that (1) the skin incision is shorter; (2) the node dissection is limited, excluding regions lateral to the femoral artery and caudad to the fossa ovalis; (3) the saphenous veins are preserved; and (4) the transposition of the sartorius muscles is eliminated.
10. The pelvic lymphadenectomy when indicated includes the distal common iliac, external iliac, and obturator groups of nodes. No further therapeutic benefit is gained from proximal iliac or para-aortic node dissection.

40 Surgery of the Penis and Urethra

Kurt A. McCammon, Jack M. Zuckerman, and Gerald H. Jordan

QUESTIONS

1. In terms of tissue transfer, which of the following statements concerning grafts is TRUE?
   a. The process of take is less than 48 hours.
   b. A graft is tissue that is excised from a donor site and reestablishes its blood supply by revascularization.
   c. During imbibition, the first phase of take, the graft exists above body temperature.
   d. Conditions of take are a reflection of only the graft host bed.
   e. Split-thickness skin grafts are less prone to contraction compared with full-thickness grafts.

2. With regard to the microanatomy of grafts, using skin as a model, which of the following statements is TRUE?
   a. The intradermal plexus is at the interface of the superficial and deep dermis.
   b. The subdermal plexus is carried at the juncture of the deep dermis and the underlying tissue.
   c. The lymphatics are most richly distributed in the adventitial dermis.
   d. The adventitial dermis, because of its collagen content, accounts for the majority of the physical characteristics.
   e. Genital and extragenital skin behaves similarly when used in genitourinary reconstruction.

3. With regard to the grafts used most commonly in genitourinary reconstructive surgery, which of the following statements is TRUE?
   a. Full-thickness skin is an optimal replacement for the tunica albuginea of the corpora cavernosa.
   b. Bladder epithelial graft is fastidious because of the nature of the superficial lamina.
   c. Buccal mucosa graft is thought to have a panlaminar plexus.
   d. Tunica vaginalis graft has proved to be a very reliable one for single-stage urethral reconstruction.
   e. Buccal mucosa grafts should not be thinned because it will adversely affect the physical and vascular properties of the graft.

4. With regard to the anatomy of the penile shaft, which of the following statements is TRUE?
   a. Throughout most of the length of the penis, the septum is a true competent septum.
   b. The erectile tissues of the normal corpora cavernosa are separated from the tunica by the space of Smith.
   c. The dorsal arteries of the penis are carried in an envelope fashion in the dartos fascia.
   d. The Buck fascia is loosely areolar and lies immediately beneath the skin.
   e. The Buck fascia attenuates on the ventrum, lateral to the corpus spongiosum.

5. According to consensus, the urethra should be divided into six entities. Which of the following statements is most accurate?
   a. The fossa navicularis is that portion of the urethra that is most dorsally displaced with regard to the surrounding spongy erectile tissue.

b. The bulbous urethral portion is invested by the thickest portion of the corpora spongiosum.
   c. The bulbous urethral at its proximal extent is part of the posterior urethra.
   d. The membranous urethra is invested by the most proximal aspect of the corpus spongiosum.
   e. The membranous urethra, throughout its length is surrounded by the external rhabdosphincter.

6. With regard to the arterial vascularization of the deep structures of the penis, which of the following statements is TRUE?
   a. The circumflex cavernosal arteries are uniform in number and distribution.
   b. The arteries to the bulb arborize into the spongy erectile tissue of the glans.
   c. The common penile artery represents the end continuation of the superficial external pudendal artery.
   d. The common penile artery divides to become the cavernosal artery and the dorsal arteries, after branching off the circumflex cavernosal arteries.
   e. The blood supply of the deep structures of the penis is derived from the common penile artery, which is the continuation of the internal pudendal artery after it branches off its perineal branch and the posterior scrotal arteries.

7. With regard to the innervation to the penis, which of the following statements is TRUE?
   a. The cavernosal nerves are purely parasympathetic and are the extensions of the nervi erigentes.
   b. The pudendal nerves accompany the dorsal artery of the penis and the dorsal vein of the penis as they run through the obturator foramen.
   c. The dorsal nerve arises in the Alcock canal as a branch of the pudendal nerve.
   d. The dorsal nerves throughout their course are prominent, large nerve bundles.
   e. The skin of the shaft of the penis is innervated by a branch of the femoral nerve.

8. Which of the following statements regarding lichen sclerosus (LS) is FALSE?
   a. Lichen sclerosus is the preferred term for what was previously known as *balanitis xerotica obliterans*.
   b. LS is the most common cause of meatal stenosis.
   c. There is a strong association with an infectious etiology for the development of LS.
   d. Circumcision may be curative if only foreskin is involved with LS.
   e. Topical steroids may help stabilize the inflammatory process early in the disease course.

9. Each of the following statements regarding complications associated with lichen sclerosus are true, EXCEPT:
   a. Urethral stricture may develop secondary to iatrogenic injury from repeat instrumentation.
   b. Genital or extragenital skin may be used for urethral reconstruction for LS-associated urethral strictures.

c. Meatal stenosis and high-pressure voiding with subsequent urinary extravasation into the glands of Littre may result in urethral stricture formation.

d. Squamous cell carcinoma may develop in patients with a long history of LS.

e. Patients under consideration for meatal reconstruction with LS must undergo retrograde urethrography to rule out proximal strictures before surgery.

10. Urethrocutaneous fistulae may develop secondary to all of the following, EXCEPT:

a. complication following hypospadias repair or other urethral surgery.

b. recurrence following fistula repair as a result of distal obstruction and high-pressure voiding.

c. extravasation of infected urine and periurethral abscess formation.

d. complication of genital herpes simplex viral infection.

e. early fistula following urethral surgery may result from hematoma, infection, or tension with the closure.

11. With regard to urethral meatal stenosis in childhood, which of the following statements is TRUE?

a. Meatal stenosis is a frequent complication of phimosis

b. Meatal stenosis is frequently associated with upper tract changes, and all patients should be evaluated with ultrasonography and voiding cystourethrography

c. When ammoniacal meatitis is noted, often a short course of meatal dilation and steroid cream application will resolve the problem.

d. When meatal stenosis is present, usually a dorsally based YV advancement flap repair is preferred

e. Meatal stenosis in childhood is frequently associated with concomitant lichen sclerosus

12. When treating a patient with penile amputation, which of the following statements is TRUE?

a. Replantation is not a consideration in self-inflicted injury, because most of these patients are chronically psychotic and will eventually try to amputate the penis again

b. If the distal part of the penis is not available, even if the amputation involves mostly skin with much of the shaft preserved, it is recommended that the remaining shaft be buried in the scrotum

c. In the case of amputation associated with avulsion, debridement to undivided tissue must precede penile replantation

d. The classic technique for replantation involves coaptation of the dorsal nerve, the deep dorsal vein, and the cavernosal arteries

e. The McRoberts technique of macroreplantation is not the preferred method of management for these patients, but when the situation warrants it, it is very successful

13. All of the following statements regarding circumcision are true, EXCEPT:

a. Circumcision may be performed in the neonatal period in newborns born with a distal hypospadias, but not in those with proximal hypospadias.

b. Young boys with recurrent urinary tract infections (UTIs) should be considered for circumcision.

c. The most common complication following newborn circumcision is bleeding.

d. Circumcision has been shown to reduce the risk of human immunodeficiency virus (HIV) transmission in heterosexual men.

e. Small skin dehiscence following circumcision may be managed conservatively with local wound care and healing by secondary intention.

14. Concerning genital lymphedema, which of the following statements is TRUE?

a. Reconstruction for lymphedema that is the consequence of the indirect effects of radiation is best accomplished with excision of the tissues and coverage with split-thickness skin grafts (STSGs).

b. In reconstruction for lymphedema, it is essential to maintain the parietal tunica vaginalis of the testes intact with grafting over that location.

c. When considering reconstruction for lymphedema, full-thickness skin grafts (FTSGs) are preferable because of the distribution of the lymphatics in the superficial (adventitial) dermis.

d. In the case of genital lymphedema, it is not unusual for the immune response of the tissues to be altered and for patients to have significant involvement with genital papillomas.

e. Not unusually, in cases where the genital lymphedema is localized, the midline of the scrotum can be preserved for reconstruction.

15. Which of the following statements is most accurate concerning anterior urethral stricture disease?

a. It causes limitation of the urethral lumen because of the bulk of the scar.

b. It most often is limited to the urethral epithelium.

c. It implies a scarring process, usually involving both the epithelium and the underlying spongy erectile tissue of the corpora cavernosa.

d. It causes limitation of the urethral lumen because of contraction and noncompliance of the scar.

e. It is a metaplastic process of the urethral epithelium.

16. Which of the following statements concerning pelvic fracture urethral injury is TRUE?

a. It involves the tissues of the epithelium as well as the underlying erectile tissues of the corpora cavernosa.

b. It involves the tissues of the epithelium as well as the underlying erectile tissue of the corpus spongiosum.

c. It is not a true stricture but rather fibrosis that results from distraction of the urethra.

d. The stricture process can often be occult because of the unpredictable involvement of the urethral tissues.

e. The defect is usually predictably proximal to the external sphincter at the junction of the prostatic urethra with the membranous urethra.

17. In determining the anatomy of the stricture, all of the following provide useful information EXCEPT:

a. magnetic resonance imaging (MRI).

b. high-resolution ultrasonography.

c. contrast studies.

d. urethroscopy.

e. calibration with bougie à boule.

18. With regard to planning of reconstruction for urethral stricture, which of the following statements is TRUE?

a. Even if a patient does not have retention, placement of a suprapubic tube may help define strictured areas.

b. Tightly stenotic areas should be dilated to pass endoscopes proximally.

c. The effects of hydrodilation are manifested most immediately distal to the area of narrowest stenosis.

d. Calibration of strictured areas to 16 Fr or greater reliably predicts the potential for segments to contract.

e. Sonourethrogram by itself accurately predicts depth of spongiofibrosis.

19. With regard to direct visual internal urethrotomy, which of the following statements is TRUE?

    a. Strictures are best incised at the 12-o-clock position.

    b. Deep incision of the corpus spongiosum has been shown to optimize long-term results.

    c. In optimally selected patients, long-term success of internal urethrotomy is approximately 90%.

    d. Internal urethrotomy should be the first procedure considered for any stricture of the anterior urethra.

    e. It can be associated with erectile dysfunction.

20. Concerning anterior urethral reconstruction, which of the following statements is TRUE?

    a. Excision and primary anastomosis reconstruction are severely limited and useful only for very proximal strictures 1 to 2 cm in length.

    b. Performance of the excision and primary anastomosis technique is facilitated by dissection of the corpus spongiosum to the level of the glans penis.

    c. Success requires total excision of the fibrosis with a widely spatulated anastomosis.

    d. Reconstruction is facilitated by development of the intracrural space with infrapubectomy.

    e. In cases of longer strictures, excision with partial anastomosis allowing one wall to granulate offers acceptable results.

21. With regard to genital skin flap operations for anterior urethral reconstruction, which of the following statements is TRUE?

    a. Flap operations are best applied as individual techniques and require the surgeon to be intimately familiar with the individual steps of each technique.

    b. The operation can conceptually become one operation with multidimensional application.

    c. The operations are all based on mobilization of the extended Buck fascia.

    d. The operations require a comfortable understanding of the extended circumflex iliac superficial vascular pattern.

    e. They are of limited value in patients who have been previously circumcised.

22. With regard to continence after reconstruction for pelvic fracture urethral distraction injuries, which of the following statements is TRUE?

    a. Location of the injury along the course of the membranous urethra is not associated with continence postoperatively.

    b. Continence can be accurately predicted by contrast studies.

    c. Continence is best predicted by the appearance of the bladder neck on endoscopy.

    d. Continence is best addressed after a procedure to reestablish urethral continuity is performed.

    e. Continence is best in patients with partial distraction injuries.

23. In dealing with the entity of chordee without hypospadias, which of the following statements is TRUE?

    a. Correction of curvature is often achieved with mobilization of the corpus spongiosum alone.

    b. It often can be corrected with maneuvers that lengthen the foreshortened ventral skin.

    c. It is best straightened by an incision and grafting operation.

    d. Division of the urethra/corpus spongiosum is virtually always indicated.

    e. It is usually present with either ventral curvature or ventral curvature associated with torsion.

24. With regard to acquired curvatures of the penis that are not Peyronie disease, which of the following statements is TRUE?

    a. Most are characterized by prominent dorsal scars.

    b. In most cases, global cavernosal veno-occlusive dysfunction (CVOD) is not a complicating factor.

    c. They are virtually never associated with "minimal" buckling trauma.

    d. Patients often have significant penile foreshortening.

    e. There is usually an association with either hypospadias or epispadias.

25. All of the following are true regarding pelvic fracture urethral injuries (PFUI), EXCEPT:

    a. Pelvic fractures are associated with urethral injuries in about 10% of cases.

    b. PFUIs most commonly occur between the prostate and membranous urethra.

    c. In the prepubescent male, PFUI's are more likely to involve the prostatic urethra.

    d. A normal anterior urethral on retrograde urethrography nearly ensures an anastomotic repair of a PFUI is feasible.

    e. The appearance of the bladder neck on preoperative contrast studies does not accurately predict continence outcomes following anastomotic repair of PFUIs.

26. In pelvic fracture urethral injuries, after excision of the traumatic scar, the distance between the two ends of healthy urethra can be minimized by all of the following, EXCEPT:

    a. mobilizing the corpus spongiosum off the corpora cavernosa up to the corona of the glans.

    b. excision of Buck fascia from the corpus spongiosum.

    c. dissection of the intracrural space down to the pubis.

    d. periosteal elevation and infrapubectomy.

    e. rerouting of the spongiosum above the crura of the corpora cavernosa.

27. Which of the following patients should be considered for penile revascularization to prevent ischemic stenosis following PFUI repair?

    a. Men with erectile dysfunction (ED) following PFUI, but normal hemodynamics on penile duplex sonography

    b. Men with normal erectile function following PFUI

    c. Men following PFUI with ED and hemodynamics on penile duplex sonography suggesting venous leak

    d. Men with arteriogenic ED following PFUI who demonstrate bilateral occlusion of the internal pudendal arteries without reconstitution

    e. Men with arteriogenic ED following PFUI who demonstrate unilateral occlusion of the internal pudendal artery

28. Which of the following statements regarding total phallic construction is FALSE?

    a. Phallic rigidity may be achieved in the neophallus by placement of a penile prosthesis before the return of tactile sensation of the phallus.

    b. Current techniques are accomplished with a variety of flap designs, which use microvascular free flap transfer.

    c. Urinary fistulae, although a common complication following phallic construction, are often resolved with conservative measures and do not routinely require operative repair.

    d. Complications following prosthesis placement into patients following total phallic construction are higher than those following placement into men with normal corporal anatomy.

e. Penile tactile and erogenous sensation can be achieved following total phallic construction via coaptation of the flap cutaneous nerves to the dorsal penile/clitoral nerve, the pudendal nerve, or the ilioinguinal nerve.

29. All of the following may be repaired with excision and primary anastomotic urethroplasty, EXCEPT:

    a. pelvic fracture urethral injury with a 3-cm gap demonstrated on preoperative urethrography.

    b. straddle injury resulting in a 1-cm bulbar urethral stricture.

    c. iatrogenic urethral trauma during a transurethral resection resulting in a 1-cm bulbar urethral stricture.

    d. idiopathic proximal 1-cm bulbar urethral stricture in a patient with a history of a prior hypospadias repair.

    e. perineal trauma resulting in a 2-cm proximal bulbar urethral stricture.

ANSWERS

1. **b. A graft is tissue that is excised from a donor site and reestablishes its blood supply by revascularization.** The term *graft* implies that tissue has been excised and transferred to a graft host bed, where a new blood supply develops by a process termed *take*. Take requires approximately 96 hours and occurs in two phases. The initial phase, imbibition, requires about 48 hours. During that phase, the graft survives by "drinking" nutrients from the adjacent graft host bed, and the temperature of the graft is less than the core body temperature. The second phase, inosculation, also requires about 48 hours and is the phase in which true microcirculation is reestablished in the graft. During that phase, the temperature of the graft rises to core body temperature. The process of take is influenced by both the nature of the grafted tissue and the conditions of the graft host bed. Processes that interfere with the vascularity of the graft host bed thus interfere with graft take.

2. **b. The subdermal plexus is carried at the juncture of the deep dermis and the underlying tissue.** The epidermal, or epithelial layer, is a covering, the barrier to the "outside," and is adjacent to the superficial dermis, or superficial lamina. At approximately that interface is the superficial plexus. In the case of skin, the plexus is the intradermal plexus. There are some lymphatics in the superficial dermal or tunica layer. On the undersurface of the deep dermal layer or deep lamina is the deep plexus. In the case of skin, this is the subdermal plexus. The deep dermis contains most of the lymphatics and greater collagen content than found in the superficial dermal layer. The deep or reticular dermis is generally thought to account for the physical characteristics of the tissue. There is a difference between genital full-thickness skin (penile and preputial skin grafts) and extragenital full-thickness skin. This is probably a reflection of the increased mass of the graft in extragenital skin grafts. This increased mass makes the graft more fastidious, and the poor results reported with urethral reconstruction with extragenital full-thickness skin grafts are probably due to poor or ischemic take.

3. **c. Buccal mucosa graft is thought to have a panlaminar plexus.** In the bladder epithelial graft, there is a superficial and a deep plexus; however, many more perforators connect the plexuses. Thus bladder epithelial grafts tend to have more favorable vascular characteristics. In the case of the oral mucosal grafts, there is a panlaminar plexus. Thus the oral mucosal graft can be thinned somewhat, provided a sufficient amount of deep lamina is carried to preserve the physical characteristics. The oral mucosal grafts are thought to have optimal vascular characteristics. The thinned graft diminishes the total graft mass while preserving the physical characteristics and not adversely affecting the vascular characteristics. Tunica vaginalis grafts have been tried for urethral reconstruction with uniformly poor results. The dermal graft (not full thickness skin) has been used for years to augment the tunica albuginea of the corpora cavernosa.

4. **b. The erectile tissues of the normal corpora cavernosa are separated from the tunica by the space of Smith.** The corpora cavernosa are not separate structures but constitute a single space with free communication through an incompetent midline septum, composed of multiple strands of elastic tissue similar to that making up the tunica albuginea. The erectile tissue is separated from the tunica albuginea by a thin layer of areolar connective tissue that was described by Smith. The Buck fascia is directly abutted to the tunica albuginea of the corpora cavernosa. The Buck fascia surrounds the adventitia of the corpora spongiosum in envelope fashion, and the dorsal neurovascular structures are contained in envelope fashion between the superficial and deep laminar of the Buck fascia on the dorsum. The Buck fascia is thus "devoted" to the deep structures. The dartos fascia is loosely areolar and lies immediately beneath the skin. It is in that fascial layer that the arborizations of the superficial external pudendal vessels and the posterior scrotal vessels are carried.

5. **b. The bulbous urethral portion is invested by the thickest portion of the corpora spongiosum.** The fossa navicularis is contained within the spongy erectile tissue of the glans penis and terminates at the junction of the urethral epithelium with the skin of the glans. The bulbous urethra is covered by the midline fusion of the ischiocavernosus musculature and is invested by the bulbospongiosum of the proximal corpus spongiosum. It becomes larger and lies closer to the dorsal aspect of the corpus spongiosum, exiting from its dorsal surface before the posterior attachment of the bulbospongiosum to the perineal body. The membranous urethra is the portion that traverses the perineal pouch and is partially surrounded by the external urethral sphincter. This segment of the urethra is unmatched to fixed structures, has the distinction of being the only portion of the male urethra that is not invested by another structure, and is lined with a delicate transitional epithelium.

6. **e. The blood supply of the deep structures of the penis is derived from the common penile artery, which is the continuation of the internal pudendal artery after it branches off its perineal branch and the posterior scrotal arteries.** The common penile artery is the continuation of the internal pudendal artery giving off perineal posterior scrotal branches. From that point onward, it is termed the *common penile artery*. As it nears the urethral bulb, the artery divides into its three terminal branches as follows: (1) the bulbourethral arteries, which enter the proximal corpus spongiosum; (2) the dorsal artery, which travels along the dorsum of the penis contained in envelope fashion between the superficial and deep lamina of the Buck fascia; and (3) the cavernosal arteries, usually a single artery, which arise and penetrate the corpora cavernosa at the hilum and run the length of the penile shaft. The circumflex cavernosal arteries are given off at varying locations along the dorsal artery, but their distribution is neither uniform nor dependable.

7. **c. The dorsal nerve arises in the Alcock canal as a branch of the pudendal nerve.** The cavernosal nerves are a combination of the parasympathetic and visceral afferent fibers that constitute the autonomic nerves of the penis. These provide the nerve supply to the erectile apparatus. The pudendal nerves enter the perineum with the internal pudendal vessels through the lesser sciatic notch at the posterior border of the ischiorectal fossa. They run in the fibrofascial pudendal canal of Alcock to the edge of the urogenital diaphragm. Each dorsal nerve of the penis arises on Alcock canal as the first branch of the pudendal nerve. On the shaft, their fascicles fan out to supply proprioceptive and sensory nerve terminals in the tunica of the corpora cavernosa and sensory terminals in the skin. The skin of the penis is innervated by branches of the genitofemoral nerve.

8. **c. There is a strong association with an infectious etiology for the development of LS.** The etiology of LS has not been well defined. Multiple potential infectious etiologies have been suggested, but recent studies have found no association. Other proposed etiologies include a Koebner phenomenon, autoimmune event, and genetic associations. The remaining answer choices are correct.

9. **b. Genital or extragenital skin may be used for urethral reconstruction for LS-associated urethral strictures.** Most surgeons now believe that LS is a disease of genital skin. For this reason, genital skin is not appropriate for reconstruction in patients with LS. Although it is technically possible to use extragenital skin for reconstruction, oral mucosal grafting has emerged as a better tissue in patients with LS associated urethral strictures. Patients with meatal stenosis from LS not infrequently also have more proximal strictures and need a complete workup prior to surgery. Patients with long-standing LS should be monitored for potential development of squamous cell carcinoma, because this has been reported.

10. **d. Complication of genital herpes simplex viral infection.** Genital HSV has not been reported to cause urethrocutaneous fistulae. Each of the remaining answers is a potential etiology for urethrocutaneous fistula formation.

11. **c. When ammoniacal meatitis is noted, often a short course of meatal dilation and steroid cream application will resolve the problem.** Meatal stenosis in the male child appears to be a consequence of circumcision, which allows for ammoniacal meatitis. Children seen with ammoniacal meatitis are usually started with meatal dilation using steroid cream. Within a week, the process seems to settle down. Anecdotally, the fusion of the ventral meatus skin, which causes meatal stenosis, seems to be avoided. Because childhood meatal stenosis truly represents a fusion of the ventral urethral meatus, dividing the thin membrane of fusion is preferred. This leaves the child with a slit-shaped meatus.

12. **e. The McRoberts technique of macroreplantation is not the preferred method of management for these patients, but when the situation warrants it, it is very successful.** Often the amputation is self-inflicted, usually during an acute psychotic break. This should not preclude replantation unless the patient adamantly refuses such treatment. Even then, with a court order and the agreement of two or more surgeons, replantation may be undertaken. If possible, microreplantation should be carried out. This technique consists of an anatomic approximation of the tunica albuginea of the corporal bodies, a spatulated two-layer anastomosis of the urethra. The dorsal nerves are coapted using an epineural technique unless the injury is distal, at which point a vesicular coaptation may be required. The dorsal vein is anastomosed, and the dorsal arteries are anastomosed. Anastomosis of the cavernosal arteries is not possible and should not be attempted. If the situation is such that microreplantation cannot be undertaken, then the technique described by McRoberts can be carried out. His series and other series show that a high degree of success can be expected after replantation without microvascular reanastomosis. In most patients, however, they will have numbness distal to the replant site. With microreplantation, it is not at all unusual for patients to have excellent sensation distal to the area of injury and to have resumption of normal erectile function.

If the patient presents with the distal part having been disposed of or otherwise unavailable, then the wound should be closed. Often the penis will have been stretched during the amputation and an excess of skin will have been removed, leaving a good length intact with denuded penile shaft structures. In that case, the corporeal bodies would be closed, the urethral meatus must be spatulated, and the penis can be immediately covered with a split-thickness skin graft. If the injury occurs because of avulsion, replantation is not an option as the stretch injury to the spermatic vessels or vessels of the penis cause unpredictable damage to the endothelium.

13. **a. Circumcision may be performed in the neonatal period in newborns born with a distal hypospadias, but not in those with proximal hypospadias.** Newborns with any concern for hypospadias (distal or proximal) should NOT undergo circumcision. It is essential to preserve the foreskin so that it may be used for the hypospadias repair if necessary. Circumcision has consistently been shown in well-conducted randomized controlled trials to reduce the risk of HIV acquisition in heterosexual men by 50% to 60%. Circumcision will reduce the risk for UTI in infants and should be considered in those with recurrent infections. Most skin dehiscence following circumcision can be managed conservatively and does not require operative intervention.

14. **a. Reconstruction for lymphedema that is the consequence of the indirect effects of radiation is best accomplished with excision of the tissues and coverage with STSGs.** Patients with lymphedema can readily undergo reconstruction. When the lymphedematous tissue has been excised, the testes will be free and, as in a degloving injury, they must be fixed in the midline in an anatomically correct position. The shaft of the penis should be covered with a STSG. If the scrotum cannot be closed, a meshed STSG is used to cover the testes, as described. Not uncommonly, these patients have hydroceles, the parietal tunica vaginalis must be excised, and grafting can be done directly onto the visceral tunica vaginalis of the testicles. Unlike the full-thickness skin flap (FTSF), split-thickness skin carries little of the reticular dermis and hence few of the lymphatic channels. Reaccumulation of lymphedema will occur within a FTSG and can recur in a thick STSG. In many cases of lymphedema limited to the genitalia, the posterior scrotal skin and the lateral scrotal skin are spared from the lymphedematous process. Thus, in some cases, primary closure after excision can be accomplished using these tissues. If grafting is required, using these tissues to blend the grafts into the groin and perineum technically is much easier. The lymphedematous process involves recurrent cellulitis, lymphedema, and the development of lymphangiectasia. Lymphangiectasia can look like genital papilloma; however, it is a very different process. If there is any question, biopsy can clarify the issue.

15. **d. It causes limitation of the urethral lumen because of contraction and noncompliance of the scar.** The term urethral stricture refers to anterior urethral disease. By virtue of the Consensus Conference, obliterative processes of the membranous urethra, such as those associated with pelvic fracture, would be referred to as pelvic fracture urethral injury (PFUI), and other narrowing processes of the posterior urethra are correctly referred to as either contractures or stenoses. Thus the term *urethral stricture* describes a process that involves the urethral epithelium along with the spongy erectile tissue of the corpus spongiosum, and this is referred to as spongiofibrosis. In some cases, the scarring process can extend through the tissues of the corpus spongiosum and into the adjacent tissues. It is contraction of the scar that reduces the urethral lumen. Squamous metaplasia is often seen involving the urothelium of the urethra proximal to a narrow caliber urethral stricture.

16. **c. It is not a true stricture but rather fibrosis that results from distraction of the urethra.** By virtue of the Consensus Conference, narrowing of the posterior urethra is not referred to as a stricture. Those obliterative processes associated with pelvic fracture are termed pelvic fracture urethral injury (PFUI). PFUI is an obliterative process of the posterior urethra that has resulted in fibrosis and is the defect of distraction of the urethra in that area. Although the distraction defect can be lengthy in some cases, the actual process involving the tissues of the urethra is usually confined.

17. **a. Magnetic resonance imaging (MRI).** To devise an appropriate treatment plan, it is important to determine the location, length, depth, and density of the stricture (spongiofibrosis). The length and location of the stricture can be determined using radiographs, urethroscopy, and ultrasonography. The depth and density of the scar in the spongy tissue can be deduced from the physical examination, the appearance of the urethra in contrast studies, the amount of elasticity noted on urethroscopy, and the depth and density of fibrosis as evidenced by ultrasonographic evaluation of the urethra, although the absolute length of spongiofibrosis may not be evident on ultrasonographic evaluation. MRI has been suggested as useful in patients with pelvic fracture urethral distraction, particularly in cases in which the anatomy of the pelvis has become significantly distorted. With regard

to anterior urethral stricture, however, MRI has not been useful, with the exception of those cases in which there is urethral carcinoma. In those cases, MRI can provide invaluable information concerning the spread of the tumor. Bougie à boule calibration can be very helpful.

18. **a. Even if a patient does not have retention, placement of a suprapubic tube may help define strictured areas**. In selected patients, we have found it useful to place a suprapubic tube to defunctionalize the urethra. After 6 to 8 weeks, if there will be a constriction of an area that was hydrodilated with voiding, the tendency for that constriction to occur should become apparent. It is imperative, however, to completely evaluate the urethra proximal and distal to the stricture with endoscopy and bougienage during surgery, to ensure that all of the involved urethra is included in the reconstruction. Whereas hydraulic pressure generated by voiding may keep segments proximal to the stricture patent, unless these segments are included in the repair, they are at risk for contraction after obstruction of the narrow-caliber segment is relieved with reconstruction. For this reason, any abnormal areas of the urethra that are proximal to a narrow-caliber segment of the stricture must be treated with suspicion. If the lumen does not appear to demonstrate evidence of diminished compliance, then we presume that area to be uninvolved in active stricture disease. However, coning down of the urethra suggests its involvement in the scar. Use of a sonourethrogram is thought by some to accurately establish length of stricture but not the extent of spongiofibrosis.

19. **e. It can be associated with erectile dysfunction**. Many surgeons have learned to perform internal urethrotomy by making a single incision at the 12-o'clock position. This location might be questioned, however, based on the location of the urethra within the corpus spongiosum. Distally, although the anterior aspect of the corpus spongiosum is thicker, a deep incision in the more distal aspects of the anterior urethra will certainly enter the corpora cavernosa, and these incisions have been associated with the creation of erectile dysfunction. The most common complication of internal urethrotomy is recurrence of stricture. Less commonly noted complications of internal urethrotomy include bleeding and extravasation of irrigation fluid into the perispongiosal tissues. One report that used the actuarial technique showed the curative success rate of internal urethrotomy to be 29% to 30% for all patients. Other evaluations have confirmed this success rate. However, a number of studies do show which strictures best respond to internal urethrotomy. These are strictures of the bulbous urethra that are less than 1.5 cm in length and are not associated with the dense or deep spongiofibrosis (i.e., straddle injuries). In those particular cases, long-term success has been shown to be 75% to 78%. For strictures outside the bulbous urethra, most studies do not show internal urethrotomy to have long-term success.

20. **c. Success requires total excision of the fibrosis with a widely spatulated anastomosis**. It has now been demonstrated with certainty that the most dependable technique of anterior urethral reconstruction is the complete excision of the area of fibrosis, with a primary reanastomosis of the normal ends of the anterior urethra. The best results are achieved when the following technical points are observed: (1) the area of the fibrosis is totally excised; (2) the urethral anastomosis is widely spatulated, creating a large ovoid anastomosis; (3) the anastomosis is tension free; (4) epithelial apposition is achieved. With vigorous mobilization, development of the intracrural space, and detachment of the bulbospongiosum from the perineal body, significant lengths of stricture can be excised and reanastomosed. For very proximal bulbous strictures, tension-free anastomosis can be facilitated by the dissection of the membranous urethra. As a rule, the closer the stricture is to the membranous urethra, the longer it can be and still be reconstructed by anastomotic techniques. The tenet that excision and primary anastomosis should be the goal for all bulbous strictures is one that is being further reinforced by current published series. Although guideline lengths of 1 to 2 cm

are valuable for planning, most would agree that if excision and primary anastomosis is possible it should be done, and, with aggressive dissection and the maneuvers described earlier, often strictures much longer than the "guideline lengths" can be so reconstructed.

21. **b. The operation can conceptually become one operation with multidimensional application**. A number of applications of genital skin islands, mobilized on either the dartos fascia of the penis or the tunica dartos of the scrotum, have been proposed for repair of urethral stricture disease. In the past, these flap operations were considered to be separate procedures. We suggest that all of these procedures are really different applications of a single concept, proposed by the microinjection studies of Quartey. Skin islands, as mentioned, can be viewed as passengers on fascial flaps, and the design of flaps for urethral reconstruction can be done parallel to the design of flaps for reconstruction in general. These procedures that use skin islands oriented on the penile dartos fascia have been also useful for reconstruction of the fossa navicularis. There are three important considerations for the use of flaps in urethral reconstruction: (1) the nature of the flap tissue, (2) the vasculature of the flap, and (3) the mechanics of flap transfer. The skin must be nonhirsute for urethral reconstruction. In addition, for donor site consideration, it is most convenient to use the areas of redundant nonhirsute genital skin. These skin islands can be reliably elevated even in patients who have been circumcised.

22. **d. Continence is best addressed after a procedure to reestablish urethral continuity is performed**. We have found, and others have reported, that the competence of the bladder neck is difficult to accurately assess before the reestablishment of urethral continuity. Even in cases in which an obvious scar is noted to involve the bladder neck, follow-up of these patients after urethral reconstruction has found many patients with more than adequate continence. Still other patients are believed to have incontinence due to scar incarceration of the bladder neck. In our experience, however, this is an infrequent occurrence, and the appearance of the bladder neck by any modality available is not predictive of continence. It is currently our practice to reestablish the continuity of the urethra and, in cases in which there are concerns about continence, to forewarn the patient before the urethral reconstruction. Colopinto and others have not shown an association of ultimate continence as related to the location of the distraction injury.

23. **e. It is usually present with either ventral curvature or ventral curvature associated with torsion**. In many cases, there are abnormalities of the ventral penile skin. In patients who have chordee without hypospadias, the photograph will reveal an erect penis commensurate with the size of the detumescent penis, whereas in the congenital curvature patient, the erect penis will be noticeably large. Because of their congenital anomaly, these patients often become relatively reclusive and have poor self and genital images and may benefit from sex therapy. Even in patients with obvious abnormalities of the corpus spongiosum (i.e., poor ventral fusion or frank bifid corpus spongiosum), wide mobilization usually reveals that it is not the corpus spongiosum that remains as the ventral limiting factor. In most patients, the penis will remain curved because of the inelasticity of the ventral aspect of the corpora cavernosa. If the epithelial tube has served as an adequate urethra (i.e., it is not stenotic), the morbidity of the urethral division and subsequent need for urethral reconstruction must be considered before undertaking such a procedure. In children, after mobilization and excision of the dysgenetic tissues, the residual chordee can usually be corrected by making a longitudinal incision with a sharp blade. If this maneuver is not sufficient, the dorsal neurovascular structures can be mobilized in concert with the Buck fascia and a small ellipse or ellipses of dorsal tunica albuginea excised and closed with watertight plicating sutures.

24. **b. In most cases, global cavernosal veno-occlusive dysfunction (CVOD) is not a complicating factor**. When a young man presents with an acquired curvature of the penis, one must always

allow for the possibility of Peyronie disease. Occasionally, however, a patient or his initial-care physician will ignore the stigmata of the trauma (often described as "minimal" by patients), and the patient will present with a noticeable lateral scar that causes both indentation of the lateral aspect of the penis and, in some cases, curvature. Patients who had preexisting lateral curvature may actually notice that their penis has been straightened by the trauma, but they are disturbed by the concavity caused by the scar. The pathology of a subclinical fracture of the penis is believed to be due to either the disruption of the outer longitudinal layer of the tunica albuginea during the buckling trauma only or the disruption of both layers of the tunica albuginea during the buckling trauma but with preservation of Buck fascia. These patients usually have normal erectile function, and there is no association with concomitant global CVOD. However, the association of CVOD and trauma of the penis continues to be seen, and some patients, after fracture-type injuries of the penis, will have significant problems with erectile dysfunction. These injuries are not associated with shortening of the penis. It is the lack of erectile dysfunction and penile shortening that help distinguish these patients from those with Peyronie disease. Although foreshortening of the penis is not a characteristic of either the injury itself or the resulting scar in either of these injuries, these patients are not thought to be best treated by approaching the opposite aspect of the scar and excising an ellipse of the tunica. This would result in bilateral scars, which will cause bilateral indentation of the penis, and although the penis will have been straightened by the correction, most patients are upset by the cosmetic and functional result of a near-circumferential indentation of the penis. Curvatures associated with hypospadias or epispadias are not acquired curvatures.

25. **b. PFUIs most commonly occur between the prostate and membranous urethra.** Pelvic fracture distraction injuries of the membranous urethra have been compared with plucking an apple (prostate) off its stem (the membranous urethra). This analogy implies that the injury most frequently occurs at the apex of the prostate. Experience shows that this is not the case, however, and the most frequent point of distraction is at the departure of the bulbous urethra from the membranous urethra. The distraction can, however, involve all or any portion of the membranous urethra between the departure of the bulbous urethra and the apex of the prostate. The remaining answer choices are correct.

26. **a. Mobilizing the corpus spongiosum off the corpora cavernosa up to the corona of the glans.** Aggressive mobilization of the corpus spongiosum is performed with caution, because it is thought to have possible ill effects on retrograde blood supply, which in the pelvic fracture patient may be tenuous. Meticulous detachment of the investment of Buck fascia from the corpus spongiosum increases the compliance of the corpus and limits the need for aggressive mobilization. It is important to try to avoid the creation of chordee during the repair of a distraction injury. To prevent chordee, the attachment cannot be carried beyond the area of the penoscrotal attachment. Development of the intracrural space, infrapubectomy, and, if needed, rerouting of the corpus spongiosum each shorten the course that the corpus spongiosum must traverse and allow reconstruction without attendant chordee.

27. **d. Men with arteriogenic ED following PFUI who demonstrate bilateral occlusion of the internal pudendal arteries without reconstitution.** Patients with an intact pudendal artery on one side are often potent and reliably cured with reconstruction. Patients with only reconstituted vessels, either unilateral or bilateral, are rarely potent but reliably reconstructed. Those patients at risk for ischemic stenosis are only those with bilateral complete obstruction of the internal pudendal vessels without reconstitution. In such a patient, we now perform penile arterial revascularization to augment the vascularity and, with that accomplished, then proceed to urethral reconstruction. Patients without ED by definition have normal penile hemodynamics and do not require further investigation before repair of a PFUI.

28. **b. Current techniques are accomplished with a variety of flap designs, which use microvascular free flap transfer.** Rigidity for intercourse in the patient with phallic construction is usually achieved by either an externally applied or a permanently implanted prosthesis. Prosthetic implantation is never undertaken until 1 year after phallic construction, because protective sensibility must be demonstrated in the flap. When the flap is transferred, it is, by definition, rendered insensate. At about 3 to 4 months after reconstruction, however, as nerve regeneration occurs, sensation becomes noticeable. In addition, before prosthetic implantation is undertaken, the urethra must be patent and proved to be durable.

29. **d. Idiopathic proximal 1-cm bulbar urethral stricture in a patient with a history of a prior hypospadias repair.** Patients with a history of hypospadias can be expected to have altered or absent retrograde blood supply to the urethra through the normal arborization in the glans. In this situation, transecting techniques to repair urethral strictures should be avoided unless performed in a "vessel-sparing" fashion to avoid the risk of ischemic urethral stenosis. Inlay or onlay graft or flap techniques may be used in these patients, as these do not disrupt the proximal blood supply to the urethra. The remaining scenarios can be reliably repaired with anastomotic urethroplasty.

CHAPTER REVIEW

1. A meshed split-thickness graft that is applied to the genitalia should not be expanded but rather placed on the recipient site without expansion to allow collections from beneath the graft to escape.
2. Split-thickness grafts may contain some lymphatics; however, full-thickness grafts have a full complement of lymphatics.
3. Split-thickness grafts are more likely to take (become vascularized) but tend to contract and become brittle when mature, whereas full-thickness grafts have more difficulty becoming vascularized but are less likely to contract and are more durable when mature.
4. Tunica vaginalis grafts result in aneurysmal dilatation when they are used for large defects.
5. The superficial dorsal penile vein usually drains to the left saphenous vein; the deep dorsal and circumflex veins lying beneath the Buck fascia drain to the periprostatic plexus.
6. The Buck fascia is adjacent to the deep structures of the penis; the dartos fascia is next to the skin.
7. Lichen sclerosus is a disease of the skin and may involve large portions of the genital skin; therefore, using the genital skin for reconstruction may result in recurrence of the disease. Oral mucosal grafting has emerged as a better tissue in patients with lichen sclerosus–associated urethral strictures.
8. Lichen sclerosus may be a premalignant lesion and often results in meatal stenosis.
9. A spontaneous urethral fistula or unexplained periurethral abscess may be the harbinger of a urethral carcinoma.
10. Circumcision provides protection for heterosexual men in areas of endemic HIV; it reduces the risk of acquiring herpes simplex type 2, papillomavirus, and genital ulcer disease.
11. Cellulitis may be a problem in patients who have genital lymphedema.
12. As a general rule in the urethra, flaps are best suited for distal reconstruction, grafts for proximal reconstruction.
13. A urethral stricture involves the epithelium as well as the corpus spongiosum (spongiofibrosis).

14. For urethral distraction injuries (posterior urethral disruptions), an aligning catheter, at the very worst, facilitates subsequent reconstruction and, at best, may leave the patient with an endoscopically manageable urethra.

15. Because paraphimosis tends to recur, a dorsal slit or circumcision should be electively planned.

16. For urethral reconstruction an onlay graft or flap has a higher success rate than tabularized grafts.

17. Vesicourethrorectal fistulae are most successfully closed when normal tissue is interposed between the rectum and the bladder/urethra. The gracilis muscle interposition flap is an excellent tissue to interpose and, when used, has a high success rate.

18. Curvature of the penis in patients with Peyronie disease who require repair are best managed with corporal plication techniques and not grafting.

19. The corpora cavernosa are not separate structures but constitute a single space with free communication through an incompetent midline septum.

20. Meatal stenosis in the male child appears to be a consequence of circumcision.

21. It is imperative to completely evaluate the urethra proximal and distal to a stricture with endoscopy and bougienage during surgery, to ensure that all of the involved urethra is included in the reconstruction.

22. The curative success rate of internal urethrotomy is 29% to 30% for all patients. The strictures that respond best to internal urethrotomy are strictures of the bulbous urethra that are less than 1.5 cm in length and are not associated with the dense or deep spongiofibrosis.

23. The best results for primary reanastomosis are achieved when the following technical points are observed: (1) the area of the fibrosis is totally excised; (2) the urethral anastomosis is widely spatulated, creating a large ovoid anastomosis; (3) the anastomosis is tension free; and (4) epithelial apposition is achieved.

24. In complete membranous urethra disruption, the most frequent point of distraction is at the departure of the bulbous urethra from the membranous urethra. The distraction can, however, involve all or any portion of the membranous urethra between the departure of the bulbous urethra and the apex of the prostate.

25. Aggressive mobilization of the corpus spongiosum is performed with caution in patients with urethral disruptions because it is thought to have possible ill effects on retrograde blood supply to the urethra.

41 Surgery of the Scrotum and Seminal Vesicles

Frank A. Celigoj and Raymond A. Costabile

QUESTIONS

1. Which of the following vessels has the least direct contribution to the arterial supply of the vas deferens?
   a. Deferential artery
   b. Internal spermatic artery
   c. Superior vesicle artery
   d. Inferior epigastric artery
   e. Inferior epididymal artery

2. The best reason for using the no-scalpel vasectomy technique is:
   a. it has a higher sterilization rate than standard vasectomy with incision.
   b. patients are rendered sterile in less time.
   c. it is easier to learn than the standard technique.
   d. it results in a lower rate of complications, including hematoma and infection.
   e. it results in a higher rate of reversibility.

3. The no-scalpel technique for vasectomy reduces the rate of:
   a. hematoma.
   b. vasectomy failures.
   c. recanalization.
   d. injury to testicular artery.
   e. chronic orchialgia.

4. Vasectomy failure rate when both the abdominal and testicular ends of the divided vas deferens are occluded with hemoclips is:
   a. less than 1%.
   b. 5% to 10%.
   c. 10% to 20%.
   d. 20% to 30%.
   e. 50% to 60%.

5. The technical aspect shown to decrease vasectomy failure rates the most is:
   a. no-scalpel technique.
   b. conventional technique.
   c. fascial interposition of dartos fascia between the divided ends of the vas deferens.
   d. occluding both ends of the divided vas deferens with hemoclips.
   e. occluding both ends of the divided vas deferens thermally with the use of intraluminal cautery.

6. The technical aspect when performing vasectomy to make vasectomy reversal easier in the future is:
   a. no-scalpel technique.
   b. not excising a long segment of vas deferens.
   c. dividing the vas deferens as close to the epididymis as possible.
   d. occluding both ends of the divided vas deferens with hemoclips.
   e. occluding both ends of the divided vas deferens thermally with the use of intraluminal cautery.

7. Vasectomy has been established as associated with:
   a. prostate cancer.
   b. dementia.
   c. cardiovascular disease.
   d. atherosclerosis.
   e. a 10% incidence of chronic scrotal pain.

8. What is the estimated percentage of men who develop antisperm antibodies after vasectomy?
   a. 0% to 20%
   b. 20% to 40%
   c. 40% to 60%
   d. 60% to 80%
   e. >80%

9. Which of the following is an indication for repeat vasectomy?
   a. Painless sperm granuloma
   b. Motile sperm found in semen analysis 3 months after vasectomy
   c. Nonmotile sperm found in semen analysis 3 months after vasectomy
   d. Persistent testicular pain 3 months after vasectomy
   e. All of the above

10. Pressure-induced injury following vasectomy occurs in:
    a. the testis.
    b. the ejaculatory duct.
    c. the epididymis.
    d. the vas deferens.
    e. the seminal vesicles.

11. In the management of chronic orchialgia, which of the following statements is TRUE?
    a. Imaging studies are not indicated.
    b. Varicocele is not a significant contributor of chronic scrotal pain.
    c. Orchiectomy usually relieves the pain.
    d. Denervation of the cord may offer relief in selected cases.
    e. Diagnostic epididymal puncture should be performed to rule out chronic bacterial epididymitis.

12. Which of the following statements is TRUE regarding hydrocelectomy?
    a. Hematoma is the least frequent complication.
    b. The Jaboulay bottleneck operation is associated with a high recurrence rate.
    c. The Lord plication is an ideal operation for long-standing postinfectious hydroceles.
    d. Sclerotherapy is often the treatment of choice for young men of reproductive age.
    e. The Jaboulay bottleneck operation is associated with a low recurrence rate.

13. A nontransilluminating, nontender mass is noted in the epididymis on physical examination and confirmed to be solid by sonography. What is the most likely diagnosis?

    a. Epididymal cyst

    b. Adenomatoid tumor

    c. Spermatocele

    d. Testicular tumor

    e. Hydrocele

14. Men who were treated with epididymectomy for chronic epididymitis responded the most favorably if:

    a. there was a palpable epididymal abnormality.

    b. there was no palpable abnormality, but there were sonographic changes of the epididymis.

    c. there were no palpable abnormalities and no sonographic changes of the epididymis.

    d. they had improvement of pain with spermatic cord block.

    e. none of the above applied.

15. Which of the following statements is TRUE regarding retractile testes in adults?

    a. As in children, surgical repair is never indicated.

    b. A dartos pouch orchidopexy is the treatment of choice.

    c. Simple three-stitch orchiopexy of the tunica albuginea to the dartos, as for torsion prophylaxis, is effective in preventing retraction.

    d. Bilateral orchiopexy is necessary for a unilateral retractile testis.

    e. Coexisting varicocele is common.

16. The most appropriate approach to a long-standing, thick-walled, loculated hydrocele is:

    a. excision of the hydrocele sac.

    b. the Jaboulay bottleneck technique.

    c. the Lord plication technique.

    d. the inguinal approach.

    e. sclerotherapy.

17. In men with chronic orchitis without an identifiable bacterial pathogen, antibiotics:

    a. decrease the length of symptoms.

    b. improve the severity of symptoms.

    c. decrease the length of time to full activity.

    d. are steadily being prescribed more frequently empirically.

    e. none of the above apply.

18. When a clinically palpable varicocele is encountered in a patient with orchialgia, varicocelectomy will resolve the pain:

    a. 10% of the time.

    b. 25% of the time.

    c. 50% of the time.

    d. 75% of the time.

    e. 90% of the time.

19. What is the embryologic origin of the seminal vesicles?

    a. Müllerian duct

    b. Ectodermal ridge

    c. Distal mesonephric duct

    d. Swelling of the distal paramesonephric duct

    e. Neural crest cells

20. What percentage of the ejaculate volume is made up of seminal vesicle secretions?

    a. 5% to 10%

    b. 20% to 30%

    c. 60% to 80%

    d. 90%

    e. The seminal vesicle does not contribute to the seminal plasma volume.

21. What artery is the major blood supply to the seminal vesicle?

    a. Hypogastric

    b. Vesiculodeferential artery

    c. Inferior vesicle

    d. Internal iliac

    e. Deep dorsal penile

22. Decreased T1 signal intensity on MRI, along with increased T2 intensity of seminal vesicles, is indicative of which process?

    a. Inflammation of the seminal vesicles

    b. Hemorrhage within the seminal vesicles

    c. Seminal vesicle tumors

    d. Seminal vesicle cysts

    e. Normal seminal vesicles

23. Agenesis of the seminal vesicle is associated with significant ipsilateral renal anomalies. What is the embryologic reason for this?

    a. A genetic defect links seminal vesicle agenesis to renal agenesis.

    b. A mutation occurs in the cystic fibrosis transmembrane regulator gene.

    c. There was an insult to the mesonephric duct at approximately 12 weeks' gestation.

    d. There was an embryologic insult to the mesonephric duct earlier than 7 weeks' gestation.

    e. There is no association between agenesis of the seminal vesicle and ipsilateral renal anomalies.

24. What disorder is frequently associated with bilateral agenesis of the seminal vesicles?

    a. Cystic fibrosis

    b. Kartagener syndrome

    c. Young syndrome

    d. Kallmann syndrome

    e. Klinefelter syndrome

25. What causes the majority of seminal vesicle cysts?

    a. Ejaculatory duct stone

    b. Obstruction of the ejaculatory duct

    c. Inflammation

    d. Renal agenesis

    e. Trisomy 21

26. What is the most common type of malignant neoplasm found in seminal vesicles?

    a. Primary adenocarcinoma

    b. Sarcoma

    c. Cystosarcoma phyllodes

    d. Metastatic tumors

    e. Amyloidosis

27. What is the best initial test for a suspected seminal vesicle abnormality?

    a. Computed tomography (CT)

    b. Transrectal ultrasonography

    c. Magnetic resonance imaging (MRI)

    d. Fine-needle biopsy

    e. Vasography

28. What is the best method to differentiate a benign from malignant seminal vesicle mass?
    a. Biopsy of the lesion
    b. Contrast medium-enhanced CT
    c. Gadolinium-enhanced MRI
    d. Transrectal ultrasonography
    e. Rectal examination

29. What is the best surgical approach to a congenital lesion of the seminal vesicle?
    a. The perineal route because this has the quickest recovery.
    b. The transcoccygeal route because these are usually large lesions.
    c. The laparoscopic route so that the ipsilateral kidney can be dealt with concomitantly and recovery may be shorter.
    d. The paravesical route because this has a lower incidence of postoperative erectile dysfunction.
    e. The transvesical route because rectal injury is much less likely.

30. What is the best indication for the transcoccygeal approach to the seminal vesicle?
    a. Need for exploration of the ipsilateral kidney
    b. Patient with previous suprapubic and/or perineal surgery
    c. Patient wishing to maintain potency
    d. Patient with bilateral large seminal vesicle lesions
    e. Patient with metastatic tumor to the seminal vesicle

31. In a patient with a seminal vesicle abscess, the treatment of choice is:
    a. laparoscopic unroofing.
    b. transvesical excision of the seminal vesicle.
    c. aspiration and antibiotic instillation.
    d. endoscopic unroofing by deep transurethral resection.
    e. retropubic approach to unroof the abscess.

ANSWERS

1. **c. Superior vesicle artery.** The superior vesicle artery does not supply the vas deferens, whereas all of the other arteries listed may have a branch to the vas deferens.
2. **d. It results in a lower rate of complications, including hematoma and infection.** This method eliminates the scalpel incision, results in fewer hematomas and infections, and leaves a much smaller wound than conventional methods of accessing the vas deferens for vasectomy.
3. **a. Hematoma.** The no-scalpel technique significantly decreases the rate of hematomas, infections, and pain during the procedure.
4. **a. Less than 1%.** Vasectomy failure rate when both the abdominal and testicular ends of the divided vas deferens are occluded with hemoclips is less than 1%.
5. **c. Fascial interposition of dartos fascia between the divided ends of the vas deferens.** Interposition of dartos fascia between the divided ends of the vas deferens is a technique for occlusion that has been reported to reduce the recanalization rate to nearly zero.
6. **b. Not excising a long segment of vas deferens.** The technical aspects when performing vasectomy to make vasectomy reversal easier in the future include not excising a long segment of vas deferens, dividing the vas deferens approximately 3 cm cephalad to the cauda of the epididymis in the straight portion of the vas deferens, and transecting the vas deferens, followed by low-voltage cautery occlusion and then by fascial interposition.
7. **e. A 10% incidence of chronic scrotal pain.** Vasectomy does not have an established association with prostate cancer, dementia, cardiovascular disease, or atherosclerosis, although it has been associated with a 10% incidence of chronic scrotal pain.

8. **d. 60% to 80%.** Vasectomy disrupts the blood-testis barrier, resulting in detectable levels of serum antisperm antibodies in 60% to 80% of men.
9. **b. Motile sperm found in semen analysis 3 months after vasectomy.** If any motile sperm are found in the ejaculate 3 months after vasectomy, consideration should be given to repeating the procedure.
10. **c. The epididymis.** The brunt of pressure-induced damage after vasectomy falls on the epididymis and efferent ductules.
11. **d. Denervation of the cord may offer relief in selected cases.** Microsurgical total denervation of the spermatic cord is a procedure used with reported success in several small series.
12. **e. The Jaboulay bottleneck operation is associated with a low recurrence rate.** The Jaboulay bottleneck operation, in which the sac edges are sewn together behind the cord, reduces the chance of recurrence caused by reapposition of the edges of the hydrocele sac.
13. **b. Adenomatoid tumor.** Most nontransilluminable solid epididymal masses are benign adenomatoid tumors.
14. **a. There was a palpable epididymal abnormality.** A retrospective review of men who underwent epididymectomy for chronic epididymitis showed that outcomes were best when the patient had a palpable epididymal abnormality on physical examination. Men in this study without a palpable abnormality, but with sonographic changes, had slightly worse outcomes, and those with neither a palpable abnormality nor a demonstrable ultrasonographic abnormality did not improve with epididymectomy.
15. **b. A dartos pouch orchidopexy is the treatment of choice.** Creation of a dartos pouch will keep the testis well down into the scrotum and permanently prevent retraction.
16. **a. Excision of the hydrocele sac.** Excising the hydrocele is recommended for long-standing, thick-walled, loculated hydroceles.
17. **d. Are steadily being prescribed more frequently empirically.** Despite evidence that up to 75% of patients with epididymitis/orchitis do not have an identifiable bacterial urinary tract infection concomitantly with their clinical epididymitis, antibiotics are routinely given. Empirical antibiotic administration in the absence of positive urine cultures has been steadily increasing, from 75% to 95% between the years of 1965 and 2005 and is not indicated.
18. **c. 50% of the time.** When a clinically palpable varicocele is encountered in a patient with orchialgia, varicocelectomy will resolve the pain 50% of the time.
19. **c. Distal mesonephric duct.** The seminal vesicle develops as a dorsolateral bulbous swelling of the distal mesonephric duct at approximately 12 fetal weeks.
20. **c. 60% to 80%.** The secretions from the seminal vesicle contribute 60% to 80% of the ejaculate volume.
21. **b. Vesiculodeferential artery.** The blood supply to the seminal vesicle is from the vesiculodeferential artery, a branch of the superior vesical artery.
22. **a. Inflammation of the seminal vesicles.** Seminal vesiculitis shows decreased signal intensity on the T1-weighted image, whereas the T2-weighted image intensity is higher than that of both fat and the normal seminal vesicle.
23. **d. There was an embryologic insult to the mesonephric duct earlier than at 7 weeks' gestation.** Unilateral agenesis of the seminal vesicles has an incidence of 0.6% to 1% and may be associated with unilateral absence of the vas deferens, as well as ipsilateral renal anomalies.
24. **a. Cystic fibrosis.** Of men with bilateral absence of the vas deferens or seminal vesicles, 70% to 80% carry the genetic mutation associated with cystic fibrosis. Conversely, 80% to 95% of men with cystic fibrosis have bilateral absence of the vas deferens or seminal vesicles.
25. **b. Obstruction of the ejaculatory duct.** Cysts of the seminal vesicles may be either congenital or acquired and are thought to be due to obstruction of the ejaculatory duct.
26. **d. Metastatic tumors.** Very few primary tumors of the seminal vesicles have been reported. It is more common for carcinoma

of the bladder, prostate, or rectum, or lymphoma to secondarily involve the seminal vesicles.

27. **b. Transrectal ultrasonography.** Transrectal ultrasonography is the preferred initial test for seminal vesicle abnormality, because of its low invasiveness, ease of performance, and ability to perform concomitant transrectal biopsies.

28. **a. Biopsy of the lesion.** Transrectal ultrasonography and biopsy of the seminal vesicle mass is accurate and easily accomplished.

29. **c. The laparoscopic route so that the ipsilateral kidney can be dealt with concomitantly and recovery may be shorter.** Although data are limited for laparoscopic excision of benign seminal vesicle disease alone, this approach appears to afford superb visualization with minimal postoperative morbidity and shorter hospitalization, compared with the open surgical alternatives.

30. **b. Patient with previous suprapubic and/or perineal surgery.** In individuals for whom the perineal or supine position may be difficult to maintain, or for those who have had multiple suprapubic or perineal surgeries, the transcoccygeal approach may be useful.

31. **d. Endoscopic unroofing by deep transurethral resection.** If the abscess is in the portion of the seminal vesicle adjacent to the prostate, a deep transurethral resection into the prostatic substance, just distal to the bladder neck at the 5-o'clock or 7-o'clock position, may be effective in relieving the problem. However, a CT-guided aspiration and drain placement is becoming the preferred least-traumatic option.

CHAPTER REVIEW

1. Because scrotal cases are considered clean rather than sterile, prophylactic antibiotics are recommended preoperatively. Hair removal should occur immediately before the procedure.

2. Fournier gangrene is a necrotizing fasciitis that involves the skin and subcutaneous tissue and is confined by the dartos fascia on the penis, Colles fascia in the perineum, and Scarpa fascia in the abdomen. Proper resuscitation requires broad-spectrum antibiotics, including a third-generation cephalosporin, an aminoglycoside, and metronidazole. These patients require fluid resuscitation and, when hemodynamically stable, debridement. Daily debridement in the operating room until all nonviable tissue is removed should be subsequently performed.

3. Ninety-seven percent of patients undergoing open-ended vasectomy develop sperm granulomas.

4. Division of the vas deferens during vasectomy should occur at least 3 cm from the epididymitis. There is no vasectomy technique that is 100% effective; more than 80% of the patients achieve azoospermia at 3 months following vasectomy.

5. When the testis is removed for orchialgia, pain relief is better achieved if the orchiectomy is performed through an inguinal incision rather than a transscrotal incision.

6. There is no level 1 evidence that orchiectomy is effective for the treatment of chronic orchialgia.

7. Any surgical manipulation of the epididymis results in azoospermia on that side.

8. Leaving a scrotal drain after scrotal procedures does not lessen the complication rate or the development of postoperative hematomas.

9. When repairing large hydroceles, the epididymis and spermatic vessels may be splayed by the hydrocele, and care must be taken to identify them to avoid injury.

10. Microsurgical denervation of the spermatic cord has been used for the treatment of orchialgia with reported success rates as high as two thirds achieving pain relief. It should only be considered if a cord block is successful.

11. Seminal vesicle cysts are associated with ipsilateral renal agenesis or dysplasia in two thirds of patients and have been associated with polycystic kidney disease.

12. *Mycobacterium tuberculosis* and *Schistosoma haematobium* may infect the seminal vesicles.

13. Vasectomy has not been established to be associated with prostate cancer, dementia, cardiovascular disease, or atherosclerosis, although it has been associated with a 10% incidence of chronic scrotal pain.

14. Vasectomy disrupts the blood-testis barrier, resulting in detectable levels of serum antisperm antibodies in 60% to 80% of men.

15. The Jaboulay bottleneck operation, in which the sac edges are sewn together behind the cord, reduces the chance of recurrence caused by reapposition of the edges of the hydrocele sac.

16. Of men with bilateral absence of the vas deferens or seminal vesicles, 70% to 80% are carriers of the genetic mutation associated with cystic fibrosis. Conversely, 80% to 95% of men with cystic fibrosis have bilateral absence of the vas deferens or seminal vesicles.

17. Very few primary tumors of the seminal vesicles have been reported. It is more common for carcinoma of the bladder, prostate, or rectum or lymphoma to secondarily involve the seminal vesicles.

42

Surgical, Radiographic, and Endoscopic Anatomy of the Kidney and Ureter

Sero Andonian and Mohamed Aly Elkoushy

QUESTIONS

1. The exact position of the kidney within the retroperitoneum varies during:
   a. different phases of respiration.
   b. presence of anatomic anomalies.
   c. body position.
   d. a, b, and c
   e. a and c

2. Gerota fascia envelops the kidney and the adrenal gland on all aspects but remains open:
   a. inferiorly.
   b. laterally.
   c. medially.
   d. inferiorly and laterally.
   e. inferiorly and medially.

3. The white line of Toldt is the lateral reflection of posterior parietal peritoneum that covers:
   a. the ascending colon.
   b. the descending colon.
   c. the transverse colon.
   d. the ascending and descending colons.
   e. the ascending and transverse colon.

4. What are the columns of Bertin?
   a. Extensions of renal medulla between the pyramids
   b. Extensions of renal cortex between the pyramids
   c. Cortical extensions between renal lobules
   d. The collecting ducts
   e. None of the above

5. Compared with the liver, the normal adult kidneys in gray-scale ultrasound appear:
   a. hyperechoic.
   b. isoechoic.
   c. hypoechoic.
   d. b and c
   e. variable, depending on the renal function.

6. Occlusion or injury to a segmental renal artery will cause:
   a. no pathologic conditions.
   b. opening of the collateral circulation.
   c. segmental renal infarction.
   d. an effect that depends on the availability of collaterals.
   e. renal atrophy.

7. Ureteropelvic junction obstruction may be commonly caused by:
   a. the lower anterior segmental artery when it passes anterior to the ureter.
   b. crossing of the ureter by any of the renal segmental arteries.
   c. the posterior segmental artery when it passes posterior to the renal pelvis.
   d. the posterior segmental artery when it passes anterior to the ureter.
   e. the lower anterior segmental artery when it passes posterior to the ureter.

8. Occlusion of a segmental renal vein results in:
   a. segmental renal congestion.
   b. segmental renal atrophy.
   c. no pathologic conditions.
   d. an effect that depends on the availability of collaterals.
   e. gross hematuria.

9. The main renal vasculature can be accurately identified with 100% sensitivity by:
   a. Doppler ultrasonography.
   b. computed tomography angiography (CTA).
   c. intravenous urography.
   d. noncontrast computed tomography.
   e. All of the above

10. Medial displacement of both pelvic ureteral segments might result from:
    a. pelvic lipomatosis.
    b. postabdominoperineal surgery.
    c. retroperitoneal fibrosis.
    d. All of the above
    e. a and c

11. If the small ureteral arteries that anastomose in the ureteral adventitia are disrupted, this may result in:
    a. ureteral ischemia.
    b. ureteral stricture.
    c. a and b
    d. no impact on ureteral blood supply.
    e. gross hematuria.

12. The blood supply of the mid-ureter is mostly:
    a. anterior.
    b. posterior.
    c. medial.
    d. lateral.
    e. any of the above.

13. What is the Mercier bar?
    a. The intramural ureter
    b. The bladder trigone
    c. The interureteral ridge
    d. Intraureteral valves
    e. None of the above

14. The higher the grade of the ureteral orifice:
    a. the greater its tendency to be laterally located.
    b. the lesser its tendency to reflux.
    c. the greater its tendency to be associated with ureterocele.
    d. the greater its tendency to reflux.
    e. None of the above

ANSWERS

1. **d. a, b, and c.** The exact position of the kidney within the retroperitoneum varies **during different phases of respiration, body position, and presence of anatomic anomalies.** For example, the kidneys move inferiorly about 3 cm (one vertebral body) during inspiration and during the changing of body position from supine to the erect position.

2. **a. Inferiorly.** Gerota fascia encasing the kidneys, adrenal glands, and abdominal ureters is closed superiorly and laterally and serves as an anatomic barrier to the spread of malignancy and a means of containing perinephric fluid collections. Superiorly, the Gerota fascia is continuous with the diaphragmatic fascia on the inferior surface of the diaphragm, whereas inferiorly, the anterior and posterior layers of Gerota fascia are loosely attached where perinephric fluid collections can track inferiorly into the pelvis without violating Gerota fascia.

3. **d. The ascending and descending colons.** To access the kidneys transperitoneally, the colon needs to be mobilized from the white line of Toldt, which is the lateral reflection of posterior parietal peritoneum **over the ascending and descending colon.**

4. **b. Extensions of renal cortex between the pyramids.** The renal cortex is about 1 cm in thickness and covers the base of each renal pyramid peripherally and **extends downwards between the individual pyramids to form the columns of Bertin.**

5. **b. Isoechoic.** In adults, the normal kidneys have smooth margins and are **isoechoic to the liver.** However, both renal cortices and pyramids are usually hypoechoic to the liver, spleen, and renal sinus. Compared with renal parenchyma, renal sinus appears hyperechoic because of the presence of hilar adipose tissue, blood vessels, and lymphatics.

6. **c. Segmental renal infarction.** After entering the hilum, each artery divides into five segmental end arteries that do not anastomose significantly with other segmental arteries. **Therefore, occlusion or injury to a segmental branch will cause segmental renal infarction.** Nevertheless, the area supplied by each segmental artery could be independently surgically resected.

7. **d. The posterior segmental artery when it passes anterior to the ureter.** The posterior segmental artery from the posterior division **passes posterior to the renal pelvis** while the others pass anterior to the renal pelvis. **If the posterior segmental branch passes anterior to the ureter, ureteropelvic junction obstruction may occur.**

8. **c. No pathologic conditions.** The renal venous drainage correlates closely with the arterial supply with the exception that unlike the arterial supply, venous drainage has extensive collateral communication through the venous collars around minor calyceal infundibula. Furthermore, the interlobular veins that drain the **post-glomerular capillaries also communicate freely with perinephric veins** through the subcapsular venous plexus of stellate veins. Therefore, occlusion of a segmental venous branch **has little effect on venous outflow.**

9. **b. Computed tomography angiography (CTA).** Doppler ultrasonography clearly identifies renal arteries at their origin from the abdominal aorta. However, the main renal artery is often difficult to identify at baseline ultrasonography. Therefore, **CTA is currently considered the gold standard to assess renal arteries** with 100% sensitivity for identification of renal arteries and veins.

10. **d. All of the above.** Medial displacement of **both pelvic ureteral segments might result from retroperitoneal fibrosis, pelvic lipomatosis, or postabdominoperineal surgery.** However, medial displacement and concavity of **a single pelvic ureter** may result from enlarged hypogastric nodes, a bladder diverticulum, or aneurismal dilatation of the hypogastric artery. Nevertheless, this may be a **normal finding in adult females** if only the right ureter is affected because of the uterine tilt to the left.

11. **c. a and b.** The abdominal portion of the ureter is supplied mainly by arterial branches medially from the main renal artery or the aorta, which form a longitudinal anastomosis on the ureteral wall. Despite this anastomotic plexus, **ureteral ischemia is not uncommon** if these small and delicate ureteral branches are disrupted. Unnecessary lateral retraction and removal of the periureteral adventitial tissues containing the blood supply can result in ureteral ischemia and subsequent stricture.

12. **b. Posterior.** Although main renal arteries or the aorta supply the abdominal ureter medially, the blood supply to the distal ureter comes laterally from the superior vesical artery, a branch of the internal iliac artery, and the mid-ureter is supplied by branches **arising posteriorly** from the common iliac arteries. Therefore, the blood supply of the ureter is medial in the proximal part, posterior in the mid portion, and lateral in the distal portion.

13. **c. The interureteral ridge.** Once the cystoscope is inside the bladder neck, the trigone can be seen as a raised, smooth triangle. The apex of that triangle is situated at the bladder neck; its base is formed by **the interureteral ridge or Mercier bar,** extending between the two ureteral orifices.

14. **a. The greater its tendency to be laterally located.** The ureteral orifices are classified according to their position or configuration. They are normally located at the medial aspect of the trigone (position A). However, they may be located at the lateral wall of the bladder or at its junction with the trigone (position C) or in between positions A and C (position B). In terms of configuration; grade 0 indicates a normal ureteral orifice that looks like a cone or a volcano. Grades 1, 2, and 3 describe stadium, horseshoe, and golf-hole orifice, respectively. **The higher the grade of the orifice, the greater its tendency to be laterally located and to reflux.**

CHAPTER REVIEW

1. The medial aspect of each kidney is rotated anteriorly 30 degrees.
2. The 12th rib overlies the right kidney; the 11th and 12th ribs overlie the left kidney.
3. The columns of Bertin contain the interlobar arteries.
4. Renal hilar structures from anterior to posterior are renal vein, renal artery, and renal pelvis.
5. The line of Brodel is an avascular plane between the anterior and posterior segments. It is variable in location and must be defined for each individual kidney.
6. Lumbar veins may drain directly into the renal veins, which occurs more commonly on the left. They may be the source of troublesome bleeding when dissecting around the renal vein.
7. Gerota fascia encasing the kidneys, adrenal glands, and abdominal ureters is closed superiorly and laterally and serves as an anatomic barrier to the spread of malignancy as well as a means of containing perinephric fluid collections. Superiorly, the Gerota fascia is continuous with the diaphragmatic fascia on the inferior surface of the diaphragm, whereas inferiorly, the anterior and posterior layers of Gerota fascia are loosely attached where perinephric fluid collections can track inferiorly into the pelvis without violating Gerota fascia.
8. Each renal artery divides into five segmental end arteries that do not anastomose significantly with other segmental arteries. They are end arteries and, when occluded, cause renal tissue ischemia and tissue atrophy.
9. The renal venous drainage has extensive collateral communication, and occlusion of a segmental vein will not impair the venous drainage to that segment.
10. Removal of the periureteral adventitial tissues containing the blood supply can result in ureteral ischemia and subsequent stricture.
11. The blood supply of the ureter is medially in the proximal part, posteriorly in the mid portion, and laterally in the distal portion.

43

Physiology and Pharmacology of the Renal Pelvis and Ureter

Robert M. Weiss and Darryl T. Martin

QUESTIONS

1. During development, the ureteral lumen is obliterated and then recanalizes. Which of the following substances appears to be involved in this recanalization process?
   a. Prostaglandin E_2
   b. c-KIT
   c. Angiotensin
   d. Calcitonin gene-related peptide (CGRP)
   e. Acetylcholine

2. Caspases are involved in:
   a. smooth muscle relaxation.
   b. smooth muscle contraction.
   c. hysteresis.
   d. apoptosis.
   e. calcium sequestration.

3. The resting membrane potential is primarily determined by the distribution of which of the following ions across the cell membrane and the preferential permeability of the cell membrane to that ion?
   a. Potassium
   b. Sodium
   c. Calcium
   d. Chloride
   e. Barium

4. With excitation of the ureteral muscle cell, an action potential is formed. Which of the following pairs of ions are primarily responsible for the upstroke of the action potential?
   a. Potassium and calcium
   b. Sodium and chloride
   c. Calcium and sodium
   d. Potassium and sodium
   e. Calcium and chloride

5. Which of the following must be phosphorylated for smooth muscle contraction to occur?
   a. Actin
   b. Myosin
   c. Calmodulin
   d. Calcium
   e. Troponin

6. The primary site for intracellular storage of calcium is:
   a. mitochondria.
   b. caveolae.
   c. the nucleolus.
   d. actin.
   e. the endoplasmic reticulum.

7. The second messenger involved in β-adrenergic agonist-induced ureteral relaxation is:
   a. cyclic adenosine monophosphate (AMP).
   b. cyclic guanosine monophosphate (GMP).
   c. nitric oxide.
   d. inositol 1,4,5-triphosphate (IP_3).
   e. diacylglycerol (DG).

8. The enzyme that degrades cyclic GMP is:
   a. guanylyl cyclase.
   b. myosin light-chain kinase.
   c. phosphodiesterase.
   d. phospholipase C.
   e. nitric oxide synthase (NOS).

9. The enzyme that degrades cyclic AMP is:
   a. adenylyl cyclase.
   b. myosin light-chain kinase.
   c. phosphodiesterase.
   d. phospholipase C.
   e. NOS.

10. Nitric oxide causes smooth muscle relaxation. In doing so, it activates which of the following enzymes?
    a. Guanylyl cyclase
    b. Myosin light-chain kinase
    c. Phosphodiesterase
    d. Phospholipase C
    e. NOS

11. The substrate for NOS is:
    a. cyclic AMP.
    b. cyclic GMP.
    c. GTP.
    d. L-Arginine.
    e. L-Citrulline.

12. Inducible NOS (iNOS) is:
    a. nicotinamide adenine dinucleotide phosphate (NADPH) independent and calcium independent.
    b. NADPH independent and calcium dependent.
    c. NADPH dependent and calcium independent.
    d. NADPH dependent and calcium dependent.
    e. nitric oxide dependent and calcium dependent.

13. The enzyme involved in the formation of DG is:
    a. adenylyl cyclase.
    b. guanylyl cyclase.
    c. phosphodiesterase.
    d. protein kinase C.
    e. phospholipase C.

14. DG increases the activity of which enzyme?
    a. Adenylyl cyclase
    b. Guanylyl cyclase
    c. Phosphodiesterase
    d. Protein kinase C
    e. Phospholipase C

15. An agent that prevents reuptake of norepinephrine in nerve terminals and thus potentiates and prolongs the activity of norepinephrine is:
    a. tyrosine.
    b. monoamine oxidase.
    c. imipramine.
    d. tetramethylammonium.
    e. tetraethylammonium.

16. Norepinephrine is synthesized from:
    a. tyrosine.
    b. arginine.
    c. choline.
    d. cocaine.
    e. imipramine.

17. Which of the following inhibits ureteral and renal pelvic contractile activity?
    a. Substance P
    b. Neurokinin A
    c. Neuropeptide K
    d. Neuropeptide Y
    e. CGRP

18. Which of the following collagen types is associated with ureteral obstruction?
    a. Type I collagen
    b. Type II collagen
    c. Type III collagen
    d. Type IV collagen
    e. Type V collagen

19. The enzyme involved in prostaglandin synthesis is:
    a. phospholipase C.
    b. cyclooxygenase.
    c. protein kinase C.
    d. phosphodiesterase.
    e. adenosine triphosphate.

20. With ureteral obstruction, prostaglandins are involved in a process that aids in the preservation of renal function. What is this process?
    a. Afferent arteriole vasoconstriction
    b. Afferent arteriole vasodilatation
    c. Efferent arteriole vasoconstriction
    d. Efferent arteriole vasodilatation
    e. Glomerular vasoconstriction

21. Which of the following agents could theoretically cause urinary retention?
    a. Bethanechol
    b. BAY K 8644
    c. Prostaglandin $F_{2\alpha}$

    d. Verapamil
    e. Substance P

22. Which of the following is a β-adrenergic agonist?
    a. Cromakalim
    b. Physostigmine
    c. Propranolol
    d. Phenoxybenzamine
    e. Isoproterenol

23. Which of the following conditions must be present for urine to pass efficiently from the ureter into the bladder?
    a. Intraluminal ureteral contractile pressure must be above 40 cm H_2O.
    b. The ureterovesical junction must relax.
    c. Intraluminal ureteral contractile pressures must be greater than intravesical baseline pressures.
    d. Intravesical contractile pressures must be less than 40 cm H_2O.
    e. The bladder must relax just before contraction of the ureter.

24. What is normal baseline or resting ureteral pressure?
    a. 0 to 5 cm H_2O
    b. 5 to 10 cm H_2O
    c. 10 to 15 cm H_2O
    d. 15 to 20 cm H_2O
    e. 20 to 25 cm H_2O

25. The Laplace equation expresses the relationship between the variables that affect intraluminal pressure. Which of the following conforms to the Laplace relationship?
    a. Tension = (radius × wall thickness)/pressure
    b. Tension = (radius × pressure)/wall thickness
    c. Tension = (wall thickness × pressure)/radius
    d. Pressure = (radius × wall thickness)/tension
    e. Pressure = (radius × tension)/wall thickness

26. Factors that facilitate ureteral stone passage include:
    a. increased hydrostatic pressures proximal to the calculus and relaxation of the ureter in the region of the stone.
    b. increased hydrostatic pressures proximal to the calculus and contraction of the ureter in the region of the stone.
    c. decreased hydrostatic pressures proximal to the calculus and relaxation of the ureter in the region of the stone.
    d. decreased hydrostatic pressures proximal to the calculus and contraction of the ureter in the region of the stone.
    e. decreased contractile pressures proximal to the calculus and contraction of the ureter in the region of the stone.

27. Which of the following hormones inhibits ureteral contractility?
    a. Bombesin
    b. Thyroxine
    c. Estrogen
    d. Aldosterone
    e. Progesterone

28. A drug that has efficacy in managing ureteral colic is:
    a. bethanechol.
    b. prostaglandin $F_{2\alpha}$.
    c. physostigmine.
    d. indomethacin.
    e. ephedrine.

29. Which of the following is a calcium-binding protein that plays a role in smooth muscle contraction?
    a. Connexin 43
    b. Calmodulin
    c. Cromakalim
    d. Survivin
    e. Myosin

30. In the ureter, the resting or the contractile force developed at any given length depends on the direction in which the change in length is occurring. This is referred to as:
    a. viscoelasticity.
    b. creep.
    c. hysteresis.
    d. stress relaxation.
    e. compensatory relaxation.

31. Which of the following is noted to be expressed before initiation of ureteral peristaltic activity?
    a. Prostanoids
    b. Nitric oxide
    c. c-KIT
    d. Myosin light chain
    e. Phosphodiesterase

32. Ureteral pacemaker activity is amplified by:
    a. prostanoids.
    b. norepinephrine.
    c. CGRP.
    d. cyclic GMP.
    e. potassium channel openers.

33. Which cells are the primary pacemaker cells for ureteral peristalsis?
    a. Interstitial cells of Cajal-like cells (ICC-like cells)
    b. c-KIT-positive mast cells
    c. c-KIT-negative typical smooth muscle cells
    d. Atypical smooth muscle cells
    e. Caveolae-containing smooth muscle cells

ANSWERS

1. **c. Angiotensin.** At a point during development, the ureteral lumen is obliterated and then recanalizes. It appears that angiotensin, acting through the AT2 receptor, is involved in the recanalization process. Knockout mice for the ATR2 gene have congenital anomalies of the kidney and urinary tract, which include multicystic dysplastic kidneys, megaureters, and ureteropelvic junction obstructions.

2. **d. Apoptosis.** Programmed cell death, or apoptosis, is involved in branching of the ureteric bud and subsequent nephrogenesis, and inhibitors of caspases, which are factors in the signaling pathway of apoptosis, inhibit ureteral bud branching.

3. **a. Potassium.** When a ureteral muscle cell is in a nonexcited or resting state, the electrical potential difference across the cell membrane, the transmembrane potential, is referred to as the *resting membrane potential* (RMP). The RMP is determined primarily by the distribution of potassium ions (K^+) across the cell membrane and by the permeability of the membrane to potassium ions.

4. **c. Calcium and sodium.** When the ureteral cell is excited, its membrane loses its preferential permeability to K^+ and becomes more permeable to calcium ions (Ca^{2+}) that move inward across the cell membrane, primarily through L-type Ca^{2+} channels, and give rise to the upstroke of the action potential.

5. **b. Myosin.** The most widely accepted theory suggests that phosphorylation of myosin is involved in the contractile process.

6. **e. The endoplasmic reticulum.** Calcium release from tightly bound storage sites (i.e., the endoplasmic or sarcoplasmic reticulum) increases the Ca^{2+} concentration in the sarcoplasm.

7. **a. Cyclic AMP.** Cyclic AMP is believed to mediate the relaxing effects of β-adrenergic agonists in a variety of smooth muscles.

8. **c. Phosphodiesterase.** Another cyclic nucleotide, cyclic GMP, also can cause smooth muscle relaxation. Cyclic GMP is synthesized from GTP by the enzyme guanylyl cyclase and is degraded to 5′-GMP by a phosphodiesterase.

9. **c. Phosphodiesterase.** Phosphodiesterase activity that can degrade both cyclic AMP and cyclic GMP has been demonstrated in the canine ureter, and various inhibitors can preferentially inhibit the breakdown of one or the other cyclic nucleotide.

10. **a. Guanylyl cyclase.** Nitric oxide released from the nerve activates the enzyme guanylyl cyclase in the smooth muscle cell, with the resultant conversion of guanosine triphosphate to cyclic GMP, with resultant smooth muscle relaxation.

11. **d. L-Arginine.** NOS converts L-arginine to nitric oxide and L-citrulline in a reaction that requires nicotinamide adenine dinucleotide phosphate (NADPH).

12. **c. NADPH dependent and calcium independent.** An inducible NOS isoform, iNOS, is NADPH dependent but Ca^{2+} independent and has been identified in ureteral smooth muscle.

13. **e. Phospholipase C.** Some actions of α_1-adrenergic and muscarinic cholinergic agonists and a number of other hormones, neurotransmitters, and biologic substances are associated with an increase in intracellular Ca^{2+} and are related to changes in inositol lipid metabolism. These agonists combine with a receptor on the cell membrane, and the agonist-receptor complex, in turn, activates an enzyme, phospholipase C, that leads to the hydrolysis of polyphosphatidylinositol 4,5-bisphosphate, with the formation of two second messengers: IP_3 and DG.

14. **d. Protein kinase C.** DG binds to an enzyme, protein kinase C, causes its translocation to the cell membrane, and, by reducing the concentration of Ca^{2+} required for protein kinase C activation, results in an increase in this enzyme's activity.

15. **c. Imipramine.** The greatest percentage of the norepinephrine is actively taken up (reuptake or neuronal uptake) into the neuron. Neuronal reuptake regulates the duration for which norepinephrine is in contact with the innervated tissue and thus regulates the magnitude and duration of the catecholamine-induced response. Agents such as cocaine and imipramine (Tofranil, Mallinckrodt, Inc., Hazelwood, MO), which inhibit neuronal uptake, potentiate the physiologic response to norepinephrine.

16. **a. Tyrosine.** Norepinephrine, the chemical mediator responsible for adrenergic transmission, is synthesized in the neuron from tyrosine.

17. **e. CGRP.** Tachykinins and CGRP are neurotransmitters released from peripheral endings of sensory nerves. Tachykinins stimulate contractile activity, and CGRP inhibits contractile activity.

18. **c. Type III collagen.** Increased amounts of type III collagen are seen in a variety of obstructed ureteral states.

19. **b. Cyclooxygenase.** The "primary" prostaglandins, PGE_1, PGE_2, and $PGF_{2\alpha}$, are synthesized from the fatty acid arachidonic acid by enzymatic reactions involving two cyclooxygenase (COX) isoforms, COX-1 and COX-2.

20. **b. Afferent arteriole vasodilatation.** Indomethacin has been used in the management of ureteral colic. The beneficial effects are probably due to indomethacin's inhibition of the prostaglandin-mediated vasodilatation that occurs subsequent to obstruction. The vasodilatation theoretically would result in an increase in glomerular capillary pressure and subsequent increase in pelviureteral pressure.

21. **d. Verapamil.** The calcium channel blockers verapamil, D-600 (a methoxy derivative of verapamil), diltiazem, and nifedipine

have been shown to inhibit ureteral activity. These inhibitory effects are accompanied by decreases in action potential duration, number of oscillations on the plateau of the guinea pig action potential, excitability, and rate of rise and amplitude of the action potential. High concentrations of verapamil and D-600 cause a complete cessation of electrical and mechanical activity. Similar inhibition of bladder activity can occur.

22. **e. Isoproterenol.** Isoproterenol, a β-adrenergic agonist, depresses contractility.

23. **c. Intraluminal ureteral contractile pressures must be greater than intravesical baseline pressures.** The theoretical aspects of the mechanics of urine transport within the ureter were described in detail by Griffiths and Notschaele in 1983.* At normal flow rates, while the renal pelvis fills, a rise in renal pelvic pressure occurs, and urine is extruded into the upper ureter, which is initially in a collapsed state. The contraction wave originates in the most proximal portion of the ureter and moves the urine in front of it in a distal direction. The urine that had previously entered the ureter is formed into a bolus. To propel the bolus of urine efficiently, the contraction wave must completely coapt the ureteral walls, and the pressure generated by this contraction wave provides the primary component of what is recorded by intraluminal pressure measurements. The bolus that is pushed in front of the contraction wave lies almost entirely in a passive, noncontracting part of the ureter.

24. **a. 0 to 5 cm H$_2$O.** Baseline or resting ureteral pressure is approximately 0 to 5 cm H$_2$O.

25. **b. Tension = (radius × pressure)/wall thickness.** The Laplace equation expresses the relationship between the variables that affect intraluminal pressure: pressure = (tension × wall thickness)/radius. The Laplace law: T = PR, where T is tension, P is pressure and R is radius.

26. **a. Increased hydrostatic pressures proximal to the calculus and relaxation of the ureter in the region of the stone.** Two factors that appear to be most useful in facilitating stone passage are an increase in hydrostatic pressure proximal to a calculus and relaxation of the ureter in the region of the stone.

27. **e. Progesterone.** Several studies have shown an inhibitory effect of progesterone on ureteral function. Progesterone has been noted to increase the degree of ureteral dilatation during pregnancy and to retard the rate of disappearance of hydroureter in postpartum women.

28. **d. Indomethacin.** Indomethacin, by reducing pelviureteral pressure and thus pelviureteral wall tension, might eliminate some of the pain of renal colic that is dependent on distention of the upper urinary tract.

29. **b. Calmodulin.** With excitation, there is a transient increase in the sarcoplasmic Ca^{2+} concentration from its steady-state concentration of 10^{-8} to 10^{-7} M to a concentration of 10^{-6} M or higher. At this higher concentration, Ca^{2+} forms an active complex with the calcium-binding protein calmodulin. Calmodulin without Ca^{2+} is inactive. The calcium-calmodulin complex activates a calmodulin-dependent enzyme, myosin light-chain kinase. The activated myosin light-chain kinase, in turn, catalyzes the phosphorylation of the 20,000-dalton light chain of myosin. Phosphorylation of the myosin light chain allows activation by actin of myosin Mg^{2+}-ATPase activity, leading to hydrolysis of ATP and the development of smooth muscle tension or shortening.

30. **c. Hysteresis.** Because the ureter is a viscoelastic structure, the resting or contractile force developed at any given length depends on the direction in which change in length is occurring and on the rate of length change. This is referred to as *hysteresis*; for the ureter, at any given length, the resting force is less and contractile force is greater when the ureter is allowed to shorten than when the ureter is being stretched.

31. **c. c-KIT.** This tyrosine kinase receptor is important in the development of pacemaker activity and peristalsis of the gut (Der-Silaphet et al, 1998). Pezzone and colleagues (2003) identified c-KIT-positive cells in the mouse ureter. The expression of c-KIT was noted to be upregulated in the embryonic murine ureter before its development of unidirectional peristaltic contractions (David et al, 2005). Incubation of isolated cultured embryonic murine ureters with antibodies that neutralize c-KIT activity alters ureteral morphology and inhibits unidirectional peristalsis. c-KIT-positive cells have been identified in the human ureter (Metzger et al, 2004).

32. **a. Prostanoids.** The ionic conduction underlying pacemaker activity in the upper urinary tract is due to the opening and slow closure of voltage-activated L-type Ca^{2+} channels, which are amplified by prostanoids (Santicioli et al, 1995a). This is opposed by the opening and closure of voltage and Ca^{2+}-dependent K^{+} channels. It has been suggested that prostaglandins and excitatory tachykinins, released from sensory nerves, help maintain autorhythmicity in the upper urinary tract through maintenance of Ca^{2+} mobilization. Tetrodotoxin and blockers of the autonomic nervous system, both parasympathetic and sympathetic, have little effect on peristalsis, suggesting that autonomic neurotransmitters play little role in maintaining pyeloureteral motility.

33. **d. Atypical smooth muscle cells.** Atypical smooth muscle cells give rise to pacemaker activity in the rat and guinea pig ureter. In contrast to typical smooth muscle cells, they have less than 40% of their cellular area occupied by contractile elements and demonstrate sparse immunoreactivity for smooth muscle actin (Klemm et al, 1999; Lang et al, 2001). ICC-like cells in the upper urinary tract do not appear to be primary pacemaker cells but rather may provide for preferential conduction of electrical signals from pacemaker cells to typical smooth muscle cells of the renal pelvis and ureter (Klemm et al, 1999). In the mouse ureteropelvic junction, c-KIT-positive ICC-like cells have been identified that showed high-frequency, spontaneous, transient inward currents that often occurred in bursts to sum and produce long-lasting large inward currents (Lang et al, 2007b). It is postulated that in the absence of a proximal pacemaker drive, these ICC-like cells could act as pacemaker cells and trigger contractions in adjacent smooth muscle cells in the ureteropelvic junction. Thus atypical smooth muscle cells and ICC-like cells both may play a pacemaker role in the initiation and propagation of pyeloureteric peristalsis (Lang et al, 2006, 2007a).

CHAPTER REVIEW

1. Efficient propulsion of the urinary bolus depends on the ability of the walls of the ureter to coapt.
2. Autonomic neurotransmitters play little role in maintaining pyeloureteral motility even though the ureter is supplied by sympathetic and parasympathetic neurons.
3. Ureteral muscle fibers are arranged in a longitudinal, circumferential, and spiral configuration.
4. The ureter is a syncytial type of smooth muscle without discrete neuromuscular junctions.
5. Ureteral peristalsis can occur without innervation; however, the nervous system does play at least a modulating role in ureteral peristalsis, particularly the sympathetic nervous system.
6. Alpha-adrenergic stimulation increases ureteral activity. Beta-adrenergic stimulation inhibits ureteral and renal pelvic activity.
7. Ureteral pressures can be as high as 20 to 80 cm of water during a contraction.
8. Pressure within the bladder during the storage phase is of paramount importance in determining the efficiency of urine transport across the ureterovesical junction (UVJ).
9. Ureteral obstruction causes a gradual increase in ureteral length and diameter.
10. Infection impairs urine transport by reducing ureteral contractions; it also reduces compliance at the UVJ, which may permit reflux.
11. Progesterone has an inhibitory effect on ureteral function. Progesterone has been noted to increase the degree of ureteral dilatation during pregnancy and to retard the rate of disappearance of hydroureter in postpartum women. The obstruction of pregnancy is primarily due, however, to mechanical factors and secondarily due to the hormonal effects of progesterone.
12. Pacemaker cells have resting potentials less negative than non-pacemaker cells and are located near the pelvicalyceal border.
13. Phosphodiesterase inhibitors and alpha 1A antagonists cause ureteral smooth muscle relaxation.
14. UPJ obstruction may be mechanical or due to a disordered propagation of peristaltic activity. Some have suggested that the latter is due to an alteration in the configuration of the muscle fibers at the UPJ.
15. Ureteral decompensation will occur when there are sustained intravesicular pressures that exceed 40 cm H_2O.

44 Renal Physiology and Pathophysiology

Daniel A. Shoskes and Alan W. McMahon

QUESTIONS

1. The AT1 receptor:
   a. has a more pronounced vasoconstriction on the afferent rather than the efferent arteriole.
   b. is the receptor for angiotensin I.
   c. protects against ischemia-reperfusion injury by intrarenal dilation.
   d. mediates increased release of aldosterone.
   e. is not expressed in the kidney.

2. Which of the following statements about endothelin is FALSE?
   a. Stimulation of endothelin-1 (ET-1) decreases sodium excretion.
   b. Endothelin is the most potent vasoconstrictor yet identified.
   c. ET-1 release is inhibited by nitric oxide.
   d. ET-1 release stimulates aldosterone secretion.
   e. ET-1 release reduces renal blood flow.

3. Which of the following is a vasodilator of the renal artery?
   a. Endothelin
   b. Carbon monoxide
   c. Atrial natriuretic peptide
   d. Norepinephrine
   e. Angiotensin II

4. Which of the following statements is FALSE regarding carbon monoxide (CO) and the enzyme hemoxygenase?
   a. Hemoxygenase-2 (HO-2) is a constitutive enzyme.
   b. HO-1 is an inducible enzyme.
   c. Increased CO increases ischemia-reperfusion injury in the kidney.
   d. HO-1 expression helps to maintain renal medullary blood flow.
   e. HO-1 produces CO through the catabolism of heme.

5. Which of the following statements regarding erythropoiesis is FALSE?
   a. Reduced erythropoiesis and anemia are common in chronic renal disease.
   b. Erythropoiesis is inhibited by low circulating oxygen tension.
   c. During chronic inflammation, erythropoiesis is decreased.
   d. The kidney makes most of the erythropoietin in the body.
   e. There are erythropoietin receptors in many organs of the body.

6. Which of the following statements is TRUE about sodium and the kidney?
   a. By definition, hypernatremia is always associated with elevated total body sodium content.
   b. Normal compensation for hyponatremia is decreased antidiuretic hormone (ADH) secretion and thirst suppression.
   c. Abnormal elevation of serum lipids can lead to a false, elevated measurement of serum sodium.

   d. If asymptomatic hyponatremia does not improve within 24 hours, intravenous hypertonic saline should be started.
   e. In therapy for symptomatic hyponatremia, the goal should be a normal serum sodium value of 135 mEq/L within 48 hours.

7. The syndrome of inappropriate antidiuretic hormone secretion (SIADH):
   a. is associated with decreased aquaporin expression in the kidney.
   b. is always seen in patients with hypervolemia.
   c. is associated with high total body sodium.
   d. is triggered by low circulating volume.
   e. may be treated with lithium or demeclocycline.

8. Which of the following statements regarding therapy for hyponatremia is FALSE?
   a. Fluid overload as a result of hypertonic saline infusion should be treated with a loop diuretic such as furosemide.
   b. Too-rapid correction can lead to a cerebral demyelination syndrome.
   c. Aggressive therapy should be discontinued when the serum sodium concentration is raised 10% or symptoms subside.
   d. Intranasal desmopressin is a useful adjuvant therapy.
   e. For acute severe hyponatremia with symptoms, a typical infusion rate of hypertonic saline would be 1 mL/kg/hr.

9. Diabetes insipidus:
   a. may be classified as nephrogenic or urogenic.
   b. is associated with inappropriately concentrated urine.
   c. is associated with hypervolemia.
   d. is associated with mutations of the genes producing aldosterone.
   e. results in impairment of maximum concentrating ability of the kidney due to loss of the medullary osmotic gradient.

10. Which of the following statements regarding potassium is FALSE?
    a. Angiotensin-converting enzyme (ACE) inhibitors may be a cause of hypokalemia.
    b. Potassium is primarily an intracellular ion.
    c. Acidosis drives potassium out of the cell into the circulation.
    d. High-sodium load in the distal tubule promotes potassium excretion.
    e. Upper limit for safe intravenous potassium infusion is 40 mEq/hr.

11. Which of the following statements regarding hyperkalemia is FALSE?
    a. Hemolysis of the blood sample may falsely elevate the measured potassium.
    b. Hyperkalemia can cause peaked T waves on the electrocardiogram (ECG).
    c. All patients with a serum potassium value greater than 5.5 mEq/L require immediate therapy.

d. Nebulized albuterol can reduce serum potassium by promoting an intracellular shift of potassium.

e. Intravenous calcium does not lower serum potassium but is given to protect the heart from the effects of hyperkalemia.

12. Which of the following statements is TRUE about acid handling?

a. Normal pH in the blood is 7.56 to 7.60.

b. Normal body metabolism produces less than 1000 mmol of acid per day.

c. All acids produced by metabolism can be excreted by the lungs.

d. Immediate response to an acid load is through buffers in the blood.

e. Ammonia (NH_4) is the most important buffer in the blood.

13. Which of the following statements regarding renal handling of acid is FALSE?

a. Most bicarbonate is reabsorbed in the distal collecting tubule.

b. Lungs can excrete volatile acid, but the kidneys must excrete fixed acid.

c. Carbonic anhydrase catalyzes the production of H^+ and $HCO_3^?$ from H_2O and CO_2.

d. Chronic respiratory acidosis should lead to increased H^+ in the kidney.

e. Ammonium ion (NH_4^+) is produced from glutamine, primarily by proximal tubular cells.

14. A patient who has a blood pH of 7.2 has:

a. pure metabolic acidosis.

b. pure respiratory acidosis.

c. acidemia.

d. a blood buffer system that is not working.

e. a mixed acid-base disturbance.

15. In a patient with acidosis:

a. increasing the blood HCO_3^- level increases the anion gap.

b. direct bicarbonate loss from the kidney would lead to metabolic acidosis and a normal anion gap.

c. lactic acidosis usually presents as a nonanion gap metabolic acidosis.

d. appropriate respiratory compensation for a metabolic acidosis is decreased respiration with an increased Pco_2.

e. It is not possible to have both a respiratory and metabolic acidosis at the same time.

16. Which of the following statements regarding renal tubular acidosis (RTA) is FALSE?

a. The hallmark of RTA type I is a hyperchloremic metabolic acidosis with a high urinary pH (>5.5) in the presence of persistently low serum HCO_3^-.

b. Type I RTA is also called distal RTA.

c. Type II RTA is more common in children.

d. The hallmark of type IV RTA is hypokalemia.

e. The form of RTA most commonly associated with renal calculi is type I.

17. Which of the following statements regarding metabolic alkalosis is FALSE?

a. Paradoxical aciduria may occur due to distal tubule injury.

b. Excessive nasogastric fluid loss can lead to metabolic alkalosis that is chloride responsive.

c. Appropriate respiratory compensation is decreased respiration and increased Pco_2.

d. Hyperaldosteronism can lead to chloride-resistant metabolic alkalosis.

e. Therapy for chloride-responsive metabolic alkalosis requires replacement of chloride AND fluid volume.

18. Which of the following is NOT a function of ADH?

a. Increased aquaporin-2 insertion into the luminal membrane of the collecting duct

b. Increased urea transporter insertion into the luminal membrane of the collecting duct

c. Increased systemic vascular resistance

d. Increased sodium reabsorption

e. Increased free water excretion in response to hypernatremia

19. Which of the following statements is TRUE about vitamin D metabolism?

a. Vitamin D deficiency is uncommon in chronic renal failure.

b. Dermally synthesized cholecalciferol is the most potent form of vitamin D.

c. Dermally synthesized cholecalciferol must be hydroxylated by both the liver and kidney for maximal potency.

d. Vitamin D activity is mediated through membrane-bound vitamin D receptors.

e. Vitamin D increases renal excretion of calcium.

20. Which of the following statements regarding parathyroid hormone (PTH) is FALSE?

a. PTH secretion is increased by hypocalcemia.

b. PTH secretion is increased by hyperphosphatemia.

c. PTH receptors are found mainly in bone and kidney.

d. PTH increases calcium and phosphorus reabsorption in the distal tubule.

e. PTH helps regulate 1,25(OH)-vitamin D levels by increasing 1α-hydroxylase activity.

21. Renal blood flow (RBF):

a. is equal in all parts of the kidney.

b. accounts for 5% to 10% of cardiac output.

c. courses through the glomerulus through the afferent arteriole and exits through the efferent venule.

d. is similar in men and women.

e. is one of the determinants of the glomerular filtration rate.

22. All of the following can increase total glomerular flow rate (GFR) EXCEPT increased:

a. RBF.

b. intraglomerular (hydraulic) pressure.

c. glomerular permeability.

d. efferent arteriolar resistance.

e. functioning nephron number.

23. All of the following are important in GFR regulation EXCEPT:

a. afferent arteriolar tone.

b. distal tubule chloride concentrations.

c. angiotensin II.

d. nitric oxide.

e. serum osmolality.

24. All of the following statements regarding GFR assessment are true EXCEPT:
    a. Plasma creatinine is an accurate marker of early reductions in GFR.
    b. Inulin clearance is an accurate but impractical measurement of GFR.
    c. Twenty-four-hour creatinine clearance overestimates GFR by 10% to 20%.
    d. Use of the four-variable modification of diet in renal disease (MDRD) formula improves the accuracy of the plasma creatinine.
    e. Plasma urea is an unreliable estimate of GFR.

25. Which of the following statements regarding glucose handling in the kidney is FALSE?
    a. Glucose is freely filtered across the glomerulus.
    b. Glucose reabsorption is facilitated by specific glucose transporters in the proximal convoluted tubule (PCT).
    c. Glucose reabsorption is linked to bicarbonate reabsorption in the PCT.
    d. Glucose reabsorption is 100% up to plasma glucose levels of 400 mg/dL.
    e. Glucose reabsorption is a passive process.

26. Which of the following statements about the proximal convoluted tubule is FALSE?
    a. It functions as a bulk transporter, rather than a fine-tuner of ultrafiltrate.
    b. It is able to increase or decrease reabsorption rates in response to changes in GFR.
    c. It has a minor role in sodium reabsorption.
    d. It reabsorbs 80% of filtered water, mainly through aquaporin-1 water channels.
    e. It is the major site of bicarbonate reabsorption.

27. All of the following statements are true regarding the loop of Henle EXCEPT:
    a. It is responsible for the generation of a hypertonic medullary interstitium, which is necessary for urinary concentration.
    b. It is able to increase or decrease reabsorption rates in response to changes in GFR.
    c. The descending limb is highly water permeable.
    d. The thin ascending limb actively reabsorbs sodium, chloride, and urea.
    e. The thick ascending limb is impermeable to water.

28. Which of the following statements about the thick ascending limb of the loop of Henle is FALSE?
    a. Twenty-five percent of filtered sodium is actively reabsorbed by the furosemide-sensitive NKCC2 cotransporter.
    b. Calcium and magnesium reabsorption is inhibited by furosemide.
    c. Potassium is reabsorbed and returned to the systemic circulation by renal outer medullary potassium (ROMK) channels.
    d. It is the site of uromodulin secretion.
    e. Ten percent to 20% of filtered bicarbonate is reabsorbed in the thick ascending limb of the Henle loop (TALH).

29. Regarding the distal convoluted tubule (DCT), all of the following statements are true EXCEPT:
    a. The DCT reabsorbs 10% of filtered sodium by the thiazide-sensitive NCC cotransporter.
    b. Sodium reabsorption is dependent solely on luminal sodium concentrations.

    c. Calcium reabsorption is paracellular and influenced by sodium reabsorption.
    d. Magnesium reabsorption is transcellular by luminal magnesium channels.
    e. Loop diuretics increase sodium reabsorption in the DCT.

30. All of the following statements are TRUE about the collecting tubule EXCEPT:
    a. The collecting tubule is designed for fine tuning, rather than bulk transport, of ultrafiltrate.
    b. Sodium reabsorption is regulated by aldosterone and occurs passively through luminal sodium channels.
    c. Potassium reabsorption is dependent on both aldosterone and luminal flow rates.
    d. The collecting tubule is impermeable to water at all times.
    e. Intercalated cells are largely responsible for acid-base regulation in the collecting tubule.

Pathology

1. See Figure 44-1. A renal biopsy is depicted in Figure 44-1 and is reported as "normal renal biopsy." The location of this biopsy is from the:
    a. cortex.
    b. medulla.
    c. hilum.
    d. papilla.
    e. capsule.

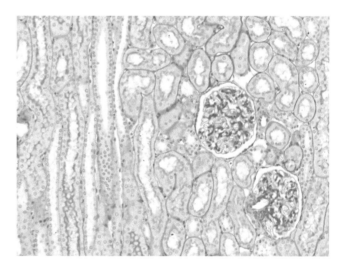

Figure 44-1. (From Bostwick DG, Cheng L. Urologic surgical pathology. 2nd ed. Edinburgh: Mosby; 2008.)

ANSWERS

1. **d. Mediates increased release of aldosterone.** AT1, the receptor for angiotensin II, mediates the release of aldosterone. Intrarenal dilatation is mediated through AT2.
2. **a. Stimulation of endothelin-1 (ET-1) decreases sodium excretion.** Despite reduction in renal blood flow, stimulation of ET-1 by endothelin increases net sodium excretion.
3. **b. Carbon monoxide.** The others are vasoconstrictors.
4. **c. Increased CO increases ischemia-reperfusion injury in the kidney.** CO is protective against renal ischemia-reperfusion injury.
5. **b. Erythropoiesis is inhibited by low circulating oxygen tension.** Erythropoiesis is increased by low circulating oxygen tension.
6. **b. Normal compensation for hyponatremia is decreased antidiuretic hormone (ADH) secretion and thirst suppression.**

7. **e. May be treated with lithium or demeclocycline.** Lithium or demeclocycline may be used to treat SIADH.
8. **d. Intranasal desmopressin is a useful adjuvant therapy.** Desmopressin is useful to treat hypernatremia caused by diabetes insipidus.
9. **e. Results in impairment of maximum concentrating ability of the kidney due to loss of the medullary osmotic gradient.** In both nephrogenic and neurogenic diabetes insipidus, maximum concentrating ability of the kidney is impaired because of loss of the medullary osmotic gradient.
10. **a. Angiotensin-converting enzyme (ACE) inhibitors may be a cause of hypokalemia.**
11. **c. All patients with a serum potassium value greater than 5.5 mEq/L require immediate therapy.** Patients with mild elevation of potassium, especially when chronic and not associated with ECG changes, do not require emergent therapy.
12. **d. Immediate response to an acid load is through buffers in the blood.**
13. **a. Most bicarbonate is reabsorbed in the distal collecting tubule.** Most bicarbonate reabsorption in the kidney occurs in the proximal tubule.
14. **c. Acidemia.** The only thing that is certain with a low pH is that there is acidemia. This may be caused by metabolic, respiratory, or mixed disorders.
15. **b. Direct bicarbonate loss from the kidney would lead to metabolic acidosis and a normal anion gap.** Direct bicarbonate loss is "measured" in the anion gap and therefore leads to metabolic acidosis with a normal anion gap.
16. **d. The hallmark of type IV RTA is hypokalemia.** RTA type IV is most commonly associated with hyperkalemia. Aldosterone deficiency or resistance leads to decreased secretion of potassium in the distal tubule.
17. **a. Paradoxical aciduria may occur due to distal tubule injury.** Metabolic alkalosis is often associated with hypovolemia and elevated aldosterone. In an attempt to conserve sodium and water, H^+ may be exchanged with sodium, leading to aciduria, despite the presence of systemic alkalosis.
18. **e. Increased free water excretion in response to hypernatremia.** ADH decreases free water excretion in response to hypernatremia in an attempt to return plasma osmolality to normal.
19. **c. Dermally synthesized cholecalciferol must be hydroxylated by both the liver and kidney for maximal potency.** Cholecalciferol is minimally active, but potency increases 100 times after it is hydroxylated at the 1- and 25-position to form calcitriol.
20. **d. PTH increases calcium and phosphorus reabsorption in the distal tubule.** PTH increases phosphorus excretion in the kidney.

21. **e. Is one of the determinants of the glomerular filtration rate.**
22. **c. Glomerular permeability.** Glomerular permeability is already maximal under normal conditions for water and small solutes, so GFR will not increase significantly with increased glomerular permeability. Rather, one sees increased filtration of larger substances such as albumin.
23. **e. Serum osmolality.** GFR is not affected significantly by serum osmolality.
24. **a. Plasma creatinine is an accurate marker of early reductions in GFR.** Plasma creatinine is a very insensitive marker of early reductions in GFR, because increases in tubular secretion of creatinine keep plasma levels from rising until there has been a significant reduction in GFR.
25. **d. Glucose reabsorption is 100% up to plasma glucose levels of 400 mg/dL.** The reabsorptive threshold for glucose is about 200 mg/dL. Plasma levels above this result in urinary glucose wasting.
26. **c. It has a minor role in sodium reabsorption.** The PCT accounts for 65% of sodium reabsorption, the most of any tubular segment.
27. **d. The thin ascending limb actively reabsorbs sodium, chloride, and urea.** Reabsorption of sodium, chloride, and urea occurs passively in the thin ascending limb.
28. **c. Potassium is reabsorbed and returned to the systemic circulation by renal outer medullary potassium (ROMK) channels.** Potassium is recycled in the thick ascending limb of the Henle loop (TALH) rather than reclaimed so that luminal potassium concentrations change very little.
29. **c. Calcium reabsorption is paracellular and influenced by sodium reabsorption.** Calcium reabsorption is transcellular through ECaC1 channels, and paracellular calcium movement is inhibited by claudin 8.
30. **d. The collecting tubule is impermeable to water at all times.** Water permeability is low in the basal state but increases markedly under the influence of ADH.

Pathology

1. **a. Cortex.** The photomicrograph reveals a normal renal biopsy from the cortex. Notice the fine-tufted glomeruli with the vessel entering. Also notice the minimal amount of interstitial tissue. The tubules with the smaller lumen and larger cells are proximal tubules; the tubules with the thinner cells and wider lumens are distal tubule cells. Glomeruli and proximal and distal tubules are located in the cortex, not in the medulla.

CHAPTER REVIEW

1. The determinants of GFR are hydraulic pressure (intra-arterial pressure), which promotes filtration; oncotic pressure, which opposes filtration; permeability of the glomerular basement membrane, which is normally maximal for water and small molecules; and pressure in Bowman space, which opposes filtration.
2. GFR is regulated through two mechanisms: autoregulation, which is an intrinsic property of arterial smooth muscle, and tubular glomerular feedback, which involves the renin-angiotensin system.
3. The ideal substance to measure GFR is freely filtered and not metabolized, secreted, or reabsorbed by the kidney. Because creatinine is secreted by the renal tubule, it is not ideal; however, because of the ease of measurement, it is practical. When bowel is placed in the urinary tract, electrolytes, water, and substances used to measure GFR are reabsorbed by the bowel, thus rendering them less than ideal agents for determining GFR in this circumstance. Also, creatinine is
a very insensitive marker of early reductions in GFR, because increases in tubular secretion of creatinine keep plasma levels from rising until there has been a significant reduction in GFR.
4. The Cockcroft-Gault, MDRD, and CKD-EPI formulae calculate GFR from serum creatinine and thus do not require a urine collection. They take into account the patient's age, sex, and race. They are generally good approximations of GFR, and in selected circumstances, one may be preferred over the other.
5. For each doubling of plasma creatinine there is an approximately 50% reduction in GFR.
6. Renal blood flow is 20% of cardiac output. Cortical blood flow is approximately 5 times as great as medullary blood flow.
7. Sixty percent to 65% of filtrate is reabsorbed in the proximal tubule.

8. The bulk of bicarbonate is reclaimed in the proximal tubule.
9. The thick ascending limb of Henle reabsorbs sodium in excess of water and is important for maintaining the medullary osmotic gradient. It is here that loop diuretics have their action.
10. The kidney secretes protons to maintain acid-base balance in the cortical collecting duct. When a proton is secreted as ammonium, its effect on urinary pH is minimal, and therefore it does not generate a significant hydrogen ion gradient, whereas when protons are secreted and coupled with sulfate and/or phosphate (titratable acid), the urine pH is lowered, thus increasing the hydrogen ion gradient and limiting the ability of the kidney to secrete additional protons by this mechanism.
11. Tamm-Horsfall protein is the matrix of renal tubule casts.
12. Atrial natriuretic peptide (ANP) is produced in the atrium and promotes natriuresis. It is useful in monitoring myocardial function.
13. Vasopressin, in addition to increasing water reabsorption, increases sodium reabsorption, promotes potassium secretion, increases adrenocorticotropic hormone (ACTH) production, and releases factor VIII and von Willebrand factor.
14. Vitamin D becomes biologically active in the kidney and (a) increases intestinal absorption of calcium, (b) regulates osteoblastic activity, (c) increases reabsorption of calcium in the kidney and, (d) suppresses PTH release.
15. Parathyroid hormone increases bone reabsorption, increases renal reabsorption of calcium and promotes phosphate secretion, and stimulates production of calcitriol, the active form of vitamin D.
16. Metabolic alkalosis is often associated with hypovolemia and elevated aldosterone. In an attempt to conserve sodium and water, H^+ may be exchanged with sodium, leading to aciduria, despite the presence of systemic alkalosis.

45 Renovascular Hypertension and Ischemic Nephropathy

Frederick A. Gulmi, Ira W. Reiser, and Samuel Spitalewitz

QUESTIONS

1. A 67-year-old male with stable renal function and a creatinine of approximately 3 mg/dL presents with peripheral vascular disease and a blood pressure of 160/70 mm Hg. He was a long-standing smoker but has recently stopped. He is referred for evaluation for treatment of "ischemic nephropathy." He has hyperlipidemia and had a myocardial infarction 3 years before presentation. His current medications are a calcium channel blocker, an adequate-dose diuretic, and a statin. Which of the following is the most appropriate next step?

   a. Refer the patient for magnetic resonance angiography (MRA) with gadolinium.

   b. Add an angiotensin-converting enzyme (ACE) inhibitor.

   c. Refer for an angiogram.

   d. Increase the diuretic.

   e. Observe for deterioration in renal function and then refer for an angiogram.

2. Which of the following is most similar to human renal vascular hypertension and is felt to be angiotensin dependent rather than volume dependent?

   a. The two-kidney, one-clip Goldblatt model

   b. The one-kidney, one-clip Goldblatt model

   c. The two-kidney, two-clip Goldblatt model

3. Since the results of the Coral trial have been published, which statement is true regarding progression to end-stage renal disease?

   a. Surgical intervention and/or percutaneous angioplasty with intervention is no longer ever indicated.

   b. Medical intervention is superior to surgical intervention

   c. Medical intervention is superior to percutaneous angioplasty with stenting.

   d. Medical intervention is equal to percutaneous angioplasty with stenting.

   e. Percutaneous angioplasty with stenting is superior to medical intervention.

4. Which of the following statements is TRUE regarding surgical revascularization of a renal artery?

   a. A kidney less than 8 cm in length can be successfully revascularized.

   b. Retrograde filling of the distal renal artery by collateral circulation on radiographic or scintigraphic imaging studies is more likely to result in a successful surgical outcome.

   c. Patients who require renal vascular surgery do not have significant vascular disease elsewhere.

   d. Correction of a renal artery lesion and an aortic aneurysm need to be done simultaneously.

   e. A renal ostial lesion always requires surgical revascularization rather than percutaneous angioplasty and stenting.

5. Ischemic nephropathy results from:

   a. a reduction in renal blood flow and perfusion.

   b. proinflammatory cytokines and/or angiotensin II.

   c. an irreversible change in perfusion pressure.

   d. a failure of autoregulation alone.

   e. failure of development of collateral circulation.

ANSWERS

1. **b. Add an angiotensin-converting enzyme (ACE) inhibitor.** According to the Coral trial, medical therapy consisted of an ACE inhibitor, a statin, and a diuretic. A calcium channel blocker was not necessarily part of the therapy unless blood pressure could not be controlled on an ACE inhibitor and a diuretic alone. With this combination, medical therapy proved to be as beneficial as more aggressive therapy with angiography and with stenting. The patient has significant renal failure, and gadolinium is relatively contraindicated because this may predispose to nephrogenic systemic fibrosis. In fact, further investigation at this point is not indicated because the patient's renal function is stable. Similarly, an angiogram is not indicated. Increasing the diuretic is not indicated because the diuretic is already on board and the presumption is that the dose is adequate. The final choice is not indicated unless there is rapid deterioration of renal function, and even then, there are no data to support that intervening with angiography and percutaneous angioplasty is helpful.

2. **a. The two-kidney, one-clip Goldblatt model.** The other choices do not allow for natriuresis/diuresis from the opposite unclipped kidney. Thus, those two models are volume-dependent causes of hypertension rather than angiotensin dependent.

3. **d. Medical intervention is equal to percutaneous angioplasty with stenting.** Surgical intervention and or percutaneous angioplasty under certain circumstances may be indicated—specifically, if blood pressure cannot be well controlled medically or there is very rapid deterioration of renal function. The results of the trial are clearly outlined in the text and require no specific explanation.

4. **b. Retrograde filling of the distal renal artery by collateral circulation on radiographic or scintigraphic imaging studies is more likely to result in a successful surgical outcome.** As stated in the text, a kidney less than 8 cm in length cannot be successfully revascularized because it has reached end-stage. Most patients with renal vascular disease have significant vascular disease elsewhere. Renal artery correction and aortic aneurysm correction need not be done simultaneously. A renal ostial lesion may be corrected by percutaneous angioplasty and stenting depending on its radiologic appearance.

5. **b. Proinflammatory cytokines and/or angiotensin II.** Renal blood flow and perfusion may sometimes be maintained at baseline in patients with ischemic nephropathy. Ischemic nephropathy can reverse, and it is is not secondary to a failure of autoregulation alone, as explained in the text. Many patients with progressive ischemic nephropathy have collateral circulation.

CHAPTER REVIEW

1. There is an extremely high morbidity and mortality rate in patients who require dialysis due to end-stage renal disease resulting from atherosclerotic renal artery occlusion.

2. There are two major pathologic causes of renal artery disease: (1) atherosclerosis and (2) fibrous dysplasia.

3. In unilateral renal artery stenosis with a normal contralateral kidney, hypertension is due to angiotensin-induced vasoconstriction.

4. In bilateral renal artery stenosis or in renal artery stenosis in a solitary kidney, hypertension is due to volume overload.

5. Computed tomographic (CT) angiography and magnetic resonance angiography do not visualize the distal renal arterial tree well.

6. Except in rare circumstances, functional testing for renal vascular hypertension has been largely replaced by anatomic imaging of the renal artery lesions.

7. Causes of renal vascular hypertension in children include fibromuscular dysplasia, vasculitis, neurofibromatosis, and neuroblastoma.

8. Widespread glomerular hyalinization indicates irreversible ischemic renal injury and suggests that there would be little benefit from relief of renal artery obstruction.

9. Extensive atherosclerotic disease precludes renal revascularization.

10. When the aorta is severely diseased, renal revascularization on the left may be accomplished with a splenorenal bypass, and on the right with a hepatorenal bypass or a supraceliac lower thoracic aorta renal bypass.

11. A transient deterioration of renal function is not infrequently seen following a contrast load in patients with significant renal artery stenosis and limited renal function.

12. Atherosclerotic renal artery disease generally involves the ostium of the proximal renal artery. Fibromuscular disease usually occurs in white females, often is bilateral, and involves the distal portion of the renal artery.

13. At least 70% to 80% renal artery occlusion is necessary to produce clinical effects.

14. The decrease in renal function occurring with renal ischemia is primarily due to proinflammatory mediators that result in fibrosis.

15. Perimedial and intimal fibroplasia, if left untreated, progress and result in loss of renal function.

16. In patients with atherosclerotic renal artery stenosis, there is no significant difference between patients treated medically and those treated with angioplasty.

17. If blood pressure cannot be well controlled medically or there is very rapid deterioration of renal function, surgical intervention and or percutaneous angioplasty may be indicated.

18. A kidney less than 8 cm in length cannot be successfully revascularized because it has reached end-stage.

46

Etiology, Pathogenesis, and Management of Renal Failure

David A. Goldfarb, Emilio D. Poggio, and Sevag Demirjian

QUESTIONS

1. A 70-kg man will have the greatest change in glomerular filtration rate (GFR) when the creatinine changes from:
   a. 0.9 to 1.2 mg/dL.
   b. 1.8 to 1.9 mg/dL.
   c. 3.2 to 3.9 mg/dL.
   d. 4.1 to 4.7 mg/dL.
   e. 7.9 to 11 mg/dL.

2. In patients with occult renal artery stenosis, angiotensin-converting enzyme (ACE) inhibitors cause acute renal failure due to:
   a. sodium retention.
   b. increased antidiuretic hormone.
   c. afferent arteriolar vasoconstriction.
   d. efferent arteriolar vasodilation.
   e. decreased sympathetic nervous system activity.

3. Six days after partial nephrectomy in a solitary kidney, the patient is oliguric. Large amounts of fluid are coming from the flank drain. The serum creatinine increases from 1.7 to 3.2 mg/dL. The next step in management is:
   a. renal angiography.
   b. computed tomography (CT) scan with intravenous contrast.
   c. renal scan.
   d. immediate surgical exploration.
   e. magnetic resonance imaging (MRI).

4. After a 7-hour-long, complex urethral reconstruction performed in the extended lithotomy position, a patient has severe thigh and buttock pain. The creatinine phosphokinase (CPK) is dramatically elevated. The next step is:
   a. dopamine infusion.
   b. plasmapheresis.
   c. dobutamine infusion.
   d. forced alkaline diuresis.
   e. dialysis.

5. The sentinel cellular change in renal ischemic injury is:
   a. loss of cell polarity.
   b. depletion of adenosine triphosphate (ATP).
   c. alteration of Na^+ metabolism.
   d. increased intracellular Ca^{2+}.
   e. increased oxidant stress.

6. The renal structure at greatest risk for ischemic injury is the:
   a. afferent arteriole.
   b. cortical collecting duct.
   c. juxtaglomerular apparatus.
   d. straight segment (S3) proximal tubule.
   e. distal convoluted tubule.

7. A patient with acute kidney injury (AKI) has a urinary sodium of 10 mEq/L, urinary osmolality of 650, and a renal failure index of <1. Urinalysis shows 10 to 20 red blood cells (RBCs) per high-power field (HPF), 3 to 5 white blood cells per HPF, 2+ proteinuria, and RBC casts. The most likely diagnosis is:
   a. acute tubular necrosis.
   b. prerenal azotemia.
   c. acute glomerulonephritis.
   d. acute interstitial nephritis.
   e. obstruction.

8. When AKI is first recognized in a patient, the initial therapeutic intervention should be to:
   a. begin low-dose dopamine.
   b. administer a cardiac inotropic agent.
   c. restore adequate circulating blood volume.
   d. administer a loop diuretic.
   e. begin a mannitol infusion.

9. Loop diuretics are of benefit in the management of AKI due to:
   a. improved patient survival.
   b. decreased metabolic demand.
   c. decreased hypoxic cell swelling.
   d. free radical scavenging.
   e. increased renal vascular resistance.

10. The major risk of MRI with gadolinium in patients with advanced chronic kidney disease (CKD) is:
    a. nephrotoxicity.
    b. anaphylaxis.
    c. nephrogenic systemic fibrosis.
    d. seizures.
    e. hepatotoxicity.

11. Dopamine therapy in acute kidney injury:
    a. causes efferent arteriolar vasodilation.
    b. is recommended for routine use after renal transplantation.
    c. is effective due to improved cardiac function.
    d. is an unproven treatment.
    e. improves patient survival.

12. A patient with AKI after partial nephrectomy has a serum potassium of 6.9 mEq/L and widening of the QRS complex on electrocardiogram (ECG). The initial step in management should be:
    a. intravenous (IV) calcium.
    b. IV insulin and glucose.
    c. sodium polystyrene sulfonate resin (Kayexalate).
    d. IV furosemide.
    e. dialysis.

13. A patient with a serum creatinine level of 2.7 mg/dL requires renal angiography. The best way to protect renal function is:
    a. saline diuresis.
    b. pre-study mannitol.
    c. furosemide before study.
    d. dopamine throughout the study.
    e. atrial natriuretic factor before study.

14. In response to a reduction in renal mass, a number of events occur within the kidney that include all of the following, except:
    a. activation of the sympathetic nervous system.
    b. hyperfiltration.
    c. glomerular hypertrophy.
    d. intrarenal vascular occlusion.
    e. interstitial fibrosis.

15. A 65-year-old man has a radical nephrectomy. The estimated GFR by the Modification of Diet in Renal Disease (MDRD) equation is 52 mL/min. Follow-up should include:
    a. low-protein diet.
    b. renal transplant evaluation.
    c. nephrology consult for stage 3 CKD.
    d. reassessment of kidney function every few months.
    e. loop diuretics.

16. A hypertensive patient with CKD should take an ACE inhibitor drug to:
    a. improve renal function.
    b. prevent progressive kidney disease.
    c. improve cardiac ejection fraction.
    d. enhance glycemic control.
    e. control blood lipids.

17. The most common cause for end-stage renal disease (ESRD) in the United States is:
    a. focal segmental glomerulosclerosis (FSGS).
    b. membranoproliferative glomerulonephritis (type 2).
    c. membranous glomerulonephritis.
    d. autosomal dominant polycystic kidney disease.
    e. diabetes mellitus.

18. The patient at lowest risk for progressive CKD is:
    a. diabetic, GFR = 86, albuminuria > 300.
    b. postnephrectomy, GFR = 62 mL/min, albuminuria = < 30 mg/g.
    c. hypertensive, GFR = 75 mL/min, albuminuria = 80 mg/g.
    d. IgA nephropathy, GFR 42 mL/min, albuminuria = 70 mg/g.
    e. autosomal dominant polycystic kidney disease (ADPKD), GFR 28 mL/min, albuminuria = < 30 mg/g.

19. A hypertensive 38-year-old man has a serum creatinine of 2.4 mg/dL. The urinalysis has 10 to 20 RBCs/HPF, 3 + protein, and RBC casts. Ultrasound shows echogenic kidneys without hydronephrosis. The best way to achieve a diagnosis is:
    a. renal angiography.
    b. renal biopsy.
    c. retrograde pyelography.
    d. magnetic resonance imaging.
    e. spiral CT scan.

20. All of the following promote fibrosis in the kidney except:
    a. angiotensin II.
    b. aldosterone.
    c. atrial natriuretic peptide.
    d. transforming growth factor–β.
    e. high-salt diet.

21. Chronic kidney disease patients treated with an ACE inhibitor may experience a decrease in residual renal function in the setting of:
    a. unilateral renal artery stenosis.
    b. concomitant treatment with an alpha-blocker.
    c. acquired renal cystic disease.
    d. left ventricular hypertrophy.
    e. ADPKD with cysts > 10 cm.

22. The best renal replacement therapy for an otherwise healthy 37-year-old woman with chronic interstitial nephritis is:
    a. preemptive transplantation.
    b. stabilize with hemodialysis 1 year, then transplant.
    c. stabilize with peritoneal dialysis 1 year, then transplant.
    d. home hemodialysis.
    e. peritoneal dialysis with an automated cycler.

23. Hospitalization in ESRD patients on hemodialysis is most commonly due to:
    a. hypertension.
    b. ileus.
    c. diabetes.
    d. hyperkalemia.
    e. access catheter infection.

24. All the following have a direct toxic effect on the kidney except:
    a. iodinated contrast agent.
    b. myoglobin.
    c. gadolinium-based contrast agents.
    d. carboplatin.
    e. aminoglycoside antibiotics.

25. The strongest predictor of hospitalization in chronic dialysis patients is:
    a. African-American race.
    b. hematocrit < 30%.
    c. glomerulonephritis.
    d. poor nutritional status.
    e. age < 30 years.

Imaging

1. See Figure 46-1. A 55-year-old woman had this abdominal radiograph 1 day after a contrast-enhanced CT scan was done for abdominal pain. Her creatinine before the CT scan was 1.9 mg/dL. The most likely diagnosis is:
   a. normal film.
   b. acute tubular necrosis.
   c. renal artery occlusion.
   d. hypertensive kidneys.
   e. nephrocalcinosis.

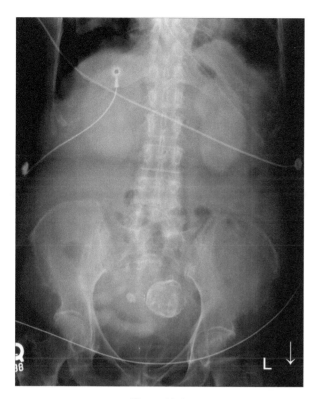

Figure 46-1.

ANSWERS

1. **a. 0.9 to 1.2 mg/dL.** The relationship between serum creatinine is not linear. Above a GFR of 60 mL/min, changes in serum creatinine are minimal. The change in serum creatinine from 0.9 to 1.2 may be associated with a large drop in GFR (120 mL/min to 60 mL/min). Below a GFR of 60, proportional increments in creatinine are associated with smaller changes in GFR. This is most notable at very high creatinine levels.

2. **d. Efferent arteriolar vasodilatation.** Angiotensin II has selectively greater vasoconstrictor effects on the efferent than on the afferent arteriole, whereas vasodilatory prostaglandins cause afferent arteriolar vasodilatation. Drugs that block angiotensin II synthesis (ACE inhibitors), block angiotensin II receptor binding (angiotensin II receptor antagonists), or inhibit vasodilatory prostaglandin synthesis (nonsteroidal anti-inflammatory drugs) may cause ARF in selected clinical settings.

3. **c. Renal scan.** There are several ways to confirm urinary extravasation. These include assessment of drain fluid for creatinine, intravenous administration of a vital dye excreted by the kidneys (such as indigo carmine or methylene blue), and radiographic demonstration of a fistula (isotope renography, retrograde pyelography, cystography, computed tomography). Renal scan can assess perfusion and also demonstrate extravasation.

4. **d. Forced alkaline diuresis.** The combination of renal hypoperfusion and the nephrotoxic insult of myoglobin or hemoglobin within the proximal tubule may result in acute tubular necrosis (ATN). Early recognition of this disorder is crucial, because a forced alkaline diuresis is indicated to minimize nephrotoxicity.

5. **b. Depletion of adenosine triphosphate (ATP).** The sentinel biochemical event in renal ischemia is the depletion of ATP, which is the major energy currency for cellular work.

6. **d. Straight segment (S3) proximal tubule.** The S3 segment of the proximal tubule is associated with the greatest ischemic damage. Other structures that sustain injury in this region include the medullary thick ascending limb, which is metabolically active and rich in the energy-requiring Na+,K+-ATPase.

7. **c. Acute glomerulonephritis.** A low fractional excretion of sodium (or renal failure index) may be associated with either prerenal azotemia or acute glomerulonephritis. These entities could be separated clinically by examination of the urinalysis results. Conditions associated with prerenal azotemia would have a bland urinalysis, whereas proteinuria, RBCs, and RBC casts would be seen with acute glomerulonephritis.

8. **c. Restore adequate circulating blood volume.** During the initial stages, a trial of parenteral hydration with isotonic fluids may correct acute renal failure (ARF) secondary to prerenal causes.

9. **b. Decreased metabolic demand.** Loop diuretics decrease active NaCl transport in the thick ascending limb of Henle and thereby limit energy requirements in the metabolically active segment, which often bears the greatest ischemic insult.

10. **c. Nephrogenic systemic fibrosis.** Recently, gadolinium-based contrast agents have been associated with the development of nephrogenic systemic fibrosis. At-risk patients include those with advanced CKD. It is important that these compounds be given to these patients only after careful consideration of the indication for the study.

11. **d. Is an unproven treatment.** Results of clinical studies have not conclusively proved that dopamine infusion improves ARF.

12. **a. Intravenous (IV) calcium.** Priorities for treatment of acute hyperkalemia with electrocardiographic changes include stabilizing the electrical membrane of the cardiac conduction system, which may be accomplished with the use of intravenous calcium salts. These have an immediate effect and a rather short duration of action.

13. **a. Saline diuresis.** A study by Solomon and coworkers confirmed that prestudy intravenous hydration with saline was crucial in limiting the nephrotoxic effect of radiocontrast agents in patients with preexisting azotemia. The addition of either a loop diuretic or mannitol did not improve outcome.

14. **d. Intrarenal vascular occlusion.** In response to reduced nephron mass, a mosaic of events occurs linking sympathetic nervous system activation, renal structural remodeling, altered gene expression and regulation, and several regulatory mechanisms for progression.

15. **c. Nephrology consult for stage 3 CKD.** According to the National Kidney Foundation (K/DOQI) guidelines, this patient indeed has stage 3 CKD. A nephrologist should be following this patient and appropriate preventive strategies instituted for preservation of kidney function and minimizing the impact of comorbidities.

16. **b. Prevent progressive kidney disease.** Angiotensin-converting enzyme (ACE) inhibitors work by hemodynamic and nonhemodynamic mechanisms to slow the progression of renal disease.

17. **e. Diabetes mellitus.** Diabetes mellitus and hypertension account for the greatest percentage of cases, followed by glomerular diseases (e.g., FSGS, membranous glomerulonephritis), and then secondary glomerulonephritis associated with systemic diseases (e.g., systemic lupus erythematosus, Wegener granulomatosis).

18. **b. Postnephrectomy, GFR = 62 mL/min, albuminuria = <30 mg/g.** The risk of progressive renal disease is based on the cause for renal function reduction, the GFR, and the albuminuria score. In a and c the GFR is higher, and there is cause for ongoing injury. One-time reduction in GFR with nephrectomy in the absence of ongoing injury (no albuminuria) should yield a more favorable prognosis.

19. **b. Renal biopsy.** For definitive diagnosis, a renal biopsy is required to aid prognosis and therapy decisions, especially in the setting of abnormal renal function.

20. **c. Atrial natriuretic peptide.** All choices promote renal fibrosis except atrial natriuretic peptide, which may have the opposite effect.

21. **e. Autosomal dominant PKD with cysts larger than 10 cm.** Individuals with bilateral renal artery stenosis and autosomal dominant PKD patients with cyst size greater than 10 cm may also experience a decrease in residual renal function while being given ACE inhibitor therapy.

22. **a. Preemptive transplantation.** A comparison of outcomes suggests that renal transplantation is the best overall treatment for ESRD patients.

23. **e. Access catheter infection.** The most recent USRDS data identify the most common reason for hospital admission in ESRD patients on hemodialysis is catheter infection.

24. **c. Gadolinium-based contrast agents.** Gadolinium is not toxic to the kidney. Its risk relates to the development of nephrogenic systemic fibrosis, which can carry a high mortality in patients with severely reduced GFR. All the others demonstrate direct toxicity to the kidney.

25. **d. Poor nutritional status.** The strongest predictors of the number of hospitalizations per year of patients at risk include low serum albumin, decreased activity level, diabetes mellitus as a primary cause of ESRD, peripheral vascular disease, white race, increasing age, and congestive heart failure. Both nutritional status (levels of serum albumin, creatinine, transferrin, and prealbumin, and lean body mass) and inflammatory response (e.g., C-reactive protein) are independent predictors of hospitalization in chronic hemodialysis patients.

Imaging

1. **b. Acute tubular necrosis.** Both kidneys are diffusely dense 24 hours after contrast administration (persistent nephrogram), with no excretion into the collecting system, making ATN the best diagnosis. The process is likely related to contrast-induced nephropathy. Renal artery occlusion is usually a unilateral process, and the nephrogram is absent in the affected kidney because of the lack of perfusion. The kidneys are small in patients with severe hypertension, and the nephrogram would have washed out at 24 hours rather than be persistent. No calcifications are seen in the kidneys, making nephrocalcinosis an unlikely diagnosis.

CHAPTER REVIEW

1. Acute renal failure is divided into prerenal, intrarenal, and postrenal.

2. Prerenal failure is the result of decreased renal blood flow or increased nitrogen load. The serum blood urea nitrogen-to-creatinine ratio is greater than 10:1. Urine volume is generally low, osmolality high, and sodium content very low.

3. Intrarenal failure is due to parenchymal disease. It may involve the glomerulus as in acute glomerulonephritis, the tubule as in ATN, or the interstitium as in acute interstitial nephritis. The serum blood urea nitrogen-to-creatinine ratio is 10:1. Urine output is variable, and urinary sodium is generally above 20 mEq/L. If the cause is ATN, urinary sodium is generally greater than 40 mEq/L.

4. Postrenal failure is due to obstruction of the entire nephron mass. Patients who are anuric should be suspected of having complete urinary tract obstruction, acute cortical necrosis, or bilateral vascular occlusion. The serum blood urea nitrogen-to-creatinine ratio is 10:1.

5. In acute tubular necrosis, renal blood flow is reduced by 50% or more with the perfusion defect most marked in the outer medulla. Tubule permeability is also increased.

6. The use of mannitol before an ischemic insult has been shown to be of benefit.

7. Hyperkalemia, as evidenced on the electrocardiogram by peaked T-waves, a prolonged PR interval, and widening of the QRS complex is initially treated with IV calcium salts to stabilize the myocardium and then transiently lower serum potassium with IV glucose and insulin or IV sodium bicarbonate, as well as to permanently lower the potassium with either Kayexalate or dialysis. Administration of Kayexalate has been associated with colonic necrosis

8. The indications for initiation of dialysis include volume overload, severe hyperkalemia, severe metabolic acidosis, pericarditis, selected poisonings, and uremic symptomatology.

9. Peritoneal dialysis is less stressful hemodynamically.

10. The mortality rate for patients with acute tubular necrosis approximates 50%. Of those who survive ATN, 5% will require chronic dialysis.

11. Patients who are to receive IV contrast and are at risk for renal failure should be given IV hydration with saline before the use of nonionic IV contrast.

12. CKD is defined as a GFR less than 60 mL/min.

13. Hyperfiltration results when a decreased number of nephrons are called on to perform the entire workload. This results in elevated glomerular hydrostatic pressure, which is a major contributor to decreased renal function.

14. A family history of ESRD is a strong predictor of future risk for renal failure.

15. The Cockcroft Gault formula, MDRD equation, and CKD-EPI equation are all used to estimate GFR from serum creatinine. These equations are inaccurate for patients who have changing renal function, are at the extremes of age or body size, are obese, have decreased muscle mass, or are sick with moderately advanced renal failure.

16. Cystatin-C, a serum protein, may be more predictive of renal function than creatinine.

17. Mortality rates secondary to sepsis are one to several hundred times higher in dialysis patients.

18. Creatinine is secreted by the renal tubule and may overestimate renal function, particularly at low GFRs. Cimetidine and trimethoprim block this secretion.

19. Drugs that block angiotensin II production or action appear to decrease the rate of decline in renal function in patients with chronic renal disease.

20. In urology, rhabdomyolysis is associated with the protracted exaggerated lithotomy and lateral decubitus positions.

21. The sentinel event in renal ischemia is depletion of ATP.

22. The presence of albumen in the urine of patients with chronic renal failure is an important predictor of the rate of decline in renal function.

23. When the GFR falls below 50% of normal, progressive loss of renal function occurs even though the cause of the renal failure is inactive or no longer present.

24. The remaining lifetime for patients on dialysis is 15% to 25% of the general population.

25. Myoglobin can be nephrotoxic to the proximal tubule and may result in acute tubular necrosis (ATN). Early recognition of muscle necrosis with resultant myoglobinuria is crucial because a forced alkaline diuresis is indicated to minimize nephrotoxicity.

26. A low fractional excretion of sodium (or renal failure index) may be associated with either prerenal azotemia or acute glomerulonephritis.

27. Gadolinium based contrast agents have been associated with the development of nephrogenic systemic fibrosis. Patients at risk are those with advanced CKD.

28. Individuals with bilateral renal artery stenosis and those with autosomal dominant PKD with cyst size greater than 10 cm may experience a decrease in residual renal function when receiving ACE inhibitor therapy.

47 Renal Transplantation

Hans Albin Gritsch and Jeremy Matthew Blumberg

QUESTIONS

1. Which of the following renal diseases has a high probability of recurrence in patients with a kidney transplant, resulting in failure of the kidney graft?
   a. Chronic glomerulonephritis
   b. Focal segmental glomerulosclerosis
   c. IgA nephropathy
   d. Alport syndrome
   e. Autosomal dominant polycystic kidney disease

2. Lymphoproliferative disorders are most commonly associated with which of the following viruses?
   a. Herpes simplex virus type 1
   b. Varicella-zoster virus
   c. Epstein-Barr virus (EBV)
   d. Cytomegalovirus (CMV)
   e. Cocksackie virus

3. Pretransplant nephrectomy is indicated for:
   a. hypertension controlled with medication.
   b. prior renal infection.
   c. symptomatic renal stones.
   d. 200 mg/dL proteinuria.
   e. most polycystic kidneys.

4. The best renal imaging protocol for a living renal donor to define renal anatomy and renal vasculature and to rule out renal stones is:
   a. kidney, ureter, bladder (KUB) radiography and selective renal arteriography.
   b. magnetic resonance nephrotomography and angiography.
   c. helical computed tomography (CT) without and with intravenous iodinated contrast.
   d. helical CT without and with intravenous iron contrast.
   e. renal ultrasonography and selective renal arteriography.

5. After living donor nephrectomy, the renal donor is expected to have what level of total renal function?
   a. 50%
   b. 60%
   c. 75%
   d. 90%
   e. 95%

6. Kidney transplant survival rates are poorest for which of the following donor categories?
   a. Sibling
   b. Parent
   c. Spouse
   d. Standard criteria deceased
   e. Expanded criteria deceased

7. Which of the following is required for the cellular sodium-potassium pump to maintain a high intracellular concentration of potassium and a low intracellular concentration of sodium?
   a. ADP
   b. ATP
   c. CMP
   d. CTP
   e. Nitric oxide

8. The best solution for preservation of all abdominal organs is:
   a. EuroCollins.
   b. Collins 2.
   c. Sach solution.
   d. University of Wisconsin (UW) solution.
   e. Histidine-tryptophan-ketoglutarate (HTK).

9. A cadaver kidney transplant recipient receives points on the national waiting list for all of the following EXCEPT:
   a. time on the waiting list.
   b. age younger than 18 years.
   c. panel reactive antibody (PRA) level greater than 80%.
   d. histocompatibility.
   e. full-time employment.

10. The standard method of urinary tract reconstruction during renal transplantation is:
    a. ureteropyelostomy.
    b. ureteroureterostomy.
    c. ureteroneocystostomy.
    d. vesicopyelostomy.
    e. cutaneous ureterostomy.

11. A woman wishes to donate a kidney to her husband who has end-stage renal disease (ESRD). She is ABO blood type A, and he is ABO blood type O. Each of the following is a possible solution to this problem EXCEPT:
    a. plasmapheresis.
    b. immunoadsorption.
    c. immunoglobulin administration.
    d. anti CD-37 antibody administration.
    e. paired kidney exchange.

12. The risk of a hyperacute rejection after kidney transplantation is high when which of the following is positive?
    a. B-cell flow cross match
    b. T-cell flow cross match
    c. B-cell complement-dependent cytotoxicity cross match
    d. T-cell complement-dependent cytotoxicity cross match
    e. DR-cell cross match

13. Which of the following immunosuppressants inhibits cell cycle progression?
    a. Azathioprine
    b. Mycophenolate mofetil
    c. Cyclosporine
    d. Tacrolimus
    e. Sirolimus

14. Which of the following paired immunosuppressants have similar mechanisms of action and toxicity?
    a. Azathioprine and cyclosporine
    b. Azathioprine and tacrolimus
    c. Basiliximab and mycophenolate mofetil
    d. Tacrolimus and cyclosporine
    e. OKT3 and mycophenolate mofetil

15. Which of the following two drugs have been used to reduce calcineurin inhibitor dosing and cost while maintaining blood levels and immunosuppressive effect?
    a. Diltiazem and ketoconazole
    b. Prednisone and azathioprine
    c. Basiliximab and daclizumab
    d. Equine antilymphocyte globulin and azathioprine
    e. Mycophenolate mofetil and azathioprine

16. Prophylaxis against *Pneumocystis* infection is best achieved with:
    a. trimethoprim-sulfamethoxazole.
    b. erythromycin.
    c. ciprofloxacin.
    d. cephalexin.
    e. minocycline.

17. Prophylaxis against cytomegalovirus infection is best done with:
    a. trimethoprim-sulfamethoxazole.
    b. erythromycin.
    c. ganciclovir.
    d. basiliximab.
    e. minocycline.

18. Five years after successful renal transplantation, a 55-year-old man is referred to you because of total gross hematuria. Each of the following is an important part of the workup EXCEPT:
    a. urine cytology.
    b. urine PCA3 determination.
    c. images of the native kidneys.
    d. images of the kidney transplant.
    e. cystourethroscopy.

19. Which of the following interferes with the tubular secretion of creatinine and can cause an increase in serum creatinine levels?
    a. Azathioprine
    b. Trimethoprim
    c. Mycophenolate mofetil
    d. Tacrolimus
    e. Basiliximab

20. Oral fluconazole is prescribed to treat cystitis caused by yeast. Which of the following medications will need to have the dose reduced?
    a. Muromonab-CD3
    b. Prednisone
    c. Tacrolimus

    d. Azathioprine
    e. Mycophenolate mofetil

21. Hemorrhagic cystitis in an immunosuppressed patient has been most commonly associated with which of the following viruses?
    a. Cytomegalovirus
    b. Adenovirus
    c. Herpes simplex virus type 1
    d. Herpes simplex virus type 2
    e. Polyoma virus

22. The most common cancer after kidney transplantation is:
    a. skin.
    b. cervix.
    c. Kaposi sarcoma.
    d. thyroid.
    e. breast.

23. Hyperlipidemia is most often associated with which of the following three-drug combinations?
    a. Prednisone, cyclosporine, sirolimus
    b. Equine antithymocyte globulin, tacrolimus, mycophenolate mofetil
    c. Mycophenolate mofetil, tacrolimus, basiliximab
    d. Cyclosporine, tacrolimus, mycophenolate mofetil
    e. Basiliximab, mycophenolate mofetil, azathioprine

24. A kidney transplant patient with chronic rejection presents with constipation. The contraindicated treatment is:
    a. oral docusate calcium
    b. oral psyllium
    c. polyethylene glycol–electrolyte solution
    d. phospho-soda enema
    e. soap suds enema

25. Patients with chronic renal insufficiency should be referred for kidney transplant evaluation when:
    a. the disease is confirmed by kidney biopsy.
    b. the estimated glomerular filtration rate is less than 20 mg/dL.
    c. the estimated glomerular filtration rate is less than 8 mg/dL.
    d. they are on dialysis.
    e. they have identified a living kidney donor.

26. The peritoneal dialysis solution containing the following compound that may lead to false point-of-care glucose readings is:
    a. dextran.
    b. icodextrin.
    c. glucose.
    d. sucrose.
    e. D-xylose.

27. A 52-year-old diabetic man with a solitary right kidney has a 7-cm mass noted on ultrasound in the lower pole. He is blood type O and has had multiple abdominal operations including previous partial nephrectomies with blood transfusions. His serum creatinine is 2.3 mg/dL and he is not aware of any potential kidney transplant donors. In preparation for partial nephrectomy he should have:
    a. referral to a vascular surgeon for creation of a dialysis fistula prior to surgery.
    b. consent for placement of a peritoneal dialysis catheter.
    c. magnetic resonance angiogram with gadolinium contrast.
    d. computed tomography with iodinated contrast.
    e. referral to a transplant surgeon.

28. A frequent symptom associated with hyperphosphatemia is:
    a. seizures.
    b. flank pain.
    c. headache.
    d. diarrhea.
    e. conjunctival itching.

29. The most common causes of death following kidney transplant in order are:
    a. kidney failure, sepsis, and cancer.
    b. cancer, sepsis, and heart disease.
    c. heart disease, sepsis, and stroke.
    d. sepsis, cancer, and heart disease.
    e. heart disease, cancer, and stroke.

30. Which of the following has been associated with a higher incidence of mortality in living donor nephrectomies?
    a. Open donor nephrectomy
    b. Ligation of the renal vein with an Endo-GIA stapling device
    c. Ligation of the renal artery with a single Hem-o-Lok® clip
    d. Insufflation with a Veress needle during laparoscopic donor nephrectomy
    e. Retroperitoneoscopic donor nephrectomy

31. A 54-year-old male with ESRD due to type 2 diabetes mellitus has been on hemodialysis for 2 years and is referred for transplant evaluation. Which of the following is an absolute contraindication to renal transplantation?
    a. Gleason 3 + 3 prostate cancer treated by radical prostatectomy 1 year ago
    b. Recent development of a gangrenous toe
    c. Gleason 3 + 4 prostate cancer treated with external beam radiation 3 years ago; prostate-specific antigen (PSA) currently 0.2 ng/mL
    d. A T1aN0Mx, Fuhrman grade 2 renal cell carcinoma treated by radical nephrectomy 1 year ago
    e. History of right below-the-knee amputation 4 years ago, currently using prosthesis and able to walk 100 yards with no difficulty

32. All of the following place a deceased donor into the Centers for Disease Control's "high-risk" category EXCEPT a:
    a. man who has had sex with another man during the previous month.
    b. donor who has smoked crack cocaine within the last year.
    c. history of intravenous heroin use 3 years ago.
    d. man who was released from prison after a 15-year sentence 5 days before the pronouncement of brain death.
    e. 23-year-old woman who was currently working as a prostitute.

33. Regarding allograft nephrectomy, which of the following statements is TRUE?
    a. Allograft nephrectomy is indicated for all failed kidney transplants.
    b. Allograft nephrectomy is a relatively simple procedure and can be performed without significant prior experience.
    c. Levels of circulating anti-human leukocyte antigen (HLA) antibodies may be reduced by allograft nephrectomy if the transplant fails within the first year.
    d. Post-transplant gross hematuria arising from the transplant is an absolute indication for allograft nephrectomy.
    e. Allograft nephrectomy is mandatory if a patient is a candidate for a second renal transplant.

34. The test that is most sensitive for finding donor-specific antibodies (DSA) is:
    a. complement dependent lymphocytotoxicity assay.
    b. B-cell flow-cytometric cross match.
    c. T-cell flow-cytometric cross match.
    d. solid-phase single-antigen bead testing.
    e. pronase-treated flow-cytometric cross match.

35. A healthy 32-year-old female with no prior history of urolithiasis wishes to donate a kidney to her 33-year-old husband, who has ESRD due to congenital reflux nephropathy. On CT scan evaluation, she is found to have a 1.5-mm calculus in the right renal pelvis. The metabolic stone workup is normal. Which of the following statements is TRUE?
    a. She cannot donate her kidney because of her renal stone.
    b. She should be accepted as a donor, and the left kidney should be removed for donation.
    c. She may be considered for donation of the right kidney.
    d. She cannot donate because of her husband's etiology of ESRD.
    e. She must undergo treatment of her stone with a 5-year stone-free interval before being considered a suitable donor.

ANSWERS

1. **b. Focal segmental glomerulosclerosis.** Patients with focal segmental glomerulosclerosis, hemolytic-uremic syndrome, or primary oxalosis should be counseled about the significant probability of disease recurrence and the risk of secondary graft failure.

2. **c. Epstein-Barr virus (EBV).** EBV titers are determined in children, and, for the EBV-seronegative child, a kidney from an EBV-seronegative donor is preferred to reduce the risk of a post-transplant lymphoproliferative disorder, the most common de novo malignancy in pediatric organ transplant recipients.

3. **c. Symptomatic renal stones.** The generally accepted recommendations for pretransplant nephrectomy, as outlined in the table, include the following: renal stones not cleared by minimally invasive techniques or lithotripsy; solid renal tumors with or without acquired renal cystic disease; polycystic kidneys that are symptomatic, extend below the iliac crest, have been infected, or have solid tumors; persistent antiglomerular basement membrane antibody levels; significant proteinuria not controlled with medical nephrectomy or angio-ablation; recurrent pyelonephritis; and grade 4 or 5 hydronephrosis.

4. **c. Helical computed tomography (CT) with and without intravenous contrast.** Three-dimensional CT angiography with and without intravenous contrast has been widely accepted for use with living renal donors because it satisfactorily excludes stone disease, demonstrates renal and vascular anatomy, and defines the urinary collecting system, all with minimal donor morbidity and at reasonable expense.

5. **c. 75%.** Hyperfiltration injury has not been a problem for living renal donors. Endogenous creatinine clearance rapidly approaches 70% to 80% of the preoperative level, and this has been shown to be sustained for more than 10 years. The development of late hypertension is nearly the same as that for the general population, and the development of proteinuria is negligible.

6. **e. Expanded criteria deceased.** Kidney transplant survival rates are poorest when the quality of the kidney is the worst. Expanded criteria deceased kidney donors are older than the age of 60 years or are older than the age of 50 years and have two of the following: death from cerebrovascular accident, hypertension, or serum creatinine greater than 1.5 mg/dL.

7. **b. ATP.** ATP is required for the cellular sodium-potassium pump to maintain a high intracellular concentration of potassium and a low intracellular concentration of sodium.

8. **d. University of Wisconsin (UW) solution.** The UW solution minimizes cellular swelling with the impermeable solutes lactobionate, raffinose, and hydroxyethyl starch. Phosphate is used for its hydrogen ion buffering qualities, adenosine is for ATP synthesis during reperfusion, glutathione is a free radical scavenger, allopurinol inhibits xanthine oxidase and the generation of free radicals, and magnesium and dexamethasone are membrane-stabilizing agents. A major advantage of this preservation solution has been its utility as a universal preservation solution for all intra-abdominal organs.

9. **e. Full-time employment.** A point system that has evolved in the United States for the selection of cadaver kidney transplant recipients includes the following variables: waiting time; human leukocyte antigen panel reactive antibody greater than 80%; age younger than 18 years; donor of kidney, liver segment, lung segment, partial pancreas, or small bowel segment; and histocompatibility.

10. **c. Ureteroneocystostomy.** Urinary tract reconstruction is usually by antireflux ureteroneocystostomy, of which there are several techniques.

11. **d. Anti-CD 37 antibody administration.** Plasmapheresis and immunoadsorption are used to remove antibodies. Immunoglobulin administration and anti CD-20 antibody (not anti CD-37 antibody) are used to prevent antibody reformation. Paired kidney exchange is an inexpensive way to deal with the problem.

12. **d. T-cell complement dependent cytotoxicity cross match.** Hyperacute rejection is rare when the T-cell microlymphocytotoxicity cross match between recipient serum and donor lymphocytes is negative.

13. **e. Sirolimus.** Sirolimus (formerly called *rapamycin*) inhibits cell cycle progression. Azathioprine and mycophenolate mofetil are purine antagonists, and they prevent lymphocyte proliferation. Tacrolimus and cyclosporine are calcineurin inhibitors. They inhibit the production of calcineurin and interleukin-2.

14. **d. Tacrolimus and cyclosporine.** These two drugs have similar mechanisms of action, effectiveness, and cost but slightly different side effect profiles, and they are not used together.

15. **a. Diltiazem and ketoconazole.** Diltiazem and ketoconazole have been used to reduce calcineurin inhibitor dosing and cost while maintaining blood levels and immunosuppressive effect.

16. **a. Trimethoprim-sulfamethoxazole.** Commonly used regimens to prevent infections and peptic ulcer disease include trimethoprim-sulfamethoxazole for 3 months for prophylaxis against *Pneumocystis* pneumonia.

17. **c. Ganciclovir.** Prophylaxis against cytomegalovirus disease is possible with ganciclovir, acyclovir, valacyclovir, or cytomegalovirus immune globulin.

18. **b. Urine PCA3 determination.** Urine PCA3 determinations have been used to screen for prostate cancer, not renal cell carcinoma or urothelial carcinomas.

19. **b. Trimethoprim.** Trimethoprim interferes with the tubular secretion of creatinine, and this can cause an increase in serum creatinine levels.

20. **c. Tacrolimus.** Cyclosporine and tacrolimus doses usually have to be reduced when fluconazole or ketoconazole is given because these drugs interfere with the metabolism of both of those immunosuppressants via the cytochrome P450 system.

21. **b. Adenovirus.** Hemorrhagic cystitis can be caused by adenovirus. The disease is usually self-limited and resolves within a few weeks.

22. **a. Skin.** Immunosuppressed patients are more likely to develop cancer than age-matched control subjects in the general population. Among several thousand tumors that occurred in renal transplant recipients, the common cancers, in order, were skin, lymphoma, Kaposi sarcoma, carcinomas of the cervix, renal tumors, and carcinomas of the vulva and perineum.

23. **a. Prednisone, cyclosporine, sirolimus.** Prednisone, cyclosporine, and sirolimus all result in hyperlipidemia.

24. **d. Phospho-soda enema.** Patients with poor renal function cannot easily eliminate a large phosphate load. If the serum calcium × phosphorus product exceeds 60 mg^2/dL^2, vascular calcium deposits can lead to arterial thrombosis and calciphylaxis.

25. **b. The estimated glomerular filtration rate is less than 20 mg/dL.** For many patients with end-stage renal disease, a kidney transplant is the optimal renal replacement. An evaluation can identify potential barriers to transplantation and facilitate the education of potential living kidney donors. The best outcomes are achieved with renal transplantation immediately prior to the need for dialysis. In the United States, a patient must have documentation of a glomerular filtration rate of less than 20 mg/dL to be placed on the national waiting list for deceased donors.

26. **b. Icodextrin.** This glucose polymer and maltose can be detected by some point-of-care devices, leading to a falsely elevated glucose reading. Inappropriate treatment of this result could lead to severe hypoglycemia and altered mental status.

27. **a. Referral to a vascular surgeon for creation of a dialysis fistula prior to surgery.** This patient is very likely to need hemodialysis because he has very marginal renal function. Early creation of a fistula is the safest vascular access for dialysis. With multiple previous abdominal operations, he is not a good candidate for peritoneal dialysis. Iodinated contrast is a relative contraindication due to the marginal renal function, and gadolinium contrast has a risk of nephrogenic fibrosis. Referral to the transplant surgeon is more appropriate once the pathology of the tumor is known.

28. **e. Conjunctival itching.** The hyperphosphatemia due to renal failure leads to severe itching, conjunctival irritation, and alterations in bone metabolism.

29. **c. Heart disease, sepsis, and stroke.** Based on the Annual Report of the United States Renal Data System in 2014, the most common causes of death in patients with renal failure are heart disease, sepsis, and stroke.

30. **c. Ligation of the renal artery with a single Hem-o-Lok® (Teleflex, Morrisville, NC) clip.** Ligation of the renal artery with Hem-o-Lok® clips, particularly when used as a single clip in an effort to increase renal artery length, has been associated with donor mortality secondary to hemorrhage.

31. **b. Recent development of a gangrenous toe.** Serious, active infection, such as a gangrenous toe or foot, is a contraindication to renal transplantation. Once the infection is completely treated, the patient may again be considered for transplantation.

32. **b. Donor who has smoked crack cocaine within the last year.** The Centers for Disease Control (CDC) does not consider inhaled or smoked drug use to be higher risk for the contraction of transmissible disease. All the other scenarios listed would place the donor in a CDC higher risk category.

33. **c. Levels of circulating anti-human leukocyte antigen (HLA) antibodies may be reduced by allograft nephrectomy if the transplant fails within the first year.** Allograft nephrectomy can be a technically challenging procedure and is reserved for few clinical situations. Removal of an allograft that has failed during the first year post-transplant can lower levels of anti-HLA antibodies that may make subsequent transplantation more difficult due to positive cross matches.

34. **d. Solid-phase single-antigen bead testing.** Very low levels of specific anti-HLA antibodies are detected by single-antigen bead testing (SAB). Because SAB is so sensitive, an antibody detected by SAB does not necessarily produce a positive flow-cytometric or complement-dependent lymphocytotoxicity cross match.

35. **c. She may be considered for donation of the right kidney.** Although urolithiasis is an important aspect of the living kidney donor evaluation, urinary stones are not an absolute contraindication to donation. Potential donors with a single, tiny stone may donate if they have a normal metabolic stone workup. In general, the kidney with the stone is used for donation.

CHAPTER REVIEW

1. The most common causes of ESRD, in order, are diabetes, hypertension, glomerulonephritis, and renal cystic disease.
2. ESRD in children may result in growth failure, poor nutrition, and psychiatric problems.
3. The major causes of death for patients with ESRD who are on dialysis or who have received a transplant are heart disease, sepsis, and stroke. Patients older than the age of 50 years have a 20% mortality in the first year of dialysis.
4. A defunctionalized bladder usually regains normal volume within weeks of transplantation.
5. Clean intermittent catheterization when necessary has been successfully used in transplant recipients.
6. Surgical treatment of the bladder outlet should not be performed in the anuric patient. If the native kidneys are producing no urine and a procedure on the bladder outlet is deemed necessary, bladder cycling should be instituted.
7. The quality of early graft function is directly correlated with cold ischemia time.
8. The routine use of a ureteral stent for all cases of renal transplantation has been shown to reduce the incidence of ureteral complications.
9. The histocompatibility antigens of greatest importance are ABO blood group and the major histocompatibility complex (MHC).
10. Class I antigens are HLA-A, HLA-B, and HLA-C. Class II antigens are HLA-DR, HLA-DQ, and HLA-DP. Class I antigens are on all nucleated cells. Class II antigens are expressed by antigen-presenting cells.
11. Lymphoma may respond to a reduction in immunosuppression.
12. Patients with focal segmental glomerulosclerosis, hemolytic-uremic syndrome, or primary oxalosis should be counseled about the significant probability of disease recurrence and the risk of secondary graft failure.
13. The recommendations for pretransplant nephrectomy include the following: renal stones not cleared by minimally invasive techniques or lithotripsy; solid renal tumors with or without acquired renal cystic disease; polycystic kidneys that are symptomatic, extend below the iliac crest, have been infected, or have solid tumors; persistent antiglomerular basement membrane antibody levels; significant proteinuria not controlled with medical nephrectomy or angio-ablation; recurrent pyelonephritis; and grade 4 or 5 hydronephrosis.
14. Hyperfiltration injury has not been a problem for living renal donors.
15. Sirolimus (formerly called *rapamycin*) inhibits cell cycle progression. Azathioprine and mycophenolate mofetil are purine antagonists, and they prevent lymphocyte proliferation. Tacrolimus and cyclosporine are calcineurin inhibitors. They inhibit the production of calcineurin and interleukin-2.
16. Cyclosporine and tacrolimus doses usually have to be reduced when fluconazole or ketoconazole is given because these drugs interfere with the metabolism of both of those immunosuppressants via the cytochrome P450 system.
17. Immunosuppressed patients are more likely to develop cancer than age-matched control subjects in the general population. Among several thousand tumors that occurred in renal transplant recipients, the common cancers, in order, were skin, lymphoma, Kaposi sarcoma, carcinomas of the cervix, renal tumors, and carcinomas of the vulva and perineum.

48 Pathophysiology of Urinary Tract Obstruction

Kirstan K. Meldrum

QUESTIONS

1. Which of the following histopathologic findings has been shown to have a negative impact on recovery of renal function at the time of pyeloplasty?
   a. Increased collagen deposition in the renal parenchyma
   b. Extensive glomerulosclerosis
   c. Mesangial cell proliferation
   d. Increased collagen deposition and extensive glomerulosclerosis
   e. Increased matrix metalloproteinase-9 (MMP-9), interleukin-18 (IL-18), and transforming growth factor-β (TGF-β)

2. Which of the following statements correctly defines the ability of magnetic resonance urography (MRU) to assess renal function?
   a. MRU with gadopentetate dimeglumine contrast accurately estimates global renal function.
   b. MRU with gadopentetate dimeglumine contrast accurately estimates differential renal function.
   c. MRU with contrast is not indicated to assess renal function in patients with renal insufficiency.
   d. MRU correlates well with renal scintigraphy.
   e. All of the above.

3. There is a low risk for development of nephrogenic systemic fibrosis after contrast MRI in patients with:
   a. obstructive uropathy.
   b. normal renal function.
   c. diabetic nephropathy.
   d. ischemic nephropathy.
   e. none of the above.

4. Internalized ureteral stent failure is more common in patients with:
   a. advanced cancer.
   b. normal renal function.
   c. solitary kidneys.
   d. horseshoe kidneys.
   e. duplicated collecting systems.

5. The fibroblasts that accumulate in the renal interstitium in response to obstruction are derived from which sources?
   a. Resident fibroblasts within the interstitium
   b. Bone marrow
   c. Transformed renal tubular epithelial cells
   d. None of the above
   e. All of the above

6. Which of these predict poor functional recovery after relief of ureteral obstruction?
   a. Absence of pyelolymphatic backflow
   b. Good compliance of the collecting system
   c. Presence of minimal obstruction
   d. Normal renal cortical thickness
   e. Absence of infection

7. Ureteral stenting is preferred versus percutaneous nephrostomy in patients with:
   a. advanced cervical cancer.
   b. uncorrected coagulopathy.
   c. ureteral stone with suspected sepsis.
   d. hydronephrosis of pregnancy.
   e. all of the above.

8. Postobstructive diuresis is:
   a. generally prolonged.
   b. usually self-limited.
   c. not associated with hypernatremia.
   d. common with unilateral obstruction in a patient with two kidneys.
   e. associated with concentrated urine initially.

9. The release of tumor necrosis factor-α (TNF-α) in obstructive uropathy is stimulated by:
   a. angiotensin II.
   b. cysteinyl aspartate-specific proteinases.
   c. cytochrome c.
   d. tissue inhibitors of metalloproteinases (TIMPs).
   e. all of the above.

10. Which of the following characterizes obstructive nephropathy when compared with hydronephrosis?
    a. Bilateral ureteral dilation
    b. Unilateral ureteral dilation
    c. Renal function impairment
    d. Calyceal blunting
    e. None of the above

11. Which of these urinary changes occur after relief of bilateral ureteral obstruction?
    a. Increased sodium excretion
    b. Water retention
    c. Decreased potassium excretion
    d. Decreased magnesium excretion
    e. None of the above

12. Which of the following is thought to play a role in postobstructive diuresis after release of bilateral ureteral obstruction?
    a. Increased renal aquaporin-2 water channels
    b. Increased renal aquaporin-3 water channels
    c. Increased antidiuretic hormone (ADH)
    d. Increased atrial natriuretic peptide (ANP)
    e. Increased aldosterone

13. After 8 hours of unilateral ureteral obstruction, which of the following occurs in the obstructed kidney?
    a. Increased renal blood flow
    b. Increased glomerular filtration
    c. Shift of blood flow from the inner to the outer cortex
    d. Decreased ureteral pressure
    e. None of the above

14. Atrial natriuretic peptide induces which of the following?
    a. Decrease in urinary sodium excretion
    b. Increase in afferent arteriolar dilation
    c. Increase in efferent arteriolar dilation
    d. Decrease in glomerular filtration rate (GFR)
    e. Increase in renin production

15. Which of the following occurs after bilateral ureteral obstruction?
    a. Shift of blood flow to the outer renal cortex
    b. Decrease in atrial natriuretic peptide
    c. Decrease in collecting system pressure during the first day
    d. Increase in renal plasma flow at 8 hours
    e. None of the above

16. Which of the following may promote tubular interstitial fibrosis in the obstructed kidney?
    a. Increase in renal metalloproteinase levels
    b. Increase in expression of transforming growth factor-β
    c. Administration of enalapril
    d. Administration of losartan
    e. Decrease in inflammatory cell infiltration

17. A difference between unilateral ureteral obstruction (UUO) and bilateral ureteral obstruction (BUO) is that:
    a. fractional excretion of sodium after relief of obstruction is greater in BUO.
    b. atrial natriuretic peptide levels are higher in UUO.
    c. risk of postobstructive diuresis is less with BUO.
    d. urinary pH is higher in UUO.
    e. new-onset hypertension is more common with UUO.

18. What is one of the earliest pathologic findings associated with urinary tract obstruction?
    a. Glomerulosclerosis
    b. Tubulointerstitial fibrosis
    c. Inflammatory cell infiltration
    d. Apoptosis
    e. Parenchymal thinning

19. Which of the following statements is TRUE of compensatory renal growth?
    a. Glomerular number increases.
    b. Insulin-like growth factor-1 is inhibitory.
    c. It increases with age.
    d. It is primarily related to cellular hypertrophy rather than hyperplasia.
    e. It is more common with partial obstruction.

20. The chance for renal recovery after ureteral obstruction is most influenced by:
    a. early relief of obstruction.
    b. presence of extrarenal pelvis.
    c. presence of a solitary kidney.
    d. uninfected urine.
    e. normal blood pressure.

21. Which of the following is expected in a kidney that has been obstructed for 1 month?
    a. Increased renal pelvic pressure
    b. Downregulation in sodium transporters
    c. Reduced urinary pH
    d. Reduced tubulointerstitial fibrosis
    e. Increased aquaporin-2 water channels

22. Hydronephrosis is most suggestive of significant obstruction in the presence of:
    a. an elevated resistive index.
    b. an increase in ureteral jet frequency.
    c. a $T_{1/2}$ of 15 minutes after Lasix administration on a MAG3 renogram.
    d. a pelvic calcification on non-contrast computed tomography (CT).
    e. a dramatic delay in radiotracer uptake on a MAG3 Lasix renogram

23. A reduction in concentrating ability of the obstructed kidney is due to:
    a. decreased ADH expression.
    b. maintenance of a medullary hypertonicity and reduced GFR.
    c. increased renal aquaproin-1 water channels.
    d. decreased renal aquaporin-2 water channels.
    e. urea backflux from the inner medullary collecting duct.

24. A persistent concentrating defect after relief of BUO is primarily due to:
    a. continued excessive secretion of atrial natriuretic peptide.
    b. decreased synthesis of aquaporins.
    c. decreased synthesis of cyclic adenosine monophosphate (AMP).
    d. persistent hypokalemia.
    e. decreased release of ADH from the posterior pituitary.

25. In studies of complete UUO for 24 hours, renal blood flow has been shown to:
    a. briefly cease with ureteral clamping and then gradually return toward control.
    b. gradually decline over the course of the constriction.
    c. increase by 25% and remain elevated during the obstruction.
    d. increase over an hour and then steadily decrease.
    e. remain unchanged during clamping and undergo reactive hyperemia on release.

26. Ureteral and tubular pressure changes in experimental unilateral ureteral occlusion over 24 hours are characterized by:
    a. a continued increase due to urine secretion.
    b. an immediate decrease as flow ceases.
    c. an increase followed by a decrease.
    d. no change due to extravasation of tubule fluid.
    e. no change due to contralateral renal compensation.

27. Which of the following have been implicated in the initial rise in renal blood flow in UUO?
    a. Adenosine and bradykinin
    b. Atrial natriuretic peptide and platelet-activating factor
    c. Dopamine and acetylcholine
    d. Prostaglandin and nitric oxide
    e. Endothelin and angiotensin II

28. Which of the following best explains the greater fractional excretion of sodium that follows the release of BUO compared with UUO?
    a. Better-preserved glomerular filtration rate with UUO than with BUO
    b. Greater expansion of extracellular volume with BUO than with UUO
    c. More contralateral compensation with BUO than with UUO
    d. Less atrial natriuretic protein production with BUO than with UUO
    e. More secretion of aldosterone with BUO than with UUO

29. Obstruction causes which of the following disturbances in the renal regulation of acid-base balance?
    a. Decreased bicarbonate reclamation in the proximal tubule
    b. Decreased H^+-adenosine triphosphate (ATP)ase expression in the collecting duct
    c. Greater buffering of acid loads by glutamine breakdown to NH_3
    d. Decreased proportion of H^+ buffered as titratable acid rather than as NH_4^+
    e. Urine pH above 7.4

30. A 5-year-old child presents to the emergency room with symptoms of acute renal colic. Which is the most appropriate initial imaging study to obtain for his evaluation?
    a. Excretory urogram
    b. Magnetic resonance urography
    c. Low-dose noncontrast CT
    d. Ultrasound
    e. Whitaker test

31. Which of the following contribute(s) to obstruction-induced tubulointerstitial fibrosis?
    a. Angiotensin II
    b. IL-18
    c. Transforming growth factor-β
    d. TNF-α
    e. All of the above

32. Obstruction induces apoptosis, or programmed cell death, of nephrons. Which key family of enzymes is involved in apoptosis?
    a. Aminopeptidases
    b. Caspases
    c. Metalloproteinases
    d. Phosphatases
    e. Reverse transcriptases

33. Which of the following studies best predicts whether renal functional recovery will occur after reconstruction of an obstructed kidney?
    a. Diuretic-mercaptoacetyltriglycine (MAG)-3 scan
    b. Diuretic-diethyltriaminepentaacetic acid (DTPA) scan
    c. Duplex ultrasonography of the kidneys
    d. Dimercaptosuccinic acid (DMSA) renogram
    e. Unenhanced magnetic resonance urogram

34. Which of the following mediators has been implicated in obstruction-induced apoptosis?
    a. TNF-α
    b. TGF-β
    c. Angiotensin II
    d. IL-18
    e. a, b, and d

35. Why are nonsteroidal anti-inflammatory drugs (NSAIDs) beneficial in managing the pain associated with renal colic?
    a. They reduce collecting system pressure.
    b. They increase renal blood flow.
    c. They can be associated with gastrointestinal bleeding.
    d. They are safe to use in patients with renal insufficiency.
    e. They provide good pain control but are inferior to opioids in managing renal colic.

36. A 10-year-old patient presents to the emergency room with abdominal pain and is found to have significant right hydronephrosis and no ureteral dilation on ultrasound. The next step in management is:
    a. Cystoscopy with a retrograde pyelogram
    b. Robotic pyeloplasty
    c. MAG3 Lasix renogram
    d. Magnetic resonance urogram
    e. Observation

37. A 55-year-old, otherwise healthy woman has a chronically obstructed left kidney and normal right kidney. Which differential renal function for the left kidney would best serve as a cutoff point below which nephrectomy should be performed and above which salvage should be considered?
    a. 5%
    b. 10%
    c. 25%
    d. 35%
    e. 45%

38. Angiotensin-converting enzyme (ACE) inhibitors or angiotensin receptor blockers attenuate the decrease in GFR caused by ureteral obstruction by reducing constriction at which level?
    a. Afferent arteriole
    b. Efferent arteriole
    c. Glomerular capillary
    d. Juxtaglomerular mesangial cell
    e. Renal artery

39. Epithelial-mesenchymal transition is a process that:
    a. involves conversion of renal tubular epithelial cells into mesangial cells.
    b. is simulated by bone morphogenetic protein-7 (BMP-7).
    c. involves conversion of renal tubular epithelial cells into matrix-producing fibroblasts.
    d. is inhibited by TGF-β1.
    e. is of little significance in obstruction-induced renal fibrosis.

40. Postobstructive diuresis and natriuresis are seen more often following relief of BUO rather than UUO because:
    a. renal sodium transporters are decreased only during BUO.
    b. third-space sequestration of fluid is greater with UUO.
    c. atrial natriuretic peptide secretion decreases during UUO.
    d. contralateral increases in transporters attenuate natriuresis of UUO.
    e. greater increases in vasopressin (ADH) with BUO inhibit sodium transport.

ANSWERS

1. **d. Increased collagen deposition and extensive glomerulosclerosis.** Histopathologic findings may predict recovery of renal function. The presence of increased collagen deposition in the renal parenchyma at the time of pyeloplasty and the presence of extensive glomerulosclerosis have both been shown to have a negative impact on recovery of renal function (Kim et al, 2005; Kiratli et al, 2008; Elder et al, 1995).*
2. **e. All of the above.** All listed techniques can be used to assess renal function. MRU has been demonstrated to have an excellent correlation with the renal isotope GFR in the adult (Abo El-Ghar-2 et al, 2008) and pediatric patients (Jones et al, 2008) with obstructed kidneys. The incorporation of intravenous administration of gadopentetate-DTPA has allowed a dynamic, functional assessment of the collecting system that correlates well with diuretic renal scintigraphy, yet provides far greater anatomic detail than nuclear studies. Differential GFR can be assessed with postimaging processing, and contrast washout can be measured to calculate renal clearance, differentiating dilated systems from obstructed systems (Rohrschneider et al, 2002; Chu et al, 2004).
3. **b. Normal renal function.** The use of gadodiamide-based magnetic resonance imaging (MRI) in patients with renal insufficiency [GFR < 30 mL/min] has been seen to increase the risk of nephrogenic systemic fibrosis (NSF). The risk of NSF is associated with the use of some gadolinium agents (especially gadodiamide) in patients with renal insufficiency [GFR < 30 mL/min], limiting the utility of contrast MRI in such patients (Broome et al, 2007; Frokaier et al, 2007; Sadowski et al, 2007; Abo El-Ghar-2 et al, 2008).
4. **a. Advanced cancer.** Ureteral stenting may not be as effective for treating patients with extrinsic ureteral obstruction. Docimo and Dewolf (1989) reported a mean 43% failure rate in ureteral stents placed for extrinsic ureteral obstruction, the majority related to malignancy. The recent development of metallic stents, however, composed of a unique continuous unfenestrated coil, has improved stent indwelling times in patients with extrinsic ureteral compression.
5. **e. All of the above.** The pathophysiology of obstruction-induced renal fibrosis involves an expansion in the number of matrix-producing fibroblasts. Although resident renal fibroblasts and bone marrow–derived fibroblasts contribute to this population, evidence suggests that the phenotypic transformation of renal tubular epithelial cells into matrix-producing fibroblasts (epithelial mesenchymal transition) is an important source of fibroblasts during renal injury (Healy et al, 1998; Strutz et al, 1995).
6. **a. Absence of pyelolymphatic backflow.** Factors that have a positive influence on functional recovery include a smaller degree of obstruction, greater compliance of the collecting system, and presence of pyelolymphatic backflow (Shokeir et al, 2002). Conversely, older age and decreased renal cortical thickness are predictors of diminished recovery of renal function (Lutaif et al, 2003).

7. **b. Uncorrected coagulopathy.** If the patient with obstructive uropathy has an uncorrectable coagulopathy or platelet abnormality, ureteral stenting is indicated. Compared with percutaneous nephrostomy placement, stent insertion may require greater x-ray exposure (Mokhmalji et al, 2001). This may be of concern in pregnant patients, particularly early in gestation when the fetus is most sensitive to radiation effects (McAleer and Loughlin, 2004). Percutaneous nephrostomy should be strongly considered if pyonephrosis is suspected.
8. **b. Usually self-limited.** Postobstructive diuresis is generally self-limited and is generally associated with initial hyposthenuric urine. Release of obstruction can result in marked diuresis and natriuresis.
9. **a. Angiotensin II.** The release of TNF-α, a potent inflammatory cytokine, is stimulated by angiotensin, especially in the first few hours of renal obstruction. It can upregulate its own expression as well as that of other inflammatory mediators, such as interleukin-1, platelet-activating factor, nitric oxide, eicosanoids, and cell adhesion molecules.
10. **c. Renal function impairment.** The term *obstructive nephropathy* should be reserved for the damage to the renal parenchyma that results from an obstruction to the flow of urine anywhere along the urinary tract. The term *hydronephrosis* implies dilatation of the renal pelvis and calyces and can occur without obstruction.
11. **a. Increased sodium excretion.** There is a profound diuresis and an increase in sodium excretion after relief of bilateral ureteral obstruction. This is due to ANP and, perhaps, reduced sodium transporters. The massive natriuresis enhances excretion of phosphate, potassium, and magnesium.
12. **d. Increased atrial natriuretic peptide (ANP).** The accumulation of extracellular volume stimulates the synthesis and release of ANP, which promotes increased GFR and sodium excretion. Decreases in the aquaporin water channels in the kidney further promote the diuresis.
13. **d. Decreased ureteral pressure.** In the late phase after UUO, there is a decline in both renal blood flow and ureteral pressure resulting in a gradual loss in renal function. In addition, there is a shift of blood flow from the outer to inner cortex with UUO that is opposite to that which is seen with BUO.
14. **b. Increase in afferent arteriolar dilation.** By promoting dilation of the afferent arteriole and constriction of the efferent arteriole, ANP increases GFR. It also decreases the sensitivity of tubuloglomerular feedback, inhibits renin release, and increases the ultrafiltration coefficient.
15. **a. Shift of blood flow to the outer renal cortex.** There is a shift of blood flow to the outer renal cortex with BUO in contrast to the reversed pattern with UUO.
16. **b. Increase in expression of transforming growth factor-β.** There is increased expression of TGF-β with obstruction that contributes to an increase in the extracellular matrix of the kidney and promotes inflammation. TGF-β is activated by angiotensin II, and animal models have demonstrated that pharmacologic methods of inhibiting angiotensin II reduce the fibrosis occurring after obstruction.
17. **a. Fractional excretion of sodium after relief of obstruction is greater in BUO.** The increased fractional excretion of sodium in BUO is due to volume expansion, resulting in increased levels of ANP and the overall increased solute load.
18. **c. Inflammatory cell infiltration.** Inflammatory cell infiltration occurs early in the course of obstruction (Diamond et al, 1994, 1998) and results in the release of a variety of cytokines and growth factors that stimulate fibroblast proliferation and activation, and an imbalance in extracellular matrix (ECM) synthesis, deposition, and degradation.
19. **d. It is primarily related to cellular hypertrophy rather than hyperplasia.** Compensatory renal growth of the unaffected kidney has been demonstrated, and studies indicate that when the kidney enlarges an increase in the number of nephrons or glomeruli does not occur, indicating that the increase in volume is primarily a consequence of cellular hypertrophy

---

*Sources referenced can be found in *Campbell-Walsh Urology, 11th Edition,* on the Expert Consult website.

(Peters et al, 1993). These growth patterns may depend on the age of the subject. Insulin-like growth factor-1 is thought to stimulate this event. It is more prominent in the immature kidney and appears to be directly proportional to the duration of obstruction and more prominent with complete obstruction.

20. **a. Early relief of obstruction.** Although the other factors influence recovery of renal function after release of obstruction, prompt eradication of obstruction provides the best approach for salvage.

21. **b. Downregulation in sodium transporters.** Obstruction results in a reduction in sodium transporters, including Na+,K+-ATPase. It also promotes tubulointerstitial fibrosis, a reduction in aquaporin channels, and acidification defects. The collecting system pressure should not be increased at this point.

22. **E. A dramatic delay in radiotracer uptake on MAG3 Lasix renogram.** Although an elevated resistive index and a pelvic calcification on noncontrast CT may suggest obstruction, the presence of a significant delay in radiotracer uptake on a MAG3 Lasix renogram is most suggestive of high-grade obstruction. A $T_{1/2}$ of 15 minutes suggests an equivocal delay in drainage from the collecting system, and obstruction is associated with a decrease, not an increase, in ureteral jet frequency.

23. **d. Decreased renal aquaporin-2 water channels.** The concentrating defect that occurs with obstruction is not due to inadequate levels of ADH. Choices b, c, and e result in enhanced concentrating ability, whereas a reduction in aquaporin-2 water channels does the opposite.

24. **b. Decreased synthesis of aquaporins.** Li and coworkers (2001) showed that the polyuria after release of BUO correlated with a decreased expression of aquaporins 1, 2, and 3. Over a 30-day period, the expressions of AQP-2 and -3 gradually normalized, but the expression of AQP-1 remained decreased. The reduced rate of synthesis and mobilization of water channels into the nephron membranes accounts for a decreased response to exogenous vasopressin or cyclic AMP.

25. **d. Increase over an hour and then steadily decrease.** Renal blood flow initially rises in the first phase, because of afferent arteriolar vasodilatation. In phase 2, efferent arteriolar constriction keeps ureteral pressure elevated, but in phase 3, both preglomerular and postglomerular vasoconstriction reduce renal blood flow and ureteral pressure.

26. **c. An increase followed by a decrease.** The first phase is characterized by a rise in both ureteral pressure and renal blood flow lasting 1 to 1.5 hours. This is followed by a decline in renal blood flow (RBF) and a continued increase in ureteral (tubular) pressure lasting until the fifth hour of occlusion. The final phase involves a further decline in RBF and a progressive decline in ureteral pressure.

27. **d. Prostaglandin and nitric oxide.** Studies during the early, vasodilatory phase of UUO have shown that the increase in RBF can be prevented by prostaglandin synthesis inhibitors, such as indomethacin or other NSAIDs. Intravenous administration of indomethacin before ureteral ligation results in a decline in renal blood flow without the initial vasodilatation. In addition, administration of nitric oxide (NO) synthesis inhibitors, such as N-nitro-L-arginine methyl ester (L-NAME) or N-monomethyl-L-arginine (L-NMMA), attenuates the initial rise in RBF with occlusion in rats, and when L-NMMA was discontinued, the rise in RBF was restored in 10 minutes. These findings provide evidence for a role of prostaglandins and nitric oxide in reducing preglomerular afferent arteriolar vascular resistance in the early phase of UUO.

28. **b. Greater expansion of extracellular volume with BUO than with UUO.** With bilateral obstruction, the contralateral renal unit does not have the opportunity for compensation as with UUO. Extracellular volume may be greatly expanded so that postobstructive diuresis is most commonly seen in this type of obstruction. After relief of BUO, the increased extracellular volume with attendant salt and water buildup, urea and other osmolytes, and increased production of atrial natriuretic peptide and potentially other natriuretic substances all contribute to a profound natriuresis and a fractional excretion for sodium that is greater than after relief of UUO.

29. **b. Decreased H+-adenosine triphosphate (ATP)ase expression in the collecting duct.** The cumulative evidence shows a major acidification defect in the distal nephron. Release of obstruction does not result in bicarbonaturia, indicating that proximal reclamation remains intact. There is a defect in the proximal handling and breakdown of glutamine, which means that a higher proportion of protons are buffered as titratable acid. The best evidence indicates a defect in the expression of H+-ATPase in the collecting duct. Even so, because there is a deficit in filtered and excreted phosphate, fewer protons can be buffered by phosphate so that the pH of the urine may be lower in spite of a total net decrease in H+ secretion.

30. **d. Ultrasound.** Because of emerging concerns about radiation exposure with CT and a documented increased risk of brain cancer and leukemia in children receiving cumulative radiation doses from CT of 50 mGy or 30 mGy, respectively (Miglioretti et al, 2013; Pearce et al, 2012), ultrasound remains the primary imaging modality of choice in children suspected to have renal obstruction. Low-dose CT is indicated if the ultrasound is inconclusive. MRU holds great promise as an imaging modality that avoids ionizing radiation, but because of cost and restricted availability, it is not a first-line imaging tool.

31. **e. All of the above.** Tubule cells, macrophages, and fibroblasts all contribute to the fibrotic process. The mediators of angiotensin II, growth factors, and cytokines contribute to the process and offer opportunities for pharmacologic intervention.

32. **b. Caspases.** Cysteinyl aspartate-specific proteinases (caspases) are known to mediate apoptotic cell death in obstructed kidneys. This is a family of 12 enzymes that cleave nuclear and cytoplasmic substrates, resulting in nuclear fragmentation and condensation. Caspases can be activated by either an intrinsic pathway involving disturbances in the mitochondrial membrane and release of cytochrome c or by a death receptor signaling pathway (i.e., Fas or TNF-α binding to their receptor on the cell membrane).

33. **d. Dimercaptosuccinic acid (DMSA) renogram.** The DMSA renogram has been shown to be superior to DTPA or MAG-3 for the prediction of renal recovery (Thompson and Gough, 2001). Although some have successfully used these other radiotracers to predict functional recovery, the cortical phase of the renogram is the critical factor. Doppler ultrasonography and MRU have not been demonstrated to predict renal recovery.

34. **e. a, b, and d.** TNF-α, TGF-β, and IL-18 have all been implicated in obstruction-induced apoptosis. The role of angiotensin II in this process is less convincing, with recent studies suggesting no benefit of either ACE inhibitors or angiotensin II type 2 receptor antagonists in preventing obstruction-induced apoptosis.

35. **a. They reduce collecting system pressure.** In clinical trails, NSAIDs have proven superior to opioids in managing renal colic, and are associated with less emesis and less potential for abuse. NSAIDs reduce the pain associated with renal colic by reducing collecting system pressure and distention. This effect appears to be primarily mediated by a reduction in renal blood flow, but NSAIDs may also reduce hydrostatic pressures in the collecting system by preventing the downregulation in aquaporin and major sodium channels in the renal tubule. Because NSAIDs reduce renal blood flow, they are contraindicated in patients with renal insufficiency, and opioids are therefore the preferred method of pain control in this patient population.

36. **c. MAG3 Lasix renogram.** Although hydronephrosis is suggestive of renal obstruction in the presence of pain, hydronephrosis alone does not indicate urinary tract obstruction, and significant hydronephrosis can be present in the absence of obstruction. The most appropriate next step in management would therefore be a Lasix renogram to evaluate the function and drainage of the kidney. Although an MRU would provide this information as well, it is considered a second-line test because of its cost and lesser availability.

37. **b. 10%.** The usual cutoff point for nephrectomy is 10% or less of total renal function being supplied by the affected kidney. This has not been prospectively studied but is based on common clinical practice, and, as such, this must be tempered by clinical insight into the overall status of the patient.
38. **a. Afferent arteriole.** Reduced preglomerular resistance increases glomerular capillary pressure and filtration rate.
39. **c. Involves conversion of renal tubular epithelial cells into matrix-producing fibroblasts.** Growing evidence suggests that under pathologic conditions, renal tubular epithelial cells can also undergo a phenotypic transformation into matrix producing myofibroblasts by a process called epithelial-mesenchymal transition (Healy et al, 1998; Strutz et al, 1995). These activated fibroblasts acquire mesenchymal markers, migrate into the interstitial space across damaged tubular basement membranes, and become capable of producing extracellular matrix. EMT appears to be a major contributing factor to tubulointerstitial fibrosis in the obstructed kidney, and a number of growth factors, cytokines, and ECM compounds regulate EMT, of which TGF-β1 is the chief and most studied mediator. BMP-7 is a member of the TGF-β family that has been shown to reverse the process of EMT and promote resolution of fibrosis and the restoration of the normal architecture of the obstructed kidney (Patel et al, 2005; Manson et al, 2011).

40. **d. Contralateral increases in transporters attenuates natriuresis of UUO.** Diuresis and natriuresis occurs primarily after release of BUO because volume expansion, release of ANP, and decreases in the tubular sodium transporters all occur. With UUO, transporter synthesis increases in the unobstructed kidney to help compensate and reduce excretory losses in the obstructed kidney.

CHAPTER REVIEW

1. With unilateral ureteral obstruction, renal blood flow increases during the first 1 to 2 hours. It begins to decrease at 3 to 4 hours and markedly declines after 5 hours of obstruction.
2. The increase in renal blood flow in unilateral ureteral obstruction is a result of relaxation of afferent arterials in which prostaglandin E_2 and nitrous oxide play a role.
3. Reduction in whole-kidney GFR after prolonged obstruction is due to afferent arteriolar vasoconstriction mediated by the renin-angiotensin system. Thus angiotensin II is an important mediator of reduced renal blood flow in the second and third phases of ureteral obstruction. Moreover, thromboxane A_2 may also contribute.
4. In bilateral ureteral obstruction, there is a modest increase in renal blood flow lasting approximately 2 hours, followed by a profound decline in renal blood flow.
5. In unilateral ureteral obstruction, there is a shift of blood flow from the outer cortex to the inner cortex. In bilateral ureteral obstruction, the shift is in the opposite direction toward the outer cortex.
6. With the release of bilateral obstruction, a postobstructive diuresis may occur that is much greater than in unilateral ureteral obstruction due to accumulated solutes and volume expansion.
7. Partial neonatal obstruction may impair nephrogenesis.
8. Following complete ureteral obstruction, urine is reabsorbed by (1) extravasation at the calyceal fornix, (2) pyelovenous backflow, (3) pyelolymphatic backflow, and (4) tubular reabsorption.
9. Following obstruction, there is a dysregulation of the aquaporin water channels in the proximal tubule, descending loop, and collecting duct, which may contribute to long-term polyuria.
10. The excretion of sodium following the relief of bilateral ureteral obstruction is greater than after unilateral ureteral obstruction, because in bilateral obstruction there is retention of sodium, water, urea, and other osmotic substances and an increase of atrial natriuretic factor, all of which stimulate a profound natriuresis.
11. Obstruction causes a defect in urinary acidification(proton secretion) in the distal tubule and collecting duct.
12. Compensatory renal growth decreases progressively with increasing age. Although the kidney does enlarge, there is not an increase in nephrons or number of glomeruli after birth.
13. Functional recovery has been reported as long as 150 days following relief of unilateral ureteral obstruction.
14. Older age and decreased cortical thickness are predictors of diminished recovery following relief of obstruction.

15. Recovery of renal function following relief of obstruction is affected by the duration, the degree, the patient's age, baseline renal function, collecting system compliance, and infection.
16. Chronic ureteral obstruction leads to renal inflammation, increased extracellular matrix formation, tubulointerstitial fibrosis, and apoptosis of renal tubules, thus limiting the potential for return of renal function.
17. Ureteral obstruction may result in prolonged decreases in concentrating ability, urinary acidification, and electrolyte transport long after the obstruction is released.
18. A Whitaker test requires a fixed rate of infusion of 10 mL/min into the renal pelvis. A catheter is placed in the bladder. After equilibration, a renal pelvic pressure less than 15 cm of water is considered normal. A pressure greater than 22 cm of water is considered obstructed, and a pressure of 15 to 22 cm of water is equivocal.
19. For diuretic renograms, a half-time of less than 10 min is normal; a half-time greater than 20 min is obstructed, and between 10 and 20 min is equivocal.
20. Postobstructive diuresis is a result of (1) a physiologic diuresis that involves volume expansion and solute accumulation and (2) a pathologic diuresis that involves derangements of the medullary gradient and transport processes for solutes in the renal tubule.
21. Distended bladders should be expeditiously decompressed. There is no role for gradual decompression, because this does not limit hematuria or postobstructive diuresis.
22. Hypertension may occur with obstruction and is probably due to upregulation of the renin-angiotensin system.
23. The pathophysiology of obstruction-induced renal fibrosis involves an expansion in the number of matrix-producing fibroblasts.
24. By promoting dilation of the afferent arteriole and constriction of the efferent arteriole, atrial natriuretic peptide increases GFR. It also decreases the sensitivity of tubuloglomerular feedback, inhibits renin release, and increases the ultrafiltration coefficient.
25. Inflammatory cell infiltration occurs early in the course of obstruction
26. NSAIDs reduce the pain associated with renal colic by reducing collecting system pressure and distention. This effect appears to be primarily mediated by a reduction in renal blood flow, but NSAIDs may also reduce hydrostatic pressures in the collecting system by preventing the downregulation in aquaporin and major sodium channels in the renal tubule. Because NSAIDs reduce renal blood flow, they are contraindicated in patients with renal insufficiency.

49 Management of Upper Urinary Tract Obstruction

Stephen Y. Nakada and Sara L. Best

QUESTIONS

1. Ureteropelvic junction (UPJ) obstruction in the neonate is most frequently found as a result of:
   a. maternal-fetal ultrasonography.
   b. voiding cystourethrography.
   c. diuretic renography.
   d. abdominal radiography.
   e. physical examination.

2. Which study is diagnostic for functional obstruction at the UPJ?
   a. Retrograde pyelography
   b. Three-dimensional helical computed tomography (CT)
   c. Diuretic renography
   d. Renal ultrasound
   e. Renal angiography

3. A 62-year-old man presents with left flank pain. Intravenous pyelography reveals delayed excretion and hydronephrosis to the level of a 2.5-cm calculus at the UPJ. Percutaneous stone extraction is accomplished without difficulty, but a postextraction nephrostogram reveals hydronephrosis to the level of the UPJ without residual stone. A follow-up nephrostogram 1 week later is unchanged. The best next step is:
   a. removal of the nephrostomy tube.
   b. diuretic renography.
   c. CT angiography.
   d. antegrade endopyelotomy.
   e. Whitaker pressure-perfusion test.

4. The condition most predictive of failure after percutaneous endopyelotomy is:
   a. renal ptosis.
   b. ipsilateral stones.
   c. ipsilateral renal function.
   d. moderate to severe hydronephrosis.
   e. chronic flank pain.

5. A 27-year-old woman has right flank pain, and her diuretic renography reveals UPJ obstruction and a differential renal function of 75:25 (L:R). The next best step is:
   a. CT angiography.
   b. stent placement.
   c. endopyelotomy.
   d. laparoscopic pyeloplasty.
   e. laparoscopic nephrectomy.

6. The highest failure rate in treating UPJ obstruction is associated with:
   a. antegrade endopyelotomy.
   b. retrograde ureteroscopic endopyelotomy.
   c. balloon dilation.
   d. pyeloplasty.
   e. cautery balloon incision.

7. The most appropriate location for endoscopic incision of a proximal ureteral stricture is:
   a. lateral.
   b. anterior.
   c. medial.
   d. posterior.
   e. anterolateral.

8. The best treatment option for a patient with a functional left ureteroenteric anastomotic stricture is:
   a. metallic stent.
   b. balloon dilation.
   c. laser endoureterotomy.
   d. cautery wire balloon incision.
   e. open repair.

9. The most common cause of retroperitoneal fibrosis is:
   a. methysergide.
   b. infection.
   c. lymphoma.
   d. breast cancer.
   e. immune-mediated aortitis.

10. Retrocaval ureter results from:
   a. persistence of posterior cardinal veins.
   b. persistence of anterior cardinal veins.
   c. duplication of inferior vena cava.
   d. aberrance of lumbar veins.
   e. retroaortic renal veins.

11. Transperitoneal laparoscopic pyeloplasty:
   a. is used rarely compared with the retroperitoneal approach.
   b. does not require water-tight, tension-free anastomosis.
   c. provides more working space than in the retroperitoneal approach.
   d. provides unfamiliar anatomy.
   e. does not require an external surgical drain.

12. Surgical repair of ureteropelvic junction obstruction requires:
   a. a funnel-shaped transition between the renal pelvis and ureter.
   b. dependent drainage.
   c. water-tight anastomosis.
   d. tension-free anastomosis.
   e. all of the above.

13. Contraindications for transureteroureterostomy include a history of:
   a. retroperitoneal fibrosis.
   b. urothelial malignancy.
   c. nephrolithiasis.
   d. a, b, and c.
   e. b and c.

14. A 25-year-old man presents with right flank pain. He underwent a laparoscopic pyeloplasty, which failed within 1 year. Consequently, he underwent failed endopyelotomy. A CT scan shows a small, intrarenal pelvis and moderate cortical loss in the right kidney with a normal-appearing left kidney. A renogram reveals 35% differential function on the affected side, and a diuretic study demonstrates functional obstruction (>30 min). The next step is:
    a. chronic internal ureteral stent.
    b. ileal ureter.
    c. Davis intubated ureterotomy.
    d. ureterocalicostomy.
    e. renal autotransplantation.

15. Spiral flap procedures for UPJ obstruction are used:
    a. to bridge a shorter length stenosis.
    b. to treat crossing vessels.
    c. to bridge a longer length stenosis.
    d. for a small, intrarenal pelvis.
    e. only in the presence of greater than 30% ipsilateral renal function.

16. Foley Y-V plasty is a suitable approach when encountering:
    a. high ureteral insertion.
    b. small intrarenal pelvis.
    c. anterior crossing vessel.
    d. duplication of collecting system.
    e. redundant renal pelvis.

17. Which type of pyeloplasty is suitable when there is an aberrant crossing vessel?
    a. Foley Y-V plasty
    b. Culp-DeWeerd spiral flap
    c. Dismembered pyeloplasty
    d. Scardino-Prince vertical flap
    e. Ligation and transection of the crossing vessel

18. Ileal ureter can be performed when the patient has:
    a. renal insufficiency (serum creatinine >2 mg/dL).
    b. inflammatory bowel disease.
    c. bladder dysfunction.
    d. radiation enteritis.
    e. small intrarenal pelvis.

19. A 55-year-old woman underwent left transperitoneal laparoscopic dismembered pyeloplasty over an internal ureteral stent. An abdominal drain was placed at surgery, and there was minimal drain output during the first 24 hours after surgery. Within 3 hours after Foley catheter removal, the patient's nurse noted a significant amount of fluid coming out of the drain site. The next step is to:
    a. change dressings frequently and continue observation.
    b. replace the urethral catheter.
    c. restrict fluid intake.
    d. remove the surgical drain.
    e. change the ureteral stent.

20. In performing a psoas hitch, additional bladder mobility can be achieved by transection of the:
    a. contralateral superior vesical artery.
    b. ipsilateral inferior vesical artery.
    c. contralateral inferior vesical artery.
    d. ipsilateral superior vesical artery.
    e. ipsilateral gonadal artery.

21. A 40-year-old woman with a history of hypertension and recurrent nephrolithiasis presents with a 5-cm proximal right ureteral stricture following an iatrogenic injury in a recent abdominal surgery. She has had an indwelling right nephrostomy tube for more than 6 months. Her baseline serum creatinine is 2.5 mg/dL. Renal scan shows split function of 65% in the right kidney. Her bladder capacity is found to be less than 300 mL. The next step is:
    a. ureteroureterostomy.
    b. Boari flap.
    c. transureteroureterostomy.
    d. ileal ureteral substitution.
    e. autotransplantation.

22. During a psoas hitch, the structure particularly susceptible to injury is the:
    a. obturator nerve.
    b. iliohypogastric nerve.
    c. ilioinguinal nerve.
    d. sacral nerve.
    e. genitofemoral nerve.

23. The technique that does not require normal bladder capacity, drainage, and function is the:
    a. ileal ureteral substitution.
    b. psoas hitch.
    c. ureteroneocystostomy.
    d. endoscopic incision of transmural ureter.
    e. Boari flap.

Imaging

1. See Figure 49-1. A 72-year-old man with malaise has this CT scan. The serum creatinine is mildly elevated. What is the best diagnosis?
    a. Retroperitoneal fibrosis
    b. Retroperitoneal hematoma
    c. Tuberculosis
    d. Retroperitoneal sarcoma
    e. Perianeurysmal fibrosis

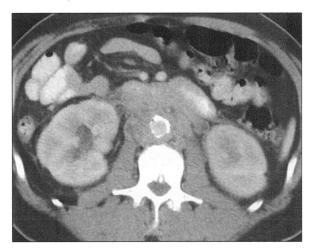

Figure 49-1.

ANSWERS

1. **a. Maternal-fetal ultrasonography.** The current widespread use of maternal ultrasonography has led to a dramatic increase in the number of asymptomatic newborns who are diagnosed with

hydronephrosis, many of whom are subsequently found to have ureteropelvic junction obstruction.

2. **c. Diuretic renography.** Provocative testing with a diuretic urogram may allow accurate diagnosis of UPJ obstruction. Renal ultrasound, CT scan, and retrograde pyelogram give anatomic assessments of the UPJ without quantitatively assessing urinary drainage and function.

3. **e. Whitaker pressure-perfusion test.** When doubt remains as to the clinical significance of a dilated collecting system, placement of percutaneous nephrostomy allows access for pressure perfusion studies. In the pressure perfusion test, first described by Whitaker in 1973 and then modified in 1978, the renal pelvis is perfused with normal saline or dilute radiographic contrast solution, and the pressure gradient across the presumed area of obstruction is determined. Renal pelvic pressures in excess of 15 to 22 cm H_2O are highly suggestive of a functional obstruction. Although diuretic renography is useful for diagnosis as well, the Whitaker test is ideal for this situation because a nephrostomy tube is already in situ.

4. **d. Moderate to severe hydronephrosis.** Consideration of any of the less invasive alternatives to open operative intervention must take into account individual anatomy including, but not limited to, the degree of hydronephrosis, overall and ipsilateral renal function, and, in some cases, the presence of crossing vessels or concomitant calculi. One study found that endopyelotomy success rates were less than 50% when significant hydronephrosis and crossing vessels were identified preoperatively.

5. **b. Laparoscopic pyeloplasty.** Evidence indicates that crossing vessels lower the success rate of endopyelotomy from several investigators. When such patients were culled from the pool of candidates available for treatment of UPJ obstruction, endopyelotomy success rates improved in most studies. A CT angiography would be necessary to assess this. However, laparoscopic pyeloplasty would be a straightforward minimally invasive option for this young patient. The kidney has too much function to remove at this stage.

6. **c. Balloon dilation.** McClinton reported long-term follow-up data on balloon dilation of the UPJ, finding a success rate of only 42%, which was significantly lower than the initial publications would indicate.

7. **a. Lateral.** Proximal ureteral strictures are incised laterally, similar to UPJ strictures. Posterior incision is offered to UPJ obstruction patients who have failed open pyeloplasty. Distal strictures are incised anteriorly, as are strictures of the middle ureter.

8. **e. Open repair.** Several studies have linked poor outcomes with endoscopic management of left ureteroenteric strictures. This may be a result of diminished blood flow to the ureter because the left ureter requires more mobilization than the right side at the time of diversion. Although metallic stents show promise in limited studies, using open repair, reports demonstrate an 80% success.

9. **e. Immune-mediated aortitis.** Growing evidence indicates that the majority of cases of retroperitoneal fibrosis are, in fact, immune-mediated aortitis. Regardless, the other conditions are relatively rare causes of retroperitoneal fibrosis.

10. **a. Persistence of posterior cardinal veins.** Retrocaval ureter results from the persistence of the posterior cardinal veins.

11. **c. Provides more working space than that in the retroperitoneal approach.** Transperitoneal laparoscopic pyeloplasty provides a larger working space relative to a retroperitoneoscopic approach. Together with more familiar anatomy, the transperitoneal approach is used most commonly in the laparoscopic urologic community to date.

12. **e. All of the above.** For any surgical repair of UPJ obstruction, the resultant anastomosis should be widely patent and completed in a watertight fashion without tension. In addition, the reconstructed UPJ should allow a funnel-shaped transition between the pelvis and the ureter that is in a position of dependent drainage.

13. **d. a, b, and c.** Relative contraindications include history of nephrolithiasis, retroperitoneal fibrosis, urothelial malignancy, chronic pyelonephritis, and abdominopelvic radiation.

14. **d. Ureterocalicostomy.** Direct anastomosis of the proximal ureter to the lower calyceal system is a well-accepted salvage technique for the failed pyeloplasty and small renal pelvis.

15. **c. To bridge a longer length stenosis.** Flap procedures can be useful in situations involving a relatively long segment of ureteral narrowing or stricture. Of the various flap procedures, a spiral flap can bridge a strictured or narrow area of longer length. The flap procedures are not appropriate in the setting of crossing vessels.

16. **a. High ureteral insertion.** The Foley Y-V-plasty is designed for repair of a UPJ obstruction secondary to a high ureteral insertion. It is specifically contraindicated when transposition of lower pole vessels is necessary. In situations requiring concomitant reduction of redundant renal pelvis, this technique is also of little value.

17. **c. Dismembered pyeloplasty.** In the presence of crossing aberrant or accessory lower pole renal vessels associated with UPJ obstruction, a dismembered pyeloplasty is the only method to allow transposition of the UPJ in relation to these vessels.

18. **e. Small intrarenal pelvis.** In ileal segment usage, a small intrarenal pelvis is not contraindicated and an ileocalycostomy can be performed successfully.

19. **b. Replace the urethral catheter.** If the drain output increases following the removal of the Foley catheter, the catheter should be replaced for several days to avoid vesicoureteral reflux up the stent in the operated ureter and decrease urinary extravasation.

20. **a. Contralateral superior vesical artery.** In psoas hitch, transection of the contralateral superior vesical artery can be helpful to bridge the gap to the ipsilateral ureteral end, thereby achieving tension-free anastomosis.

21. **e. Autotransplantation.** Ureteroureterostomy is inappropriate for a 5-cm upper ureteral defect. Boari flap is inappropriate for a small bladder capacity. Transureteroureterostomy is contraindicated in the patient with a history of recurrent nephrolithiasis. Ileal ureter is contraindicated in the presence of elevated serum creatinine above 2 mg/dL. Autotransplant is appropriate for this particular patient.

22. **e. Genitofemoral nerve.** The genitofemoral nerve courses over the psoas muscle.

23. **d. Endoscopic incision of transmural ureter.** Normal bladder function without significant outlet obstruction is crucial to the success of ileal ureteral substitution, psoas hitch, Boari flap, and ureteroneocystostomy.

Imaging

1. **a. Retroperitoneal fibrosis.** There is increased soft tissue in the retroperitoneum, which obscures and effaces the planes between the inferior vena cava and the aorta. Tuberculosis causes calcification and stricturing in the kidneys and collecting systems, and tuberculous iliopsoas abscess extends along the iliopsoas muscles. Retroperitoneal hematoma and sarcoma are not centered solely around the aorta and the inferior vena cava. In perianeurysmal fibrosis, a retroperitoneal fibrosis-like picture occurs in association with an abdominal aortic aneurysm; the aorta is of normal caliber in this case.

CHAPTER REVIEW

1. Intrinsic UPJ obstruction is a result of an aperistaltic segment in which the normal spiral arrangement of the muscle bundles is replaced by longitudinal muscle bundles and fibrous tissue.
2. A crossing vessel has the most detrimental effect on the success of an endopyelotomy.
3. UPJ obstruction may coexist with vesicoureteral reflux.
4. A multicystic kidney is distinguished from a UPJ obstruction on ultrasound by the "cyst" being connected in hydronephrosis as opposed to being distinct in a multicystic dysplastic kidney.
5. A Whittaker test is performed by perfusing the renal pelvis at 10 mL/min. Pressures less than 15 cm H_2O suggest a nonobstructed system. Pressures greater than 22 cm H_2O suggest an obstructed system, and pressures between the two are indeterminate.
6. The indications for repair of a UPJ include symptoms, impairment of renal function, stones, infection, and hypertension.
7. In neonates, unilateral hydronephrosis when carefully followed results in 7% of patients requiring a pyeloplasty.
8. Generally, kidneys with less than 15% function are not salvageable in adult patients.
9. A long segment stricture (>2 cm) is generally not successfully managed by the endopyelotomy method. An endopyelotomy cannot be performed safely by any route until access across the UPJ is established.
10. The majority of endopyelotomy failures occur within the first year. Success rates for endopyelotomy in properly selected patients range between 60% and 80%.
11. High-grade hydroureteronephrosis and crossing vessels have a detrimental effect on the success rate of endopyelotomy.
12. When bleeding occurs following an endopyelotomy, one should have a low threshold to precede to angiography to thrombose the severed vessel.
13. Seventy percent of failures following laparoscopic pyeloplasty occur in the first 2 years.
14. When repairing a retrocaval ureter, the ureter is transected and relocated ventral to the vena cava.
15. Lower ureteral strictures are incised in an anterior medial direction; upper ureteral strictures are incised in a lateral or posterior lateral direction.
16. With ureteral strictures, one must always rule out malignancy.
17. There is no significant difference in preserving renal function in the adult when reimplanting the ureter into the bladder by either a refluxing or antirefluxing method.
18. Most patients with long-term urinary conduits will have an element of hydronephrosis that is not secondary to obstruction.
19. Retroperitoneal fibrosis secondary to malignancy is often indistinguishable from idiopathic retroperitoneal fibrosis and can be identified only with appropriate biopsy that identifies islands of tumor cells.
20. The initial management of retroperitoneal fibrosis is generally with steroids. Steroids are more likely to be beneficial if there is evidence of active inflammation as indicated by an elevated erythrocyte sedimentation rate, leukocytosis, and infiltration of lymphocytes on biopsy.
21. In addition to steroids, azathioprine, cyclophosphamide, cyclosporine, colchicine, and tamoxifen have been used to treat retroperitoneal fibrosis with some success.
22. Generally, 25% renal function is required to keep a repair of the UPJ or ureter open.
23. For any surgical repair of UPJ obstruction, the resultant anastomosis should be widely patent and completed in a watertight fashion without tension. In addition, the reconstructed UPJ should allow a funnel-shaped transition between the pelvis and the ureter that is in a position of dependent drainage.

50 Upper Urinary Tract Trauma

Richard A. Santucci and Mang L. Chen

QUESTIONS

1. What method is used to perform "one-shot" intraoperative intravenous pyelography (IVP) in a 50-kg woman?
   a. Inject a 50-mL bolus of intravenous contrast agent followed by a full IVP series including abdominal compression to evaluate the ureters.
   b. Inject a 100-mL bolus of intravenous contrast agent followed in exactly 10 minutes by a flat plate of the abdomen on the operating room table.
   c. Inject a 50-mL bolus of intravenous contrast agent followed in exactly 10 minutes by a flat plate of the abdomen on the operating room table.
   d. Determine the patient's serum creatinine level before administration of intravenous contrast agent to make sure that he or she will not experience renal failure as a result of reaction to the contrast agent.
   e. Inject 100 mL of intravenous contrast and obtain a kidney, ureter, bladder (KUB) film 20 minutes following injection.

2. What is the best option for repair of midureteral transection after a stab wound?
   a. Ureteroureterostomy
   b. Transureteroureterostomy
   c. Boari flap
   d. Nephrectomy
   e. Cutaneous ureterostomy

3. When ureteroureterostomy is performed, which of the following is required?
   a. Postoperative retroperitoneal Penrose drain
   b. Postoperative nephrostomy drain
   c. Spatulated, watertight repair
   d. Nonabsorbable sutures
   e. Intraperitonealization of the ureteral anastomosis

4. Which maneuver is cited as a cause of ureteral injury during stone basketing?
   a. Ureteroscopy without dilating the ureteral orifice first
   b. Ureteroscopy in nondilated systems
   c. Use of the holmium laser
   d. Pulsatile saline irrigation to assist visualization
   e. Persistence in stone basketing attempts in the face of a ureteral tear

5. Which of the following is a contraindication to transureteroureterostomy for repair of significant lower ureter injury?
   a. History of urolithiasis
   b. History of ureteral trauma
   c. Obesity
   d. Neurogenic bladder
   e. Spinal fracture

6. What is the treatment of choice for a ureteral contusion caused by a high-velocity bullet?
   a. Observation
   b. Ureteral stent placement
   c. Transureteroureterostomy
   d. Ureteroureterostomy
   e. Oversewing the contusion with healthy ureteral tissue

7. Which imaging technique is most useful for detecting ureteral injuries after trauma?
   a. Computed tomography (CT) without use of contrast material
   b. CT with use of contrast agent, obtained immediately after injection of the contrast agent
   c. CT with the use of contrast material, obtained 20 minutes after injection of the contrast agent
   d. Intravenous pyelography
   e. Furosemide (Lasix) renography

8. Which of the following statements is TRUE about ureteral injuries during laparoscopy?
   a. The total number of injuries has stayed steady over the years.
   b. Surgery for endometriosis greatly increases the risk.
   c. Bipolar cautery use during tubal ligation eliminates risk.
   d. Most ureteral injuries are recognized immediately.
   e. Indigo carmine dye eliminates the risk of injury.

Imaging

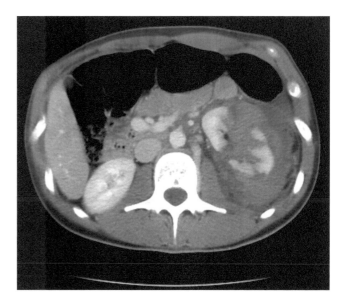

Figure 50-1.

1. A 22-year-old woman has a CT scan (Figure 50-1) after a motor vehicle accident. Her vital signs are stable, and there are no other significant injuries.

   The next step is:

   a. open surgical repair of the kidney.

   b. delayed imaging to evaluate the collecting system.

   c. left nephrectomy to avoid future complications.

   d. renal artery embolization.

   e. intravenous urogram.

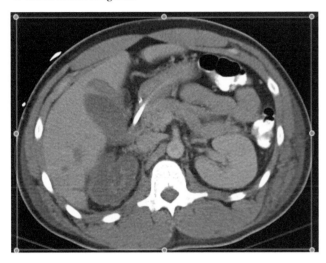

Figure 50-2.

2. A 24-year-old man had a CT scan (Figure 50-2) 36 hours after a motor vehicle accident. The most likely diagnosis is:

   a. ureteral injury.

   b. segmental renal artery transection.

   c. main renal artery occlusion.

   d. ureteropelvic junction disruption.

   e. traumatic renal vein occlusion.

ANSWERS

1. **b. Inject a 100-mL bolus of intravenous contrast agent followed in exactly 10 minutes by a flat plate of the abdomen on the operating room table.** Only a single film is taken 10 minutes after intravenous injection (IV push) of 2 mL/kg of contrast material.

2. **a. Ureteroureterostomy.** Ureteroureterostomy, so-called end-to-end repair in injuries to the upper two thirds of the ureter, is common (up to 32% of one large series) and has a reported success rate as high as 90%.

3. **c. Spatulated, watertight repair.** Repair ureters under magnification with spatulated, tension-free, stented, watertight anastomosis and place a retroperitoneal closed suction drain.

4. **e. Persistence in stone basketing attempts in the face of a ureteral tear.** One factor cited as a cause of injury was the persistence in stone basketing attempts after recognition of a ureteral tear. Current recommendations are to stop and place a ureteral stent.

5. **a. History of urolithiasis.** This operation is contraindicated in patients with a history of urothelial calculi.

6. **d. Ureteroureterostomy.** Ureteral contusions, although the most "minor" of ureteral injuries, often heal with stricture or break down later if microvascular injury results in ureteral necrosis. Severe or large areas of contusion should be treated with excision and ureteroureterostomy.

7. **c. CT with the use of contrast material, obtained 20 minutes after injection of the contrast agent.** Because modern helical CT scanners can obtain images before intravenous contrast dye is excreted in the urine, delayed images must be obtained (5 to 20 minutes after contrast material injection) to allow contrast material to extravasate from the injured collecting system, renal pelvis, or ureter.

8. **b. Surgery for endometriosis greatly increases the risk.** A large percentage of ureteral injuries after gynecologic laparoscopy occur during electrosurgical or laser-assisted lysis of endometriosis.

Imaging

1. **b. Delayed imaging to evaluate the collecting system.** When blunt renal trauma results in deep parenchymal lacerations, delayed imaging at the time of the CT is essential to evaluate the collecting system for injury. In a stable patient with this type of injury, neither surgical repair nor angiographic embolization is indicated. Most renal injuries heal well with conservative and expectant management, making options a and c incorrect. Intravenous urography no longer plays a role in the acute evaluation of blunt renal trauma.

2. **c. Main renal artery occlusion.** There is complete absence of enhancement of the entire right kidney, which is caused only by main renal artery occlusion. Segmental occlusion would cause abnormality only in a portion of the right renal nephrogram. Ureteral injury and UPJ disruption may cause delay in the nephrogram but not complete absence of enhancement.

CHAPTER REVIEW

1. The best indication of significant urinary system injury is gross or microscopic hematuria.
2. Evaluation of urologic trauma in children differs from adults in that children: (1) are at greater risk for renal trauma, (2) often do not become hypotensive with major blood loss, and (3) have a higher propensity for renal anomalies.
3. Rapid deceleration involving high-velocity impact may result in injuries at points of fixation such as the ureteral pelvic junction and the renal hilum (renal artery intimal disruption).
4. The degree of hematuria and the severity of renal injury are not consistently correlated.
5. Criteria for radiologic imaging include (1) all penetrating trauma, (2) high-impact rapid deceleration trauma, (3) all blunt trauma with gross hematuria, (4) all blunt trauma with microhematuria and hypotension, and (5) all pediatric patients with microscopic hematuria.
6. Adult patients with microscopic hematuria without shock may be observed without imaging studies.
7. Findings suggestive of a major renal injury on CT include medial hematoma, medial urinary extravasation, and lack of contrast enhancement of the entire kidney.
8. Nonoperative management for renal injuries is preferred in the hemodynamically stable patient, particularly with grades I to III renal injuries.
9. Exploration of renal gunshot wounds is no longer mandatory in selected cases. Those patients with grade I to IV parenchymal lacerations with well-contained hematomas who are hemodynamically stable may be observed expectantly.

10. Absolute indications for renal exploration are (1) hemodynamic instability with shock, (2) expanding pulsatile hematoma, (3) suspected renal pedicle avulsion, and (4) ureteral pelvic junction disruption.

11. Surgical exploration of the acutely injured kidney is best performed through a transabdominal incision with early isolation of the renal artery to the affected kidney.

12. "Damage control" involves packing the wound around the injured kidney with laparotomy pads to control bleeding and a planned return to the operating room in 24 hours. This is rarely indicated but is a management strategy in the multiply injured patient in whom an attempt to salvage the kidney is necessary when the additional time required to do this is inadvisable during initial post-trauma exploration.

13. Hypertension as a result of renal trauma is due to renal vascular injury or compression of the renal parenchyma by a circumferential hematoma (Page kidney).

14. When repairing ureteral injuries, the ureteral tissue should be debrided back to bleeding tissue to remove all traumatized microvascular damaged tissue.

15. Placement of a vascular graft anterior to the ureter and aneurysms may cause a periureteral inflammatory reaction and ureteral injury/stenosis.

16. In emergent situations when a ureteral repair in the multiply traumatized patient cannot be adequately performed, the ureter may be tied off and the kidney drained postoperatively through a percutaneous nephrostomy with planned reconstruction at a later date, or a single J stent may be placed up the ureter to the renal pelvis, secured to the ureter, and brought out through the flank.

17. Intravenous methylene blue and indigo carmine should be avoided in pregnant patients or those taking a serotonin reuptake inhibitor.

18. When anastomosing the ureter to the bladder for a traumatic distal ureteral injury, the ureter should be spatulated and sewn to the bladder in a nontunneled (refluxing) fashion.

19. Ureteral transections should be repaired within 3 days of the injury, or the repair should be delayed for 6 weeks.

20. It is prudent to isolate the ureteral repair from other organs with omentum or peritoneum.

21. The uterine artery may be a significant source of the blood supply to the distal ureter in females and, when ligated during a hysterectomy, may lead to ureteral ischemia, resulting in ureteral stenosis, urinoma, or ureterovaginal fistula.

22. Ureteral injury occurring during vascular surgery should be repaired and isolated from the graft with normal tissue such as omentum.

51 Urinary Lithiasis: Etiology, Epidemiology, and Pathogenesis

Margaret S. Pearle, Jodi A. Antonelli, and Yair Lotan

QUESTIONS

1. The ethnic/racial group with the highest prevalence of stone disease is:
   a. African-Americans.
   b. Hispanics.
   c. Whites.
   d. Asians.
   e. American Indians.

2. The geographic area in the United States associated with the highest incidence of calcium oxalate stone disease is the:
   a. northeast.
   b. southeast.
   c. southwest.
   d. west.
   e. northwest.

3. Which of the following occurs when the concentration product of urine is in the metastable range?
   a. Urine is supersaturated.
   b. Homogeneous nucleation occurs.
   c. Solubility product is reduced.
   d. Urinary inhibitors decrease the formation product.
   e. Nucleation never occurs.

4. The process by which nucleation occurs in pure solutions is:
   a. homogeneous nucleation.
   b. heterogeneous nucleation.
   c. epitaxy.
   d. aggregation.
   e. agglomeration.

5. The proteinaceous portion of stones is composed of:
   a. concentric lamination.
   b. protein-crystal complex.
   c. matrix.
   d. nephrocalcin.
   e. osteocalcin.

6. Citrate inhibits calcium oxalate stone formation by:
   a. binding urinary inhibitors.
   b. lowering urine magnesium levels.
   c. increasing urinary saturation of sodium urate.

   d. complexing calcium.
   e. lowering urine pH.

7. Stone-forming propensity is best described by:
   a. formation product.
   b. ionic activity.
   c. saturation index.
   d. solubility product.
   e. relative saturation ratio.

8. The most common abnormal urinary finding in patients undergoing Roux-en-Y gastric bypass surgery is:
   a. hypercalciuria.
   b. low urine pH.
   c. low urine volume.
   d. hypocitraturia.
   e. hyperoxaluria.

9. The vitamin D metabolite that stimulates intestinal calcium absorption is:
   a. 7-dehydrocholesterol.
   b. cholecalciferol.
   c. 25-dihydroxyvitamin D_3.
   d. 1,25-dihydroxyvitamin D_3.
   e. calcitonin.

10. Which of the following factors increases intestinal oxalate absorption?
    a. High dietary calcium intake
    b. Low dietary calcium intake
    c. *Oxalobacter formigenes* colonization in the colon
    d. *Helicobacter pylori* colonization in the stomach
    e. Irritable bowel syndrome

11. The primary determinant of urinary citrate excretion is:
    a. acid-base status.
    b. urinary sodium excretion.
    c. citric acid intake.
    d. insulin sensitivity.
    e. urinary calcium excretion.

12. The underlying abnormality of renal hypercalciuria is:
    a. enhanced calcium filtration.
    b. enhanced calcium secretion.
    c. enhanced calcium reabsorption.

d. primary renal wasting of calcium.

e. primary renal storage of calcium.

13. Hypercalciuria associated with sarcoidosis is a result of:

    a. absorptive hypercalciuria.

    b. renal hypercalciuria.

    c. resorptive hypercalciuria.

    d. acidosis.

    e. medical induction.

14. Enteric hyperoxaluria occurs as a result of:

    a. excessive intake of oxalate.

    b. reduced excretion of oxalate.

    c. increased dietary fat.

    d. low calcium intake.

    e. fat malabsorption.

15. The most likely mechanism accounting for low urinary pH in uric acid stone formers with type 2 diabetes mellitus is:

    a. defective ammoniagenesis.

    b. impaired urinary bicarbonate excretion.

    c. lactic acidosis.

    d. glucosuria.

    e. ketoacidosis.

16. In idiopathic calcium oxalate stone formers, Randall plaques originate in the:

    a. basement membrane of the thin loops of Henle.

    b. terminal collecting ducts.

    c. medullary interstitium.

    d. vasa recta.

    e. papillary tip.

17. In calcium oxalate stone formers, Randall plaques are composed of:

    a. calcium oxalate.

    b. brushite.

    c. calcium carbonate.

    d. calcium apatite.

    e. uric acid.

18. Urinary saturation of calcium oxalate is most strongly dependent on:

    a. Urinary calcium concentration

    b. Urinary oxalate concentration

    c. Both urinary calcium and oxalate concentrations

    d. Urinary pH

    e. Urinary citrate concentration

19. *O. formigenes* reduces urinary oxalate by:

    a. reducing intestinal calcium absorption, leading to decreased luminal free oxalate and reduced oxalate absorption.

    b. degrading urinary oxalate in infected urine.

    c. binding oxalate in the intestinal lumen and preventing its reabsorption.

    d. inhibiting the intestinal oxalate transporter.

    e. using oxalate as a substrate in the intestine, thereby reducing intestinal oxalate absorption.

20. Which of the following organisms is most likely to produce urease?

    a. *Staphylococcus aureus*

    b. *Escherichia coli*

    c. *Streptococcus pneumoniae*

    d. *Serratia marcescens*

    e. *Chlamydia*

21. The mechanism responsible for type 1 (distal) renal tubular acidosis (RTA) is:

    a. impaired bicarbonate reabsorption in the proximal tubule.

    b. defective H^+-ATPase in the distal tubule that is unable to excrete excess acid.

    c. defective ammoniagenesis.

    d. impaired excretion of nontitratable acids.

    e. hypoaldosteronism.

22. Patients with Lesch-Nyhan syndrome treated with high doses of allopurinol are at risk for formation of stones of which of the following compositions?

    a. Hypoxanthine

    b. Uric acid

    c. Xanthine

    d. 2,8-Dihydroxyadenine

    e. Calcium apatite

23. The etiology of ammonium acid urate stone formation in patients abusing laxatives is:

    a. recurrent infections with urease-producing bacteria.

    b. chronic dehydration and excessive uric acid excretion.

    c. increased ammoniagenesis.

    d. urinary phosphate deficiency and intracellular acidosis.

    e. chronic dehydration, intracellular acidosis, and low urinary sodium.

24. The primary mechanism of action of citrate in preventing stone formation is:

    a. reducing urinary calcium excretion.

    b. reducing urinary oxalate excretion.

    c. complexing calcium in urine.

    d. complexing oxalate in urine.

    e. complexing phosphate in urine.

25. Type 1 (distal) RTA is characterized by which abnormality?

    a. Hyperkalemia

    b. Hypochloremia

    c. Alkalosis

    d. Hypercitraturia

    e. Hypokalemia

26. The primary defect in type 2 (proximal) RTA is failure of bicarbonate reabsorption in the:

    a. glomerulus.

    b. proximal tubule.

    c. loop of Henle.

    d. distal tubule.

    e. collecting duct.

27. The most common abnormality identified in patients with uric acid stones is:

    a. acidic urine.

    b. alkaline urine.

    c. low uric acid concentration.

    d. high uric acid concentration.

    e. distal renal tubular acidosis.

28. The etiology of stone formation in patients with cystic fibrosis is:
    a. absorptive hypercalciuria.
    b. renal leak hypercalciuria.
    c. renal tubular acidosis.
    d. reduced or absent *O. formigenes.*
    e. chronic diarrheal syndrome.

29. Carbonic anhydrase inhibitors are associated with formation of stones composed of:
    a. calcium oxalate.
    b. calcium phosphate.
    c. struvite.
    d. cystine.
    e. uric acid.

30. Which of the following physiologic changes occurs in the kidney during pregnancy?
    a. Decreased uric acid excretion
    b. Decreased citrate excretion
    c. Increased calcium excretion
    d. Decreased glomerular filtration rate (GFR)
    e. Increased magnesium excretion

ANSWERS

1. **c. Whites.** The highest prevalence of stone disease in both men and women occurs in whites. In men the lowest prevalence occurs in African-Americans, whereas Asian women have been found to have the lowest prevalence in one series.

2. **b. Southeast.** According to hospital discharge rates among U.S. veterans, calcium oxalate stone disease is most prevalent in the southeast.

3. **a. Urine is supersaturated.** The solubility product refers to the point of saturation where dissolved and crystalline components in solution are in equilibrium. Addition of more crystals to the solution will result in precipitation of crystals. In this supersaturated urine (metastable state), crystallization can occur on preexisting crystals, but spontaneous crystallization occurs only when the concentration product exceeds the formation product. In the metastable state, the presence of inhibitors prevents or delays crystallization.

4. **a. Homogeneous nucleation.** The process by which nuclei form in pure solutions is called *homogeneous nucleation.* Heterogeneous nucleation occurs when microscopic impurities or other constituents in the urine promote nucleation by providing a surface on which the crystal components can grow.

5. **c. Matrix.** Depending on their type, kidney stones contain between 2.5% and 65% of noncrystalline material or matrix. Extensive investigations have characterized matrix as a derivative of several of the mucoproteins of urine and serum.

6. **d. Complexing calcium.** Citrate inhibits stone formation by complexing calcium, thereby lowering urinary saturation of calcium oxalate. In addition it inhibits spontaneous precipitation of calcium oxalate and agglomeration of calcium oxalate crystals. It also inhibits calcium oxalate and calcium phosphate crystal growth, with its effect on calcium phosphate crystal growth more pronounced than on calcium oxalate crystal growth. Last, it prevents heterogeneous nucleation of calcium oxalate by monosodium urate.

7. **c. Saturation index.** The state of saturation of the urine with respect to particular stone-forming salts indicates the stone-forming propensity of the urine. The state of saturation is determined by pH and the ionic strength of the major ions in solution. Relative saturation ratio, determined by the EQUIL 2 computer program, has been the standard for determining stone-forming propensity. However, the newer *JESS* computer program takes into account several soluble complexes not recognized by the EQUIL 2 program and is likely a more accurate measure of stone-forming propensity, although it has not yet gained widespread use.

8. **e. Hyperoxaluria.** Hyperoxaluria has been described in both stone-forming and non-stone-forming patients who have undergone Roux-en-Y gastric bypass surgery, with urinary oxalate levels in some patients exceeding 100 mg/day. A mild decrease in urinary calcium compared with stone-forming control subjects has been described by some investigators but is a less consistent and severe finding.

9. **d. 1,25-Dihydroxyvitamin D_3.** It is generally accepted that 1,25-dihydroxyvitamin D_3 is the vitamin D metabolite that is the most potent stimulator of intestinal calcium absorption. The other metabolites, except for calcitonin, are precursors of 1,25-dihydroxyvitamin D_3.

10. **b. Low dietary calcium intake.** Intestinal oxalate absorption is modulated by dietary oxalate and calcium intake and by the presence or absence of *O. formigenes.* In the setting of a high calcium intake, oxalate absorption decreases, and during calcium restriction, oxalate absorption increases because of reduced formation of a soluble calcium oxalate complex and increased availability of oxalate for absorption. *H. pylori*, which can colonize the stomach, has no effect on intestinal oxalate absorption. *O. formigenes*, an oxalate-degrading bacterium, uses oxalate as a substrate in the intestinal lumen, thereby reducing oxalate absorption. Irritable bowel syndrome, unless it is associated with chronic diarrhea, does not affect intestinal oxalate absorption.

11. **a. Acid-base status.** Acid-base status determines urinary citrate excretion. Metabolic acidosis reduces citrate excretion by augmenting citrate reabsorption and mitochondrial oxidation, whereas alkalosis enhances citrate excretion. Citric acid intake has a limited effect on urinary citrate excretion because only a small portion of dietary citrate is excreted into the urine unmetabolized. The majority of absorbed citrate is metabolized to bicarbonate, which is neutralized by the free proton from citric acid, thereby providing no net alkali load that would increase urinary citrate excretion.

12. **d. Primary renal wasting of calcium.** In this condition, the underlying abnormality is a primary renal leak of calcium due to impaired renal tubular calcium reabsorption.

13. **a. Absorptive hypercalciuria.** The sarcoid granuloma produces 1,25-dihydroxyvitamin D_3, causing increased intestinal calcium absorption, hypercalcemia, and hypercalciuria.

14. **e. Fat malabsorption.** Malabsorption from any cause, including small bowel resection, intrinsic disease, or jejunoileal bypass, increases luminal fatty acids and bile salts. Calcium, which normally complexes with oxalate to form a soluble complex that is lost in the stool, instead binds to fatty acids, thereby increasing luminal oxalate available for absorption. In addition, poorly absorbed bile salts increase colonic permeability to oxalate, further increasing oxalate absorption.

15. **a. Defective ammoniagenesis.** Patients with type 2 diabetes mellitus typically exhibit characteristics of the metabolic syndrome, including insulin resistance. Although peripherally, insulin resistance leads to typical symptoms of diabetes, insulin resistance at the level of the kidney leads to impaired ammoniagenesis, by way of reduced production of ammonia from glutamine and reduced activity of the Na^+/H^+ exchanger in the proximal tubule that is responsible for either the direct transport or trapping of ammonium in the urine. The result is reduced urinary ammonium and low urine pH.

16. **a. Basement membrane of the thin loops of Henle.** In idiopathic calcium oxalate stone formers, Randall plaques have been found to originate in the basement membrane of the thin loops of Henle. From there, they extend through the medullary interstitium to a subepithelial location, where they serve as an anchoring site for calcium oxalate stone formation.

17. **d. Calcium apatite.** Randall plaques are invariably composed of calcium apatite, which serve as an anchoring site onto which calcium oxalate crystals can adhere and grow.

18. **c. Both urinary calcium and oxalate concentrations.** Urinary saturation of calcium oxalate is strongly, positively correlated with urinary calcium and oxalate concentrations. Both contribute equally to urinary saturation of calcium oxalate.

19. **e. Using oxalate as a substrate in the intestine, thereby reducing intestinal oxalate absorption.** *O. formigenes* is an oxalate-degrading bacterium found in the intestinal lumen that uses oxalate as an energy source, thereby reducing luminal oxalate and intestinal oxalate absorption. *Oxalobacter* is not found in urine.

20. **a. *Staphylococcus aureus*.** Although *Proteus* species are most commonly associated with struvite stones, more than 90% of *S. aureus* organisms produce urease and are therefore associated with struvite stone formation.

21. **b. Defective H⁺-ATPase in the distal tubule that is unable to excrete excess acid.** A defective H^+-ATPase in the distal tubule has been implicated in the inability to excrete excess acid in the presence of an oral acid load among patients with distal RTA. Type 2, or proximal RTA, is characterized by impaired bicarbonate reabsorption in the proximal tubule, and type 4 RTA is common in diabetics with chronic renal damage who demonstrate aldosterone resistance.

22. **c. Xanthine.** Patients with Lesch-Nyhan syndrome suffer from an inherited deficiency of the purine salvage enzyme hypoxanthine-guanine phosphoribosyltransferase, which leads to the accumulation of hypoxanthine, which is ultimately converted to uric acid. Allopurinol inhibits xanthine oxidase, which is responsible for converting hypoxanthine to xanthine and xanthine to uric acid. High doses of allopurinol in these patients lead to the accumulation of hypoxanthine and xanthine, but because xanthine is less soluble in urine than is hypoxanthine, xanthine stones form.

23. **e. Chronic dehydration, intracellular acidosis, and low urinary sodium.** Subjects who abuse laxatives are chronically dehydrated, resulting in intracellular acidosis. In addition, urinary sodium is low from sodium loss as a result of the laxatives. In this environment, urate preferentially complexes with the abundant ammonium rather than sodium and produces ammonium acid urate stones.

24. **c. Complexing calcium in urine.** The primary mechanism of action of citrate is as a complexing agent for calcium, thereby reducing ionic calcium and urinary saturation of calcium oxalate.

25. **e. Hypokalemia.** Distal RTA is characterized by hypokalemic, hyperchloremic, nonanion gap metabolic acidosis and a urinary pH consistently above 6.0.

26. **b. Proximal tubule.** The primary defect in type 2 or proximal RTA is a failure of bicarbonate reabsorption in the proximal tubule, leading to excessive urinary bicarbonate excretion and metabolic acidosis.

27. **a. Acidic urine.** Patients with uric acid stones often have prolonged periods of acidity in the urine.

28. **d. Reduced or absent *O. formigenes*.** Cystic fibrosis patients on chronic antibiotic therapy have been shown to have reduced or absent *O. formigenes* colonization, which potentially leads to increased intestinal oxalate absorption and reduced secretion.

29. **b. Calcium phosphate.** Carbonic anhydrase inhibitors such as acetazolamide and topiramate block reabsorption of bicarbonate in the renal proximal and distal tubules, thereby preventing urinary acidification and inducing a metabolic acidosis. Similar to RTA, carbonic anhydrase inhibition results in the formation of calcium phosphate stones because of the high urine pH, hypercalciuria, and hypocitraturia.

30. **c. Increased calcium excretion.** During pregnancy, increased renal blood flow increases GFR, thereby increasing the filtered load of calcium, sodium, and uric acid. Placental production of 1,25-dihydroxyvitamin D_3 increases intestinal calcium absorption, further increasing urinary calcium.

CHAPTER REVIEW

1. Renal calculi are two to three times more common in men than women, and in this country whites have the highest prevalence. They are uncommon before the age of 20 years, and the peak incidence occurs in the fourth to sixth decades of life.

2. The prevalence and incidence of stone disease is directly correlated with body mass index; patients with high body mass index excrete increased levels of oxalate, uric acid, sodium, and phosphorus, and are more likely to have urinary supersaturation for uric acid. The incidence and prevalence of stone disease has been increasing around the world.

3. Concentration product is the product of the concentrations of the chemical components.

4. Solubility product is the concentration at which precipitation of the components occurs.

5. A solution is saturated when the solubility product is exceeded.

6. When the solubility product is exceeded and precipitation does not occur, the solution is said to be metastable. When precipitation occurs, the concentration at that point is called *formation product*.

7. Magnesium and citrate inhibit crystal aggregation (the former complexes with oxalate and the latter with calcium); nephrocalcin inhibits nucleation, growth, and aggregation; Tamm-Horsfall glycoprotein inhibits aggregation; and osteopontin inhibits crystal growth, nucleation, and aggregation of calcium oxalate crystals.

8. Nanobacteria have been implicated in calcifying nanoparticles and serving as a nidus for stone formation.

9. Most stone-forming salts are found in the urine in a supersaturated state. Inhibitors keep them in solution.

10. The noncrystalline component of stones is called *matrix* and generally accounts for about 2.5% of the weight of the stone. It is composed of mucoproteins, carbohydrates, and urinary inhibitors.

11. Parathormone increases renal calcium reabsorption and enhances phosphate excretion.

12. Patients with small bowel disease or a history of intestinal resection and an intact colon have an increased oxalate absorption.

13. Calcium absorption occurs primarily in the small intestine at a rate that is dependent on calcium intake.

14. Calcium oxalate accounts for 60% of stones; mixed calcium oxalate and hydroxyapatite, 20%; brushite, 2%; uric acid, 10%; struvite, 10%; and cystine, 1%.

15. Hypercalciuria is the most common abnormality identified in calcium stone formation. Hypercalciuria is defined as a urinary excretion greater than 4 mg/kg/day.

17. Absorptive hypercalciuria is defined as an increased urinary calcium excretion after an oral calcium load and is due to increased intestinal absorption of calcium. Alteration of vitamin D receptors and/ or sensitivity has been suggested as the etiology. Renal hypercalciuria is due to impaired renal tubular reabsorption of calcium and leads to secondary hyperparathyroidism.

18. Reabsorptive hypercalciuria is due to hyperparathyroidism. The administration of thiazides to patients with primary hyperparathyroidism exacerbates hypercalcemia. Parathormone-like hormone resulting in hypercalcemia is produced by lung, breast, renal, penile, and head and neck tumors; lymphoma; and myeloma.

19. Hyperoxaluria is defined as greater than 40 mg/day excreted in the urine. Foods that are oxalate rich include nuts, chocolate, brewed tea, spinach, broccoli, strawberries, and rhubarb.

20. Hyperuricosuria is defined as urinary uric acid excretion exceeding 600 mg/day.
21. Hyperuricosuria promotes sodium urate formation, which promotes calcium oxalate stone formation through heterogenous nucleation.
23. Citrate inhibits stone formation by complexing with calcium and thereby preventing spontaneous nucleation of calcium oxalate; it inhibits agglomeration and growth of the crystal, and it enhances the inhibitory effect of Tamm-Horsfall glycoprotein. It prevents heterogeneous nucleation of calcium oxalate by monosodium urate.
24. Hypocitraturia is defined as urinary citrate excretion of less than 320 mg/day.
24. Renal tubular acidosis, type 1 (distal tubular RTA) is characterized by calcium phosphate stone formation, hypercalciuria, hypocitraturia, and an increased urinary pH.
25. Low magnesium levels result in reduced inhibitory activity and are often associated with decreased urinary citrate levels.
26. Cystine stones form due to a defect in the transport of four amino acids: cystine, lysine, ornithine, and arginine. It is inherited as an autosomal recessive and accounts for up to 10% of stones in children. There are two genes involved in the inheritance of the disease. There are three types based on urine excretion amounts: types A, B, and AB.
27. Stones of infection (struvite stones) are composed of magnesium ammonium phosphate and may contain carbonate apatite; they occur in association with urea-splitting bacteria. Urease-producing pathogens include *Proteus, Klebsiella, Pseudomonas,* and *Staphylococcus.*
28. The cause of stones associated with horseshoe kidneys and ureteropelvic junction obstructions is due to both the anatomic abnormality resulting in stasis and an underlying metabolic abnormality.
29. Medullary sponge kidney is characterized by ectasia of the renal collecting ducts and leads to stones through renal acidifying defects, hypercalciuria, and hypocitraturia.
30. Most stones in pregnancy pass spontaneously.
31. The most important determinate of uric acid stone formation is low urinary pH. Low urinary pH in uric acid stone formers is likely due to impaired ammoniagenesis associated with insulin resistance.
32. Medications which may precipitate as stones include triampterine, silica, indinavir, ephedrine, and ciprofloxacin.
33. Heterogeneous nucleation occurs when microscopic impurities or other constituents in the urine promote nucleation by providing a surface on which the crystal components can grow.
34. Intestinal oxalate absorption is modulated by dietary oxalate and calcium intake and by the presence or absence of *O. formigenes.*
35. Acid-base status determines urinary citrate excretion. Metabolic acidosis reduces citrate excretion.
36. The sarcoid granuloma produces 1,25-dihydroxyvitamin D_3, causing increased intestinal calcium absorption, hypercalcemia, and hypercalciuria.
37. Malabsorption from any cause, including small bowel resection, intrinsic disease, or jejunoileal bypass, increases luminal fatty acids and bile salts. Calcium, which normally complexes with oxalate, forming a soluble complex that is lost in the stool, instead binds to fatty acids, thereby increasing luminal oxalate available for absorption. In addition, poorly absorbed bile salts increase colonic permeability to oxalate, further increasing oxalate absorption.
38. Type 1 or distal tubule RTA is characterized by an impairment in hydrogen ion secretion. Type 2, or proximal RTA, is characterized by impaired bicarbonate reabsorption in the proximal tubule. Type 4 RTA is common in diabetics with chronic renal damage who demonstrate aldosterone resistance.

52 Evaluation and Medical Management of Urinary Lithiasis

Michael E. Lipkin, Michael N. Ferrandino, and Glenn M. Preminger

QUESTIONS

1. Patients with enteric hyperoxaluria are most likely to form stones composed of:
   a. calcium phosphate.
   b. calcium oxalate.
   c. magnesium ammonium phosphate.
   d. uric acid.
   e. cystine.

2. The risk factor most associated with recurrent stone formation in patients with inflammatory bowel disease is:
   a. hyperabsorption of oxalate in the jejunum.
   b. hyperexcretion of calcium from the distal tubule.
   c. diminished citrate absorption in the terminal ileum.
   d. hyperabsorption of calcium in the small bowel.
   e. increased colonic absorption of free oxalate.

3. Hypocitraturia in patients with inflammatory bowel disease or chronic diarrhea syndrome is due to:
   a. persistent bicarbonate losses.
   b. hypokalemia.
   c. metabolic acidosis.
   d. intracellular acidosis.
   e. All of the above

4. The optimum treatment for patients with enteric hyperoxaluria includes:
   a. calcium supplements, potassium citrate, and increased oral fluid intake.
   b. dietary restriction of oxalate.
   c. thiazides and potassium citrate.
   d. allopurinol.
   e. pyridoxine.

5. The most important factor predisposing patients to gouty diathesis is:
   a. hypercalciuria.
   b. low urinary pH.
   c. hypocitraturia.
   d. low urine volumes.
   e. hyperuricosuria.

6. The initial laboratory test that provides the most important diagnostic clue in patients with uric acid calculi is:
   a. urine pH.
   b. serum uric acid levels.
   c. urine sodium.
   d. urine calcium.
   e. urine uric acid levels.

7. The most appropriate medical treatment of a patient with gouty diathesis is:
   a. allopurinol.
   b. thiazides.
   c. increased fluids.
   d. dietary calcium restriction.
   e. potassium citrate.

8. A patient with recurrent uric acid calculi is placed on oral medical treatment and returns for follow-up 3 months later. He is noted to have significantly elevated urinary uric acid levels as compared with his first 24-hour urine collection. This finding is due to:
   a. increased production of endogenous uric acid.
   b. failure to avoid high-sodium foods.
   c. increased solubility of uric acid.
   d. increased consumption of red meat.
   e. inhibition of xanthine oxidase.

9. A patient with uric acid calculi is placed on alkali therapy but returns 1 year later having passed two calcium phosphate stones. A repeat 24-hour urine demonstrates a urine pH of 7.4, a urinary citrate of 450 mg/day, and a urinary uric acid of 875 mg/day. The most likely cause for recurrent stone formation is:
   a. cessation of potassium citrate.
   b. increase in oral purine intake.
   c. decrease in solubility of uric acid.
   d. excess alkalization.
   e. increase in saturation of oxalate.

10. A patient with gouty diathesis is started on sodium bicarbonate therapy, and urinary pH is maintained between 6.3 and 6.7. Calcium oxalate stones may form due to:
    a. sodium-inhibiting calcium reabsorption in the proximal tubule.
    b. homogeneous nucleation of calcium oxalate.
    c. undiagnosed hypercalciuria.
    d. lack of allopurinol in medical management regimen.
    e. reduction in monosodium urate.

11. A 58-year-old Hispanic female with a history of recurrent urinary tract infections treated three to four times in the past 18 months is seen by her family physician. At present she is asymptomatic. She has no history of nephrolithiasis. Renal ultrasound demonstrates moderate left hydronephrosis and a large density within the renal pelvis with posterior shadowing. A kidney-ureter-bladder (KUB) view with tomography reveals a poorly opacified dendritic stone in the renal pelvis and lower pole calyces. Prior urine cultures have *Proteus* and *Klebsiella* species. The stone composition of this patient is most likely:
    a. calcium oxalate.
    b. uric acid.
    c. magnesium ammonium phosphate.
    d. cystine.
    e. hydroxyapatite.

12. The most significant factor contributing to stone formation in patients with struvite calculi is:
    a. gouty diathesis.
    b. recurrent urinary tract infections.
    c. family history.
    d. hyperoxaluria.
    e. hypercalciuria.

13. Which of the following treatments is contraindicated for patients with recurrent struvite calculi?
    a. Orthophosphate
    b. Fluoroquinolones
    c. Thiazide diuretics
    d. Acetohydroxamic acid
    e. Calcium channel blockers

14. Acetohydroxamic acid contributes to reducing infection stone formation by:
    a. reversing associated metabolic defects.
    b. preventing recurrent urinary tract infections.
    c. alkalization of the urine.
    d. irreversibly inhibiting urease.
    e. All of the above

15. A 12-year-old boy is seen for evaluation of recurrent nephrolithiasis. He has spontaneously passed three stones over the previous 4 years and has recently undergone shockwave lithotripsy twice without success. He has been treated in the past with an unknown medication, but this was discontinued because the parents believed it was of no benefit. Urinalysis demonstrates hexagonal crystals. The likely metabolic diagnosis contributing to this patient's recurrent stone formation is:
    a. hypocitraturia.
    b. hyperoxaluria.
    c. low urine volumes.
    d. gouty diathesis.
    e. cystinuria.

16. First-line medical treatment for the prevention of recurrent cystine stones would be aimed at:
    a. urinary acidification.
    b. increasing the solubility of cystine.
    c. decreasing urinary sodium.
    d. decreasing the solubility of cystine.
    e. binding of cystine within the intestines.

17. α-Mercaptopropionylglycine (α-MPG, Thiola Mission Pharmacal Company, San Antonio, TX) may be helpful in the management of cystinuria because it:
    a. acts as a diuretic, further decreasing urinary cystine concentration.
    b. is significantly more effective than D-penicillamine.
    c. can be used as both an oral and intrarenal chemolytic agent.
    d. has equivalent efficacy at increasing solubility with reduced toxicity compared with D-penicillamine.
    e. adequately alkalizes the urine, obviating the need for potassium citrate.

18. Three years after initiating treatment for cystine stones with α-MPG, 800 mg/day, a patient returns with a follow-up, 24-hour urine collection demonstrating a significant reduction in cystine excretion from 740 to 250 mg/day. Urine volume is 775 mL/day. He has two additional stones. The reason for recurrent stone formation is:
    a. increased age, thereby exacerbating the disorder.
    b. decreased efficacy of α-MPG.

    c. continued supersaturation of urinary cystine.
    d. continued hypocitraturia.
    e. increased urine acidity.

19. A 19-year-old white woman with a 6-year history of recurrent stone disease is found to have multiple bilateral renal calculi by renal ultrasound during an evaluation for recurrent flank pain. She reports having passed more than 10 stones in the previous 2 years. Review of the renal ultrasound indicates no evidence of hydronephrosis. KUB film and tomograms demonstrate five stones on the left and eight stones on the right, all less than 4 mm. She has a strong family history of stones with three first-degree relatives and two cousins with nephrolithiasis. Urine pH is consistently above 6.8. Stone compositions have been mixed calcium phosphate and calcium oxalate. The most definitive test to identify this disorder would demonstrate:
    a. decreased serum parathyroid hormone (PTH) levels.
    b. persistently elevated urine calcium.
    c. inability to reduce the urine pH below 5.3.
    d. normalization of hypercalciuria.
    e. marked increase in urinary uric acid levels with initiation of treatment.

20. Which of the following is NOT a cause of hypocitraturic calcium nephrolithiasis?
    a. Thiazide-induced hypocitraturia
    b. Absorptive hypercalciuria type I
    c. Distal renal tubular acidosis
    d. Metabolic acidosis
    e. Chronic diarrheal syndrome

21. The most appropriate treatment for patients with renal tubular acidosis is:
    a. thiazides.
    b. allopurinol.
    c. sodium alkali.
    d. acetohydroxamic acid.
    e. potassium alkali.

22. Renal tubular acidosis may be associated with nephrolithiasis due to:
    a. hypercalciuria and hypocitraturia.
    b. hyperoxaluria and hypercalcemia.
    c. hyperuricosuria.
    d. hypocitraturia with normal urine magnesium.
    e. hypercitraturia and hypercalciuria.

23. Chronic metabolic acidosis may cause:
    a. increased PTH levels.
    b. significantly reduced bone density.
    c. hypercalcemia.
    d. increased intestinal calcium absorption.
    e. All of the above

24. To accurately diagnose a patient with renal leak hypercalciuria, one must identify both:
    a. increased intestinal calcium absorption and hyperthyroidism.
    b. renal leak of calcium and normal intestinal calcium absorption.
    c. hypoparathyroidism and increased intestinal calcium absorption.
    d. secondary hyperparathyroidism and renal calcium leak.
    e. primary hyperparathyroidism and increased intestinal calcium absorption.

25. Which of the following findings would support the diagnosis of renal leak hypercalciuria?

    a. Hypocitraturia

    b. Low urinary pH

    c. Normocalciuria on a calcium-restricted diet

    d. Decreased urinary sodium with thiazide challenge

    e. Low or low/normal radial bone density

26. The primary abnormality in patients with renal leak hypercalciuria is considered to be:

    a. impairment of renal tubular reabsorption of calcium.

    b. excessive mobilization of calcium from bone.

    c. increased 1,25-(OH)$_2$ vitamin D levels.

    d. elevation of serum PTH levels.

    e. hyperabsorption of intestinal calcium.

27. Which of the following mechanisms explains the effectiveness of thiazides in treating patients with renal leak hypercalciuria? Thiazides:

    a. bind calcium in the intestinal tract.

    b. cause intracellular volume depletion.

    c. augment calcium reabsorption in the proximal tubule.

    d. directly inhibit calcium absorption.

    e. restore normal serum 1,25-(OH)$_2$ vitamin D levels.

28. Which of the following are potential side effects of treatment with thiazides?

    a. Hypokalemia

    b. Hypocitraturia

    c. Hyperuricemia

    d. Hypomagnesuria

    e. All of the above

29. The primary defect in patients with absorptive hypercalciuria is considered to be:

    a. hyperabsorption of intestinal calcium.

    b. hypersecretion of PTH.

    c. renal leak of calcium.

    d. bone disease.

    e. excessive dietary intake of calcium-containing foods.

30. After 18 months of chlorthalidone treatment, a patient with hypercalciuria is doing well with no further stone formation. However, 8 months later, while still on thiazides, she passed a small stone. The most likely cause of her recurrent stone formation is:

    a. excessive intake of dietary calcium.

    b. inappropriate fluid management.

    c. excessive sodium intake.

    d. thiazide-induced hypocitraturia.

    e. cessation of medications.

31. A patient with absorptive hypercalciuria is continued on chlorthalidone and potassium citrate without problems for 18 months and then passes two stones spontaneously. She claimes that she is still on her medications. The most likely cause of her continued stone formation is:

    a. excessive calcium intake.

    b. heterogeneous nucleation of calcium oxalate.

    c. high dietary sodium intake.

    d. bone mobilization of calcium.

    e. exacerbation of intestinal calcium absorption.

32. The metabolic condition in a patient with absorptive hypercalciuria type II is:

    a. a less severe form of absorptive hypercalciuria type I.

    b. controlled by a calcium-restricted diet.

    c. not characterized by a renal leak of calcium.

    d. characterized by an increased intestinal absorption of calcium.

    e. all of the above.

33. The most appropriate treatment in a patient with absorptive hypercalciuria type II may include all of the following EXCEPT:

    a. moderate intake of high calcium-containing foods.

    b. limit sodium intake.

    c. increase fluids to maintain urine volumes greater than 2 L/day.

    d. restrict dietary oxalate.

    e. begin potassium citrate.

34. The metabolic abnormality most commonly seen after Roux-en-Y gastric bypass surgery is:

    a. hypercalcuria.

    b. gouty diathesis.

    c. hyperuricosuria.

    d. hyperoxaluria.

    e. hypomagnesemia.

Imaging

1. A 50-year-old woman with chronic left back pain undergoes an intravenous urogram (IVU) depicted in Figure 52-1A (Scout film) and Figure 52-1B (3 minute excretory film). A spiral computed tomography (CT) scan (not shown) shows the filling defects depicted to measure 400 Hounsfield units. These findings are most suggestive of:

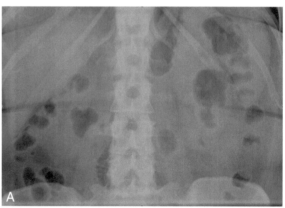

Scout

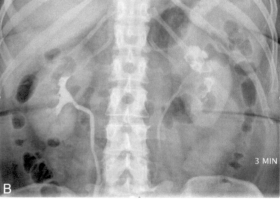

Excretory phase

Figure 52-1.

a. urothelial carcinoma.

b. uric acid calculi.

c. calcium oxalate calculi.

d. blood clots.

e. drug calculi.

ANSWERS

1. **b. Calcium oxalate.** Patients with enteric hyperoxaluria are more likely to form calcium oxalate stones, owing to increased urinary excretion of oxalate and decreased inhibitory activity from hypocitraturia, secondary to chronic metabolic acidosis and hypomagnesuria. In addition, fluid loss from persistent diarrhea from inflammatory bowel disease may cause an extremely concentrated environment suitable for stone formation.

2. **e. Increased colonic absorption of free oxalate.** Intestinal hyperabsorption of oxalate in patients with enteric hyperoxaluria is the most significant risk factor leading to recurrent calculus formation. Intestinal transport of oxalate is primarily increased because of the effects of bile salts and fatty acids on the permeability of colonic intestinal mucosa to oxalate. The total amount of oxalate absorbed may also be increased because of an enlarged intraluminal pool of oxalate available for absorption. Intestinal fat malabsorption characteristic of ileal disease will exaggerate calcium soap formation, limit the amount of "free" calcium to complex to oxalate, and thereby raise the oxalate pool available for absorption.

3. **e. All of the above.** Acid-base status is probably the most important factor in the renal handling of citrate. Hypokalemia with its induced intracellular acidosis (caused by bicarbonate loss from chronic diarrhea) will reduce urinary citrate by both enhancing renal tubular resorption and reducing the synthesis of citrate. Therefore, in patients with enteric hyperoxaluria in whom bicarbonate loss and hypokalemia both contribute to metabolic acidosis, the hypocitraturia is often profound.

4. **a. Calcium supplements, potassium citrate, and increased oral fluid intake.** The initial goals of medical management are to rehydrate and reverse metabolic acidosis. Hydration is at times difficult in some patients because an increase in oral fluids may exacerbate diarrhea. Hydration and potassium citrate will contribute to the reversal of the metabolic acidosis, as well as enhance the excretion of citrate to increase its inhibitory effects on stone formation. Calcium supplements will bind excess oxalate within the intestine, thereby reducing intestinal oxalate absorption. Calcium citrate may offer an ideal calcium supplement in this condition because it should reduce urinary oxalate and increase urinary citrate. Thiazides may worsen metabolic acidosis and hypokalemia through their diuretic effects and renal potassium losses. Colon resection may be of benefit in those patients refractory to medical management because the primary site of intestinal absorption of oxalate is the large bowel.

5. **b. Low urinary pH.** Although low urine volumes and hyperuricosuria contribute to the possibility of uric acid stone formation, the most critical determinant of the crystallization of uric acid remains urinary pH. In addition, uric acid stones may be formed in patients with primary gout with associated severe hyperuricosuria and other secondary causes of purine overproduction such as myeloproliferative states, glycogen storage disease, and malignancy.

6. **a. Urine pH.** Patients with gouty diathesis and uric acid stones will characteristically have urinary pH lower than the dissociation constant for uric acid (5.5). In fact, many will have a urine pH consistently close to 5. Whereas serum and urine uric acid levels may be elevated in patients with uric acid calculi, the urine pH remains the most cost-effective means of screening for this condition and monitoring therapy.

7. **e. Potassium citrate.** Allopurinol will decrease the production of uric acid by inhibiting xanthine oxidase in the purine metabolic pathway but is most effective in patients with extremely elevated levels of uric acid (urinary uric acid >1500 mg/day). In addition, increasing total urine volume will decrease the concentration of uric acid to assist in preventing stone formation. However, raising the urinary pH above the dissociation constant of uric acid is the key to preventing recurrent uric acid stone formation and correcting gouty diathesis. The urine pH should be maintained between 6.0 and 6.5. Thiazides and calcium restriction have limited roles in the medical treatment of uric acid stone patients.

8. **c. Increased solubility of uric acid.** With adequate alkali therapy, this patient has been able to raise the urine pH above the dissociation constant of uric acid. The solubility of uric acid is more than 10 times greater at a pH of 7 than at a pH of 5. Therefore patients may initially present with low/normal 24-hour urinary uric acid levels because the uric acid will precipitate out of solution in the acid urinary environment. Once the urine has been alkalized, all of the uric acid will come back into solution, causing a significant increase in the measured urinary uric acid.

9. **d. Excess alkalization.** Excessive alkalization with urinary pH values above 7.0 may result in calcium phosphate stone formation. Alkali therapy with potassium citrate should aim to keep the urinary pH between 6.5 and 7.0 when treating patients with gouty diathesis.

10. **a. Sodium-inhibiting calcium reabsorption in the proximal tubule.** Patients treated with sodium alkali will occasionally begin forming calcium oxalate stones due to an excess sodium load that will inhibit reabsorption of calcium in the proximal tubule, thereby causing hypercalciuria. In addition, heterogeneous nucleation of calcium oxalate induced by monosodium urate may occur in those individuals with hyperuricosuria. Thus potassium-based alkali, usually in the form of potassium citrate, is the treatment of choice for patients with gouty diathesis.

11. **c. Magnesium ammonium phosphate.** Ascending urinary tract infections with urea-splitting organisms such as *Proteus* species will metabolize urea to ammonia. Ammoniuria, in conjunction with a matrix composed of organic compounds, carbonate apatite, inflammatory cells, and bacteria, results in the rapid formation of an "infection" calculus, eventually progressing into a mineralized, dense stone. Bacteria trapped within the stone perpetuate the recurrent urinary tract infections, and further stone formation eventually develops into the classic staghorn calculus.

12. **b. Recurrent urinary tract infections.** Etiologic factors involved with infection calculi include a history of recurrent urinary tract infections and potential anatomic or physiologic abnormalities. It is important to remember that these patients may also have underlying metabolic disorders such as hypercalciuria, which could contribute to the stone formation. These disorders are most commonly found in patients with mixed stone composition (i.e., struvite and calcium calculi). A comprehensive metabolic evaluation is warranted in these patients.

13. **a. Orthophosphate.** "Struvite stones," "infection stones," or "triple-phosphate stones" all refer to calculi composed of magnesium ammonium phosphate or carbonate apatite. Because phosphate is a major component of these two salts, phosphate therapy would be contraindicated in cases of infection calculi because this medication may promote further stone formation.

14. **d. Irreversibly inhibiting urease.** Acetohydroxamic acid (AHA), a competitive inhibitor of the bacterial enzyme urease, will reduce the urinary saturation of struvite and retard stone formation. When given at a dose of 250 mg orally three times a day, this medication can prevent the recurrence of new stones and inhibit the growth of existing stones in patients with chronic urea-splitting infections. AHA can also cause dissolution of

small stones. However, up to 30% of patients will experience minor side effects including headache, nausea, vomiting, anemia, rash, and alopecia. In addition, 15% of patients have developed deep venous thrombosis while on long-term treatment. Therefore careful monitoring is required when using this medication.

15. **e. Cystinuria.** Cystinuria is a complex autosomal recessive disorder of amino acid transport involving cystine, ornithine, lysine, and arginine (COLA). Supersaturation of the urine will occur in patients with the homozygous state. Therefore it is unusual to see a family history with cystine stones, and the age at onset is often in the first or second decade.

16. **b. Increasing the solubility of cystine.** Increasing the solubility of cystine is the mainstay of treating this disorder. Therefore medical therapy is aimed at dissociating cystine into cysteine, which is 200 times more soluble than cystine. Solubility increases dramatically when this disulfide exchange occurs, effectively preventing further stone formation.

17. **d. Has equivalent efficacy at increasing solubility with reduced toxicity compared with D-penicillamine.** D-Penicillamine and α-MPG are equally effective in their ability to decrease urinary cystine levels. However, studies have demonstrated that α-MPG is significantly less toxic than D-penicillamine. Moreover, the side effects that may occur with α-MPG are also less severe. However, if a patient has been doing well on D-penicillamine with no significant complications, there is no need to switch medications.

18. **c. Continued supersaturation of urinary cystine.** The primary goal of medical therapy is to reduce the urinary cystine concentration below the solubility limit of 200 to 250 mg/L of urine. Because many of these patients present at a young age, compliance may be difficult. Even though this patient's cystine excretion has been reduced to 250 mg/day by the α-MPG therapy, his cystine concentration remains greater than 300 mg/L. Therefore a combination of medication along with an increased urine output is essential to reduce the urinary cystine concentration. Long-term follow-up is necessary to ensure urinary cystine beneath the saturation concentration.

19. **c. Inability to reduce the urine pH below 5.3.** Renal tubular acidosis is a clinical syndrome of chronic metabolic acidosis resulting from renal tubular abnormalities while glomerular filtration is relatively well preserved. Although patients may present with many different symptoms and physical findings, renal stone formation is a well-recognized manifestation of distal renal tubular acidosis (dRTA). Patients with the incomplete form of dRTA are not persistently acidemic despite their inability to lower urinary pH with an acid load. These patients are able to compensate for their acidification defect and remain in acid-base balance by increasing ammonia synthesis and ammonium excretion as a buffering mechanism. The initial identification of incomplete dRTA is often a chance finding. Many of these patients will present with recurrent nephrolithiasis or may be referred for evaluation after the discovery of nephrocalcinosis after routine abdominal radiographs. Most patients will have normal serum electrolytes, yet they will have a high-normal urine pH along with significant hypocitraturia. The diagnosis of incomplete dRTA can be confirmed by inadequate urinary acidification after an ammonium chloride loading test.

20. **b. Absorptive hypercalciuria type I.** Urinary citrate is a potent inhibitor of stone formation, particularly in excess of 600 mg/day on a 24-hour urine collection. Hypocitraturia can be a result of any acidotic state because acidosis will cause both decreased endogenous renal citrate production and increased renal tubular absorption of citrate. Hypokalemia induced by thiazide wasting of potassium will cause intracellular metabolic acidosis, thus using citrate and reducing excretion in a manner similar to metabolic acidosis. Chronic diarrheal syndromes promote intestinal loss of alkali and dehydration, resulting in metabolic acidosis and reduced urinary citrate levels.

21. **e. Potassium alkali.** In the past, sodium alkali has been the treatment of choice for chronic therapy in patients with distal renal tubular acidosis. It was given in the form of either sodium bicarbonate or Shohl solution (a combination of sodium citrate and citric acid). Although sodium alkali is beneficial in correcting the acidosis, excess sodium may be detrimental to calcium metabolism, especially with respect to nephrolithiasis. Sodium alkali therapy has been complicated by the development of calcium stones (calcium phosphate or calcium oxalate), especially when the urinary pH is above 7. Potassium citrate has been shown to reduce the excretion of urinary calcium, whereas sodium alkali has no effect on urinary calcium. Therefore potassium alkali, usually in the form of potassium citrate (POLYCITRA-K, ALVA Pharmaceuticals, Mountain View, CA; Urocit-K, Mission Pharmacal Company, Mountain View, CA), is the recommended first-line therapy.

22. **a. Hypercalciuria and hypocitraturia.** Hypocitraturia, commonly seen in patients with distal renal tubular acidosis, promotes the formation of nephrolithiasis due to reduced inhibitory action of urinary citrate. In addition, hypercalciuria will occur due to mobilization of calcium from bone and impaired renal tubular absorption of calcium, both as a result of chronic acidosis.

23. **b. Significantly reduced bone density.** It is well established that metabolic acidosis may cause a negative calcium balance as a result of impaired renal tubular reabsorption of calcium in the proximal tubule, leading to excessive renal loss of calcium. In addition, intestinal calcium absorption is diminished in patients with persistent acidosis. Slow dissolution of bone mineral can also be identified as calcium and phosphate act as buffering mechanisms to correct the acidosis. Chronic acidosis has been cited as a major factor in the genesis of bone disease.

24. **d. Secondary hyperparathyroidism and renal calcium leak.** To confirm the diagnosis of renal hypercalciuria, evidence for secondary hyperparathyroidism and renal leak of calcium must be present. Both of these values can be obtained during the fasting urinary calcium test. Before arrival at the physician's office, it is essential that patients adhere to a calcium- and sodium-restricted diet for at least 12 hours before testing to eliminate the effects of absorbed calcium on fasting calcium excretion. Three hundred mL of distilled water is consumed 12 and 9 hours before the fasting urine collection to ensure adequate hydration. At 7 AM, patients empty their bladder completely, discard the urine, and drink another 600 mL of distilled water. Urine is then collected as a pooled sample for a 2-hour period (7 AM to 9 AM). A fasting serum blood is obtained at the end of the 2-hour period. The serum sample is analyzed for PTH levels. The fasting urine sample is assayed for calcium and creatinine. Fasting urinary calcium is expressed as milligrams per deciliter of glomerular filtrate because it is reflective of renal function. To obtain this value, urinary calcium in milligrams per milligram of creatinine is multiplied by serum creatinine in milligrams per deciliter. Normal fasting urinary calcium is less than 0.11 mg/dL glomerular filtrate.

25. **e. Low or low/normal radial bone density.** Patients with renal hypercalciuria may display a low or low/normal radial bone density. The diminished bone density is a result of the secondary hyperparathyroidism, which causes stimulation of PTH and subsequent production of 1,25-$(OH)_2$ vitamin D. Both PTH and vitamin D will act on bone to mobilize calcium and cause a loss in bone density. Calcium restriction has no effect in managing renal hypercalciuria.

26. **a. Impairment of renal tubular reabsorption of calcium.** The primary abnormality in renal hypercalciuria is an impairment in proximal renal tubular calcium reabsorption. This urinary calcium wasting and subsequent reduction in serum calcium concentration stimulates the production of PTH. As a result, vitamin D synthesis in the kidney is stimulated. Both PTH and vitamin D will increase bone resorption and absorption of intestinal calcium, increasing the circulating concentration and filtered load of calcium. This often causes significant hypercalciuria.

Unlike primary hyperparathyroidism, serum calcium is normal and the state of hyperparathyroidism is secondary.

27. **c. Augment calcium reabsorption in the proximal tubule.** Thiazide is the primary medical treatment of renal hypercalciuria and has been shown to correct the renal leak of calcium by augmenting calcium reabsorption in the distal tubule. In addition, thiazides cause extracellular volume depletion, thereby stimulating proximal tubular reabsorption of calcium. A positive calcium balance ensues, with correction of the secondary hyperparathyroidism.

28. **e. All of the above.** Thiazide diuretics can cause hypokalemia. Symptoms of hypokalemia include muscle cramps and weakness. Consideration should be given to starting patients concurrently on potassium supplementation with potassium citrate, as patients can also become hypocitraturic. It is reasonable to check a basic metabolic panel 1 to 2 weeks after initiating a thiazide to monitor potassium levels. Thiazides can also cause low urinary citrate and magnesium. In addition, they can lead to impaired carbohydrate metabolism and hyperuricemia. A small percentage of patients may also have sexual side effects including decreased libido or erectile dysfunction.

29. **a. Hyperabsorption of intestinal calcium.** The basic abnormality in absorptive hypercalciuria type I is the intestinal hyperabsorption of calcium. The consequent increase in the circulating concentration of calcium enhances the renal filtered load and suppresses parathyroid function. Hypercalciuria results from the combination of increased filtered load and reduced renal tubular reabsorption of calcium, a function of parathyroid suppression. The excessive renal loss of calcium compensates for the high calcium absorption from the intestinal tract and helps to maintain serum calcium in the normal range.

30. **d. Thiazide-induced hypocitraturia.** Intracellular acidosis resulting from thiazide-induced hypokalemia will augment renal tubular reabsorption of citrate with resultant hypocitraturia. The reduction in the inhibitory effects of hypocitraturia may promote further stone formation. Therefore potassium repletion is necessary if long-term thiazide treatment is anticipated. Our potassium supplement of choice is potassium citrate, in either pill or liquid preparations.

31. **c. High dietary sodium intake.** A high dietary sodium intake has two deleterious effects in this case. An excess sodium load will inhibit reabsorption of calcium in the proximal tubule, thereby causing hypercalciuria. Moreover, sodium will block the hypocalciuric action of thiazides. Therefore patients placed on thiazide diuretics for management of hypercalciuria should also be placed on a dietary sodium restriction.

32. **e. All of the above.** Absorptive hypercalciuria type II is believed to be a less severe form of absorptive hypercalciuria type I. Placing a patient on a calcium-restricted diet will normalize his or her urinary calcium excretion. However, patients with hypercalciuria type I have a high urinary calcium excretion despite dietary modifications. Appropriate therapy for absorptive hypercalciuria type II would be to moderate calcium intake and maintain a high fluid intake to maintain urine output greater than 2 L/day. A severe dietary calcium restriction is not indicated because significant dietary modifications may exacerbate stone disease.

33. **d. Restrict dietary oxalate.** Initial treatment of patients diagnosed with absorptive hypercalciuria type II includes moderating dietary calcium intake to reduce the filtered calcium load, increasing fluid intake to maintain urine output greater than 2 L/day, limiting sodium intake to reduce the calciuric effects of sodium on proximal tubular reabsorption of calcium, and initiating potassium citrate to alkalize the urine and reduce calcium stone formation.

34. **d. Hyperoxaluria.** Roux-en-Y gastric bypass has been shown to lead to significantly increased urinary oxalate. Other metabolic abnormalities seen in patients with Roux-en-Y gastric bypass include low urine volumes and hypocitraturia. In contrast, restrictive bariatric surgery such as gastric band or sleeve do not lead to hyperoxaluria. These patients have low urine volumes as their primary metabolic abnormality.

Imaging

1. **b. Uric acid calculi.** The scout radiograph from the IVU (Fig. 52-1A) shows no densely radiopaque calculi. On the excretory images (Fig. 52-1B), there are well-demarcated filling defects with a staghorn configuration in the left renal pelvis and detached round calculi in the mildly hydronephrotic upper pole calyces. Calcium oxalate or cystine calculi should be much more radiopaque on the scout radiograph and would have Hounsfield units above 600. Uric acid calculi are often not seen on a KUB and have densities in the 400 to 600 Hounsfield range, thus making b the most likely possibility. Urothelial carcinoma will not have a smooth and rounded configuration to the filling defects in the collecting system, and their density will be similar to tissue. Drug calculi occur in patients on protease inhibitor therapy for human immunodeficiency virus (HIV) infections. They tend to be tiny in size, cause ureteral obstruction, and are unlikely to be visible on an IVU.

CHAPTER REVIEW

1. First-time stone formers are at a 50% risk for recurrence. Males have both a higher incidence of calculi and a higher recurrence rate.
2. Infection calculi may contain large quantities of endotoxin.
3. A complete urine collection is confirmed by the 24-hour excretion of creatinine. On average 1 mg/kg/hour is excreted.
4. As the phosphate content of the stone increases from calcium oxalate to calcium oxalate/calcium apatite to calcium apatite, the incidence of renal tubular acidosis increases from 5% to 39% and the incidence of primary hyperthyroidism from 2% to 10%. Thus higher phosphate content in stones correlates with an increased incidence of renal tubular acidosis and primary hyperparathyroidism.
5. Obesity increases the risk of nephrolithiasis.
6. Hypercalciuria not associated with hypercalcemia may be subdivided into (1) excess gastrointestinal absorption, (2) renal tubular leak, or (3) normocalcemic hyperparathyroidism.
7. Patients with hyperuricosuria have increased calcium oxalate urolithiasis due to heterogeneous nucleation.
8. Increased protein intake increases the likelihood of renal stones due to increased urinary calcium, oxalate, and uric acid excretion. Moderate calcium ingestion and a reduced sodium diet, when combined with animal protein restriction, reduce calcium stone episodes by approximately 50%.
9. Thiazides may unmask primary hyperparathyroidism by causing a marked rise in serum calcium. They also cause hypocitraturia.
10. Indinavir stones may not be visible on CT.
11. Furosemide-induced nephrolithiasis should always be considered in neonates who develop nephrolithiasis.
12. Children with stones should always be worked up because inborn errors of metabolism may be responsible for the stones in a significant number of patients. The inborn errors of metabolism most commonly found in this circumstance include cystinuria, renal tubular acidosis, and primary hyperoxaluria.
13. Patients with diabetes mellitus may have altered ammonium metabolism resulting in acidic urine that predisposes them to calcium oxalate and/or uric acid calculi.

14. Sulfate content in a 24-hour urine is an indication of the amount of protein intake. Protein intake increases calcium, oxalate, and uric acid excretion.
15. Intestinal fat malabsorption characteristic of ileal disease will exaggerate calcium soap formation, limit the amount of "free" calcium to complex to oxalate, and thereby raise the oxalate pool available for absorption.
16. Acid-base status is probably the most important factor in the renal handling of citrate.
17. The primary site of intestinal absorption of oxalate is the large bowel.
18. The solubility of uric acid is more than 10 times greater at a pH of 7 than at a pH of 5.
19. Sodium alkali therapy has been complicated by the development of calcium stones (calcium phosphate or calcium oxalate), especially when the urinary pH is above 7.

53

Strategies for Nonmedical Management of Upper Urinary Tract Calculi

Brian R. Matlaga and James E. Lingeman

QUESTIONS

1. The best predictor of post–percutaneous nephrolithotomy (PNL) urosepsis is:
   a. preoperative bladder urine culture.
   b. intraoperative bladder urine culture.
   c. stone culture.
   d. preoperative blood culture.
   e. intraoperative blood culture.

2. What is the risk of mortality from an untreated struvite staghorn stone?
   a. Less than 10%
   b. 10% to 30%
   c. 30% to 50%
   d. 50% to 70%
   e. Greater than 70%

3. The increased risk of residual fragments after extracorporeal shockwave lithotripsy (SWL) of large-volume calculi is of particular importance for patients with stones composed of:
   a. brushite.
   b. uric acid.
   c. struvite.
   d. calcium oxalate monohydrate.
   e. calcium oxalate dihydrate.

4. What is the single most important factor when choosing among SWL, ureteroscopic stone removal, and PNL for renal calculi?
   a. Stone composition
   b. Stone location
   c. Anatomic abnormalities
   d. Stone burden
   e. Body habitus

5. What is the preferred treatment for a known brushite stone former harboring a lower pole renal calculus 25 mm in diameter?
   a. SWL
   b. SWL with ureteral stenting
   c. Flexible ureteroscopy with holmium laser lithotripsy
   d. PNL
   e. Laparoscopic pyelolithotomy

6. What is the preferred initial treatment for staghorn calculi?
   a. SWL with ureteral stenting
   b. Flexible ureteroscopy with holmium laser lithotripsy
   c. PNL
   d. Extended pyelolithotomy
   e. Anatrophic nephrolithotomy

7. Which of the following is the most difficult stone composition to fragment with SWL?
   a. Calcium oxalate dihydrate
   b. Calcium oxalate monohydrate
   c. Struvite
   d. Hydroxyapatite
   e. Uric acid

8. What is the preferred treatment approach for a symptomatic 1.5-cm stone in a lower pole calyceal diverticulum?
   a. SWL
   b. Flexible ureteroscopy
   c. PNL
   d. PNL with fulguration of the diverticulum
   e. Laparoscopic diverticulectomy

9. What is the preferred initial treatment for a 10-mm stone in the renal pelvis of a horseshoe kidney with minimal hydronephrosis?
   a. SWL
   b. Flexible ureteroscopy
   c. PNL
   d. Laparoscopic pyelolithotomy
   e. Symphysiotomy with pyelolithotomy

10. What is the preferred treatment approach for a 10-mm renal calculus in a patient who weighs 375 lb?
   a. SWL
   b. Flexible ureteroscopy
   c. PNL
   d. SWL using the "blast path" technique
   e. Open surgery

11. What is the preferred treatment option for a patient with a symptomatic 1.5-cm renal calculus and a coagulopathy?
   a. SWL
   b. SWL after administration of fresh-frozen plasma
   c. Indwelling ureteral stent
   d. Flexible ureteroscopy
   e. PNL

12. Residual fragments after SWL have been associated with which of the following?
   a. Hypertension
   b. An increased rate of recurrent stones
   c. A decreased rate of recurrent stones
   d. Perinephric hematomas
   e. Hematuria

13. What is the most sensitive test for identifying residual fragments after PNL?

    a. Nephrotomography

    b. Magnetic resonance imaging (MRI)

    c. Ultrasonography

    d. Noncontrast computed tomography (CT)

    e. Contrast-enhanced CT

14. Factors affecting the probability of spontaneous passage of ureteral calculi include all of the following EXCEPT:

    a. stone size.

    b. stone location at presentation.

    c. stone composition.

    d. degree of hydronephrosis.

    e. duration of symptoms.

15. Irreversible loss of renal function can occur within what time period when a completely obstructing ureteral stone is present?

    a. 1 week

    b. 2 to 4 weeks

    c. 4 to 6 weeks

    d. More than 6 weeks

    e. 3 months

16. A first-time stone former is diagnosed with a 4-mm proximal ureteral calculus. The best initial management is:

    a. ureteroscopic laser lithotripsy.

    b. ureteral stent placement.

    c. SWL.

    d. expectant management.

    e. SWL with ureteral stent placement.

17. Large-volume matrix calculi, which form as a consequence of urinary tract infection, are:

    a. effectively fragmented with SWL.

    b. best approached in a ureteroscopic fashion.

    c. generally sterile.

    d. radiopaque and well visualized on plain radiographic studies.

    e. most efficiently treated with PNL.

18. Ureteral stent placement when SWL is performed for ureteral stones is appropriate for all of the following reasons EXCEPT:

    a. solitary kidney.

    b. relief of severe symptoms.

    c. enhancement of stone fragmentation.

    d. relief of obstruction.

    e. aid in localization of difficult-to-visualize stones.

19. The preferred single agent for medical expulsive therapy for distal ureteral calculi is:

    a. nifedipine.

    b. tamsulosin.

    c. Solu-Medrol.

    d. ibuprofen.

    e. terazosin.

20. The treatment modality associated with the greatest stone-free rates and the least morbidity for patients with distal ureteral stones of any size is:

    a. PNL.

    b. SWL.

    c. ureteroscopy.

    d. open ureterolithotomy.

    e. laparoscopic ureterolithotomy.

ANSWERS

1. **c. Stone culture.** The best predictor of post-PNL urosepsis is stone culture or renal pelvic urine culture results.

2. **b. 10% to 30%.** The 10-year mortality rate of untreated staghorn stones was 28%, versus 7.2% in patients treated with surgery.

3. **c. Struvite.** Struvite stones must be removed completely to minimize the risk of continued urea-splitting bacteriuria.

4. **d. Stone burden.** Stone burden (size and number) is perhaps the single most important factor in deciding the appropriate treatment modality for a patient with kidney calculi.

5. **d. PNL.** The Lower Pole Stone Study Group compared ureteroscopy and PNL for patients with 10- to 25-mm lower pole stones and found a significant difference in stone clearance, with only 40% of the ureteroscopic cohort stone free at 3 months versus 76% of the PNL cohort.

6. **c. PNL.** The management of staghorn stones with a combined approach must be viewed as primarily percutaneous, with SWL being used only as adjunct to minimize the number of accesses required.

7. **b. Calcium oxalate monohydrate.** Cystine and brushite are the stones most resistant to SWL, followed by calcium oxalate monohydrate. Next, in descending order, are hydroxyapatite, struvite, calcium oxalate dihydrate, and uric acid stones.

8. **d. PNL with fulguration of the diverticulum.** The percutaneous approach for the management of patients with calyceal diverticular stones provides the patient with the best chance of becoming stone and symptom free. Fulguration of the diverticulum will reduce the risk of recurrence of the diverticulum.

9. **a. SWL.** SWL can achieve satisfactory results in properly selected patients, such as those with small stones (<1.5 cm) in the presence of normal urinary drainage. For larger stones, or when there is evidence of poor urinary drainage, PNL should be used as the primary approach.

10. **b. Flexible ureteroscopy.** Retrograde ureteroscopic intrarenal surgery may be the preferred modality of treatment for morbidly obese patients when the stone burden is not excessively large.

11. **d. Flexible ureteroscopy.** When anticoagulation cannot be temporarily discontinued, the use of ureteroscopy in combination with holmium laser lithotripsy is preferred. One study reported that even when patients' coagulopathies were not fully corrected the stones could be successfully treated with no increase in hemorrhagic complications.

12. **b. An increased rate of recurrent stones.** At follow-up (1.6 to 85.4 months), 43% of the patients with residual fragments had a significant symptomatic episode or required intervention.

13. **d. Noncontrast computed tomography (CT).** Although flexible nephroscopy is often considered the "gold standard" for assessing

residual stones after PNL, the routine use of flexible nephroscopy has been challenged by studies showing the high sensitivity of noncontrast CT in detecting residual stones. Noncontrast CT had 100% sensitivity for detecting residual stones after PNL in 36 patients evaluated by both CT and flexible nephroscopy.

14. **c. Stone composition.** One study analyzed 75 patients with ureteral calculi and found that the interval to stone passage was highly variable and dependent on stone size, location, and side. Stones that were smaller, more distal, and on the right side were more likely to pass spontaneously. In another study, duration of symptoms before presentation was the most influential factor, followed by the degree of hydronephrosis.

15. **b. 2 to 4 weeks.** Even with complete ureteral obstruction, irreversible loss of renal function does not occur for more than 2 weeks but can progress to total renal unit loss at up to 6 weeks.

16. **d. Expectant management.** The majority of ureteral stones less than 5 mm will pass spontaneously and therefore can be treated with expectant management.

17. **e. Most efficiently treated with PNL.** Matrix stones are most effectively treated with PNL. SWL is usually ineffective because of the stone's gelatinous nature, and ureteroscopy may be compromised by the large volume of stone material present.

18. **c. Enhancement of stone fragmentation.** Although early reports supported the routine use of a ureteral stent to bypass ureteral stones before SWL, data analyzed by the American Urological Association Ureteral Calculi Guidelines Panel showed no improvement in fragmentation with stenting, and therefore routine stent placement before SWL was discouraged. However, ureteral stent placement is appropriate for other indications, such as management of pain, relief of obstruction, and stones that are difficult to visualize, and is mandatory in a patient who has a solitary obstructed kidney.

19. **b. Tamsulosin.** Tamsulosin, a selective α-adrenergic blocker, is the preferred agent for medical expulsive therapy, owing to its reported efficacy and superior side effect profile.

20. **c. Ureteroscopy.** The stone-free rate for distal ureteral stones approached with ureteroscopy was 91% in the American Urological Association/European Association of Urology Ureteral Stones Guidelines document, an outcome superior to SWL.

CHAPTER REVIEW

1. Determinants of poor stone clearance rates after SWL include large renal calculi, lower pole or obstructed portions of the collecting system, very hard stones, and obesity.
2. Most calyceal stones in the absence of intervention are likely to increase in size and cause pain or infection.
3. If left untreated, staghorn calculi are likely to be associated with a progressive decrease in renal function.
4. Patients with cystinuria are more likely to have decreased renal function than other stone formers.
5. There is a linear correlation between Hounsfield units (density) and success of SWL.
6. Complete stone clearance from lower pole calyces is less likely than from other calyces for reasons that are not totally clear.
7. Spontaneous passage of a distal ureteral stone is more likely than that of a proximal ureteral stone.
8. For patients with proximal ureteral stones, there is no difference between treating the stone in situ or pushing it back into the renal pelvis when utilizing SWL.
9. In humans, there is no clear time threshold for irreversible damage in complete ureteral obstruction. It is clear, however, that patients with compromised vasculature, decreased renal reserve, poor nutrition, and other comorbid diseases such as diabetes, tolerate obstruction less well than patients with normal kidneys. Most agree that a significantly obstructing stone should not be allowed to persist beyond 2 to 4 weeks.
10. Untreated staghorn calculi are associated with recurrent urinary tract infections, urosepsis, renal function deterioration, and increased mortality.
11. Renal stones <1 cm are best treated with SWL or ureterorenoscopic extraction; stones between 1 and 2 cm which are not in the lower pole are best treated with SWL or PNL; stones >2 cm are best treated with PNL.
12. Matrix renal stones are best removed with PNL.
13. Alpha blockers increase the rate of spontaneous passage of ureteral stones. Tamsulosin, a selective α-adrenergic blocker, is the preferred agent for medical expulsive therapy.
14. Bacteria may reside deep in the stone and may be impossible to eradicate without complete stone removal.
15. Medications responsible for producing stones include ephedrine, indinavir, triamterene, magnesium trisilicate, ciprofloxacin, and sulfa drugs.
16. The best predictor of post-PNL urosepsis is stone culture or renal pelvic urine culture results.
17. Stone burden (size and number) is perhaps the single most important factor in deciding the appropriate treatment modality for a patient with kidney calculi.
18. Cystine and brushite are the stones most resistant to SWL, followed by calcium oxalate monohydrate.
19. The percutaneous approach for the management of patients with calyceal diverticular stones provides the patient with the best chance of becoming stone and symptom free.
20. When anticoagulation cannot be temporarily discontinued, the use of ureteroscopy in combination with holmium laser lithotripsy is preferred.
21. The majority of ureteral stones less than 5 mm will pass spontaneously.
22. Pregnant women who require admission and require treatment for renal colic have a greater risk of preterm delivery.
23. Pregnancy induces a state of absorptive hypercalciuria and mild hyperuricosuria that is offset by increased excretion of urinary inhibitors such as citrate and magnesium, as well as increased urinary output.
24. SWL is now known to induce acute structural changes in the treated kidney in most, if not all, patients. The insult is primarily a vascular injury.
25. Uncorrected coagulopathy and an active, untreated urinary tract infection are two absolute contraindications to PNL.
26. Physiologic solutions should be used for irrigation during PNL to minimize the risk of dilutional hyponatremia in the event of large-volume extravasation.

54

Surgical Management for Upper Urinary Tract Calculi

Brian R. Matlaga, Amy E. Krambeck, and James E. Lingeman

QUESTIONS

1. Renal colic during pregnancy is associated with which of the following?
   a. Increased risk of preterm delivery
   b. Urinary tract infection
   c. Renal dysfunction
   d. Increased rate of spontaneous stone passage
   e. A lack of clinical symptoms

2. Metabolic changes associated with pregnancy that are relevant to urolithiasis include all of the following EXCEPT:
   a. absorptive hypercalciuria.
   b. hypercalcemia.
   c. hyperuricosuria.
   d. increased citrate excretion.
   e. increased magnesium excretion.

3. What is the preferred initial diagnostic study for suspected urolithiasis in pregnant patients?
   a. Kidney, ureter, and bladder radiograph (KUB)
   b. Tailored intravenous pyelography (i.e., two or three films)
   c. Renal ultrasonography
   d. Spiral computed tomography (CT)
   e. magnetic resonance imaging (MRI)

4. All of the following treatments of an obstructing ureteral calculus in a pregnant woman are acceptable EXCEPT:
   a. ureteroscopy.
   b. placement of a double-J ureteral stent.
   c. placement of a nephrostomy drain.
   d. shockwave lithotripsy (SWL).
   e. All of the above are acceptable interventions.

5. The risk of ureteral perforation is greatest with which of the following intracorporeal lithotripsy technologies?
   a. Electrohydraulic lithotripsy (EHL)
   b. Holmium laser
   c. Pulsed-dye laser
   d. Ultrasonic lithotripsy
   e. Ballistic lithotripsy

6. The risk of retrograde stone propulsion is greatest with which of the following intracorporeal lithotripsy technologies?
   a. EHL
   b. Holmium laser
   c. Pulsed dye laser
   d. Ultrasonic lithotripsy
   e. Ballistic lithotripsy

7. What are the preferred initial power settings for holmium laser lithotripsy of ureteral stones?
   a. 0.6 J, 6 Hz
   b. 0.6 J, 10 Hz

   c. 1.0 J, 10 Hz
   d. 1.2 J, 10 Hz
   e. 1.0 J, 15 Hz

8. Which intracorporeal lithotripsy technology will most efficiently fragment and evacuate renal calculi?
   a. Ultrasonic lithotripsy
   b. Ballistic lithotripsy
   c. Combination ultrasonic/ballistic lithotripsy
   d. Holmium laser
   e. EHL

9. Which intracorporeal lithotripsy technology has the least risk of ureteral perforation?
   a. Ultrasound
   b. Ballistic
   c. Holmium laser
   d. EHL
   e. Erbium laser

10. Energy sources for SWL include all of the following EXCEPT:
    a. electrohydraulic.
    b. holmium laser.
    c. piezoelectric.
    d. electromagnetic.
    e. microexplosive.

11. What is a major disadvantage of ultrasound imaging for SWL?
    a. Inability to visualize ureteropelvic junction (UPJ) stones
    b. Exposure to ionizing radiation
    c. Inability to visualize radiolucent stones
    d. Expense of ultrasonography systems
    e. Inability to visualize ureteral stones

12. Factors influencing the amount of pain during SWL include all but which of the following?
    a. Power level applied
    b. Stone composition
    c. Type of shockwave generator
    d. Shockwave energy density at the point of skin penetration
    e. Stone location

13. Which lithotripter produces the highest stone-free rates?
    a. Wolf Piezolith 2300
    b. Siemens Lithostar
    c. Modified Dornier HM3
    d. Unmodified Dornier HM3
    e. HealthTronics LithoTron

14. Possible mechanisms producing stone fragmentation during SWL include all of the following EXCEPT:
    a. compression fracture.
    b. spallation.

c. acoustic cavitation.

d. dynamic fatigue.

e. vaporization.

15. What percentage of kidneys experience trauma during SWL?

   a. 0% to 20%

   b. 20% to 40%

   c. 40% to 60%

   d. 60% to 80%

   e. 80% to 100%

16. Risk factors that will enhance the bioeffects of shockwaves include all of the following EXCEPT:

   a. patient age older than 60 years.

   b. pediatric age.

   c. stone burden.

   d. preexisting hypertension.

   e. reduced renal mass.

17. The primary insult to the kidney exposed to shockwaves occurs in which of the following tissues?

   a. Blood vessels

   b. Proximal tubule

   c. Renal papillae

   d. Glomerulus

   e. Renal capsule

18. Which anesthetic technique is associated with the greatest likelihood of a successful SWL treatment outcome?

   a. General endotracheal

   b. Intravenous sedation

   c. Epidural

   d. Sedation

   e. Topical anesthetic

19. Which of the following is an absolute contraindication to PNL?

   a. Morbid obesity

   b. Uncorrected coagulopathy

   c. Neurogenic bladder

   d. Pelvic kidney

   e. Horseshoe kidney

20. Which treatment maneuver will reduce the likelihood of SWL-induced renal injury?

   a. Begin treatment at a high energy level

   b. Treat at a rate of 120 shocks per minute

   c. Treat with a topical local anesthetic

   d. Pretreat the targeted kidney at a low energy level and then ramp up treatment to a high energy level

   e. Pretreat the contralateral kidney at a high energy level and then ramp up treatment of the target kidney to a high energy level

21. What is the most common secondarily infecting organism after percutaneous stone removal?

   a. *Proteus mirabilis*

   b. *Klebsiella oxytoca*

   c. *Pseudomonas aeruginosa*

   d. *Staphylococcus epidermidis*

   e. *Enterococcus (Streptococcus) faecalis*

22. Which of the following is the antimicrobial of choice for ureteroscopy?

   a. First-generation cephalosporin

   b. Second-generation cephalosporin

   c. Aminoglycoside

   d. Fluoroquinolone

   e. Nitrofurantoin

23. What is the preferred site of puncture into the renal collecting system during access for PNL?

   a. Upper pole infundibulum

   b. Anterior lower pole calyx

   c. Posterior lower pole calyx

   d. Upper pole calyx

   e. Renal pelvis

24. Risk factors for colon injury during PNL include all of the following EXCEPT:

   a. horseshoe kidney.

   b. kyphoscoliosis.

   c. access lateral to the posterior axillary line.

   d. previous jejunoileal bypass for obesity.

   e. upper pole puncture.

25. To minimize the risk of lung and pleura injury during supracostal upper pole access for PNL:

   a. the puncture should be performed during full expiration.

   b. the puncture should be performed during full inspiration.

   c. CO_2 should be injected through the ureteral catheter to identify the upper pole calyx.

   d. the puncture should be done with local anesthesia.

   e. the puncture should be performed by a radiologist.

26. Indications for supracostal access during PNL include all of the following EXCEPT:

   a. predominant stone distribution in the upper pole.

   b. access to the UPJ or proximal ureter required.

   c. cystine stones.

   d. multiple lower pole infundibula and calyces containing stone material.

   e. horseshoe kidneys.

27. When performing PNL and endopyelotomy in the same setting, the optimal point of entry is:

   a. posterior upper pole calyx.

   b. posterior lower pole calyx.

   c. anterior upper pole calyx.

   d. anterior lower pole calyx.

   e. renal pelvis.

28. During access for PNL, what is the preferred initial wire?

   a. Amplatz Super-stiff

   b. Benson

   c. Hydrophilic glide

   d. Lunderquist

   e. J-tipped movable core

29. What is the most common serious error in PNL access?

   a. Not using an Amplatz sheath

   b. Overadvancement of the dilator/sheath

   c. Anterior calyceal puncture

d. Ultrasonographically guided puncture

e. The use of telescoping metal dilators

30. What is the appropriate irrigating solution for PNL?

a. 3% sorbitol

b. Sterile water

c. Glycine

d. Dilute contrast material

e. 0.9% saline

31. Middle or upper pole access for PNL in horseshoe kidneys is preferred for all of the following reasons EXCEPT:

a. a higher incidence of retrorenal colon.

b. malrotation of the renal collecting system.

c. incomplete ascent of horseshoe kidneys.

d. anterior medial location of lower pole calyces.

e. facilitated access to the UPJ or upper ureter.

32. What is the most significant complication of PNL?

a. Hemorrhage

b. Extravasation of irrigation fluid

c. Incomplete stone removal

d. Urinary tract infection

e. Pleural effusion

33. What is the risk of arteriovenous fistula formation after PNL?

a. 1 in 10

b. 1 in 100

c. 1 in 200

d. 1 in 500

e. 1 in 1000

34. If uncontrolled bleeding persists after nephrostomy tube placement after PNL, what would the preferred approach be?

a. Insertion of a double-J stent

b. Administration of furosemide (Lasix) to promote diuresis

c. Surgical exploration

d. Immediate angiography

e. Insertion of a Kaye tamponade balloon

35. If a retroperitoneal injury to the colon is diagnosed after PNL, what is the preferred management?

a. Surgical exploration and repair

b. Diverting colostomy with later definitive repair

c. Leaving the nephrostomy tube in for 2 weeks to allow the tract to mature

d. Insertion of a double-J stent and withdrawal of the nephrostomy tube into the colon

e. Immediate removal of the nephrostomy tube

36. The use of double-J stents to reduce the risk of steinstrasse after SWL has been demonstrated to be beneficial for what size of stones?

a. Greater than 5 mm

b. Greater than 10 mm

c. Greater than 15 mm

d. Greater than 20 mm

e. Greater than 25 mm

37. Proper management of a stone trapped in a basket, with an avulsed ureter all in continuity and no safety guidewire in place, is:

a. immediate surgical exploration and primary repair.

b. cystoscopy to place a guidewire and ureteral stent.

c. placement of a percutaneous nephrostomy drain.

d. immediate ureteral reimplantation.

e. immediate ileal ureter.

38. During the course of a ureteroscopic laser lithotripsy procedure for a 1-cm proximal ureteral stone, a ureteral perforation is noted after fragmentation and removal of the calculus. On inspection of the perforation, a stone fragment is noted outside the ureter in the retroperitoneum. The most appropriate management is to:

a. terminate the procedure and place a ureteral stent.

b. advance the ureteroscope into the retroperitoneum and remove the stone fragment with a basket device.

c. place a nephrostomy tube.

d. perform laparoscopic exploration and removal of the residual fragment.

e. advance the ureteroscope into the retroperitoneum and fragment the stone with the holmium:YAG laser.

ANSWERS

1. **a. Increased risk of preterm delivery.** Pregnant women who require admission and require treatment for renal colic have a greater risk of preterm delivery compared with pregnant women who do not suffer from renal calculi.

2. **b. Hypercalcemia.** Pregnancy induces a state of absorptive hypercalciuria and mild hyperuricosuria that is offset by increased excretion of urinary inhibitors such as citrate and magnesium, as well as increased urinary output. The metabolic changes in pregnancy do not influence the rate of new stone occurrence. However, paradoxically, it has been suggested that metabolic alterations in urine may contribute to accelerated encrustation of stents during pregnancy.

3. **c. Renal ultrasonography.** To avoid the small risk of radiation, ultrasonography has become the first-line diagnostic study for urolithiasis in pregnancy.

4. **d. Shockwave lithotripsy.** Shockwave lithotripsy is not an appropriate treatment for a pregnant woman and should not be performed.

5. **a. Electrohydraulic lithotripsy (EHL).** The major disadvantage of EHL is its propensity to damage the ureteral mucosa and its association with ureteral perforation.

6. **e. Ballistic lithotripsy.** Ballistic lithotripsy is accompanied by a relatively high rate of stone propulsion of between 2% and 17% when ureteral stones are treated. The holmium laser has been associated with a reduced potential for causing retropulsion owing to the weak shockwave that is typically induced during holmium laser lithotripsy.

7. **a. 0.6 J, 6 Hz.** It is recommended to begin treatment using low pulse energy (i.e., 0.6 J) with a pulse rate of 6 Hz and increase the pulse frequency (in preference to increasing the pulse energy) as needed to speed fragmentation.

8. **c. Combination ultrasonic/ballistic lithotripsy.** Combination ultrasonic and ballistic lithotrites have been reported to provide greater stone clearance rates than do conventional ultrasonic or ballistic lithotrites.

9. **b. Ballistic.** When compared with EHL or ultrasonic or laser lithotripsy, ballistic devices have a significantly lower risk of ureteral perforation.

10. **b. Holmium laser.** There are three primary types of shockwave generators: electrohydraulic (spark gap), electromagnetic, and piezoelectric. Microexplosive generators have also been produced but have not gained mainstream acceptance.

11. **e. Inability to visualize ureteral stones.** Sonographic localization of a kidney stone requires a highly trained operator. Furthermore, localization of stones in the ureter is difficult or impossible.

12. **b. Stone composition.** The discomfort experienced during SWL is related directly to the energy density of the shockwave as it

passes through the skin as well as the size of the focal point, parameters that are affected by all of the choices listed except for stone composition.

13. **d. Unmodified Dornier HM3 (Dornier MedTech).** To date, despite the proliferation of lithotripters and the variety of solutions devised for stone targeting and shockwave delivery, no other lithotripter system has convincingly equaled or surpassed the results produced by the unmodified Dornier HM3 device.

14. **e. Vaporization.** Several potential mechanisms for SWL stone breakage have been described: (1) spall fracture, (2) squeezing, (3) shear stress, (4) superfocusing, (5) acoustic cavitation, and (6) dynamic fatigue.

15. **e. 80% to 100%.** SWL is now known to induce acute structural changes in the treated kidney in most, if not all, patients. Morphologic studies using both MRI and quantitative radionuclide renography have suggested that 63% to 85% of all SWL patients treated with an unmodified Dornier HM3 lithotripter exhibit one or more forms of renal injury within 24 hours of treatment.

16. **c. Stone burden.** Patients with existing hypertension are at increased risk for the development of perinephric hematomas as a consequence of SWL. Age is a factor on both ends of the scale in that children and the elderly both appear to be at a greater risk for structural and functional changes after exposure to shockwaves. These responses are probably related to a reduction in the large renal reserve present in most healthy adult patients.

17. **a. Blood vessels.** Macroscopically, the acute changes noted in dog and pig kidneys treated with a clinical dose of shockwaves are strikingly similar to those described for patients. This lesion is predictable in size, is focal in location, and is unique in the types of injuries (primarily vascular insult) induced. Regions of damage reveal rupture of nearby thin-walled veins, walls of small arteries, and glomerular and peritubular capillaries, which correlates with the vasoconstriction measured in both treated and untreated kidneys. These observations show that both the microvasculature and the nephron are susceptible to shockwave damage; however, the primary injury appears to be a vascular insult.

18. **a. General endotracheal.** Patients undergoing SWL with general endotracheal anesthesia experience a significantly greater stone-free outcome than do patients undergoing SWL with alternative anesthetics.

19. **b. Uncorrected coagulopathy.** Uncorrected coagulopathy and an active, untreated urinary tract infection are two absolute contraindications to PNL.

20. **d. Pretreat the targeted kidney at a low energy level and then ramp up treatment to a high energy level.** A number of studies have demonstrated that pretreating the target kidney with low-energy shockwaves, followed by a full clinical treatment dose, will attenuate the renal injury associated with SWL.

21. **d. *Staphylococcus epidermidis.*** Cephalosporins are the most appropriately used antibiotics for prophylaxis of surgical procedures in noninfected stone cases, because the most common secondarily infecting organism is *S. epidermidis.*

22. **d. Fluoroquinolone.** The prophylactic antimicrobial agent of choice for ureteroscopy is a fluoroquinolone.

23. **c. Posterior lower pole calyx.** Because the posterior calyces are generally oriented so that the long axis points to the avascular area of the renal cortex, a posterolateral puncture directed at a posterior calyx would be expected to traverse through the avascular zone.

24. **e. Upper pole puncture.** A puncture placed too laterally may injure the colon. The position of the retroperitoneal colon is usually anterior or anterolateral to the lateral renal border. Therefore, risk of colon injury is usually only with a very lateral (lateral to the posterior axillary line) puncture. Posterior colonic displacement is more likely in thin female patients with very little retroperitoneal fat and/or elderly patients, as well as in patients with jejunoileal bypass resulting in an enlarged colon. Other factors increasing the risk of colon injury include anterior

calyceal puncture, previous extensive renal operation, horseshoe kidney, and kyphoscoliosis. A retrorenal colon is more frequently noted on the left side.

25. **a. The puncture should be performed during full expiration.** A supracostal puncture should be performed only during full expiration.

26. **c. Cystine stones.** A supracostal puncture is indicated when the predominant distribution of stone material is in the upper calyces, when there is an associated UPJ stricture requiring endopyelotomy, in cases of multiple lower pole infundibula and calyces containing stone material or an associated ureteral stone, in staghorn calculi with substantial upper pole stone burden, and in horseshoe kidneys.

27. **a. Posterior upper pole calyx.** A posterior upper pole calyx puncture, typically through a supracostal approach, aligns the axis of puncture with the UPJ. This allows the treating urologist to perform endopyelotomy with a rigid nephroscope, while exerting minimal torque on the instrument.

28. **c. Hydrophilic glide.** The hydrophilic glide wire is preferred for entering the collecting system, because it is the most flexible and maneuverable wire available.

29. **b. Overadvancement of the dilator/sheath.** Overadvancement of the dilator/sheath is the most common serious error in access for PNL and may result in significant trauma to the renal collecting system and/or excessive hemorrhage.

30. **e. 0.9% saline.** Physiologic solutions should be used for irrigation during PNL to minimize the risk of dilutional hyponatremia in the event of large-volume extravasation.

31. **a. A higher incidence of retrorenal colon.** The optimal point of entry for a horseshoe kidney is through a posterior calyx, which is typically more medial than in the normal kidney because of the altered renal axis and rotation associated with the midline fusion. An upper pole collecting system puncture is often appealing, because the entire kidney is usually subcostal. In most cases the lower pole calyces are anterior and inaccessible percutaneously.

32. **a. Hemorrhage.** Bleeding is the most significant complication of PNL, with transfusion rates varying from less than 1% to 10%.

33. **c. 1 in 200.** Bleeding from an arteriovenous fistula or pseudoaneurysm requiring emergency embolization is seen in less than 0.5% of patients.

34. **e. Insertion of a Kaye tamponade balloon.** If bleeding is not controlled by nephrostomy tube placement and clamping, a Kaye nephrostomy tamponade balloon catheter should be placed (Cook Urological, Spencer, IN). The Kaye nephrostomy tube incorporates a low-pressure 12-mm balloon that may be left inflated for prolonged periods to tamponade bleeding from the nephrostomy tract.

35. **d. Insertion of a double-J stent and withdrawal of the nephrostomy tube into the colon.** Colonic injury is an unusual complication often diagnosed on a postoperative nephrostogram. Typically, the injury is retroperitoneal; thus signs and symptoms of peritonitis are infrequent. If the perforation is extraperitoneal, management may be expectant with placement of a ureteral catheter or double-J stent to decompress the collecting system and by withdrawing the nephrostomy tube from an intrarenal position to an intracolonic position, thus serving as a colostomy tube. The colostomy tube is left in place for a minimum of 7 days and is removed after a nephrostogram or a retrograde pyelogram showing no communication between the colon and the kidney.

36. **d. Greater than 20 mm.** Stents may be particularly advantageous with stones larger than 20 mm.

37. **c. Placement of a percutaneous nephrostomy drain.** Should a ureteral avulsion occur, the patient should undergo immediate diversion of the renal unit with the placement of a percutaneous nephrostomy drain.

38. **a. Terminate the procedure and place a ureteral stent.** When an extruded stone is noted outside the ureter, the procedure should be terminated and a ureteral stent placed.

CHAPTER REVIEW

1. EHL produces a hydraulic shockwave and cavitation bubble. It may be used in normal saline solutions.
2. Holmium laser lithotripsy causes stone vaporization by a photothermal mechanism, and when it is used the stone should be painted.
3. Cyanide may be produced when the holmium laser is used to fragment uric acid calculi. To date no untoward effects due to this have been reported.
4. Ultrasound breaks the stone by causing the stone to resonate at a high frequency. Considerable heat may develop at the interface.
5. Stone comminution occurs by two basic mechanisms: mechanical stresses produced by the incident shockwave and collapse of cavitation bubbles adjacent to the surface of the stone.
6. The entire ureter can be more easily accessed in the female with a rigid ureteroscope.
7. For uncomplicated ureteroscopies, a ureteral stent may be safely omitted.
8. There is a 3% to 6% incidence of ureteral stricture following ureteroscopy; therefore, follow-up imaging should be performed.
9. Struvite stones must be removed completely to minimize the risk of continued urea-splitting bacteriuria.
10. Cystine and brushite are the stones most resistant to SWL, followed by calcium oxalate monohydrate. Next, in descending order, are hydroxyapatite, struvite, calcium oxalate dihydrate, and uric acid stones.
11. When anticoagulation cannot be temporarily discontinued, the use of ureteroscopy in combination with holmium laser lithotripsy is preferred.
12. The majority of ureteral stones less than 5 mm will pass spontaneously.
13. There are three primary types of shockwave generators: electrohydraulic (Spark Gap), electromagnetic, and piezoelectric. Microexplosive generators have also been produced but have not gained mainstream acceptance.
14. Patients with existing hypertension are at increased risk for the development of perinephric hematomas as a consequence of SWL.
15. Cephalosporins are the most appropriately used antibiotics for prophylaxis of surgical procedures in noninfected stone cases, because the most common secondarily infecting organism is *S. epidermidis*.
16. Transvaginal ultrasonography may be used in the pregnant female to observe the lower ureters.
17. Fifty percent to 80% of pregnant patients will spontaneously pass the calculus.
18. Pregnancy induces a state of absorptive hypercalciuria and mild hyperuricosuria that is offset by increased excretion of urinary inhibitors such as citrate and magnesium, as well as increased urinary output. The metabolic changes in pregnancy do not influence the rate of new stone occurrence. However, paradoxically, it has been suggested that metabolic alterations in urine may contribute to accelerated encrustation of stents during pregnancy.

55 Lower Urinary Tract Calculi

Brian M. Benway and Sam B. Bhayani

QUESTIONS

1. Vesical calculus disease is usually associated with what condition in the United States?
   a. Foreign bodies
   b. Urinary tract infections
   c. Catheterization
   d. Bladder outlet obstruction
   e. None of the above

2. Magnesium ammonium phosphate stones are most often formed in association with infection with which bacteria?
   a. *Pseudomonas*
   b. *Providencia*
   c. *Klebsiella*
   d. *Staphylococcus*
   e. *Proteus*

3. Urease-producing bacteria hydrolyze urea into:
   a. uric acid.
   b. carbon monoxide.
   c. carbon dioxide.
   d. ammonium.
   e. carbon dioxide and ammonium.

4. Which continent diversion has the highest risk of stone formation?
   a. Mainz pouch
   b. Kock pouch
   c. Orthotopic hemi-Kock pouch
   d. Indiana pouch
   e. Cecal reservoir

5. Risk factors for the formation of stones in patients with urinary diversions include all of the following EXCEPT:
   a. hypocitruria.
   b. hyperchloremic metabolic acidosis.
   c. hypercalciuria.
   d. hyperoxaluria.
   e. urinary tract infection.

6. What is the most accurate examination to document the presence of a bladder stone?
   a. Ultrasonography
   b. Excretory urography
   c. Computed tomography
   d. Cystoscopy
   e. Plain (kidney/ureter/bladder) radiography

7. Appropriate treatment options for bladder calculi include all of the following EXCEPT:
   a. irrigation with Suby solution G.
   b. shockwave lithotripsy.
   c. electrohydraulic lithotripsy.
   d. ultrasonic lithotripsy.
   e. holmium laser lithotripsy.

8. Urethral calculi in women are associated with which of the following?
   a. Metabolic disturbances
   b. Urethral stricture
   c. Urethral diverticulum
   d. Foreign bodies
   e. None of the above

9. All of the following regarding primary bladder calculi in children are true EXCEPT:
   a. the peak incidence is between the ages of 2 and 4 years.
   b. patients usually present with multiple calculi.
   c. the incidence is much higher in males than females.
   d. formation is associated with low-phosphate diets.
   e. formation is generally not associated with urinary tract infection.

10. Endoscopic management of bladder calculi is considered an acceptable intervention in:
    a. a 26-year-old man with a history of neurogenic bladder who underwent augmentation cystoplasty at the age of 12 years and performs transurethral clean intermittent catheterization.
    b. a 12-year-old girl with myelomeningocele who underwent bladder neck closure and creation of a Mitrofanoff catheterizable stoma at the age of 8 years.
    c. a 76-year-old man with a history of bladder cancer who underwent cystectomy with Indiana pouch diversion.
    d. a 65-year-old woman with a history of bladder cancer who underwent cystectomy with Kock pouch diversion.
    e. a and d.

11. All of the following are true about bladder calculi in augmented bladders EXCEPT:
    a. mean time to first stone formation is 2 to 6 years after augmentation.
    b. catheterization through a Mitrofanoff stoma is associated with an increased risk of stone formation.
    c. males are 3 to 10 times more likely to develop stones than females.
    d. autoaugmentation is associated with a comparatively low risk of bladder stone formation.
    e. All of the above are true.

12. Bladder stone formation in patients who have undergone kidney or pancreatic transplantation has been associated with:
    a. nonabsorbable suture material used for the anastomosis.
    b. incomplete bladder emptying due to diabetic cystopathy.
    c. bacteriuria associated with included duodenal segments.
    d. metabolic acidosis due to bicarbonate leak.
    e. all of the above.

13. Which of the following is(are) typically associated with preputial calculi?

    a. Stranguria

    b. Phimosis

    c. Voided urine culture positive for enterococcus or *Escherichia coli*

    d. a and b.

    e. b and c.

14. Which of the following statements about prostatic calculi is (are) TRUE?

    a. Most prostatic calculi are asymptomatic

    b. Large prostatic calculi most commonly involve the central zone of the prostate

    c. Serum prostate-specific antigen and intraprostatic stone volume are directly correlated

    d. Uric acid is the predominant component of prostatic calculi

    e. All of the above

ANSWERS

1. **d. Bladder outlet obstruction.** Bladder outlet obstruction may be an etiologic factor in more than 75% of bladder calculi cases and is most often related to benign prostatic hyperplasia.

2. **e. *Proteus.*** Whereas all these organisms produce urease, infection with *Proteus* species is most commonly associated with bladder calculi.

3. **e. Carbon dioxide and ammonium.** Urease hydrolyzes urea, forming ammonium and carbon dioxide, which increases urinary pH. Alkaline urine promotes supersaturation and precipitation of crystals of magnesium ammonium phosphate and carbonate apatite.

4. **b. Kock pouch.** The Kock pouch has a 4% to 43% incidence of stone formation. The predominant location of calculi in the Kock pouch is along staple lines of the afferent nipple valve. Substituting polyglycolic mesh for Marlex mesh in collar construction and limiting the number of staples has reduced the incidence of pouch calculi.

5. **d. Hyperoxaluria.** Patients with augments and diversions often have reabsorption of urinary solutes, especially sulfate and ammonium, through the intestinal segment with resultant metabolic disturbances. Chronic hyperchloremic metabolic acidosis may develop that, in turn, can result in hypercalciuria, hyperphosphaturia, hypermagnesuria, and hypocitraturia, predisposing the patient to urinary tract calculi.

6. **d. Cystoscopy.** Cystoscopy is the single most accurate examination to document the presence of a bladder calculus. Cystoscopy also assists in surgical planning by identifying prostatic enlargement, bladder diverticulum, or urethral stricture that may need correction before or in conjunction with the treatment of the stone.

7. **a. Irrigation with Suby solution G (B. Braun Melsungen AG, Bethlehem, PA).** Dissolution as primary treatment for bladder calculi can be protracted and is now rarely used.

8. **c. Urethral diverticulum.** Urethral calculi in females are exceptionally rare because of low rates of bladder calculi and a short urethra that permits passage of many smaller calculi. Calculi in the female urethra are typically associated with urethral diverticulum or urethrocele.

9. **b. Patients usually present with multiple calculi.** Primary bladder calculi in children are generally solitary and, once removed, recurrence is rare. Primary bladder calculi are 9 to 33 times more common in boys and are generally not associated with anatomic, functional, or infectious abnormalities. Cereal diets low in phosphate and animal protein are considered an important risk factor. Dietary modification results in a sharp decrease in stone formation.

10. **e. a and d.** Endoscopic instrumentation is not advised in patients who have undergone continent diversion with Indiana or Penn pouches, or for those with Mitrofanoff catheterizable stomas, because there is a significant risk of injury to the continence mechanisms and the narrow limbs themselves. Although percutaneous intervention is generally advised for the treatment of stones in patients with pouch diversions, the large caliber of the catheterizable limb and the nipple valve of the Kock pouch will tolerate endoscopic instrumentation. Transurethral endoscopic management is generally considered safe in augmented bladders, regardless of the type of substitution performed.

11. **c. Males are 3 to 10 times more likely to develop stones than females.** Unlike the nonaugmented population, females who have undergone augmentation cystoplasty are more likely to develop bladder calculi than males, likely owing to the higher incidence of cloacal abnormalities, which require additional procedures to establish continence. Bladder stone formation is more common in patients who have undergone intestinal substitution, as opposed to gastric and ureteric substitution or autoaugmentation, although the role of intestinal mucus in stone formation remains a matter of debate.

12. **e. All of the above.** All of the above have been found to be associated with bladder stone formation after renal transplantation, as well as pancreatic allografts, which are drained via the bladder. Although scant reports have noted stone formation on absorbable suture, the overwhelming majority of stone formation occurs in the presence of nonabsorbable suture or clip material.

13. **e. b and c.** Stranguria is a common presenting complaint in patients with migratory urethral calculi but is rarely associated with preputial calculi. Rather, progressive voiding complaints are the norm, with rare progression to urinary retention.

14. **a. Most prostatic calculi are asymptomatic.** The vast majority of prostatic calculi are asymptomatic and are an infrequent cause of lower urinary tract symptomatology. The majority of stones are found in the posterior and posterolateral zones of the prostate, and large stones are rarely found within the central zone. Serum prostate-specific antigen levels are unaffected by the presence of prostate calculi. Prostatic calculi are generally composed of calcium phosphate and calcium carbonate, which form on nidi of inspissated prostatic secretions.

CHAPTER REVIEW

1. Clean intermittent catheterization is associated with a significant reduction in risk of bladder stone formation compared with an indwelling catheter.

2. If a spinal cord injury patient has a bladder stone, the risk of a subsequent bladder calculus is markedly increased.

3. The holmium laser is the safest instrument to use to fragment bladder calculi.

4. Bladder outlet obstruction may be an etiologic factor in over 75% of bladder calculi cases and is most often related to benign prostatic hyperplasia.

5. *Proteus* species is the most commonly found organism associated with bladder calculi.

6. Patients with augments and diversions often have reabsorption of urinary solutes, especially sulfate and ammonium, through the intestinal segment with resultant metabolic disturbances. Chronic hyperchloremic metabolic acidosis may develop, which can, in turn, result in hypercalciuria, hyperphosphaturia, hypermagnesuria, and hypocitraturia, predisposing the patient to urinary tract calculi.

7. Primary bladder calculi in children are generally solitary and, once removed, recurrence is rare; cereal diets low in phosphate and animal protein are considered an important risk factor.

8. Endoscopic instrumentation is not advised in patients who have undergone continent diversion with Indiana or Penn pouches or for those with Mitrofanoff catheterizable stomas because there is a significant risk of injury to the continence mechanisms.

9. Prostatic calculi are generally composed of calcium phosphate and calcium carbonate, which form on nidi of inspissated prostatic secretions.

56 Benign Renal Tumors

Vitaly Margulis, Jose A. Karam, Surena F. Matin, and Christopher G. Wood

QUESTIONS

1. The most accurate imaging study to characterize a renal mass is:
   a. intravenous pyelography.
   b. ultrasonography.
   c. computed tomography (CT) with and without contrast enhancement.
   d. magnetic resonance imaging (MRI).
   e. renal arteriography.

2. A hyperdense renal cyst may also be termed a:
   a. probable malignancy.
   b. Bosniak II cyst.
   c. Bosniak III cyst.
   d. Bosniak IV cyst.
   e. probable angiomyolipoma.

3. The primary indication for fine-needle aspiration of a renal mass is which suspected clinical diagnosis?
   a. Renal cell carcinoma
   b. Renal oncocytoma
   c. Renal adenoma
   d. Renal metastasis
   e. Renal angiomyolipoma

4. All of the following statements are TRUE about renal cysts EXCEPT:
   a. They are the most common benign renal lesions found in the kidney.
   b. They are best characterized using the Bosniak criteria to assess risk that the patient harbors a malignancy.
   c. They are best imaged using ultrasound to allow classification with the Bosniak criteria.
   d. They can harbor internal septa, calcifications, and internal debris and still be considered benign according to the Bosniak classification.
   e. They rarely require treatment.

5. Which of the following is TRUE about renal adenoma?
   a. There is uniform agreement regarding the clinical and pathologic classification of renal adenoma.
   b. Recent studies suggest that renal adenoma may be a premalignant precursor of papillary renal cell carcinoma (RCC).
   c. They are most common in young females.

   d. They can be high grade or low grade, as long as they are smaller than 3 cm.
   e. They are usually of clear cell histology but can also be found with chromophobe and papillary cells.

6. A diagnosis of renal adenoma:
   a. can be made primarily on the basis of histologic criteria.
   b. can be rendered only if tumor is smaller than 1 cm.
   c. is commonly made at autopsy.
   d. requires specific immunohistochemical staining.
   e. can be confirmed by electron microscopy.

7. A healthy 62-year-old man is scheduled to undergo surgery for a 3.0-cm enhancing renal mass; CT shows it to be interpolar, exophytic, and with a central stellate scar. Which of the following best describes the most appropriate surgical strategy?
   a. A radical nephrectomy with adrenalectomy
   b. A radical nephrectomy without adrenalectomy
   c. Renal exploration with biopsy and intraoperative frozen section analysis determining radical versus partial nephrectomy
   d. Renal exploration and partial nephrectomy with intraoperative frozen section analysis of histology (if malignant, a radical nephrectomy)
   e. Partial nephrectomy

8. A 48-year-old woman with a history of seizure disorder presents with recurrent gross hematuria and left flank pain. Abdominal CT shows a large left perinephric hematoma associated with a 3.0-cm left renal angiomyolipoma. There are also multiple right renal angiomyolipomas ranging in size from 1.5 to 6.5 cm. The next best step in management of the left renal lesion is:
   a. selective embolization.
   b. radical nephrectomy.
   c. observation.
   d. partial nephrectomy.
   e. laparoscopic exposure and renal cryoablation.

9. Which of the following statements is TRUE regarding multiloculated cystic nephromas?
   a. They are complex cystic lesions that are typically classified as Bosniak II.
   b. They are malignant 2% to 5% of the time.
   c. They are more common in men than in women.
   d. They are characterized by bimodal age distribution.
   e. They are readily differentiated from RCC on the basis of appropriate imaging studies.

10. Metanephric adenoma is differentiated from RCC based on all the following features EXCEPT:

    a. female predominance.

    b. benign clinical course.

    c. specific pattern on immunostain marker panel.

    d. characteristic appearance on MRI.

    e. peak incidence in the fifth decade of life.

11. Which of the following would be considered diagnostic for renal angiomyolipoma?

    a. Hyperechoic pattern on ultrasonography

    b. Enhancement of more than 30 Hounsfield units (HU) on CT

    c. Small area of less than −20 HU on nonenhanced CT

    d. Aneurysmal changes on renal arteriogram

    e. Positive signal on T2-weighted images of MRI

12. Which of the following features is typically required for the diagnosis of renal adenoma in a clinical setting?

    a. Tumor size smaller than 3 cm

    b. Low to moderate grade

    c. Papillary architecture

    d. Nonconventional histology

    e. Noncentral location

13. Which of the following tumors is most likely to be a malignant RCC?

    a. A 2.5-cm hyperechoic complex cyst, with no enhancement after intravenous administration of a contrast agent

    b. A 6.0-cm complex cyst with four thin septa

    c. A 5.0-cm cyst with thin, curvilinear calcification

    d. An 11-cm cyst with water density and a homogeneous nature

    e. A 3.0-cm tumor with fat associated with calcification

14. A reliable finding for the diagnosis of renal oncocytoma is:

    a. trisomy of chromosomes 7 and 17.

    b. a central, stellate scar on CT.

    c. a spoke-wheel pattern on renal angiography.

    d. multiple mitochondria on electron microscopy.

    e. a hypervascular pattern.

15. A distinctive finding for renal angiomyolipoma is:

    a. positive staining for vimentin.

    b. a unique cytokeratin expression pattern.

    c. positive staining for human melanoma black-45.

    d. multiple microsomes on electron microscopy.

    e. occasional aneuploidy.

16. All of the following statements accurately describe mixed epithelial and stromal tumors of the kidney EXCEPT:

    a. There is a female predilection.

    b. They are associated with estrogen replacement therapy in women or with androgen ablation therapy in men.

    c. Radiologic diagnostic criteria exist for reliable differentiation from RCC.

    d. Nephron sparing with partial nephrectomy when technically feasible is appropriate.

    e. A benign clinical course is expected.

17. A 44-year-old man undergoes left laparoscopic partial nephrectomy for a 2-cm exophytic renal mass. Final pathologic review reveals intersecting fascicles of smooth muscle with no evidence of hypercellularity, pleomorphism, or mitotic activity. Surgical margins are negative. The next step in management is:

    a. complete radical nephrectomy.

    b. adjuvant chemotherapy.

    c. adjuvant targeted therapy.

    d. observation.

    e. retroperitoneal external-beam radiation therapy.

Pathology

1. A nephrectomy is performed in a 67-year-old man for a solid renal mass; the gross specimen is depicted in Figure 56-1A and the microscopic findings are shown in Figure 56-1B. The pathology report states that this neoplasm has oncocytic features. The next step in management is:

    a. biopsy opposite kidney.

    b. ask the pathologist for a subclassification.

    c. no further follow-up required.

    d. chest CT scan.

    e. endocrine workup.

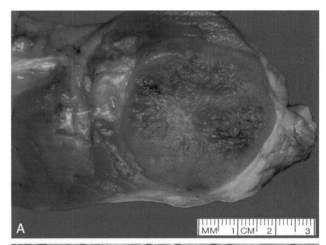

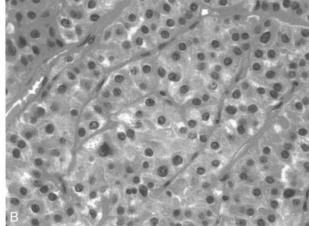

Figure 56-1. (From Bostwick DG, Cheng L. Urologic surgical pathology. 2nd ed. Edinburgh: Mosby; 2008. **A**, Courtesy Philip Bomeisl, MD.)

2. A 35-year-old man has a renal mass incidentally discovered. He is asymptomatic and a left nephrectomy is planned. A biopsy is obtained and the pathologic findings are depicted in Figure 56-2 and reported as metanephric adenoma. The next step in management is:

a. proceed with nephrectomy.

b. perform a partial nephrectomy.

c. stain for Wilms tumor marker WT1.

d. observation.

e. obtain a chest CT scan.

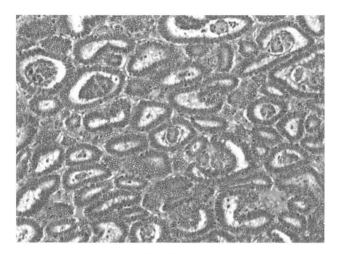

Figure 56-2. (From Bostwick DG, Cheng L. Urologic surgical pathology. 2nd ed. Edinburgh: Mosby; 2008.)

Imaging

1. See Figure 56-3. A CT scan is obtained in a 23-year-old woman with hematuria. In this patient:

a. selective renal embolization may be indicated in symptomatic lesions.

b. there is an associated high risk for urothelial neoplasms.

c. the renal lesions contain microscopic fat.

d. the renal lesions commonly calcify.

e. the renal lesions are premalignant.

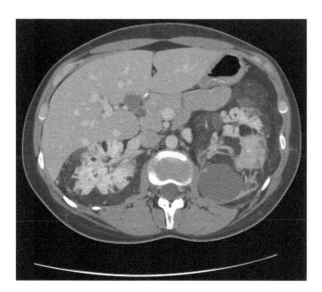

Figure 56-3.

ANSWERS

1. **c. Computed tomography (CT) with and without contrast enhancement.** A dedicated (thin-slice) renal CT scan remains the single most important radiographic image for delineating the nature of a renal mass. In general, any renal mass that enhances with administration of intravenous contrast material on CT should be considered a renal cell carcinoma (RCC) until proved otherwise.

2. **b. Bosniak II cyst.** Category II lesions are minimally complicated cysts that are benign but have some radiologic findings that cause concern. Classic hyperdense renal cysts are small (<3 cm), round, and sharply marginated and do not enhance after administration of contrast material.

3. **d. Renal metastasis.** Fine-needle aspiration or biopsy is of limited value in the evaluation of renal masses. The major problem with this technique is the high incidence of false-negative findings in patients with renal malignancy. The primary indication for needle aspiration or biopsy of a renal mass occurs when a renal abscess or infected cyst is suspected or when differentiating RCC from metastatic malignancy or renal lymphoma.

4. **c. They are best imaged using ultrasound to allow classification with the Bosniak criteria.** Contrast enhancement using imaging that utilizes contrast (CT, MRI) is critical to the Bosniak classification criteria.

5. **b. Recent studies suggest that renal adenoma may be a premalignant precursor of papillary renal cell carcinoma (RCC).** Recent immunohistochemical studies suggest that renal adenomas are commonly associated with papillary RCC and may represent a premalignant precursor along a biologic continuum.

6. **c. Is commonly made at autopsy.** Small, evidently benign, solid renal cortical lesions have been found at autopsy with an incidence of 7% to 23% and have been designated *renal adenomas*.

7. **e. Partial nephrectomy.** Most renal oncocytomas cannot be differentiated from malignant RCCs on the basis of clinical or radiographic means, nor can they be reliably differentiated on frozen section at the time of surgery. Given these uncertainties about a diagnosis, and the excellent outcomes obtained with partial nephrectomy of either benign or malignant tumors, most authors have emphasized the need to treat these tumors with nephron-sparing surgery depending on the clinical circumstances.

8. **a. Selective embolization.** Most patients with acute or potentially life-threatening hemorrhage will require total nephrectomy if exploration is done. If the patient has tuberous sclerosis, bilateral disease, preexisting renal insufficiency, or other medical or urologic disease that could affect renal function in the future, selective embolization should be considered. In such circumstances, selective embolization can temporize and in many cases will prove to be definitive treatment.

9. **d. They are characterized by bimodal age distribution.** Multiloculated cystic nephroma is a characteristic renal lesion with a bimodal age distribution and a benign clinical course.

10. **d. Characteristic appearance on MRI.** Metanephric adenoma is radiographically indistinguishable from RCC and is typically a diagnosis made postoperatively. All other answers are distinguishing features of metanephric adenoma.

11. **c. Small area of less than −20 HU on nonenhanced CT.** The presence of even a small focus of fat, as evidenced by less than −20 HU on a nonenhanced CT scan, is diagnostic for angiomyolipoma. The findings described in a, b, and d are all suggestive, but not diagnostic, for renal angiomyolipoma.

12. **c. Papillary architecture.** Most pathologists will not make the diagnosis of renal adenoma in a nonautopsy setting unless the lesion is low grade, small (<1.0 cm), and of papillary architecture.

13. **e. A 3.0-cm tumor with fat associated with calcification.** Tumors with calcification associated with fat are uncommon but are almost always malignant RCC. In this setting the fat is thought to be a reactive process related to tumor necrosis. Calcification is virtually never seen in association with angiomyolipoma. The lesions described in a to c are Bosniak II renal cysts, with risk of malignancy of less than 10%. The lesion described in d is a simple cyst and highly likely to be benign despite its large size.

14. **d. Multiple mitochondria on electron microscopy.** A distinctive and diagnostic feature of renal oncocytoma is the presence of multiple mitochondria on electron microscopy. Suggestive radiographic findings including a central stellate scar on CT or spoke-wheel pattern on renal angiography have been described but can be seen with RCC and are absent in many oncocytomas. Trisomy of chromosomes 7 and 17 is found in papillary RCC, not renal oncocytoma.

15. **c. Positive staining for human melanoma black (HMB)-45.** Angiomyolipoma will stain positive for HMB-45 in most cases, and this can be used to confirm the diagnosis in challenging cases. This antigen, which was originally found in association with melanoma, is expressed by most angiomyolipomas.

16. **c. Radiologic diagnostic criteria exist for reliable differentiation from RCC.** Conclusive differentiation of mixed epithelial/stromal tumor from RCC or cystic Wilms tumor is not possible based on current imaging modalities. The other answers are characteristic for mixed epithelial/stromal tumors.

17. **d. Observation.** Pathologic diagnosis is of renal leiomyoma with a benign clinical course. Observation is appropriate.

Pathology

1. **b. Ask the pathologist for a subclassification.** Both oncocytoma and chromophobe RCC have oncocytic features. Notice the central scar on the gross specimen and the eosinophilic cytoplasm, and also the low mitotic activity on the photomicrograph. These are the hallmarks of oncocytoma. The pathology report should state with clarity what it is because the management for the two is very different.

2. **b. Perform a partial nephrectomy.** Metanephric adenoma is benign and may stain positive for the Wilms tumor marker WT1. Notice the uniformity of the cells, scant cytoplasm, and no nuclear mitotic activity. The three elements of a Wilms tumor are not present.

Imaging

1. **a. Selective renal embolization may be indicated in symptomatic lesions.** The CT scan demonstrates multiple bilateral low-attenuation lesions. The attenuation of the majority of the lesions is similar to the low density of retroperitoneal fat and lower than the fluid in the gallbladder. This indicates that the lesions are composed of macroscopic fat and represent angiomyolipomas. There are also large cysts in the left kidney. Calcification in angiomyolipomas is unusual, and bilateral angiomyolipomas are often seen in patients with tuberous sclerosis. There is no association with urothelial neoplasms. Angiomyolipomas that are larger than 4 cm have a propensity to bleed spontaneously, and angiographically directed selective embolization of such lesions is indicated when they are symptomatic. Microscopic fat is not visible on CT.

CHAPTER REVIEW

1. Loss of PKD1 and PKD2 leads to cyst formation.
2. Simple renal cysts increase in both size and number with time. The risk factors for development of cysts include age, male gender, hypertension, and renal insufficiency.
3. There is a higher incidence of RCC in acquired renal cystic disease. These patients also have a higher incidence of papillary adenomas. Papillary adenomas may be linked to the development of papillary renal cell carcinoma.
4. The diagnosis of oncocytoma may be made on biopsy with reasonable assurance if the features are classic; however, on occasion it may be difficult to differentiate an RCC with oncocytic features from an oncocytoma. Under these circumstances, the lesion should be treated as though it were an RCC.
5. Oncocytomas are derived from distal renal tubule cells. Chromophobe RCCs also originate from distal renal tubule cells.
6. Angiomyolipomas may be difficult to differentiate from RCCs when they are lipid poor and appear more solid on CT.
7. Multiloculated cystic nephroma is a characteristic renal lesion with a bimodal age distribution and a benign clinical course.
8. Tumors with calcification associated with fat are uncommon but are almost always malignant RCC. In this setting the fat is thought to be a reactive process related to tumor necrosis. Calcification is virtually never seen in association with angiomyolipoma.
9. A distinctive and diagnostic feature of renal oncocytoma is the presence of multiple mitochondria on electron microscopy.

57

Malignant Renal Tumors

Steven C. Campbell and Brian R. Lane

QUESTIONS

1. What is the most accurate imaging study for characterizing a renal mass?
   a. Intravenous pyelography
   b. Ultrasonography
   c. Computed tomography (CT) with and without contrast enhancement
   d. Magnetic resonance imaging (MRI)
   e. Renal arteriography

2. A hyperdense renal cyst may also be termed a:
   a. probable malignancy.
   b. Bosniak II cyst.
   c. Bosniak III cyst.
   d. Bosniak IV cyst.
   e. probable angiomyolipoma.

3. The most generally accepted indication for fine-needle aspiration of a renal mass is a suspected clinical diagnosis of:
   a. renal cell carcinoma (RCC).
   b. renal oncocytoma.
   c. renal cyst.
   d. renal metastasis.
   e. renal angiomyolipoma.

4. Recommended postoperative radiographic surveillance of the chest after radical nephrectomy for T1N0M0 RCC is:
   a. no imaging studies.
   b. chest radiograph at 1 year.
   c. chest radiograph annually for 3 years.
   d. chest CT at 1 year and then chest radiograph annually for 2 years.
   e. chest radiograph annually for 5 years.

5. The European Organisation for Research and Treatment of Cancer 30904 study randomly assigned patients to radical versus partial nephrectomy. Which of the following was an inclusion criterion?
   a. Clinical T1a tumor (<4.0 cm)
   b. Tumor size <5.0 cm
   c. Estimated glomerular filtration rate (GFR) >60 mL/min/1.73 m^2
   d. No hypertension
   e. Age <70 years

6. Following partial nephrectomy for pathologic stage T3aN0M0 RCC, it is recommended to perform surveillance abdominal CT scanning with what frequency?
   a. Never
   b. Every 6 months for at least 3 years and then annually to year 5
   c. Every year to year 5
   d. Every 2 years
   e. Every year for 2 years and then at year 5

7. Following partial nephrectomy of a solitary kidney, what is the most effective method of screening for hyperfiltration nephropathy?
   a. Urinary dipstick test for protein
   b. 24-hour urinary protein measurement
   c. Iothalamate GFR measurement
   d. Serum creatinine measurement
   e. Renal biopsy

8. The most accurate and practical assessment of renal function for routine use after nephrectomy is:
   a. serum creatinine measurement.
   b. urinary dipstick test for protein.
   c. 24-hour urinary protein measurement.
   d. iothalamate GFR measurement.
   e. serum creatinine–based estimation of GFR, such as CKD-EPI formula.

9. What is an important prerequisite for successful cryoablation of a renal tumor?
   a. Slow freezing
   b. Rapid thawing
   c. A single freeze-thaw cycle
   d. A double freeze-thaw cycle
   e. Freezing of tumor to a temperature of −10° C

10. Which two imaging modalities are the preferred and most accurate for demonstrating the presence and extent of an inferior vena caval tumor thrombus?
    a. Abdominal ultrasonography and CT
    b. MRI and renal artery angiography
    c. CT and MRI
    d. MRI and contrast venacavography
    e. Contrast venacavography and transesophageal ultrasonography

11. In patients undergoing complete surgical excision of an RCC, the lowest 5-year survival rate is associated with which factor?
    a. Perinephric fat involvement
    b. Microvascular renal invasion
    c. Subdiaphragmatic inferior vena caval involvement
    d. Intra-atrial tumor thrombus
    e. Lymph node involvement

12. A 45-year-old man has a 5-cm RCC in the upper pole of a solitary left kidney and a single 2-cm left lower lung metastasis. What is the best treatment?
    a. Initial targeted therapy, then partial nephrectomy
    b. Partial nephrectomy, then targeted therapy
    c. Staged partial nephrectomy and pulmonary lobectomy
    d. Simultaneous partial nephrectomy and pulmonary lobectomy
    e. Simultaneous radical nephrectomy and pulmonary lobectomy

13. A healthy 79-year-old man is referred after renal biopsy of a 3.0-cm centrally located renal mass. The biopsy is definitive for renal oncocytoma. The other kidney is normal, the serum creatinine level is 1.0 mg/dL, and there is no evidence of metastatic disease. What is the best next step?
    a. Open radical nephrectomy
    b. Laparoscopic nephroureterectomy
    c. Percutaneous thermal ablation
    d. Partial nephrectomy
    e. Observation with follow-up renal imaging in 6 to 12 months

14. Tuberous sclerosis is similar to von Hippel-Lindau disorder in which of the following respects?
    a. Propensity toward development of seizure disorders
    b. Similarity of cutaneous lesions
    c. Common development of adrenal tumors
    d. Frequent involvement of cerebral cortex with vascular lesions
    e. Mode of genetic transmission

15. A 48-year-old woman with a history of seizure disorder presents with recurrent gross hematuria and left flank pain. Abdominal CT shows a large left perinephric hematoma associated with a 3.0 cm left renal angiomyolipoma. There are also multiple right renal angiomyolipomas ranging in size from 1.5 to 6.5 cm. What is the best management of the left renal lesion?
    a. Selective embolization
    b. Radical nephrectomy
    c. Observation
    d. Partial nephrectomy
    e. Laparoscopic exposure and renal cryoablative therapy

16. Which of the following statements is TRUE regarding cystic nephromas occurring in adults?
    a. They are complex cystic lesions that are typically classified as Bosniak II to III.
    b. They are malignant 2% to 5% of the time.
    c. They are more common in men than in women.
    d. When suspected, they should be treated by radical nephrectomy.
    e. They are readily differentiated from cystic RCC on the basis of appropriate imaging studies.

17. Which environmental factor is most commonly accepted as a risk factor for RCC?
    a. Radiation therapy
    b. Antihypertensive medications
    c. Tobacco use
    d. Diuretics
    e. High-fat diet

18. Which of the following manifestations is restricted to certain families with the von Hippel-Lindau disorder?
    a. RCC
    b. Pancreatic cysts or tumors
    c. Epididymal tumors
    d. Pheochromocytoma
    e. Inner ear tumors

19. RCC develops in what percentage of patients with the von Hippel-Lindau disorder?
    a. 0% to 20%
    b. 21% to 40%
    c. 41% to 60%

    d. 61% to 80%
    e. 81% to 100%

20. What is the most common cause of death in patients with the von Hippel-Lindau syndrome?
    a. Renal failure
    b. Cerebellar hemangioblastoma
    c. Unrelated medical disease
    d. Pheochromocytoma
    e. RCC

21. The von Hippel-Lindau syndrome tumor suppressor protein regulates the expression of which of the following mediators of biologic aggressiveness for RCC?
    a. Basic fibroblast growth factor
    b. Vascular endothelial cell growth factor
    c. Epidermal growth factor receptor
    d. Hepatocyte growth factor (scatter factor)
    e. P-glycoprotein (multiple drug resistance efflux protein)

22. What do the hereditary papillary RCC syndrome and von Hippel-Lindau syndrome have in common?
    a. The mode of genetic transmission
    b. Chromosome 3 abnormalities
    c. A propensity toward tumor formation in multiple organ systems
    d. Inactivation of a tumor suppressor gene
    e. Nearly complete penetrance

23. Mutation of the *met* proto-oncogene in hereditary papillary RCC leads to:
    a. increased expression of hepatocyte growth factor.
    b. increased sensitivity to vascular endothelial growth factor.
    c. inactivation of a tumor suppressor gene that regulates cellular proliferation.
    d. constitutive activation of the receptor for hepatocyte growth factor.
    e. increased expression of vascular endothelial growth factor.

24. P-glycoprotein is a transmembrane protein that is involved in:
    a. immunotolerance.
    b. resistance to high-dose interleukin-2 (IL-2) therapy.
    c. resistance to cisplatin therapy.
    d. resistance to radiation therapy.
    e. efflux of large hydrophobic compounds, including many cytotoxic drugs.

25. Pathology demonstrates venous involvement limited to the main renal vein along with contralateral adrenal involvement with RCC. There is also a 6-cm bulky retroperitoneal lymph node replaced with cancer. What is the stage?
    a. pT3aN1M0
    b. pT3aN2M0
    c. pT3aN1M1
    d. pT3bN1M1
    e. pT4N2M0

26. Which of the following is most likely to demonstrate an infiltrative growth pattern?
    a. Clear cell RCC
    b. Sarcomatoid variants of RCC
    c. Papillary RCC
    d. Chromophobe RCC
    e. Oncocytoma

27. What is the most common mutation identified in sporadic clear cell RCC?

    a. Activation of the *met* proto-oncogene

    b. Activation of the von Hippel-Lindau tumor suppressor gene

    c. Inactivation of the von Hippel-Lindau tumor suppressor gene

    d. Inactivation of *p53*

    e. Inactivation of genes on chromosome 9

28. Which of the following cytogenetic abnormalities is among those commonly associated with papillary RCC?

    a. Trisomy of chromosome 7

    b. Trisomy of the Y chromosome

    c. Loss of chromosome 17

    d. Loss of all or parts of chromosome 3

    e. Loss of chromosome 7

29. What percentage of RCCs are chromophobe cell carcinomas?

    a. 0% to 2%

    b. 4% to 5%

    c. 8% to 10%

    d. 12% to 15%

    e. 18% to 25%

30. Most renal medullary carcinomas are:

    a. found in patients with sickle cell disease.

    b. diagnosed in the fifth decade of life.

    c. responsive to high-dose chemotherapy.

    d. genetically and histologically similar to papillary RCC.

    e. metastatic at the time of diagnosis.

31. Which paraneoplastic syndrome associated with RCC can often be managed or palliated medically?

    a. Polycythemia

    b. Stauffer syndrome

    c. Neuropathy

    d. Hypercalcemia

    e. Cachexia

32. A healthy 64-year-old man is found to have a 6.0-cm solid, heterogeneous mass in the hilum of the right kidney. CT of the abdomen and pelvis shows interaortocaval lymph nodes enlarged to 2.5 cm. A chest radiograph and a bone scan are negative, and the contralateral kidney is normal. The serum creatinine level is 1.0 mg/dL. What is the best next step?

    a. Right radical nephrectomy and regional or extended lymph node dissection

    b. Abdominal exploration, sampling of the enlarged lymph nodes, and possible radical nephrectomy pending frozen section analysis

    c. CT-guided percutaneous biopsy of the lymph nodes

    d. CT-guided percutaneous biopsy of the tumor mass

    e. Systemic therapy followed by radical nephrectomy

33. Which of the following patients would be the best candidate for percutaneous biopsy or fine-needle aspiration of a renal mass?

    a. A 42-year-old man with a 2.5-cm Bosniak III complex renal cyst

    b. An 88-year-old man with unstable angina and a 1.7-cm solid, enhancing renal mass

    c. A 32-year-old woman with bilateral solid, enhancing renal masses ranging in size from 1.5 to 4.0 cm

    d. A 48-year-old woman with a 3.5-cm solid, enhancing renal mass with fat density present

    e. A 38-year-old woman with a fever, a urinary tract infection, and a 3.5-cm solid/cystic, enhancing renal mass

34. A 67-year-old man undergoes radical nephrectomy and inferior vena caval thrombectomy (level 2 tumor thrombus). The primary tumor is otherwise confined to the kidney, and the lymph nodes are not involved. What is the approximate 5-year cancer-free survival rate?

    a. 15% to 25%

    b. 26% to 35%

    c. 36% to 45%

    d. 46% to 65%

    e. 66% to 80%

35. Which of the following is NOT a predictor of cancer-specific survival after nephrectomy for RCC?

    a. Pathologic stage

    b. Tumor size

    c. Fuhrman nuclear grade

    d. Patient age

    e. Histologic necrosis

36. Which of the following statements about renal lymphoma is TRUE?

    a. Five percent to 10% of all lymphomas involving the kidney are primary tumors

    b. The radiographic patterns manifested by renal lymphoma are diverse and can be difficult to differentiate from RCC

    c. Percutaneous biopsy is rarely indicated if renal lymphoma is suspected

    d. Renal failure associated with renal lymphoma is most often due to extensive parenchymal replacement by the malignancy

    e. The most common pattern of renal involvement is from direct extension from adjacent retroperitoneal lymph nodes

37. Which of the following would be considered diagnostic for renal angiomyolipoma (AML)?

    a. Hyperechoic pattern on ultrasonography

    b. Enhancement of >30 Hounsfield units on CT scan

    c. Small area measuring less than −20 Hounsfield units on nonenhanced CT

    d. Aneurysmal changes on renal arteriogram

    e. Positive signal on T2 images of MRI

38. The main limitation of renal mass biopsy is:

    a. risk of needle tract seeding.

    b. difficulty differentiating the eosinophilic variants of RCC from renal oncocytoma.

    c. risk of pneumothorax.

    d. risk of hemorrhage.

    e. high incidence of inadequate tissue sampling.

39. Which of the following tumors is most likely to be a malignant RCC?

    a. 2.5-cm hyperechoic complex cyst, with no enhancement with IV contrast

    b. 6.0-cm complex cyst with four thin septae

    c. 5.0-cm cyst with thin, curvilinear calcification

    d. 11-cm cyst with water density and homogeneous nature

    e. 3.0-cm solid lesion with fat associated with calcification

40. A common and pathogenic cytogenetic finding in children with RCC is:
    a. *VHL* mutation.
    b. *B cMET* oncogene mutation.
    c. *p53* mutation.
    d. *TFE3* gene fusions.
    e. *PTEN* mutations.

41. The central mediator for loss of VHL protein function is:
    a. hypoxia-inducible factor (HIF) alpha.
    b. platelet derived growth factor (PEGF).
    c. erythropoietin.
    d. vascular endothelial growth factor (VEGF).
    e. *p53*.

42. Most tumors at various sites in the von Hippel-Lindau syndrome share the following characteristic:
    a. Malignant behavior
    b. Hypervascularity
    c. Rapid growth rate
    d. High nuclear grade
    e. Symptomatic presentation

43. One major difference between hereditary papillary RCC syndrome and von Hippel-Lindau syndrome is:
    a. pattern of genetic inheritance.
    b. age of onset.
    c. gender distribution.
    d. incidence of metastasis.
    e. incidence of associated tumors in nonrenal organ systems.

44. Which syndrome is most likely to exhibit aggressive behavior of RCC?
    a. von Hippel-Lindau syndrome
    b. Hereditary papillary RCC syndrome
    c. Hereditary leiomyomatosis and RCC syndrome
    d. Birt-Hogg-Dubé syndrome
    e. Familial oncocytosis

45. Spontaneous pneumothorax is occasionally observed in which of the following?
    a. von Hippel-Lindau syndrome
    b. Hereditary papillary RCC syndrome
    c. Hereditary leiomyomatosis and RCC syndrome
    d. Birt-Hogg-Dubé syndrome
    e. Familial oncocytosis

46. Chromophobe RCC shares many characteristics with:
    a. oncocytoma.
    b. type 2 papillary RCC.
    c. clear cell RCC.
    d. mesoblastic nephroma.
    e. mixed epithelial and stromal tumor of the kidney.

47. A finding that is diagnostic for collecting duct carcinoma is:
    a. central location and infiltrative growth pattern.
    b. aggressive clinical course.
    c. *p53* mutation.
    d. positive staining for *Ulex europaeus* lectin.
    e. sensitivity to chemotherapy.

48. Sarcomatoid differentiation is most commonly observed with which histologic subtypes of RCC?
    a. Clear cell and papillary
    b. Papillary and chromophobe
    c. Clear cell and collecting duct
    d. Clear cell and chromophobe
    e. Chromophobe and collecting duct

49. Which of the following factors has greatest utility for predicting bone metastasis from RCC?
    a. Tumor size
    b. Tumor grade
    c. Performance status
    d. Elevated alkaline phosphatase
    e. Invasion of the perinephric fat

50. The prognosis for a 3-cm tumor infiltrating the renal sinus fat is:
    a. similar to a pT1bN0 tumor.
    b. similar to a pT2aN0 tumor.
    c. similar to a pT3a tumor with invasion of the perinephric fat laterally.
    d. worse than a pT3a tumor with invasion of the perinephric fat laterally.
    e. similar to a tumor with ipsilateral adrenal involvement.

51. The single most important prognostic factor for RCC is:
    a. tumor size.
    b. tumor grade.
    c. tumor stage.
    d. histologic subtype.
    e. performance status.

52. The most accurate assessment of prognosis for patients with RCC is usually provided by:
    a. tumor size.
    b. clinician judgment.
    c. tumor stage.
    d. integrated analysis of prognostic factors.
    e. performance status.

53. Which of the following indicates a tumor that is NOT correctly staged according to the 2009 TNM staging system for RCC?
    a. Localized RCC, 8.5 cm: *pT2a*
    b. RCC with direct ipsilateral adrenal involvement: *pT3a*
    c. RCC with metastatic involvement of the adrenal gland: *pM1*
    d. RCC with tumor thrombus within a segmental branch of the renal vein: *pT3a*
    e. RCC with three lymph node metastases: *pN1*

54. Risk of local recurrence is highest in which of the following situations?
    a. *pT3b* tumor after radical nephrectomy and inferior vena cava (IVC) thrombectomy
    b. von Hippel-Lindau patient after partial nephrectomy with wedge resection of a single tumor
    c. 4.5-cm tumor after partial nephrectomy with focal positive parenchymal margin
    d. 3.5-cm tumor after cryoablation
    e. 2.5-cm centrally located tumor after radiofrequency ablation

55. What is the most common form of renal sarcoma?
    a. Liposarcoma
    b. Rhabdomyosarcoma
    c. Fibrosarcoma
    d. Leiomyosarcoma
    e. Angiosarcoma

56. The most useful prognostic factors for renal sarcoma are:
    a. tumor size and grade.
    b. tumor stage and grade.
    c. histologic subtype and stage.
    d. tumor stage and ploidy status.
    e. margin status and grade.

57. Which of the following renal tumors has the best prognosis?
    a. Sarcoma
    b. Carcinoid
    c. Adult Wilms
    d. Primitive neuroectodermal tumor
    e. Small cell

58. Patients with which RCC subtype are most likely to benefit from targeted therapy, such as tyrosine kinase inhibitors?
    a. Papillary RCC
    b. Clear cell RCC
    c. Renal medullary carcinoma
    d. Collecting duct carcinoma
    e. Chromophobe RCC

59. Standard postoperative adjuvant therapy for patients at high risk of recurrence following nephrectomy includes which of the following?
    a. High-dose IL-2
    b. Targeted molecular therapy
    c. Autologous tumor vaccine
    d. Observation
    e. Interferon-α (IFN-α)

60. Agents targeting which of the following signaling pathways in clear cell RCC have significant antitumor effects in patients with metastatic disease?
    a. VEGF and epidermal growth factor receptor (EGFR)
    b. *p53* and EGFR
    c. VEGF and mammalian target of rapamycin (mTOR)
    d. mTOR and transforming growth factor-α (TGF-α)
    e. All of the above

61. Of the following, which is the greatest determinant of renal function after partial nephrectomy?
    a. Surgical approach (open vs. minimally invasive)
    b. Tumor size
    c. Absence of a functioning contralateral kidney
    d. Renal function before partial nephrectomy
    e. Gender

62. Which of the following statements is TRUE regarding chronic kidney disease (CKD)?
    a. CKD due to surgery has the same impact as CKD due to medical causes
    b. Serum creatinine below 1.4 mg/dL excludes the possibility of CKD

c. CKD can be diagnosed based on a single estimated GFR value less than 60 mL/min/1.73 m^2
    d. Increasing CKD stage has been associated with an increase in morbid cardiovascular events for subjects in the general population
    e. Choice of intervention for localized renal malignancy has little impact on development or progression of CKD

63. Which of the following is an indication for adrenalectomy at the time of partial nephrectomy?
    a. 6-cm upper pole renal tumor
    b. 4-cm adrenal lesion measuring −20 Hounsfield units on noncontrast CT scan
    c. Bilateral adrenal hyperplasia
    d. 3-cm renal tumor adjacent to the adrenal gland on CT scan, but readily separable from the adrenal gland at surgery
    e. 1.5-cm adrenal lesion that is bright on T2-weighted MRI

Pathology

1. A 49-year-old man has a biopsy of a peripheral lower pole exophytic 4-cm mass of the right kidney. The histology is depicted in Figure 57-1 and is read as clear cell carcinoma. Metastatic workup is negative. He should be advised to:
   a. receive targeted chemotherapy.
   b. have a radical nephrectomy.
   c. have the tumor ablated with cryotherapy.
   d. have a partial nephrectomy.
   e. receive radiation therapy.

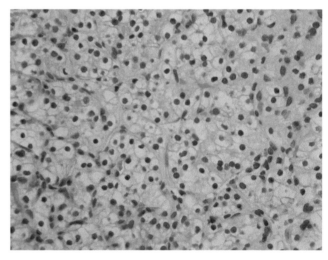

Figure 57-1. (From Bostwick DG, Cheng L. Urologic surgical pathology. 2nd ed. Edinburgh: Mosby; 2008.)

2. A 48-year-old woman has a right radical nephrectomy for a 6-cm mass. Preoperative metastatic workup was negative. The pathology is illustrated in Figure 57-2 and is read as collecting duct carcinoma. She should be advised to:
   a. receive targeted chemotherapy.
   b. receive radiation therapy to the nephrectomy bed.
   c. receive platinum-based chemotherapy.
   d. follow up with her primary care physician.
   e. be followed closely because the development of metastatic disease is likely.

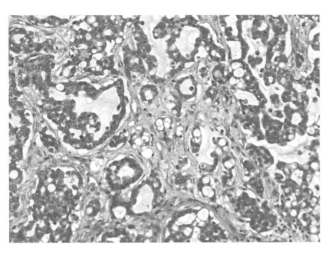

Figure 57-2. (From Bostwick DG, Cheng L. Urologic surgical pathology. 2nd ed. Edinburgh: Mosby; 2008.)

Imaging

1. See Figure 57-3. A 55-year-old man with hematuria has this contrast-enhanced CT scan for evaluation. The most appropriate therapy is:

a. laparoscopic nephron-sparing surgery.

b. radical nephrectomy.

c. open nephron-sparing surgery.

d. radiofrequency ablation.

e. cryoablation.

2. See Figure 57-4. A 45-year-old man with no urinary symptoms has this axial contrast-enhanced CT scan. What is the most likely diagnosis?

a. Bosniak II-F lesion—short-interval imaging follow-up

b. Bosniak IV—cystic RCC

c. Bosniak II cyst

d. Bosniak III cyst

e. Bosniak I cyst

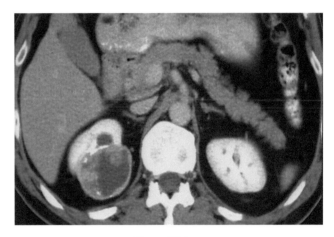

Figure 57-4.

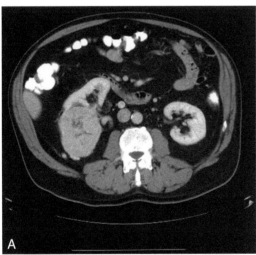

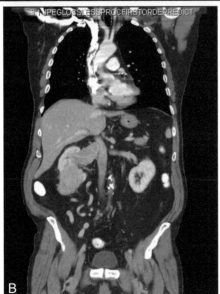

Figure 57-3.

ANSWERS

1. **c. Computed tomography (CT) with and without contrast enhancement.** A dedicated (thin-slice) renal CT scan remains the single most important radiographic image to delineate the nature of a renal mass. In general, any renal mass that enhances with administration of intravenous contrast material on CT scanning should be considered a renal cell carcinoma until proved otherwise.

2. **b. Bosniak II cyst.** Category II lesions are minimally complicated cysts that are benign but have some radiologic findings that cause concern. Classic hyperdense renal cysts are small (<3 cm), round, sharply marginated, and do not enhance after administration of contrast material. Hyperdense cysts that are 3 cm or larger are classified as *Bosniak II-F* lesions.

3. **d. Renal metastasis.** The traditionally accepted indications for needle aspiration or biopsy of a renal mass are when a renal abscess or infected cyst is suspected, or when differentiating RCC from metastatic malignancy or renal lymphoma. Fine-needle aspiration or biopsy is now performed with increased frequency for the evaluation of renal masses in other circumstances, particularly for patients in whom a wide variety of treatment options are under consideration.

4. **c. Chest radiograph annually for 3 years.** Surveillance for recurrent malignancy after radical nephrectomy for RCC can be tailored according to the initial pathologic tumor stage. This patient is low risk (pT1N0M0) and the American Urological Association (AUA) Guidelines recommend an annual chest radiograph for 3 years and only as clinically indicated beyond that time period.

5. **b. Tumor size <5.0 cm.** A solitary tumor and a normal contralateral kidney were also required, but criteria for the latter were not well defined.

6. **b. Every 6 months for at least 3 years and then annually to year 5.** Surveillance for recurrent malignancy after nephron-sparing surgery for RCC can be tailored according to the initial pathologic tumor stage. This patient is intermediate to high risk and the AUA Guidelines recommend a baseline abdominal scan (CT or MRI) within 3 to 6 months following surgery with continued imaging (ultrasonography, CT, or MRI) every 6 months for at least 3 years and annually thereafter to year 5. Imaging beyond 5 years may be performed at the discretion of the clinician.

7. **b. 24-hour urinary protein measurement.** Patients who undergo nephron-sparing surgery for RCC may be left with a relatively small amount of renal tissue. These patients are at risk for long-term renal functional impairment from hyperfiltration renal injury. Because proteinuria is the initial manifestation of the phenomenon, a 24-hour urinary protein measurement should be obtained yearly in patients with a solitary remnant kidney to screen for hyperfiltration nephropathy.

8. **e. Serum creatinine–based estimation of GFR, such as CKD-EPI formula.** At present, there are several formulas in clinical use, including the MDRD, Cockcroft-Gault, and CKD-EPI formulas, each of which is an improvement over using serum creatinine alone for identification of patients with or at risk for chronic kidney disease. Serum levels of creatinine are dependent on gender, muscle mass, and other factors and can therefore lead to an underappreciation of kidney disease in certain populations, such as thin, elderly women. Urinary creatinine measurement is impractical and provides only marginally more valuable information than serum creatinine. Urinary protein measurement can identify patients with early signs of kidney disease (proteinuria) but is not the best screening test. Direct measurement of GFR using iothalamate (or other agents) is costly and not routinely available; it is therefore impractical in most settings.

9. **d. A double freeze-thaw cycle.** Renal cryosurgery is an ablative nephron-sparing treatment option for RCC that can be performed percutaneously under radiographic guidance or laparoscopically under direct vision and ultrasound guidance. The aim of cryosurgery is to ablate the same predetermined volume of tissue that would have been removed had a conventional surgical excision been performed. Established critical prerequisites for successful cryosurgery include rapid freezing, gradual thawing, and a repetition of the freeze-thaw cycle.

10. **c. CT and MRI.** Both CT and MRI are noninvasive and accurate modalities for demonstrating both the presence and the distal extent of vena caval involvement. Although MRI has been recommended as the test of choice at most centers, several recent studies have demonstrated that multiplanar CT also provides sufficient information for surgical planning, and it has become the preferred diagnostic study at many centers.

11. **e. Lymph node involvement.** In most studies, the presence of lymph node or distant metastases has carried a dismal prognosis that is much more pronounced than the other distractors.

12. **d. Simultaneous partial nephrectomy and pulmonary lobectomy.** The subset of patients with metastatic RCC and a solitary metastasis, estimated at between 1.6% and 3.2% of patients, may benefit from nephrectomy with resection of the metastatic lesion. This patient also needs partial nephrectomy to preclude the need for dialysis.

13. **e. Observation with follow-up renal imaging in 6 to 12 months.** Renal mass biopsy is now performed with increased frequency and should be considered in an elderly patient such as this. For those in whom nonextirpative options are being considered, biopsy can provide important information, such as a definitive nonmalignant diagnosis (as in this example). Given the benign nature of renal oncocytomas, the best answer is observation with follow-up imaging in 6 to 12 months.

14. **e. Mode of genetic transmission.** Approximately 20% of angiomyolipomas are found in patients with the tuberous sclerosis (TS) syndrome, an autosomal dominant disorder characterized by mental retardation, epilepsy, and adenoma sebaceum, a distinctive skin lesion. TS, similar to von Hippel-Lindau, is transmitted in an autosomal dominant manner.

15. **a. Selective embolization.** Most patients with acute or potentially life-threatening hemorrhage will require total nephrectomy if exploration is performed, and if the patient has TS, bilateral disease, preexisting renal insufficiency, or other medical or urologic disease that could affect renal function in the future, selective embolization should be considered. In such circumstances, selective embolization can temporize by controlling hemorrhage and in many cases will prove to be definitive treatment.

16. **a. They are complex cystic lesions that are typically classified as Bosniak II to III.** Cystic nephromas are benign renal neoplasms that occur most commonly in middle-aged women. They appear to be genetically related to mixed epithelial and stromal tumors (MESTs) but generally have a somewhat different radiographic appearance. Unlike MESTs, which contain a solid stromal component and often appear as solid or Bosniak IV lesions on cross-sectional imaging, cystic nephromas are typically characterized as complex cystic lesions without a solid component.

17. **c. Tobacco use.** The most generally accepted environmental risk factor for RCC is tobacco use, although the relative associated risks have been modest, ranging from 1.4 to 2.3 when compared with controls. All forms of tobacco use have been implicated, with risk increasing with cumulative dose or pack-years. Other well-established risk factors include obesity and hypertension.

18. **d. Pheochromocytoma.** The familial form of the common clear cell variant of RCC is the von Hippel-Lindau syndrome. Major manifestations include the development of RCC, pheochromocytoma, retinal angiomas, and hemangioblastomas of the brainstem, cerebellum, or spinal cord. Penetrance for all of these traits is far from complete, and some, such as pheochromocytomas, tend to be clustered in certain families but not in others.

19. **c. 41% to 60%.** RCC develops in about 50% of patients with von Hippel-Lindau syndrome and is distinctive for early age at onset, often developing in the third, fourth, or fifth decades of life, and for bilateral and multifocal involvement.

20. **e. RCC.** With improved management of the central nervous system manifestations of the disease, RCC has now become the most common cause of mortality in patients with von Hippel-Lindau syndrome.

21. **b. Vascular endothelial cell growth factor.** Inactivation or mutation of the von Hippel-Lindau gene leads to dysregulated expression of hypoxia inducible factor-1, an intracellular protein that plays an important role in regulating cellular responses to hypoxia, starvation, and other stresses. This in turn leads to a severalfold upregulation of the expression of vascular endothelial growth factor (VEGF), the primary proangiogenic growth factor in RCC, contributing to the pronounced neovascularity associated with this carcinoma.

22. **a. The mode of genetic transmission.** Studies of families with hereditary papillary renal cell carcinoma (HPRCC) have demonstrated an autosomal dominant mode of transmission, similar to von Hippel-Lindau syndrome. Von Hippel-Lindau syndrome is caused by inactivation or mutation of a tumor suppressor gene, whereas HPRCC is caused by activation of an oncogene.

23. **d. Constitutive activation of the receptor for hepatocyte growth factor.** Missense mutations of the *met* proto-oncogene at 7q31 were found to segregate with the disease, implicating it as the relevant genetic locus. The protein product of this gene is the receptor tyrosine kinase for the hepatocyte growth factor (also known as scatter factor), which plays an important role in regulating the proliferation and differentiation of epithelial and endothelial cells in a wide variety of organs, including the kidney. Most of the mutations in hereditary papillary RCC have been found in the tyrosine kinase domain of *met* and lead to constitutive activation.

24. **e. Efflux of large hydrophobic compounds, including many cytotoxic drugs.** P-glycoprotein is a 170-kDa transmembrane protein expressed by 80% to 90% of RCCs that acts as an energy-dependent efflux pump for a wide variety of large hydrophobic compounds, including several cytotoxic drugs.

25. **c. pT3aN1M1.** Isolated renal vein involvement is now classified as T3a and nodal classification has been simplified such that all nodal involvement is now classified as N1. Contiguous invasion of the ipsilateral adrenal is now classified as T4, but metastatic involvement of the contralateral (or ipsilateral) adrenal gland is classified as M1, reflecting a likely hematogenous pattern of dissemination.

26. **b. Sarcomatoid variants of RCC.** Most RCCs are round to ovoid and circumscribed by a pseudocapsule of compressed parenchyma and fibrous tissue rather than a true histologic capsule. Unlike upper tract transitional cell carcinomas, most RCCs are not grossly infiltrative, with the notable exception of some sarcomatoid variants.

27. **c. Inactivation of the von Hippel-Lindau tumor suppressor gene.** Chromosome 3 alterations and von Hippel-Lindau mutations are common in conventional RCC, and mutation or inactivation of this gene has been found in over 75% of sporadic cases.

28. **a. Trisomy of chromosome 7.** The cytogenetic abnormalities associated with papillary RCC are characteristic and include trisomy of chromosomes 7 and 17 and loss of the Y chromosome.

29. **b. 4% to 5%.** Chromophobe cell carcinoma is a distinctive histologic subtype of RCC that appears to be derived from the cortical portion of the collecting duct. It represents 4% to 5% of all RCCs.

30. **e. Metastatic at the time of diagnosis.** Renal medullary carcinoma is a rare histologic subtype of RCC that occurs almost exclusively in association with sickle cell trait. It is typically diagnosed in young African Americans, often in the third decade of life. Many cases are both locally advanced and metastatic at the time of diagnosis. Most patients have not responded to therapy and have succumbed to their disease in a few to several months.

31. **d. Hypercalcemia.** Hypercalcemia has been reported in up to 13% of patients with RCC and can be due to either paraneoplastic phenomena or osteolytic metastatic involvement of the bone. The production of parathyroid hormone–like peptides is the most common paraneoplastic etiology, although tumor-derived 1,25-dihydroxyvitamin D_3 and prostaglandins may contribute in a minority of cases. Medical management includes vigorous hydration followed by diuresis with furosemide and the selective use of bisphosphonates, corticosteroids, and/or calcitonin.

32. **a. Right radical nephrectomy and regional or extended lymph node dissection.** An aggressive surgical approach is still preferred because it will likely prolong survival and represents the only realistic chance for a cure. Lymph nodes in this size range are most likely malignant, and this patient will likely need to consider adjuvant clinical trials. An extended lymph node dissection includes the interaortocaval nodes and nodes alongside and behind the ipsilateral great vessel from the crus of the diaphragm to the ipsilateral common iliac artery.

33. **e. A 38-year-old woman with a febrile urinary tract infection and a 3.5-cm solid/cystic, enhancing renal mass.** Patients with flank pain, a febrile urinary tract infection, and a renal mass may be considered for percutaneous biopsy or aspiration to establish a diagnosis of renal abscess rather than malignancy.

34. **d. 46% to 65%.** Venous involvement was once thought to be a poor prognostic finding for RCC, but more recent studies suggest that most patients with tumor thrombi can be salvaged with an aggressive surgical approach. These studies document 45% to 69% 5-year survival rates for patients with venous tumor thrombi as long as the tumor is otherwise confined to the kidney.

35. **d. Patient age.** Although patient age and comorbidity are important predictors of overall survival in patients with RCC and strongly affect the choice of treatment in these patients, they have no effect on the likelihood of dying of cancer-specific causes. Each of the other factors has been incorporated into one or more RCC prognostic algorithms for cancer-specific outcomes.

36. **b. The radiographic patterns manifested by renal lymphoma are diverse and can be difficult to differentiate from RCC.** Five different radiographic patterns have been described for lymphoma involving the kidney, including a solitary mass that can be difficult to differentiate from RCC.

37. **c. Small area measuring less than −20 Hounsfield units on nonenhanced CT.** The presence of even a small focus of fat, as evidenced by a density less than −20 HU on a nonenhanced CT scan, is diagnostic for AML. The findings described in a, b, and d are all suggestive but not diagnostic for renal AML.

38. **b. Difficulty differentiating the eosinophilic variants of RCC from renal oncocytoma.** The main limitation of renal mass biopsy is difficulty differentiating renal oncocytoma, the most common benign renal mass, from eosinophilic variants of conventional, papillary, and chromophobe RCC on biopsy material. The risk of complications is low in the modern era with the use of smaller gauge needles, and needle tract seeding with RCC appears to be a rare event.

39. **e. 3.0-cm solid lesion with fat associated with calcification.** Tumors with calcification associated with fat are uncommon but are almost always malignant RCC. In this setting the fat is thought to be a reactive process related to tumor necrosis. Calcification is virtually never seen in association with AML. The lesions described in a–c are Bosniak II renal cysts, with risk of malignancy of <10%. The lesion described in d is a simple cyst and highly likely to be benign despite its large size.

40. **d. *TFE3* gene fusions.** Mutations or translocations resulting in *TFE3* gene fusions are common in RCC occurring in the pediatric population. Although these cancers often present with advanced stage, the t(X;17) variant frequently follows an indolent course while t(X;1) cancers can recur with late lymph node metastases.

41. **a. Hypoxia-inducible factor (HIF) alpha.** Inactivation of the VHL protein or loss of its function allows HIF-2 alpha to accumulate, leading to a variety of downstream events including upregulation of VEGF, erythropoietin, and PEGF. HIF-2 alpha is the primary mediator of these events.

42. **b. Hypervascularity.** Tumors in the von Hippel-Lindau syndrome include adrenal pheochromocytoma, retinal angiomas, cerebellar and brainstem hemangioblastoma, RCC, and others. Most are relatively slow growing and asymptomatic if patients are evaluated and screened in a proactive manner. The common feature is that almost all are hypervascular.

43. **e. Incidence of associated tumors in nonrenal organ systems.** The incidence of nonrenal tumors is low in the hereditary papillary RCC syndrome in contrast to von Hippel-Lindau syndrome, in which patients commonly develop tumors in the eyes, spinal cord, cerebellum, adrenal glands, inner ear, epididymis, and pancreas.

44. **c. Hereditary leiomyomatosis and RCC syndrome.** Malignant behavior is particularly common in the hereditary leiomyomatosis and RCC syndrome, and proactive and aggressive surgical management is recommended.

45. **d. Birt-Hogg-Dubé syndrome.** Lung cysts and spontaneous pneumothoraces are well described and relatively common findings in the Birt-Hogg-Dubé syndrome.

46. **a. Oncocytoma.** Both chromophobe RCC and renal oncocytoma are derived from the distal tubules and both are commonly observed in the Birt-Hogg-Dubé syndrome. There are also some overlapping cytogenetic changes, all suggesting a potential relationship between these renal tumors.

47. **d. Positive staining for *Ulex europaeus* lectin.** *Ulex europaeus* lectin is expressed by the normal collecting duct, and tumor staining suggests origin from this structure. Most collecting duct carcinomas are centrally located and exhibit an infiltrative growth pattern and aggressive clinical course, but this is also true for

poorly differentiated transitional cell carcinomas (TCCs) of the renal pelvis or centrally located sarcomatoid RCC.

48. **d. Clear cell and chromophobe.** Sarcomatoid differentiation is most commonly found in association with clear cell and chromophobe RCC.

49. **c. Performance status.** Poor performance status (PS) can be used to segregate patients when deciding whether to obtain a bone scan for metastatic RCC. Shvarts and colleagues (2004)* have shown that patients with good performance status (ECOG performance status = 0), no evidence of extraosseous metastases, and no bone pain were extremely low risk for bone metastasis and did not benefit from bone scanning. They recommended a bone scan for all other patients, and the incidence of bone metastasis in this group was >15%.

50. **d. Worse than a pT3a tumor with invasion of the perinephric fat laterally.** Invasion of the perisinus fat medially has been shown to be a poor prognostic sign. Medial invasion places the tumor in proximity to the venous system and likely increases the risk of metastatic dissemination. Ipsilateral adrenal involvement is even worse, and these are now classified as pT4 if due to direct local extension, or pM1 otherwise, consistent with a hematogenous route of dissemination.

51. **c. Tumor stage.** Although not truly a single factor because it combines tumor size with several other pieces of information obtained from final pathologic analysis, tumor stage is the most powerful individual predictor of oncologic outcomes. When incorporated into a multi-predictor analysis, such as a nomogram or other multivariable analysis, the predictive ability increases further.

52. **d. Integrated analysis of prognostic factors.** Integrated analysis of a variety of factors such as tumor size, stage, and grade, performance status, and histologic subtype has yielded the most accurate prognostication for RCC. Several studies have documented that nomograms and other algorithms outperform traditional staging systems, clinical opinion, individual risk factors, and chance.

53. **b. RCC with direct ipsilateral adrenal involvement: *pT3a*.** Several studies have demonstrated that RCC directly invading the adrenal gland is associated with poorer prognosis than RCC with perinephric or renal sinus fat invasion. Direct ipsilateral adrenal involvement is now grouped with other RCCs that extend beyond Gerota fascia as pathologic stage T4 *(pT4)*. These patients have a high risk for disease recurrence or progression.

54. **b. von Hippel-Lindau patient after partial nephrectomy with wedge resection of a single tumor.** Local recurrence after partial nephrectomy for von Hippel-Lindau disease is common if patients are followed long-term due to multifocal tumor diathesis. These kidneys have been shown to harbor several hundred incipient tumors, and the risk of local recurrence is thus high during longitudinal follow-up after partial nephrectomy.

55. **d. Leiomyosarcoma.** Leiomyosarcoma is the most common histologic subtype of renal sarcoma, accounting for 50% to 60% of such tumors. The most common type of sarcoma in the retroperitoneum is liposarcoma.

56. **e. Margin status and grade.** Margin status and tumor grade are the primary prognostic factors for sarcoma. Patients with high-grade disease are at risk for systemic metastasis and those with low-grade disease are at risk for local recurrence. Wide local excision with negative margins is essential for minimizing the risk of recurrence for sarcomas because these tumors are derived from the mesenchymal tissues and are typically infiltrative, and thus do not respect natural barriers.

57. **b. Carcinoid.** All of these tumor types have a relatively poor prognosis except for renal carcinoid, which tends to be associated with good outcomes in most patients.

58. **b. Clear cell RCC.** Targeted molecular therapies, such as tyrosine kinase inhibitors, mostly target VEGF and thus the pathways that are typically upregulated in clear cell RCC. Most objective responses have been observed in individuals with clear cell RCC. Standard of care for the treatment of metastatic non–clear cell RCC is not well defined at present.

59. **d. Observation.** All randomized postoperative adjuvant trials in patients with resected RCC have failed to demonstrate an improvement in survival or time to progression. Several ongoing clinical trials are evaluating whether targeted molecular therapy will show a benefit, but the results are not available at present. The standard of care continues to be surveillance with periodic radiographic and clinical observations, although enrollment in a clinical trial is highly preferred.

60. **c. VEGF and mammalian target of rapamycin (mTOR).** Several clinical trials indicate that agents targeting VEGF signaling, including sunitinib, sorafenib, and pazopanib, and mTOR pathway signaling, including temsirolimus and everolimus, demonstrate substantial tumor responses or significant improvement in progression-free or overall survival.

61. **d. Renal function prior to partial nephrectomy.** When compared with radical nephrectomy, partial nephrectomy has been associated with better renal functional outcomes. The main determinants of renal function after partial nephrectomy are the quality of the kidney prior to surgery and the quantity of vascularized parenchymal mass that is preserved after excision of the tumor and reconstruction of the kidney. Warm ischemia time, if prolonged, can also contribute to a decline in renal function after partial nephrectomy.

62. **d. Increasing chronic kidney disease (CKD) stage has been associated with an increase in morbid cardiovascular events, hospitalization and death on a longitudinal basis for subjects in the general population.** In this setting, CKD is predominantly due to medical causes. CKD due to surgical causes appears to be more stable than that due to medical causes.

63. **e. 1.5-cm adrenal lesion that is bright on T2-weighted MR imaging.** Several pathologic adrenal lesions can be diagnosed based on their radiographic characteristics without histologic confirmation. Lesions that are bright on T2-weighted MR imaging are suspicious for pheochromocytomas and should be surgically removed. Careful preoperative and intraoperative management are essential for safe management in this circumstance.

Pathology

1. **d. Have a partial nephrectomy.** Notice the clear cytoplasm due to glycogen characteristic of clear cell carcinoma of the kidney. Because of the patient's young age, a nephron-sparing approach is preferred. Because the tumor is located in the lower pole, is peripheral, and is exophytic, it is ideal for this approach. These tumors are not sensitive to radiation therapy, cryotherapy does not have long-term extended follow-up, and targeted chemotherapy is not appropriate for a surgically curable lesion.

2. **e. Be followed closely because the development of metastatic disease is likely.** Collecting duct cancers have a high likelihood of being metastatic at diagnosis. None of the other therapies listed are helpful in this disease.

Imaging

1. **b. Radical nephrectomy.** The images demonstrate a large mass in the lower pole of the right kidney, with tumor extension into the right renal vein, extending to the junction of the right renal vein with the inferior vena cava. The renal vein is enlarged, and tumor vessels are seen within the thrombus in the renal vein. These findings make radical nephrectomy the best option.

2. **b. Bosniak IV—cystic RCC.** Notice the enhancing nodules within the cyst wall with foci of dystrophic calcification making cystic renal cell carcinoma the most likely diagnosis.

---

*Sources referenced can be found in *Campbell-Walsh Urology, 11th Edition,* on the Expert Consult website.

CHAPTER REVIEW

1. A solid mass on CT scan that enhances more than 15 Hounsfield units is suggestive of RCC.
2. Twenty percent of small solid enhancing masses on CT are benign.
3. Hyperdense cysts (Bosniak II) contain old blood and are benign.
4. Clear cell RCCs originate from the proximal tubule; oncocytomas and chromophobe RCCs originate from the distal tubule.
5. There is ample evidence for impaired immune surveillance in RCC.
6. Bilateral involvement in RCC either synchronously or metachronously occurs in 2% to 4% of patients.
7. RCC pathologically is classified as clear cell: 70% to 80%; papillary: 10% to 15%; chromophobe: 3% to 5%; collecting duct: less than 1%; and medullary: rare.
8. Alterations in chromosome 3 are common in clear cell renal carcinoma.
9. Papillary renal cell cancer has a tendency to multifocality.
10. Paraneoplastic syndromes include hypercalcemia, hypertension, polycythemia, and hepatic dysfunction (Stauffer syndrome).
11. Stauffer syndrome is a perineoplastic syndrome associated with RCC that results in elevated liver function tests. If hepatic function does not normalize after nephrectomy, persistent hepatic dysfunction is indicative of persistent disease.
12. Enlarged perirenal lymph nodes noted on CT may be inflammatory, particularly if they are less than 2 cm in diameter. Lymph nodes larger than 2 cm generally contain metastases.
13. Extended lymphadenectomy for renal cell carcinoma has not been shown to be beneficial for the majority of patients over conventional lymphadenectomy, which includes the renal hilar and adjacent paracaval or para-aortic lymph nodes.
14. Fuhrman grading system from 1 to 4 is used to grade the renal tumor and is based on nuclear characteristics.
15. There is an increased incidence of renal cell carcinoma in patients with acquired renal cystic disease.
16. RCC involving the vena cava that infiltrates the wall of the vena cava has an extremely poor prognosis.
17. A patient with a tumor thrombus involving the vena cava associated with metastatic regional nodal disease has a very poor prognosis.
18. A patient with a tumor thrombus involving the vena cava in which the nodes are negative and there is no invasion of the vein wall (except the ostia) has a good prognosis.
19. Ipsilateral adrenalectomy as part of a radical nephrectomy is not necessary unless there is CT evidence of adrenal involvement, contiguous spread of the tumor to the adrenal, or large upper pole renal masses that are adjacent to the adrenal gland.
20. The risk for developing recurrent malignant disease is greatest in the first 3 years after surgery.
21. In a partial nephrectomy, the amount of renal parenchyma taken with the tumor appears to be immaterial provided the margin itself is negative.
22. RCCs less than 3.5 cm in general grow less than 0.5 cm per year; some may grow up to 1 cm per year.
23. Incomplete excision of a large primary tumor or debulking is rarely indicated as a sole treatment.
24. Sarcomas typically have a pseudocapsule that cannot be relied on for a plane of dissection because tumor will be left behind.
25. Metastatic tumors to the kidney are common, appearing in 12% of patients who die of other cancers; the most common primary lesions are those of the lung, breast, or gastrointestinal tract, melanoma, or hematologic.
26. Positron emission tomography scanning using radiolabeled anticarbonic anhydrase IX is taken up by clear cell renal carcinoma.
27. Major poor prognostic indicators include tumors that extend beyond Gerota fascia, involve contiguous organs, have lymph node involvement, or are metastatic.
28. Patients with von Hippel-Lindau disease should have their tumors treated when they reach 3 cm in size.
29. Patients with a significant reduction in renal mass are at risk for developing long-term renal functional impairment from hyperfiltration renal injury. These patients should have their urinary protein excretion monitored because proteinuria is the initial manifestation of hyperfiltration injury.
30. Established critical prerequisites for successful cryosurgery include rapid freezing, gradual thawing, and a repetition of the freeze-thaw cycle.
31. Approximately 20% of angiomyolipomas are found in patients with the tuberous sclerosis (TS) syndrome, an autosomal dominant disorder characterized by mental retardation, epilepsy, and adenoma sebaceum, a distinctive skin lesion. TS, similar to VHL, is transmitted in an autosomal dominant manner.
32. Cystic nephromas are benign renal neoplasms that occur most commonly in middle-aged women.
33. The von Hippel–Lindau syndrome's major manifestations include the development of renal cell carcinoma, pheochromocytoma, retinal angiomas, and hemangioblastomas of the brain stem, cerebellum, or spinal cord.
34. Inactivation or mutation of the von Hippel–Lindau gene leads to dysregulated expression of hypoxia inducible factor-1, an intracellular protein that plays an important role in regulating cellular responses to hypoxia, starvation, and other stresses. This in turn leads to a several-fold upregulation of the expression of vascular endothelial growth factor (VEGF).
35. Hereditary papillary renal cell carcinoma has an autosomal dominant mode of transmission.
36. Chromosome 3 alterations and von Hippel–Lindau mutations are common in conventional renal cell carcinoma, and mutation or inactivation of this gene(VHL) has been found in over 75% of sporadic cases.
37. Renal medullary carcinoma is a rare histologic subtype of RCC that occurs almost exclusively in association with sickle cell trait.
38. Most collecting duct carcinomas are centrally located and exhibit an infiltrative growth pattern and aggressive clinical course.
39. Direct ipsilateral adrenal involvement is now grouped with other RCC's that extend beyond Gerota fascia as pathologic stage T4 (pT4).

Thomas W. Jarrett, Armine K. Smith, and Surena F. Matin

QUESTIONS

1. Which of the following factors would raise the possibility of hereditary upper tract urothelial cancer and prompt microsatellite instability evaluation or genetic testing?
   a. Young age
   b. Personal history of colon cancer
   c. Two first-degree relatives with endometrial cancer
   d. All of the above
   e. None of the above

2. Which environmental factor has NOT been shown to be associated with development of upper tract urothelial carcinoma?
   a. Long-term use of phenacetin
   b. Smoking
   c. Obesity
   d. Aristolochic acid ingestion
   e. Exposure to aromatic amines

3. The majority of ureteral tumors occur in the:
   a. proximal ureter.
   b. midureter.
   c. distal ureter.
   d. proximal and midureter.
   e. distal and mid ureter.

4. The most important determinant of oncologic outcome in upper tract urothelial carcinoma is:
   a. stage and grade.
   b. number of tumors.
   c. location.
   d. tumor size.
   e. tumor architecture.

5. The most frequent presenting symptom of upper tract urothelial carcinoma is:
   a. dysuria.
   b. flank pain.
   c. weight loss.
   d. hematuria.
   e. abdominal mass.

6. Computed tomography (CT) urography outperforms intravenous pyelography in detection of upper tract tumors.
   a. True
   b. False

7. At the time of nephroureterectomy, the ureteral stump can be safely left in place for patients with urothelial tumors of the renal pelvis.
   a. True
   b. False

8. Initial evaluation of positive cytology should include which of the following?
   a. Cystoscopy
   b. Ureteroscopy
   c. CT urography
   d. a, b, and c
   e. a and b
   f. a and c

9. All of the following agents have been used in instillation therapy EXCEPT:
   a. bacille Calmette-Guérin (BCG).
   b. cisplatin.
   c. mitomycin C (MMC).
   d. thiotepa.
   e. gemcitabine.

10. Neoadjuvant chemotherapy is the standard of care in patients with locally advanced upper tract urothelial carcinoma.
    a. True
    b. False

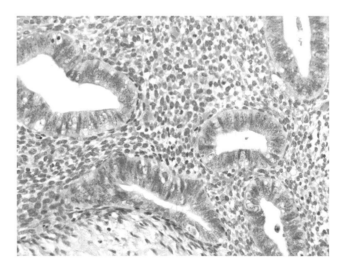

Figure 58-1. (From Bostwick DG, Cheng L. Urologic surgical pathology. 2nd ed. Edinburgh: Mosby; 2008.)

Pathology

1. A 38-year-old woman has right flank pain and microscopic hematuria. Cytology is atypical. CT scan shows a mass in the distal right ureter with hydronephrosis. Cystoscopy is negative, and attempted ureteroscopy is unsuccessful. The distal ureter is excised, and the pathology is depicted in Figure 58-1 and is reported as endometriosis. The patient should be advised to:

a. have a diagnostic laparoscopy.

b. receive ablative hormonal therapy.

c. have periodic upper tract imaging.

d. have cystoscopy and cytology twice yearly for the next 2 years.

e. have a hysterectomy and bilateral salpingo-oophorectomy.

2. A 60-year-old man has a right ureteral mass excised. The pathology is low-grade noninvasive transitional cell carcinoma (TCC) (Figure 58-2). He has no prior history of upper tract disease or bladder cancer. Management should consist of:

a. interval cystoscopies and cytology.

b. instillation of BCG into the right upper tract.

c. systemic platinum chemotherapy.

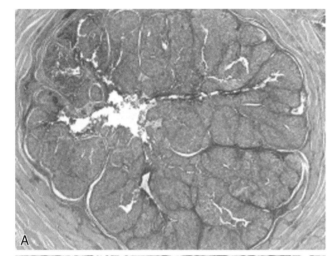

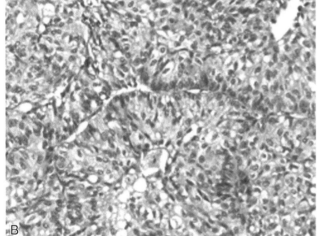

Figure 58-2. (From Bostwick DG, Cheng L. Urologic surgical pathology. 2nd ed. Edinburgh: Mosby; 2008.)

d. periodic ureteroscopies of the left system.

e. no further follow-up.

Imaging

1. See Figure 58-3. A CT scan of a 62-year-old man with hematuria is shown. The most likely diagnosis is:

a. renal cell carcinoma.

b. urinary obstruction.

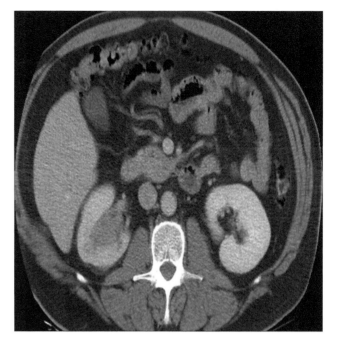

Figure 58-3.

c. urothelial carcinoma.

d. lymphoma.

e. metastatic disease.

ANSWERS

1. **d. All of the above.** Patients with hereditary nonpolyposis colorectal carcinoma (HNPCC) or Lynch syndrome present at a younger age and are more likely to be female. In addition, the presence of either a personal history or having two first-degree relatives with an HNPCC-associated cancer (particularly colon and endometrial) should raise suspicion for a hereditary component, and these patients should be referred for microsatellite or genetic testing.

2. **c. Obesity.** Of all the listed environmental insults, obesity has not been associated with upper tract urothelial cancers (UTUCs). Aristolochic acid has been implicated in the etiology of Balkan endemic and Chinese herb nephropathy because of its mutagenic action. The effect of smoking has been linked to generation of aromatic amines, which are metabolized into carcinogenic *N*-hydroxyalanine. Notably, this risk is dose dependent and can be modified by smoking cessation. Analgesic abuse is a well-documented risk factor, and experimental evidence supports phenacetin-induced papillary necrosis as a cofactor in renal failure and carcinogenesis. Aromatic amines account for carcinogenicity of β-naphthylamine and benzidine, which have been implicated as occupational hazards in the chemical, petroleum, and plastic industries, among others. Similar to smoking, the duration of exposure is important in determining the risk for UTUC development.

3. **e. Distal and midureter.** Ureteral tumors occur more commonly in the lower than in the upper ureter. Overall, approximately 70% of ureteral tumors occur in the distal ureter, 25% in the midureter, and 5% in the proximal ureter.

4. **a. Stage and grade.** The most well-established current predictors of survival in patients with upper tract urothelial tumors are stage and grade. The most significant decrease in survival is seen in T3 tumors, and higher-grade tumors are more likely to invade the surrounding tissues, hence presenting with higher stage. Although there have been studies showing differences

in prognosis based on the tumor number, location, size, and architecture, these criteria are evolving and warrant further investigation.

5. **d. Hematuria.** The most common presenting symptom of upper tract urothelial tumors is hematuria, either gross or microscopic; this occurs in 56% to 98% of patients. Flank pain is the second most common symptom, occurring in 30% of patients with tumors. Approximately 15% of patients are asymptomatic at presentation and are diagnosed when an incidental lesion is found on radiologic evaluation.

6. **a. True.** Although intravenous pyelography has been the traditional means for diagnosis of upper tract lesions, this has largely been replaced by CT urography, which is easier to perform and less labor intensive. With CT urography, the sensitivity for detecting upper tract malignant disease has been reported to approach 100%, with a specificity of 60% and a negative predictive value of 100%. It also has a higher degree of accuracy in determining the presence of renal parenchymal lesions.

7. **b. False.** Complete removal of the distal ureter and bladder cuff offers oncologic outcomes superior to those for incomplete resection. The risk of tumor recurrence in a remaining ureteral stump is 30% to 75%. In addition, adequate cystoscopic surveillance of a residual distal ureter stump after nephroureterectomy is virtually impossible, contributing to high rates of local recurrence. Therefore the entire distal ureter, including the intramural portion and the ureteral orifice, must be removed.

8. **f. a and c.** Ureteroscopy should be reserved for situations in which the diagnosis remains in question after conventional radiographic studies, and for patients in whom the treatment plan may be modified on the basis of the ureteroscopic findings. Although the risks of tumor seeding, extravasation, and dissemination are low in experienced hands, these risks are real and should preclude ureteroscopy when it is unnecessary. Because upper urinary tract tumors are often associated with bladder cancers, cystoscopy is mandatory in the evaluation to exclude coexistent bladder lesions.

9. **b. Cisplatin.** The largest experience of instillation therapy for UTUC is from use of BCG via a nephrostomy tube for primary treatment of carcinoma in situ (CIS), and favorable responses are seen. Although the experience with thiotepa, MMC, and gemcitabine is limited, a few small retrospective series have described their use in this setting.

10. **b. False.** There are no randomized trials evaluating the effects of neoadjuvant and adjuvant chemotherapy on patients with UTUC, and the small number of cases treated with adjuvant chemotherapy precludes definitive conclusions of efficacy. However, given the significant influence of renal function on eligibility to receive effective chemotherapy, the focus is shifting toward a neoadjuvant approach, with several trials underway.

Pathology

1. **c. Have periodic upper tract imaging.** With no symptoms, no further workup is indicated. The patient should be followed for possible development of a ureteral vesicle stricture at the site of the anastomosis.

2. **a. Interval cystoscopies and cytology.** Patients who have upper tract TCC have as high as a 30% incidence of bladder tumors and should be followed as for bladder cancer. Moreover, periodic upper tract imaging is necessary.

Imaging

1. **c. Urothelial carcinoma.** There is an enhancing mass centered in the renal sinus. The appearance is typical for a urothelial neoplasm of the renal pelvis.

CHAPTER REVIEW

1. Upper tract urothelial tumors are rarely diagnosed at autopsy; they present clinically during the patient's lifetime much as bladder tumors do. The peak incidence occurs between ages 70 and 80, and they occur twice as frequently in men as in women.
2. Upper tract recurrence is more likely with high-grade tumors and those associated with carcinoma in situ. Multifocality and the incidence of bilateral disease increases with the presence of CIS.
3. Upper tract tumors develop in 2% to 4% of patients with bladder cancer. Patients with upper tract tumors develop bladder cancer 30% of the time.
4. Bilateral upper tract tumors occur either synchronously or metachronously in 2% to 6% of patients.
5. In renal pelvic tumors, parenchyma invasion is the most significant predictor of metastases.
6. Inverted papillomas may be associated with upper tract tumors; it is not likely that cancers arise from them.
7. Squamous cell carcinoma and adenocarcinoma, although rare in the upper tract, are usually associated with long-term obstruction, inflammation, and occasionally calculi.
8. Tumor stage and grade, lymphovascular invasion, and lymph node spread are predictors of poor prognosis. The single most important predictor of outcome is stage.
9. A significant problem with ureteroscopic biopsy is that grade may be accurate, but accurate staging can be extremely difficult.
10. There is a 30% to 50% recurrence rate in ureteral tissue left distal to an invasive ureteral cancer.
11. Upper tract ureteral tumors after radial cystectomy for bladder cancer occur in 4% to 7% of patients.
12. Patients with Balkan nephropathy, those with analgesic abuse, and those who have ingested arsenic in endemic

regions of Taiwan have a higher tendency for multiple and bilateral recurrences than do those with sporadic tumors.
13. Patients with T3 tumors located in the renal pelvis have a better survival than those with T3 tumors located in the ureter. Of renal pelvic tumors, 50% are invasive at diagnosis.
14. An adrenalectomy is not indicated for patients undergoing a nephroureterectomy for upper tract tumors.
15. After percutaneous resection of a tumor of the renal pelvis, the nephrostomy is left indwelling to allow for revisualization several weeks later to be certain that all tumors have been removed.
16. Hydronephrosis in the presence of urothelial carcinoma predicts invasion 80% of the time.
17. Tumor cell implantation has been reported to occur in wounds, port sites, and nephrostomy tracks.
18. Lymphadenectomy has prognostic and possible therapeutic value in patients with T2 to T4 disease.
19. Hereditary TCC should be suspected in patients with hereditary nonpolyposis colorectal carcinoma (HNPCC) or Lynch syndrome. Additionally, the presence of either a prior history of or two first-degree relatives with an HNPCC-associated cancer (particularly colon and endometrial) should raise suspicion for hereditary TCC, and these patients should be referred for microsatellite or genetic testing.
20. Aristolochic acid has been implicated in etiology of Balkan endemic and Chinese herb nephropathy.
21. About 70% of ureteral tumors occur in the distal ureter, 25% in the midureter, and 5% in the proximal ureter.
22. The largest experience of instillation therapy for upper tract urothelial carcinoma is with the use of BCG via a nephrostomy tube for primary treatment of CIS. Favorable responses have been reported.

59 Retroperitoneal Tumors

Louis L. Pisters, Philippe E. Spiess, and Dan Leibovici

QUESTIONS

1. Which of the following is NOT considered an etiologic factor for soft tissue sarcoma?
   a. Viral infection
   b. Previous radiation exposure
   c. Scar tissue from previous injury
   d. Retroperitoneal fibrosis
   e. Gardner syndrome

2. Which of the following considerations does NOT support the dormant embryonal stem-cell origin theory of sarcoma pathogenesis?
   a. Occasional malignant transformation of hemangiopericytoma into hemangiosarcoma
   b. The occasional occurrence of heterotopic tissue in a retroperitoneal sarcoma
   c. The occurrence of dedifferentiated liposarcoma
   d. The fact that mesenchymal tissue turnover is much slower than that of mucosal linings
   e. The possible occurrence of sarcoma in very young children

3. Genetic aberrations associated with soft tissue sarcomas include which of the following?
   a. Ring chromosome 12 is commonly found in malignant fibrous histiocytoma
   b. Deletions of suppressor gene pRb are detected in pleomorphic liposarcoma
   c. Translocation between chromosomes 12 and 16 is observed in myxoid liposarcoma
   d. Translocation of chromosome 7p to 12q is observed in leiomyosarcoma
   e. Aneuploidy is a normal finding in schwannomas

4. A patient undergoes surgical resection of a poorly differentiated retroperitoneal liposarcoma. There was macroscopic residual tumor. In terms of surgical staging, the patient would be considered:
   a. Rx.
   b. R0.
   c. R1.
   d. R2.
   e. R3.

5. Which of the following may represent a malignant lesion if greater than 6 cm?
   a. Rhabdomyoma
   b. Aggressive fibromatosis
   c. Pelvic lipomatosis
   d. Lipoblastoma
   e. Leiomyoma

6. Any fat-containing retroperitoneal mass, until proven otherwise, should be considered:
   a. a renal angiomyolipoma.
   b. an adrenal myelolipoma.
   c. a well-differentiated liposarcoma.
   d. an adrenal pheochromocytoma.
   e. an osteosarcoma.

7. A pretreatment retroperitoneal mass biopsy should be obtained using:
   a. an image-guided biopsy, preferably using a retroperitoneal approach.
   b. an open or laparoscopic guided biopsy if possible.
   c. a fine-needle aspiration technique as more diagnostic.
   d. any technique necessary as required to diagnose a retroperitoneal sarcoma in all cases.
   e. an endoscopic technique in all cases because it avoids potential seeding of the peritoneum.

8. Postoperative radiotherapy should be considered:
   a. if it can compensate for an incomplete resection or positive surgical margins.
   b. based on careful review of an individual case and not solely on the margin status at the time of the initial or re-resection.
   c. if negative margins have been obtained at the time of the original resection.
   d. if positive microscopic surgical margins have been obtained but the surgeon feels that all gross disease has been resected.
   e. if a radiation oncologist deems it to beneficial.

9. The adjuvant systemic regimen best studied in the management of retroperitoneal soft tissue sarcoma following surgical resection is:
   a. single-agent gemcitabine.
   b. targeted therapy using pazopanib.
   c. single-agent doxorubicin.
   d. combination therapy using epirubicin and ifosfamide.
   e. single-agent trabectedin.

10. The most important determinant of the likelihood of sarcoma recurrence following surgical status is:
    a. sarcoma histologic subtype.
    b. tumor grade.
    c. tumor ploidy.
    d. presence of lymphovascular invasion.
    e. final surgical margin status.

ANSWERS

1. **d. Retroperitoneal fibrosis.** Of the clinical parameters listed, only retroperitoneal fibrosis is not an etiologic factor associated with development of a soft-tissue sarcoma. When a patient presents with retroperitoneal fibrosis, a malignancy such as a soft-tissue sarcoma is in the differential diagnosis, but that does not mean it constitutes an etiologic factor. The remaining choices—viral infection, previous radiation exposure, scar tissue from a previous injury, and Gardner syndrome—are all etiologic factors with soft-tissue sarcomas.

2. **a. Occasional malignant transformation of hemangiopericy-toma into hemangiosarcoma.** It is rare for a benign entity such as a hemangioma or hemangiopericytoma to differentiate into a malignant hemangiosarcoma; therefore this does not support the dormant embryonal stem-cell origin theory. The remaining choices are all correct and support this theory.

3. **c. Translocation between chromosomes 12 and 16 is observed in myxoid liposarcoma.** Genetic aberrations including a balanced translocation of chromosomes 12 and 16 t(12:16) (q13: p11) appear in 90% of myxoid liposarcoma cases and are pathognomonic of this sarcoma (Eneroth et al, 1990).* The remaining choices are all incorrect.

4. **d. R2.** The presence of macroscopic residual tumor following surgical resection renders the patient R2. R0 represents tumor that was entirely resected with no residual tumor and negative surgical margins; R1 represents microscopic residual tumor (i.e., a positive surgical margin); R2 represents macroscopic residual tumor; and R3 represents tumor spillage and dissemination at the time of resection.

5. **e. Leiomyoma.** Distinguishing a leiomyoma from a leiomyosarcoma can be difficult under rigorous microscopic pathology review, but parameters suggestive of malignancy include tumor size, pleomorphism, cellularity, necrosis, atypia, and mitosis. Hence, of the choices given, leiomyoma is the correct answer.

6. **c. A well-differentiated liposarcoma.** Retroperitoneal liposarcomas are the most common type of retroperitoneal soft tissue sarcomas. Based in large part on this important fact, any fat-containing retroperitoneal mass should be considered a well-differentiated liposarcoma until proven otherwise. All other choices are incorrect.

7. **a. An image-guided biopsy, preferably using a retroperitoneal approach.** Many experts feel that a pretreatment biopsy should be obtained (whenever feasible) using an image-guided and, if possible, a retroperitoneal approach to minimize the risk of cancer spillage/dissemination. The other choices are incorrect because they are not the preferred diagnostic approach to obtaining a pretreatment biopsy, although they are occasionally obtained when an image-guided biopsy is not technically feasible.

8. **b. Based on careful review of an individual case and not solely on the margin status at the time of the initial or re-resection.** Postoperative radiotherapy should be offered to patients based not solely on their margin status at the time of surgical resection (either primary or redo) but rather on the individual characteristics of the case. All other choices are incorrect.

9. **d. Combination therapy using epirubicin and ifosfamide.** The combination of the systemic agents epirubicin and ifosfamide are the best studied in the management of retroperitoneal soft-tissue sarcomas (and overall soft-tissue sarcomas for that matter). This systemic chemotherapy combination has been used in pivotal trials of perioperative systemic therapy. Other systemic agents such as single-agent gemcitabine, doxorubicin, and trabectedin as well as targeted agents (e.g., pazopanib) have not been as well studied in the management of retroperitoneal sarcomas and hence are incorrect choices to this question.

10. **e. Final surgical margin status.** The final surgical margin status is the most important prognostic factor of the likelihood of recurrence. Although other options listed, such as tumor grade and ploidy, have prognostic importance for retroperitoneal sarcomas, they are of lesser importance in predicting the likelihood of recurrence following surgical resection; hence the remaining choices are incorrect.

CHAPTER REVIEW

1. Retroperitoneal sarcomas have a propensity for hematogenous spread—usually to the lung and liver.
2. Pelvic lipomatosis is a hyperplastic rather than a neoplastic process.
3. Myelolipoma usually occurs in the adrenal gland but may be found in the retroperitoneum.
4. Sarcomas have a tendency to recur, in part owing to pseudoencapsulation and the false gross appearance of complete surgical resection. Surgical margin status is the most important prognostic indicator for local recurrence and survival.
5. Rhabdomyosarcomas are classified as embryonal, alveolar, and undifferentiated.
6. Sarcomas arise de novo and not from malignant transformation of a benign tumor.
7. Liposarcoma, leiomyosarcoma and malignant fibrous histiocytoma make up 80% of retroperitoneal sarcomas.

Liposarcoma is the most common type of retroperitoneal soft tissue sarcoma.

8. Radiation therapy has been shown to be beneficial in selected circumstances and may be given preoperatively, intraoperatively, or postoperatively.
9. Tumor involvement of neural foramina suggests unresectability.
10. Staging of retroperitoneal sarcomas: R0 represents tumor that was entirely resected with no residual tumor and negative surgical margins; R1 represents microscopic residual tumor (i.e., a positive surgical margin); R2 represents macroscopic residual tumor; and R3 represents tumor spillage and dissemination at the time of resection.
11. Surgical margin status is the most important prognostic factor of the likelihood of recurrence. Tumor grade and ploidy also have prognostic importance, but to a lesser degree.

---

*Sources referenced can be found in *Campbell-Walsh Urology, 11th Edition*, on the Expert Consult website.

60 Open Surgery of the Kidney

Aria F. Olumi, Mark A. Preston, and Michael L. Blute, Sr.

QUESTIONS

1. A healthy 45-year-old man with no family history of cancer is found to have a 6-cm enhancing mass in the upper pole of his right kidney. A 2-cm solitary nodule is noted on preoperative chest radiography. Computed tomography (CT) confirms a solitary nodule in the lower lobe of the right lung. What is the most appropriate treatment course?

   a. Systemic chemotherapy alone

   b. Radical right nephrectomy and postoperative chemotherapy

   c. Biopsy of pulmonary nodule

   d. Radical nephrectomy and simultaneous pulmonary metastectomy

   e. Radical nephrectomy with staged resection of pulmonary nodule 6 weeks postoperatively

2. What is the preferred technique for radical nephrectomy and removal of tumor thrombus above the level of the diaphragm in the absence of significant metastatic disease?

   a. Flank incision with extensive liver mobilization and removal of tumor through an incision in the diaphragm

   b. Flank incision with cardiopulmonary bypass and deep hypothermic circulatory arrest (CPB-DHCA)

   c. Chevron incision with CPB-DHCA

   d. Chevron incision with Pringle maneuver

   e. Midline incision with CPB-DHCA

3. Deep hypothermic circulatory arrest (DHCA) can have irreversible neurologic effects after what period of time?

   a. 10 minutes

   b. 20 minutes

   c. 40 minutes

   d. 60 minutes

   e. 90 minutes

4. In a 45-year-old man with a normal contralateral kidney and no family history of kidney cancer, in which of the following clinical scenarios would partial nephrectomy be indicated?

   a. Two tumors less than 3 cm each in the upper and lower pole

   b. Single 8-cm tumor in the upper pole

   c. Single 2-cm tumor in a hilar location with small renal vein tumor thrombus

   d. Single 4-cm tumor in any location

   e. All of the above

5. What is the strongest modifiable risk factor for renal insufficiency after partial nephrectomy?

   a. Duration of renal ischemia

   b. Surgical approach

   c. Administration of nephrotoxins

   d. Resection margin

   e. Administration of heparin

6. During a posterior right lumbotomy approach, what is the order of appearance of the renal artery, renal vein, and renal pelvis?

   a. Artery, renal pelvis, vein

   b. Artery, vein, renal pelvis

   c. Renal pelvis, artery, vein

   d. Vein, renal pelvis, artery

   e. Renal pelvis, vein, artery

7. Match the following T stage with the tumor characteristics:

   1. T3c
   2. T1a
   3. T3a
   4. T4
   5. T2b

   a. Greater than 10 cm confined to capsule

   b. Less than 4 cm confined to capsule

   c. 6 cm invading adrenal gland

   d. 5 cm with renal sinus fat invasion

   e. 13 cm with renal vein thrombus invading the wall of the inferior vena cava

8. Five days after left partial nephrectomy for a hilar tumor, there is persistent drainage from the Penrose drain site. Laboratory analysis of the drain fluid demonstrates elevated amylase levels. Imaging studies demonstrate small bowel dilation consistent with ileus and fluid around the tail of pancreas. What is the ideal management?

   a. Antibiotics

   b. Immediate surgical exploration

   c. Percutaneous drain placement

   d. Nasogastric tube placement, parenteral nutrition, and conservative management

   e. Nasogastric tube placement, low-fat diet, and conservative management

9. Which segmental branch of the renal artery is most consistent and supplies 25% of the arterial supply to the renal unit?

   a. Apical (superior) segmental artery

   b. Anterior superior segmental artery

   c. Posterior segmental artery

   d. Anterior inferior segmental artery

   e. The basilar (inferior) segmental artery

10. What maneuver refers to the reflection of the second and third portions of the duodenum in a medial direction to expose the right renal vessels and ventral inferior vena cava?

    a. Cattell maneuver

    b. Langenbeck maneuver

    c. Sorcini maneuver

    d. Kocher maneuver

    e. Pringle maneuver

11. What partial nephrectomy technique should be used as a last resort in a solitary kidney?
    a. Enucleation
    b. Wedge resection
    c. Cryotherapy
    d. Polar resection
    e. Extracorporeal repair and autotransplantation

12. The subcostal nerve may be inadvertently transected during an anterior subcostal incision for a radical nephrectomy. Between what two layers does this nerve run?
    a. Posterior peritoneum and transversalis fascia
    b. Scarpa fascia and external oblique muscle
    c. External oblique and internal oblique
    d. Internal oblique and transversalis
    e. Skin and Scarpa fascia

13. What is the motor deficit resulting from transaction of the subcostal nerve?
    a. Winged scapula
    b. Hemidiaphragmatic paralysis
    c. Paresis of the flank musculature and flank bulge
    d. Inability to flex ipsilateral adductor muscle
    e. Weakness of contralateral rectus abdominis muscle

14. What percentage of patients have multiple renal arteries?
    a. 0% to 2%
    b. 2% to 10%
    c. 10% to 20%
    d. 20% to 30%
    e. More than 30%

15. Which of the following is NOT an indication for simple nephrectomy?
    a. Nonfunctional chronically infected kidney
    b. Nonfunctional persistently hydronephrotic kidney causing pain
    c. Renovascular hypertension refractory to medical and nephron-sparing surgical intervention
    d. Polycystic kidney with minimal function and recurrent infections
    e. Kidney with 8-cm enhancing upper pole hilar mass

16. Two days after cardiopulmonary bypass and circulatory arrest (20 minutes) for an extensive right-sided renal mass with thrombus extending into the atrium, using traditional median sternotomy, a relatively healthy 36-year-old patient is unable to be extubated and has no purposeful right-sided movement. Imaging reveals a large left-sided cerebrovascular infarct. What clinical scenario can explain this event?
    a. Pulmonary air embolism
    b. Cerebral ischemia from bypass and circulatory arrest
    c. Tension pneumothorax
    d. Right main stem bronchial intubation
    e. Unrecognized paradoxical embolism

17. Which form of therapy has been considered the "gold standard" for localized renal cell carcinoma?
    a. Chemotherapy
    b. Immunotherapy
    c. Radiation
    d. Hormonal therapy
    e. Surgical resection

18. On postoperative day 2 after radical nephrectomy for a 14-cm complex left renal tumor using an anterior midline incision, there are overt signs of peritonitis. The patient is 72 years old with significant atherosclerotic disease. At exploration, the entire small bowel is necrotic and nonviable. What artery was inadvertently ligated?
    a. Celiac
    b. Left gastric
    c. Inferior mesenteric
    d. Superior mesenteric
    e. Right gastroepiploic

19. During resection of a large right renal mass, the main renal artery is identified, ligated, and divided, but the renal vein fails to decompress. What is the most likely explanation for this?
    a. Renal vein tumor thrombus
    b. Subclinical renal arteriovenous malformation
    c. Bleeding disorder
    d. Arterial collateral branch vessels
    e. Extensive venous collateral obstruction

20. What is most appropriate setting for a thoracoabdominal incision?
    a. Large right upper pole renal mass with tumor thrombus in the renal vein
    b. 5-cm right renal tumor in a hilar location
    c. Large left lower pole tumor with extensive lymphadenopathy
    d. Large right renal mass with tumor thrombus to the retrohepatic level
    e. A 10-cm right lower pole tumor with arteriovenous malformation

21. What is the most common complication associated with performing CPB-DHCA for the removal of large renal cell tumor thrombus?
    a. Pulmonary air emboli
    b. Intestinal ischemia
    c. Bleeding and coagulopathy
    d. Lower extremity tumor emboli
    e. Tumor emboli

22. Which of the following is NOT a proposed benefit of renal artery embolization (RAE)?
    a. Shrinkage of an arterialized tumor thrombus to ease surgical removal
    b. Reduced blood loss
    c. Facilitation of dissection due to tissue plane edema
    d. Ability to ligate the renal vein before the renal artery at time of nephrectomy
    e. Modulation of the immune response
    f. None of the above

23. What is the most common complication after RAE?
    a. Groin hematoma from puncture site
    b. Paraplegia from spinal artery occlusion
    c. Coil migration
    d. Postinfarction syndrome (pain, nausea, and fever)
    e. Adrenal insufficiency

24. What is the most common complication after partial nephrectomy for nonexophytic renal masses?
    a. Hemorrhage
    b. Renal failure

c. Rhabdomyolysis

d. Hydronephrosis

e. Urinary leak

25. Ten days after a left partial nephrectomy for a 4.5-cm hilar tumor, there is persistent fluid output from the surgical drain. No ureteral stent was placed at the time of surgery, and a small opening in the collecting system was oversewn. The creatinine concentration of the drain fluid is 34.5 mg/dL, consistent with urine. Despite conservative management, the volume fails to decline. A retrograde pyelogram demonstrates a moderate amount of contrast extravasation, confirming the urinary fistula. What is the most appropriate management at this time?

a. Immediate reexploration and repair

b. Percutaneous nephrostomy tube placement

c. Removal of surgical drain

d. Internalized ureteral stent placement

e. Internalized ureteral stent placement, continued surgical drain monitoring, and placement of Foley catheter

ANSWERS

1. **d. Radical nephrectomy and simultaneous pulmonary metastectomy.** This patient would be best managed with a radical nephrectomy and simultaneous removal of the pulmonary nodule. Systemic therapy is not a primary treatment unless there is extensive metastatic disease at presentation. Given his age and lack of medical problems, there is no reason to delay the removal of his kidney and the pulmonary nodule. The tumor location and pulmonary nodule both can be accessed through one incision (i.e., thoracoabdominal).

2. **c. Chevron incision with CPB-DHCA.** CPB-DHCA has been established as the most prudent course for the removal of these tumor thrombi. The chevron incision provides the best exposure. Alternatives to CPB, including extensive liver mobilization and intrapericardial resection, carry an increased risk of bleeding.

3. **c. 40 minutes.** The duration of DHCA can vary depending on the degree of tumor thrombus. Vena cava resection and substitution can add additional time if there is significant tumor invasion into the wall of the vena cava. Studies have suggested that irreversible neurologic effects may be observed after 40 minutes of DHCA.

4. **d. Single 4-cm tumor in any location.** In patients with a normal contralateral kidney, the current literature supports elective partial nephrectomy for single T1 tumors.

5. **a. Duration of renal ischemia.** Duration of renal ischemia is the strongest modifiable risk factor for renal insufficiency after partial nephrectomy.

6. **c. Renal pelvis, artery, vein.** The renal pelvis is the first structure one encounters with the posterior right lumbotomy incision, followed by the artery and vein. This approach can be used to repair ureteropelvic junction obstruction, especially in children or patients with multiple prior abdominal and/or flank surgeries.

7. **a:** T2b; **b:** T1a; **c:** T4; **d:** T3a; **e:** T3c.

8. **d. Nasogastric tube placement, parenteral nutrition, and conservative management.** Conservative management of a pancreatic fistula should be the first approach in this patient. Initial nasogastric tube placement can help resolve the ileus. Parenteral nutrition will limit any pancreatic secretions from oral intake.

9. **c. Posterior segmental artery.** The posterior division is the first and most consistent branch point of the renal artery and supplies roughly one fourth of the blood supply.

10. **d. Kocher maneuver.** Mobilization of the second and third portions of the duodenum is referred to as a *Kocher maneuver*. The Pringle maneuver is the temporary occlusion of the porta hepatis. The Langenbeck maneuver is the division of the coronary and right triangular ligaments, providing medial rotation of the right lobe of the liver and exposure of the suprarenal inferior vena cava.

11. **e. Extracorporeal repair and autotransplantation.** All patients with solitary kidneys are high-risk candidates for partial nephrectomy and may have transient renal impairment postoperatively. The degree and duration of renal impairment may be increased owing to risks associated with renal autotransplantation (hemorrhage, thrombosis, lymphocele, stenosis).

12. **d. Internal oblique and transversalis.** The subcostal nerve runs between these two layers. Caution must be taken not to sever this nerve during flank incisions.

13. **c. Paresis of the flank musculature and flank bulge.** Damage to the subcostal nerve results in denervation and paresis of the flank musculature, leading to chronic postoperative pain or flank bulge.

14. **d. 20% to 30%.** Multiple postmortem and radiographic studies estimate that 25% of the general population have supernumerary renal arteries.

15. **e. Kidney with 8-cm enhancing upper pole hilar mass.** There should be little reservation about performing a radical nephrectomy for an enhancing mass, especially in the upper pole. Almost all nonmalignant disease affecting the kidney can be treated via a simple approach.

16. **e. Unrecognized paradoxical embolism.** This rare but devastating clinical situation occurs in patients with a patent foramen ovale. An embolism may originate from tumor thrombus manipulation or from deep venous thromboembolism.

17. **e. Surgical resection.** There have been numerous studies to suggest that surgical resection is the mainstay of therapy for kidney cancer.

18. **d. Superior mesenteric.** Ligation of the superior mesenteric artery produces ischemia in the bowel distribution above. The superior mesenteric artery can be mistaken for the left renal artery from the anterior approach. Visualizing the artery from a posterior position as it enters the hilum will help to minimize this complication.

19. **d. Arterial collateral branch vessels.** Failure of the renal vein to decompress after ligation of the main renal artery indicates additional arterial inflow, which may be secondary to a missed lower or upper pole artery or extensive collateral arteries.

20. **a. Large right upper pole renal mass with tumor thrombus in the renal vein.** The thoracoabdominal incision is ideal for larger tumors involving the upper pole. The incision is also ideal for managing tumor thrombus extending into the renal vein. The inferior vena cava can be nicely exposed via this approach.

21. **c. Bleeding and coagulopathy.** Intraoperatively, the administration of heparin in addition to hypothermia leads to significant coagulopathy. The bleeding from heparin is typically limited to an "ooze" intraoperatively and should not consume time and energy during the operation. After tumor removal, the rewarming process helps to promote coagulation.

22. **f. None of the above.** Proposed benefits of preoperative RAE include shrinkage of an arterialized tumor thrombus to ease surgical removal, reduced blood loss, facilitation of dissection due to tissue plane edema, ability to ligate the renal vein before the renal artery at time of nephrectomy, and modulation of the immune response.

23. **d. Postinfarction syndrome (pain, nausea, and fever).** The triad of fever, flank pain, and nausea occurs in up to 75% of patients after angioembolization. Fevers can often exceed 39.4 ° C (103 ° F) and are best managed with antipyretics.

24. **e. Urinary leak.** Partial nephrectomy for nonexophytic masses has an increased risk of entering the collecting system. Even when the collecting system is closed under direct vision, there may still be extravasation of urine that collects in the perirenal space. The use of postoperative surgical drains is imperative in the management of these collections to reduce the risk of infections. In addition, the drain output volume can be observed to determine if collections are resolving. Renal failure is rare unless operating on a solitary kidney or on a patient with marginal renal function. Rhabdomyolysis can be encountered secondary to patient positioning and increased body mass index.

25. **e. Internalized ureteral stent placement, continued surgical drain monitoring, and placement of Foley catheter.** Placement of a ureteral stent can promote urine drainage into the bladder. Keeping a Foley catheter in place reduces urine reflux.

CHAPTER REVIEW

1. The right renal artery is posterior to the inferior vena cava.
2. Renal arteries are end arteries; ligation results in infarction of the segment that they supply.
3. The renal venous network intercommunicates.
4. Lumbar veins often enter the left renal vein and, not infrequently, the right renal vein. They enter posteriorly. Care must be taken when encircling the renal vein not to tear one of these lumbar veins.
5. There is no conclusive evidence that renal artery embolization has any immunologic therapeutic benefit.
6. The renal artery is always ligated before the renal vein when performing a nephrectomy; each vessel is ligated individually.
7. Patients with a glomerular filtration rate of less than 60 mL/min or those with significant proteinuria are at risk for postoperative renal failure following renal surgery—particularly when a nephrectomy is performed.
8. Adrenalectomy is not recommended as part of a radical nephrectomy unless imaging shows adrenal involvement with tumor or an upper pole tumor is contiguous with the adrenal.
9. Transesophageal echocardiography is an excellent modality to determine the level of the vena cava tumor thrombus immediately before the surgical event.
10. In patients with vena cava tumor thrombi cephalad to the hepatic venous outflow who require CPB, either mild hypothermia and no circulatory arrest or significant hypothermia with circulatory arrest may be performed. Each technique has its advantages and disadvantages. The method used is at the discretion of the surgeon.
11. The addition of a lymphadenectomy to a radical nephrectomy for renal cell carcinoma has a questionable impact on progression-free and overall survival. It may be considered in patients who have enlarged lymph nodes on preoperative imaging, those in whom cytoreductive surgery is being performed, and those with ominous pathologic findings of the primary renal tumor.
12. Ligation of the right renal vein will result in failure of the right renal unit due to lack of venous collateral vessels.
13. Ligation of the left renal vein is possible because collateral venous drainage may occur through lumbar and gonadal vessels.
14. The renal vein ostium of the vena cava should be excised in patients with vena cava tumor thrombi, as invasion of the vena cava vein wall at this site is not uncommonly found.
15. 25% of the general population have supernumerary renal arteries.
16. The superior mesenteric artery can be mistaken for the left renal artery from the anterior approach. Rarely, the hepatic artery can be mistaken for the right renal artery. Visualizing the artery from a posterior position relative to the renal vein as it enters the hilum will help identify the renal artery.
17. Proposed benefits of preoperative renal artery embolization include shrinkage of an arterialized vena cava tumor thrombus to ease surgical removal, reduced blood loss, facilitation of dissection due to tissue plane edema, and the ability to ligate the renal vein before the renal artery at time of nephrectomy. These patients may develop the postinfarction syndrome (pain, nausea, and fever). The triad of fever, flank pain, and nausea occurs in up to 75% of patients after angioembolization.

61 Laparoscopic and Robotic Surgery of the Kidney

Michael J. Schwartz, Soroush Rais-Bahrami, and Louis R. Kavoussi

QUESTIONS

1. A 22-year-old woman presents with severe intermittent, positional left flank pain. Her medical and surgical histories are unremarkable, and her body mass index (BMI) is 19 kg/m². Renal ultrasound shows no evidence of stones or hydronephrosis. What is the best next step in evaluation?

   a. Cystoscopy and retrograde pyelogram
   b. Computed tomography (CT) urogram
   c. Flat and upright intravenous pyelogram
   d. Nuclear renal scan
   e. Observation

2. A laparoscopic renal biopsy is performed for a 53-year-old man with chronic renal insufficiency of unclear etiology and a BMI of 47 kg/m². A prior percutaneous approach did not obtain adequate tissue. Using a two-port retroperitoneal approach, copious retroperitoneal fat is encountered and there is difficulty with orientation and localizing the kidney. The best next step is to:

   a. abort the procedure. Recommend a repeat percutaneous image-guided approach to the nephrology service.
   b. advance a biopsy needle under laparoscopic guidance through the fat to the presumed location of the kidney.
   c. convert to an open retroperitoneal procedure using a mini flank incision.
   d. intraoperative renal ultrasound to localize the kidney.
   e. place a third port to aid in dissection.

3. The following are preferred methods of renal hilar ligation during laparoscopic/robotic nephrectomy EXCEPT:

   a. en bloc stapling of the renal artery together with the renal vein.
   b. stapling the renal artery and vein separately.
   c. multiple titanium clips on the artery, stapler ligation of the vein.
   d. multiple Hem-o-lok clips on the artery, stapler ligation of the vein.
   e. all of the above are preferred methods of renal hilar ligation.

4. Absolute contraindications to laparoscopic partial nephrectomy include:

   a. aspirin therapy for cardiac stents.
   b. multiple prior abdominal surgeries.
   c. prior ipsilateral renal surgery.
   d. untreated infection.
   e. body mass index greater than 50 kg/m².

5. On postoperative day 3 following robotic-assisted laparoscopic right partial nephrectomy, a 54-year-old man presents to the emergency room with nausea, low-grade fever, right-sided abdominal pain, and foul-smelling discharge from a right lateral trocar site. CT scan with oral contrast demonstrates extravasation of contrast from the ascending colon with an adjacent fluid collection. The most likely etiology of the injury is:

   a. trocar injury.
   b. blunt dissection.
   c. sharp dissection.
   d. bowel ischemia.
   e. electrocautery scatter.

6. A 65-year-old man underwent an uncomplicated robot-assisted left laparoscopic partial nephrectomy and was discharged home on postoperative day 2, voiding clear yellow urine. He presents to the emergency room a week later with new-onset gross hematuria and flank pain. He is mildly tachycardic and hypotensive. Hematocrit is 22%. One hour after fluid resuscitation, his vital signs have normalized, but the hematuria persists and he is requiring continuous bladder irrigation (CBI). The best next step is:

   a. CT scan with intravenous (IV) contrast.
   b. intensive care unit (ICU) admission, blood transfusion, and serial hematocrits.
   c. echocardiogram.
   d. renal angiography with angioembolization.
   e. cystoscopy, placement of left ureteral stent.

7. A 53-year-old woman who underwent a laparoscopic heminephrectomy for a 5-cm central kidney tumor continues to have drain output greater than 150 mL per day on postoperative day 3. Drain fluid assessment demonstrates a creatinine level of 19 mg/dL while the patient's serum creatinine is within normal limits (1.1 mg/dL). The best way to resolve the leakage is to:

   a. continue the drain and observe.
   b. insert an indwelling ureteral stent.
   c. insert an indwelling ureteral stent and Foley catheter.
   d. insert a percutaneous nephrostomy tube.
   e. consider a completion nephrectomy.

8. A 50-year-old man presents with 4+ proteinuria and intermittent milky-white urine after recent travel. Retrograde pyelogram demonstrates a lymphorenal fistula. Complete blood count (CBC) demonstrates eosinophilia, and urine culture is positive for *Wuchereria bancrofti*. Treatment options recommended prior to laparoscopic nephrolysis include all of the following EXCEPT:

   a. treatment course of diethylcarbamazine.
   b. low-fat diet.
   c. nonsteroidal anti-inflammatory drug (NSAID) administration.
   d. observation.
   e. retrograde instillation of silver nitrate into the collecting system.

9. A robotic-assisted laparoscopic left partial nephrectomy is performed to resect a local recurrence following laparoscopic radio-frequency ablation of an anterior renal tumor. During exposure of the left renal vessels, dense adhesions and scar tissue are encountered and a deep injury to the pancreatic tail is identified. This scenario is best managed by:

   a. application of biologic glue or sealant over the tail of the pancreas.
   b. distal pancreatectomy with an endoscopic GIA stapler.
   c. routine completion of the case, drain placement, and postoperative bowel rest.

d. routine completion of the case with administration of somatostatin postoperatively.

e. routine completion of the case with postoperative bowel rest and parenteral nutrition.

10. Standard trocar placement for renal surgery may need to be adjusted based on which of the following patient characteristics?

a. Obese body habitus

b. Prior abdominal surgery

c. Renal tumor size

d. Robotic assistance

e. All of the above

11. Laparoscopic unilateral simple nephrectomy is indicated in all of the following clinical scenarios EXCEPT:

a. 40-year-old woman with renovascular hypertension refractory to medical and angiographic repair.

b. 58-year-old man with left-sided xanthogranulomatous pyelonephritis and differential renal function of 8%.

c. 69-year-old man with 7-cm endophytic right renal mass with 25 Hounsfield unit enhancement on abdominal CT.

d. 63-year-old man with left renal tuberculosis recalcitrant to medical management.

e. 34-year-old woman with chronic right flank pain, right hydronephrosis not amenable to surgical repair, and dramatic thinning of the right renal parenchyma.

12. When obtaining access for laparoscopic renal surgery, which of the following technique(s) is/are employed to minimize the risk of bowel injury?

a. Insertion of a Veress needle (Ethicon US, LLC) away from prior surgical scars

b. Hasson technique of open trocar placement

c. Retroperitoneal approach

d. a and b.

e. a, b, and c

13. During laparoscopic renal cyst decortication for a large, symptomatic left perihilar cyst, a major portion of the cyst wall is noted to be adjacent to the vessels and collecting system. The best next step in management to prevent cyst recurrence is:

a. complete the removal of the cyst wall. Repair any vascular or collecting system injuries as necessary.

b. place a pedicle of autologous fat in the defect.

c. fill the cystic space with talc.

d. plan to leave a drain in the defect for 6 to 8 weeks, periodically instilling a sclerosis agent.

e. all of the above are equally viable options.

14. Routine lymphadenectomy when performing laparoscopic radical nephrectomy for node-negative patients by preoperative imaging has been shown to yield:

a. increased overall survival.

b. higher complication rates.

c. 10% rate of lymph node metastasis.

d. increased cancer-specific survival.

e. none of the above.

15. A patient clinically suited to undergo cytoreductive nephrectomy may benefit from the laparoscopic approach to cytoreductive nephrectomy over open cytoreductive nephrectomy in regard to all of the following EXCEPT:

a. decreased blood loss.

b. shorter perioperative hospitalization.

c. shortened convalescence with similar survival.

d. shorter time interval to commencing systemic therapy.

e. improved overall survival.

16. A mesenteric defect is recognized during medial reflection of the descending colon in a laparoscopic left partial nephrectomy. Before completion of the case, the mesenteric defect should be repaired to prevent:

a. internal hernia.

b. formation of adhesions.

c. postoperative hemorrhage.

d. colonic injury.

e. none of the above.

17. An area of serosal denudation is noticed by the bedside assistant while performing colonic mobilization bluntly with a suction-irrigation device during a robotic-assisted laparoscopic left nephrectomy. The best choice in management of this injury is:

a. routine completion of the case with postoperative bowel rest and parenteral nutrition

b. placement of imbricating stiches to repair the area of serosal disruption.

c. segmental colon resection and primary reanastomosis.

d. end colostomy.

e. diverting loop ileostomy.

18. Laparoscopy is now the preferred method for addressing most surgical renal pathology based on widely reproducible findings in comparative studies with open approaches showing:

a. equivalent outcomes.

b. superior cosmesis.

c. reduced analgesic requirement.

d. shorter convalescence.

e. all of the above.

19. When compared with traditional laparoscopic renal surgery, robotic-assisted laparoscopic renal surgery has been shown to provide:

a. improved oncologic outcomes.

b. reduced cost.

c. more surgeons the ability to offer a laparoscopic approach.

d. improved operative times.

e. shorter hospital stay.

ANSWERS

1. **c. Flat and upright intravenous pyelogram.** Ptotic kidneys often present with a history similar to that of a ureteropelvic junction obstruction, with the primary exception that the associated pain is often positional and relieved after a period of lying down. The supine position often eliminates the transient renal ischemia or urinary obstruction that may be the cause of discomfort. The demographic most commonly afflicted with renal ptosis is a young, thin female similar to the patient described. Determining renal descent of approximately two lumbar vertebral bodies with supine and erect intravenous pyelograms makes the diagnosis of a ptotic kidney. A secondary evaluation option is power Doppler sonography performed with the patient in both the supine and erect positions. Nephropexy should not proceed before definitively establishing the diagnosis of a ptotic kidney.

2. **d. Intraoperative renal ultrasound to localize the kidney.** In this case, the patient's obese body habitus and associated retroperitoneal fat pose a challenge in proper orientation and identification of the kidney from the retroperitoneoscopic approach.

In obese patients, intraoperative ultrasonography may be required to localize the kidney when copious retroperitoneal or perinephric fat is present. Beyond simply assisting in identification of the kidney, it may allow for precise tissue sampling, particularly in the setting of a failed prior percutaneous biopsy attempt.

3. **d. Multiple Hem-o-lok clips on the artery, stapler ligation of the vein.** There are multiple safe and acceptable methods of ligating the renal vessels during a laparoscopic nephrectomy. Commonly, an endovascular gastrointestinal anastomosis stapler is used to ligate the renal hilar vessels separately, first ligating the artery followed by ligation of the vein. En bloc stapling of the renal hilar vessels has not been shown to result in significantly different blood pressures, presence of bruits, or rates of arteriovenous fistulization in a randomized control trial compared to separate staple ligation. In cases where clips are employed, multiple titanium clips are recommended on the remnant patient side of the vessels. Based on safety data derived in the laparoscopic donor nephrectomy population, the use of Hem-o-lok clips (Weck Closure Systems, Research Triangle Park, NC) is contraindicated for the ligation of the renal artery per recommendations of the manufacturer as well as the Food and Drug Administration.

4. **d. Untreated infection.** Untreated infection is an absolute contraindication for laparoscopic renal surgery, as are uncorrected coagulopathy and hypovolemic shock. Laparoscopic partial nephrectomy has been reported as a feasible, safe approach in appropriately selected patients with intravascular stents on aspirin therapy, multiple prior abdominal operations, history of prior ipsilateral renal surgery (open and laparoscopic), and morbid obesity.

5. **e. Electrocautery scatter.** The clinical scenario described represents a classic presentation of an unrecognized bowel injury. Although blunt dissection, sharp dissection, and transmission of thermal energy from electrocautery are each responsible for approximately equal proportions of bowel injuries, electrocautery scatter is the most frequent cause of unrecognized bowel injury. Delayed necrosis and perforation of the bowel wall from electrocautery may lead to atypical or delayed presentation and most commonly presents between postoperative days 3 and 5. Trocar placement and bowel ischemia are both infrequent causes of bowel injury.

6. **d. Renal angiography with angioembolization.** A patient who has recently undergone traditional laparoscopic or robot-assisted laparoscopic partial nephrectomy presenting with gross hematuria and hemodynamic changes likely has a postoperative bleed resulting from an arteriovenous fistula or pseudoaneurysm formation. Although a CT scan with intravenous contrast may help diagnose and localize a postoperative bleed, this will ultimately delay treatment. Immediate renal angiogram with selective arterial embolization allows for diagnosis, localization, and definitive treatment in the same setting. Furthermore, immediate angiography avoids the systemic contrast bolus required for CT angiography.

7. **a. Continue the drain and observe.** This patient with continued drain output with elevated drain fluid creatinine following laparoscopic heminephrectomy likely has a perinephric urinary extravasation. Urinary extravasation after laparoscopic partial nephrectomy is more common in cases of centrally located tumors or larger resections requiring more extensive reconstruction. These urinary leaks will almost always resolve with observation. If the drain output does not decrease, then ureteral obstruction is likely to be present, and placement of a ureteral stent is indicated. There is no indication at this point for either a nephrostomy tube or completion nephrectomy.

8. **c. Nonsteroidal anti-inflammatory drug (NSAID) administration.** Chyluria is caused by lymphatic rupture or fistulous connection into the pyelocalyceal system, often diagnosed as described in the clinical scenario posed. Most cases are self-limited and improve with no intervention. Laparoscopic nephrolysis should only be undertaken after attempts at more conservative management methods, including changing to a low-fat diet, treatment course of diethylcarbamazine, and retrograde injection of sclerosing agents into the collecting system.

9. **b. Distal pancreatectomy with an endoscopic GIA stapler.** Deep injuries to the pancreas should be intraoperatively addressed because pancreatic leak may lead to significant postoperative morbidity. The distal pancreas is most often manipulated during the medial mobilization of the spleen, pancreas, and descending colon during transperitoneal laparoscopic or robotic left-sided renal or adrenal surgery. The best approach is typically to isolate the injury and seal it using an endovascular GIA stapling device (Medtronic, Minneapolis, MN). This is the same approach used with much success during intentional distal pancreatectomy and closes both the pancreatic stump and duct, if injured. Application of a biologic glue or sealant may be used as an adjuvant but should not be the primary means of addressing the pancreatic injury. Drain placement and observation may be used for superficial but not deep pancreatic injuries. Bowel rest and use of somatostatin are not sufficient treatment to prevent sequelae of a deep pancreatic injury that may have resulted in leakage from the pancreatic duct.

10. **e. All of the above.** Trocar placement for renal surgery should be individualized based on patient characteristics and surgical approach planned. Patient body habitus, prior surgical history, intraoperative findings (including adhesions), renal pathology, surgical indication, and surgical approach (transperitoneal vs. retroperitoneal, robotic-assistance vs. conventional laparoscopy vs. laparoendoscopic single-site surgery [LESS]) are all factors to consider to optimize trocar placement.

11. **c. 69-year-old man with 7-cm endophytic right renal mass with 25 Hounsfield unit enhancement on abdominal CT.** Laparoscopic simple nephrectomy is removal of the entire kidney for the treatment of a variety of benign renal diseases. Of the clinical scenarios provided, all are indications for laparoscopic simple nephrectomy except that of the 69-year-old male with a contrast-enhancing renal mass on abdominal CT imaging. This is likely representative of a malignant renal cortical neoplasm, and a laparoscopic simple nephrectomy should not be pursued for management of a suspected malignancy.

12. **e. a, b, and c.** In cases of prior abdominal surgery, obtaining access for laparoscopic renal surgery should be performed with care. Insertion of a Veress needle away from prior surgical scars is one method to avoid potential adhesions and injury to the bowel. Also, other options to help decrease the risk of bowel injury in the setting of prior abdominal surgery include open trocar placement by using a Hasson technique or avoiding the peritoneal space by developing the retroperitoneal space and performing retroperitoneoscopic renal surgery.

13. **b. Place a pedicle of autologous fat in the defect.** Laparoscopic cyst decortication may be challenging in cases of central or perihilar cysts, in which it is often not feasible to remove a portion of the cyst wall adjacent to the hilar vessels or renal collecting system. In such cases, a portion of the cyst wall may be retained and a pedicle of autologous fat can be draped within the defect to serve as a wick.

14. **c. 10% rate of lymph node metastasis.** In a study of patients without suspicion for lymph node involvement on preoperative imaging, a 10% rate of lymph node metastases was noted in patient undergoing laparoscopic radical nephrectomy. Those with positive lymph nodes were found to harbor higher-grade lesions, with T3 or T4 disease on pathology. Although there may be potential benefit of lymphadenectomy for a portion of clinically node-negative patients, lymphadenectomy in the setting of laparoscopic radical nephrectomy with clinically negative lymph nodes has not been shown to improve overall or cancer-specific survival.

15. **e. Improved overall survival.** Laparoscopic cytoreductive nephrectomy provides the benefits of a minimally invasive surgical approach with decreased blood loss, shorter perioperative

hospitalization, shortened convalescence, and, in some studies, shortened interval duration to commencement of systemic therapy. Studies of laparoscopic and open approaches to cytoreductive nephrectomy have demonstrated no significant difference in survival.

16. **a. Internal hernia.** Formation of a mesenteric defect during colonic reflection should be managed with careful closure of the defect to prevent an internal hernia through which loops of small bowel may pass and incarcerate. Care should be taken during repair of a mesenteric defect to not compromise the blood supply to the colon, which traverses the mesentery. Degree of adhesion formation, risk of postoperative hemorrhage, and rates of colonic injury are not reportedly different in the setting of colonic mesenteric defects.

17. **b. Placement of imbricating stiches to repair the area of serosal disruption.** When recognized intraoperatively, the area of a suspected bowel injury should be carefully examined to ensure that a deeper defect into the muscular layers or a full-thickness bowel wall defect is not present.

Serosal disruption, particularly as a result of blunt or sharp dissection without risk of electrocautery scatter, may be oversewn to repair and reinforce the area. There is no need for segmental resection, diversion, or colostomy formation. Conservative management without intraoperative repair is not recommended in these cases as the depth of injury may potentially be more significant than what is intraoperatively recognized.

18. **e. All of the above.** All of the above are well-established benefits of laparoscopy compared with open surgery for a variety of renal surgeries.

19. **c. More surgeons the ability to offer a laparoscopic approach.** Data support the proposition that introduction of robotic assistance has increased the number of surgeons who are providing laparoscopic renal surgical options to their patients in the form of robotic-assisted laparoscopy. The use of the Da Vinci Robotic System (Intuitive Surgical, Sunnyvale, CA) has not consistently demonstrated improvement in operative times, cost, length of hospitalization, or oncologic outcomes.

CHAPTER REVIEW

1. Obesity is associated with an increased risk of open conversion.
2. Transperitoneal laparoscopy provides the largest working space with greater versatility of angles and instrumentation
3. When a laparoscopic nephrectomy is performed, the renal artery should be divided first, followed by division of the renal vein. The vascular stapler will provide three rows of staples left on the stump.
4. In obese patients, intraoperative ultrasonography may be helpful in localizing the kidney.
5. One must be careful not to mistake the inferior vena cava for the renal vein, particularly when using retroperitoneal access, in which anatomic landmarks may be more subtle.
6. En bloc hilar stapling (artery and vein together) has not been shown to result in arteriovenous fistula formation.
7. In patients undergoing partial nephrectomy (open or laparoscopic), there is no demonstrated difference in long-term outcome for those who have positive surgical margins versus those who do not. Nonetheless, negative surgical margins should always be the goal of any oncologic renal surgery.
8. Patients with unrecognized bowel injury following laparoscopy typically present with persistent and increased trocar-site pain at the site closest to the bowel injury.
9. Port-site tumor implantation is usually associated with high-grade renal transitional-cell carcinoma and less commonly with renal cell carcinoma. It is often associated with intraoperative tumor spillage.
10. When renal hilar vascular clamping is used during partial nephrectomy, there may be less injury to the kidney when artery-only clamping is performed rather than artery and vein clamping.
11. Blunt dissection, sharp dissection, and transmission of thermal energy from electrocautery are each responsible for approximately equal proportions of bowel injuries; electrocautery scatter is the most frequent cause of unrecognized bowel injury.
12. Chyluria is caused by lymphatic rupture or fistulous connection into the pyelocalyceal system. Most cases are self-limited and improved with no intervention.

62 Nonsurgical Focal Therapy for Renal Tumors

Chad R. Tracy and Jeffrey A. Cadeddu

QUESTIONS

1. Nephron-sparing surgery (partial nephrectomy):
   a. is the predominant treatment modality used in the United States for the management of small renal masses.
   b. offers equivalent cancer-specific and overall survival compared with radical nephrectomy.
   c. when performed laparoscopically, it is associated with fewer complications than radiofrequency ablation (RFA) or cryoablation.
   d. offers metastatic recurrence-free survival and cancer-specific survival similar to that of radiofrequency ablation and cryoablation.
   e. was not impacted by the advent of hand-assisted laparoscopic radical nephrectomy.

2. With regard to deciding on a particular ablation modality, which of the following should be considered?
   a. RFA is associated with less postoperative hemorrhage than cryoablation.
   b. Both RFA and cryoablation are subject to "heat sink."
   c. The American Urological Association (AUA) guidelines currently recommend consideration of ablation for primary treatment of T1a renal tumors, even for younger, healthier patients, with the understanding that recurrence rates may be higher and salvage procedure more difficult.
   d. All of the above
   e. Both a and b are true

3. The critical treatment temperature threshold during cryoablation at which irreparable cell damage is achieved is:
   a. 0° C.
   b. −60° C.
   c. −20° C.
   d. −40° C.
   e. −19.4° C.

4. Critical parameters for successful renal cryosurgery include:
   a. a double freeze-thaw cycle.
   b. achieving a critical target temperature.
   c. treatment under real-time image guidance.
   d. treatment to beyond 1 cm of the targeted lesion.
   e. all of the above.

5. Compared with renal cryoablation, the primary disadvantage of RFA is:
   a. higher risk of hemorrhage following RFA.
   b. inability to use RFA laparoscopically.
   c. inability to monitor treatment under image guidance.
   d. inferior cancer-specific survival.
   e. none of the above.

6. Recent meta-analyses have demonstrated:
   a. higher local recurrence rates with ablative technologies when compared with partial or radical nephrectomy.
   b. no evidence for the superiority of one ablation technology versus the other with regard to oncologic outcomes or complications.
   c. a lack of uniformity regarding evaluation, patient selection, treatment, and follow-up of patients undergoing renal tumor ablation.
   d. fewer complications with renal tumor ablation compared with extirpative treatments.
   e. all of the above.

7. The most important technique to increase the size of RF lesions is:
   a. using higher RF currents.
   b. applying RF currents faster to achieve better heating.
   c. clamping hilar vessels.
   d. reducing impedance by improving current conductivity.
   e. using "dry" RFA.

8. Regarding high-intensity focused ultrasonography (HIFU), which of the following is TRUE?
   a. Preliminary data suggest equivalent oncologic outcomes with HIFU when compared with alternative ablative technologies or extirpative options.
   b. HIFU acts through local thermal and cavitary processes to generate tissue temperatures in excess of 65° C.
   c. Animal and human studies have demonstrated consistent tissue necrosis following treatment.
   d. The most commonly cited complication following HIFU for the treatment of renal lesions is post-treatment hemorrhage.
   e. Because renal HIFU is performed under real-time image guidance, targeting is not significantly impacted by respiratory movement.

9. Following tumor ablation, the most reliable method of documenting treatment success is:
   a. biopsy of the treatment area with hematoxylin and eosin (H&E) staining.
   b. biopsy of the treatment area with reduced nicotinamide adenine dinucleotide (NADH) diaphorase staining.
   c. follow-up computed tomography (CT) or magnetic resonance imaging (MRI) with contrast that demonstrates complete loss of contrast enhancement and stable or decreased size of the treated area.
   d. follow-up CT or MRI without contrast that demonstrates a decrease in size of the treated area.
   e. all of the above.

ANSWERS

1. **d. Offers metastatic recurrence-free survival and cancer-specific survival similar to that of radiofrequency ablation and cryoablation.** Nephron-sparing surgery is considered the gold standard treatment for small renal masses but is underused in the United States. Partial nephrectomy offers equivalent oncologic outcomes when compared with radical nephrectomy and demonstrates superior renal functional preservation. Laparoscopic partial nephrectomy offers excellent cancer-specific end points but is technically challenging and is associated with significant complications. Cryoablation and radiofrequency ablation are associated with significantly fewer complications than laparoscopic partial nephrectomy. There is no significant difference in metastatic recurrence-free survival between extirpative and ablative treatments. Cancer-specific survival (CSS) following RFA is comparable to laparoscopic partial nephrectomy. CSS is comparable between open partial nephrectomy and both RFA and cryoablation. Preliminary studies suggest that the technical ease and minimal morbidity of hand-assisted laparoscopic nephrectomy may ultimately lead to fewer nephron-sparing procedures.

2. **e. Both a and b are true.**

3. **d. −40° C.** Experimental evidence suggests that irreversible cellular damage is achieved in normal renal parenchyma at −19.4° C. However, tumor cells require lower treatment temperatures to achieve uniform cellular necrosis. The recommended treatment temperature during renal cryosurgery is −40° C.

4. **e. All of the above.** Animal studies have demonstrated that a single freeze-thaw cycle is inferior to a double freeze-thaw cycle with respect to adequacy of tissue ablation and local tumor control. As mentioned, complete cellular necrosis is consistently achieved at a targeted temperature of −40° C. Campbell and colleagues (1998)* demonstrated that the aforementioned threshold temperature of −40° C was achieved 3.1 mm inside the edge of the evolving ice ball. To guarantee that the tumor is completely ablated with a margin of normal tissue, the ice ball is generally carried 5 to 10 mm beyond the edge of the tumor when viewed under real-time imaging.

5. **c. Inability to monitor treatment under image guidance.** The primary disadvantage when employing RFA for the treatment of renal lesions is difficulty in monitoring treatment under real-time image guidance. The risk of hemorrhage is higher with cryoablation. RFA may be employed laparoscopically, percutaneously, or openly. Cancer-specific survival is equivalent between RFA and cryoablation.

6. **e. All of the above.** Three recent meta-analyses evaluated outcomes following partial nephrectomy, radical nephrectomy, cryoablation, and RFA for the treatment of small renal masses. Both RFA and cryoablation demonstrated higher local recurrence rates when compared with partial or radical nephrectomy. However, the majority of published studies on cryoablation and RFA have enrolled small numbers of patients and used disparate operative and follow-up protocols. The pathology is either not obtained or is difficult to interpret, and the reliability of radiographic imaging remains unknown. Although the aggregate duration of follow-up is too short to derive irrefutable conclusions, treatment outcomes with cryoablation and RFA appear comparable. In general, complications occur with equal or less frequency with tumor ablation when compared with partial or radical nephrectomy.

7. **d. Reducing impedance by improving current conductivity.** The electrically conductive agent facilitates the delivery of energy from the electrode to surrounding tissue, rendering it a much larger, "virtual" electrode. Impedance remains lower, and larger volumes are ablated. One technique to accomplish this is to employ saline-cooled electrodes, which reduce charring at the tip of the electrode and thereby reduce impedance.

8. **b. HIFU acts through local thermal and cavitary processes to generate tissue temperatures in excess of 65° C.** The use of HIFU in the treatment of small renal masses remains investigational. Experimental data has demonstrated "skip" lesions following treatment, which have been attributed to targeting obstacles, including acoustic interference and respiratory movement. Skin burns have been reported in as many as 10% of patients.

9. **c. Follow-up computed tomography (CT) or magnetic resonance imaging (MRI) with contrast that demonstrates complete loss of contrast enhancement and stable or decreased size of the treated area.** Complete loss of contrast enhancement on follow-up CT or MRI has been considered a sign of complete tissue destruction. Following cryoablation, the treated area demonstrates a decrease in size of approximately 50% in the year following treatment. Following RFA, the treated area may not demonstrate a decrease in size. Any increase in size following treatment should be viewed as an ominous sign, and intervention should be directed accordingly. Postablative biopsy, although helpful, yields ambiguous results following RFA. Its use and interpretation remain controversial.

CHAPTER REVIEW

1. Currently, a double freeze-thaw cycle is suggested for cryotherapy with a period of time during each cycle in which the temperature is maintained at −40° C.

2. Radiofrequency waves generate heat by causing ionic agitation in the tissue through which they pass; charring at the probe tip prevents adequate conduction of the wave from the probe into tissue; to prevent heat at the probe becoming excessive with resultant charring, the probes are cooled.

3. CT or MRI is used to follow patients after ablative therapy. There should be a complete lack of contrast enhancement at the tumor site. Successful cryoablation on follow-up imaging often reveals up to a 50% reduction in size of the lesion. RF ablation followed over the long term often shows a slight reduction in size and cavitation.

4. The tumor should be biopsied to confirm its malignant nature before ablative therapy is performed.

5. The most common complication following cryoablation is hemorrhage; a serious complication following radiofrequency ablation is ureteral/collecting system injury. Bleeding is less common following radiofrequency ablation.

6. High-intensity focused ultrasonography generates heat by focusing the ultrasound waves at a point; unfortunately, skin burns are a common complication of this technology.

7. There is no significant difference in metastatic recurrence-free survival between extirpative and ablative treatments. Cancer-specific survival (CSS) following RFA is comparable to laparoscopic partial nephrectomy. CSS is comparable between open partial nephrectomy and both RFA and cryoablation.

---

*Sources referenced can be found in *Campbell-Walsh Urology, 11th Edition*, on the Expert Consult website.

63 Treatment of Advanced Renal Cell Carcinoma

W. Marston Linehan and Ramaprasad Srinivasan

QUESTIONS

1. What is the approximate overall objective response rate to interleukin-2 (IL-2) monotherapy in patients with metastatic renal cell carcinoma (RCC)?
   a. 5%
   b. 10%
   c. 15%
   d. 25%
   e. 35%

2. Which of the following regarding IL-2 therapy for metastatic RCC is TRUE?
   a. IL-2 has demonstrable efficacy in clear cell as well as papillary RCC.
   b. Randomized studies have demonstrated a survival benefit associated with high-dose IL-2.
   c. Low-dose subcutaneous and high-dose intravenous IL-2 have comparable efficacy.
   d. Durable complete responses are seen in a small proportion of patients receiving high-dose IL-2.
   e. Newer formulations have led to better tolerability of high-dose IL-2.

3. In the Memorial Sloan-Kettering Cancer Center (MSKCC) prognostic scheme for patients with metastatic RCC undergoing therapy with cytokine or chemotherapy, which of the following is NOT a predictor of poor outcome?
   a. Karnofsky performance status greater than 80%
   b. Elevated lactate dehydrogenase
   c. Elevated calcium
   d. Decreased hemoglobin
   e. Absence of prior nephrectomy

4. In which of the following patients with metastatic RCC is cytoreductive nephrectomy most appropriate?
   a. A 50-year-old male with an Eastern Cooperative Oncology Group (ECOG) performance status of 0, a large 12-cm right renal mass, and four small pulmonary metastases
   b. A 67-year-old female with an ECOG performance status of 0, a 7-cm left renal mass, retroperitoneal adenopathy, and hepatic metastases that have doubled in size over 4 weeks
   c. An 81-year-old man with an asymptomatic 6-cm right renal mass and multiple hepatic metastases who has declined systemic therapy
   d. A 72-year-old man with an ECOG performance status of 2, a 5-cm right renal mass, and mild dyspnea associated with numerous pulmonary metastases

5. The rationale for cytoreductive nephrectomy followed by immunotherapy with cytokines in patients with synchronous metastatic RCC includes all of the following EXCEPT:
   a. removal of tumor burden.
   b. removal of source of tumor-associated immunosuppressive factors.
   c. reversal of acquired immune dysfunction.
   d. improved tolerance to cytokine therapy.
   e. improved T-lymphocyte function.

6. Which of the following statements about cytokine therapy for metastatic renal cell carcinoma is TRUE?
   a. Lymphokine-activated killer (LAK) cells augment the efficacy of both interferon-α (IFN-α) and IL-2.
   b. Randomized trials have demonstrated a significant survival advantage for combined IL-2 and interferon versus either agent given as monotherapy.
   c. The combination of IL-2 and interferon leads to higher overall response rates than either agent alone.
   d. The complete response rate with interferon-α monotherapy is 10%.

7. Which of the following metastatic RCC tumors is most likely to benefit from cytokine therapy?
   a. Papillary carcinoma
   b. Clear cell carcinoma
   c. Medullary carcinoma
   d. Collecting duct carcinoma
   e. Chromophobe carcinoma

8. A 58-year-old woman had a nephrectomy 6 years previously for a grade 2 clear cell carcinoma. She was incidentally found to have three left-sided pulmonary nodules (two <1.0 cm, other 2.5 cm). A physical examination is normal, as are all blood chemistries. Computed tomography (CT) of the brain, lungs, abdomen, and pelvis show three pulmonary nodules with no associated hilar or mediastinal adenopathy, and a bone scan is normal. Which of the following is the most appropriate next step in her management?
   a. Therapy with high-dose IL-2
   b. Biopsy of a pulmonary nodule
   c. Mediastinoscopy followed by resection of the pulmonary nodules
   d. Observation
   e. IFN-α therapy

9. The sirolimus analogues temsirolimus and everolimus act primarily on which of the following pathways?
   a. vascular endothelial growth factor (VEGF)
   b. Platelet-derived growth factor (PDGF)
   c. Raf-1
   d. mechanistic target of rapamycin (mTOR)
   e. c-met

10. The overall RECIST response rate in metastatic clear cell RCC patients receiving front-line therapy with sunitinib is:
    a. 15% to 20%.
    b. 30% to 40%.
    c. 60% to 70%.
    d. less than 10%.
    e. greater than 70%.

11. In patients with previously untreated metastatic clear cell RCC, sunitinib is:

    a. associated with a higher response rate compared with interferon-α.

    b. associated with a longer progression free survival compared with interferon-α.

    c. associated with a better quality of life compared with interferon-α.

    d. all of the above.

    e. none of the above.

12. Which of the following agents has been shown to prolong progression-free survival in patients with metastatic clear cell RCC who have progressed on first-line therapy with VEGFR antagonists?

    a. Axitinib

    b. Bevacizumab + interferon-α

    c. High-dose IL-2

    d. Everolimus

    e. Low-dose subcutaneous IL-2

13. Randomized trials in patients with previously untreated metastatic clear cell RCC have demonstrated that sorafenib is:

    a. associated with better overall survival compared with interferon-α.

    b. associated with a longer progression free survival compared with interferon-α.

    c. associated with a better quality of life compared with interferon-α.

    d. all of the above.

    e. none of the above.

14. Which of the following agents has been shown in randomized phase 3 trials to prolong survival in "poor risk" metastatic RCC patients?

    a. IL-2

    b. Sunitinib

    c. Sorafenib

    d. Temsirolimus

    e. IFN-α

15. Which of the following molecules is NOT known to be upregulated as a consequence of VHL dysfunction?

    a. VEGF

    b. PDGF

    c. TGF-α

    d. Glut-1

    e. Raf-1

16. In what proportion of sporadic clear cell tumors are mutations or promoter hypermethylation of the *VHL* gene seen?

    a. 70% to 90%

    b. 10% to 20%

    c. 100%

    d. Less than 10%

17. A 47-year-old man presents with multiple metastatic lesions to the lungs and liver 8 months following a radical nephrectomy for a 9-cm papillary type I renal tumor. Which of the following statements about his systemic treatment options is TRUE?

    a. Sunitinib is associated with a 30% to 40% overall RECIST response rate in this subtype of RCC.

    b. Sorafenib is associated with better long-term outcomes than sunitinib in papillary type I RCC.

    c. mTOR inhibitors improve survival in patients with metastatic papillary RCC.

    d. Enrollment in a phase 2 trial evaluating a novel inhibitor of MET activity is a reasonable consideration in this patient.

18. Which of the following statements about agents targeting components of the VHL pathway is TRUE in patients with metastatic clear cell RCC?

    a. The combination of sunitinib and temsirolimus is associated with higher progression-free and overall survival than sunitinib alone.

    b. The addition of IFN-α to bevacizumab has been shown in randomized trials to improve progression free survival compared with bevacizumab alone.

    c. Overlapping toxicity may limit maximal tolerated doses when two agents targeting this pathway are combined.

    d. MET is an important target in clear cell renal cancer due to the presence of MET mutations in approximately 90% of clear cell renal tumors.

ANSWERS

1. **c. 35%.** Although response rates of 30% or more were reported in early phase 2 studies with IL-2, the overall response rate with this agent was determined to be approximately 15% in larger studies and meta-analysis.

2. **d. Durable complete responses are seen in a small proportion of patients receiving high-dose IL-2.** Complete responses are seen in 7% to 9% of metastatic clear cell RCC patients receiving high-dose IL-2, with the majority of these remaining disease-free for long periods. The efficacy of IL-2 has not been adequately evaluated in patients with non–clear cell histologies, and the use of this agent is largely restricted to clear cell RCC patients. There are no randomized phase 3 studies demonstrating survival benefit with IL-2.

3. **a. Karnofsky performance status greater than 80%.** A Karnofsky performance score below 80% was determined to be an adverse prognostic feature and is one of the factors used to predict outcome in the MSKCC prognostic system for patients with metastatic RCC. All other factors listed have been associated with poor outcome.

4. **a. A 50-year-old male with an Eastern Cooperative Oncology Group (ECOG) performance status of 0, a large 12-cm right renal mass, and four small pulmonary metastases.** Cytoreductive nephrectomy is most likely to benefit patients who are good surgical candidates as well as candidates for postnephrectomy systemic therapy, such as those with a good performance status, those with a relatively slow rate of disease progression, and those with relatively low metastatic burden (as demonstrated in a randomized phase III study where interferon was offered post-nephrectomy). Patients described in b-d are less likely to benefit from this approach because they do not satisfy one or more of the above criteria.

5. **d. Improved tolerance to cytokine therapy.** Studies suggest patients with synchronous metastatic RCC have a high frequency of acquired immune dysfunction involving T lymphocytes. The abnormalities described include increased T-cell apoptosis, impaired proliferative responses, and tumor-associated immunosuppressive factors. Cytoreductive nephrectomy may improve these abnormalities. No data demonstrate better patient tolerance to cytokine therapy.

6. **c. The combination of IL-2 and interferon leads to higher overall response rates than either agent alone.** In a randomized phase 3 study, the combination of IL-2 and interferon was associated with a higher response rate than either agent given alone, although this did not translate to an improved long-term outcome (overall survival) in the combination arm. The addition of LAK cells to cytokine therapy does not appear to improve outcome.

7. **b. Clear cell carcinoma.** Clear cell RCC is the histology most likely to respond to cytokine therapy. Although there are inadequate data to make definitive determinations about the activity of cytokines such as IL-2 or interferons in other histologic subtypes, these agents do not appear particularly effective in non–clear cell RCC variants.

8. **c. Mediastinoscopy followed by resection of the pulmonary nodules.** Patients with metachronous pulmonary nodules related to remote renal tumors may have prolonged survival following resection of the nodule(s) as demonstrated by several retrospective studies.

9. **d. mTOR.** mTOR (mammalian target of rapamycin) is the primary target of sirolimus (rapamycin) and its analogues.

10. **b. 30% to 40%.** Objective overall RECIST response rates in metastatic clear cell RCC patients undergoing sunitinib therapy is approximately 30% to 40%, as demonstrated in a randomized phase 3 study comparing sunitinib with interferon.

11. **d. All of the above.** A randomized phase 3 study demonstrated that sunitinib was associated with a higher response rate, longer progression free survival and better quality of life compared with interferon-α in the front-line treatment of patients with metastatic clear cell RCC.

12. **d. Everolimus.** In a randomized phase 3 trial, everolimus has been shown to prolong progression-free survival compared with placebo (median PFS 4.0 vs. 1.9 months) in patients with metastatic clear cell RCC who have progressed on sunitinib and/or sorafenib.

13. **e. None of the above.** In a randomized phase 2 study, sorafenib was not superior to interferon-α in previously untreated patients with metastatic clear cell RCC.

14. **d. Temsirolimus.** In a randomized phase 3 study, temsirolimus was associated with better overall survival than interferon-α (median 10.9 vs. 7.3 months) in metastatic RCC patients presenting with three or more predefined factors predictive of poor-prognosis.

15. **e. Raf-1.** Raf-1 is a mediator of growth factor signaling pathways but has not been shown to be upregulated in RCC as a consequence of VHL inactivation/HIF upregulation.

16. **a. 70% to 90%.** Based on numerous recent studies, it is estimated that VHL inactivation by mutation or promoter hypermethylation occurs in 70% to 90% of clear cell renal tumors.

17. **d. Enrollment in a phase 2 trial evaluating a novel inhibitor of MET activity is a reasonable consideration in this patient.** There is no conclusive evidence suggesting that standard agents with activity in clear cell RCC (including VEGF pathway inhibitors and mTOR inhibitors) have a favorable impact on outcome in patients with metastatic papillary RCC, and patients with these tumors are appropriate candidates for rational targeted therapy approaches. The presence of activating c-met mutations in some papillary tumors has kindled interest in the evaluation of c-met pathway antagonists in this patient population.

18. **c. Overlapping toxicity may limit maximal tolerated doses when two agents targeting this pathway are combined.** Agents targeting different components of the VHL/HIF pathway often share an overlapping adverse event profile and dictate the need for dose reduction of individual agents when used in combination. Although this is an area under active investigation, there is currently no evidence to suggest that combined therapy with VEGF pathway and mTOR antagonists is superior to either class of agents administered alone. C-met mutations have been identified in some papillary tumors but not in clear cell RCC.

CHAPTER REVIEW

1. Metastatic RCC is almost always fatal, with a 10-year survival of less than 5%.

2. In patients with metastatic RCC, long-term survival is generally associated with a long interval between the initial diagnosis and the appearance of metastatic disease and the development of limited sites of metastatic disease.

3. Nephrectomy as the sole treatment for metastatic RCC is unlikely to affect survival. However, when combined with cytokine therapy in carefully selected patients, there is an improvement in overall survival but not necessarily in cancer-specific survival.

4. Isolated pulmonary nodules are the most common metastatic site amenable to resection with curative intent.

5. After nephrectomy, the incidence of spontaneous regression of metastases is less than 1%.

6. High dose IL-2 causes the vascular leak syndrome.

7. Patients who overexpress carbonic anhydrase IX are most likely to benefit from IL-2 therapy.

8. The *VHL* gene is a tumor suppressor gene. Mutations of this gene promote accumulation of hypoxia-inducible factor, which upregulates a variety of growth factors.

9. Conventional cytotoxic chemotherapy is generally ineffective for metastatic RCC.

10. Hormonal therapy for metastatic RCC has no role.

11. Targeted chemotherapy in clear cell RCC is directed at vascular endothelial growth factor.

12. Performance status, lactate dehydrogenase, hemoglobin, calcium, and prior nephrectomy may be used to stratify patients as to survival.

13. The efficacy of IL-2 has not been adequately evaluated in patients with non-clear cell histologies, and the use of this agent is largely restricted to clear cell RCC patients.

14. The addition of LAK cells to cytokine therapy does not appear to improve outcome.

15. Patients with metastatic RCC have a high frequency of acquired immune dysfunction involving T-lymphocytes. The abnormalities include increased T-cell apoptosis, impaired proliferative responses, and tumor-associated immunosuppressive factors. Cytoreductive nephrectomy may improve these abnormalities; however, there are no data to demonstrate that cytoreductive nephrectomy improves the patient's tolerance to cytokine therapy.

16. There is no conclusive evidence suggesting that standard agents with activity in clear cell RCC (including VEGF pathway inhibitors and mTOR inhibitors) have a favorable impact on outcome in patients with metastatic papillary RCC.

17. Agents targeting different components of the VHL/HIF pathway often share an overlapping adverse event profile and dictate the need for dose reduction of individual agents when used in combination.

64 Surgical and Radiologic Anatomy of the Adrenals

Ravi Munver, Jennifer K. Yates, and Michael C. Degen

QUESTIONS

1. Which of the following statements is (are) TRUE?
   a. The weight of each of the glands is approximately 10 g.
   b. The adrenal glands are in close proximity to the crus of the diaphragm.
   c. The right gland is crescentic in shape.
   d. The left adrenal gland lies adjacent to the splenic vessels.
   e. Both b and d.

2. Which of the following statements is (are) TRUE?
   a. The right renal vein is longer than the left renal vein.
   b. The right adrenal vein is longer than the left adrenal vein.
   c. The right kidney is typically located lower in the retroperitoneum than the left kidney.
   d. The right adrenal gland is typically located higher in the retroperitoneum than the left adrenal gland.
   e. Both c and d.

3. The adrenal arteries are branches from:
   a. the aorta.
   b. the inferior phrenic arteries.
   c. the renal arteries.
   d. the celiac arterial trunk.
   e. a, b, and c.

4. In cases of renal ectopia, the ipsilateral adrenal gland is typically:
   a. absent.
   b. found in its normal anatomic position in the upper retroperitoneum.
   c. found in association with the contralateral adrenal gland.
   d. found closely applied to the superior pole of the ectopic kidney.
   e. found closely associated with the ipsilateral renal artery.

5. In cases of unilateral renal agenesis, the ipsilateral adrenal gland is commonly:
   a. absent.
   b. found in its normal anatomic position in the upper retroperitoneum.
   c. found in association with the contralateral adrenal gland.
   d. found just inside the ipsilateral internal inguinal ring.
   e. found in an ectopic, intrathoracic location.

6. As one proceeds outward from the adrenal medulla, the three separate functional layers of the adrenal cortex are, in correct order:
   a. zona reticularis, zona fasciculata, and zona glomerulosa.
   b. zona fasciculata, zona reticularis, and zona glomerulosa.
   c. zona glomerulosa, zona fasciculata, and zona reticularis.
   d. zona glomerulosa, zona reticularis, and zona fasciculata.
   e. zona reticularis, zona glomerulosa, and zona fasciculata.

7. Which of the following statements is (are) FALSE?
   a. The adrenal medulla produces catecholamines in response to stimulation from the sympathetic nervous system.
   b. The zona glomerulosa produces aldosterone in response to angiotensin II.
   c. The zona fasciculata of the adrenal cortex produces glucocorticoids in response to adrenocorticotropic hormone (ACTH).
   d. The zona reticularis of the adrenal cortex produces androgens in response to luteinizing hormone (LH).
   e. Both b and c.

8. Which of the following statements is TRUE?
   a. Ultrasound imaging cannot differentiate between solid and cystic masses of the adrenal gland.
   b. Contrast resolution of magnetic resonance imaging (MRI) is inferior to that of computed tomography (CT) in enabling differentiation of adrenal masses.
   c. CT is the most widely used modality for imaging the adrenal glands.
   d. Normal adrenal tissue has a density of greater than 10 Hounsfield units on noncontrast CT imaging.
   e. MRI, via T1-weighted and T2-weighted images, can provide functional data about adrenal masses.

ANSWERS

1. **e. Both b and d.** Both adrenal glands are in close proximity to the crus of the diaphragm. The left adrenal gland is in contact with the medial aspect of the upper pole of the left kidney. The adjacent structures include the splenic vessels and body of the pancreas anteriorly, the aorta medially, and the psoas muscle posteriorly.

2. **e. Both c and d.** The right kidney is typically located lower in the retroperitoneum than the left kidney. The right adrenal gland lies more superiorly in the retroperitoneum than the left adrenal gland.

3. **e. a, b, and c.** The three main adrenal arteries each branch into cascades of 10 to 50 smaller arteries which then supply each adrenal gland. The three major arterial sources for each gland are: (1) superior branches from the inferior phrenic artery, (2) middle branches directly from the aorta, and (3) inferior branches from the ipsilateral renal artery.

4. **b. Found in its normal anatomic position in the upper retroperitoneum.** In cases of renal ectopia, the adrenal gland is usually found in approximately its normal anatomic position.

5. **b. Found in its normal anatomic position in the upper retroperitoneum.** In cases of renal agenesis, the adrenal gland on the involved side is typically present.

6. **a. Zona reticularis, zona fasciculata, and zona glomerulosa.** The adult adrenal gland consists of an outer cortex, which makes up approximately 90% of the adrenal mass, and an inner medulla. The adrenal cortex consists of three concentric zones: the outer zona glomerulosa comprising approximately 15% of the cortex, the middle zona fasciculata 80% of the cortex, and the inner zona reticularis 5% to 7% of the cortex. The zona glomerulosa produces aldosterone, zona fasciculata produces glucocorticoids, and zona reticularis produces sex steroids.

7. **d. The zona reticularis of the adrenal cortex produces androgens in response to luteinizing hormone (LH).** The production of androgen by the zona reticularis is regulated by pituitary release of ACTH.

8. **c. CT is the most widely used modality for imaging the adrenal glands.** Ultrasound imaging can be used to differentiate between solid and cystic adrenal masses. Normal adrenal tissue has a density of less than or equal to 10 Hounsfield units (HU) on noncontrast CT imaging. MRI, via T1-weighted and T2-weighted images, is superior to CT and enables differentiation of adrenal masses. Although CT and MRI provide excellent morphologic information, these studies cannot provide functional data.

CHAPTER REVIEW

1. The adrenals are enclosed within Gerota fascia.
2. The right adrenal vein is short and enters the vena cava posterolaterally.
3. Adrenal rests are found in proximity to the celiac axis and along the path of gonadal descent. In patients with congenital adrenal hyperplasia, adrenal rests along the spermatic cord may become quite large.
4. The right kidney is typically located lower in the retroperitoneum than the left kidney. The right adrenal gland lies more superiorly in the retroperitoneum than the left adrenal gland. Both adrenal glands are in close proximity to the crus of the diaphragm.
5. In cases of renal ectopia, the adrenal gland is usually found in approximately its normal anatomic position.
6. The zona glomerulosa produces aldosterone, zona fasciculata produces glucocorticoids, and zona reticularis produces sex steroids.
7. The production of androgen by the zona reticularis is regulated by pituitary release of adrenocorticotropic hormone (ACTH).
8. Normal adrenal tissue has a density of less than or equal to 10 Hounsfield units (HU) on noncontrast CT imaging.

Pathophysiology, Evaluation, and Medical Management of Adrenal Disorders

Alexander Kutikov, Paul L. Crispen, and Robert G. Uzzo

QUESTIONS

1. At birth the adrenal cortex:
   a. is completely developed.
   b. weighs half as much as the adrenal cortex in adults.
   c. is composed of fetal and adult components.
   d. will continue to enlarge until 12 months of age.
   e. is composed of a single histologic zone.

2. Adrenal rest tissue within the testis can mimic testicular cancer in patients with:
   a. neuroblastoma.
   b. pheochromocytoma.
   c. primary aldosteronism.
   d. congenital adrenal hyperplasia.
   e. cryptorchidism.

3. In cases of renal agenesis, the ipsilateral adrenal gland is typically:
   a. absent.
   b. in the normal location.
   c. located at the level of the eighth thoracic vertebral body.
   d. located at the level of the first lumbar vertebral body.
   e. at a location dependent on the cause of renal agenesis.

4. The most abundant product of the adrenal cortex is:
   a. mineralocorticoids.
   b. glucocorticoids.
   c. adrenal androgens.
   d. catecholamines.
   e. adrenocorticotropic hormone (ACTH).

5. Aldosterone synthase (CYP11B2) is unique to:
   a. the zona glomerulosa.
   b. the zona fasciculata.
   c. the zona reticularis.
   d. the adrenal medulla.
   e. the distal renal tubule.

6. The only zone of the adrenal cortex that does not atrophy upon pituitary failure is:
   a. the zona glomerulosa.
   b. the zona fasciculata.
   c. the zona reticularis.
   d. the adrenal medulla.
   e. none of the above.

7. Presence of the phenylethanolamine-*N*-methyltransferase (PNMT) enzyme in the adrenal medulla is significant because:
   a. the enzyme catalyzes degradation of catecholamines to metanephrines.
   b. the enzyme catalyzes conversion of catecholamines to vanillylmandelic acid (VMA).
   c. the enzyme converts tyrosine to dopamine.
   d. the enzyme catalyzes the conversion of norepinephrine to epinephrine.
   e. all of the above.

8. Metanephrines:
   a. refers to the term used for catecholamines and their byproducts.
   b. refers to the combined term for methylated metabolites of norepinephrine (normetanephrine) and epinephrine (metanephrine).
   c. refers to precursors to normetanephrines.
   d. are rarely helpful in establishing a diagnosis of pheochromocytoma.
   e. refers to the term used to describe epinephrine and norepinephrine in the context of pheochromocytoma symptomatology.

9. The term *free metanephrines*:
   a. is interchangeable with the term *total metanephrines*.
   b. is interchangeable with the term *fractionated metanephrines*.
   c. refers to normetanephrine and metanephrine that are not conjugated by a sulfate moiety.
   d. refers to normetanephrine and metanephrine that are not bound to albumin.
   e. refers to all of the above.

10. The most common cause of Cushing syndrome (exclusive of exogenous steroid intake) is:
    a. Cushing disease.
    b. a cortisol-producing adrenal adenoma.
    c. ectopic ACTH production by a lung malignancy.
    d. an adrenal carcinoma.
    e. a pheochromocytoma.

11. What common urologic ailment can be found in up to 50% of patients with Cushing syndrome?
    a. Testicular cancer
    b. Torsion of the appendix testis
    c. Urolithiasis
    d. Fournier gangrene
    e. Stress urinary incontinence

12. How does one perform a low-dose dexamethasone suppression test (LDDST)?
    a. Admit the patient and measure serum cortisol levels every 6 hours while the patient is on a dexamethasone drip.
    b. Measure the patient's saliva cortisol level at midnight.
    c. Obtain a 24-hour urine cortisol measurement after the patient receives 1 mg of dexamethasone with the first void.

d. Have the patient take 10 mg of dexamethasone at 11 PM and measure urinary cortisol the next morning.

e. Have the patient take 1 mg of dexamethasone at 11 PM and measure serum cortisol the next morning.

13. The adrenal surgeon plays no role in the management of Cushing disease.

a. True

b. False

14. What percentage of patients presenting with primary aldosteronism are hypokalemic?

a. 5% to 12%

b. 9% to 37%

c. 33% to 50%

d. 55% to 75%

e. 63% to 91%

15. Elevated aldosterone in patients with familial hyperaldosteronism type I is mediated by:

a. renin.

b. sodium.

c. angiotensin II.

d. cortisol.

e. ACTH.

16. What percentage of patients with a positive screening test will be diagnosed with primary aldosteronism after confirmatory testing?

a. 2% to 10%

b. 20% to 40%

c. 30% to 50%

d. 50% to 70%

e. 75% to 90%

17. What is the most common subtype of primary aldosteronism?

a. Idiopathic hyperplasia

b. Aldosterone-producing adenoma

c. Unilateral adrenal hyperplasia

d. Familial hyperaldosteronism type I

e. Adrenocortical carcinoma

18. The primary determinant of potentially surgically correctable primary aldosteronism is:

a. blood pressure.

b. patient age.

c. demonstration of lateralized aldosterone secretion.

d. response to medical therapy.

e. plasma aldosterone levels.

19. Which class of antihypertensives is contraindicated during the evaluation of primary aldosteronism?

a. Calcium channel blockers

b. Alpha blockers

c. Beta blockers

d. Aldosterone-receptor blockers

e. Angiotensin-converting enzyme inhibitors

20. What percentage of patients with incidental adrenal masses prove to have pheochromocytoma?

a. 1%

b. 5%

c. 10%

d. 25%

e. 35%

21. What subtype is assigned to patients with a von Hippel-Lindau (*VHL*) mutation and a history of pheochromocytoma but no other stigmata of the VHL syndrome?

a. Type 1

b. Type 2A

c. Type 2B

d. Type 2C

e. None of the above

22. What genetic abnormality is strongly linked with malignant pheochromocytoma?

a. *RET* mutation

b. *VHL* mutation

c. *SDHB* mutation

d. *SDHD* mutation

e. All of the above

23. What test is considered the cornerstone for modern pheochromocytoma biochemical testing?

a. Plasma catecholamines

b. Plasma-free metanephrines or fractionated urinary metanephrines

c. Vanillylmandelic acid testing

d. Fasting morning urinary norepinephrine

e. Adrenal vein sampling for catecholamines

24. With regard to preoperative pheochromocytoma blockade, β-blockers should be started:

a. 2 weeks prior to adrenalectomy.

b. at least several days prior to α-blockers.

c. to control tachycardia and arrhythmias that can result upon initiation of α blockade.

d. in conjunction with metyrosine.

e. never, because β-blockers can be lethal in patients with pheochromocytomas.

25. Patients with adrenal crisis can exhibit all of the following symptoms EXCEPT:

a. hypotension unresponsive to fluid resuscitation.

b. abdominal pain.

c. nausea.

d. fever.

e. priapism.

26. All of the following lesions can be extra-adrenal EXCEPT:

a. myelolipoma.

b. ganglioneuroma.

c. aldosteronoma.

d. pheochromocytoma.

e. oncocytoma.

27. A 25-year-old woman is diagnosed with a left adrenal mass, with abundant stippled calcifications, that exhibits imaging features inconsistent with adrenal adenoma. The patient complains of a severe bout of diarrhea that started approximately 8 months ago. Adrenalectomy reveals a ganglioneuroma. At her postoperative visit she is grateful, because her gastrointestinal (GI) complaints vanished following surgery. The substance responsible for diarrhea in this patient is most likely:

a. metanephrine.

b. epinephrine.

c. norepinephrine.

d. VMA.

e. vasoactive intestinal polypeptide (VIP).

28. What percentage of adrenal cysts is associated with malignancy in surgical series?

a. 1%

b. 3%

c. 7%

d. 12%

e. 15%

29. Adrenocortical carcinoma in children:

a. has a more favorable 5-year survival rate compared with adults.

b. uses the same pathologic staging system as adults.

c. is rarely associated with virilization.

d. has equal female and male incidence in children older than 10 years.

e. is frequently metastatic to the central nervous system.

30. The most common hormone secreted by adrenocortical carcinoma is:

a. aldosterone.

b. testosterone.

c. dehydroepiandrosterone (DHEA).

d. cortisol.

e. androstenedione.

31. The Weiss criteria for identifying malignant adrenal tumors should be applied with caution in tumors with:

a. necrosis.

b. high mitotic index.

c. inferior vena cava (IVC) invasion.

d. liver metastasis.

e. oncocytic features.

32. In patients presenting with metastatic adrenocortical carcinoma, the systemic agent of choice is:

a. valrubicin.

b. mitotane alone or in combination with additional cytotoxic agents.

c. gemcitabine and cisplatin.

d. docetaxel (Taxotere).

e. bleomycin, etoposide, and cisplatin.

33. In the treatment of pathologically localized adrenocortical carcinoma:

a. adjuvant radiation therapy decreases systemic progression.

b. complete surgical resection offers the best chance of cure.

c. increased Ki-67 expression has been associated with improved survival.

d. the tumor's functional status is an independent predictor of survival.

e. adjuvant therapy with mitotane has no proven benefit.

34. A 50% false-positive rate can be seen during low-dose dexamethasone suppression testing in:

a. men with testicular cancer.

b. women taking oral contraceptives.

c. men with history of orchiopexy.

d. patients with brain malignancy.

e. patients with pheochromocytoma.

35. The adrenal gland should be resected whenever one performs a radical nephrectomy.

a. True

b. False

36. What common over-the-counter medication can produce a false-positive result during plasma free metanephrine testing?

a. Ibuprofen

b. Aspirin

c. Omeprazole

d. Diphenhydramine

e. Acetaminophen

37. A 55-year-old woman presents for the evaluation of an adrenal mass. Past medical history is significant for severe hypertension requiring four oral medications for adequate blood pressure control. A noncontrast computed tomography (CT) scan of the abdomen reveals a 3-cm left adrenal mass, with an average attenuation of 7 Hounsfield units (HU). Appropriate initial screening should include:

a. free-fractionated plasma metanephrines, plasma aldosterone concentration, and plasma renin activity.

b. low-dose dexamethasone suppression test and serum catecholamines.

c. late-night salivary cortisol test, plasma aldosterone concentration, plasma renin activity, and plasma free metanephrines.

d. plasma aldosterone concentration and plasma renin activity.

e. 24-hour urinary-fractionated metanephrines and serum cortisol concentration.

38. A 62-year-old man presents for postoperative surveillance of renal cell carcinoma. Three years prior, a right nephrectomy was performed for T2N0M0 grade III clear cell renal cell carcinoma. A current abdominal CT scan reveals a 3.5-cm right adrenal mass with an average attenuation of 32 HU prior to contrast administration. A CT washout study is performed, and absolute percent washout is calculated to be 52%. No other suspicious lesions are noted within the chest, abdomen, or pelvis. The next step in management should be:

a. observation.

b. adrenalectomy.

c. percutaneous biopsy.

d. initiation of an oral tyrosine kinase inhibitor.

e. assessment of the adrenal tumor's functional status.

39. A 58-year-old woman has been diagnosed with primary aldosteronism based on appropriate screening and confirmatory testing. A CT scan of the abdomen reveals a 1.0-cm left adrenal mass. Adrenal vein sampling is performed with the results outlined below. Results of adrenal vein sampling:

Right cortisol gradient 2.7:1

Left cortisol gradient 3.4:1

Aldosterone ratio (left:right) 2.5:1

The next step in management would be:

a. Repeat adrenal vein sampling with ACTH stimulation

b. Counseling for left adrenalectomy

c. Counseling for right adrenalectomy

d. Initiation of medical management based on diagnosis of bilateral adrenal hyperplasia

e. ^{131}I-Iodomethyl-norcholesterol (NP-59) scintigraphy to confirm lateralization

40. A 43-year-old woman undergoes an uneventful right laparoscopic adrenalectomy for a 4.5-cm pheochromocytoma. The pathology report states that the lesion is benign and that the margins are negative. On postoperative day 1, she is ready for discharge and wants to know if any additional follow-up is necessary. You inform her that the following is required:

   a. Consideration of genetic screening

   b. Repeat metabolic testing in 2 weeks

   c. Cross-sectional imaging in 6 months

   d. Biochemical testing in 6 months and then lifelong biochemical testing

   e. All of the above

Pathology

1. A 60-year-old woman is noted to have a 4-cm left adrenal mass on an abdominal CT scan. The endocrine workup is negative, and the mass is excised laparoscopically. The pathology depicted in Figure 65-1 is reported as a myolipoma. The next step in management is:

   a. no additional therapy is indicated because this is a benign tumor.

   b. ask the pathologist to grade the tumor.

   c. the patient should receive mitotane.

   d. the patient should be followed carefully for development of hypertension.

   e. a metaiodobenzylguanidine (MIBG) scan should be obtained.

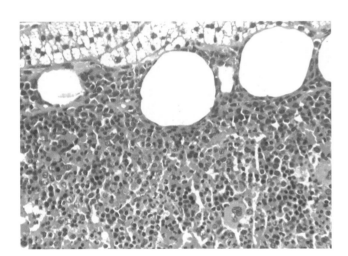

Figure 65-1. (From Bostwick DG, Cheng L. Urologic surgical pathology. 2nd ed. Edinburgh: Mosby; 2008.)

2. A 45-year-old man has an incidentally discovered 6-cm adrenal mass. Hormonal workup is negative. The mass is laparoscopically removed. The pathology is depicted in Figure 65-2 and is read as adrenal corticocarcinoma. On separate stains the lesion stains positive for Ki-67. The next step in management is:

   a. request a pathologic grade.

   b. stain for catecholamines.

   c. inquire as to whether any fat was observed in the specimen.

   d. short-term follow-up with imaging.

   e. adjuvant mitotane.

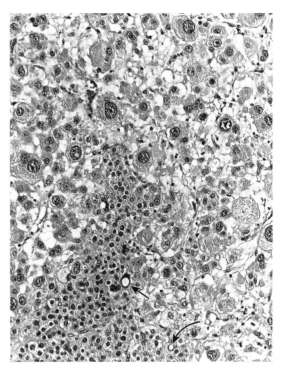

Figure 65-2. (From Bostwick DG, Cheng L. Urologic surgical pathology. 2nd ed. Edinburgh: Mosby; 2008.)

Imaging

1. See Figure 65-3. A 42-year-old man with lung cancer has this CT scan. The right adrenal nodule has attenuation measurements of 7 HU. The most likely diagnosis is:

   a. adrenal adenoma.

   b. adrenal metastasis.

   c. indeterminate adrenal nodule.

   d. pheochromocytoma.

   e. adrenal myelolipoma.

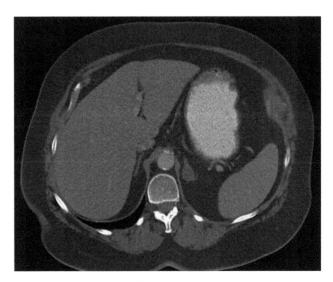

Figure 65-3.

ANSWERS

1. **c. Is composed of fetal and adult components.** The adrenal gland weighs twice as much as the adult gland and begins to atrophy at birth. Development of the gland continues during the first 3 years of life, with the zona reticularis developing last.

2. **d. Congenital adrenal hyperplasia.** Testicular adrenal rests must be remembered when evaluating patients with congenital adrenal hyperplasia and testicular masses to avoid an unnecessary orchiectomy.

3. **b. In the normal location.** Reports of adrenal agenesis are extremely rare.

4. **c. Adrenal androgens.** Although adrenal androgens are arguably the least physiologically significant compounds produced by the adrenals, the glands produce more than 20 mg of these compounds per day. Meanwhile, only 100 to 150 mcg/day of aldosterone and approximately 10 to 20 mg/day of cortisol are produced by the glands.

5. **a. The zona glomerulosa.** The zona glomerulosa cells are the sole source of aldosterone in humans.

6. **a. The zona glomerulosa.** Production of aldosterone in the zona glomerulosa is primarily regulated by angiotensin II through the renin-angiotensin-aldosterone system and potassium levels. Elevation of ACTH can also increase aldosterone secretion, but this is a much less potent stimulus. Therefore, in pituitary failure, when ACTH levels fall, the zona glomerulosa fails to atrophy.

7. **d. The enzyme catalyzes the conversion of norepinephrine to epinephrine.** PNMT is virtually unique to the adrenal medulla (the brain and organ of Zuckerkandl also express the protein). Therefore the presence of PNMT results in epinephrine being virtually a unique product of the adrenal gland.

8. **b. Refers to the combined term for methylated metabolites of norepinephrine (normetanephrine) and epinephrine (metanephrine).** The enzyme catechol-O-methyltransferase catalyzes the methylation of norepinephrine to normetanephrine and epinephrine to metanephrine. The term normetanephrines is not used.

9. **c. Refers to normetanephrine and metanephrine that are not conjugated by a sulfate moiety.** Free metanephrines are unsulfonated normetanephrine and metanephrine, whereas total metanephrines refers to both conjugated and free compounds. The term *fractionated metanephrines* refers to laboratory reports that differentiate between metanephrine and normetanephrine concentrations (i.e., instead of only reporting metanephrine concentration, state the concentration of metanephrine and normetanephrine separately).

10. **a. Cushing disease.** Cushing disease, which describes overproduction of ACTH by the pituitary, accounts for some 70% of endogenous Cushing syndrome.

11. **c. Urolithiasis.** Urolithiasis is seen in up to 50% of patients with Cushing syndrome; therefore stone formers with cushingoid features deserve a hypercortisolemia workup. The astute urologist should also remember that Cushing patients can also exhibit hypogonadal hypogonadism and should have a low threshold for a hypercortisolism workup in men with low testosterone and low gonadotropin levels.

12. **e. Have the patient take 1 mg of dexamethasone at 11 PM and measure serum cortisol the next morning.** Despite its intimidating name and rather complex physiologic underpinnings, the test is remarkably simple to administer. Write the patient a prescription for 1 mg of dexamethasone and ask that it be taken by mouth at 11 PM. The next morning, determine the patient's serum cortisol level. If the cortisol level is 5 mcg/dL or higher (i.e., not suppressed), then the patient likely has hypercortisolemia. Be aware that women on birth control will have false-positive results.

13. **b. False.** ACTH-secreting pituitary adenomas are treated with transsphenoidal surgical resection. However, a cure is seen in only 60% to 80% of patients. Among those who are cured, there is approximately 25% relapse. One option for patients who are refractory to neurosurgical treatment is a bilateral adrenalectomy. However, this treatment should not be performed hastily. It is crucial that a thoughtful multidisciplinary decision be made. Up to 30% of patients with Cushing disease who undergo bilateral adrenalectomy may develop Nelson syndrome—progressive growth of the pituitary adenoma causing increased intracranial pressure and compression of the ocular chiasm.

14. **b. 9% to 37%.** Although hypokalemia has been classically described as a common finding in primary aldosteronism, only 9% to 37% of newly diagnosed patients are hypokalemic.

15. **e. ACTH.** Because of the chimeric fusion of the promoter region of 11β-hydroxylase and the coding region of aldosterone synthase, aldosterone production is mediated by ACTH in familial hyperaldosteronism type I.

16. **d. 50% to 70%.** Fifty percent to 70% of patients with a positive screening test will be diagnosed with primary aldosteronism following confirmatory testing.

17. **a. Idiopathic hyperplasia.** This subtype of primary aldosteronism accounts for approximately 60% of cases.

18. **c. Demonstration of lateralized aldosterone secretion.** Lateralization of aldosterone secretion is the primary determinant of successful surgical treatment of primary aldosteronism.

19. **d. Aldosterone-receptor blockers.** Aldosterone-receptor blockers (spironolactone and eplerenone) are contraindicated during the evaluation of primary aldosteronism. Patients requiring these agents for blood pressure control should be transitioned to other medications during testing for at least 6 weeks.

20. **b. 5% (approximately).** Incidentally discovered lesions account for 10% to 25% of all pheochromocytomas.

21. **d. Type 2C.** Type 1 = VHL patient with no evidence or family history of pheochromocytoma. Type 2 patients are those with evidence or family history of pheochromocytoma. Type 2 is further subdivided. Type 2A = patients with concomitant RCC; type 2B = no evidence of renal malignancy; type 2C = patients with pheochromoctyoma and evidence of a *VHL* gene mutation but no other stigmata of VHL.

22. **c. *SDHB* mutation.** Patients with multiple endocrine neoplasia (types 2A and 2B) possess a mutation in the *RET* proto-oncogene. Approximately half of these patients develop pheochromocytoma, but only about 3% of those with pheochromocytoma exhibit malignant potential. Ten percent to 20% of patients with VHL develop pheochromocytomas, but only 5% of those with pheochromocytoma have malignant disease. Pheochromocytoma among patients with neurofibromatosis type 1 is rare (1%), but malignant disease can be seen in more than 10%. Familial paraganglioma syndrome type 4 (*SDHB* mutation) carries the highest risk of malignancy (30% to 50%) among patients with the condition who develop pheochromocytoma (≈20%). Its pathologic cousin, familial paraganglioma syndrome type 1 (*SDHD* mutation), carries a negligible risk (<3%) of malignancy among patients who develop pheochromocytomas (≈20%).

23. **b. Plasma-free metanephrines or fractionated urinary metanephrines.** Methylated metabolites of catecholamines are known as *metanephrines*. Therefore normetanephrine (from norepinephrine) and metanephrine (from epinephrine) are collectively known as *metanephrines*. The vast majority of methylation occurs within the adrenal medulla or pheochromocytoma, when present. Because this conversion of catecholamines to metanephrines is an uninterrupted process within pheochromocytomas, testing for these compounds is a much more sensitive means of tumor detection than the measurement of catecholamine levels, which may be paroxysmal. Furthermore, measurement of levels of metanephrines is rather specific. Controversy exists regarding whether measurement of plasma-free metanephrines versus fractionated urinary metanephrine should be used as the initial test. The term "free" indicates that the metanephrines being measured are not conjugated by a sulfate

moiety, whereas the term "fractionated" simply indicates that normetanephrine and metanephrine levels are reported as separate values.

24. **c. To control tachycardia and arrhythmias that can result upon initiation of α blockade.** Beta-blockade should never be started prior to appropriate α blockade. In the absence of α blockade, β antagonists cause a potentiation of the action of epinephrine on the α_1 receptor, due to blockade of the arteriolar dilation at the β_2 receptor. Nevertheless, β blockade is at times necessary to control reflex tachycardia and arrhythmias that can result from α blockade.

25. **e. Priapism.** Patients with adrenal crisis are easily misdiagnosed with an acute abdomen. Children can exhibit hypoglycemic seizures. Persistent painful erections are generally not associated with adrenal insufficiency.

26. **c. Aldosteronoma.** All listed lesions, other than an aldosterone-producing adenoma, can develop outside of the adrenal gland.

27. **e. Vasoactive intestinal polypeptide (VIP).** Ganglioneuromas are rare lesions that can arise in the adrenal glands and can secrete VIP, causing profound diarrhea in some patients. Nevertheless, most ganglioneuromas are asymptomatic.

28. **c. 7%.** In a meta-analysis accounting for 515 adrenal cysts, the incidence of associated adrenal malignancy was 7%.

29. **a. Has a more favorable 5-year survival rate compared with adults.** The 5-year survival rate in children with adrenal cortical carcinoma is 54% compared with only 20% to 47% in adults.

30. **d. Cortisol.** Up to 74% of functional adrenocortical tumors produce excess cortisol.

31. **e. Oncocytic features.** The Weiss criteria should be applied with caution in pediatric cases and in those with oncocytic features.

32. **b. Mitotane alone or in combination with additional cytotoxic agents.** Mitotane has adrenolytic activity and is the first-line agent of choice in patients with metastatic adrenocortical carcinoma. The addition of streptozotocin or etoposide, doxorubicin, and cisplatin to mitotane is potentially beneficial and is currently being investigated in a randomized trial.

33. **b. Complete surgical resection** (including en bloc resection of locally advanced disease) **offers the best chance of cure.** Adjuvant radiation therapy has demonstrated a decreased rate of local recurrence but has not been shown to improve overall survival. Adjuvant mitotane therapy has been shown to significantly improve recurrence-free and overall survival. A tumor's functional status has not been consistently demonstrated to impact survival.

34. **b. Women taking oral contraceptives.** The urologist must be aware that the low-dose dexamethasone suppression test can yield as high as a 50% false-positive rate in women using oral contraceptives, because the contraceptives increase total (but not bioavailable) cortisol levels by raising the patient's cortisol-binding globulin concentrations.

35. **b. False.** The classic description by Robson in the 1950s suggested that radical nephrectomy should include adrenalectomy. Today, however, adrenalectomy is believed to be necessary only for large (T2) upper pole tumors, in cases in which an abnormality in the gland can be seen on preoperative imaging and in cases in which a vein thrombus is present to the level of the adrenal gland.

36. **e. Acetaminophen.** Prior to plasma-free metanephrine testing, ideally patients should not consume food or liquids after midnight. Caffeinated beverages, especially, must be avoided. Acetaminophen can produce a false-positive result due to cross reactivity in the assay and should be stopped for at least 5 days

prior to testing. Tricyclic antidepressants and phenoxybenzamine should also be stopped, because these have been shown to be responsible for false-positive results (Eisenhofer et al, 2003).* Usual antihypertensive therapy can be continued. Although β blockade can potentially result in a false-positive test result, the current recommendation is to stop the medication only on repeat testing (Eisenhofer et al, 2003). Ideally, the serum sample should be drawn in the supine position following at least 20 minutes of supine rest. Position is especially important if a positive result has been obtained and confirmatory testing is being performed.

37. **c. Late-night salivary cortisol test, plasma aldosterone concentration, plasma renin activity, and plasma-free metanephrines.** All patients presenting with an adrenal mass should be evaluated for cortisol and catecholamine hypersecretion. Given the patient's history of hypertension, evaluation of primary aldosteronism should also be undertaken. Choice c is the best answer.

38. **e. Assessment of the adrenal tumor's functional status.** Although there is a high probability that the adrenal lesion, in this case, represents a recurrence of the patient's renal cell carcinoma, the functional status of the adrenal mass should be assessed. A pheochromocytoma may always be lurking.

39. **b. Counseling for left adrenalectomy.** Both the right and left cortisol gradients suggest proper catheter placement for adrenal vein sampling. The aldosterone ratio of 2.5:1 demonstrates left lateralization of autonomous aldosterone secretion, and counseling for left adrenalectomy is appropriate.

40. **e. All of the above.** The patient is less than 50 years old; therefore genetic screening is recommended. Up to 25% of patients who appear to have sporadic pheochromocytoma on presentation turn out to have germline mutations upon genetic testing. Repeat metabolic testing at 2 weeks after resection is prudent. Most experts recommend additional biochemical testing at 6 months, followed by annual lifelong screening. More than 15% of patients will demonstrate recurrence of pheochromocytoma in the first 10 years after a successful resection. Recurrent disease has been reported more than 15 years following adrenalectomy; therefore lifelong annual biochemical screening is advised. Although cross-sectional imaging is not absolutely required in the face of a negative biochemical workup, most surgeons obtain at least one study at some point during the postoperative follow-up.

Pathology

1. **a. No additional therapy is indicated because this is a benign tumor.** This is a benign myolipoma. Notice that it consists of fat mixed with hematopoietic elements.

2. **d. Short-term follow-up with imaging.** The marked nuclear variability, increased mitotic figures, and positive staining for Ki-67 all strongly suggest adrenal corticocarcinoma. No further pathologic information is necessary. These patients have a high risk of developing metastatic disease, at which time mitotane would be considered.

Imaging

1. **a. Adrenal adenoma.** Adrenal nodules that are less than 10 HU in density are almost always benign nodules, most often adrenal adenomas.

---

*Sources referenced can be found in *Campbell-Walsh Urology, 11th Edition*, on the Expert Consult website.

CHAPTER REVIEW

1. The right adrenal gland is triangular in shape; the left is crescent shaped.
2. The zona glomerulosa secretes mineralocorticoids, the zona fasciculata secretes glucocorticoids, and the zona reticularis secretes sex steroids.
3. The production of cortisol is circadian, with the peak occurring in the early morning and the nadir at 11:00 PM.
4. Adrenal androgens are under the control of ACTH.
5. Ectopic ACTH production almost always originates from malignant tissue.
6. Renin release is stimulated by low renal perfusion pressure, increased renal sympathetic nervous activity, and low sodium.
7. Mineralocorticoid production results in sodium retention and volume expansion initially; however, with continued production, the kidney escapes from the sodium-retentive action of the hormone.
8. Sodium loading reduces endogenous aldosterone and renin production in those patients who do not have autonomous aldosterone secretion from aldosterone producing tumors.
9. The predictors of persistent hypertension following adrenalectomy for primary aldosteronism include (1) age older than 50 years, (2) the requirement for more than two antihypertensive agents preoperatively, (3) a first-degree relative with hypertension, (4) prolonged duration of hypertension prior to adrenalectomy, and (5) renal insufficiency.
10. Ki-67 staining of adrenal tissue is perhaps the best indicator of malignancy.
11. Chromogranin A elevation in the serum has been used as a confirmatory test in patients with pheochromocytoma.
12. Restoration of intravascular volume is the most important component of preoperative preparation in patients with pheochromocytoma.
13. The most frequent cause of adrenal insufficiency in the United States is autoimmune adrenalitis; in developing countries, it is tuberculosis.
14. Patients with congenital adrenal hyperplasia have a high risk for developing benign adrenal corticoadenomas.
15. The Weiss criteria distinguish benign from malignant adrenal tumors. The presence of three or more of the Weiss criteria is associated with malignancy. When oncocytic features are present, the criteria should be used with caution.
16. An attenuation of less than 10 Hounsfield units on unenhanced CT scan is strongly suggestive of an adrenal adenoma.
17. There are four histologic types of adrenal cysts: (1) pseudocyst, (2) endothelial, (3) epithelial, and (4) parasitic.
18. Positron emission tomography (PET) scan is the preferred imaging modality for pheochromocytoma.
19. Pheochromocytomas recur in up to 16% of patients who have had a complete surgical resection; 50% of the recurrences are malignant.
20. Metastases to the adrenal are common.
21. Production of aldosterone in the zona glomerulosa is primarily regulated by angiotensin II through the renin-angiotensin-aldosterone system and potassium levels.
22. Epinephrine is virtually a unique product of the adrenal gland, and when it is the dominant catechol produced by a tumor, an adrenal origin is suggested.
23. Cushing disease is a result of an overproduction of ACTH by the pituitary. It accounts for some 70% of endogenous Cushing syndrome.
24. Urolithiasis is seen in up to 50% of patients with Cushing syndrome.
25. Up to 30% of patients with Cushing disease who undergo bilateral adrenalectomy may develop Nelson syndrome—progressive growth of the pituitary adenoma causing increased intracranial pressure and compression of the ocular chiasm.
26. Although hypokalemia has been classically described as a common finding in primary aldosteronism, only 9% to 37% of newly diagnosed patients are hypokalemic.
27. Conversion of catecholamines to metanephrines is an uninterrupted process within pheochromocytomas; testing for these compounds is a much more sensitive means for tumor detection than the measurement of catecholamine levels, which may be paroxysmal.
28. Ganglioneuromas are rare lesions that can arise in the adrenal glands and can secrete the vasoactive intestinal polypeptide (VIP), causing profound diarrhea in some patients.
29. All patients presenting with an adrenal mass should be evaluated for cortisol and catecholamine hypersecretion.

66 Surgery of the Adrenal Glands

Hoon Ho Rha and Sey Kiat Lim

QUESTIONS

1. Which of the following statements regarding the anatomy of the right adrenal gland is TRUE?
   a. Its vein drains into the right renal vein.
   b. It is usually located on the upper pole and lateral border of the right kidney.
   c. The medulla is innervated by preganglionic sympathetic nerve fibers.
   d. It is usually located more caudal than the left adrenal gland and is closely related to the diaphragm.
   e. The right adrenal gland only receives arterial supply from the right renal artery.

2. What is the risk of malignancy in an incidentaloma of more than 6 cm?
   a. 2%
   b. 6%
   c. 10%
   d. 25%
   e. 50%

3. Absolute contraindications to laparoscopic adrenalectomy include:
   a. significant abdominal adhesions.
   b. adrenal mass greater than 12 cm in size.
   c. invasive adrenal cortical carcinoma with thrombus in the inferior vena cava.
   d. malignant pheochromocytoma.
   e. all of the above.

4. Which of the following statements regarding the perioperative management of pheochromocytoma is FALSE?
   a. Preoperative sympatholytic therapy with alpha-adrenergic blockers should be started for at least 2 weeks before surgery.
   b. Phenoxybenzamine may lead to tachycardia, and beta-adrenergic blockade should be started before phenoxybenzamine administration.
   c. α-Methylparatyrosine (metyrosine) can be used preoperatively in patients with cardiomyopathies or resistant to α-blockers.
   d. The adrenal vein should be ligated early during surgical excision of a pheochromocytoma.
   e. Intravenous drugs with short half-lives are preferred versus longer acting drugs for controlling blood pressure fluctuations during surgical excision of a pheochromocytoma.

5. The lumbodorsal posterior approach to open adrenalectomy is not ideal in any of the following circumstances EXCEPT:
   a. large adrenal tumors.
   b. bilateral adrenal hyperplasia.
   c. bilateral small adrenocortical carcinoma.

   d. patients with ventilatory difficulties.
   e. b and c.

6. In bilateral adrenalectomy, steroids replacement should be started:
   a. on induction of general anesthesia.
   b. after ligation of the right adrenal vein.
   c. after excision of both adrenal glands.
   d. during closing of the abdominal incision.
   e. in the recovery room after surgery.

7. A 57-year-old male with no significant medical problems presented with a right-sided abdominal mass. Computed tomographic (CT) imaging showed an 18-cm right adrenal tumor with invasion of the upper pole of the right kidney and tumor thrombus extending into the retrohepatic inferior vena cava. Which is the best surgical approach for this patient?
   a. Open lumbodorsal posterior approach
   b. Open anterior transabdominal approach
   c. Open thoracoabdominal approach
   d. Laparoscopic transperitoneal approach
   e. Robot-assisted laparoscopic transperitoneal approach

8. Which of the following is NOT a possible approach to the left adrenal gland in the anterior transabdominal approach?
   a. Through the gastrocolic ligament
   b. Through the lienorenal ligament
   c. Through the transverse mesocolon
   d. Through the lesser omentum
   e. All the above are possible approaches

9. Which of the following statements on partial adrenalectomy is FALSE?
   a. The adrenal gland is usually exposed but not mobilized.
   b. The arterial supply of the adrenal gland can be ligated without devascularizing the gland.
   c. It is generally safe to ligate the main adrenal vein if the adrenal gland is not mobilized.
   d. A repeat partial adrenalectomy is indicated in a small local recurrence of an adrenal mass previously treated with partial adrenalectomy.
   e. Partial adrenalectomy may be indicated in multiple endocrine neoplasia type IIA.

10. During a right adrenalectomy, severe bleeding is encountered. The possible causes include all of the following EXCEPT:
    a. right adrenal vein avulsion at the origin on the inferior vena cava.
    b. avulsion of the right hepatic vein branch.
    c. disruption of the adrenal capsule.
    d. inadvertent ligation of the upper pole renal artery.
    e. all of the above.

ANSWERS

1. **c. The medulla is innervated by preganglionic sympathetic nerve fibers.** The right adrenal vein drains directly into the inferior vena cava and derives its arterial supply through the superior, middle, and inferior adrenal arteries from the inferior phrenic artery, the abdominal aorta, and the renal artery, respectively. It is usually more cephalad than the left adrenal gland and is located at the upper pole and medial border of the right kidney. It is closely related to the diaphragm posteriorly, and thus extra care should be taken during surgical dissection, especially of large tumors.

2. **d. 25%.** Of adrenal lesions larger than 6 cm, 25% are adrenal cortical carcinomas, and these larger lesions should be resected. Risk of malignancy in lesions smaller than 4 cm is 2%. Approximately 6% of adrenal lesions between 4 and 6 cm are malignant, and surgical resection can be considered in appropriate individuals.

3. **c. Invasive adrenal cortical carcinoma with thrombus in the inferior vena cava.** Previous abdominal surgeries may result in dense intra-abdominal adhesions that may make surgery difficult. With improved laparoscopic techniques and equipment, large adrenal tumors are no longer considered absolute contraindication to the laparoscopic approach. Literature had described the feasibility of resecting large adrenal tumors laparoscopically. However, the risk of open conversion is greater in such large tumors. Invasion of adrenal cortical carcinoma into surrounding structures will make laparoscopic resection very difficult, and extension of tumor into the inferior vena cava should be considered an absolute contraindication to the laparoscopic approach.

4. **b. Phenoxybenzamine may lead to tachycardia, and beta-adrenergic blockade should be started before phenoxybenzamine administration.** Preoperative sympatholytic therapy with alpha-adrenergic blockers for at least 2 weeks before surgery helps in both hemodynamic and glucose control and should be continued until the day of surgery. Phenoxybenzamine, being nonselective, may lead to tachycardia, and beta-adrenergic blockade may be necessary. Because phenoxybenzamine is an irreversible noncompetitive alpha-adrenergic blocker, prolonged hypotension in the immediate postoperative period and central nervous system effects such as somnolence may be expected. Beta-adrenergic blockade, if needed, must be given with caution in patients with myocardial depression and started only after phenoxybenzamine therapy. α-Methylparatyrosine decreases the rate of catecholamine synthesis and might be useful in patients with cardiomyopathies or resistant to α-blockers. The adrenal vein should be ligated early during the resection of pheochromocytoma to avoid the systemic release of catecholamines during manipulation of the adrenal gland. Lastly, drugs with rapid onset and short half-lives, such as nitroprusside, phentolamine, nitroglycerin, or nicardipine, are generally preferred in intraoperative hypertensive episodes, because hypotension can occur after ligation of the adrenal vein or excision of the pheochromocytoma.

5. **b. Bilateral adrenal hyperplasia.** Although the posterior approach is the most direct route to the adrenal glands and no major muscles are divided, surgical exposure is limited. In addition, access to the adrenal vein and great vessels is more difficult, which may be problematic in event of excessive intraoperative bleeding. Thus this approach is not ideal in large adrenal tumors or adrenocortical carcinoma. The prone position will also make ventilating the patient difficult. However, this approach provides ready access to both adrenal glands through two separate incisions and is ideal for bilateral adrenal hyperplasia or small adrenal tumors.

6. **c. After excision of both adrenal glands.** It is generally recommended that steroid replacement be started as soon as the both adrenal glands are excised to minimize acute adrenal insufficiency. Patients can present with back/abdominal pain, nausea, vomiting, diarrhea, hypotension, fever, hypoglycemia, and hyperkalemia.

7. **c. Open thoracoabdominal approach.** Surgical exposure is limited with the lumbodorsal posterior approach, and this approach should not be used for large tumors or adrenocortical carcinoma. Although the open anterior transabdominal approach using the subcostal or chevron incision gives a fairly good and adequate exposure for most cases, this approach might not be adequate in this case in view of the involvement of the retrohepatic inferior vena cava. The open thoracoabdominal approach is generally reserved for large and invasive tumors with extensive involvement of surrounding structures or vena cava that cannot be safely removed via the anterior transabdominal approach. The thoracoabdominal approach is particularly useful in right-sided tumors, because the liver and inferior vena cava can limit exposure, whereas on the left side, the spleen and pancreas can generally be elevated to provide adequate exposure. Minimally invasive approaches such as conventional laparoscopic or robot-assisted laparoscopic approach are usually contraindicated in such large tumors with extensive involvement of the great vessels.

8. **e. All the above are possible approaches.**

9. **d.** A repeat partial adrenalectomy is indicated in a small local recurrence of an adrenal mass previously treated with partial adrenalectomy. The arterial supply of the adrenal gland forms a plexus circumferentially around the gland and can usually be taken without fear of devascularizing the adrenal cortex, and the gland will remain viable as long it remains attached to the kidney or to an area of unmobilized connective tissue. The venous system drains into a central adrenal vein, and the main adrenal vein can be taken as long as the remnant adrenal gland remains in situ without mobilization. However, it would be prudent to preserve the main adrenal vein as long as it is safe and adequate margins can be obtained. A local recurrence after a previous partial adrenalectomy, regardless of size of recurrence, is an absolute contraindication to a repeat partial adrenalectomy. Multiple endocrine neoplasia type IIA is associated with adrenal tumors, and therefore partial adrenalectomy may be indicated in these patients.

10. **d. Inadvertent ligation of the upper pole renal artery.** All of the vascular injuries noted cause bleeding except ligation of an upper pole renal artery. Ligation of this artery would result in upper pole devascularization, not hemorrhage.

CHAPTER REVIEW

1. The right adrenal vein enters the inferior vena cava in a posterior lateral position. When torn, the vena cava must be rotated to gain access to suture the defect.
2. Local regional recurrence in the adrenal cortical carcinoma occurs in 60% of cases.
3. It is important to note that the tail of the pancreas can lie adjacent to the upper pole of the left kidney and adrenal. Care must be taken not to injure this organ.
4. In a thoracoabdominal incision, the diaphragm should not be incised radially but, rather, circumferentially because the former results in a phrenic nerve injury with an atonic diaphragm lateral to the incision.
5. An Addisonian crisis is most commonly seen after excision of an adrenal tumor that secretes cortisol as the contralateral adrenal is suppressed.
6. In removing large adrenal masses, it is important to be careful not to ligate an upper pole renal artery branch because this will result in an infarction of the renal segment that is served by this artery.
7. The most common sites from which metastases occur to the adrenal are lung, breast, kidney, and melanoma.
8. Before resecting aldosterone-secreting tumors, consideration should be given to preoperative administration of spironolactone and correction of hypokalemia and hypomagnesemia if they exist.
9. Twenty-five percent of adrenal lesions greater than 6 cm are adrenal cortical carcinomas, and these larger lesions should be resected. The risk of malignancy in lesions less than 4 cm is 2%.
10. Preoperative sympatholytic therapy with alpha-adrenergic blockers for at least 2 weeks before surgery in patients with a pheochromocytoma is necessary because it restores vascular volume and helps in both hemodynamic and glucose control. If a beta blocker is necessary to control cardiac arrthymias, it should be begun after full alpha blockade has been achieved.

67

Surgical, Radiographic, and Endoscopic Anatomy of the Female Pelvis

Larissa V. Rodriguez and Leah Yukie Nakamura

QUESTIONS

1. Relative to the ureter, the uterine vessels are found:
   a. laterally.
   b. posteriorly.
   c. anteriorly.
   d. medially.
   e. running together in a common sheath.

2. In contrast to that of the male, the female bladder neck:
   a. has extensive adrenergic innervation.
   b. has a thickened middle smooth muscle layer.
   c. is largely responsible for urinary continence.
   d. is surrounded by type I (slow-twitch) fibers.
   e. has longitudinal smooth muscle fibers that extend to the external meatus.

3. To avoid denervation of the striated urethral sphincter, incisions through the vaginal wall to enter the retropubic space should be made:
   a. perpendicular to the urethra.
   b. over the urethra.
   c. close to the lateral margins of the urethra.
   d. cephalad to the bladder neck.
   e. far lateral in the vaginal wall, parallel to the urethra.

4. A Martius (labial fat pad) rotational flap used in the repair of a vesicovaginal fistula receives blood supply from the:
   a. terminal branches of the internal pudendal artery and vein.
   b. superficial inferior epigastric vessels.
   c. inferior epigastric vessels.
   d. accessory pudendal vessels.
   e. external pudendal vessels.

5. The round ligament:
   a. terminates in the uterus.
   b. is the main source of blood supply to the ovaries.
   c. is the male homologue of the spermatic cord.
   d. terminates in the labia.
   e. is NOT part of the broad ligament.

6. The transversalis fascia is:
   a. part of the inner stratum.
   b. part of the outer stratum.
   c. continuous with the endopelvic fascia.
   d. part of the intermediate stratum.
   e. b and c.

7. After a sacrospinous ligament fixation, the patient wakes up with pain in the posterior and lower leg. The nerve that was likely compromised is the:
   a. femoral nerve.
   b. pudendal nerve.
   c. sacral plexus.
   d. obturator nerve.
   e. a and b.

8. The arcus tendineus fascia pelvis:
   a. is present only in females.
   b. attaches from the ischial spine to the sacrum.
   c. is also known as the *tendinous arc*.
   d. is present only in males.
   e. all of the above.

9. Squamous metaplasia of the bladder:
   a. is a premalignant lesion.
   b. is a sign of an underlying serious infection.
   c. should always be treated with surgical resection.
   d. is a normal finding in premenopausal females.
   e. is none of the above.

10. The ureter can be injured during a hysterectomy:
    a. at the time of division of the ovarian artery.
    b. at the time of division of the uterine artery.
    c. at the time of division of the cardinal ligament.
    d. while dissecting out the cervix.
    e. all of the above.

11. During a sacrospinous ligament vault suspension, significant bleeding is encountered. The bleeding vessels most likely originates from the:
    a. anterior division of internal iliac.
    b. posterior division of internal iliac.
    c. perineal artery.
    d. mesenteric artery.

12. The cavernous nerve, responsible for clitoral engorgement during sexual activity, is derived from:
    a. the pudendal nerve.
    b. the dorsal nerve of the clitoris.
    c. the superior hypogastric plexus.
    d. the inferior hypogastric plexus.

ANSWERS

1. **c. Anteriorly.** In women, the ureter first runs posterior to the ovary, then turns medially to run deep to the base of the broad ligament before entering a loose connective tissue tunnel through the substance of the cardinal ligament.
2. **e. Has longitudinal smooth muscle fibers that extend to the external meatus.** At the female bladder neck, the inner longitudinal fibers converge radially to pass downward as the inner longitudinal layer of the urethra. The middle circular layer does not appear to be as robust as that of the male. The female bladder neck differs strikingly from the male in possessing little adrenergic innervation.
3. **e. Far lateral in the vaginal wall, parallel to the urethra.** Somatic and autonomic nerves to the urethra travel on the lateral walls of the vagina near the urethra. During transvaginal incontinence surgery, the anterior vaginal wall should be incised laterally to avoid these nerves and prevent type III urinary incontinence.
4. **e. External pudendal vessels.** The labial fat pads receive blood supply from the external pudendal branches of the femoral vessels.
5. **d. Terminates in the labia.** The round ligament lies in the base of the broad ligament and arises from the uterus, then travels through the femoral canal to terminate in the labia. It is not a vital support structure to the uterus and does not carry blood supply to the ovaries.
6. **e. b and c.** The transversalis fascia is part of the outer stratum and is continuous with the endopelvic and lateral pelvic fascia. Both the transversalis and endopelvic fascia play important roles at the exit points of the pelvic organs. The endopelvic fascia extends from the uterine artery down to where the vagina and levator ani fuse.
7. **c. Sacral plexus.** During a sacrospinous ligament fixation, the sacral plexus is at jeopardy of being injured because it lies immediately posterior to the sacrospinous ligament as it leaves through the greater sciatic foramen. The pudendal nerve may also be injured during this repair.
8. **c. Is also known as the *tendinous arc*.** The arcus tendineus fascia pelvis or tendinous arc is a thickened band of the pelvic fascia that runs from the ischial spine to the pubic bone. It originates from the pubic bone laterally and is connected to the pubovesical ligament medially and the tendinous arch of the levator ani.
9. **d. Is a normal finding in premenopausal females.** Premenopausal women can have normal signs of squamous metaplasia at the trigone and base of the bladder. This is a nonkeratanizing metaplasia or vaginal metaplasia that is hormonally responsive and is a normal variant.
10. **e. All of the above.** The ureter is vulnerable to injury because it comes in close proximity to many of the structures that are dissected and divided during a radical hysterectomy. It crosses the infundibulopelvic ligament under the ovarian artery and is just medial to the uterine artery. It also passes through the cardinal ligament and lies in close proximity to the cervix.
11. **b. Posterior division of the internal iliac artery.**
12. **d. The inferior hypogastric plexus.**

CHAPTER REVIEW

1. The pubovesical (pubourethral or puboprostatic in the male) ligaments that attach to the bladder neck and pubis hold the bladder neck in place and provide a hammock-like support to the midurethra.
2. The uterosacral ligaments originate from the sciatic foramen and insert into the lateral aspect of the fascia that encircles the cervix.
3. The lymphatic drainage of the vulva, clitoris, and labia minora is to the inguinal nodes.
4. The anterior vagina provides support to the urethra.
5. At the female bladder neck, the inner longitudinal fibers converge radially to pass downward as the inner longitudinal layer of the urethra. The middle circular layer does not appear to be as robust as that of the male. The female bladder neck differs strikingly from the male in possessing little adrenergic innervation.
6. Somatic and autonomic nerves to the urethra travel on the lateral walls of the vagina near the urethra.
7. During a sacrospinous ligament fixation, the sacral plexus is in jeopardy of being injured as it lays immediately posterior to the sacrospinous ligament as it leaves through the greater sciatic foramen. The pudendal nerve may also be injured during this repair.
8. Squamous metaplasia at the trigone and base of the bladder is a nonkeratanising metaplasia that is hormonally responsive and is a normal variant.
9. The ureter crosses the infundibulopelvic ligament under the ovarian artery and is just medial to the uterine artery. It also passes through the cardinal ligament and lies in close proximity to the cervix.

68 Surgical, Radiographic, and Endoscopic Anatomy of the Male Pelvis

Benjamin I. Chung and James D. Brooks

QUESTIONS

1. The greater and lesser sciatic foramina are separated by the:
   a. sacrotuberous ligament.
   b. Cooper (pectineal) ligament.
   c. arcuate line.
   d. sacrospinous ligament.
   e. piriformis muscle.

2. During inguinal incisions, the vessels invariably encountered in Camper fascia are the:
   a. superficial inferior epigastric artery and vein.
   b. superficial circumflex iliac artery and vein.
   c. external pudendal artery and vein.
   d. gonadal artery and veins.
   e. accessory obturator vein.

3. Rupture of the penile urethra at the junction of the penis and scrotum can result in urinary extravasation into all of the following structures EXCEPT the:
   a. anterior abdominal wall up to the clavicles.
   b. scrotum.
   c. penis, deep to the dartos fascia.
   d. perineum in a "butterfly" pattern.
   e. buttock.

4. Accessory obturator veins (from the external iliac artery) and accessory obturator arteries (from the inferior epigastric artery) are encountered in:
   a. 50% and 25% of patients, respectively.
   b. 5% and 50% of patients, respectively.
   c. 50% and 75% of patients, respectively.
   d. 25% and 50% of patients, respectively.
   e. 25% and 5% of patients, respectively.

5. A retractor blade has rested on the psoas muscle during a prolonged procedure, resulting in a femoral nerve palsy. Postoperatively, the patient will experience:
   a. inability to flex the hip and numbness over the anterior thigh.
   b. inability to flex the knee and numbness over the thigh.
   c. numbness over the anterior thigh only.
   d. inability to extend the knee and numbness over the anterior thigh.
   e. inability to flex the knee only.

6. Autonomic nerves contributing to the pelvic plexus include the:
   a. superior hypogastric nerves from the para-aortic plexuses.
   b. pelvic sympathetic trunks.
   c. pelvic parasympathetic neurons from the sacral spinal cord.
   d. a and c only.
   e. a, b, and c.

7. To preserve the vascular supply to the ureter, incisions in the peritoneum should be made:
   a. medially in the abdomen and laterally in the pelvis.
   b. laterally in the abdomen and medially in the pelvis.
   c. always medial to the ureter.
   d. always lateral to the ureter.
   e. directly over the ureter.

8. All of the following features of the ureterovesical junction cooperate to prevent vesicoureteral reflux EXCEPT:
   a. fixation of the ureter to the superficial trigone.
   b. sphincteric closure of the ureteral orifice.
   c. detrusor backing.
   d. telescoping of the bladder outward over the ureter.
   e. passive closure of the intramural ureter caused by bladder filling.

9. Which of the following statements about the trigone is TRUE?
   a. Epithelium is thicker than the rest of the bladder and densely adherent.
   b. Superficial smooth muscle is a continuation of Waldeyer sheath.
   c. Smooth muscle enlarges to form thick fascicles.
   d. Smooth muscle of the ureter forms the interureteric ridge (Mercier bar).
   e. When the bladder empties, the trigone is thrown into thick folds.

10. Arterial supply to the bladder includes:
    a. the superior vesical artery.
    b. the inferior vesical artery.
    c. the obturator artery.
    d. the inferior hemorrhoidal artery.
    e. all of the above.

11. Which of the following statements concerning the male striated urethral sphincter is TRUE?
    a. It is composed of type I (slow-twitch) and type II (fast-twitch) fibers.
    b. It is bounded above by the superior fascia.
    c. It receives motor blanches from the dorsal nerve of the penis.
    d. It is shaped like a signet ring and is 2 to 2.5 cm in length.
    e. It is densely supplied with proprioceptive muscle spindles.

12. The first branch of the pudendal nerve in the perineum is the:
    a. dorsal nerve of the penis.
    b. inferior rectal nerve(s).
    c. perineal nerve.
    d. posterior femoral cutaneous branches.
    e. posterior scrotal branches.

13. Lymphatic drainage from the scrotum travels:
    a. through perianal nodes to reach the pelvis.
    b. directly to the deep pelvic lymph nodes.
    c. through the superficial and deep inguinal lymph nodes.
    d. to prepubic nodes.
    e. to para-aortic lymph nodes along with testicular drainage.

14. Which layers of the scrotum and testicular tunics usually need to be debrided in patients with Fournier gangrene?
    a. The scrotal skin only
    b. The scrotal skin and dartos layer
    c. The scrotal skin, dartos layer, and external spermatic fascia
    d. The scrotal skin, dartos layer, and external cremasteric and internal spermatic fasciae, leaving the tunica vaginalis intact
    e. All tissues, including the tunica vaginalis

15. Lymphatic drainage from the bladder passes through the:
    a. external iliac lymph nodes.
    b. obturator and internal iliac lymph nodes.
    c. internal and common iliac lymph nodes.
    d. common iliac, periureteral, and para-aortic lymph nodes.
    e. a, b, and c.

16. To preserve potency during a radical cystectomy, ligation of the lateral and posterior vascular pedicles is best carried out:
    a. close to their origin from the internal iliac vessels.
    b. near the bladder.
    c. from beneath the bladder after rotating the prostate cephalad.
    d. as they cross the ureter.
    e. lateral to the rectum.

ANSWERS

1. **d. Sacrospinous ligament.** The sacrospinous ligament separates the greater and lesser sciatic foramina.
2. **a. Superficial inferior epigastric artery and vein.** The superficial inferior epigastric vessels are encountered during inguinal incisions and can cause troublesome bleeding during placement of pelvic laparoscopic ports.
3. **e. Buttock.** Blood and urine can accumulate in the scrotum and penis deep to the dartos fascia after an anterior urethral injury. In the perineum, their spread is limited by the fusions of Colles fascia to the ischiopubic rami laterally and to the posterior edge of the perineal membrane; the resulting hematoma is therefore butterfly shaped. These processes will not extend down the leg or into the buttock, but they can freely travel up the anterior abdominal wall deep to Scarpa fascia to the clavicles and around the flank to the back.
4. **a. 50% and 25% of patients, respectively.** In half of patients, one or more accessory obturator veins drain into the underside of the external iliac vein and can easily be torn during lymphadenectomy. In 25% of people, an accessory obturator artery arises from the inferior epigastric artery and runs medial to the femoral vein to reach the obturator canal.
5. **d. Inability to extend the knee and numbness over the anterior thigh.** The femoral nerve (L2, L3, L4) supplies sensation to the anterior thigh and motor innervation to the extensors of the knee.
6. **e. a, b, and c.** The presynaptic sympathetic cell bodies reach the pelvic plexus by two pathways: (1) the superior hypogastric plexus and (2) the pelvic continuation of the sympathetic trunks. Presynaptic parasympathetic innervation arises from the intermediolateral cell column of the sacral cord.
7. **b. Laterally in the abdomen and medially in the pelvis.** Blood supply to the pelvic ureter enters laterally; thus the pelvic peritoneum should be incised only medial to the ureter.
8. **b. Sphincteric closure of the ureteral orifice.** The intravesical portion of the ureter lies immediately beneath the bladder urothelium and is therefore quite pliant; it is backed by a strong plate of detrusor muscle. With bladder filling, this arrangement is thought to result in passive occlusion of the ureter, like a flap valve.
9. **d. Smooth muscle of the ureter forms the interureteric ridge (Mercier bar).** Fibers from each ureter meet to form a triangular sheet of muscle that extends from the two ureteral orifices to the internal urethra meatus. The edges of this muscular sheet are thickened between the ureteral orifices (the interureteric crest, or Mercier bar) and between the ureters and the internal urethral meatus (Bell muscle).
10. **e. All of the above.** In addition to the vesical branches, the bladder may be supplied by any adjacent artery arising from the internal iliac artery.
11. **d. It is shaped like a signet ring and is 2 to 2.5 cm in length.** The membranous urethra spans on average 2 to 2.5 cm (range: 1.2 to 5 cm). In the male it is surrounded by the striated (external) urethral sphincter, which is often incorrectly depicted as a flat sheet of muscle sandwiched between two layers of fasciae. The striated sphincter is actually shaped like a signet ring, broad at its base and narrowing as it passes through the urogenital hiatus of the levator ani to meet the apex of the prostate.
12. **a. Dorsal nerve of the penis.** The pudendal nerve follows the vessels in their course through the perineum. Its first branch, the dorsal nerve of the penis, travels ventral to the main pudendal trunk in the Alcock canal.
13. **c. Through the superficial and deep inguinal lymph nodes.** The penis, scrotum, and perineum drain into the inguinal lymph nodes. These nodes can be divided into superficial groups and deep groups.
14. **b. The scrotal skin and dartos layer.** The external, cremasteric, and internal spermatic fasciae are embryologically distinct from the scrotal and dartos layers and have their own blood and nerve supplies. It is uncommon for them to be involved in the necrotic process in Fournier gangrene; therefore they can be spared. (In practice in patients with Fournier gangrene, all scrotal tissue is debrided to the tunica vaginalis.)
15. **e. a, b, and c.** In the bladder, the bulk of the lymphatic drainage passes to the external iliac lymph nodes. Some anterior and lateral drainage may go through the obturator and internal iliac nodes, and portions of the bladder base and trigone may drain into the internal and common iliac groups. Complete lymph node dissection during radical cystectomy should encompass all of these lymph node groups.
16. **b. Near the bladder.** The bladder vasculature pierces the pelvic autonomic plexuses near the origin of the arteries from the internal iliac arteries. Ligation of these vessels proximally will injure the pelvic autonomic nervous plexuses. Ligation is best carried out near the bladder to avoid nerve damage.

CHAPTER REVIEW

1. Scarpa fascia on the abdomen forms a distinct layer and is continuous with Colles fascia in the perineum medially. It fuses with the deep fascia of the thigh laterally. Colles fascia is continuous with the dartos fascia of the penis. Thus, urinary extravasation and infections confined by these fascia attachments do not allow for extension down the legs or into the buttocks but may allow for it to travel to the clavicles.

2. The internal oblique and the transversalis fascia fuse to form the conjoin tendon. The conjoin tendon reinforces the posterior wall of the inguinal canal.

3. A direct hernia of the inguinal canal occurs medial to the inferior epigastric vessels; an indirect hernia occurs lateral to these vessels.

4. The superior vesicle artery arises from the proximal portion of the obliterated umbilical artery. The obliterated umbilical artery may be used to find the superior vesicle artery.

5. In 25% of people there is an accessory obturator artery that arises from the inferior epigastric artery and courses medial to the femoral vein.

6. The genitofemoral nerve courses along the ventral surface of the psoas muscle; the femoral nerve runs in the substance of the psoas muscle. Retractors compressing the muscle may result in nerve palsy. Sutures placed perpendicular to the muscle fibers may entrap the nerves.

7. The obturator nerve supplies the adductors of the thigh.

8. The male bladder neck receives abundant sympathetic innervation. The female bladder neck receives little sympathetic innervation.

9. The blood supply to the prostate enters at the 4 and 8 o'clock positions. It is important to understand this in an open prostatectomy when securing hemostasis.

10. Although lymphatic supply from the prostate is primarily to the obturator and internal iliac nodes, it may drain directly to the presacral and external iliac nodes.

11. Denonvilliers fascia separates the prostate from the rectum.

12. Scrotal lymphatics do not cross the median raphe; drainage is to the ipsilateral inguinal nodes. Lymphatics from the penis cross over extensively and may drain to either or both groin nodes irrespective of the side of the penis involved.

13. The cavernosal nerves pass by the tips of the seminal vesicles and lie within the leaves of the lateral endopelvic fascia and course very close to the apex of the prostate, where they are most vulnerable to injury.

14. The ureter is anterior (ventral) to the common iliac artery.

15. The blood supply to the pelvic ureter enters laterally.

16. The bladder is an intra-abdominal organ in the infant and may project above the umbilicus.

17. The muscle of the trigone has three layers: (1) the superficial layer, derived from the longitudinal muscle of the ureter; (2) the deep layer, which arises from Waldeyer sheath on the ureter and inserts at the bladder neck; and (3) the detrusor layer.

18. The bladder has a lateral pedicle that is lateral to the ureter and a posterior pedicle that is posteromedial to the ureter.

69 Physiology and Pharmacology of the Bladder and Urethra

Toby C. Chai and Lori A. Birder

QUESTIONS

1. The lower urinary tract is innervated by three sets of peripheral nerves. Which of the following is correct?
   a. Pelvic parasympathetic nerves arise at the sacral spinal cord level and excite the bladder and urethra.
   b. Sympathetic nerves inhibit the bladder body and excite the bladder neck and urethra
   c. Pudendal (somatic) nerves excite the bladder body and the external urethral sphincter.
   d. All of the above are true.
   e. None of the above are true.

2. "Sensing" bladder volume is relevant during bladder storage. Which of the following is correct?
   a. It has been speculated the sense of imminent micturition arises in the urethra.
   b. Bladder filling has been shown to correlate with episodic bursts of sensation and afferent discharge.
   c. Nathan first described sensations of awareness during bladder filling.
   d. Sensations of awareness during bladder distension can be mapped to the urinary bladder.
   e. All are correct.

3. Bladder afferents can be:
   a. characterized by responses to receptive field stimulation.
   b. classified according to ability to respond to a diverse range of chemical mediators.
   c. silent initially but sensitized during inflammatory processes.
   d. variable in both morphology and function depending upon species.
   e. All of the above.

4. Sensitization of afferents in bladder pathology can:
   a. open ion channels in the nerve terminals.
   b. release a number of inflammatory mediators.
   c. develop rapidly and be relatively short lived.
   d. be resolved easily.
   e. a-c only.

5. Patients with irritable bowel syndrome (IBS) often report changes in bladder function. Which of the following statements is correct?
   a. This is an example of cross-organ sensitization.
   b. In animal models colonic inflammation rarely leads to bladder dysfunction.
   c. Cross-organ sensitization only occurs between the gastrointestinal tract and the urinary bladder.
   d. The mediators, which are responsible for these conditions, have been well described.
   e. None are true.

6. In terms of nerves innervating the detrusor:
   a. the majority express acetylcholinesterase enzyme.
   b. acetylcholine and adenosine triphosphate (ATP) appear to provide the majority of the excitatory input.
   c. release of both acetylcholine and ATP result in smooth muscle contraction.
   d. additional substances released from efferent nerves include nitric oxide and vasoactive intestinal polypeptide.
   e. all are correct.

7. In terms of adrenergic influences:
   a. reflex bladder activity can be modulated by alpha-1 adrenergic mechanisms.
   b. alpha-1 adrenergic mechanisms control blood pressure and tissue blood flow.
   c. the beta-3 adrenergic receptors are present at a number of sites (both peripherally and centrally).
   d. beta-3 receptor agonists, via effects on a number of sites, are a promising treatment for overactive bladder.
   e. all are correct.

8. Which of the following is TRUE about ATP?
   a. It is the main excitatory neurotransmitter for bladder contraction in humans.
   b. It can activate two main families of purinergic receptors: P2X and P2Y
   c. Purinergic neurotransmission plays an important role in bladder overactivity and bladder pain
   d. b and c are true
   e. All are correct

9. During bladder storage:
   a. bladder accommodation is dependent upon activation of sympathetic pathways.
   b. bladder accommodation is dependent upon quiescence of parasympathetic efferent pathways.
   c. intravesical pressure measurements are low when below the voiding threshold.
   d. the sympathetic reflex provides negative feedback.
   e. all are true.

10. During storage phase of the bladder:
    a. the urothelium plays an important role in accommodating urine storage.
    b. the urothelium is only a barrier and exhibits no other functions.
    c. increase of urothelial-mediators during bladder filling can influence smooth muscle tone.
    d. the urothelial surface cells change shape during bladder filling.
    e. a, c, and d are correct.

11. The guarding reflex is a mechanism for maintaining continence and is characterized by:
    a. activation of pudendal motoneurons.
    b. increased outlet resistance.
    c. activation of external urethral sphincter motoneurons.
    d. activation of afferent input from the urethra or pelvic floor that leads to closure of the urethral outlet.
    e. all of the above.

12. Electrical stimulation of the sacral nerve roots is known to be:
    a. an effective treatment for refractory overactive bladder
    b. an effective treatment for non-obstructive urinary retention
    c. effective by modulation of central nervous system pathways
    d. a better treatment compared with posterior tibial nerve stimulation.
    e. a-c are correct.

13. In terms of bladder emptying:
    a. switching between bladder storage and emptying can occur involuntarily (reflex emptying) or voluntarily.
    b. reflex voiding only occurs in the normal adult.
    c. initial expulsion of urine consists of initial contraction of the urethral sphincter.
    d. relaxation of the urethral smooth muscle during micturition is achieved by release of acetylcholine.
    e. none are true.

14. The facilitatory urethra to bladder reflex was characterized by:
    a. Barrington
    b. Delancey
    c. de Groat
    d. increased urethral afferent activation promoting bladder emptying.
    e. a and d are correct

15. An essential control center for micturition in healthy individuals is:
    a. the dorsal pontine tegmentum.
    b. Barrington nucleus.
    c. the pontine micturition center.
    d. the M region.
    e. all of the above.

16. In terms of cerebral control of voiding in humans:
    a. coordinated relaxation and contraction of urethra and bladder is driven by a long-loop spinobulbospinal reflex.
    b. afferents activated during bladder filling synapse in the central PAG and PMC regions.
    c. spinobulbospinal voiding-reflex pathway functions as a "switch."
    d. absence of the "switch" would lead to incontinence.
    e. all of the above.

17. In terms of continence and brain-bladder control:
    a. it involves limbic areas associated with basic emotion and safety.
    b. it involves cortical circuits concerned with social propriety.
    c. the PAG and PMC form the main brainstem "switch."
    d. all of the above.

18. The contraction of detrusor by cholinergic muscarinic receptor agonists is characterized by:
    a. IP3 hydrolysis and release of intracellular calcium.
    b. decreased calcium flux through nifedipine-sensitive calcium channels.
    c. involvement of the muscarinic M1 subtype only.
    d. stimulation of the Rho-kinase pathway.
    e. none of the above.

19. Stimulation of beta-adrenergic receptors in human detrusor is characterized by:
    a. relaxation of detrusor smooth muscle.
    b. involvement of beta 2 and beta 3 subtype receptors.
    c. accumulation of cyclic adenosine monophosphate (cAMP).
    d. all of the above.

20. Urethral tone and intraurethral pressure are influenced by:
    a. alpha adrenergic receptors.
    b. sympathetic innervation.
    c. number of intramural ganglia.
    d. parasympathetic innervation.
    e. a and b are correct

21. Which transgenic animal models has (have) been published showing detrusor overactivity?
    a. Increased M3
    b. Decreased P2X3/P2X2
    c. Decreased BK
    d. Decreased β1-integrin
    e. c and d are correct

22. The lamina propria (LP) of the bladder is thought to be the critical compartment because of which cell(s) that can mediate interaction between urothelium and nerves within the LP?
    a. Fibroblasts
    b. Ganglion cells
    c. Myofibroblasts
    d. Interstitial cells
    e. c and d are correct

23. The primary mechanism of action of onabotulinumtoxinA is:
    a. blockade of intracellular vesicle fusion in presynaptic nerves.
    b. suppression of afferent nerves in the lamina propria.
    c. blockade of M3 receptor on detrusor myocyte.
    d. opening of BK channel on detrusor myocyte.
    e. blockade of voltage dependent calcium channels on detrusor myocyte.

24. What distinguishing feature(s) in the bladder urothelium distinguish(es) it from the lamina propria, detrusor and serosal compartments?
    a. Presence of connexin-43 (Cx43)
    b. Presence of purinergic receptors
    c. Presence of tight junction proteins
    d. Presence of uroplakins
    e. c and d are correct

25. During acute bacterial cystitis, uropathogenic bacteria induce a host immune response due to their interaction with which of the following receptors on the urothelial cell?
    a. TRPV1
    b. M2
    c. NK-A
    d. TLR4
    e. P2X3

26. Maintenance of normal bladder compliance during urinary storage is (are) due to:
    a. passive viscoelastic properties.
    b. active neural signaling.
    c. modulation of filling rate.
    d. all of the above.
    e. a and b are correct.

27. Connexin-43 (Cx43) is important in regulating detrusor contractility because:
    a. it regulates acetylcholine release by efferent nerves.
    b. it breaks down acetylcholine in the neuromuscular junction.
    c. it allows for passage of ions between adjoining detrusor myocytes.
    d. it has a circadian rhythm of expression.
    e. c and d are correct.

28. Which urethral mechanisms are involved in maintenance of continence in the female?
    a. Network of submucosal vascularity
    b. Guarding reflex
    c. Hammock hypothesis
    d. Sympathetic tone
    e. All are correct

29. G-coupled proteins:
    a. mediate many different receptor functions.
    b. enzymatically cleave ATP to adenosine monophosphate (ADP).
    c. regulate protein folding in the endoplasmic reticulum (ER).
    d. help regulate intracellular calcium concentrations.
    e. a and d are correct.

30. Urothelial barrier function is maintained by which of the following?
    a. Gap junctions
    b. Uroplakins
    c. TLR4 receptor
    d. Aquaporin channels
    e. Mucinous layer

31. In supraspinal SCI (spinal cord injury), the mechanisms mediating neurogenic detrusor overactivity include that it:
    a. is mediated by C-fiber afferent fibers.
    b. involves NGF in pathophysiology.
    c. can be blocked by?-blockers.
    d. is associated with external sphincter contractions.
    e. all are correct.

32. Membrane potential of a cell:
    a. requires energy to maintain, even at rest.
    b. at rest, is maintained by low intracellular potassium and high extracellular potassium.
    c. at rest, is maintained by low intracellular sodium and high intracellular chloride.
    d. becomes electrically more negative during an action potential in a neuron.
    e. changes during an action potential due to influx of anions into the detrusor myocyte.

33. Which of the following mechanisms is unique to M2 muscarinic receptor activation when compared to M3 muscarinic receptor activation?
    a. Mediates rise in intracellular calcium when activated
    b. Uses G-coupled proteins
    c. Involves cAMP downstream
    d. Causes detrusor contraction
    e. Causes detrusor relaxation

34. Isolated nocturia complaints are due to:
    a. nocturnal polyuria.
    b. sleep apnea.
    c. detrusor overactivity.
    d. peripheral edema.
    e. a, b, and d are correct.

35. Which of the following declines with aging?
    a. Bladder sensation
    b. ATP content of bladder
    c. Detrusor contractile responses to α-adrenergic stimulation
    d. Detrusor contractile responses to cholinergic or electrical stimulation
    e. Bladder capacity

36. Urine from BPS/IC patients has been found to contain:
    a. a protein that inhibits urothelial cell growth in culture.
    b. a virus that induces T-cell mediated inflammation.
    c. a protozoan that invades the urothelial cell.
    d. an increased level of ATP.
    e. a and d are correct.

37. The "motor-sensory" hypothesis is used to explain mechanism of action in treating:
    a. bladder underactivity with a muscarinic agonist.
    b. neurogenic detrusor overactivity with TRPV1 blocker.
    c. idiopathic detrusor overactivity with onabotulinumtoxin A.
    d. urinary urgency with antimuscarinics.
    e. urinary frequency with α-blockers.

38. The reason that some women void without measureable increase in Pdet is because:
    a. the detrusor does not need to contract during voiding in women.
    b. the urethra contains smooth, in addition to striated, muscle fibers.
    c. there is a reduced parasympathetic innervation to the female bladder.
    d. Pdet is not the only measure of the bladder's mechanical work ability.
    e. the female bladder has increased viscoelastic properties.

39. Differences between smooth and striated muscles include:
    a. actinomyosin cross-bridge cycling in smooth muscle only.
    b. visible striations in striated muscle only.
    c. release of acetylcholine by pre-junctional motor neurons in smooth muscle only.

d. lack of intermediate filaments in skeletal muscles only.

e. b and d are correct.

40. Bladder outlet obstruction results in:

a. change in collagen subtype proportions.

b. afferent and efferent neuronal hypertrophy.

c. urothelial hyperplasia.

d. C-fiber mediated micturition reflex.

e. a, b, and d are correct.

41. The principle behind neuromodulation in treating overactive bladder is:

a. inhibition of detrusor interstitial cell activity.

b. block of release of postganglionic neuronal acetylcholine.

c. activation of C-fiber afferents.

d. inhibition of somatic afferent processing in spinal cord.

e. excitation of sacral sympathetic nerve fibers.

42. Which of the following animal models best mimics human BPS/IC?

a. Social stress model

b. Water avoidance stress model

c. Acetic acid infusion into bladder

d. Cyclophosphamide intraperitoneal injection

e. Bowel radiation model

43. Etiologic causes for stress urinary incontinence may include:

a. decreased urethral support.

b. loss of urothelial seal.

c. decreased serotonin in sacral spinal cord.

d. shortened urethra.

e. a, b, and c are correct.

44. The neurotransmitter released by sympathetic preganglionic neurons at the ganglia is:

a. acetylcholine.

b. norepinephrine.

c. adenosine triphosphate.

d. epinephrine.

e. nitric oxide.

45. The action potential in either an afferent or efferent neuron is due to:

a. influx of Na.

b. influx of K.

c. influx of Cl.

d. influx of Ca.

e. efflux of Ca.

ANSWERS

1. b. Sympathetic nerves inhibit the bladder body and excite the bladder neck and urethra.
2. e. All are correct.
3. e. All are correct.
4. e. a-c only.
5. a. This is an example of cross-organ sensitization.
6. e. All are correct.
7. e. All are correct.
8. d. b and c are true.
9. e. All are true.
10. e. a, c, and d are correct.
11. e. All of the above.
12. e. a-c are correct.
13. a. Switching between bladder storage and emptying can occur involuntarily (reflex emptying) or voluntarily.
14. e. a and d are correct.
15. e. All of the above.
16. e. All of the above.
17. d. All of the above.
18. a. IP3 hydrolysis and release of intracellular calcium.
19. d. All of the above.
20. e. a and b are correct.
21. e. c and d are correct.
22. e. c and d are correct.
23. a. Blockade of intracellular vesicle fusion in presynaptic nerves.
24. e. c and d are correct.
25. d. TLR4
26. e. a and b are correct.
27. e. c and d are correct.
28. e. All are correct.
29. e. a and d are correct.
30. b. Uroplakins.
31. e. All are correct.
32. a. Requires energy to maintain, even at rest.
33. c. Involves cAMP downstream.
34. e. a, b, and d are correct.
35. a. Bladder sensation.
36. e. a and d are correct.
37. d. Urinary urgency with antimuscarinics.
38. d. Pdet is not the only measure of bladder's mechanical work ability.
39. e. b and d are correct.
40. e. a, b, and d are correct.
41. d. Inhibition of somatic afferent processing in spinal cord.
42. b. Water avoidance stress model.
43. e. a, b, and c are correct.
44. a. Acetylcholine.
45. a. Influx of Na.

CHAPTER REVIEW

1. The bladder has two parts: the body, which lies above the ureteral orifices, and the base, consisting of the trigone and bladder neck.
2. Smooth muscle is able to adjust its length over a much wider range than skeletal muscle. Thus, an empty bladder has a small intravesical space despite the amount of smooth muscle it contains.
3. There is a complete, competent ring of smooth muscle around the bladder neck in the male. This does not occur in the female.
4. In women the density of adrenergic innervation in the bladder neck is less than in men.
5. Myofibroblasts in the lamina propria modulate physiologic interactions between the urothelium and detrusor.
6. Bladder wall blood flow is reduced by distention; in patients with decreased compliance, this effect is pronounced.
7. In the female, the external urethral sphincter covers the ventral surface of the urethra in a horseshoe configuration.
8. The levator ani pelvic floor muscle does not surround the ventral aspect of the urethra in either the male or the female.

9. The external urethral sphincter is composed of (1) periurethral striated muscle of the pelvic floor and (2) striated muscle within the urethra.

10. The bladder urothelium serves a barrier function but is permeable to water to a limited degree and can actively transport sodium.

11. There is no definite evidence that the GAG layer acts as a primary epithelial barrier.

12. Urothelial cells release chemical mediators such as NO, ATP, acetylcholine, and substance P that have excitatory and inhibitory actions on afferent nerves in the bladder wall.

13. Prostaglandins are released from the urothelium.

14. Uroplakin and tight junction proteins are important in maintaining the urothelial barrier function.

15. The normal bladder at rest may be spontaneously active.

16. A low voiding pressure in women does not equate with impaired detrusor contractility.

17. The parasympathetic nerves from S2-4 excite the bladder and relax the urethra. They have afferent fibers. The lumbar sympathetic nerves inhibit the bladder body and excite the bladder base and urethra. They also have afferent fibers. The pudendal nerves (S2-4) excite the external urethral sphincter. Afferent nerve fibers travel with the pudendal nerve as well.

18. There may be parasympathetic afferent and efferent nerve interconnections at the level of the intramural ganglia.

19. Pelvic nerve afferents monitor bladder volume and amplitude of the bladder contraction.

20. The bladder neck and proximal urethra contain the largest density of bladder nerves.

21. Decreased afferent sensitivity or excitability in certain pathologic conditions as well as aging may be an important cause of impaired voiding.

22. Activation of the parasympathetic pathway during voiding triggers the release of NO, which is a major inhibitor of urethral smooth muscle.

23. Cross organization may occur between bladder and bowel, uterus, pelvic urethra, vagina, and prostate. This may contribute to the chronic pelvic pain syndrome.

24. A substantial proportion of the C-fiber afferent population is silent; pathologic conditions may recruit mechanosensitive C-fibers to form a new functional afferent pathway.

25. Activation of the central serotonergic system can suppress voiding by inhibiting the parasympathetic excitatory input to the urinary bladder.

26. The bladder sympathetic reflex promotes closure of the urethral outlet and inhibits neurally mediated contractions of the bladder.

27. While the bladder fills, the external sphincter activity increases (guarding reflex)—that is, pudendal motor neurons are activated by bladder afferent input.

28. The dorsal pontine tegmentum is the control center for micturition.

29. Stimulation of beta 2 and beta 3 receptors relaxes the detrusor.

30. Sex steroids modulate receptors and influence growth of bladder tissues.

31. After spinal cord injury, a C-fiber–mediated spinal reflex develops and may play a role in the development of detrusor overactivity.

32. Alterations of neural networks occur in the central nervous system following obstruction of the lower urinary tract.

33. Obstruction-induced detrusor overactivity may be due to denervation supersensitivity.

34. With aging detrusor contractility, bladder sensation and urethral pressure decline.

35. Sacral neuromodulation is thought to have its beneficial effect by somatic inhibition of sensory processing in the spinal cord.

36. The hammock hypothesis of urinary continence suggests that the urethra has a fixed dorsal surface due to its attachments to the pubis, pelvic muscles, and fascia, which allows ventral wall compression of the urethra against the fixed dorsal wall.

70

Pathophysiology and Classification of Lower Urinary Tract Dysfunction: Overview

Alan J. Wein

QUESTIONS

1. Which of the following best describes normal bladder behavior during the filling-storage phase of the micturition cycle?
   a. Low compliance due to elastic properties
   b. High compliance due to elastic properties
   c. Low compliance due to elastic and viscoelastic properties
   d. High compliance due to elastic and viscoelastic properties
   e. High compliance due to a low relaxation coefficient of the lamina propria

2. A patient who has significantly and urodynamically dangerous decreased compliance because of a replacement by collagen of other components of the stroma is generally best managed by:
   a. pharmacologic regimen.
   b. hydraulic distention.
   c. nerve section.
   d. augmentation cystoplasty.
   e. neuromodulation.

3. The "guarding reflex" refers to the:
   a. abrupt increase in striated sphincter activity seen with a cough during normal bladder filling/storage.
   b. spinal sympathetic inhibition of parasympathetic ganglion activity.
   c. gradual increase in striated sphincter activity seen during normal bladder filling/storage.
   d. gradual inhibition of the pontine-mesencephalic micturition center by the cerebral cortex during normal bladder filling/storage.
   e. gradual inhibition of the sacral spinal cord ventral nuclei by the pontine-mesencephalic brainstem during normal bladder filling/storage.

4. The primary effect of the spinal sympathetic reflexes that are evoked in animals during bladder filling and that facilitate bladder filling/storage is:
   a. neurally mediated stimulation of the α-adrenergic receptors in the area of the smooth sphincter.
   b. neurally mediated stimulation of the β-adrenergic receptors in the bladder body smooth musculature.
   c. direct inhibition of detrusor motor neurons in the sacral spinal cord.
   d. neurally mediated inhibition of cholinergic receptors in the area of the bladder body.
   e. neurally mediated sympathetic modulation of cholinergic ganglionic transmission.

5. The organizational center for the micturition reflex in an intact neural axis is the:
   a. pontine mesencephalic formation in the brainstem.
   b. frontal area of the cerebral cortex.
   c. parietal area of the cerebral cortex.
   d. cerebellum.
   e. sacral spinal cord.

6. Involuntary bladder contractions are most commonly seen in association with:
   a. sacral spinal cord neurologic disease or injury.
   b. infrasacral neurologic disease or injury.
   c. suprasacral neurologic disease or injury.
   d. peripheral nerve neurologic disease or injury.
   e. interstitial cystitis.

7. Using the functional classification system, the usual lower urinary tract dysfunction seen after a stroke would be categorized as:
   a. failure to store because of the bladder (overactivity).
   b. combined deficit (failure to store because of the bladder, failure to empty because of striated sphincter dyssynergy).
   c. combined deficit (failure to store because of the bladder, failure to empty because of a nonrelaxing outlet).
   d. failure to store because of the bladder (hypersensitivity).
   e. failure to store because of the outlet.

8. In the International Continence Society (ICS) classification system, the disorder described in question 7 would be characterized as:
   a. during storage, overactive neurogenic detrusor activity increased sensation, low bladder capacity, and incompetent urethral closure mechanism and during voiding, normal detrusor activity and abnormal urethral function (dysfunctional voiding).
   b. during storage, normal detrusor function, increased sensation, low bladder capacity, and normal urethral closure mechanism and during voiding, normal detrusor activity and abnormal urethral function (dysfunctional voiding).
   c. during storage, overactive neurogenic detrusor activity, normal sensation, normal bladder capacity, and incompetent urethral closure mechanism and during voiding, normal detrusor activity and normal urethral function.
   d. during storage, stable detrusor activity, reduced sensation, low bladder capacity, and normal urethral closure mechanism and during emptying, normal detrusor activity and abnormal urethral function (dysfunctional voiding).
   e. during storage, overactive neurogenic detrusor activity, normal sensation, low capacity, normal compliance, and normal urethral closure function and during emptying, normal detrusor activity and normal urethral function.

9. In the current ICS terminology, "detrusor hyperreflexia" has been replaced by:
   a. detrusor instability.
   b. idiopathic detrusor overactivity.
   c. hyperactive bladder.
   d. neurogenic detrusor overactivity.
   e. neurogenic detrusor instability.

10. In the Krane-Siroky urodynamic classification system, a patient with post–cerebrovascular accident voiding dysfunction characterized by urgency, frequency, and urge incontinence would most commonly be characterized as having:
    a. detrusor areflexia, striated sphincter dyssynergia, and smooth sphincter dyssynergia.
    b. detrusor hyperreflexia, striated sphincter synergia, and smooth sphincter dyssynergia.
    c. detrusor hyperreflexia, striated sphincter dyssynergia, and smooth sphincter synergia.
    d. detrusor areflexia, striated sphincter synergia, and smooth sphincter dyssynergia.
    e. detrusor hyperreflexia, striated sphincter synergia, and smooth sphincter dyssynergia.

11. In the Lapides classification system, a patient with post–cerebrovascular accident voiding dysfunction characterized by urgency, frequency, and urge incontinence would most commonly be characterized as having:
    a. sensory neurogenic bladder.
    b. motor paralytic bladder.
    c. uninhibited neurogenic bladder.
    d. reflex neurogenic bladder.
    e. autonomous neurogenic bladder.

12. A reflex neurogenic bladder, as described in the Lapides system classification, is characteristically seen in which of the following?
    a. Traumatic spinal cord injury between the sacral spinal cord and the brainstem
    b. Traumatic spinal cord injury between the sacral spinal cord and conus medullaris
    c. Cerebrovascular accident and insulin-dependent diabetes mellitus
    d. Non-insulin-dependent diabetes mellitus
    e. Multiple sclerosis

13. In the Bors-Comarr system of classification, the term *unbalanced*, when applied to a patient with an upper motor neuron (UMN) lesion, implies:
    a. cerebellar lesion.
    b. involuntary bladder contractions during filling.
    c. areflexic bladder.
    d. decreased bladder compliance during filling.
    e. sphincter dyssynergia.

14. In the Bors-Comarr system, a patient with post–cerebrovascular accident voiding dysfunction characterized by urgency, frequency, and urge incontinence would most commonly be characterized as having:
    a. a UMN lesion, complete, and balanced.
    b. a UMN lesion, complete, and imbalanced.
    c. a lower motor neuron (LMN) lesion, complete, and imbalanced.
    d. an LMN lesion, incomplete, and balanced.
    e. a UMN lesion/LMN lesion, complete, and balanced.

15. Which of the following is an absolute requirement for a patient to be included in the symptom syndrome of overactive bladder?
    a. Nocturia
    b. Urinary frequency
    c. Urgency
    d. Urgency incontinence
    e. Detrusor overactivity

16. Which of the following pathophysiologic factors is shared by men and women with urinary incontinence (failure to store) due to outlet underactivity?
    a. Bladder neck hypermobility
    b. Intrinsic sphincter dysfunction
    c. Proximal urethral hypermobility
    d. Nonrelaxing striated sphincter
    e. Bladder neck dysfunction

ANSWERS

1. **d. High compliance due to elastic and viscoelastic properties.** The normal adult bladder response to filling at a physiologic rate is an almost imperceptible change in intravesical pressure. During at least the initial stages of bladder filling, after unfolding of the bladder wall from its collapsed state, this high compliance ($\Delta V/\Delta P$) of the bladder is due primarily to its elastic and viscoelastic properties. Elasticity allows the constituents of the bladder wall to stretch to a certain degree without any increase in tension. Viscoelasticity allows stretch to induce a rise in tension followed by a decay (stress relaxation) when the filling (stretch stimulus) slows or stops.

2. **d. Augmentation cystoplasty.** The viscoelastic properties of the stroma (bladder wall less smooth muscle and epithelium) and the urodynamically relaxed detrusor muscle account for the passive mechanical properties and normal bladder compliance seen during filling. The main components of stroma are collagen and elastin. When the collagen component increases, compliance decreases. This can occur with various types of injury, chronic inflammation, bladder outlet obstruction, and neurologic decentralization. Once decreased compliance occurs because of a replacement by collagen of other components of the stroma, it is generally unresponsive to pharmacologic manipulation, hydraulic distention, or nerve section. Most often, under those circumstances, augmentation cystoplasty is required to achieve satisfactory reservoir function.

3. **c. Gradual increase in striated sphincter activity seen during normal bladder filling/storage.** There is a gradual increase in urethral pressure during bladder filling, contributed to by at least the striated sphincter element and perhaps by the smooth sphincteric element as well. The rise in urethral pressure seen during the filling/storage phase of micturition can be correlated with an increase in efferent pudendal nerve impulse frequency and in electromyographic activity of the periurethral striated musculature. This constitutes the efferent limb of a spinal somatic reflex, the so-called *guarding reflex*, which results in a gradual increase in striated sphincter activity during normal bladder filling and storage.

4. **e. Neurally mediated sympathetic modulation of cholinergic ganglionic transmission.** Does the nervous system affect the normal bladder response to filling? At a certain level of bladder filling, spinal sympathetic reflexes facilitatory to bladder filling/storage are clearly evoked in animals, a concept developed over the years by deGroat and colleagues, who have also cited indirect evidence to support such a role in humans. This inhibitory effect is thought to be mediated primarily by sympathetic modulation of cholinergic ganglionic transmission. Through this reflex mechanism, two other possibilities exist for promoting filling/storage. One is neurally mediated stimulation of the predominantly α-adrenergic receptors in the area of the smooth sphincter, the net result of which would be to cause an increase in resistance in that area. The second is neurally mediated stimulation of the predominantly β-adrenergic receptors (inhibitory) in the bladder body smooth musculature, which would cause a decrease in bladder wall tension. McGuire has also cited evidence for direct inhibition of detrusor motor neurons in the sacral spinal cord during bladder filling that is due to increased afferent pudendal nerve activity generated by receptors in the

striated sphincter. Good evidence also seems to exist to support a tonic inhibitory effect of other neurotransmitters on the micturition reflex at various levels of the neural axis. Bladder filling and consequent wall distention may also release autocrine-like factors that influence contractility (e.g., nitric oxide, prostaglandins, peptides).

5. **a. Pontine mesencephalic formation in the brainstem.** Although the origin of the parasympathetic neural outflow to the bladder, the pelvic nerve, is in the sacral spinal cord, the actual organizational center for the micturition reflex in an intact neural axis is in the brainstem, and the complete neural circuit for normal micturition includes the ascending and descending spinal cord pathways to and from this area and the facilitatory and inhibitory influences from other parts of the brain.

6. **c. Suprasacral neurologic disease or injury.** Involuntary contractions (IVCs) are most commonly seen associated with suprasacral neurologic disease or after suprasacral neurologic injury; however, they may also be associated with aging, inflammation or irritation of the bladder wall, bladder outlet obstruction, or stress urinary incontinence, or they may be idiopathic.

7. **a. Failure to store because of the bladder (overactivity).** The classic symptoms of poststroke lower urinary tract dysfunction are urgency, frequency, and possible urgency incontinence. The urodynamic findings are generally detrusor overactivity during filling/storage with normal sensation and synergic sphincter activity during voluntary or involuntary emptying, unless the patient attempts to inhibit the involuntary contractions with striated sphincter contraction. This translates simply in the functional system to a failure to store because of the bladder.

8. **e. During storage, overactive neurogenic detrusor activity, normal sensation, low capacity, normal compliance, and normal urethral closure function and during emptying, normal detrusor activity and normal urethral function.** The micturition dysfunction of a stroke patient with urgency incontinence would most likely be classified during storage as overactive neurogenic detrusor function, normal sensation, low capacity, normal compliance, and normal urethral closure function. During voiding, the dysfunction would be classified as normal detrusor activity and normal urethral function, assuming that no anatomic obstruction existed.

9. **d. Neurogenic detrusor overactivity.** The Standardization Subcommittee of the ICS made some changes in definitions of terms (published as a committee report in 2002). One change was to eliminate the terms *detrusor hyperreflexia* and *instability* and replace them with the terms *neurogenic detrusor overactivity* and *idiopathic detrusor over-activity* (Abrams P et al, 2003).*

10. **b. Detrusor hyperreflexia, striated sphincter synergia, and smooth sphincter dyssynergia.** When exact urodynamic classification is possible, this system provides a truly precise description of the voiding dysfunction that occurs. If a normal or hyperreflexic detrusor exists with coordinated smooth and striated sphincter function and without anatomic obstruction, normal bladder emptying should occur. *Detrusor hyperreflexia* is most commonly associated with neurologic lesions above the sacral spinal cord. Striated sphincter dyssynergia is most common after complete suprasacral spinal cord injury, following the period of spinal shock. Smooth sphincter dyssynergia is seen most classically in autonomic hyperreflexia, when it is characteristically associated with detrusor hyperreflexia and striated sphincter dyssynergia. *Detrusor areflexia* may be secondary to bladder muscle decompensation or to various other conditions that produce inhibition at the level of the brainstem micturition center, sacral spinal cord, bladder ganglia, or bladder smooth muscle. Patients with a voiding dysfunction secondary to detrusor areflexia generally attempt bladder emptying by abdominal straining, and their continence status and the efficiency of their emptying efforts are determined by the status of their smooth and striated sphincter mechanisms.

11. **c. Uninhibited neurogenic bladder.** Lapides contributed significantly to the classification and care of the patient with neuropathic voiding dysfunction by slightly modifying and popularizing a system originally proposed by McLellan in 1939. Lapides' classification differs from that of McLellan in only one respect, and that is the division of the group "atonic neurogenic bladder" into sensory neurogenic bladder and motor neurogenic bladder. This remains one of the most familiar systems to urologists and nonurologists because it describes in recognizable shorthand the clinical and cystometric conditions of many types of neurogenic voiding dysfunction. An uninhibited neurogenic bladder was described originally as resulting from injury or disease to the "corticoregulatory tract." The sacral spinal cord was presumed to be the micturition reflex center, and this corticoregulatory tract was believed to normally exert an inhibitory influence on the sacral micturition reflex center. A destructive lesion in this tract would then result in overfacilitation of the micturition reflex. Cerebrovascular accident, brain or spinal cord tumor, Parkinson disease, and demyelinating disease were listed as the most common causes in this category. The voiding dysfunction is most often characterized symptomatically by frequency, urgency, and urge incontinence, as well as urodynamically by normal sensation with IVC at low filling volumes. Residual urine is characteristically low unless anatomic outlet obstruction or true smooth or striated sphincter dyssynergia occurs. The patient can generally initiate a bladder contraction voluntarily but is often unable to do so during cystometry because sufficient urine storage cannot occur before the IVC is stimulated.

12. **a. Traumatic spinal cord injury between the sacral spinal cord and the brainstem.** Reflex neurogenic bladder describes the post-spinal shock condition that exists after complete interruption of the sensory and motor pathways between the sacral spinal cord and the brainstem. Most commonly, this occurs in traumatic spinal cord injury and transverse myelitis, but it may occur with extensive demyelinating disease or any process that produces significant spinal cord destruction as well. Typically, there is no bladder sensation and there is inability to initiate voluntary micturition. Incontinence without sensation generally results because of low-volume IVC. Striated sphincter dyssynergia is the rule. This type of lesion is essentially equivalent to a complete UMN lesion in the Bors-Comarr system.

13. **e. Sphincter dyssynergia.** This system applies only to patients with neurologic dysfunction and considers three factors: (1) the anatomic localization of the lesion; (2) the neurologic completeness or incompleteness of the lesion; and (3) a designation as to whether lower urinary tract function is balanced or unbalanced. The latter terms are based solely on the percentage of residual urine relative to bladder capacity. Unbalanced signifies the presence of greater than 20% residual urine in a patient with a UMN lesion or 10% in a patient with an LMN lesion. This relative residual urine volume was ideally meant to imply coordination (synergy) or dyssynergia between the smooth and striated sphincters of the outlet and the bladder, during bladder contraction or during attempted micturition by abdominal straining or the Credé method.

14. **a. A UMN lesion, complete, and balanced.** In this system, UMN bladder refers to the pattern of micturition that results from an injury to the suprasacral spinal cord after the period of spinal shock has passed, assuming that the sacral spinal cord and the sacral nerve roots are intact and that the pelvic and pudendal nerve reflexes are intact. LMN bladder refers to the pattern resulting if the sacral spinal cord or sacral roots are damaged and the reflex pattern through the autonomic and somatic nerves that emanate from these segments is absent. This system implies that if skeletal muscle spasticity exists below the level of the lesion, the lesion is above the sacral spinal cord and is by definition a UMN lesion. This type of lesion is characterized by IVCs during filling. If flaccidity of the skeletal musculature below the level of

---

*Sources referenced can be found in *Campbell-Walsh Urology, 11th Edition,* on the Expert Consult website.

a lesion exists, an LMN lesion is assumed to exist, implying detrusor areflexia. Exceptions occur and are classified in a mixed lesion group characterized either by IVCs with a flaccid paralysis below the level of the lesion or by detrusor areflexia with spasticity or normal skeletal muscle tone neurologically below the lesion level. UMN lesion, complete, and imbalanced implies a neurologically complete lesion above the level of the sacral spinal cord that results in skeletal muscle spasticity below the level of the injury. IVC occurs during filling, but a residual urine volume of greater than 20% of the bladder capacity is left after bladder contraction, implying obstruction in the area of the bladder outlet during the involuntary detrusor contraction. This obstruction is generally due to striated sphincter dyssynergia, typically occurring in patients who are paraplegic and quadriplegic with lesions between the cervical and the sacral spinal cord. Smooth sphincter dyssynergia may be seen as well in patients with lesions above the level of T6, usually in association with autonomic hyperreflexia. LMN lesion, complete, and imbalanced implies a neurologically complete lesion at the level of the sacral spinal cord or of the sacral roots, resulting in skeletal muscle flaccidity below that level. Detrusor areflexia results,

and whatever measures the patient may use to increase intravesical pressure during attempted voiding are not sufficient to decrease residual urine to less than 10% of bladder capacity.

15. **c. Urgency.** Overactive bladder is defined (ICS) as urgency, with or without urinary urgency incontinence, usually with frequency and nocturia. One third of the patients have incontinence, but two thirds do not. Frequency and nocturia are usually but not always present. Detrusor overactivity (DO) is a urodynamic term indicating an involuntary bladder contraction. Urgency may or may not be associated with DO on a urodynamic study.

16. **b. Intrinsic sphincter dysfunction.** Failure to store because of outlet underactivity in the female is due to a combination of a failure of support, generally accompanied by hypermobility of the bladder outlet and intrinsic sphincter dysfunction (ISD). It is impossible to have effort-related incontinence in the woman without some element of ISD. Outlet-related incontinence in the male is most commonly seen after prostatectomy, and there is no pathophysiologic factor of hypermobility involved. The condition is essentially ISD. A nonrelaxing striated sphincter would not produce urinary incontinence, nor would bladder neck dysfunction.

CHAPTER REVIEW

1. The spinal sympathetic reflexes are facilatatory to bladder filling/storage.
2. The micturition cycle is divided into two phases: (1) bladder filling/urine storage and (2) bladder empting/voiding.
3. There are two urethral sphincters: (1) the smooth urethral sphincter is the smooth musculature of the bladder neck and proximal urethra; the smooth sphincter is not under voluntary control; and (2) the striated sphincter, which has two parts—the striated intramural sphincter, called the rhabdosphincter, and the external striated sphincter, which is part of the levator musculature. This sphincter is under voluntary control.
4. While collagen content of the bladder wall increases, compliance decreases.
5. There is increased afferent input when inflammation or irritation occurs, causing hypersensitivity to pain.
6. The hammock hypothesis of continence proposes that there is a fixed dorsal portion of the urethra due to fascial attachments against which the ventral aspect of the urethra is compressed.

7. Increases in intra-abdominal pressure are transmitted to the proximal urethra (as well as the mid-urethra in females).
8. The bladder response to filling at a physiologic rate is an almost imperceptible change in intravesical pressure.
9. Elasticity allows the constituents of the bladder wall to stretch to a certain degree without any increase in tension. Viscoelasticity allows stretch to induce a rise in tension followed by a decay (stress relaxation) when the filling (stretch stimulus) slows or stops.
10. Involuntary contractions (IVCs) are most commonly seen associated with suprasacral neurologic disease or after suprasacral neurologic injury; however, they may also be associated with aging, inflammation, or irritation of the bladder wall, bladder outlet obstruction, or stress urinary incontinence, or they may be idiopathic.
11. Overactive bladder is defined (ICS) as urgency, with or without urinary urgency incontinence, usually with frequency and nocturia.
12. It is impossible to have effort-related incontinence in the woman without some element of ISD.

71 Evaluation and Management of Women with Urinary Incontinence and Pelvic Prolapse

Kathleen C. Kobashi

QUESTIONS

1. Which of the following is *not* a risk factor for urinary incontinence?
   a. Increased body mass index (BMI)
   b. Male gender
   c. Fecal incontinence
   d. Smoking
   e. increased age

2. Based on the CARE trial, patients without stress incontinence undergoing a sacrocolpopexy should undergo sacrocolpopexy:
   a. only.
   b. with urethral bulking injection.
   c. with Burch colposuspension.
   d. with Burch only if occult stress incontinence is noted.
   e. followed by urodynamics if de novo stress incontinence develops postoperatively.

3. A 49-year-old woman has a POP-Q score that is recorded as Aa-3, Ba-3, Ap-3, Bp-3. She has:
   a. no prolapse.
   b. stage 1 prolapse.
   c. stage 2 prolapse.
   d. stage 3 prolapse.
   e. stage 4 prolapse.

4. A patient is suspected of having a urinary tract–vaginal fistula. Which method would be the best dye test method to facilitate diagnosis of an isolated ureterovaginal fistula?
   a. Oral pyridium
   b. Intravesical indigo carmine
   c. Intravenous indigo carmine
   d. Simultaneous oral pyridium and intravenous indigo carmine
   e. Simultaneous oral pyridium and intravesical indigo carmine

5. A healthy 65-year-old woman has bothersome prolapse and stress urinary incontinence (SUI). Exam shows stage 3 anterior prolapse and no apical or posterior prolapse or stress incontinence. On urodynamics she has a stable bladder and no SUI. The next step is repeat stress testing with:
   a. the urethral catheter removed.
   b. the prolapse reduced.
   c. the prolapse reduced and the urethral catheter removed.
   d. both the rectal and urethral catheters removed.
   e. a smaller caliber urethral catheter.

6. The POP-Q (Pelvic Organ Prolapse Quantification) system:
   a. is a simple six-point quantification system for pelvic prolapse.
   b. was created in an effort to quantify pelvic organ prolapse and urinary incontinence.
   c. includes six specific points of position measurement in relation to the introitus.
   d. includes a simplified five-level staging system that does not require listing each of the points specifically.
   e. includes measurement of the total vaginal length performed *without* reduction of the prolapse.

7. A 34-year-old female is undergoing urodynamics for symptoms of urinary hesitancy. She is noted to have an absence of electromyelogram (EMG) recruitment with a squeezing of the clitoris. This represents a:
   a. disruption at the level of sacral nerve roots 2-4.
   b. dysfunction in the cauda equina.
   c. positive bulbocavernosus reflex (BCR).
   d. normal finding in 30% of normal females.
   e. problem with technique in assessing for the BCR.

8. The Food and Drug Administration (FDA) released a safety statement regarding the use of mesh in the pelvic floor that applied to:
   a. slings only.
   b. transvaginal prolapse repairs only.
   c. transabdominal prolapse repairs only.
   d. all prolapse repairs.
   e. all slings and pelvic prolapse repairs.

9. A 62-year-old man has bothersome urinary frequency and urgency associated with rare leakage. He has no obstructive symptoms, and postvoid residual (PVR) is 20 mL. Urinalysis is negative. The only therapy he has tried is a 2-week course of oxybutynin, but he is currently on no medications. The next step is:
   a. behavioral therapy, including dietary modification, fluid management, and bladder training.
   b. alpha-blocker therapy.
   c. repeat a trial of antimuscarinic therapy.
   d. beta-3 agonist therapy.
   e. combination of antimuscarinic and beta-3 agonist therapy.

10. "Eyeball urodynamics" can provide information regarding:
    a. detrusor compliance.
    b. bladder outlet obstruction.
    c. abdominal leak point pressure.
    d. detrusor leak point pressure.
    e. detrusor-sphincter coordination.

11. Multichannel urodynamics:
    a. is the most accurate diagnostic tool available for the evaluation of incontinence.
    b. should be used in all patients with incontinence.
    c. includes three directly measured values: detrusor pressure (Pdet), vesical pressure (Pves), and abdominal pressure (Pabd).
    d. is not helpful in determining if a patient is at risk of developing upper tract deterioration.
    e. all of the above.

12. Urodynamics should be considered in which of the following circumstances?

    a. In patients in whom conservative measures have failed

    b. In patients in whom the clinical picture is unclear

    c. In patients in whom the symptoms cannot be confirmed by the clinician

    d. In patients who have undergone previous pelvic floor reconstruction

    e. All of the above

13. Electromyelography should:

    a. be performed on all patients undergoing urodynamics.

    b. demonstrate recruitment during the filling phase.

    c. be active during coughing.

    d. be silent with BCR.

    e. be active during the voiding phase.

ANSWERS

1. **b. Male gender.** Obesity, advanced age, female gender, smoking, and associated pelvic floor disorders are risk factors for the development of urinary incontinence.

2. **c. With Burch colposuspension.** The CARE (Colpopexy and Urinary Reduction Efforts) trial was designed to evaluate whether a Burch colposuspension performed at the time of sacrocolpopexy for prolapse in women who did not have preoperative SUI reduced postoperative SUI. The study demonstrated a significantly higher incontinence rate at all points of follow-up in the women who did not undergo a Burch (Brubaker et al., 2006).* This landmark study was performed with the Burch as the anti-incontinence procedure of choice, though one may deduce that a sling could be substituted for the Burch colposuspension. One would not choose urethral injection in light of the fact that the patient is already proceeding with surgery, particularly given the higher success rates and durability of response with available surgical options.

3. **a. No prolapse.** The Pelvic Organ Prolapse-Quantification ("POP-Q") system (Bump et al., 1996) is a nine-measure system that was created in an effort to provide objectivity to POP quantification. Six vaginal points labeled Aa, Ba, C, D, Ap, and Bp are measured in relation to the hymenal ring during Valsalva maneuver. Aa and Ba represent points along the anterior vaginal wall, whereas Ap and Bp represent the posterior wall. Point C is the most distal point of the vaginal cuff or cervix, and D is the distance to the posterior fornix and is measured only if the cervix is still present. Points above the hymen are considered negative, and points below the hymen are positive with a maximal established range of −3 to +3. The remaining three points are the genital hiatus (gh), which represents the size of the vaginal opening; the perineal body (pb), which represents the distance between the vagina and the anus; and the total vaginal length (tvl), which is measured by reducing the prolapse and measuring the depth of the vagina. A staging system based on these measurements ranges from stage 0 (no prolapse), in which all A and B points are −3, to stage 4, in which the leading edge is represented by an absolute number which is equal to or greater than (tvl-2) cm. This number is preceded by a + sign as it is below the hymen.

4. **e. Simultaneous oral pyridium and intravesical indigo carmine.** Oral pyridium will be excreted in the urine, so it will discolor a vaginal tampon whether the fistula is vesicovaginal or ureterovaginal or both. Intravenous indigo carmine would also demonstrate tampon staining in a similar pattern, but this is not practical as it involves the need for intravenous access. Presumably, staining higher on the tampon would indicate a ureterova-

ginal fistula, whereas lower staining would suggest a vesicovaginal fistula; however, it can be difficult to differentiate with certainty because the dye can diffuse, and 12% of patients with a vesicovaginal fistula have a concomitant ureteral fistula. Direct placement of dye (i.e., indigo carmine or methylene blue) into the bladder would only discolor the tampon if there is involvement of the bladder, but an isolated ureterovaginal fistula would be missed with this method. The best dye administration to evaluate for an isolated ureterovaginal fistula would be simultaneous intravesical blue dye and oral pyridium that would reveal orange staining only.

5. **b. The prolapse reduced.** When a patient who has subjective SUI and high grade prolapse does not elicit SUI on urodynamic studies (UDS), the American Urological Association/SUFU urodynamics guidelines recommend reduction of the prolapse and repeat stress testing. In patients who have SUI with no prolapse, the next step in such a situation would be to repeat stress testing with the urethral catheter removed. In this situation, one would first repeat stress testing with the prolapse adequately reduced, followed by removal of the urethral catheter. Although downsizing the catheter or removing all catheters might result in demonstration of the leakage, this is not necessary nor is it the recommendation of the guidelines.

6. **d. Includes a simplified five-level staging system that does not require listing each of the points specifically.** POP-Q is a nine-point system that was created to objectify the assessment of pelvic organ prolapse. It measures six specific points in the vagina in relation to the hymen. The remaining three points include the total vaginal length, measured with the vagina completely reduced; the perineal body; and the genital hiatus. It has been simplified into a five-stage system that does not require specific listing of each of the nine points.

7. **d. Normal finding in 30% of normal females.** BCR represents S2-4 and is present in all normal males and 70% of normal females. It is elicited by squeezing the glans penis or clitoris. During urodynamics, a positive BCR is represented by increased EMG activity.

8. **b. Transvaginal prolapse repairs only.** In 2011, the FDA released a safety communication (FDA website) regarding mesh placed transvaginally specifically for the repair of pelvic prolapse. Although the communication specifically excluded slings and transabdominally placed mesh for prolapse repair, unfortunately, subsequent media communication regarding mesh litigation created patient confusion and concern about the use of mesh in the pelvic floor in general. This prompted a joint response from the Society of Urodynamics, Female Pelvic Medicine and Urogenital Reconstruction (SUFU) and the American Urogynecology Society (AUGS) in 2014 (SUFU and AUGS websites).

9. **a. Behavioral therapy, including dietary modification, fluid management, and bladder training.** This patient has technically not yet tried the first line of therapy according to the OAB guidelines. The best response is behavioral therapy, which entails bladder exercises to train the bladder to overcome the sense of urgency when it occurs, pelvic floor exercises, fluid management, and avoidance of bladder irritants. Responses c, d, and e are all reasonable options to try subsequently in conjunction with behavioral therapy. Alpha-blockade would not be expected to be helpful in this situation, in which the patient has no obstructive symptoms.

10. **a. Detrusor compliance.** "Eyeball UDS" is a simple alternative to full multichannel UDS that can provide ample information in selected patients. The study can determine bladder sensation, compliance, stability, and capacity as well as outlet competence and PVR. A 60-mL catheter tip syringe with the barrel removed is placed into the end of the catheter, through which the bladder is filled by gravity. The height of the meniscus above the bladder represents the intravesical pressure. During the filling phase, a rise and fall in the meniscus may represent bladder overactivity, whereas a consistent gradual rise suggests compromised detrusor compliance. Because of the absence of the abdominal pressure (Pabd) channel, no information about the contribution of

abdominal pressure is gleaned, and it is therefore not possible to definitively establish the presence or absence of significant outlet obstruction. Similarly, no information about urethral function or EMG is afforded by this method, thereby making c, d, and e incorrect responses.

11. **a. Is the most accurate diagnostic tool available for the evaluation of incontinence.** Multichannel urodynamics is currently the most accurate diagnostic tool available for the evaluation of urinary incontinence. Whether it is necessary in the assessment of all patients with urinary incontinence remains controversial. Findings on urodynamics, which include direct measurements of vesical and abdominal pressures (Pves and Pabd, respectively) and a calculated measure of detrusor pressure (Pdet), can provide helpful information, including findings such as elevated Pdet that may suggest a patient is at increased risk of developing upper tract deterioration.

12. **e. All of the above.** Although a clinician may reasonably forego performing UDS on the index patient with SUI and no urinary urgency, the guidelines state that UDS may be considered in patients who are considering undergoing invasive, potentially morbid or irreversible treatments. This is left to the clinician, and the philosophy is that if the study may answer an unanswered question or somehow change the course of care, it may be considered. However, any patient with a picture complicated by issues such as previous pelvic or anti-incontinence surgery, radiation therapy, neurologic disease, or difficult or unclear diagnosis should be considered for urodynamics.

13. **c. Be active during coughing.** EMG should be used in selected patients. Recruitment should occur with BCR in all men and 70% of women and in the face of increased intra-abdominal pressure, such as with coughing. It should be silent during voiding to allow passage of urine without outlet resistance.

CHAPTER REVIEW

1. Pelvic organ prolapse is categorized according to the affected compartment: anterior (cystocele), posterior (rectocele), and apical (descent of the uterus or bowel-enterocele).
2. Hypermobility is defined as a Q tip angle of greater than 30 degrees from horizontal on abdominal straining.
3. In the pelvic organ prolapse quantification system, positions cephalad to the hymen are considered negative. Positions caudad to the hymen are considered positive.
4. Pad use per day is an unreliable indicator of the quantity of incontinence.
5. A postvoid residual of less than 50 mL represents adequate emptying. Ninety percent of normal individuals will have a PVR less than 100. A PVR greater than 200 represents inadequate emptying.
6. Stress urinary incontinence may be unmasked by the reduction of prolapse.
7. Apical prolapse is treated with uterosacral ligament suspension or a sacrospinous ligament fixation.
8. Connective tissue support for the pelvis is divided into three levels: level I, the uterosacral and cardinal ligaments support the vaginal vault; level II, the anterior and posterior endopelvic fascia to the lateral side wall support the mid-vagina; and level III, the fusion of the endopelvic fascia to the pubic symphysis and perineal body supports the distal vagina.
9. Obesity, advanced age, female gender, smoking, and associated pelvic floor disorders are risk factors for the development of urinary incontinence.
10. A Burch colpopsusension performed at the time of sacrocolpopexy for prolapse in women who do not have preoperative SUI reduces postoperative SUI.
11. Any patient with a picture complicated by issues—such as previous pelvic or antiincontinence surgery, radiation therapy, neurologic disease, or difficult or unclear diagnosis—should be considered for urodynamics.

Evaluation and Management of Men with Urinary Incontinence

Hashim Hashim and Paul Abrams

QUESTIONS

1. Which of the following is the definition of stress urinary incontinence?
   a. Leakage of urine with urgency
   b. Leakage of urine with an increase in intra-abdominal pressure
   c. Leakage of urine while asleep
   d. Leakage of urine with urgency and effort
   e. Leakage of urine without being aware of it

2. Initial assessment of men with urinary incontinence includes all of the following EXCEPT:
   a. flow test.
   b. invasive urodynamics.
   c. frequency/volume chart.
   d. urinalysis.
   e. quality-of-life questionnaire.

3. Which of the following is NOT a treatment for urgency urinary incontinence (UUI)?
   a. Bladder training
   b. Pelvic floor muscle training
   c. Antimuscarinics
   d. Duloxetine
   e. Botox

4. Which of the following is NOT a treatment for stress urinary incontinence in men?
   a. Pelvic floor muscle training
   b. Penile clamp
   c. Antimuscarinics
   d. Male sling
   e. Artificial urinary sphincter

5. Which of the following is NOT measured by the International Prostate Symptom Score (AUA-SI)?
   a. Urgency
   b. Frequency
   c. Nocturia
   d. Incontinence
   e. Straining

ANSWERS

1. **b. Leakage of urine with an increase in intra-abdominal pressure.** Leakage of urine with urgency is known as urgency urinary incontinence. Leakage of urine while asleep is nocturnal enuresis. Leakage of urine on urgency and effort is mixed urinary incontinence, and leakage of urine without being aware of it is insensible urinary incontinence.

2. **b. Invasive urodynamics.** Men with urinary incontinence should be assessed with noninvasive baseline investigations including a flow test, frequency/volume chart or bladder diary, urinalysis to exclude infection and blood in the urine, and a quality-of-life questionnaire to assess the impact of the incontinence on quality of life. Invasive urodynamics, including filling cystometry and pressure flow studies, is reserved after failure of conservative and medical therapies and when it will alter the management of the patient.

3. **d. Duloxetine.** Bladder training, pelvic floor muscle training, and antimuscarinics are first-line treatments of patients with UUI. If these fail, then patients can be treated with cystoscopic intra-detrusor botulinum toxin-A injections. Duloxetine is a serotonin, norepinephrine reuptake inhibitor that has been licensed for the treatment of stress urinary incontinence in women, and not UUI.

4. **c. Antimuscarinics.** Antimuscarinics are licensed for the treatment of overactive bladder syndrome and not stress urinary incontinence.

5. **d. Incontinence.** The IPSS or American Urological Association Symptom Index assesses three storage symptoms (urgency, frequency, nocturia), three voiding symptoms (intermittency, weak stream, straining), and one postmicturition symptom (incomplete emptying). It does not assess for urinary incontinence.

CHAPTER REVIEW

1. In men, stress incontinence is usually a consequence of prostatectomy.
2. When enuresis occurs later in life, one should suspect high-pressure chronic urinary retention.
3. A 3-day bladder diary is extremely useful in evaluating urinary incontinence.
4. Patients receiving Botox should be warned of the risk of urinary retention and the possible need for intermittent catheterization.
5. Postmicturition incontinence is treated by pelvic floor muscle training and urethral milking.
6. Men with urinary incontinence should be assessed with non-invasive baseline investigations including a flow test, frequency/volume chart or bladder diary, urinalysis to exclude infection and blood in the urine, and a quality of life questionnaire to assess the impact of the incontinence on quality of life.
7. The IPSS or AUA-SI assesses three storage symptoms (urgency, frequency, nocturia), three voiding symptoms (intermittency, weak stream, straining), and one post-micturition symptom (incomplete emptying).

73 Urodynamic and Video-Urodynamic Evaluation of the Lower Urinary Tract

Victor W. Nitti and Benjamin M. Brucker

QUESTIONS

1. Indications for urodynamic studies (UDS):
   a. are supported by high-quality, level 1 evidence for most conditions.
   b. are better defined for men than for women.
   c. are best defined by the clinician who has clear-cut reasons for performing the study and will use the information obtained to guide treatment.
   d. are of little value in assessing a patient with neurogenic lower urinary tract dysfunction.
   e. are only useful in women when incontinence is seen clinically.

2. The American Urological Association/Society for Urodynamics and Female Urology Urodynamics Guideline findings and recommendations:
   a. are all supported by level 1 or 2 evidence.
   b. do not apply to patients with neurogenic lower urinary tract dysfunction.
   c. are intended to assist the clinician in the appropriate selection of urodynamic tests, following evaluation and symptom characterization.
   d. include recommendations on standardization of urodynamic equipment.
   e. do not consider expert opinion.

3. Which of the following tests assesses bladder compliance?
   a. Cystometrogram
   b. Micturitional urethral pressure profile
   c. Postvoid residual volume
   d. Voiding pressure flow study
   e. Electromyogram

4. Detrusor pressure:
   a. can be measured directly via a transurethral catheter.
   b. should remain low (near zero) during bladder filling.
   c. rises abruptly and does not return to baseline with detrusor overactivity.
   d. rises before the external sphincter relaxes in normal voluntary micturition.
   e. is obtained by adding the abdominal pressure to the vesicle pressure.

5. Detrusor overactivity (DO):
   a. is synonymous with overactive bladder.
   b. is necessary to make a diagnosis of urodynamic bladder outlet obstruction.
   c. can be seen on UDS of asymptomatic men and women.
   d. is commonly associated with renal deterioration.
   e. is a diagnosis made based on history alone.

6. The hallmark of bladder outlet obstruction is:
   a. incomplete bladder emptying.
   b. low pressure–low flow voiding dynamics.
   c. high pressure–low flow voiding dynamics.
   d. impaired detrusor contractility.
   e. elevated postvoid residual.

7. The external urethral sphincter should normally:
   a. relax with an involuntary bladder contraction in a neurologically normal person.
   b. relax prior to a voluntary detrusor contraction in a neurologically normal person.
   c. progressively relax while the bladder fills.
   d. always contract when the detrusor contracts.
   e. contract during urination in a neurologically normal person.

8. Videourodynamics (VUDS):
   a. is the most precise measure of lower urinary tract function and should be used in all cases in which UDS is to be performed.
   b. is required to assess obstruction in a man.
   c. is the procedure of choice for documenting bladder neck dysfunction in men and women.
   d. is impractical to perform in spinal cord–injured patients.
   e. is needed to confirm detrusor overactivity.

9. Urethral function tests such as abdominal leak point pressure (ALPP) and maximum urethral closure pressure (MUCP):
   a. can precisely define intrinsic sphincter deficiency (ISD).
   b. should be done routinely before all surgery for stress incontinence.
   c. are the most important part of the UDS assessment of women with stress urinary incontinence.
   d. should not be used as a single factor to grade the severity of incontinence.
   e. can only be performed during ambulatory urodynamics.

10. Which of the following conditions/factors may result in inaccurate measurement of bladder compliance?
    a. Prior radiation to the pelvis
    b. Use of fluid-filled urodynamic catheters
    c. Presence of vesicoureteral reflux
    d. Bladder outlet obstruction
    e. History of genitourinary (GU) tuberculosis (TB)

11. According to the Functional Classification System, the symptom of stress incontinence can be classified as:
    a. failure to store secondary to an overactive bladder outlet.
    b. failure to store secondary to an overactive bladder.
    c. failure to store secondary to an underactive bladder outlet.

  d. failure to empty secondary to an underactive bladder outlet.

  e. failure to empty secondary to an overactive bladder outlet.

12. During multichannel urodynamics, what is the best measure that allows the clinician to look for abdominal straining occurring during micturition?

  a. Rectal or vaginal catheter pressure

  b. Bladder catheter pressure

  c. Uroflow pattern

  d. Electromyogram activity and uroflow velocity

  e. Postvoid residual

13. For women with stress incontinence, UDS has its most useful role in which of the following scenarios?

  a. In women who are considering surgical correction who also have urgency incontinence symptoms or difficulty emptying the bladder

  b. In predicting outcomes of surgery for women with pure stress incontinence

  c. In predicting the likelihood of voiding dysfunction in women with pure stress incontinence

  d. In predicting outcomes of conservative, nonsurgical treatments for women with mixed incontinence

  e. Prior to starting conservative, nonsurgical treatments for women with pure incontinence

ANSWERS

1. **c. Are best defined by the clinician who has clear-cut reasons for performing the study and will use the information obtained to guide treatment.** UDS has been used for decades, yet clear-cut, level 1 evidenced-based "indications" for its use are surprisingly lacking. There are a number of reasons for this. It is difficult to conduct proper randomized controlled trials on UDS for conditions in which lesser levels of evidence and expert opinion strongly suggest clinical utility and in which "empiric treatment" is potentially harmful or even life-threatening (e.g., neurogenic voiding dysfunction). In addition, symptoms can be caused by a number of different conditions, and it is difficult to study pure or homogeneous patient populations. Given the current state of evidence for UDS studies, what is most important is that the clinician has clear-cut reasons for performing the study and that the information obtained will be used to guide treatment of the patient. Despite having established nomograms for bladder outlet obstruction in men, the indications for UDS in men are no more clear-cut than they are in women. UDS probably has its most important role in the diagnosis and management of patients with neuropathic voiding dysfunction. In straightforward cases of pure stress urinary incontinence (SUI) where incontinence is seen clinically, urodynamics may not needed.

2. **c. Are intended to assist the clinician in the appropriate selection of urodynamic tests, following evaluation and symptom characterization.** The intent of the guideline was to assist clinicians in the appropriate selection of tests rather than to provide absolute indications for UDS. The review of literature produced few articles offering a high level of evidence, and most of the recommendations are based on lower levels of evidence, expert opinion, and clinical principles.

3. **a. Cystometrogram (CMG).** Compliance is the change in bladder volume/change in bladder pressure. Bladder pressure during filling is assessed by CMG.

4. **b. Should remain low (near zero) during bladder filling.** Detrusor pressure normally remains low during filling, as the bladder is highly compliant. It cannot be measured directly with a transurethral catheter, but must be obtained via subtraction of abdominal pressure from vesicle pressure. With detrusor overactivity, pressure usually returns to baseline after the involuntary contraction abates.

5. **c. Can be seen on UDS of asymptomatic men and women.** DO is defined as involuntary bladder contractions on CMG. Overactive bladder is a symptom complex with the hallmark symptom of urinary urgency and is not diagnosed on UDS. Detrusor overactivity has been reported to occur in studies on asymptomatic men and women. Impaired compliance, not DO, is associated with renal deterioration. DO is an observation made during urodynamics.

6. **c. High pressure–low flow voiding dynamics.** Obstruction is defined by high pressure low flow voiding. It may or may not be accompanied by incomplete bladder emptying. Impaired detrusor contractility may sometimes, but not always, be a long-term consequence of obstruction.

7. **b. Relax prior to a voluntary detrusor contraction in a neurologically normal person.** In a neurologically normal person, the external sphincter progressively contracts with bladder filling and will also contract during an involuntary bladder contraction (guarding reflex). External sphincter relaxation is the first step in the micturition cycle and precedes the detrusor contraction. In detrusor external sphincter dyssynergia, an abnormal neurologic condition, the external sphincter contracts when the detrusor does. Intermittent or fluctuating flow rate of urine due to intermittent contractions of the external sphincter in a neurologically normal person is considered dysfunctional voiding.

8. **c. Is the procedure of choice for documenting bladder neck dysfunction in men and women.** Although VUDS provides the most precise evaluation of voiding function and dysfunction and is particularly useful when anatomic structure and function are important, it is not practical or necessary for all centers to have VUDS capabilities. VUDS is useful for a number of conditions when an accurate diagnosis cannot otherwise be obtained (e.g., by conventional UDS) including complicated voiding dysfunction or known or suspected neuropathic voiding dysfunction (adults and children), unexplained urinary retention in women, prior radical pelvic surgery, urinary diversion, preceding or following renal transplant, or prior pelvic radiation. VUDS is the procedure of choice for documenting bladder neck dysfunction in men and women. VUDS is not specifically needed to diagnose DO.

9. **d. Should not be used as a single factor to grade the severity of incontinence.** Urethral function tests such as ALPP and MUCP have not been shown to be consistently useful in defining "ISD" or outcomes of treatments for SUI. They may be useful for some clinicians, but are by no means mandatory. According to the International Continence Society, "Urethral function measurements of leak point pressures and urethral closure pressures are not used as a single factor to grade the severity of incontinence." UDS is not necessary before surgical treatment of SUI for all women, but if it is done, the AUA/SUFU Guideline states that ALPP or MUCP should be preformed. ALPP can be reported as part of ambulatory UDS; however, it is not a measure that is unique to this method.

10. **c. Presence of vesicoureteral reflux.** Bladder outlet obstruction and radiation can cause a decrease in compliance, but should not affect its accurate measurement. GU TB also can cause significant bladder fibrosis and impaired compliance. Reflux can make compliance look worse that it actually is secondary to the "pop-off" it creates. Fluoroscopy or VUDS is necessary in some cases (e.g., neurogenic bladder) to assess for reflux during filling. In addition, filling rate and involuntary detrusor contractions can also make compliance look worse than it actually is. There are no data to support the proposition that fluid-filled catheters or air charge catheters will result in inaccurate measures of compliance, which is a measure of change volume over pressure.

11. **c. Failure to store secondary to an underactive bladder outlet.** Stress incontinence is a symptom caused by failure to store urine during increases in abdominal pressure. It can be caused by a loss of outlet resistance or an underactive bladder outlet.

12. **a. Rectal or vaginal catheter pressure.** Rectal and or vaginal pressure are used to measure abdominal pressure throughout UDS. Patients who are straining to void will exhibit increases in abdominal pressure measurements. Flow patterns can be suggestive of abdominal straining, but are not as accurate as measuring abdominal pressure. Postvoid residual may allow clinicians to understand how well the patient is emptying his or her bladder but does not give information about how voiding is accomplished. Similarly, EMG may be increased from abdominal straining, but there are many other causes of increased EMG activity during voiding. Bladder catheter pressure will increase with abdominal straining. The difference between the bladder catheter and the rectal or vaginal catheter allows for calculation of the detrusor pressure.

13. **a. In women who are considering surgical correction who also have urgency incontinence symptoms or difficulty emptying the bladder.** UDS in women with pure stress or stress-predominant mixed incontinence and normal emptying has not been shown in randomized controlled trials to be more beneficial than office evaluation alone and has not been shown to predict outcomes of surgery in the same population. Women with significant mixed incontinence and emptying problems have not been studied in randomized controlled trials, and it is felt that UDS is beneficial in these women.

CHAPTER REVIEW

1. UDS is performed in an unnatural setting and therefore does not always predict the findings with normal activity.
2. Normal uroflow is a bell-shaped curve.
3. EMG patch electrodes measure perineal muscle function with the assumption that it is reflective of urethral external sphincter function.
4. To specifically measure external sphincter function, needle electrodes must be used.
5. Mean values for compliance are 40 to 120 mL/cm H_2O.
6. Measurement of compliance is difficult to interpret; therefore, pressures during filling are more often used to predict outcome.
7. There are two types of leak-point pressures: (a) abdominal leak-point pressure, which is defined as the intravesical pressure at which urine leakage occurs due to increased abdominal pressure; and (b) detrusor leak-point pressure, which is a measure of detrusor pressure at which urine leakage occurs in the absence of a detrusor contraction or increased abdominal pressure. This measure is generally used in patients with decreased compliance or lower motor neuron disease.
8. Detrusor pressures that are sustained above 40 cm H_2O lead to deterioration of the upper tracts.
9. Maximum urethra closure pressure is defined as the difference between peak urethral pressure and intravesical pressure and is normally between 40 and 60 cm H_2O.
10. Bladder outlet obstruction index is defined by the equation: $BOOI = Pdet\ Qmax - 2(Qmax)$. In men, a value greater than 40 is considered obstructed; a value less than 20 is considered unobstructed.
11. A uroflow less than 12 mL/sec and Pdet greater than 25 cm H_2O predicts outlet obstruction in women.
12. Detrusor external sphincter dyssynergia can be due to a neurologic lesion (above the sacral micturition center) or a learned disorder. The latter is considered dysfunctional voiding.
13. Internal sphincter dyssynergia must be diagnosed by VUDS.
14. Stress incontinence, which is observed only when a coexisting prolapse is reduced, is referred to as occult or latent stress incontinence.
15. For internal sphincter dyssynergia to occur, the spinal cord lesion must be above the sympathetic outflow (T-10-L-1).
16. Videourodynamics is the procedure of choice for documenting bladder neck dysfunction in men and women.
17. In a neurologically normal person, the external sphincter progressively contracts with bladder filling and will also contract during an involuntary bladder contraction (guarding reflex). External sphincter relaxation is the first step in the micturition cycle and precedes the detrusor contraction.

74 Urinary Incontinence and Pelvic Prolapse: Epidemiology and Pathophysiology

Gary E. Lemack and Jennifer Tash Anger

QUESTIONS

1. An example of a sign of lower urinary tract (LUT) dysfunction is:
   a. incontinence while playing tennis.
   b. urodynamic stress incontinence with Valsalva leak point pressure (VLPP) of 60 cm H_2O.
   c. a symptom score of 19 on AUA Symptom Index.
   d. the finding of urinary incontinence on supine stress test.
   e. the presence of stage 2 anterior pelvic organ prolapse on cystogram.

2. Which of the following is most consistent with the diagnosis of mixed urinary incontinence?
   a. Leakage of urine with coughing and a VLPP of 60 cm H_2O
   b. Leakage of urine with urgency and detrusor overactivity incontinence
   c. Leakage of urine while coughing and detrusor leak point pressure of 50 cm H_2O
   d. Leakage of urine while coughing and leakage of urine with urgency
   e. Leakage of urine and feces while straining

3. The most common form of urinary incontinence (UI) in a woman aged 40 years is:
   a. stress incontinence.
   b. urgency incontinence.
   c. mixed incontinence.
   d. detrusor overactivity incontinence.
   e. continuous incontinence.

4. A 73-year-old white woman is G2P2 with two prior cesarean deliveries. She is taking glucophage. She has a 20-pack-year smoking history. The aspect of her history that does NOT predispose her to the development of stress urinary incontinence (SUI) is:
   a. her age.
   b. her race.
   c. mode of delivery.
   d. history of depression.
   e. smoking history.

5. Remission of incontinence would most likely be noted in a:
   a. 42-year-old woman.
   b. 41-year-old man.
   c. 65-year-old woman.
   d. 73-year-old man.
   e. 74-year-old woman.

6. The symptom most closely associated with the presence of advanced pelvic organ prolapse is the sensation of:
   a. pelvic pressure.
   b. pelvic pain.

   c. constipation.
   d. voiding difficulty.
   e. vaginal bulge.

7. Which of the following Pelvic Organ Prolapse Quantification System (POP-Q) scores is implausible?
   a. Aa of −2
   b. Ap of +4
   c. Ba of +5
   d. Bp of 0
   e. C of −7

8. A woman with POP-Q scores of Aa −1, Ba −1, C −5, Ap +1, Bp +2 would be considered to have what stage prolapse?
   a. Stage 0
   b. Stage 1
   c. Stage 2
   d. Stage 3
   e. Stage 4

9. A patient with a POP-Q score of Aa +2, Ba +2, Ap −2, Bp −2, and C 0 should be counseled to undergo:
   a. anterior colporrhaphy.
   b. posterior colporrhaphy.
   c. anterior and posterior colporrhaphy.
   d. anterior colporrhaphy and sacrospinous fixation.
   e. sacrospinous fixation.

10. During bladder storage, which is (are) most quiescent?
    a. pelvic nerve
    b. hypogastric nerve
    c. pudendal nerve
    d. A delta nerves
    e. Onuf nucleus

ANSWERS

1. **d. The finding of urinary incontinence on supine stress test.** A sign of LUT dysfunction is one that is observable by the clinician. A report of incontinence while playing tennis is a urinary symptom. A VLPP result is a urodynamic observation, whereas a cystogram report of a cystocele is a radiologic observation.

2. **d. Leakage of urine while coughing and leakage of urine with urgency.** Mixed incontinence is the symptomatic complaint of both stress urinary incontinence and urgency incontinence.
   A VLPP of 60 cm H_2O is an observation of urodynamic stress incontinence. Detrusor overactivity incontinence is a urodynamic observation. Detrusor leak point pressure is a urodynamic observation that typically indicates altered compliance.

3. **a. Stress incontinence.** Stress urinary incontinence (SUI) is the most common form of UI in young women. In contrast, urge UI and mixed UI appear to become more prevalent forms of UI

with aging. Continuous incontinence is uncommon—often associated with iatrogenic injuries to the lower urinary tract resulting in fistulae.

4. **c. Mode of delivery.** Of the risk factors noted in her history, only the mode of delivery has not been associated with an increased risk of SUI later in life. Age is strongly correlated with the development of UI of all types. White women appear to be at greater risk for UI compared with African-American and Asian women in particular. Depression, regardless of concurrent treatment, appears to be associated with a greater likelihood of UI. A history of smoking has been linked to the development of UI, particularly in women selecting surgical treatment.

5. **b. 41-year-old man.** Remission rates as high as 40% have been noted in men, whereas remission rates are considerably lower in women (less than 5%). This speaks to the transient causes of UI that are more prevalent in men, particularly younger men.

6. **e. Vaginal bulge.** Although all of the symptoms described can be associated with POP, only the specific complaint of a vaginal bulge has been consistently demonstrated to be associated with the presence of POP. All others can be associated with other conditions distinct from the presence of POP. For example, pelvic pressure can be related to pelvic floor dysfunction or a variety of other conditions, and pelvic pain can be associated with various forms of pelvic pathology including adnexal pathology.

7. **b. Ap of +4.** POP-Q points are measured by their distance from the hymenal ring (in centimeters). By definition, Aa and Ap are the points 3 cm from the hymen on the anterior and posterior vaginal walls, respectively. It would be impossible for this point to be greater than 3 cm proximal (or distal) to the hymen. In advanced prolapse, this point could be up to 3 cm distal to the hymen. C point represents the distance from the hymen to the cervix or vaginal cuff (post hysterectomy). Ba and Bp point represent the leading edge of the most advanced aspect of the prolapse on the anterior and posterior vaginal walls, respectively. As such, they can be well beyond +3 in advanced prolapse.

8. **d. Stage 3.** Staging in POP-Q is based on the leading edge of prolapse. This equates to the highest (positive) number associated with the points listed (Aa, Ba, Ap, Bp, C). The leading edge of the most advanced POP is greater than 1 cm proximal to the hymen in patients with stage 1 prolapse. Stage 2 patients will have their leading edge between 1 cm proximal to and distal to the hymen. Stage 3 indicates a leading edge greater than 1 cm beyond the hymen but not completely everted (stage 4).

9. **d. Anterior colporrhaphy and sacrospinous fixation.** This patient has both anterior compartment prolapse (based on Aa and Ba points beyond the hymen) and apical prolapse (C point at the hymen) based on the POP-Q score. Therefore, the patient should be counseled to have both anterior repair of some type (anterior colporrhaphy in this example) and apical repair (sacrospinous fixation in this example).

10. **a. Pelvic nerve.** During bladder storage, parasympathetic transmission (via the pelvic nerve) is suppressed and sympathetic transmission (via the hypogastric nerve) is active. Pudendal innervation to the external sphincter is active. Pudendal innervation is derived from Onuf nucleus in the sacral cord. A delta nerves (afferent) are active during storage and are involved in the spinal reflex mechanism that promotes closure of the bladder neck.

CHAPTER REVIEW

1. Pelvic organ prolapse may mask incontinence.
2. The prevalence of urinary incontinence in women is between 25% and 40%. Ten percent of women experience weekly incontinence episodes. Fecal incontinence occurs in 17% of women with pelvic organ prolapse.
3. The female bladder neck is weaker than the male bladder neck and is often incompetent.
4. In women the majority of the urethra should be considered an active area of sphincter control; however, in the female the most important portion of continence is the mid-urethra.
5. A Valsalva leak point pressure of less than 60 cm H_2O indicates but does not confirm intrinsic sphincter dysfunction.
6. Twelve percent of men report terminal dribbling.
7. Rates of overactive bladder increase with age.
8. Oral estrogen treatment is associated with the development of incontinence. Topical estrogen therapy is not linked to stress incontinence.
9. Intrinsic properties of the urethra mucosa and urethra wall are important in maintaining continence in women.
10. The anterior vaginal wall provides posterior support of the urethra allowing for compression of the mid-urethra. The urethra is attached laterally to the arcus tendineus by the urethra pelvic ligaments.
11. Urge UI and mixed UI appear to become more prevalent forms of UI with aging.
12. Age is strongly correlated with the development of UI of all types. White women appear to be at greater risk for UI when compared with African-American and Asian women in particular.
13. POP-Q points are measured by their distance from the hymenal ring (in centimeters). By definition, Aa and Ap are the points 3 cm from the hymen on the anterior and posterior vaginal walls, respectively. Ba and Bp point represent the leading edge of the most advanced aspect of the prolapse on the anterior and posterior vaginal walls, respectively. Thus they can be well beyond +3 in advanced prolapse. C point represents the distance from the hymen to the cervix or vaginal cuff (post hysterectomy)
14. The leading edge of the most advanced POP is greater than 1 cm proximal to the hymen in patients with stage 1 prolapse. Stage 2 patients will have their leading edge between 1 cm proximal to and distal to the hymen. Stage 3 indicates a leading edge greater than 1 cm beyond the hymen but not completely everted.

75 Neuromuscular Dysfunction of the Lower Urinary Tract

Alan J. Wein and Roger R. Dmochowski

QUESTIONS

1. What is the general pattern of voiding dysfunction secondary to neurologic lesions above the level of the brainstem?
   a. Involuntary bladder contractions, smooth sphincter dyssynergia, striated sphincter synergy
   b. Involuntary bladder contractions, smooth sphincter synergy, striated sphincter synergy
   c. Involuntary bladder contractions, smooth sphincter synergy, striated sphincter dyssynergia
   d. Detrusor hypocontractility, smooth sphincter synergy, striated sphincter synergy
   e. Detrusor areflexia, smooth sphincter synergy, striated sphincter synergy

2. What is the general pattern of voiding dysfunction that results from complete lesions of the spinal cord above the level of S2 after recovery from spinal shock?
   a. Involuntary bladder contractions, smooth sphincter dyssynergia, striated sphincter synergy
   b. Involuntary bladder contractions, smooth sphincter synergy, striated sphincter synergy
   c. Involuntary bladder contractions, smooth sphincter synergy, striated sphincter dyssynergia
   d. Detrusor hypocontractility, smooth sphincter synergy, striated sphincter synergy
   e. Detrusor areflexia, smooth sphincter synergy, striated sphincter synergy

3. Which of the following is the most common long-term expression of lower urinary tract dysfunction after a cerebrovascular accident (CVA)?
   a. Detrusor areflexia
   b. Lack of sensation of filling
   c. Impaired bladder contractility
   d. Striated sphincter dyssynergia
   e. Detrusor overactivity

4. Urinary incontinence is most likely to occur in a patient after a CVA if which of the following areas is affected?
   a. Internal capsule
   b. Basal ganglia
   c. Thalamus
   d. Cerebellum
   e. Hypothalamus

5. In a post-CVA patient who exhibits urgency and frequency but no incontinence, the state of striated sphincter activity can most commonly be best described as:
   a. uninhibited relaxation.
   b. dyssynergia.
   c. fixed voluntary tone.
   d. pseudodyssynergia.
   e. myotonus.

6. A 65-year-old man who has sustained a stroke but is otherwise in good health has symptoms of hesitancy, straining to void, urgency, and frequency. The optimal next step in management is:
   a. anticholinergic therapy.
   b. transurethral resection of the prostate (TURP).
   c. transurethral incision of the bladder neck and prostate.
   d. clean intermittent catheterization.
   e. full urodynamic evaluation.

7. When considering the subject of voiding dysfunction associated with brain tumors, which of the following areas is more likely to be associated with urinary retention than with urinary incontinence?
   a. Pituitary gland
   b. Cerebellum
   c. Posterior fossa
   d. Hypothalamus
   e. Frontal cortex

8. The most common pattern of micturition in children and adults who have cerebral palsy (CP) and no other complicating neurologic condition is:
   a. abnormal filling/storage because of detrusor overactivity; normal emptying.
   b. normal filling/storage; normal emptying.
   c. normal filling/storage; abnormal emptying because of smooth sphincter dyssynergia.
   d. normal filling/storage; abnormal emptying because of striated sphincter dyssynergia.
   e. abnormal filling/storage because of detrusor overactivity; abnormal emptying because of striated sphincter dyssynergia.

9. The most common urodynamic findings in individuals with CP who do exhibit lower urinary tract dysfunction are:
   a. detrusor areflexia, coordinated sphincters.
   b. detrusor overactivity, smooth sphincter dyssynergia, striated sphincter dyssynergia.
   c. detrusor overactivity, smooth sphincter synergy, striated sphincter dyssynergia.
   d. decreased detrusor compliance, coordinated sphincters.
   e. detrusor overactivity, coordinated sphincters.

10. Deficiency of which of the following compounds in the nigrostriatal pathway accounts for most of the classic clinical motor features of Parkinson disease (PD)?
    a. Dopamine
    b. Norepinephrine
    c. Acetylcholine
    d. Serotonin
    e. L-Dopa

11. The most common urodynamic abnormality found in patients with voiding dysfunction secondary to PD is:
    a. impaired sensation during filling.
    b. striated sphincter dyssynergia.

c. striated sphincter bradykinesia.

d. detrusor overactivity.

e. impaired detrusor contractility.

12. Which of the following is more common in patients with PD than in patients with multiple system atrophy (MSA)?

a. Intrinsic sphincter deficiency

b. Evidence of striated sphincter denervation on an electromyogram

c. Decreased compliance

d. Incontinence after TURP

e. Disease diagnosis preceding voiding and erectile symptoms

13. The lesions seen in multiple sclerosis most commonly affect which of the following locations in the nervous system?

a. Thoracic spinal cord

b. Sacral spinal cord

c. Cervical spinal cord

d. Lumbar spinal cord

e. Midbrain

14. Which of the following urodynamic findings is least common in patients with multiple sclerosis and voiding dysfunction?

a. Detrusor overactivity

b. Detrusor areflexia

c. Impaired detrusor contractility

d. Striated sphincter dyssynergia

e. Smooth sphincter dyssynergia

15. The incidence of upper urinary tract deterioration is greatest in which of the following?

a. Multiple sclerosis

b. Multiple system atrophy

c. PD

d. Spinal cord injury (SCI)

e. Diabetes

16. Which of the following most accurately reflects the number of patients with HIV/AIDS, overall, with moderate or severe voiding problems?

a. 15% or less

b. 15% to 25%

c. 25% to 40%

d. 40% to 60%

e. 60% to 80%

17. The sacral spinal cord terminates in the cauda equina at approximately the spinal column level of:

a. T10.

b. L1.

c. L2.

d. L3.

e. S1.

18. In spinal shock, findings generally include all of the following EXCEPT:

a. acontractile bladder.

b. areflexic bladder.

c. open bladder neck.

d. absent guarding reflex.

e. maximal urethral closure pressure above normal.

19. All of the following are risk factors for upper urinary tract deterioration in a patient with a suprasacral SCI EXCEPT:

a. high-pressure storage.

b. high detrusor leak-point pressure.

c. chronic bladder overdistention.

d. high abdominal leak-point pressure.

e. vesicoureteral reflux with infection.

20. The presence of true detrusor-striated sphincter dyssynergia implies a neurologic lesion between the:

a. pons and the sacral spinal cord.

b. cerebral cortex and the pons.

c. cervical and the sacral spinal cord.

d. sacral spinal cord and the striated sphincter.

e. cauda equina and the striated sphincter.

21. An SCI at which of the following cord levels would be most likely to be associated with autonomic hyperreflexia?

a. Cervical

b. Thoracic

c. Lumbar

d. Sacral

e. Cauda equina

22. Which of the following is least characteristic as a finding in autonomic hyperreflexia?

a. Headache before bladder contraction

b. Hypertension

c. Flushing above the level of the lesion

d. Tachycardia

e. Sweating above the level of the lesion

23. The most common urodynamic findings in a male with autonomic hyperreflexia include all EXCEPT:

a. detrusor overactivity.

b. decreased compliance.

c. striated sphincter dyssynergia.

d. smooth sphincter dyssynergia.

e. decreased bladder capacity.

24. Which of the following is NOT among the treatments for, or prophylaxis of, autonomic hyperreflexia?

a. α-Adrenergic blockade

b. β-Adrenergic blockade

c. Ganglionic blockade

d. Spinal anesthesia

e. General anesthesia

25. In a male patient with detrusor-striated sphincter dyssynergia, a high detrusor leak-point pressure, high-pressure vesicoureteral reflux, and beginning upper urinary tract deterioration, which of the following is least likely, as an isolated procedure, to halt or reverse the upper tract changes?

a. Ureteral reimplantation

b. Augmentation cystoplasty

c. Dorsal root ganglionectomy

d. Anticholinergic therapy and intermittent catheterization

e. Sphincterotomy

26. The American Paraplegic Society guidelines for urologic care of SCI include all EXCEPT:

a. annual follow-up after injury for 5 to 10 years, then every other year if doing well.

   b. upper and lower urinary tract evaluation initially and yearly for 5 to 10 years, then every other year.

   c. cystoscopy annually for those with an indwelling catheter.

   d. urodynamic evaluation initially, yearly for 5 to 10 years, then every other year.

   e. neurologic evaluation initially and yearly for an indefinite period.

27. In a patient with voiding dysfunction secondary to myelomeningocele who has slightly decreased compliance, detrusor areflexia, and low-pressure moderate to severe vesicoureteral reflux, which of the following urodynamic changes would be most likely after ureteral reimplantation alone?

   a. Compliance increased

   b. Voiding pressure decreased

   c. Valsalva leak-point pressure decreased

   d. Maximum urethral closure pressure decreased

   e. Maximum bladder capacity decreased

28. The symptoms of voiding dysfunction in a child with tethered cord syndrome present most commonly after which of the following precipitating factors?

   a. Urinary tract infection

   b. Meningitis

   c. Puberty

   d. Cystoscopy

   e. Growth spurt

29. A classic "sensory neurogenic bladder" (Lapides classification system) is most commonly produced by:

   a. herpes zoster.

   b. herpes simplex.

   c. transverse myelitis.

   d. pernicious anemia.

   e. sacral SCI.

30. Patients who have voiding dysfunction secondary to lumbar disk disease most commonly present with which of the following symptoms and urodynamic findings?

   a. Retention; involuntary bladder contractions

   b. Incontinence; involuntary bladder contractions

   c. Retention; decreased bladder compliance

   d. Difficulty voiding; normal bladder compliance

   e. Incontinence; normal bladder compliance

31. The combination that best describes the type of permanent voiding dysfunction that can occur after radical pelvic surgery is:

   a. exertional (or stress) incontinence; detrusor areflexia.

   b. urgency incontinence; detrusor overactivity.

   c. reflex incontinence; detrusor areflexia.

   d. urgency incontinence; detrusor overactivity.

   e. exertional (or stress) incontinence; detrusor overactivity.

32. What is optimal management for a 65-year-old man who has had a first occurrence of urinary retention after radical pelvic surgery?

   a. Anticholinergic therapy

   b. Clean intermittent catheterization

   c. TURP

   d. External sphincterotomy

   e. Bethanechol chloride

33. The urodynamic parameter most likely to distinguish urinary retention due to prostatic obstruction from urinary retention due to "classic diabetic cystopathy" is:

   a. uroflow.

   b. residual urine volume.

   c. bladder compliance.

   d. vesical pressure.

   e. detrusor pressure.

34. Detrusor-striated sphincter dyssynergia is least expected to occur with which of the following conditions?

   a. Multiple sclerosis

   b. SCI

   c. Stroke

   d. Autonomic hyperreflexia

   e. Transverse myelitis

35. Differentiation of bladder neck obstruction from dysfunctional voiding is most easily and accurately made by:

   a. filling cystometry.

   b. voiding cystometry.

   c. cystourethroscopy.

   d. flowmetry and residual urine determination.

   e. video-urodynamic study.

36. Which of the following is not a typical finding in a patient with Fowler syndrome?

   a. Female younger than 30 years

   b. Unable to void for a day or more with no urgency

   c. Bladder capacity of less than 1 L

   d. Increasing lower abdominal discomfort

   e. Electromyographic (EMG) abnormalities

37. Which of the following with the typical history is the most specific study to make the diagnosis of Fowler syndrome?

   a. Striated sphincter needle EMG recording

   b. Striated sphincter patch EMG recording

   c. Neurologic examination

   d. Spinal magnetic resonance imaging (MRI) examination

   e. Detrusor pressure/urinary flow recording

38. Which of the following has proved to be successful in treating the urologic manifestations of Fowler syndrome?

   a. Estrogen therapy

   b. Progesterone therapy

   c. Baclofen therapy

   d. Botulinum toxin injection therapy

   e. Neuromodulation

39. There is an increased incidence of urinary incontinence after prostatectomy in men with:

   a. hyperthyroidism.

   b. myasthenia gravis.

   c. schizophrenia.

   d. gastroparesis.

   e. Isaacs syndrome.

40. Traumatic brain injury is:

   a. the most common form of neurologic impairment resulting from trauma.

   b. associated with an initial detrusor areflexia.

c. associated with detrusor overactivity if the lesion occurs above the pons.

d. noted to have sphincter synergia as the most common finding.

e. all of the above.

41. PD may be increasing in incidence. It represents a neurodegenerative disorder that is associated with which of the following?

a. Dopamine increases in the nigrostriatal pathway

b. Symptoms such as tremor, skeletal rigidity, and bradykinesia occur

c. Positron emission tomography scanning shows no alterations in brain activation associated with bladder filling

d. Selective stimulation of dopamine receptors with specific agonists is not beneficial for this disorder

e. PD cannot be demonstrated on neuropathologic examination

42. Increasing numbers of individuals with myelomeningocele are surviving into adulthood and older age. Critical for stability of function is recognition that the spinal cord may be tethered. Regarding the tethered spinal cord:

a. the level of tethering as demonstrated by MRI is predictive of findings on urodynamics.

b. urodynamics often shows improvement after detethering.

c. tethered cord syndrome is not usually associated with bowel or leg dysfunction.

d. there are no predictors for social continence after detethering.

e. the symptomatic tethered cord, associated with worsening ambulation, can be managed nonoperatively.

43. Cauda equina syndrome often has effects on lower urinary tract function. Cauda equina syndrome:

a. occurs in the posterior lateral disk direction and is associated in a high degree of dysfunction in patients with cauda equina syndrome.

b. presents with most common neurologic findings of L3/L4 neurologic dysfunction.

c. is caused by disk protrusions occurring at the L5 S1 levels in the majority of cases.

d. is not usually associated with other etiologies other than disk disease.

e. is universally improved after laminectomy in regards to bladder function.

44. Guillain-Barré syndrome is a demyelinating disorder. It is:

a. not usually identified as a clinical entity having sporadic clinical manifestation.

b. not caused by an acute inflammatory disorder.

c. not usually associated with an antecedent acute infectious illness.

d. associated with lower urinary tract function, usually in less than 5% of cases.

e. associated with voiding dysfunction, which is usually reversible.

ANSWERS

1. **b. Involuntary bladder contractions, smooth sphincter synergy, striated sphincter synergy.** Neurologic lesions above the level of the brainstem that affect micturition generally result in involuntary bladder contractions with smooth and striated sphincter synergy. Sensation and voluntary striated sphincter function are generally preserved. Areflexia may occur either initially or as a permanent dysfunction.

2. **c. Involuntary bladder contractions, smooth sphincter synergy, striated sphincter dyssynergia.** Patients with complete lesions of the spinal cord between spinal cord levels T6 and S2, after they recover from spinal shock, generally exhibit involuntary bladder contractions without sensation of the contraction, smooth sphincter synergy, but striated sphincter dyssynergia. Those with lesions above T6 may experience, in addition, smooth sphincter dyssynergia and autonomic hyperreflexia.

3. **e. Detrusor overactivity.** The most common long-term expression of lower urinary tract dysfunction after a CVA is detrusor hyperreflexia. Sensation is variable but is classically described as generally intact, and thus the patient has urgency and frequency with hyperreflexia.

4. **a. Internal capsule.** Previous descriptions of voiding dysfunction after a CVA have all cited the preponderance of detrusor hyperreflexia with coordinated sphincter activity. It is difficult to reconcile this with the relatively high incontinence rate that occurs, even considering the probability that a percentage of these patients had an incontinence problem before the CVA. Tsuchida and colleagues (1983)* and Khan and colleagues (1990) made early significant contributions in this area by correlating the urodynamic and computed tomography (CT) pictures after CVA. They reported that patients with lesions in only the basal ganglia or thalamus have normal sphincter function. This means that when an impending involuntary contraction or its onset was sensed, these patients could voluntarily contract the striated sphincter and abort or considerably lessen the effect of an abnormal micturition reflex. The majority of patients with involvement of the cerebral cortex and/or internal capsule were unable to forcefully contract the striated sphincter under these circumstances.

5. **d. Pseudodyssynergia.** Some authors have described striated sphincter dyssynergia in 5% to 21% of patients with brain disease and voiding dysfunction. This is incompatible with accepted neural circuitry. The authors agree with those who believe that true detrusor-striated sphincter dyssynergia does not occur in this situation. Pseudodyssynergia may indeed occur during urodynamic testing of these patients. This refers to an EMG sphincter "flare" during filling cystometry, which is secondary to attempted inhibition of an involuntary bladder contraction by voluntary contraction of the striated sphincter.

6. **e. Full urodynamic evaluation.** Poor flow rates and high residual urine volumes in a male with pre-CVA symptoms of prostatism generally indicate prostatic obstruction, but a full urodynamic evaluation is advisable before committing a patient to mechanical outlet reduction primarily to exclude detrusor hyperactivity with impaired contractility as a cause of symptoms.

7. **c. Posterior fossa.** The areas that are most frequently involved with associated micturition dysfunction are the superior aspects of the frontal lobe. When voiding dysfunction occurs, it generally consists of detrusor hyperreflexia and urinary incontinence. These individuals may have a markedly diminished awareness of all lower urinary tract events and, if so, are totally unable to even attempt suppression of the micturition reflex. Smooth and striated sphincter activity is generally synergic. Pseudodyssynergia may occur during urodynamic testing. Fowler (1999) reviewed the literature on frontal lobe lesions and bladder control. She cited instances of resection of a tumor relieving the micturition symptoms for a period of time, raising the question of whether the phenomenon of tumor-associated bladder hyperreflexia was a positive one (activating some system) rather than a negative one (releasing a system from control). Urinary retention has also been described in patients with space-occupying lesions of the frontal cortex, in the absence of other associated remarkable neurologic deficits. Posterior fossa tumors may be associated with voiding dysfunction (32% to 70%, based on references cited

---

*Sources referenced can be found in *Campbell-Walsh Urology, 11th Edition*, on the Expert Consult website.

by Fowler). Retention or difficulty voiding is the rule, with incontinence rarely reported.

8. **b. Normal filling/storage; normal emptying.** Most children and adults with only CP have urinary control and what seems to be normal filling/storage and normal emptying. The actual incidence of voiding dysfunction is somewhat vague because the few available series report findings predominantly in those who present with voiding symptoms. One study estimated that a third or more of children with CP are so affected. When an adult with CP presents with an acute or subacute change in voiding status, however, it is most likely unrelated to CP.

9. **e. Detrusor overactivity, coordinated sphincters.** In those individuals with CP who exhibit significant dysfunction, the type of damage that one would suspect from the most common urodynamic abnormalities seems to be localized above the brainstem. This is commonly reflected by detrusor overactivity and coordinated sphincters. Spinal cord damage can occur, however, and probably accounts for those individuals with CP who seem to have evidence of striated sphincter dyssynergia.

10. **a. Dopamine.** PD is a neurodegenerative disorder of unknown cause that affects primarily the dopaminergic neurons of the substantia nigra but also heterogeneous populations of neurons elsewhere. The most important site of pathology is the substantia nigra pars compacta, the origin of the dopaminergic nigrostriatal tract to the caudate nucleus and putamen. Dopamine deficiency in the nigrostriatal pathway accounts for most of the classic clinical motor features of PD.

11. **d. Detrusor overactivity.** The most common urodynamic finding is detrusor overactivity. The pathophysiology of detrusor overactivity most widely proposed is that the basal ganglia normally have an inhibitory effect on the micturition reflex, which is abolished by the cell loss in the substantia nigra.

12. **e. Disease diagnosis preceding voiding and erectile symptoms.** One study compared the clinical features of 52 patients with probable MSA and 41 patients with PD. Of patients with MSA, 60% had their urinary symptoms precede or present with their symptoms of parkinsonism. Of patients with PD, 94% had been diagnosed for several years before the onset of urinary symptoms. In patients with MSA, urinary incontinence was a significant complaint in 73%, whereas 19% had only frequency and urgency without incontinence. Sixty-six percent of the patients with MSA had a significant postvoid residual volume (100 to 450 mL). In patients with PD, frequency and urgency were the predominant symptoms in 85% and incontinence was the primary complaint in 15%. It was significant in only 5 of 32 patients with PD in whom residual urine volume was measured. Ninety-three percent of the men with MSA who were questioned about erectile function reported erectile failure, and in 13 of 27 the erectile dysfunction preceded the diagnosis of MSA. Seven of the 21 men with PD had erectile failure, but in all of these men the diagnosis of erectile dysfunction followed the diagnosis of PD by 1 to 4 years. The initial urinary symptoms of MSA are urgency, frequency, and urge incontinence, which occur as long as 4 years before the diagnosis is made, as does erectile failure. Cystourethrography or videourodynamic studies generally reveal an open bladder neck (intrinsic sphincter deficiency), and many patients exhibit evidence of striated sphincter denervation on motor unit electromyography. The smooth and striated sphincter abnormalities predispose women to sphincteric incontinence and make prostatectomy hazardous in men.

13. **c. Cervical spinal cord.** The demyelinating process most commonly involves the lateral corticospinal (pyramidal) and reticulospinal columns of the cervical spinal cord.

14. **e. Smooth sphincter dyssynergia.** Detrusor overactivity is the most common urodynamic abnormality detected, occurring in 34% to 99% of cases in reported series. Of the patients with overactivity, 30% to 65% have coexistent striated sphincter dyssynergia. As many as 60% of those with overactivity may have impaired detrusor contractility, a phenomenon that can considerably complicate treatment efforts. Bladder areflexia may also

occur; reports of its frequency vary but generally average from 5% to 20%. Generally, the smooth sphincter is synergic.

15. **d. Spinal cord injury (SCI).** Progressive neurologic diseases cause upper tract damage much less commonly than SCI, even when associated with severe disability and spasticity (Wyndaele et al, 2005).

16. **a. 15% or less.** How common are voiding problems overall in patients with HIV infection and AIDS? One study prospectively investigated voiding function in 77 men and 4 women with HIV infection or AIDS consecutively attending an outpatient clinic. Eight patients (10%) had moderate subjective voiding problems, whereas two (2%) had severe problems. The authors thought that the nature of the disturbance warranted urodynamic examination in only 4% of patients and concluded that urinary voiding symptoms are only a modest problem; overall in an HIV/AIDS population, neuropathic bladder dysfunction is rare and mostly occurs in the late stages of the disease (Gyrtrup et al, 1995).

17. **c. L2.** Spinal column (bone) segments are numbered by the vertebral level, and these have a different relationship to the spinal cord segmental level at different locations. The sacral spinal cord begins at approximately spinal column level T12-L1. The spinal cord terminates in the cauda equina at approximately the spinal column level of L2.

18. **c. Open bladder neck.** Spinal shock includes a suppression of autonomic activity and somatic activity, and the bladder is acontractile and areflexic. Radiologically, the bladder has a smooth contour with no evidence of trabeculation. The bladder neck is generally closed and competent unless there has been prior surgery or, in some cases, thoracolumbar and presumably sympathetic injury. The smooth sphincter mechanism seems to be functional. Some EMG activity may be recorded from the striated sphincter, and the maximum urethral closure pressure is lower than normal but still maintained at the level of the external sphincter zone; however, the normal guarding reflex is absent and there is no voluntary control.

19. **d. High abdominal leak-point pressure.** As with all patients with neurologic impairment, a careful initial evaluation and periodic follow-up evaluation must be performed to identify and correct the following risk factors and potential complications: bladder overdistention, high pressure storage, high detrusor leak-point pressure, vesicoureteral reflux, stone formation (lower and upper tracts), and complicating infection, especially in association with reflux.

20. **a. Pons and the sacral spinal cord.** A diagnosis of striated sphincter dyssynergia implies a neurologic lesion that interrupts the neural axis between the pontine-mesencephalic reticular formation and the sacral spinal cord.

21. **a. Cervical.** Autonomic hyperreflexia represents an acute massive disordered autonomic (primarily sympathetic) response to specific stimuli in patients with SCI above the level of T6 to T8 (the upper level of the sympathetic outflow). It is more common with cervical (60%) than thoracic (20%) injuries.

22. **d. Tachycardia.** Symptomatically, autonomic hyperreflexia is a syndrome of exaggerated sympathetic activity in response to stimuli below the level of the lesion. The symptoms are pounding headache, hypertension, and flushing of the face and body above the level of the lesion with sweating. Bradycardia is a usual accompaniment, and an arrhythmia may be present.

23. **b. Decreased compliance.** In autonomic hyperreflexia, the urodynamic picture is that of a suprasacral SCI. Smooth sphincter dyssynergia is generally found as well, at least in men.

24. **b. β-Adrenergic blockade.** Acutely the hemodynamic effects may be managed with parenteral ganglionic or α-adrenergic blockade. Any endoscopic procedure in susceptible patients ideally should be done with the patient under spinal or carefully monitored general anesthesia.

25. **a. Ureteral reimplantation.** The best initial treatment for reflux in a patient with voiding dysfunction secondary to neurologic disease or injury is to normalize lower urinary tract urodynamics

as much as possible. Depending on the clinical circumstances, this may be by pharmacotherapy, urethral dilatation (in the myelomeningocele patient), neuromodulation, deafferentation, augmentation cystoplasty, or sphincterotomy. If this fails, the question of whether to operate on such patients for correction of the reflux or to correct the reflux while performing another procedure (e.g., augmentation cystoplasty) is not an easy one because correction of reflux in an often thickened bladder may not be an easy task.

26. **e. Neurologic evaluation initially and yearly for an indefinite period.** All but e were specific recommendations (Linsenmeyer and Culkin, 1999).

27. **e. Maximum bladder capacity decreased.** One must remember the potential artifact that significant reflux can introduce into urodynamic studies. Measured bladder capacity may be more, and measured pressures at given inflow volumes may be less, than those after reflux correction. The apparent significance of detrusor overactivity may thus be underestimated.

28. **e. Growth spurt.** One study pointed out that although children often develop symptoms of tethered cord after growth spurts, in adults the presenting symptoms often follow activities that stretch the spine, such as sports or motor vehicle accidents.

29. **d. Pernicious anemia.** Although syphilitic myopathy is disappearing as a major neurologic problem, involvement of the spinal cord dorsal columns and posterior sacral roots can result in a loss of bladder sensation and large residual urine volumes and therefore can be a cause of sensory neurogenic bladder. Another spinal cord cause of the classic sensory bladder is the now uncommon pernicious anemia. The most common cause is diabetes.

30. **d. Difficulty voiding; normal bladder compliance.** A study reported on findings in 114 patients with lumbar disk protrusion who were prospectively studied. The authors found detrusor areflexia in 31 (27.2%) and normal detrusor activity in the remaining 83. All 31 patients with detrusor areflexia reported difficulty voiding with straining. Patients with voiding dysfunction generally present with these symptoms or in urinary retention. The most consistent urodynamic finding is that of a normally compliant areflexic bladder associated with normal innervation or findings of incomplete denervation of the perineal floor musculature.

31. **a. Exertional (or stress) incontinence; detrusor areflexia.** When permanent voiding dysfunction occurs after radical pelvic surgery, the pattern is generally one of a failure of voluntary bladder contraction, or impaired bladder contractility, with obstruction by what seems urodynamically to be residual fixed striated sphincter tone, which is not subject to voluntarily induced relaxation. Often, the smooth sphincter area is open and nonfunctional. Decreased compliance is common in these patients, and this, with the "obstruction" caused by fixed residual striated sphincter tone, results in both storage and emptying failure. These patients often experience leaking across the distal sphincter area and, in addition, are unable to empty the bladder because although intravesical pressure may be increased, there is nothing that approximates a true bladder contraction. The patient often presents with urinary incontinence that is characteristically most manifest with increases in intra-abdominal pressure. This is usually most obvious in females because the prostatic bulk in males often masks an equivalent deficit in urethral closure function. Alternatively, patients may present with variable degrees of urinary retention.

32. **b. Clean intermittent catheterization.** The temptation to perform a prostatectomy should be avoided unless a clear demonstration of outlet obstruction at this level is possible. Otherwise, prostatectomy simply decreases urethral sphincter function and thereby may result in the occurrence or worsening of sphincteric urinary incontinence. Most of these dysfunctions will be transient, and the temptation to "do something" other than perform clean intermittent catheterization initially after surgery in these patients, especially in those with little or no preexisting history of voiding dysfunction, cannot be too strongly discouraged.

33. **e. Detrusor pressure.** Detrusor contractility is classically described as being decreased in the end-stage diabetic bladder. Current evidence points to both sensory and motor neuropathy as being involved in the pathogenesis, the motor aspect per se contributing to the impaired detrusor contractility. The typically described classic urodynamic findings include impaired bladder sensation, increased cystometric capacity, decreased bladder contractility, impaired uroflow, and, later, increased residual urine volume. The main differential diagnosis, at least in men, is generally bladder outlet obstruction because both conditions commonly produce a low flow rate. Pressure/flow urodynamic studies easily differentiate the two.

34. **c. Stroke.** True detrusor sphincter dyssynergia should exist only in patients who have an abnormality in pathways between the sacral spinal cord and the brainstem pontine micturition center, generally due to neurologic injury or disease.

35. **e. Video-urodynamic study.** Objective evidence of outlet obstruction in these patients is easily obtainable by urodynamic study. Once obstruction is diagnosed, it can be localized at the level of the bladder neck by video-urodynamic study, cystourethrography during a bladder contraction, or micturitional urethral profilometry.

36. **c. Bladder capacity of less than 1 L.** The criteria (Swinn and Fowler, 2001; Fowler, 2003) include a bladder capacity of more than 1 L with no sensation of urgency.

37. **a. Striated sphincter needle EMG recording.** *Fowler syndrome* refers particularly to a syndrome of urinary retention in young women in the absence of overt neurologic disease. The typical history is that of a woman younger than 30 years, who has found herself unable to void during the preceding day but with no sensation of urgency. MRI studies of the brain and the entire spinal cord are normal. On concentric needle electrode examination of the striated muscle of the urethral sphincter, however, Fowler and colleagues described a unique EMG abnormality. This abnormal activity, localized to the urethral sphincter, consists of a type of activity that would be expected to cause inappropriate contraction of the muscle. Sphincter activity consists of two components: complex repetitive discharges and decelerating bursts. This abnormal activity impairs sphincter relaxation.

38. **e. Neuromodulation.** Fowler reports that efforts to treat this condition by hormonal manipulation, pharmacologic therapy, or injections of botulinum toxin have been unsuccessful. This condition is highly responsive to neuromodulation, even in women who have had retention for many months or years.

39. **b. Myasthenia gravis.** Any neuromuscular disease that affects the tone of the smooth or striated muscle of the distal sphincter mechanism can predispose an individual patient to a greater chance of urinary incontinence even after a well-performed transurethral or open prostatectomy. Myasthenia gravis is an autoimmune disease caused by autoantibodies to acetylcholine nicotinic receptors. This leads to neuromuscular blockade and hence weakness in a variety of striated muscle groups. The incidence of incontinence after prostatectomy is indeed greatly increased in patients with this disease.

40. **e. All of the above.** Traumatic brain injury has now risen to the most common etiologic factor for neurologic voiding dysfunction. Depending on the level of the injury, there may be detrusor sphincter synergia or dyssynergia. In recent studies, urinary incontinence, on a chronic basis associated with this injury, is associated with poor functional status and bilaterality of lesion. Patients who are in chronic retention are more commonly noted to have diabetes mellitus or bowel-related issues as comorbidities. Rehabilitation results in some improvement for patients, but it depends on the magnitude of injury.

41. **b. Symptoms such as tremor, skeletal rigidity, and bradykinesia occur.** The symptom complex of PD is classic for its presentation, and these symptoms are often followed longitudinally for benefit of therapy. The diagnosis of PD is classically made by neuropathologic examination; however, there is a constellation of symptoms that is consistent with

the syndrome and leads to therapeutic intervention during life. Positron emission tomography (PET) scanning shows brain responses with bladder filling. These responses are found most prominently with detrusor overactivity. The cerebellum seems to be actively involved in these increased responses. Dopaminergic agonists are used therapeutically for the management of this disorder.

42. **b. Urodynamics often show improvement after detethering.** Despite efforts at improved radiographic visualization of the spinal cord, imaging does not correlate with physical findings or connote overall responsiveness to surgical intervention because detethering remains a critical aspect of management and control of tethered cord. Cord tethering affects both bowel and leg function, as well as bladder function. Urodynamics is improved by detethering, and this parallels functional improvement in those individuals who have undergone the surgical procedure. The successful management of the tethered cord remains a critical aspect of long-term care in the myelomeningocele population.

43. **c. Is caused by disk protrusions occurring at the L5 S1 levels in the majority of cases.** Cauda equina is most commonly associated with low lumbar, high sacral disk lesions that compress the nerve roots while they ramify from the spinal cord. It can be caused by a variety of etiologies other than disk disease, which may or may not affect long-term function after laminectomy. Although urologic findings associated with cauda equina are often indications for surgery, laminectomy may not improve overall function. Posterolateral disk disease does not usually result in cauda equina syndrome.

44. **e. Associated with voiding dysfunction, which is usually reversible.** Guillain-Barré syndrome is an acute inflammatory disorder thought to be due to some inflammatory process because most patients do have evidence of acute inflammatory conditions before development of the syndrome. The syndrome is characterized by a distinct presenting scenario (ascending paralysis). Lower urinary tract dysfunction has been reported in as few as 25% to as many as 80% of cases and is usually reversible with resolution of the disorder.

CHAPTER REVIEW

1. Neurologic lesions above the brainstem generally result in involuntary bladder contractions and a coordinated sphincter.
2. Spinal cord lesions between T6 and S2 result in involuntary bladder contractions, smooth sphincter synergy, and striated sphincter dyssynergia; spinal cord lesions above T7 or T8 may have smooth sphincter dyssynergia as well.
3. Lesions below S2 result in areflexia.
4. Traumatic brain injury results in an initial period of detrusor areflexia.
5. Parkinson disease commonly results in detrusor overactivity with possible impaired detrusor contractility.
6. For a true Parkinson disease patient, a TURP is not contraindicated. However, in multisystem atrophy with Parkinson-like symptoms, smooth and striated sphincter abnormalities may result in incontinence after a TURP.
7. Spinal shock includes a suppression of autonomic activity and somatic activity, and the bladder is acontractile and areflexic. The bladder neck is generally closed.
8. Autonomic hyperreflexia is primarily a sympathetic response and occurs in patients with SCI above the level of T6; it is a syndrome of exaggerated sympathetic activity in response to stimuli below the level of the lesion. The symptoms are pounding headache, hypertension, and flushing of the face and body above the level of the lesion with sweating. Bradycardia is a usual accompaniment, and an arrhythmia may be present. Drugs commonly used to treat the manifestations include nifedipine, nitrates, and captopril.
9. In patients with SCI, bacteriuria should only be treated when there are signs or symptoms.
10. In SCI patients the incidence of bladder cancer is comparable with the general population; however, 60% of those affected present with T2 or greater disease versus 20% in the general population.
11. Tethered cord syndrome results from fixation of the spinal cord caudally with stretch as the individual grows. Presenting symptoms are back pain, leg weakness, foot deformities, scoliosis, sensory loss, and bowel and lower urinary tract dysfunction.
12. Radical pelvic surgery may result in failure of voluntary bladder contraction and residual fixed striated sphincter tone, which is not subject to voluntary control.
13. Diabetic cystopathy is a result of peripheral and autonomic neuropathy that affects both sensory and motor nerves. It is primarily a problem of overdistention, and therefore timed voidings may be helpful.
14. True detrusor sphincter dyssynergia occurs when pathways between the sacral spinal cord and the brainstem are interrupted. Therefore traumatic SCI, multiple sclerosis, and transverse myelitis are the usual causes. In patients without a neurologic lesion, the diagnosis should be suspect.
15. Radiation results in decreased cystometric capacity, decreased compliance, and a reduction in the volume at which the first urge to void is noted.
16. In patients with multiple sclerosis or voiding dysfunction secondary to radical pelvic surgery, conservative measures are preferred and irreversible treatments should be avoided.
17. Urinary retention may be secondary to herpes zoster and herpes simplex.
18. Syphilitic myopathy, pernicious anemia, and diabetes may cause the classic sensory neurogenic bladder; poliomyelitis may cause the classic motor neurogenic bladder.
19. The most common long-term expression of lower urinary tract dysfunction after a CVA is detrusor hyperreflexia.
20. Pseudodyssynergia refers to an EMG sphincter "flare" during filling cystometry, which is secondary to attempted inhibition of an involuntary bladder contraction by voluntary contraction of the striated sphincter.
21. Most children and adults with only cerebral palsy have urinary control and what seems to be normal filling/storage and normal emptying.
22. The sacral spinal cord begins at approximately spinal column level T12-L1. The spinal cord terminates in the cauda equina at approximately the spinal column level of L2.
23. Measured bladder capacity may be more, and measured pressures at given inflow volumes may be less than those after reflux correction.

76 Overactive Bladder

Marcus John Drake

QUESTIONS

1. Which definition or definitions appear in the current International Continence Society (ICS) terminology (2002)?
   a. Detrusor hyperreflexia
   b. Overactive bladder
   c. Idiopathic detrusor overactivity
   d. Detrusor instability
   e. b and c

2. Which symptoms are included in overactive bladder syndrome (OAB)?
   a. Dysuria
   b. Straining
   c. Urgency incontinence
   d. Bladder pain
   e. Stress incontinence

3. In the community, what percentage of adults have overactive bladder symptoms?
   a. Less than 5%
   b. 5% to 10%
   c. 10% to 20%
   d. 20% to 50%
   e. More than 50%

4. Mixed incontinence includes:
   a. stress urinary incontinence.
   b. continuous incontinence.
   c. postmicturition leakage.
   d. incontinence during sexual intercourse.
   e. giggle incontinence.

5. Which features are characteristics of urgency?
   a. A normal sensation.
   b. It builds up slowly.
   c. It is usually felt suprapubically.
   d. It develops quickly and may lead to incontinence.
   e. a and b

6. Which statements are TRUE for detrusor overactivity (DO)?
   a. It is characterized by phasic involuntary detrusor contractions during bladder filling.
   b. It is always accompanied by a feeling of urgency.
   c. It is a urodynamic diagnosis.
   d. It is a feature of the voiding phase of micturition.
   e. a and c

7. Detrusor overactivity can be diagnosed:
   a. only if involuntary filling phase contractions are greater than 15 cm H_2O in amplitude.
   b. if an involuntary contraction is seen during bladder filling, irrespective of size.
   c. if there is urgency incontinence but no contraction.
   d. if leakage occurs during exercise.
   e. before urodynamics if the patient has overactive bladder syndrome.

8. Which statement is FALSE with respect to the hypotheses of detrusor pathophysiology?
   a. Afferent sensitization signifies an increased afferent firing rate in response to a standardized stimulus.
   b. The myogenic and integrative hypotheses require abnormal propagation of excitation in the bladder wall.
   c. Synaptic reorganization in the spinal cord may contribute to neurogenic detrusor overactivity.
   d. Detrusor overactivity requires volitional control.
   e. Synergic coordination of bladder and outlet are determined at the brainstem/midbrain level.

9. Which of the following statements is correct regarding symptom assessment tools?
   a. OAB can be diagnosed from the frequency volume chart.
   b. A validated questionnaire is mandatory for diagnosis of OAB.
   c. Modular components of the International Consultation on Incontinence Questionnaire system (ICIQ) have undergone formal validation.
   d. A high urgency score is diagnostic of detrusor overactivity.
   e. a and b

ANSWERS

1. **e. b and c.** Detrusor hyperreflexia has been replaced by neurogenic detrusor overactivity. The concept of tone is poorly understood; hence, the term *detrusor instability* is not recommended.

2. **c. Urgency incontinence.** Urgency incontinence is experienced by a large proportion of patients with OAB.

3. **c. 10% to 20%.** Two large prevalence surveys in North America and Europe have shown the prevalence at 16%, whereas the EPIC study put the figure at nearly 12%. Prevalence of at least one lower urinary tract symptom is greater than 50% according to the EPIC study.

4. **a. Stress urinary incontinence.** This is one of the two constituents of mixed incontinence, along with urgency urinary incontinence.

5. **d. Develops quickly and may lead to incontinence.** Urgency is thought to be a symptom of rapid onset. Urgency leads to urgency incontinence in the susceptible patient, but not invariably.

6. **e. a and c.** Involuntary contractions seen on urodynamic assessment are characteristic of detrusor overactivity.

7. **b. If an involuntary contraction is seen during bladder filling, irrespective of size.**

8. **d. Detrusor overactivity requires volitional control.** Patients are unable to inhibit overactive contractions voluntarily.

9. **c. Modular components of the International Consultation on Incontinence Questionnaire system (ICIQ) have undergone formal validation.** The ICIQ generates new tools and adopts established tools for a system that allows selection of appropriate symptom assessment for specific clinical contexts.

CHAPTER REVIEW

1. DO is a urodynamic diagnosis. OAB is a symptom-based diagnosis, defined as urgency with or without urgency incontinence, usually with frequency and nocturia with no proven infection or other obvious pathology.
2. The pattern of voided volumes in patients with OAB is erratic.
3. Urgency with at least one other symptom is essential to the diagnosis of OAB.
4. The etiology of DO has been hypothesized to be due to neurogenic or myogenic disorders. Neurogenic disorders may involve (1) reduced suprapontine inhibition, (2) overexpression of primitive spinal bladder reflexes, (3) synaptic plasticity in which new reflexes develop as a response to C-fiber afferent neurons, and (4) sensitization of peripheral afferent terminals. Myogenic disorders involve spontaneous excitation, which may be a result of upregulation of surface membrane receptors.
5. A frequency voiding chart or voiding diary is essential for assessing OAB.
6. The two main urodynamic findings with overactive bladder are DO and increasing filling sensation.
7. Treatment of OAB should begin with conservative management, including lifestyle changes, followed by pharmacotherapy and, finally, for intractable cases, surgical therapy that involves either nerve stimulation or surgical procedures on the bladder itself.
8. Aging, neurologic disease, female gender, bladder outlet obstruction, and the metabolic syndrome are potential contributors to OAB.

77 Underactive Detrusor

Christopher R. Chapple and Nadir I. Osman

QUESTIONS

1. Which of the following is NOT part of the International continence society's definition of detrusor underactivity (DUA)?
   a. A contraction of reduced duration
   b. Prolonged bladder emptying
   c. Incomplete bladder emptying
   d. A contraction of reduced strength
   e. A contraction of reduced speed

2. A symptom syndrome of "underactive bladder" (UAB) is defined as:
   a. reduced desire to void, usually accompanied by urinary frequency or nocturia, with or without incontinence that predominates at night.
   b. reduced desire to void, associated with incomplete bladder emptying.
   c. symptoms of impaired bladder emptying in the absence of bladder outlet obstruction.
   d. infrequent voiding, associated with voiding symptoms and increased postvoid residual.
   e. There is currently no recognized definition for UAB.

3. What is the ultrastructural pattern associated with DUA, according to the classification of Elbadawi?
   a. Dense band pattern
   b. Degeneration pattern
   c. Dysfunction pattern
   d. Dysjunction pattern
   e. Myelohypertrophy pattern

4. Most current diagnostic criteria estimate which aspect of detrusor contraction?
   a. Efficiency
   b. Sustainability
   c. Speed
   d. Strength
   e. Duration

5. Which of the following criteria is not thought to be affected by the presence of bladder outlet obstruction?
   a. Detrusor contraction duration
   b. Bladder contractility index
   c. Detrusor contraction coefficient
   d. Projected isovolumetric pressure
   e. Watt factor

6. Which of the following statements regarding parasympathomimetic agents in DUA is TRUE?
   a. Muscarinic agonists show good efficacy in restoring contractility.
   b. Muscarinic agonists are more likely to be effective in patients with complete bladder denervation.
   c. Muscarinic agonists can cause severe cardiac depression.
   d. Anticholinesterases can cause uterine contraction.
   e. None of the above.

7. What is the proposed mechanism of action of intravesical electrotherapy (IVE)?
   a. Direct stimulation of detrusor myocytes
   b. Stimulation of mechanoreceptive afferent nerves
   c. Direct stimulation of efferent nerves
   d. Inhibition of pathologic urethral afferent signaling
   e. None of the above

8. Which of the following features appears to be associated with more positive outcomes in the treatment of DUA?
   a. Neurogenic etiology
   b. Older age
   c. Intact bladder sensation
   d. Myogenic etiology
   e. Acontractile bladder

9. Which of these neurologic disorders is most frequently associated with DUA on urodynamics?
   a. Parkinson disease
   b. Multiple sclerosis
   c. Multisystem atrophy
   d. Cerebrovascular accident—postacute phase
   e. Brain tumor

10. What is the natural history of DUA in men without known neurogenic bladder dysfunction?
    a. Deterioration in symptoms but not urodynamic parameters
    b. No significant change in urodynamic parameters for at least 10 years
    c. Improvement in contractility in at least 50% of individuals
    d. Most will require bladder outlet surgery by 10 years
    e. No studies are available

ANSWERS

1. **e. A contraction of reduced speed.** The 2002 standardization report of the ICS defines DUA as "a contraction of reduced strength and/or duration, resulting in prolonged bladder emptying and/or failure to achieve complete bladder emptying within a normal time span." An acontractile detrusor is separately defined as "one that cannot be demonstrated to contract during urodynamic studies."

2. **e. There is currently no recognized definition for UAB.** A symptom syndrome of "underactive bladder" is difficult to rationally define because of the absence of studies correlating individual symptoms to the underlying detrusor abnormality. Even then, empirical evidence would suggest that symptoms of DUA are very diverse and overlap significantly with those of OAB.

3. **b. Degeneration pattern.** The "degeneration" pattern is associated with DUA and consists of widespread disrupted detrusor

myocytes and axonal degeneration. Elbadawi proposed that distinct ultrastructural patterns observed by electron microscopy characterized the normally contractile ageing detrusor and different bladder dysfunctions. Although the applicability of this classification system is disputed, other groups have noted similar findings.

4. **d. Strength.** Most criteria focus on contraction strength as derived from detrusor pressure at maximal flow.

5. **e. Watt factor.** The watt factor is a mathematical calculation and provides a measure of bladder power. Its major advantages are that it minimally depends on volume and is not affected by increased outlet resistance. However, it is a complex calculation with no validated cutoffs.

6. **c. Muscarinic agonists can cause severe cardiac depression.** Muscarinic agonists have been associated with reports of severe myocardial depression leading to cardiac arrest. This, and their lack of efficacy, has led to their nonuse in clinical practice.

7. **b. Stimulation of mechanoreceptive afferent nerves.** IVE activates mechanosensitive bladder afferents (myelinated Aδ fibers) and restores bladder sensation. It is postulated that repeat activation of this pathway upregulates its performance during volitional voiding.

8. **c. Intact bladder sensation.** Intact bladder sensation is necessary to normally trigger the micturition reflex. Its presence suggests some residual bladder innervation and was found to be associated with better responses to some treatments of DUA (e.g., urethral sphincter botulinum neurotoxin A and muscarinic agonists)

9. **c. Multisystem atrophy.** Multisystem atrophy is a neurodegenerative disease that may be confused with Parkinson disease. It is associated with autonomic dysfunction and DUA in at least half of patients because of atrophy of parasympathetic nerves.

10. **b. No significant change in urodynamic parameters for at least 10 years.** There are very few data on the natural history of DUA. A longitudinal follow-up study (10 years) by Thomas et al showed no significant symptomatic or urodynamic deterioration in men with DUA managed conservatively at 10 years.

CHAPTER REVIEW

1. Detrusor underactivity (DUA) is a contraction of reduced strength and/or duration, resulting in prolonged bladder emptying and/or failure to achieve complete bladder emptying within a normal time span.

2. DUA often coexists with other lower urinary tract dysfunctions in the elderly.

3. Normal aging results in a reduction in autonomic innervation and a decline in sensory function in the lower urinary tract.

4. Diabetes mellitus impairs detrusor function through both myogenic and autonomic dysfunction.

5. Lumbosacral spinal cord trauma or disk disease and pelvic surgery can lead to injury of the pelvic plexus.

6. Afferent nerves play a central role in the initiation and maintenance of a detrusor contraction.

7. Treatment strategies to address DUA include timed voiding, double voiding, pelvic floor physiotherapy, and self intermittent catheterization.

8. Intravesical electrotherapy activates mechanosensitive bladder afferents (myelinated Aδ fibers) and restores bladder sensation. It is postulated that repeat activation of this pathway upregulates its performance during volitional voiding.

78 Nocturia

Jeffrey Paul Weiss and Stephen David Marshall

QUESTIONS

1. Nocturnal polyuria is defined as:
   a. nocturnal polyuria index greater than 0.33.
   b. nocturnal urine volume greater than 6.4 mL/kg.
   c. nocturnal urine volume greater than 54 mL/hr.
   d. a and b
   e. a, b, and c

2. All of the following statements are true about nocturia EXCEPT:
   a. nocturia is voiding that is preceded and followed by sleep.
   b. the prevalence of nocturia increases with age.
   c. nocturia impairs sleep efficiency, sleep latency, and slow-wave sleep and is associated with increased mortality.
   d. one or more voids per night appear to be clinically significant.
   e. nocturia is associated with falls.

3. When instructing a patient how to complete a frequency-volume chart, it is essential to:
   a. tell the patient to record what time he goes to sleep.
   b. tell the patient to record what time he awakens.
   c. tell the patient to record how much he drinks during the day.
   d. a and b
   e. a, b, and c

4. Factors that inhibit antidiuretic hormone (ADH) secretion include all of the following EXCEPT:
   a. hyperkalemia.
   b. atrial natriuretic peptide (ANP).
   c. hypercalcemia.
   d. prostaglandin E2 (PGE2).
   e. lithium.

5. A 75 year-old obese man (100 kg) with a short neck reports frequent urination during the nighttime and completes a voiding diary. His 24-hour voided volume is 2000 mL, and his nocturnal urine volume is 1000 mL. Based on these diary findings, this man has:
   a. global polyuria.
   b. nocturnal polyuria.
   c. diminished nocturnal bladder capacity.
   d. diminished global bladder capacity.
   e. none of the above.

6. According to a recent study, which of the following showed the greatest decline in nocturia severity and greatest improvement of health-related quality of life (HRQL) in men with benign prostatic hyperplasia (BPH) and nocturia?
   a. Watchful waiting.
   b. α-Blockers.
   c. Transurethral resection of the prostate (TURP).
   d. Transurethral microwave treatment (TUMT).
   e. There was no difference among these treatments.

7. When bound to V2 receptors in the renal collecting tubules, desmopressin:
   a. increases water permeability.
   b. enhances water reabsorption.
   c. dilutes extracellular fluid.
   d. concentrates urine.
   e. All of the above.

8. Current thinking is that desmopressin is most appropriate to treat:
   a. nocturnal polyuria.
   b. global polyuria.
   c. decreased global bladder capacity.
   d. decreased nocturnal bladder capacity.
   e. all of the above.

9. Which of the following have caused statistically but minimally clinically significant reductions in nocturia episodes?
   a. α-Blockers
   b. 5α-Reductase inhibitors
   c. Antimuscarinics
   d. α-Blockers and antimuscarinics
   e. All of the above

10. Regarding the frequency volume chart (voiding diary), which of the following statements is FALSE?
    a. Nocturnal urine volume is defined as the total volume of all voids preceded and followed by sleep.
    b. The first morning void counts towards total number of daily voiding episodes.
    c. Nighttime may be during daylight hours.
    d. Maximum voided volume is the single greatest urine volume measured during a 24-hour period.
    e. Nocturia or enuresis occurs when the nocturia index (Ni) is greater than 1.

ANSWERS

1. **e. a, b, and c.** Nocturnal polyuria is defined as nocturnal polyuria index (NPi) greater than 0.20 in young adults and greater than 0.33 in adults older than 65 years when 24-hour urine production is within normal limits. Other definitions include nocturnal urine volume (NUV) greater than 0.9 mL/min (54 mL/hr) and NUV greater than 1.5 mL/min (90 mL/hr). A universally accepted definition of nocturnal polyuria has yet to be identified.

2. **d. One or more voids per night appear to be clinically significant.** Several studies have shown that two or more voids per night generate bother and impair quality of life.

3. **d. a and b.** Although having the patient record how much he drinks during the day may be helpful, it is essential that the patient record the time he went to sleep and the time he awakens to know the number of nocturnal voids and nocturnal urine volume.

4. **a. Hyperkalemia.** Factors that inhibit ADH and cause diuresis (inhibit water reabsorption) include prostaglandin E2, ANP, hypercalcemia, hypokalemia, lithium, and tetracyclines. Reversal of water diuresis, accordingly, may occur through stimulation of V2 receptors, either by endogenous arginine vasopressin or a congener thereof, such as desmopressin.

5. **b. Nocturnal polyuria.** This patient suffers from nocturnal polyuria as defined by his nocturnal polyuria index (NPi). His NPi can be calculated by dividing his nocturnal urine volume by his 24-hour voided volume:

$$NPi = NUV/24\text{-hour voided volume}$$
$$= 1000\,mL/2000\,mL = 0.5$$

He has nocturnal polyuria because his NPi is greater than 0.33. Global polyuria is defined as 24-hour urine volume greater than 40 mL/kg. Diminished nocturnal bladder capacity and global bladder capacity cannot be determined by the information provided in this scenario.

6. **c. Transurethral resection of the prostate (TURP).** After 6 to 12 months, watchful waiting, α-blockers, TURP, and TUMT

yielded reduction in nocturia episodes by 7%, 17%, 75%, and 32%, respectively. Improvements in HRQL were most strongly associated with treatment-associated declines in nocturia severity.

7. **e. All of the above.** When bound to V2 receptors in the renal collecting tubules, desmopressin increases water permeability, enhances water reabsorption, dilutes extracellular fluid, and concentrates urine.

8. **a. Nocturnal polyuria.** Current thinking is that desmopressin would be the most appropriate therapy for patients with nocturia related to nocturnal polyuria.

9. **e. All of the above.** α-Blockers, 5α-reductase inhibitors, antimuscarinics, and antimuscarinics+α-blockers have been found to produce a statistically significant reduction in nocturia episodes, yielding minimal clinical significance.

10. **a. Nocturnal urine volume is defined as the total volume of all voids preceded and followed by sleep.** This is incorrect. Nocturnal urine volume is the total volume of urine passed during the night and the first morning void.

CHAPTER REVIEW

1. There is a clear impact of aging on the prevalence of nocturia. Younger people are more likely to manifest decreased nocturnal bladder capacity, whereas older people manifest overproduction of urine.
2. Accumulation of fluid in the dependent parts of the body (third spacing) and return of fluid to the circulating volume when the patient is recumbent may be the underlying cause of the nocturia.
3. The pathophysiology of nocturia may be related to increased mean arterial blood pressure when supine and an alteration of circadian rhythm of ADH (ordinarily there is an increased production of ADH at night during the hours of sleep).
4. Twenty percent of people 20 to 40 years awake to void two or more times compared with 60% of those 70 years or older.
5. Two or more voids a night is clinically significant.
6. Obstructive sleep apnea is a common cause of nocturia.
7. Desmopressin may result in hyponatremia; women are more sensitive to the drug than are men.

79 Pharmacologic Management of Lower Urinary Tract Storage and Emptying Failure

Alan J. Wein

QUESTIONS

(Multiple answers are possible throughout.)

1. The effects of administration of antimuscarinic agent to an individual with an overactive bladder (OAB) include all of the following EXCEPT:
   a. increased total bladder capacity.
   b. depressed amplitude of involuntary bladder contractions.
   c. increased outlet resistance.
   d. increased volume to the first involuntary bladder contraction.
   e. increased mean volume voided.

2. Which of the following muscarinic receptor subtypes is the most common in human detrusor smooth muscle?
   a. M_1
   b. M_2
   c. M_3
   d. M_4
   e. M_5

3. Which of the following muscarinic receptor subtypes is predominantly responsible for the mediation of bladder contraction in human detrusor smooth muscle?
   a. M_1
   b. M_2
   c. M_3
   d. M_4
   e. M_5

4. The use of antimuscarinic agents to treat OAB is limited by their lack of uroselectivity. Which of the following is NOT a recognized side effect of antimuscarinic agents?
   a. Dry mouth
   b. Constipation
   c. Cognitive dysfunction
   d. Bradycardia
   e. Blurred vision

5. Which of the following characteristics increases the possibility for an antimuscarinic agent to pass the blood-brain barrier?
   a. High lipophilicity
   b. Large molecular size
   c. Low electrical charge
   d. Quaternary ammonium structure
   e. Small molecular size

6. Anticholinergics exert their favorable effects on OAB by affecting:
   a. peripheral afferent (sensory) transmission.
   b. ganglionic transmission.
   c. central neural afferent transmission.
   d. muscarinic receptors on the detrusor smooth muscle.
   e. nicotinic receptors on the detrusor smooth muscle.

7. The Committee on Pharmacologic Treatment of the Fifth (2013) International Consultation on Incontinence assessed agents according to the Oxford Guideline, according to level of evidence and grade of recommendation with respect to treatment of detrusor overactivity (DO). Which of the following (multiple answers are possible) did NOT receive a level of evidence rating of 1 and a grade of recommendation of A?
   a. Fesoterodine
   b. Flavoxate
   c. Trospium
   d. Solifenacin
   e. Oxybutynin

8. Which of the following is NOT a class effect of antimuscarinics?
   a. Accommodation paralysis
   b. Constipation
   c. Increased heart rate
   d. Prolongation of the QT interval
   e. Dry mouth

9. Of the following choices, which are correct? The bladder contains how many β-receptor subtypes (answer 1) _____ with the (answer 2) _____ having the most important functional role.
   a. One; β_2
   b. Two; β_2
   c. Three; β_3
   d. Four; β_2
   e. Five; β_5

10. Which of the following pharmacologic actions is or are most probably responsible for the effects of oxybutynin when given systemically?
    a. Antimuscarinic, direct muscle relaxant, and local anesthetic actions, equally
    b. Direct muscle relaxant effect alone
    c. Direct muscle relaxant effect and local anesthetic action
    d. Antimuscarinic and direct muscle relaxant effects
    e. Antimuscarinic effect

11. Which of the following muscarinic receptor subtypes are NOT known to be involved in the potential antimuscarinic side effects of dry mouth, constipation, tachycardia, drowsiness, and blurred vision?
    a. M_1
    b. M_2
    c. M_3
    d. M_4
    e. M_5

12. The primary adverse event reported with the usage of oxybutynin-transdermal has been:
    a. tachycardia.
    b. dry mouth.
    c. constipation.
    d. application site reactions.
    e. blurred vision.

13. Which of the following agents is relatively selective for M_3 receptor blockade?
    a. Darifenacin
    b. Oxybutynin
    c. Solifenacin
    d. Tolterodine
    e. Trospium

14. Mirabegron probably exerts its favorable effect on OAB by:
    a. activating the β_3 adrenergic receptor.
    b. competitive blockade of the β_3 receptor.
    c. inhibiting filling induced activity in bladder afferent nerves.
    d. activating the alpha-adrenergic receptor.
    e. inhibiting the α-adrenergic receptor.

15. Of the following agents, which is actively excreted by the kidney in the proximal convoluted tubules?
    a. Darifenacin
    b. Oxybutynin
    c. Solifenacin
    d. Tolterodine
    e. Trospium

16. Which is (are) TRUE about tadalafil?
    a. It improves International Index of Erectile Function (IIEF) scores.
    b. It improves inferior petrosal sinus sampling (IPSS) scores.
    c. It improves peak flow rates.
    d. It is approved for the treatment of LUTS (lower urinary tract symptoms) due to BPO (benign prostatic obstruction).
    e. It decreases detrusor pressure at peak flow.

17. Which of the following is NOT listed as a common side effect of imipramine?
    a. Systemic antimuscarinic effects
    b. Weakness, fatigue
    c. Priapism
    d. Cardiac arrhythmia
    e. Hepatic dysfunction

18. In men with BPO and OAB, adding an antimuscarinic to an α-adrenergic blocking agent will:
    a. significantly increase residual urine volume.
    b. significantly decrease detrusor pressure at peak flow.
    c. significantly decrease peak and mean flow rate.
    d. cause a, b, and c.
    e. none of the above.

19. Intravesical botulinum toxin subtype A:
    a. activates synaptosomal-associated protein (SNAP) 25 and the soluble N-ethylmaleimide-sensitive factor attachment *protein* (SNARE) complex.
    b. acts only on smooth muscle.
    c. inhibits the peripheral release of acetylcholine.

    d. is effective only in patients with both OAB and DO.
    e. reduces firing from bladder afferents.

20. Vaginal estrogen is effective in the treatment of:
    a. urogenital atrophy.
    b. stress urinary incontinence.
    c. urgency urinary incontinence.
    d. mixed urinary incontinence.
    e. anterior vaginal prolapse.

21. The side effects of the alpha-adrenergic agonists include all of the following EXCEPT:
    a. tremor.
    b. palpitations.
    c. hypertension.
    d. somnolence.
    e. respiratory difficulties.

22. Which of the following has been reported to increase stroke risk in women younger than 50 years?
    a. Phenylpropanolamine
    b. Ephedrine
    c. Pseudoephedrine
    d. Midodrine
    e. Clenbuterol

23. In theory, which of the following agents, from the standpoint of potential efficacy and safety, would be preferred for the treatment of stress urinary incontinence (SUI) in a hypertensive individual?
    a. Ephedrine
    b. Propranolol
    c. Phenylpropanolamine
    d. Pseudoephedrine
    e. Clenbuterol

24. Which of the following statements is NOT true with respect to duloxetine hydrochloride?
    a. It significantly increases sphincteric muscle activity during filling/storage in an animal model.
    b. It is a serotonin-norepinephrine reuptake inhibitor.
    c. It is lipophilic and well absorbed.
    d. It is effective in decreasing SUI episodes in women.
    e. It is not metabolized by the liver.

25. Oral estrogen with or without progesterones in postmenopausal women:
    a. improves mixed urinary incontinence.
    b. worsens the risk of incontinence.
    c. worsens urinary incontinence in women with incontinence.
    d. improves stress urinary incontinence.
    e. improves urgency incontinence.

26. A 75-year old man placed on desmopressin therapy 3 days previously presents with a change of mental status and mental confusion. The most likely cause is:
    a. cognitive dysfunction due to antimuscarinic effect.
    b. hyponatremia.
    c. hypernatremia.
    d. hypokalemia.
    e. hyperkalemia.

27. With regard to bethanechol chloride, the least objective evidence exists to support which of the following statements?
    a. It has relatively selective in vitro action on urinary bladder and bowel.
    b. It has little or no nicotinic action.
    c. It is cholinesterase resistant.
    d. It causes in vitro contraction of bladder and smooth muscle.
    e. It facilitates bladder emptying.

28. What oral dose of bethanechol chloride is required to produce the same urodynamic effects, at least in a denervated bladder, at the subcutaneous dose of 5 mg?
    a. 200 mg
    b. 100 mg
    c. 50 mg
    d. 25 mg
    e. 10 mg

29. Prostaglandins have been hypothesized to affect bladder activity through all of the following actions EXCEPT:
    a. neuromodulation of efferent and afferent neurotransmission.
    b. sensitization to sensory stimuli (activation occurs with a lower degree of filling).
    c. activation of certain sensory nerves.
    d. potentiation of acetylcholine release from cholinergic nerve terminals.
    e. potentiation of adenosine triphosphate release from bladder mucosa.

30. With respect to α- and β – adrenergic receptors in the lower urinary tract and prostate, all the following are true EXCEPT:
    a. α receptors outnumber β receptors in the smooth muscle of the bladder base and proximal urethra.
    b. β receptors outnumber α receptors in the bladder body.
    c. α_1 receptors are more common than α_2.
    d. Lower urinary tract and prostate adrenergically induced smooth muscle contraction is mediated largely by α_1 receptors.
    e. Proximal urethral smooth muscle contraction is mediated primarily by α_1 receptors.

31. Which of the following α-adrenergic blocking agents has significant antagonistic properties at both α_1 and α_2 receptor sites?
    a. Prazosin
    b. Terazosin
    c. Phenoxybenzamine
    d. Doxazosin
    e. Tamsulosin

32. Available data suggest that which of the following side effects is more common with tamsulosin than with either terazosin or doxazosin?
    a. Dizziness
    b. Asthenia
    c. Postural hypotension
    d. Palpitations
    e. Retrograde ejaculation

33. Which of the following agents or classes of agents, when administered systemically, will selectively relax the striated musculature of the pelvic floor?
    a. Benzodiazepines
    b. Dantrolene
    c. Baclofen
    d. Botulinum toxin
    e. None of the above

34. Which of the following is the most widely distributed inhibitory neurotransmitter in the mammalian central nervous system?
    a. γ-Aminobutyric acid (GABA)
    b. Glycine
    c. Glutamate
    d. Dopamine
    e. Norepinephrine

35. Baclofen (Lioresal) acts to decrease striated sphincter activity by which of the following mechanisms?
    a. Facilitating neuronal hyperpolarization through the $GABA_A$ receptor
    b. Activating the $GABA_B$ receptor and depressing monosynaptic and polysynaptic excitation of motor neurons and interneurons in the spinal cord
    c. Inhibiting excitation-contraction coupling in skeletal muscle by decreasing calcium release from the sarcoplasmic reticulum
    d. Inhibiting excitation-contraction coupling by preventing calcium entry into the cell
    e. Inhibiting acetylcholine release at the neuromuscular junction

36. All of the following statements are true with regard to botulinum toxin EXCEPT:
    a. It has been reported to be useful in the treatment of striated sphincter dyssynergia via direct sphincteric injection.
    b. It has been reported to be useful in the treatment of DO by direct intradetrusor injection.
    c. It inhibits the release of acetylcholine and other transmitters at the neuromuscular junction of somatic nerve and striated muscle and the autonomic nerves in smooth muscle.
    d. It has been reported to be of use, via periurethral striated muscle injections, in the treatment of SUI.
    e. The immunologic subtype utilized for urologic use has primarily been type A.

37. All of the following statements are true regarding the action of atropine and atropine-like agents (antimuscarinic agents) in patients with OAB and DO EXCEPT:
    a. Volume to first involuntary contraction increases.
    b. Total bladder capacity increases.
    c. Heart rate decreases.
    d. Urgency episodes decrease.
    e. Amplitude of the DO contractions decreases.

38. Which of the following statements is FALSE with respect to atropine resistance?
    a. It is secondary to release of norepinephrine from pelvic nerve in addition to acetylcholine.
    b. It is of little importance in normal human detrusor function.
    c. Its importance in treatment of DO in humans remains to be established.
    d. It applies to the response of the whole bladder to pelvic nerve stimulation, but not to the response of the detrusor to exogenous cholinergic stimulation.
    e. It is commonly invoked as a cause for only partial clinical improvement in the treatment of OAB with antimuscarinic agents.

39. Which statement is FALSE regarding M_3 receptors?
    a. They are less common than M_2 receptors in detrusor smooth muscle.

b. They are more common than M_2 receptors in urothelium.

c. They are the most important muscarinic receptor for detrusor contraction.

d. They are blocked by atropine.

e. When activated, they lead to an increase in intracellular calcium in detrusor smooth muscle cells.

40. All of the following are well-known potential adverse events of antimuscarinic therapy EXCEPT:

a. constipation.

b. cognitive dysfunction.

c. increased heart rate.

d. blurred vision.

e. hyperhidrosis.

41. Match the side effects with the predominate muscarinic receptor subtype:

    1. M1

    2. M2

    3. M3

    4. M4

    5. M5

    6. None

a. Constipation

b. Dry mouth

c. Cognitive dysfunction

d. Increased heart rate

e. Increased QT interval

42. When used in the usual dosages for the treatment of OAB in a patient who is not on clean intermittent catheterization, antimuscarinic agents act primarily by (more than one response may be correct):

a. reducing detrusor voiding contraction.

b. decreasing activity in C fibers.

c. decreasing activity in Aδ fibers.

d. reducing the micromotions caused by the release of small packets of acetylcholine.

e. reducing excitation of afferent nerves from the urothelium and detrusor.

43. An 80-year old man has OAB-wet and cognitive dysfunction. Theoretically the antimuscarinic drug that would be expected to be the safest with respect to worsening his cognition is:

a. solifenacin.

b. oxybutynin ER.

c. fesoterodine.

d. trospium.

e. tolterodine.

44. Activation of detrusor smooth muscle by both acetylcholine and adenosine triphosphate requires:

a. increase in intracellular potassium concentration.

b. decrease in intracellular potassium concentration.

c. increase in intracellular calcium concentration.

d. increase in intracellular cyclic guanosine monophosphate.

e. increase in intracellular cyclic adenosine monophosphate.

45. Which of the following have 1A or 1B ratings (modified Oxford System) for treatment of DO?

a. Flavoxate

b. Dicyclomine

c. Estrogen

d. Tamsulosin

e. Tolterodine

f. Fesoterodine

g. Darifenacin

h. Solifenacin

i. Propiverine

j. Oxybutynin

k. Trospium

46. Which of the following drugs can produce or aggravate SUI in a woman?

a. Alfuzosin

b. Nifedipine

c. Tamsulosin

d. Oxybutynin

e. Propantheline

f. Flavoxate

g. Fesoterodine

h. Duloxetine

47. Intravesical DMSO is:

a. generally used in a 70% solution.

b. generally used in a 50% solution.

c. useful for the treatment of neurogenic DO.

d. useful for the treatment of bladder pain syndrome (interstitial cystitis).

e. useful for the treatment of idiopathic DO.

48. Regarding the vanilloids, which of the following is/are TRUE?

a. They act primarily to render C fibers insensitive.

b. They act primarily to render Aδ fibers insensitive.

c. When delivered intravesically, they cause a biphasic (excitation then blockade) effect.

d. Resiniferatoxin is much more potent than capsaicin for desensitization but proportionately less so for excitation.

e. Capsaicin is more potent than resiniferatoxin for desensitization.

49. A 30-year-old paraplegic man is wet between intermittent catheterizations (catheterizes five times per day). He is on solifenacin, 10 mg daily, and reports moderate dry mouth and increased difficulty in his bowel regimen. A reasonable next step in treatment is:

a. to increase dose of solifenacin.

b. to add oxybutynin ER, 10 mg daily.

c. to add darifenacin, 7.5 mg daily.

d. to add darifenacin, 15 mg daily.

e. to use intradetrusor botulinum toxin.

50. Generally, treatment with intradetrusor botulinum toxin:

a. must be repeated every 3 to 12 months.

b. improves quality of life in patients incontinent due to neurogenic DO.

c. loses efficacy with repeat treatments.

d. can cause urinary retention.

e. requires general anesthesia.

51. The Heart and Estrogen/Progestin Replacement Study (HERS), Women's Health Initiative, and Nurses' Health Study compositely showed that:

a. oral estrogen plus progesterone worsened urinary incontinence in older postmenopausal women with incontinence.

b. oral estrogen plus progesterone increased the incidence of SUI and urgency urinary incontinence in those continent at baseline.

c. oral estrogen and progesterone worsened the frequency of incontinence in those incontinent at baseline.

d. transvaginal estrogen improves SUI in postmenopausal women.

e. the risk of developing incontinence was increased in postmenopausal women taking estrogen alone or estrogen with progestin.

52. Adrenergically induced smooth muscle contraction in the human lower urinary tract is mediated primarily by which receptor?

a. α_{1D}

b. β_3

c. β_2

d. α_{1A}

e. α_2

ANSWERS

1. **c. Increased outlet resistance.** Atropine and atropine-like agents will depress normal bladder contractions and involuntary bladder contractions of any cause. In such patients, the volume to the first involuntary bladder contraction will generally be increased, the amplitude of the involuntary bladder contraction decreased, and the total bladder capacity increased. Outlet resistance, at least as reflected by urethral pressure measurements, does not seem to be clinically affected.

2. **b. M_2.** On the basis of existing knowledge, it is now recommended that the designations M_1 to M_5 be used to describe both the pharmacologic subtypes and the molecular subtypes of muscarinic acetylcholine receptors. The human urinary bladder smooth muscle contains a mixed population of M_2 and M_3 subtypes, with M_2 receptors predominant (M_2 receptors predominate at least 3:1 versus M_3 receptors not only on detrusor cells but also on other bladder structures, which may be of importance for detrusor activation).

3. **c. M_3.** The minor population of M_3 receptors is generally accepted at this time as primarily responsible for the mediation of bladder contraction.

4. **d. Bradycardia.** In general, drug therapy for lower urinary tract dysfunction is hindered by a concept that can be expressed in one word: uroselectivity. The clinical utility of available antimuscarinic agents is limited by their lack of selectivity, responsible for the classic peripheral antimuscarinic side effects of dry mouth, constipation, blurred vision, tachycardia, and effects on cognitive function.

5. **a, c, and e.** High lipophilicity, small molecular size, and low electrical charge increase the possibilities for an antimuscarinic agent to pass the blood-brain barrier. Quaternary ammonium compounds pass into the central nervous system to a limited extent. Tertiary amines pass the blood brain barrier to a greater extent.

6. **a and d.** The traditional view was that in OAB/detrusor overactivity, antimuscarinics act by blocking the muscarinic receptors on the detrusor muscle that are stimulated by acetylcholine released from the activated cholinergic (parasympathetic) nerves. However, antimuscarinic drugs act mainly during the storage phase of micturition, decreasing urgency and increasing bladder capacity, and during this phase there is normally no parasympathetic input to the lower urinary tract. There is good experimental evidence that antimuscarinics decrease the activity in both C and A delta afferent fibers during the filling/storage phase of micturition.

7. **b. Flavoxate.** A level of 1 implies the presence of systematic reviews, meta-analysis, and good-quality randomized controlled clinical trials. A grade of recommendation of A means that the agent is highly recommended based on level 1 evidence. Flavoxate received a level of evidence of 2, meaning that either randomized control trials and/or good-quality prospective cohort studies existed regarding its use, but a grade of recommendation of D, meaning that no recommendation for use is possible because of inconsistent/inconclusive evidence.

8. **d. Prolongation of the QT interval.** Well-known peripheral antimuscarinic side effects include blurred vision due to accommodation paralysis, constipation due to impaired bowel motility, increase in heart rate due to some blockade of M_2 cardiac receptors, and dry mouth due primarily to blockade of M_3 receptors in the salivary glands. QT prolongation is not related to muscarinic blockade but rather linked to inhibition of the hERG potassium channel in the heart. Some antimuscarinic drugs may in fact cause this, but this is not a class effect.

9. **c. Three; β_3.** Three cloned subtypes of β-adrenergic receptors, β_1, β_2, β_3, have been identified in the detrusor of most species, including humans. Studies have revealed a predominant expression of the β_3 receptor, and there is functional evidence for an important role in both normal and neurogenic bladders. The β_3 agonist mirabegron represents the first drug in this class to be developed for treatment of overactive bladder.

10. **e. Antimuscarinic effect.** Oxybutynin has several pharmacologic effects, some of which seem difficult to relate to its effectiveness in the treatment of DO. It has antimuscarinic, direct muscle relaxant, and local anesthetic actions. The local anesthetic action and direct muscle relaxant effect may be of importance when the drug is administered intravesically but probably play no role when it is given orally. In vitro, oxybutynin was shown to be 500 times weaker as a smooth muscle relaxant than as an antimuscarinic agent. Most probably, when given systematically, oxybutynin acts mainly as an antimuscarinic drug.

11. **d and e.** The M_3 receptor has a primary role in salivation, bowel motility, and visual accommodation. The M_1 receptor is thought to be involved in cognition. The M_2 receptor is the primary cholinergic receptor in the heart, causing bradycardia when activated and, potentially, tachycardia, when blocked. The M_4 and M_5 receptors do not at this time seem to have a primary role in any of these organ systems.

12. **d. Application site reactions.** The transdermal delivery of oxybutynin alters oxybutynin metabolism, reducing production of the primary metabolite, responsible for most of the side effects, to an even greater extent than extended-release oxybutynin. The primary adverse event for this preparation has been application-site reaction: pruritus in 14% and erythema in 8.3%.

13. **a. Darifenacin.** Darifenacin is relatively selective for M_3 receptor blockade, meaning that, in vitro, the affinity for M_3 receptors is greater than for the other muscarinic receptors. This is only a relative selectivity, however, and whether this translates into either greater efficacy or greater tolerability has yet to be established.

14. **a and c.** Mirabegron is a β_3 agonist, the first commercially available and approved drug of its type, approved for the treatment of overactive bladder. It acts not only by stimulating the B_3 receptors in the bladder (causing detrusor relaxation) but also by inhibiting filling induced activity in both mechanosensitive Aδ and C-fiber primary bladder afferents, at least in an animal model.

15. **e. Trospium.** Darifenacin, oxybutynin, solifenacin, and tolterodine are all actively metabolized in the liver by the cytochrome P450 enzyme system. Trospium chloride is not metabolized to any significant degree in the liver. It is actively excreted by the proximal convoluted tubules in the kidney.

16. **a, b, and d.** Tadalafil is a phosphodiesterase (PDE)-5 inhibitor. Phosphodiesterase inhibitors enhance the presumed cyclic adenosine monophosphate (AMP) and cyclic guanosine monophosphate (GMP) relaxation of lower urinary tract smooth muscles as well as blood vessels in the penis. It was originally developed for the treatment of erectile dysfunction and

improved International Index of Erectile Function scores. The observation that patients treated for erectile dysfunction with PDE-5 inhibitors had an improvement of their lower urinary tract symptoms led to interest in use of these drugs to treat LUTS and OAB. PDE-5 inhibitors significantly improve IPSS scores but do not improve peak flow rates compared with placebo. Similarly, they do not change detrusor pressure at peak flow. The mechanism behind the beneficial effect of these substances on LUTS/OAB and their site(s) of action largely remains to be elucidated. They are effective, however, and in fact tadalafil, at the time of this writing, has been approved for the treatment of LUTS due to benign prostatic obstruction.

17. **c. Priapism.** The most frequent side effects of the tricyclic antidepressants are those attributable to their systemic antimuscarinic activity. Allergic phenomena (including rash), hepatic dysfunction, obstructive jaundice, and agranulocytosis may also occur, but rarely. Central nervous system side effects may include weakness, fatigue, parkinsonian effect, fine tremor noted most in the upper extremities, manic or schizophrenic picture, and sedation, probably from an antihistaminic effect. Postural hypotension may also be seen, presumably on the basis of selective blockade (a paradoxic effect) of α_1-adrenergic receptors in some vascular smooth muscle. Tricyclic antidepressants can also cause excess sweating of obscure cause and a delay of orgasm or orgasmic impotence, the cause of which is likewise unclear. They can also produce arrhythmias and interact in deleterious ways with other drugs, and so caution must be observed in their use in patients with cardiac disease. They have not been reported to cause priapism.

18. **e. None of the above.** Several randomized control trials have demonstrated that the combination treatment of antimuscarinic drugs and α_1-adrenergic receptor antagonist is more effective at reducing male lower urinary tract symptoms than α-blockers alone in men with BPO and OAB. Used in the recommended doses, and in men whose voiding was not significantly compromised previously, none of the parameters related to emptying changed appreciably (detrusor pressures, flow rates, residual voided volume).

19. **c and e.** Botulinum toxin-A cleaves SNAP 25 and renders the SNARE complex inactive as its primary mechanism of action. It acts on both striated muscle and smooth muscle and in fact was first studied in striated muscle. It blocks acetylcholine release and reduces firing from bladder afferents. It is effective in both neurogenic and idiopathic DO and also in patients with overactive bladder. Successful OAB treatment does not appear to be related to the existence of DO.

20. **a. Urogenital atrophy.** The evidence supporting the use of estrogens in lower urinary tract dysfunction remains controversial, but considerable data support the use of vaginal estrogen in urogenital atrophy. The vaginal route improves dryness, pruritus, and dyspareunia and provides a greater improvement in physical findings than oral administration.

21. **d. Somnolence.** Potential side effects of all of these agents include blood pressure elevation, anxiety, and insomnia due to stimulation of the central nervous system; headache; tremor; weakness; palpitations; cardiac arrhythmias; and respiratory difficulties. They should be used with caution in patients with hypertension, cardiovascular disease, or hyperthyroidism.

22. **a. Phenylpropanolamine.** The risk of hemorrhagic stroke in women younger than 50 years has been reported to be 16 times higher in those who have been taking phenylpropanolamine, an α-adrenergic agonist, as an appetite suppressant, and three times higher in women who had been taking the drug for less than 24 hours as a cold remedy, although the latter was not statistically significant (the former was). Phenylpropanolamine has been removed from the market in the United States.

23. **b. Propranolol.** Theoretically, β-adrenergic blocking agents, such as propranolol, might be expected to "unmask" or potentiate an α-adrenergic effect, thereby increasing urethral

resistance. Such treatment has been suggested as an alternative treatment to α-adrenergic agonists in patients with sphincteric incontinence and hypertension. Some studies support such usage, but they are not randomized or controlled. The other compounds listed are α-adrenergic agonists and are a risk factor for increased blood pressure.

24. **e. It is not metabolized by the liver.** Duloxetine hydrochloride is a serotonin-norepinephrine reuptake inhibitor that has been shown, in an animal model, to significantly increase urethral sphincteric muscle activity during the filling/storage phase of micturition. It is lipophilic, well absorbed, and extensively metabolized by the liver. It is still approved as a treatment for stress urinary incontinence in some countries. It was withdrawn from the FDA approval process in the United States but is licensed in the European Union for the treatment of SUI in women with moderate to severe incontinence, defined as 15 or more episodes per week.

25. **b and c.** The results of the HERS study, the Women's Health Initiative (WHI) study, and the Nurses' Health Study all suggest that there is no evidence that estrogens with or without progesterone should be used in the treatment of urinary incontinence. In fact, estrogen with or without progesterone increases the risk of urinary incontinence among continent postmenopausal women and worsens urinary incontinence in those already with incontinence.

26. **b. Hyponatremia.** Side effects are relatively uncommon during desmopressin treatment, but there is a risk of water retention and hyponatremia. It is recommended that serum sodium concentration be measured in elderly patients before and after a few days of treatment.

27. **e. It facilitates bladder emptying.** Many acetylcholine-like drugs exist, but only bethanechol chloride (Urecholine, Duvoid, others) exhibits a relatively selective in vitro action on the urinary bladder and gut with little or no nicotinic action. Bethanechol chloride is cholinesterase resistant and causes in vitro contraction of smooth muscle from all areas of the bladder. Although it has been reported to increase gastrointestinal motility and has been used in the treatment of gastroesophageal reflux, and although anecdotal success in specific patients with voiding dysfunction seems to occur, there is no evidence to support its success in facilitating bladder emptying in a series of patients when the drug was the only variable.

28. **a. 200 mg.** It is generally agreed that, at least in a "denervated" bladder, an oral dose of 200 mg is required to produce the same urodynamic effects as a subcutaneous dose of 5 mg.

29. **e. Potentiation of adenosine triphosphate release from bladder mucosa.** Prostanoids are synthesized both locally in bladder muscle and mucosa, with synthesis initiated by various physiologic stimuli such as detrusor muscle stretch, mucosal injury, and neural stimulation; directly by adenosine triphosphate; and by mediators of inflammation. Prostanoids have been variably reported to be useful in facilitating bladder emptying with intravesical administration. Possible roles include (1) neuromodulators of efferent and afferent transmission; (2) sensitization; (3) activation of certain sensory nerves; and (4) potentiation of acetylcholine (but not ATP) release from cholinergic nerve terminals through prejunctional prostanoid receptors.

30. **c. α_1 receptors are more common than α_2.** The human lower urinary tract contains more α_2 than α_1 receptors, but adrenergically induced human lower urinary tract smooth muscle contraction and prostate smooth muscle contraction are mediated largely, if not exclusively, by α_1 adrenergic receptors. The remainder of the statements are true.

31. **c. Phenoxybenzamine.** Phenoxybenzamine (Dibenzyline) was the α-adrenolytic agent originally used for the treatment of voiding dysfunction. It and phentolamine have blocking properties at both α-adrenergic receptor sites. Prazosin hydrochloride (Minipress) was the first potent selective α-adrenergic antagonist

used to lower outlet resistance. Terazosin (Hytrin) and doxazosin (Cardura) are two highly selective postsynaptic α_1-adrenergic blockers. Most recently, alfuzosin and tamsulosin (Flomax), both highly selective α_1-adrenergic blockers, have appeared and are marketed solely for the treatment of benign prostatic hyperplasia because of some reports suggesting preferential action on prostatic rather than vascular smooth muscle.

32. **e. Retrograde ejaculation.** Available data suggest that retrograde ejaculation and rhinitis are more common with tamsulosin, whereas dizziness and asthenia are more common with terazosin and doxazosin.

33. **e. None of the above.** There is no class of pharmacologic agents that will selectively relax the striated musculature of the pelvic floor. Botulinum toxin-A when injected directly into the striated sphincter will relax it, but this "relative selectivity" is because of where it is locally injected.

34. **a. γ-Aminobutyric acid (GABA).** GABA and glycine have been identified as major inhibitory transmitters in the central nervous system. GABA is the most widely distributed inhibitory neurotransmitter in the mammalian central nervous system. It appears to mediate the inhibitory actions of local interneurons in the brain and presynaptic inhibition within the spinal cord.

35. **b. Activating the GABA$_B$ receptor and depressing monosynaptic and polysynaptic excitation of motor neurons and interneurons in the spinal cord.** Benzodiazepines potentiate the action of GABA by facilitating neuronal hyperpolarization through the GABA$_A$ receptor. Baclofen (Lioresal) depresses monosynaptic and polysynaptic excitation of motor neurons and interneurons in the spinal cord by activating GABA$_B$ receptors. Dantrolene (Dantrium) exerts its effects by a direct peripheral action on skeletal muscle. It is thought to inhibit the excitation-induced release of calcium ions from the sarcoplasmic reticulum of striated muscle fibers, thereby inhibiting excitation-contraction coupling and diminishing the mechanical force of contraction. Botulinum A toxin (Botox) is an inhibitor of acetylcholine release at the neuromuscular junction of somatic nerves on striated muscle.

36. **d. It has been reported to be of use, via periurethral striated muscle injections, in the treatment of SUI.** Intrasphincteric injection of botulinum toxin A was first reported useful in the treatment of striated sphincteric dyssynergia in 1990. The toxin blocks the release of acetylcholine and other transmitters from presynaptic nerve endings by interacting with the protein complex necessary for docking vesicles. This results in decreased muscle contractility and muscle atrophy at the injection site. The drug has been reported to be of use as well in the treatment of neurogenic DO and cases of non-neurogenic DO. There are seven immunologically distinct antigenic subtypes. Types A and B are in clinical use in urology, but most studies and treatments have been carried out with botulinum toxin type A (Botox). Intrasphincteric injections of botulinum toxin are not useful for SUI. In fact, they can cause SUI in females.

37. **c. Heart rate decreases.** Those with an M$_2$ receptor blockade profile can increase heart rate, but the clinical significance of this is unknown.

38. **a. It is secondary to release of norepinephrine from pelvic nerve in addition to acetylcholine.** The most common neurotransmitter mentioned as the prime alternate in atropine resistance is adenosine triphosphate. Norepinephrine is released by postganglionic sympathetic nerves (e.g., hypogastric), not by parasympathetic ones (e.g., pelvic).

39. **b. They are more common than M$_2$ receptors in urothelium.** M$_2$ receptors outnumber M$_3$ in urothelium as well as detrusor smooth muscle. All other statements are true.

40. **e. hyperhidrosis.** If anything, antimuscarinic agents can cause decreased sweating. All the others are antimuscarinic side effects.

41. **a: 3; b: 3; c: 1; d: 2; e: 6.** Increased QT interval, caused by some antimuscarinic compounds, is not an antimuscarinic property. All the others are and are caused primarily by blockade of the indicated receptor subtype.

42. **b, c, d, and e.** At the dose employed for OAB treatment, antimuscarinic agents do not cause significant reduction in the voiding contraction of voluntary micturition. They have been implicated in all the others. C and Aδ fibers refer to afferent nerves carrying noxious and "normal" stimuli, respectively.

43. **d. Trospium.** Trospium, as a quaternary amine, is lipophobic and does not penetrate well through the blood-brain barrier. The others, all tertiary amines, do pass the blood-brain barrier to a greater extent.

44. **c. Increase in intracellular calcium concentration.** This occurs through both extracellular influx and mobilization of intracellular calcium.

45. **e, f, g, h, i, j, and k.** Propiverine is a drug with "mixed action" and currently is not available in the United States but is in Europe.

46. **a and c.** The α-adrenergic antagonists can decrease outlet resistance and thereby irritate or worsen SUI. Nifedipine is a calcium antagonist; fesoterodine and propantheline are anticholinergic agents; duloxetine is a serotonin-norepinephrine reuptake inhibitor; oxybutynin is primarily an antimuscarinic agent with some direct smooth muscle relaxant effects on the bladder; and flavoxate has mixed actions and questionable effects.

47. **b and d.** DMSO is a naturally occurring compound with multiple pharmacologic actions used in a 50% solution for the treatment of bladder pain syndrome (including interstitial cystitis). It is not useful for the treatment of DO.

48. **a, c, and d.** It is possible that vanilloids have some effects on Aδ fibers as well. They cause an initial excitation followed by a long-lasting blockade. Resiniferatoxin is 1000 times more potent than capsaicin for desensitization and a few hundred times more potent for excitation.

49. **e. To use intradetrusor botulinum toxin.** Adding or increasing antimuscarinic medication will simply increase the severity of the adverse events already experienced. Intradetrusor botulinum toxin has been shown to be very effective in neurogenic DO and should be considered if following failure of, or intolerance to, antimuscarinic therapy.

50. **a, b, and d.** Repeat injections (two to nine) have not lost efficacy over time. The injections can be done without general anesthesia (local). Intravesical botulinum toxin A is effective in reducing neurogenic DO and does improve quality of life in such patients.

51. **a, b, c, and e.** a is from the Heart and Estrogen/Progestin Replacement Study, b and c from the Women's Health Initiative, and e from the Nurses' Health Study. Although many clinicians prescribe transvaginal estrogen or estrogen plus progestin cream for symptoms of OAB or/and SUI, there is no real evidence that estrogen, with or without progesterone, is useful in the treatment of urinary incontinence.

52. **d. α$_{1A}$.** More α$_2$ than α$_1$ receptors are present, but adrenergically induced contraction is mediated largely by the α$_{1A}$ (and in the detrusor, α$_{1D}$). β receptors cause smooth muscle relaxation. The β$_3$ subtype is the predominant β receptor in the human detrusor.

CHAPTER REVIEW

1. The major neurohumoral stimulus for physiologic bladder contraction is acetylcholine-induced stimulation of postganglionic parasympathetic muscarinic cholinergic receptor sites in the bladder.
2. The muscarinic receptor functions may be changed in different urologic disorders without an overt neurogenic cause.
3. Behavioral therapy should always be used in conjunction with drug therapy for OAB.
4. Calcium channel antagonists are not effective in treating OAB.
5. Potassium channel openers available today are not effective in treating OAB.
6. The use of estrogens to treat SUI has resulted in worsening of preexisting urinary incontinence in patients with SUI and urgency urinary incontinence and new-onset incontinence in patients who have not had it. The use of vaginal estrogen in the treatment of urogenital atrophy improves dryness, pruritus, dyspareunia, and physical findings. The vaginal route is more effective than oral administration.
7. Intravesical oxybutynin has shown some efficacy in treating OAB as well as in treating intestinal augmented OABs.
8. Antimuscarinics may have effects on cognitive function, particularly in the elderly.
9. Antimuscarinics may be divided into tertiary and quaternary amines. The latter are not well absorbed and have limited ability to enter the central nervous system, unlike the tertiary amines.
10. Antimuscarinics may have adverse cardiac effects.
11. α_1-adrenergic blockers are not effective in women.
12. The human urinary bladder smooth muscle contains a mixed population of M_2 and M_3 subtypes, with M_2 receptors predominant (M_2 receptors predominant at least 3:1 versus M_3). M_3 receptors are primarily responsible for the mediation of bladder contraction.
13. Mirabegron is a β_3 agonist, the first commercially available drug of its type approved for the treatment of overactive bladder.
14. PDE-5 inhibitors significantly improve IPSS scores but do not improve peak flow rates when compared with placebo.
15. Urinary tract smooth muscle contraction and prostate smooth muscle contraction are mediated largely, if not exclusively, by α_1-adrenergic receptors.

80

Conservative Management of Urinary Incontinence: Behavioral and Pelvic Floor Therapy, Urethral and Pelvic Devices

Diane K. Newman and Kathryn L. Burgio

QUESTIONS

1. A person with cognitive impairment may not be a candidate for which behavioral interventions?
   a. Prompted voiding
   b. Timed voiding
   c. Bladder training
   d. Habit training

2. A bladder diary is integral to behavioral therapy because it can:
   a. determine functional bladder capacity.
   b. provide information about symptom improvement.
   c. determine adherence to pelvic floor muscle training.
   d. provide understanding of patient's voiding pattern.
   e. b and d.

3. Which of the following statements is TRUE about pelvic floor muscle training?
   a. Pelvic floor muscle training is effective for treating stress, urge, or mixed incontinence in men and women of any age.
   b. Pelvic floor muscle training is appropriate for stress or mixed incontinence, but not for urge incontinence.
   c. Pelvic floor muscle training works for women, but not for men.
   d. Pelvic floor muscle training is not effective for older people.
   e. Pelvic floor muscle training is only useful for mild-moderate incontinence, but not severe incontinence.

4. When teaching the urge suppression technique, patients are encouraged to:
   a. stay near a bathroom as much as possible, so they won't have far to go when they feel an urge to void.
   b. stay away from the bathroom until they feel an urge to void. Then get to the bathroom as soon as possible.
   c. stay away from the bathroom until they feel the urge to void. Then stay still and wait until the urge has passed before going to the bathroom.
   d. wait as long as possible to go to the bathroom to increase bladder capacity.

5. When patients are trying to calm down urgency and prevent leakage, which of the following works BEST?
   a. Crossing the legs
   b. Squeezing the pelvic floor muscles (PFMs) while rushing to the bathroom
   c. Squeezing the PFMs while sitting still until the urgency goes away, then walking to the bathroom
   d. Relaxing the pelvic floor muscles to help relax the bladder

6. When using fluid management as a treatment for urgency incontinence, patients are told to:
   a. consume a normal amount of fluid to avoid dehydration as well as sudden urgency.

   b. increase fluid intake to ensure adequate hydration and train the bladder.
   c. decrease fluid intake to minimize bladder filling.
   d. increase fluid intake to prevent the loss of functional bladder capacity

7. When attempting to reduce dietary bladder irritants, patients should be told to:
   a. avoid spicy foods, tomatoes, and citrus fruits.
   b. eliminate caffeine.
   c. keep a diary to see which foods or beverages increase urgency.
   d. all of the above.

8. When conducting PFM training, clinicians should:
   a. ensure that patients are contracting the PFMs selectively.
   b. prescribe a specific set of exercises for the patients to do each day.
   c. teach patients to contract PFMs whenever they engage in activities that precipitate leakage.
   d. all of the above.

9. Which of the following statements is TRUE of caffeine reduction as a lifestyle modification for the treatment of incontinence?
   a. Patients should be told to eliminate caffeine gradually.
   b. Patients should be encouraged to try eliminating caffeine for a few days to see how it affects their bladder.
   c. Patients should be encouraged to reduce caffeine gradually.
   d. Patients should be advised to eliminate coffee only, as it the main source of caffeine.

ANSWERS

1. **c. Bladder training.** Bladder training is an example of "patient-dependent" interventions: It relies on active patient participation. There must be adequate function, learning capability, and motivation of the individual. Bladder training involves patient education regarding lower urinary tract function, setting incremental voiding schedules, and teaching urge control techniques to help patients postpone voiding and adhere to the schedule.

2. **e. b and d.** A bladder diary provides information on the type and amount of fluid intake, type and frequency of symptoms such as incontinence episodes, frequency of urination, the urgency associated with each, and the circumstances or reasons for incontinence episodes, which helps the provider plan appropriate components of behavioral intervention. A bladder diary is also the best noninvasive tool available to objectively monitor the patient's voiding habits and the effect of treatment on symptoms guiding the use of various treatment components.

3. **a. Pelvic floor muscle training is effective for treating stress, urge, or mixed incontinence in men and women of any age.** Behavioral interventions are well established for treating stress and urgency urinary incontinence and overactive bladder. Because behavioral treatments are effective and essentially risk free, they

are the mainstay of conservative treatment and are recommended by several guidelines and consensus panels as first-line therapy for both men and women of all ages.

4. **c. Stay away from the bathroom until they feel the urge to void. Then stay still and wait until the urge has passed before going to the bathroom.** Patients are taught not to feel compelled to rush to the nearest bathroom when they feel the urge to void, believing that they are about to lose control. With behavioral training, they learn how this natural "gotta go" response is actually counterproductive, because it increases physical pressure on the bladder, increases the feeling of fullness, exacerbates urgency, and triggers detrusor contraction. Further, while the patient approaches the toilet, visual cues can trigger urgency and incontinence. To avoid this conditioned response, patients are taught not to rush to the bathroom when they feel the urge to void. Instead, they are advised to stay away from the bathroom, so as to avoid exposure to cues that trigger urgency. They are taught strategies to suppress urgency before walking to the toilet.

5. **c. Squeezing the PFM while sitting still until the urgency goes away, then walking to the bathroom.** Patients are taught not to rush to the bathroom when they feel the urge to void. Instead, they are advised to stay away from the bathroom, so as to avoid exposure to cues that trigger urgency. They are encouraged to pause, sit down if possible, relax the entire body, and contract PFMs repeatedly, without relaxing in between contractions, to diminish urgency, inhibit detrusor contraction, and prevent urine loss. They focus on inhibiting the urge sensation, giving it time to pass. Once the sensation subsides, they walk at a normal pace to the toilet.

6. **a. Consume a normal amount of fluid to avoid dehydration as well as sudden urgency.** Fluid intake modifications depend on the patients' pattern of intake, which can be assessed by asking each patient to complete a 24- to 48-hour diary of intake and output, including voided volumes when possible. Reviewing such a diary can reveal excessive fluid intake, inadequate fluid intake, and diurnal patterns of intake that may be contributing to lower urinary tract symptoms. Although it may seem counterintuitive, it is usually good advice to encourage patients to consume at least six 8-ounce glasses of fluid each day to maintain adequate hydration. Fluid intake should be regulated to six to eight 8-ounce glasses or 30 mL/kg body weight per day with a 1500 mL/day minimum at designated times, unless contraindicated by a medical condition. The Institute of Medicine issued a report in 2004 with guidelines for total water intake for healthy people.

7. **c. Keep a diary to see which foods or beverages increase urgency.** A diary of food and beverage intake is useful for identifying which substances are in fact irritants for individual patients; a trial period of eliminating these substances one at a time can be used to confirm the relationship.

8. **d. All of the above.** It is important to verify that patients have identified and can contract the PFMs properly before initiating an exercise regimen. Specific exercise regimens vary considerably in frequency and intensity, and the ideal exercise regimen has not yet been determined. However, good results have been achieved in several trials with the use of 45 to 60 paired contractions and relaxations per day. We use an "exercise prescription" to prescribe the daily exercise program. It is important to teach patients how to prevent urine loss in daily life by occluding the urethra by using active contraction of PFMs. Although exercise alone can improve urethral pressure and structural support and reduce incontinence, this motor skill enables patients to consciously occlude the urethra at specific times when urine loss is imminent. A careful history or examination of a bladder diary can alert the provider and patient of the circumstances during which each individual patient commonly experiences urine loss. Patients then learn to anticipate these activities and prevent leakage by contracting the PFMs to occlude the urethra prior to and during coughing, sneezing, lifting, or any other physical activities that have precipitated urine leakage.

9. **b. Patients should be encouraged to try eliminating caffeine for a few days to see how it affects their bladder.** Many patients are reluctant initially to forgo their caffeine-containing products, but they may be convinced to try it for a short period of time, such as 3 to 5 days, to determine whether they are sensitive to its effects. If they experience relief from their symptoms, they are often more willing to reduce or eliminate caffeine from their diet.

CHAPTER REVIEW

1. When conservative measures are used to treat voiding dysfunction, improvement is gradual.
2. Contracting certain abdominal muscles when performing pelvic floor muscle training can be counterproductive.
3. Well-timed contractions of the external urethral sphincter can abort a detrusor contraction, defer a contraction, and suppress the sensation of urgency.
4. Patients who retain fluid during the day may benefit from support stockings, daytime elevation of the legs, and selective late-afternoon use of a diuretic to reduce nighttime voiding.
5. Caffeine is a diuretic and bladder irritant.
6. Dietary bladder irritants include caffeine, sugar substitutes, citrus fruits, highly spiced foods, and tomato products.
7. Constipation may play a significant role in voiding dysfunction.
8. Obesity is a risk factor for urinary incontinence.
9. A bladder diary is the best noninvasive tool available to objectively monitor the patient's voiding habits and the effect of treatment on symptoms guiding the use of various treatment components.
10. It is important to verify that patients have identified and can contract the pelvic floor muscles properly before initiating an exercise regimen.

81 Electrical Stimulation and Neuromodulation in Storage and Emptying Failure

Sandip P. Vasavada and Raymond R. Rackley

QUESTIONS

1. The current approved indications for sacral neuromodulation include all of the following EXCEPT:
   a. urinary urgency.
   b. urinary frequency.
   c. urgency urinary incontinence.
   d. interstitial cystitis.
   e. idiopathic nonobstructive urinary retention.

2. Which patient is NOT well suited for current neuromodulation therapies?
   a. A 65-year-old insulin-dependent diabetic man with bladder areflexia and nonobstructive urinary retention
   b. A 67-year-old woman who has had a cerebrovascular accident and now has urinary urgency and frequency
   c. A 41-year-old woman with urgency urinary incontinence
   d. A 55-year-old woman who has had vaginal sling surgery and urgency urinary incontinence
   e. A 36-year-old woman with a history of interstitial cystitis with minimal pain who voids between 20 and 25 times per day

3. What reflex or reflexes are responsible for modulation of bladder function?
   a. Guarding
   b. Bladder afferent loop
   c. Bladder bladder
   d. Bladder urethral
   e. a and b

4. Which of the following is(are) considered the major clinical concern(s) associated with performing a sacral rhizotomy?
   a. Pelvic pain
   b. Creation of bladder areflexia
   c. Abnormal sexual function
   d. Pelvic and lower extremity sensory or motor abnormalities
   e. c and d

5. The S3 sensory and motor response pattern to electrical stimulation is best described as having which one of the following?
   a. Plantarflexion of the entire foot with sensation in the leg and buttock
   b. Levator reflex (bellows reflex) and sensations in the leg and buttock
   c. Dorsiflexion of the great toe and bellows reflex and pulling sensation in the rectum, scrotum, or vagina
   d. Plantarflexion of the first three toes of the foot and sensation of pulling in the rectum or vagina
   e. Bellows reflex (levator contraction) and sensation of pulling of the rectum

6. What is the main concern when performing magnetic resonance imaging (MRI) in the setting of neuromodulation and pacemaker-type devices?
   a. Potential of dislodgement of the pacemaker
   b. Heating of the electrical leads
   c. Heating of the pacemaker
   d. Potentially fatal arrhythmias
   e. Significant neuromuscular injury risk

7. Which of the following represents the best clinical scenario for use of neuromodulation therapy in a patient with multiple sclerosis (MS)?
   a. Detrusor sphincter dyssynergy
   b. Bedridden with significant functional incontinence
   c. Mild symptoms with no potential need for future MRI
   d. A poorly compliant bladder
   e. Areflexic bladder

8. What skeletal landmarks are associated with the S3 nerve foramen?
   a. 9 cm from the tip of the coccyx
   b. 11 cm from the tip of the coccyx
   c. 13 cm from the tip of the coccyx
   d. The inferior aspect of the sacral iliac joints
   e. a and d

9. Perhaps the main reason why neuromodulation devices are not currently approved for use in the United States by the Food and Drug Administration in pediatric patients is due to:
   a. lack of efficacy.
   b. potential worsening of neuromuscular function due to bony abnormalities (spina bifida and myelomeningocele).
   c. lack of data on growth of the spinal cord and nerve roots in the setting of neuromodulation devices.
   d. worsening of bowel function (Hinman bladder syndrome).
   e. excellent results with noninvasive therapies (transcutaneous electrical nerve stimulation) and therefore no reason to perform more invasive sacral neuromodulation in the long term.

10. The best option for a patient who has undergone a failed stage I sacral neuromodulation for severe refractory urgency urinary incontinence (Medtronic [Minneapolis, MN] InterStim stage I) is:
    a. anticholinergic therapy.
    b. bilateral stimulation.
    c. radical cystectomy and ileal conduit.
    d. vaginal sling procedure.
    e. bladder augmentation.

11. Which of the following statements is FALSE about the dorsal genital nerve?

    a. Specific branches include the dorsal nerve of the penis in males and clitoral nerve in females.

    b. It is an afferent nerve that carries sensory information.

    c. Proximally, it carries sensory information from the hypogastric nerve.

    d. It is a pure sensory afferent nerve branch of the pudendal nerve.

    e. It has been proposed as a contributor to the pudendal pelvic nerve reflex.

12. An implantable pulse generator (IPG) infection would be best treated by:

    a. intravenous antibiotics.

    b. oral antibiotics.

    c. irrigation of the pocket.

    d. removal of the entire device.

    e. a and b.

13. Which of the following statements about impedances is FALSE?

    a. Impedance is best described as the resistance of flow of electrons through a circuit.

    b. If there is too much resistance, no current will flow (open).

    c. If there is too little resistance, excessive current will flow.

    d. If there is a broken circuit, electrons cannot flow, and this will result in low impedance measurements.

    e. Unipolar measurements are most useful for identifying open circuits during impedance testing.

14. Which of the following statements is FALSE about the Brindley device?

    a. It requires intact neuron pathways between the sacral cord and nuclei, pelvic nerve, and bladder to function.

    b. It works best in a state of long-term areflexic bladder function.

    c. It is used most often in patients with insufficient or nonreflex micturition after spinal cord injury.

    d. It is usually coupled with sacral posterior rhizotomy.

    e. Electrodes are applied extradurally to S2, S3, and S4 nerve roots.

15. Direct electrical stimulation of the bladder often results in all of the following EXCEPT:

    a. pelvic musculature contraction.

    b. erection.

    c. defecation.

    d. bladder neck opening.

    e. ejaculation.

16. Which one of the following statements regarding the use of the Brindley device is FALSE?

    a. It requires intact neural pathways between the sacral cord and the bladder.

    b. Sacral posterior rhizotomy is generally performed.

    c. Myogenic decompensation is a contraindication.

    d. Electrodes are applied extradurally to sacral roots S2 to S4.

    e. It utilizes the principle of poststimulation voiding.

17. Which of the following statements regarding neurostimulation or neuromodulation is FALSE?

    a. The desired effect of neurostimulation is through direct stimulation of nerves and muscles.

    b. Neurostimulation is mainly reserved for neurogenic conditions.

    c. Neurostimulation produces a delayed clinical response.

    d. The effect of neuromodulation is achieved through alteration of neurotransmission processes.

    e. Neuromodulation may be useful for neurogenic as well as non-neurogenic conditions.

18. Which of the following studies is (are) the most useful in predicting which patients will or will not respond to sacral neuromodulation?

    a. Uroflow/postvoid residual monitoring

    b. Voiding diary

    c. Urodynamics/electromyography

    d. Percutaneous lead placement and trial stimulation

    e. c and d

19. Which of the following is(are) relative clinical contraindications for excluding potential candidates for neuromodulation and neurostimulation therapies?

    a. Patients with significant anatomic abnormalities in the spine or sacrum that may present challenges to gaining access

    b. Patients who cannot manage their devices or judge the clinical outcomes due to mental incapacitation

    c. Patients with physical limitations that prevent them from achieving normal pelvic organ function such as functional urinary incontinence

    d. Patients who are noncompliant

    e. All of the above

20. Which of the following statements best characterizes bilateral S3 nerve root stimulation for sacral neuromodulation therapy?

    a. It is a rational consideration for salvage therapy or added benefit as the bladder receives bilateral innervation.

    b. It is an approach alternative to failed unilateral stimulation in patients with urinary retention.

    c. Initial basis for this approach produced in spinal cord–injured animal models suggests this may be a potential approach in humans.

    d. All of the above.

    e. a and c only.

21. Potential sites of selective nerve stimulation other than the S3 sacral root for neuromodulation therapies for pelvic health conditions include which of the following?

    a. S4 sacral root

    b. Pudendal nerve

    c. Dorsal genital nerve

    d. Posterior tibial nerve

    e. All of the above

22. When troubleshooting the complication of IPG site discomfort or pain, which of the following statements best describes the necessary action(s) needed?

    a. Rule out IPG site infection by physical examination.

    b. Turn off the device and ask the patient if the discomfort is still present to differentiate IPG pocket site issues from IPG electrical output-related causes.

    c. If the IPG discomfort is output related, check whether bipolar stimulation is better than unipolar stimulation.

    d. If IPG site discomfort is output related, check impedances because a current leak may be present from the neuroelectrode to extension lead connection.

    e. All of the above.

23. When patients report recurrent symptoms after reduction or improvement of symptoms with sacral neuromodulation therapy, which of the following should be undertaken to evaluate the reason for the loss of clinical efficacy?

    a. Check the device settings for inadvertent on/off changes and battery performance.

    b. Evaluate the stimulation perception and anatomic localization for changes.

    c. Check for intermittent stimulation perception via positional changes of the patient because this may suggest lead migration or a loose lead connection.

    d. Obtain a radiograph to detect macro changes in the neuroelectrode position if findings in b and c are evident.

    e. All of the above.

ANSWERS

1. **d. Interstitial cystitis.** Although used commonly for interstitial cystitis (IC) symptoms, urgency/frequency IC is not truly an indication for the sacral neuromodulation devices. Several groups have seen benefits of sacral neuromodulation in IC patients, and there may be an expanding indication for this in the future.

2. **a. A 65-year-old insulin-dependent diabetic man with bladder areflexia and nonobstructive urinary retention.** It is implied that the end organ response (bladder in this case) should have good function for sacral neuromodulation and, for that matter, any form of neuromodulation to work. Neurostimulation may be different, but even if neurostimulation were used, simultaneous relaxation of the outlet would be required for a coordinated contraction and emptying phase to ensue.

3. **e. a and b.** Two important reflexes may play an important role in modulation of bladder function: the guarding reflex and the bladder afferent loop reflex. Both reflexes promote urine storage under sympathetic tone. The guarding reflex guards or prevents urine loss from times of cough or other physical stress that would normally trigger a micturition episode. Suprapontine input from the brain turns off the guarding reflex during micturition to allow efficient and complete emptying. The bladder afferent reflex works through sacral interneurons that then activate storage through pudendal nerve efferent pathways directed toward the urethral sphincter. Similar to the guarding reflex, the bladder afferent reflex promotes continence during periods of bladder filling and is quiet during micturition.

4. **e. c and d.** Bilateral anterior and posterior sacral rhizotomy or conusectomy converts a hyperreflexic bladder to an areflexic one. This alone may be inappropriate therapy because it also adversely affects the rectum, anal and urethral sphincters, sexual function, and the lower extremities. In an attempt to leave sphincter and sexual function intact, selective motor nerve section was originally introduced as a treatment to increase bladder capacity by abolishing only the motor supply responsible for involuntary contractions.

5. **c. Dorsiflexion of the great toe and bellows reflex and pulling sensation in the rectum, scrotum, or vagina.** The characteristic response of the S3 nerve distribution based on its lower innervation is to the levator musculature (bellows contraction) of the anus and ipsilateral great toe contraction. The other answers suggest either S2 stimulation (leg rotation) or S4 levator contraction.

6. **b. Heating of the electrical leads.** Although many concerns exist for MRI and pacemaker devices, it has been shown that the main concern is heating of the electrical leads. This may, in turn, traumatize blood vessels, nerve roots, or other structures that the leads themselves are next to. Currently, MRI is contraindicated in the presence of a pacemaker.

7. **c. Mild symptoms with no potential need for future MRI.** It is unknown whether subcategories of MS patients (delayed emptying/storage dysfunction, areflexia, poor compliance) would be very good candidates for sacral neuromodulation, although it is doubtful based on disease severity alone. A mildly symptomatic patient without functional issues (e.g., can get to the bathroom in time with no major mobility issues) probably would be the best patient.

8. **e. a and d.** The measurements for the rough vicinity of the S3 nerve foramen have been tested by using the "cross hair" technique (Chai et al, 2000)* and simple measurements. The answers b and c are incorrect because they represent measurements from the anal verge (11 cm), and 13 cm is too far in general from the coccyx and would likely place one near S2 or S1.

9. **c. Lack of data on growth of the spinal cord and nerve roots in the setting of neuromodulation devices.** Pediatric patients have undergone sacral neuromodulation in off-label trials, but large-scale use has been limited by lack of data on the growth of the pediatric patient and the relation of the sacral lead with regard to the sacral nerve roots, and so on. Although noninvasive therapies have worked, they are limited by the need for continued repeat therapy to maintain durability of result.

10. **e. Bladder augmentation.** The patient should have tried and failed anticholinergic therapy before having the sacral neuromodulation therapy. Scheepens and coworkers have shown that bilateral stimulation, although logical, has not been shown in urgency incontinent patients to lead to much improvement (Scheepens et al, 2002). One could argue that contralateral lead placement should be attempted, but no prospective trials have shown that this makes a difference in outcomes. The vaginal sling procedure and radical cystectomy are not indicated per se in this condition (the vaginal sling is for stress urinary incontinence, and cystectomy is too radical).

11. **c. Proximally, it carries sensory information from the hypogastric nerve.** The dorsal genital nerve is a terminal branch of the pudendal nerve and is being investigated for functional neuromodulation outcomes via a percutaneous approach. It does not carry information directly from the hypogastric nerve.

12. **d. Removal of the entire device.** Because an IPG is a foreign body, it could harbor bacteria within a biofilm created by the infection. Accordingly, it is best to have it removed in its entirety. Antibiotics and irrigation for the most part are temporizing measures. Furthermore, there is risk of an infection tracking along the sacral lead, which may create a sacral infection.

13. **d. If there is a broken circuit, electrons cannot flow, and this will result in low impedance measurements.** Impedance describes the resistance to the flow of electrons through a circuit. Impedance or resistance is an integral part of any functioning circuit; however, if there is too much resistance, no current will flow (open). If there is too little resistance, excessive current flow resulting in diminished battery longevity occurs (short). If the circuit is broken somehow, electrons cannot flow. This is called an "open" circuit, and impedance measurements are high. Open circuits can be caused by a fractured lead or extension wires, loose connections, and so on.

14. **b. It works best in a state of long-term areflexic bladder function.** The chief applications of the Brindley device are in patients with inefficient or nonreflex micturition after spinal cord injury. Prerequisites for use are described by Fischer et al (1993) as the following: (1) intact neural pathways between the sacral cord nuclei of the pelvic nerve and the bladder and (2) a bladder that is capable of contracting.

15. **d. Bladder neck opening.** The spread of current to other pelvic structures the stimulus thresholds of which are lower than that of the bladder has often resulted in (1) abdominal, pelvic, and perineal pain; (2) a desire to defecate or defecation; (3) contraction of the pelvic and leg muscles; and (4) erection and ejaculation in males. It has also been noted that the increase in intravesical pressure was generally not coordinated with bladder neck opening or with pelvic floor relaxation and that other measures to accomplish voiding may be necessary.

---

*Sources referenced can be found in *Campbell-Walsh Urology, 11th Edition,* on the Expert Consult website.

16. **d. Electrodes are applied extradurally to sacral roots S2 to S4.** Prerequisites for such use were described in one study as (1) intact neural pathways between the sacral cord nuclei of the pelvic nerve and the bladder and (2) a bladder that is capable of contracting. The chief application is in patients with inefficient or no reflex micturition after spinal cord injury. Simultaneous bladder and striated sphincter stimulation is obviated by sacral posterior rhizotomy, usually complete, which also (1) eliminates reflex incontinence and (2) improves low bladder compliance, if present. Electrodes are applied intradurally to the S2, S3, and S4 roots, but the pairs can be activated independently. The current Brindley stimulator uses the principle of *poststimulus voiding*, a term first introduced by Jonas and Tanagho (1975). Relaxation time of the striated sphincter after a stimulus train is shorter than the relaxation time of the detrusor smooth muscle. Therefore, when interrupted pulse trains instead of continuous stimulus trains are used, poststimulus voiding is achieved between the pulse trains because of the higher sustained intravesical pressure when compared with the striated sphincter.

17. **c. Neurostimulation produces a delayed clinical response.** In neurostimulation, the use of electrical stimuli on nerves and muscles has mainly been developed for achieving immediate clinical responses in neurogenic conditions of pelvic organ dysfunction, whereas in neuromodulation, the use of electrical stimuli to nerves has been developed for altering neurotransmission processes in cases of non-neurogenic as well as neurogenic conditions.

18. **d. Percutaneous lead placement and trial stimulation.** Despite all the studies done to date, there are no defined preclinical factors such as urodynamic findings that can predict which patients will or will not have a response to sacral neuromodulation. Thus, a trial of stimulation via a temporary or percutaneous lead placement is the best predictor of long-term clinical responsiveness.

19. **e. All of the above.** Whereas most patients who have failed more conservative therapies are considered candidates for neurostimulation and neuromodulation therapies, all of the above clinical considerations for excluding patients from this therapy should be considered. Furthermore, relative contraindications for patients who may be considering or who have an implantable electrical stimulation device are the issues of MRI and pregnancy.

20. **d. All of the above.** Bilateral stimulation has been suggested as an alternative, particularly in failed unilateral lead placements, for potential salvage or added benefit as the bladder receives bilateral innervation. The initial basis to consider bilateral stimulation was based on animal studies demonstrating that bilateral stimulation yielded a more profound effect on bladder inhibition than did unilateral stimulation. Only one clinical study has been performed to demonstrate the potential differences in unilateral versus bilateral stimulation (Scheepens et al, 2002). This study showed no significant difference in outcomes for unilateral versus bilateral stimulation with regard to urgency urinary incontinence, frequency, or severity of leakage in the overactive bladder group, although, overall, results were impressive in both categories. The patients in the retention group had better parameters of emptying (volume per void) in bilateral as compared with unilateral stimulation.

21. **e. All of the above.** The introduction of new stimulation methods as well as application of these methods to all the different nerve locations listed will continue to provide improved treatment alternatives, as shown in animal models and human applications. In addition, these innovations will provide the ability to further develop testable hypotheses of more basic questions on electrical neurostimulation, neuromodulation, and neurophysiology of the autonomic, somatic, and central pathways that regulate pelvic organ function.

22. **e. All of the above.** The probable causes of IPG site discomfort or pain are IPG pocket related or IPG output related. Pocket-related causes of discomfort include infection, pocket location (waistline), pocket dimension (too tight, too loose), seroma, and erosion. One should turn off the IPG and determine if the discomfort is still present to differentiate pocket-related from output-related cause. If the discomfort is persistent, the cause is not related to the IPG electrical output. In the absence of clinical signs of infection, IPG pocket-related causes such as pocket size, seroma, and erosion should be considered. If the discomfort disappears, the IPG electrical output is likely causing discomfort or pain. Output-related causes include sensitivity to unipolar stimulation if this mode is used or a current leak as demonstrated by abnormal impedances.

23. **e. All of the above.** When the patient presents with recurrent symptoms, one should evaluate the stimulation perception. The possibilities are that the patient perceives the stimulation in a wrong location as compared with baseline, has no stimulation, or has intermittent stimulation based on lead migration or mechanical issues related to a loose connection or elevated impedances.

CHAPTER REVIEW

1. The mechanism of neuromodulation may be activation of neurons that cause inhibition at spinal and supraspinal levels.
2. For neuromodulation to work, there must be at least some communication between sacral outflow and the pontine micturition center so as to allow for processing of reflexes that may be inhibited by the brain.
3. Neuromodulation has been used in fecal incontinence and constipation as well as bladder dysfunction.
4. Suppression of interneuronal transmission in the bladder reflex may be how sacral neuromodulation affects detrusor overactivity.
5. The detrusor is usually innervated primarily by S3; rectal stimulation occurs in S2, S3, and S4; and erectile stimulation is mainly a function of S2.
6. Transcutaneous electrical stimulation demonstrates good efficacy but has a limited role because of the constant need to administer the therapy.
7. Sympathetic tone, for the most part, is dominant for the majority of time and provides for continence and storage of urine; parasympathetic stimulation results in a detrusor contraction and emptying of the bladder.
8. There are no preclinical factors that can predict which patients will or will not respond to neuromodulation.
9. Two important reflexes may play an important role in modulation of bladder function: the guarding reflex and the bladder afferent loop reflex. Both reflexes promote urine storage under sympathetic tone.
10. Direct electrical stimulation of the bladder has often resulted in (1) abdominal, pelvic, and perineal pain; (2) a desire to defecate or defecation; (3) contraction of the pelvic and leg muscles; and (4) erection and ejaculation in males. An increase in intravesical pressure has also been noted.

QUESTIONS

1. Urodynamic stress urinary incontinence (SUI) refers to:
   a. incontinence that is demonstrated during a cough on clinical examination.
   b. incontinence occurring in the absence of urgency.
   c. incontinence occurring in combination with detrusor overactivity.
   d. incontinence associated on coughing in association with urgency and demonstrable detrusor overactivity.
   e. incontinence occurring on coughing in the absence of urgency and of urgency incontinence and with no demonstrable detrusor overactivity.

2. Anti-incontinence surgery via the retropubic route:
   a. is an effective approach for primary intrinsic sphincter deficiency.
   b. works by restoring the same mechanism of continence that was present before the onset of incontinence.
   c. aims to improve the support to the urethrovesical junction and correct deficient urethral closure.
   d. is the most effective form of anti-incontinence surgery.
   e. is carried out laparoscopically as effectively as via an open approach.

3. The most important determinant affecting the outcome of retropubic surgery is:
   a. increasing age.
   b. postoperative activity.
   c. coexisting medical morbidity.
   d. previous surgery.
   e. obesity.

4. Intrinsic sphincter deficiency is:
   a. present only in 30% of patients presenting with SUI.
   b. most likely present in the majority of women presenting with SUI.
   c. accurately identified on the basis of Valsalva leak point pressure.
   d. an absolute contraindication to a retropubic suspension procedure.
   e. clearly defined in the current literature.

5. Retropubic colposuspension procedures may act via which of the following mechanisms?
   a. Re-creating the normal continence mechanism
   b. Elevating the anterior vaginal wall and paravesical tissues toward the iliopectineal line
   c. Anchoring the obturator internus fascia to the iliopectineal line
   d. Suspending the bladder onto the periosteum of the symphysis pubis
   e. Strengthening the pubourethral ligaments

6. In assessing the outcome of retropubic suspension surgery, which of the following is most important?
   a. Using objective urodynamic-based outcome criteria
   b. Improving symptoms from the patient's perspective
   c. Achieving complete continence
   d. Identifying the degree of improvement in the urethral closure pressure
   e. Having follow-up data of at least 6 months' duration

7. Which of the following is not an indication for retropubic repair of SUI?
   a. A patient who needs a concomitant hysterectomy that cannot be performed vaginally
   b. A patient with urethral descent with straining and SUI
   c. A patient with limited vaginal access
   d. A patient who frequently generates high intra-abdominal pressure due to a chronic cough
   e. A patient with inadequate vaginal length or mobility of the vaginal tissues

8. Which of the following statements is TRUE regarding retropubic procedures for incontinence?
   a. It is important to avoid dissecting the old retropubic adhesions from prior incontinence procedures because these may contribute to continence.
   b. Nonabsorbable sutures are better than absorbable sutures for retropubic suspension procedures.
   c. It may be necessary to open the bladder to facilitate identification of the bladder margins and bladder neck.
   d. A urethral Foley catheter is preferred for bladder drainage because it is more comfortable and associated with fewer urinary tract infections and earlier resumption of voiding.
   e. The retropubic space must be drained after the procedure to prevent bleeding.

9. Which of the following statements is TRUE regarding the Marshall-Marchetti-Krantz (MMK) procedure?
   a. It is important to elevate the mid-urethra and external sphincter in particular.
   b. It carries little risk of causing urethral obstruction.
   c. It is associated with osteitis pubis.
   d. A better than 90% cure rate can be expected in the long term.
   e. The sutures should incorporate a full thickness of the vaginal wall and lateral urethral wall.

10. Which of the following is TRUE of the Burch colposuspension?
    a. It is appropriate only for patients with adequate vaginal mobility and capacity.
    b. The repair is performed between the vagina and the arcus tendineus fasciae pelvis bilaterally.
    c. It is less effective than a tension-free vaginal tape procedure.
    d. It is less effective than a paravaginal repair.
    e. It is more effectively performed via a vaginal approach.

11. Laparoscopic retropubic colposuspension is advantageous versus open colposuspension because:

a. it is technically simple to perform.

b. it provides access for repair of an associated central defect cystocele.

c. it is more effective than an open colposuspension.

d. it is associated with shorter hospitalization and recovery times.

e. it is associated with shorter operating times.

12. Common complications specific to retropubic suspension procedures include:

a. bladder denervation.

b. detrusor sphincter dyssynergia.

c. postoperative voiding difficulty.

d. detrusor underactivity.

e. genitourinary tract fistulae.

13. Postoperative voiding difficulty after a retropubic suspension procedure:

a. is more likely if there is preexisting detrusor dysfunction.

b. may be due to detrusor sphincter dyssynergia.

c. is most likely to occur with undercorrection of the urethral axis.

d. should be managed by urethrolysis within 1 month.

e. occurs in less than 1% of patients.

14. Which of the following statements is TRUE regarding detrusor overactivity (DO) and retropubic suspension procedures?

a. Preoperative DO is a contraindication to a retropubic suspension because it increases the risk of postoperative DO.

b. New-onset DO after a suspension procedure performed for stress urinary incontinence invariably resolves within 3 months.

c. DO occurs de novo, on average in fewer than 2% of the patients reported in the literature.

d. A history of voiding symptoms and new-onset storage symptoms as well as a retropubically angulated urethra usually suggests obstruction.

e. DO is not causally related.

15. Prolapse as a reported complication of retropubic repairs:

a. is rarely associated with a central defect cystocele.

b. results in genitourinary prolapse as a sequel to Burch colposuspension to occur in less than 10% of women.

c. may aggravate posterior vaginal wall weakness, predisposing to enterocele.

d. will be prevented by a synchronous hysterectomy.

e. occurs only rarely after a paravaginal repair.

16. From comparative studies in the literature, which is correct about open retropubic colposuspension?

a. It is not as effective as a pubovaginal sling.

b. It is not effective in patients with a low leak point pressure.

c. It is no more effective than an anterior colporrhaphy.

d. It is less effective than a tension-free vaginal tape procedure.

e. It is no more effective than a paravaginal repair.

ANSWERS

1. **e. Incontinence occurring on coughing in the absence of urgency and of urgency incontinence and with no demonstrable detrusor overactivity.** Stress urinary incontinence (SUI) is the symptom of involuntary loss of urine during situations of increased intra-abdominal pressure such as coughing or sneezing. The International Continence Society defines *urodynamic stress incontinence* as the involuntary loss of urine during increased intra-abdominal pressure during filling cystometry, in the absence of detrusor (bladder wall muscle) contraction (Abrams et al, 2002).* Thus, urodynamic evaluation is a prerequisite for the diagnosis of urodynamic SUI. It is not clear, however, especially from the clinical management standpoint, whether a urodynamic diagnosis is imperative for successful treatment of SUI.

2. **c. Aims to improve the support to the urethrovesical junction and correct deficient urethral closure.** Surgical procedures to treat SUI generally aim to improve the support to the urethrovesical junction and correct deficient urethral closure. There is disagreement, however, regarding the precise mechanism by which continence is achieved in the "normal asymptomatic female" and therefore, not surprisingly, how restoration of "normality" is reestablished via surgical manipulation. Anti-incontinence surgery is generally used to address the failure of normal anatomic support of the bladder neck and proximal urethra and intrinsic sphincter deficiency (ISD). Anti-incontinence surgery does not necessarily work by restoring the same mechanism of continence that was present before the onset of incontinence. Rather, it works by a compensatory approach, creating a new mechanism of continence (Jarvis, 1994). The surgeon's preference, coexisting problems, and the anatomic features of the patient and her general health condition often influence the choice of procedure.

Current evidence would suggest that in adequately experienced hands, there is no difference in overall safety and efficacy between laparoscopic and open colposuspension. Clearly, another concern is how generalizable the data are on laparoscopic colposuspension because the majority of reported studies are from expert laparoscopists or surgeons working in specialized units. The evidence base on both laparoscopic and open colposuspension is limited by relatively short-term follow-up (robust data are needed out to 5 years) and the tendency toward small numbers, and poor methodology limits the interpretation of most studies with the exception of those reported by Carey and coworkers (2006) and Kitchener and colleagues (2006).

3. **d. Previous surgery.** Surgery for recurrent SUI has a lower success rate. One study has reported that Burch colposuspension has an 81% success rate after one previous surgical procedure has failed, but this drops to 25% after two previous repairs and 0% after three previous operations (Petrou and Frank, 2001). Other series report excellent results for colposuspension performed after prior failed surgery. Maher and associates (1999) and Cardozo and colleagues (1999) have both shown good objective (72% and 79%) and subjective (89% and 80%) success rates with repeat colposuspension at a mean follow-up of 9 months. Nitahara and coworkers (1999) reported a 69% subjective success at a mean follow-up of 6.9 years.

The evidence on the duration of symptoms as a predictor of outcome is conflicting. Age may not be a contraindication to colposuspension (with equivalent success rates in the elderly at long-term follow-up), although others reported less success with increasing age. The influence of levels of postoperative activity has been inadequately studied, so no recommendations can be made. There is limited evidence that medical comorbidity may affect on surgical outcomes depending on the outcomes selected. Obesity as a confounding variable is the subject of conflicting evidence in the literature and has not been studied in a prospective fashion. Approximately a fourth of women undergoing urodynamic study have mixed urodynamic SUI and detrusor overactivity. It is likely that the presence of concomitant detrusor overactivity lessens the success rate of surgery. There is no consensus in the literature as to whether the presence of intrinsic sphincter deficiency as assessed by ure-

*Sources referenced can be found in *Campbell-Walsh Urology, 11th Edition*, on the Expert Consult website.

thral pressure profilometry has any influence in outcome of colposuspension.

4. **b. Most likely present in the majority of women presenting with SUI.** Hypermobility of the bladder neck and proximal urethra results from a weakening or loss of the supporting elements (ligaments, fasciae, and muscles), which in turn may result from aging, hormonal changes, childbirth, and prior surgery. It seems likely that the majority of women with SUI will also have an element of intrinsic sphincteric weakness with a variable degree of loss of the normal anatomic support of the bladder neck and proximal urethra, resulting in hypermobility.

A standardized test is not, however, available to differentiate the relative contributions of intrinsic sphincter deficiency and hypermobility, and therefore few studies have been able to accurately differentiate their individual contributions to the incontinence. Retropubic procedures act to restore the bladder neck and proximal urethra to a fixed, retropubic position and are used when hypermobility is thought to be an important factor in the development of that woman's SUI. This may facilitate the function of a marginally compromised intrinsic urethral sphincter mechanism, but if significant intrinsic sphincter deficiency is present, SUI will persist despite efficient surgical repositioning of the bladder neck and proximal urethra.

5. **b. Elevating the anterior vaginal wall and paravesical tissues toward the iliopectineal line.** Retropubic colposuspension urethral repositioning can be achieved by three distinctly different procedure principles. These are all based on a similar underlying principle but in a spectrum in relation to the degree of the support/elevations they achieve, and their outcomes differ somewhat in the longer term. The Burch colposuspension is the elevation of the anterior vaginal wall and paravesical tissues toward the iliopectineal line of the pelvic side wall using two to four sutures on either side (Burch, 1961). The vaginoobturator shelf repair aims to anchor the vagina to the obturator internus fascia and is a modification of a combination of the Burch colposuspension and paravaginal defect repair with placement of the sutures laterally anchored to the obturator internus fascia rather than hitching the vagina up to the iliopectineal line (Turner Warwick, 1986). The paravaginal defect repair aims to close a presumed fascial weakness laterally at the site of attachment of the pelvic fascia to obturator internus fascia (Richardson et al, 1976). The Marshall-Marchetti-Krantz procedure is the suspension of the vesicourethral junction (bladder neck) onto the periosteum of the symphysis pubis (Marshall et al, 1949). It aims to close the fascial defect rather than elevate the tissues in the paravesical area.

6. **b. Improving symptoms from the patient's perspective.** One or more high-quality validated symptom and quality-of-life instruments should be chosen at the outset of a clinical trial representing the patient's viewpoint, accurately defining baseline symptoms as well as any other areas in which treatment may be beneficial' and assessing the objective severity and subjective impact of bother. Although many, including the author, believe that urodynamic studies are helpful in defining the underlying pathophysiology in cases with incontinence, these tests have not been proven to have adequate sensitivity, specificity, or predictive value (Chapple et al, 2005). The International Consensus Meeting on Incontinence concluded that although urodynamic studies such as frequency-volume charts and pad tests were useful, there was inadequate evidence to justify pressure-flow studies for routine testing as either entry criteria or outcome measures in clinical trials, and they recommended that most large-scale clinical trials should enroll patients by carefully defined symptom-driven criteria when the treatment will be given on an empirical basis (Abrams et al, 2005).

7. **e. A patient with inadequate vaginal length or mobility of the vaginal tissues.** Although it has been suggested that a retropubic colposuspension should be considered in patients who frequently generate high intra-abdominal pressure (e.g., those with chronic cough from obstructive pulmonary disease and women in strenuous occupations), it has also been argued that

these patients may be better served by a pubovaginal sling as well. There may be specific indications for a retropubic approach for the correction of anatomic SUI, namely:
- A patient undergoing a laparotomy for concomitant abdominal surgery that cannot be performed vaginally.
- In cases with limited vaginal access.

Conversely, contraindications include:
- If there is a history of prior failed incontinence procedures, the existence of significant sphincteric deficiency must be suspected, even if hypermobility exists, and consideration given to performing a pubovaginal sling.
- In cases with a pan-pelvic floor weakness, a colposuspension should not be used in isolation but should be used as part of a comprehensive approach to the pelvic floor and be combined as appropriate with other alternative pelvic floor repair procedures. Although lateral defect cystocele and enterocele lend themselves to retropubic repair, central defect cystocele, rectocele, and introital deficiency do not.
- In cases in which there is an inadequate vaginal length or mobility of the vaginal tissues, such as after previous vaginal surgery or irradiation or after a previous vaginal incontinence procedure, a colposuspension should not be used.
- A retropubic colposuspension does not always adequately correct the associated vaginal prolapse that frequently coexists with bladder neck hypermobility.

8. **c. It may be necessary to open the bladder to facilitate identification of the bladder margins and bladder neck.** In open retropubic suspension procedures, good access to the retropubic space is crucial. This is best performed with the patient in the supine position with the legs abducted, in either a low or a modified dorsal lithotomy position using stirrups, allowing access to the vagina during the procedure and a perineoabdominal progression. A urethral Foley catheter is inserted; the catheter balloon is used for subsequent identification of the urethra and bladder neck and is invaluable in allowing palpation of the edges of the bladder by appropriate manipulation. A Pfannenstiel or lower midline abdominal incision is made, separating the rectus muscles in the midline and sweeping the anterior peritoneal reflection off the bladder. It is essential to optimize the access to the retropubic space, and if a Pfannenstiel skin incision is made, it is advisable to utilize the suprapubic V modification described by Turner-Warwick and colleagues (1974). Likewise, whatever incision is made, extra valuable access to the retropubic space is obtained by extending the division of the rectus muscles right down to the pubic bone and elevating the aponeurotic insertion of the rectus muscle right off the upper border of the pubic bone.

The retropubic space is then developed by teasing away the retropubic fat and underlying retropubic veins from the back of the pubic bone. The bladder neck, anterior vaginal wall, and urethra are then easy to identify—often facilitated by the presence of the Foley catheter balloon. In patients who have had previous retropubic surgery, the dissection is performed sharply, and it is important to take down all old retropubic adhesions, particularly in the presence of a prior failed repair. If difficulty is encountered in the identification of the bladder neck, the bladder may be partially filled or even opened to identify its limits; an examining finger in the vagina is invaluable in aiding the dissection (Symmonds, 1972; Gleason et al, 1976).

It is important to identify the lateral limits of the bladder as it reflects off the vaginal wall, because only in this manner can one avoid inadvertent suturing of the bladder itself. Dissection over the bladder neck and urethra in the midline is to be avoided so as to not damage the intrinsic musculature. The lateral bladder wall may be "rolled off" medially and cephalad from the vaginal wall using a mounted swab and by using countertraction with a finger in the vagina. In the author's experience, it is necessary to incise the endopelvic fascia. Occasional venous bleeding from the large vaginal veins is controlled by suture ligature, although it often resolves with tying of elevating sutures. To aid in the identification of the lateral margin of the bladder, it is helpful to displace the balloon of the Foley catheter into the lateral recess, where it can be easily palpated through the bladder wall.

Absorbable sutures were used in the original descriptions of the MMK procedure (chromic catgut), Burch colposuspension (chromic catgut), and vagino-obturator shelf procedure (polyglycolic acid or polydioxanone), whereas the original paravaginal repair used nonabsorbable sutures (silicon-coated Dacron). Fibrosis during subsequent healing is likely to be the most important factor in providing continued fixation of the perivaginal fascia to the suspension sites (Tanagho, 1996); nevertheless, some surgeons believe that a nonabsorbable suture material is better because of the risk of suture dissolution before the development of adequate fibrosis (Penson and Raz, 1996). Clearly the choice of suspension suture material is personal, but it must be remembered that nonabsorbent sutures eroding into the lumen of the bladder are a not-uncommon complication and a not-uncommon source of medical litigation (Woo et al, 1995).

Some degree of immediate postoperative voiding difficulty can be expected after retropubic suspensions (Lose et al, 1987; Colombo et al, 1996). Immediately postoperatively, bladder drainage may take the form of a urethral or a suprapubic catheter, generally based on surgeon preference. A voiding trial is usually performed around the fifth day postoperatively. However, there is some evidence that a suprapubic catheter may be advantageous with respect to a lower incidence of asymptomatic and febrile urinary tract infection and earlier resumption of normal bladder function (Andersen et al, 1985; Bergman et al, 1987). In addition, the use of a suprapubic tube is generally more comfortable, allows the patient to participate in catheter management, and avoids the need for clean intermittent catheterization. Catheterization can be discontinued when efficient voiding has resumed, which is usually indicated by a postvoid residual volume either less than 100 mL or less than 30% of the functional bladder volume.

A tube drain may be placed in the retropubic space when there is concern about ongoing bleeding from perivaginal veins that may prove difficult to control with suture and electrocautery. Often, tying the suspension sutures is sufficient to stop this bleeding, but when it persists, drainage of the retropubic space is indicated. The drain is generally removed on the first to third day, when minimal output is noted.

9. **c. It is associated with osteitis pubis.** Complications occur in up to 21% of cases (Mainprize 1988), and the placement of sutures through the pubic symphysis incurs the risk of osteitis pubis, a potentially devastating complication of the MMK procedure that has been reported in 0.9% to 3.2% of patients (Lee et al, 1979; Mainprize 1988; Zorzos and Paterson, 1996). Patients usually present 1 to 8 weeks postoperatively with acute pubic pain radiating to the inner thighs and aggravated by moving. Physical examination reveals tenderness over the pubic symphysis, and radiography demonstrates haziness to the borders of the pubic symphysis and possibly lytic changes. Treatment is with bed rest, analgesics, and possibly corticosteroids (Lee et al, 1979).

10. **a. It is appropriate only for patients with adequate vaginal mobility and capacity.** The Burch retropubic colposuspension, which has undergone few modifications since its original description, is appropriate only if the patient has adequate vaginal mobility and capacity to allow the lateral vaginal fornices to be elevated toward and approximated to the Cooper ligament on either side.

11. **d. It is associated with shorter hospitalization and recovery times.** Proposed advantages to the laparoscopic approach include improved intraoperative visualization, less postoperative pain, shorter hospitalization, and quicker recovery times (Liu, 1993). Disadvantages include greater technical difficulty with resultant longer operating times and higher operating costs (Paraiso et al, 1999).

The last major publication in this field was a meta-analysis of all of the comparative studies published between 1995 and 2006 of laparoscopic versus open colposuspension (Tan et al, 2007).

End points evaluated were operative outcomes and subjective/objective cure. A random-effect model was used and sensitivity analysis performed to account for bias in patient selection. Sixteen studies matched the selection criteria, reporting on 1807 patients, of whom 861 (47.6%) underwent laparoscopic and 946 (52.4%) underwent open colposuspension. Length of hospital stay and return to normal life were significantly reduced after laparoscopic surgery. These findings remained consistent on sensitivity analysis. Bladder injuries occurred more often in the laparoscopic group, but only with marginal statistical significance. Comparable bladder injury rates were found when studies were matched for quality, year, and randomized trials. Cure rates were similar between the two procedures at 2-year follow-up.

12. **c. Postoperative voiding difficulty.** As with any major abdominal or pelvic surgical procedure, intraoperative and perioperative complications that may occur after a retropubic suspension include bleeding, injury to genitourinary organs (bladder, urethra, ureter), pulmonary atelectasis and infection, wound infection or dehiscence, abscess formation, and venous thrombosis/embolism. Other common complications more specific to retropubic suspension procedures include postoperative voiding difficulty, detrusor overactivity, and vaginal prolapse.

Nevertheless, the reported incidence of these problems is relatively low. In their meta-analysis, Leach and associates (1997) noted a 3% to 8% transfusion rate for retropubic suspensions and no significant difference in the overall medical and surgical complication rates among retropubic suspensions, needle suspensions, anterior colporrhaphy, and pubovaginal slings.

Ureteral obstruction has been reported rarely after Burch colposuspension, and it usually results from ureteral kinking after elevation of the vagina and bladder base, although direct suture ligation of the ureter can occur (Applegate et al, 1987). If identified intraoperatively, it is best remedied by removal of the offending ligature and temporary placement of a ureteral stent. The so-called *post-colposuspension syndrome*, which has been described as pain in one or both groins at the site of suspension, has been noted in as many as 12% of patients after a Burch colposuspension (Galloway et al, 1987). More recently, Demirci and associates (2001) reported the occurrence of groin or suprapubic pain in 15 of 220 women (6.8%) after Burch colposuspension with a follow-up of 4.5 years.

13. **a. Is more likely if there is preexisting detrusor dysfunction.** Postoperative voiding difficulty after any type of retropubic suspension is not uncommon, and undoubtedly its occurrence is more likely if there is preexisting detrusor dysfunction or denervation resulting from extensive perivesical dissection. In most cases, however, it is the result of overcorrection of the urethral axis, owing to sutures being inappropriately placed or excessively tightened. If they are placed too medially, sutures may also transfix the urethra or distort it.

Preoperatively, at-risk patients may be identified by their history of prior voiding dysfunction or episodes of urinary retention. Preoperatively, these women should be counseled carefully about the potential for postoperative voiding difficulty and the possible need for self-catheterization. Their incontinence should be of sufficient magnitude that its correction offsets the risk of the need for self-catheterization.

Women with post-cystourethropexy voiding problems who have obstruction often do not exhibit the classic urodynamic features of obstruction. However, the history of postoperative voiding symptoms and associated new-onset bladder irritative symptoms and a finding of a retropubically angulated and fixed urethra generally indicate that obstruction does exist (Carr and Webster, 1997). In such cases, revision of the retropubic suspension by releasing the urethra into a more anatomic position resolves voiding symptoms in as many as 90% of cases (Webster and Kreder, 1990; Nitti and Raz, 1994; Carr and Webster, 1997).

The meta-analysis by Leach and coworkers (1997) noted that the risk of temporary urinary retention lasting more than 4 weeks postoperatively was 5% for all retropubic suspensions, the risk for permanent retention was estimated to be less than

5%, and these risks were not significantly different from those for needle suspensions or pubovaginal slings.

14. **d. A history of voiding symptoms and new-onset irritative symptoms as well as a retropubically angulated urethra usually suggests obstruction.** Bladder hyperactivity commonly accompanies anatomic SUI, and its incidence preoperatively has been reported to be as high as 30% in patients undergoing either first correction or repeated operations (McGuire, 1981). Provided that it is considered as a diagnosis, urodynamic study is performed to show whether detrusor overactivity is present, an attempt at treatment of the related overactive bladder symptoms has been made (with or without success), and the patient has been advised that the presence of detrusor overactivity will increase the risk of continuing storage symptoms postoperatively, then preoperative bladder overactivity does not contraindicate a retropubic suspension procedure, provided that anatomic SUI has also been demonstrated. In the majority of cases the bladder overactivity symptoms resolve after surgical repair (McGuire, 1988). Leach and coworkers' meta-analysis (1997) found the risk of urgency after a retropubic suspension was 66% if urgency and detrusor overactivity were present preoperatively, 36% if there was urgency but no documented overactivity preoperatively, and only 11% if there was neither urgency nor overactivity preoperatively. There was no significant difference in the incidence of postoperative urgency among retropubic suspensions, needle suspensions, and pubovaginal slings. Postoperative urgency was noted in only 0.9% of MMK procedures in Mainprize and Drutz's meta-analysis of 15 series (1988), although Parnell and associates (1982) reported that 28.5% of their patients developed postoperative storage symptoms. Jarvis' meta-analysis (1994) of Burch colposuspensions found the incidence of de novo bladder overactivity to be 3.4% to 18%. More recently Smith and associates quote a figure for postoperative detrusor overactivity of 6.6% for colposuspension (range 1.0% to 16.6%), whereas the incidence of postoperative urgency or urgency incontinence after the paravaginal/vagino-obturator shelf repair has been reported to be 0% to 6% (Shull and Baden, 1989; German et al, 1994; Colombo et al, 1996).

For those patients in whom postoperative storage symptoms persist, proven to be associated with detrusor overactivity and intractable to management with anticholinergic therapy and behavioral modification, surgical techniques including intravesical botulinum toxin therapy, neuromodulation, augmentation cystoplasty, or detrusor myectomy may be indicated.

Bladder storage symptoms arising de novo after retropubic suspension may be associated with bladder outlet obstruction. This premise is supported by the frequent coexistence of these symptoms with impaired voiding after suspension procedures and confirmed by the finding that urethrolysis, by freeing the urethra from an obstructed position, often resolves both storage and voiding symptoms (Raz, 1981; Webster and Kreder, 1990).

15. **c. May aggravate posterior vaginal wall weakness, predisposing to enterocele.** Retropubic suspensions alter vaginal and bladder base anatomy, and, thus, postoperative vaginal prolapse is a potential complication. Genitourinary prolapse has been reported as a sequel to Burch colposuspension in 22.1% of women (range 9.5% to 38.2%) by Smith and colleagues (2005) in their review of the literature. The Burch colposuspension, because of lateral vaginal elevation, may aggravate posterior vaginal wall weakness, predisposing to enterocele. The incidence varies between 3% and 17% (Burch, 1961, 1968; Galloway et al, 1987; Wiskind et al, 1992); and, because of this, prophylactic obliteration of the cul-de-sac of Douglas is sometimes considered when performing retropubic suspensions (Shull and Baden, 1989; Turner-Warwick and Kirby, 1993). However, simultaneous hysterectomy is not recommended prophylactically because it does not enhance the outcome of a retropubic suspension and should be performed only if there is concomitant uterine pathology (Milani et al, 1985; Langer et al, 1988). Although the Burch colposuspension and paravaginal/vagino-obturator shelf repair both correct lateral defect cystourethroceles, recurrent cystourethroceles were noted in 11% and 39% of Burch colposuspensions and paravaginal repairs, respectively (Colombo et al, 1996). In Mainprize and Drutz's review (1988), postoperative cystocele was noted in only 0.4% of patients after an MMK procedure.

Wiskind and coworkers (1992) noted that 27% of patients who had undergone a Burch colposuspension developed prolapse requiring surgery: rectocele in 22%, enterocele in 11%, uterine prolapse in 13%, and cystocele in 2%. More recently, it has been suggested that most women are asymptomatic and fewer than 5% have been reported to request further surgery (Smith et al, 2005). Ward and associates (2004) reported 4.8% of women needing a posterior repair whereas Kwon and coworkers (2003) reported 4.7% requiring subsequent pelvic reconstruction.

Because retropubic suspensions are unable to correct central defect cystoceles, patients must be carefully examined preoperatively to exclude their presence.

16. **a. It is not as effective as a pubovaginal sling.** A total of 655 women were randomly assigned to study groups: 326 to undergo the sling procedure and 329 to undergo the Burch colposuspension; 520 women (79%) completed the outcome assessment (Aldo et al, 2007). At 24 months, success rates were higher for women who underwent the sling procedure than for those who underwent the Burch colposuspension for both the overall category of success (47% vs. 38%, $P = .01$) and the category specific to SUI (66% vs. 49%, $P < .001$). There was no significant difference between the sling and Burch colposuspension groups in the percentage of patients who had serious adverse events (13% and 10%, respectively; $P = .20$). However, more women who underwent the sling procedure had adverse events than in the Burch colposuspension group, with 415 events among 206 women in the sling group as compared with 305 events among 156 women in the Burch colposuspension group. This difference was due primarily to urinary tract infections: 157 women in the sling group (48%) had 305 events and 105 women in the Burch colposuspension group (32%) had 203 events. When urinary tract infections were excluded, although the rates of adverse events were similar in the two groups, there was more difficulty voiding. The distribution of time to return to normal voiding differed significantly between the two groups: Voiding dysfunction was more common in the sling group than in the Burch colposuspension group (14% vs. 2%, $P < .001$). Consequently, surgical procedures to reduce voiding symptoms or improve urinary retention were performed exclusively in the sling group, in which 19 patients underwent 20 such procedures (63% vs. 47%, $P < .001$). Treatment satisfaction rates for the 480 subjects who answered the satisfaction question at 24 months were significantly higher in the sling group than in the Burch colposuspension group (86% vs. 78%, $P = .02$). A further analysis of this study focused on sexual activity as assessed by the Pelvic Organ Prolapse/Urinary Incontinence Sexual Questionnaire (PISQ-12) among those sexually active at baseline and 2 years after surgery (Brubaker et al, 2009). This report demonstrated that sexual function improves after successful surgery and does not differ between Burch colposuspension and sling procedures.

It can therefore be reliably concluded that in specialist centers working in a standardized fashion, the autologous fascial sling results in a higher rate of successful treatment of SUI but also greater morbidity than the Burch colposuspension.

Comparisons between the MMK and the Burch colposuspension procedures have generally yielded similar results. Three articles that reviewed the literature on incontinence procedures all found retropubic suspensions to be more effective than either needle suspensions or anterior colporrhaphies (Jarvis, 1994; Black and Downs, 1996; Leach et al, 1997). Most studies in the literature have not demonstrated a significant difference in cure rates between retropubic suspensions (generally a Burch colposuspension) and pubovaginal slings (Jarvis, 1994; Black and Downs, 1996; Leach et al, 1997). The literature on the paravaginal repair is sparse. The only randomized study that compared the Burch colposuspension with a paravaginal repair found significantly greater subjective and objective cure with the Burch colposuspension (Colombo et al, 1996). At this point, the tension-free vaginal tape procedure appears to be at least equivalent to the Burch colposuspension.

CHAPTER REVIEW

1. Anti-incontinence surgery does not work by restoring the normal mechanism of continence but, rather, by a compensatory approach creating a new mechanism of continence.

2. Intrinsic sphincter deficiency is suggested by a leak point pressure less than 60 cm H_2O or a maximum urethral closure pressure of less than 20 cm H_2O.

3. Approximately 40% of nulliparous 30- to 49-year-old women experience some degree of incontinence with exercise.

4. If nonabsorbable sutures are used in a retropubic suspension, they may migrate into the bladder and serve as a foreign body nidus for stone formation and infection.

5. The postoperative risk of SUI in continent women undergoing an abdominal sacrocolpopexy is substantially reduced by the addition of a Burch colposuspension.

6. A maximum urethral closing pressure of less than 20 cm H_2O is a contraindication to the Burch colposuspension.

7. All patients, before any colposuspension, should be advised about the potential need for intermittent self-catheterization.

8. The Burch colposuspension is regarded as the standard open retropubic procedure for incontinence.

9. If intrinsic sphincter deficiency is the primary problem, a fascial sling procedure should be performed rather than a colposuspension.

10. A Marshall-Marchetti-Krantz procedure, a paravaginal defect repair, and needle suspension procedures are not recommended for the treatment of stress urinary incontinence.

11. The majority of women with SUI will also have an element of intrinsic sphincteric weakness with a variable degree of loss of the normal anatomic support of the bladder neck and proximal urethra, resulting in hypermobility.

12. Contraindications for a retropubic colposuspension include significant sphincteric deficiency, pan-pelvic floor weakness, and inadequate vaginal length or mobility. Moreover, it may not correct the associated vaginal prolapse.

13. Bladder hyperactivity commonly accompanies anatomic SUI, and its incidence preoperatively has been reported to be as high as 30%. In the majority of cases, the bladder overactivity symptoms resolve after surgical repair.

14. Simultaneous hysterectomy is not recommended prophylactically because it does not enhance the outcome of a retropubic suspension and should be performed only if there is concomitant uterine pathology.

Vaginal and Abdominal Reconstructive Surgery for Pelvic Organ Prolapse

J. Christian Winters, Ariana L. Smith, and Ryan Krlin

QUESTIONS

1. Which of the following statements is FALSE?
   a. Pelvic organ prolapse occurs because of defects in the supporting tissues.
   b. Pelvic organ prolapse is a manifestation of discrete descent of the female pelvic viscera.
   c. Pelvic organ prolapse occurs as compartmental defects, and multiple compartments may be affected.
   d. The aim of surgical management is restoration of normal anatomy while maintaining visceral and sexual function.
   e. Pelvic organ prolapse essentially represents hernias within the pelvic floor.

2. Which structure does not insert onto the spinous process?
   a. Arcus tendineus fasciae pelvis
   b. Sacrospinous ligament
   c. Coccygeus muscle
   d. Arcus tendineus levator ani

3. With regard to three levels of vaginal support as described by DeLancey, which of the following is TRUE?
   a. Level I support provides a primarily vertical support of the upper vagina and cervix by the cardinal uterosacral ligament complex.
   b. Level II support includes the shortest fibers and anchors the mid-vagina.
   c. Level III support has intervening paracolpium and supports the most distal portion of the vagina.
   d. Level I support originates from the greater sciatic foramen, the medial sacrum, and the sacroiliac region.
   e. Level III support does not fuse the urethra anteriorly and the perineal body posteriorly.

4. Which statement about the endopelvic fascia is FALSE?
   a. The endopelvic fascia is a composite of fibrous tissues, embedded in a matrix.
   b. The tissues are supportive and contractile.
   c. The endopelvic fascia is easily divided into the various regions, which are readily identified at surgery.
   d. The endopelvic fascia lacks the organization of the fascial coverings of skeletal muscle.
   e. The endopelvic fascia has different regions that are specifically named.

5. Which structure does not attach to the perineal body?
   a. Rectovaginal fascia
   b. Levator ani muscles
   c. Transverse perinei muscles
   d. Pubocervical fascia
   e. External anal sphincter

6. Which of the following statements about apical compartment prolapse is FALSE?
   a. Vaginal vault prolapse can occur after hysterectomy if support is not reconstituted to the cardinal uterosacral ligament complex.
   b. An apical defect may result in uterine prolapse, vaginal vault prolapse, and prolapse of the peritoneum cul-de-sac.
   c. Failure to reconstitute the vaginal vault at the time of hysterectomy will lead to immediate vault prolapse.
   d. Total procidentia includes apical prolapse of the vagina in addition to multiple compartment defects.
   e. Enteroceles may occur with or without vaginal vault prolapse.

7. Patient satisfaction is NOT highly correlated with which of the following?
   a. Patient readiness to undergo surgery
   b. Objective measures of surgical success
   c. Resolution of the symptoms of pelvic organ prolapse
   d. Lack of patient-perceived complications
   e. Achievement of patient-selected goals

8. Preoperative patient preparation does NOT include which of the following?
   a. Asking the patient to state what the planned procedure(s) is and its purpose
   b. Administering preoperative antibiotics
   c. Deep venous thrombosis prophylaxis
   d. Local estrogen therapy in women with vaginal atrophy
   e. Routine use of vaginal douches

9. Which statement is FALSE regarding biologic and synthetic grafts?
   a. Wound healing follows a stepwise cascade regardless of material type.
   b. All synthetic grafts are biologically inert.
   c. There is no ideal prosthetic implant.
   d. Biologic grafts are classified as autologous, allografts, and xenografts.
   e. Synthetic grafts may be absorbable.

10. Which statement is FALSE regarding wound healing and grafts/mesh?
    a. The amount of foreign body reaction is proportional to the surface area of the material exposed to the host.
    b. The degree of response and amount of tissue ingrowth is determined by the nature of the material.
    c. The graft functions as a permanent mechanical support.
    d. Host tissue integration leads to long-term graft function.
    e. The graft/mesh acts as a scaffold to facilitate tissue ingrowth.

11. Which of the following processes must occur for long-term graft survival?

    a. Rejection

    b. Degeneration

    c. Encapsulation

    d. Absorption

    e. Remodeling

12. Which tissue-processing technique causes the least amount of variability in tissue quality of allografts and xenografts?

    a. Tissue harvesting

    b. Cross-linking

    c. Freeze drying

    d. Tissue fenestration

    e. Solvent dehydration

13. The most important characteristic of a synthetic mesh is:

    a. type of mesh (synthetic or absorbable).

    b. pore size.

    c. filament type (monofilament or multifilament).

    d. mesh construct (woven or knitted).

    e. flexibility.

14. Which of the following statements regarding anterior colporrhaphy is FALSE?

    a. Anterior colporrhaphy is not used to treat stress incontinence.

    b. Recent series report a 40% recurrence rate for standard anterior colporrhaphy.

    c. The most likely contributing factor for failure of anterior compartment repairs is the concomitant presence of other compartmental defects.

    d. Cystoscopy with indigo carmine is not routinely necessary.

    e. Ensuring that the bladder is drained before perforating the endopelvic fascia may decrease bladder injuries.

15. Paravaginal repairs are used to repair which of the following anterior compartment defects?

    a. Lateral

    b. Central

    c. Anterior

    d. Posterior

    e. Distal

16. Which of the following statements is FALSE regarding high-grade anterior compartment prolapse?

    a. Urethral kinking or compression may occur.

    b. Occult stress urinary incontinence may be unmasked by reducing the prolapse.

    c. No method to reduce the prolapse is superior in evaluating occult stress urinary incontinence.

    d. All women with high-grade anterior compartment prolapse should undergo a prophylactic anti-incontinence procedure.

    e. Intervention for complications of mid-urethral slings equals the risk of having to perform a secondary sling.

17. A 50-year-old woman presents with symptoms of voiding difficulty and vaginal bulging. She has had no prior pelvic surgery. In the supine position she demonstrates anterior vaginal wall prolapse that extends 4 cm beyond the hymen. The cervix does not descend with straining during the supine examination. The least likely diagnosis is:

    a. cystocele only.

    b. uterine prolapse and cystocele.

    c. uterine prolapse and enterocele.

    d. uterine prolapse, enterocele, and cystocele.

    e. uterine prolapse, widened genital hiatus, and enterocele.

18. Which statement is FALSE regarding apical defects?

    a. Failure to recognize an apical defect at the time of prolapse repair will increase the risk of recurrence.

    b. Apical defects may involve the bladder and rectum.

    c. Hysterectomy with suspension of the vaginal apex to the cardinal uterosacral ligaments and attaching the pubocervical fascia to the rectovaginal fascia will ensure the apical support.

    d. Enteroceles always contain small bowel.

    e. Enteroceles are thought to occur by several mechanisms.

19. Which of the following statements is TRUE regarding uterosacral ligament suspensions?

    a. The ureter courses closer to the uterosacral ligament proximally.

    b. Suture placement in the most medial portion of the uterosacral ligament will avoid fibers of the sacral plexus.

    c. The ureters are found consistently in the same location regardless of the degree of prolapse.

    d. The sutures should be tied before performing a cystoscopy.

    e. The suspensory sutures should be trimmed before the cystoscopy.

20. What method is NOT used to identify the cardinal uterosacral ligaments?

    a. Traction of the dimples of the vaginal apex

    b. Placing an Allis clamp at the 5-o'clock and 7-o'clock positions of the vaginal vault

    c. Direct visualization

    d. Tugging on the suture tied to the cardinal uterosacral ligaments at the time of hysterectomy

    e. Randomly grasping a condensation of tissue along the pelvic side wall

21. Which of the following statements about apical repairs is TRUE?

    a. Uterosacral suspension restores the vaginal apex.

    b. With respect to durability, abdominal sacrocolpopexy has not been shown to be superior to sacrospinous ligament suspension.

    c. Sacrospinous ligament suspension does not change the vaginal axis.

    d. With abdominal uterosacral ligament suspension, one does not need to place as many sutures on the ligament.

    e. Iliococcygeus repairs always foreshorten the vaginal length.

22. A disadvantage of sacrospinous ligament fixation is:

    a. it requires a retroperitoneal approach.

    b. the sacrospinous ligament is not a reliable structure on which to anchor the vaginal apex.

    c. the procedure may only be approached anteriorly.

    d. the hospital stay is equivalent compared with abdominal sacrocolpopexy.

    e. there may be posterior or caudal displacement of the vagina.

23. Which structure is at risk of injury with sacrospinous ligament suspensions?

    a. Genitofemoral nerve

    b. Pudendal nerve

    c. Obturator vessels

    d. Ilioinguinal nerve

    e. Hypogastric vessels

24. Which statement is FALSE regarding the anatomy around the sacrospinous ligament?

    a. The pudendal nerves and vessels are in close proximity while they course around the ischial spine.

    b. The gluteal vessels course behind the sacrospinous ligament.

    c. The highest concentration of sacral nerves is by the ischial spine.

    d. The fibers of the sacrospinous ligament fan out closer to the sacrum.

    e. The optimal position to place suture for fixation is 1.5 to 2 cm medial to the ischial spine.

25. Which of the following is FALSE regarding pain from the sacrospinous ligament suspension?

    a. Gluteal pain generally resolves spontaneously in 2 to 3 months.

    b. Injection of the nerve with local anesthetic can be done to relieve the pain.

    c. Pudendal nerve entrapment causes gluteal pain.

    d. Pain may occur in 15% of patients on the ipsilateral side.

    e. Pain is musculoskeletal in origin.

26. All of the following statements regarding the iliococcygeus suspension are true EXCEPT:

    a. The site of fixation may be reached by an anterior or posterior approach.

    b. Fixation is 1 cm distal to the ischial spine near the insertion of the arcus tendineus fasciae pelvis.

    c. The dissection for the iliococcygeus suspension is as extensive as for the sacrospinous ligament fixation.

    d. The iliococcygeus suspension maintains the vagina in the normal axis.

    e. Neuropathy has been reported as a postoperative complication.

27. Key elements of the abdominal sacrocolpopexy do NOT include:

    a. use of permanent monofilament mesh.

    b. secure fixation to the sacral promontory.

    c. secure fixation to the vaginal cuff.

    d. use of a biologic graft.

    e. complete enterocele reduction and culdoplasty.

28. Which structures are the sources of severe bleeding with the abdominal sacrocolpopexy?

    a. Presacral veins

    b. Internal iliac vein

    c. Mesenteric veins

    d. Middle sacral vein

    e. a and d

29. Which statement is TRUE regarding culdoplasty?

    a. Halban culdoplasty involves placing purse-string sutures.

    b. Moschowitz culdoplasty involves placing longitudinal sutures.

    c. The risk of the Moschowitz culdoplasty is ureteral obstruction due to angulation.

    d. Culdoplasties prevent rectocele formation.

    e. Downward retraction of the end-to end anastomosis sizer may help delineate the cul-de-sac.

30. Which of the following factors is FALSE regarding advantages of colpocleisis?

    a. Shorter operative time

    b. Ability to use either regional anesthesia or local anesthesia with sedation

    c. Minimal complication rates

    d. Appropriate choice for those wishing to maintain sexual activity

    e. Decreased recuperative time

31. Which postoperative complication of both colpocleisis and partial colpocleisis, if identified preoperatively, may be reduced?

    a. Stress urinary incontinence

    b. Urinary retention

    c. Regret over loss of sexual function

    d. Recurrence

    e. Infection

32. Uterine prolapse represents the loss of:

    a. apical support from the broad ligament.

    b. anterior support from the arcus tendineus fasciae pelvis.

    c. apical support from the cardinal uterosacral ligament.

    d. posterior support from the rectovaginal fascia.

    e. apical support from the round ligaments.

33. Contraindications to performing a vaginal hysterectomy do NOT include:

    a. endometriosis of unknown extent.

    b. obliteration of the cul-de-sac.

    c. size disproportion of the uterus to the introitus.

    d. grade II uterine prolapse or greater.

    e. malignancy of the uterus or ovaries.

34. Which maneuver performed during vaginal hysterectomy is essential to prevent recurrent prolapse?

    a. Leaving an adequate stump on the uterine artery

    b. Culdoplasty

    c. Leaving an adequate stump on the cardinal uterosacral ligament complex

    d. Closure of the cul-de-sac

    e. b and d

35. Which surgical technique of rectocele repair is most associated with postoperative dyspareunia?

    a. Levator plication

    b. Site-specific repair

    c. Site-specific repair with biologic interposition graft

    d. Transanal repair of rectocele

    e. Perineorrhaphy

36. Which symptom changes the least following site-specific posterior colporrhaphy?

    a. Dyspareunia

    b. Constipation

    c. Vaginal mass

    d. Splinting

    e. Vaginal pressure or pain

37. Which statement regarding vaginal kits is TRUE?

    a. There is ample evidence to support their use.

    b. The presence of total vaginal mesh turns a single compartment repair into a multicompartmental repair.

    c. The volume of mesh used is less than that for traditional interposition repairs.

    d. The use of trocars reduces the complication rates.

    e. Complications associated with kit repairs are the same as those associated with traditional repairs.

38. Which structure is NOT used as a fixation point or point of reference for vaginal kits?

    a. Sacrospinous ligament

    b. Cardinal uterosacral ligament complex

    c. Ischial spine

    d. Obturator internus fascia

    e. Arcus tendineus fasciae pelvis

39. Complications that seem more likely when utilizing vaginal kits to repair pelvic organ prolapse include all of the following EXCEPT:

    a. pelvic hematoma.

    b. recurrent prolapse.

    c. vaginal extrusion of mesh.

    d. groin pain.

    e. visceral perforation.

40. Failure rates of standard anterior colporrhaphy:

    a. are less than those for augmented mesh repairs.

    b. are the same as those for mesh augmented repairs.

    c. are less than those for abdominal sacrocolpopexy.

    d. are the same as those for abdominal sacrocolpopexy.

    e. depend on the definition of failure used.

ANSWERS

1. **b. Pelvic organ prolapse is a manifestation of discrete descent of the female pelvic viscera.** Pelvic organ prolapse occurs because of defects within the support structures of the pelvic floor. Because the support is contiguous and boundaries are often difficult to delineate, conceptualizing the various regions of the vagina as compartments facilitates the current understanding of the pelvic floor. Multiple compartments are often involved in pelvic organ prolapse, and multiple defects can be seen in a single compartment.

2. **d. Arcus tendineus levator ani.** The spinous process serves as an anchoring point for the first three structures and is an important landmark for surgeons who operate on the pelvic floor.

3. **a. Level I support provides a primarily vertical support of the upper vagina and cervix by the cardinal uterosacral ligament complex.** Level I support originates from the greater sciatic foramen, the sacroiliac region, and the lateral sacrum. It has vertical support suspending the upper vagina and cardinal uterosacral ligament complex. Level II support has mid-length fibers and supports the mid-vagina. Level III support has no intervening paracolpium, fuses the urethra anteriorly, and blends into the perineal body posteriorly.

4. **c. The endopelvic fascia is easily divided into the various regions, which are readily identified at surgery.** The endopelvic fascia is one contiguous unit, in which distinct areas are named. However, it is often difficult to identify where one region ends and the other begins. It should be considered as a unit. The challenge of the endopelvic fascia in its use as a supportive structure is that there is inherent weakness created by its structure of fibrous tissue embedded in a matrix in contrast to the fascial covering of skeletal muscle.

5. **d. Pubocervical fascia.** The perineal body is a condensation of fibromuscular tissue and collagen. It is located in the midline between the vagina and the anus. The pubocervical fascia is an anterior structure that does not insert into the perineal body.

6. **c. Failure to reconstitute the vaginal vault at the time of hysterectomy will lead to immediate vault prolapse.** The upper vagina is supported by two structures: the cardinal uterosacral ligament complex and the broad ligament. Therefore vaginal vault prolapse does not occur immediately after hysterectomy if the cardinal uterosacral ligaments are not reattached to the vaginal vault at the time of hysterectomy, owing to the support of the broad ligaments.

7. **b. Objective measures of surgical success.** In their study, Kenton and colleagues (2007)* found that patient perception of perioperative events and bother from recurrent symptoms resulted in dissatisfaction with prolapse surgery in the presence of high objective cure rates. Patient-perceived complications included postoperative pain, minor effects of anesthesia, hospital discharge with a catheter, constipation, and urgency incontinence. Preoperative counseling is a key time in which one may educate and affect postoperative patient satisfaction.

8. **e. Routine use of vaginal douches.** The Agency for Healthcare Research and Quality identified perioperative interventions to improve patient safety, which include asking the patient to recall and state what was discussed during informed consent, administering appropriate preoperative antibiotics, and deep venous thrombosis prophylaxis. Postmenopausal patients may be treated with local estrogen therapy, which may increase vascularity and promote wound healing. Most surgeons do not use vaginal douches preoperatively.

9. **b. All synthetic grafts are biologically inert.** Synthetic grafts are not biologically inert. All grafts will become involved in the wound healing process. Physical factors of each biologic graft or synthetic mesh will have different effects on the resultant scar tissue matrix.

10. **c. The graft functions as a permanent mechanical support.** Tissue incorporation must occur for long-term success of a biologic graft or synthetic mesh. The important concept is that the graft, synthetic or biologic, serves as a scaffold to facilitate tissue ingrowth, rather than functioning as permanent mechanical support.

11. **e. Remodeling.** Incorporation through a process called *graft remodeling* is needed for long-term graft survival.

12. **a. Tissue harvesting.** The other techniques can all induce variability in tissue strength and incorporation. Aldehyde cross-linking is cytotoxic in high concentrations, attracting gelatinases to the wound that may increase the rate of graft degradation. Fenestrations may decrease seroma formation and increase both angiogenesis and tissue ingrowth. Freeze drying demonstrated reduced maximum load to failure and stiffness of cadaveric fascia lata, in addition to variability of strength and stiffness throughout the graft.

13. **b. Pore size.** Increased pore size results in greater flexibility. Pore size of 75 μm is the size that allows for the optimal tissue ingrowth with fibroblasts, blood vessels, and collagen fibrils. Monofilament knitted materials are able to assume a macroporous configuration.

14. **d. Cystoscopy with indigo carmine is not routinely necessary.** Cystoscopy after the administration of indigo carmine or methylene blue is recommended as a routine practice after anterior colporrhaphy. If blue-tinged urine is not seen effluxing from each ureteral orifice, catheterization may be considered before taking down the plication sutures. Appropriate steps must be performed to ensure ureteral patency, including takedown of the sutures.

15. **a. Lateral.** Lateral defects are repaired with paravaginal repairs. This defect may be approached transvaginally or transabdominally.

16. **d. All women with high-grade anterior compartment prolapse should undergo a prophylactic anti-incontinence procedure.** The risks and benefits of prophylactic anti-incontinence procedure on continent women should be reviewed with each patient. The literature supports selective use of an anti-incontinence procedure at the time of pelvic organ prolapse repair. All women with advanced-stage anterior compartment prolapse should be screened for occult stress urinary incontinence.

17. **a. Cystocele only.** The patient has grade 4 anterior vaginal wall prolapse and the likelihood that the prolapse is bladder only is

---

*Sources referenced can be found in *Campbell-Walsh Urology, 11th Edition*, on the Expert Consult website.

very low. She has a high likelihood of concomitant uterine prolapse.

18. **d. Enteroceles always contain small bowel.** Enteroceles may involve omentum and small bowel. Large vaginal vault prolapse may involve the bladder and rectum. Enteroceles can occur from causes that may be congenital, from pulsion, from traction, or iatrogenically.

19. **d. The sutures should be tied before performing a cystoscopy.** The sutures of the uterosacral ligament suspension should be tied before cystoscopy to evaluate the patency of the ureters. If cystoscopy is performed before tying the sutures, there may not be enough traction or compression from the sutures to appreciate ureteral obstruction. However, if the sutures need to be taken down, leaving them untrimmed until after the cystoscopy is practical because the tails will facilitate identification of the most lateral suture. They will need to be taken down one at a time until the offending suture is identified. While the ureter courses distally, it gets closer to the cardinal uterosacral ligament complex, becoming the closest at the level of the cervix. Location of the ureters may vary considerably depending on the degree of prolapse.

20. **e. Randomly grasping a condensation of tissue along the pelvic side wall.** The cardinal uterosacral ligament complex should be identified by tenting this structure either at the dimples of the vaginal apex or by placing Allis clamps at the vaginal vault, or by tugging on the sutures. Alternatively, they can be directly visualized intra-abdominally. Random grasping of a condensation of tissue places the ureter at risk.

21. **a. Uterosacral suspension restores the vaginal apex.** The uterosacral suspension restores the normal anatomy of the vaginal apex. In contrast, right-sided unilateral sacrospinous ligament fixation often results in the vagina being displaced posteriorly and to the right. The abdominal sacrocolpopexy has been demonstrated to be superior to sacrospinous ligament suspension with respect to durability. Although the iliococcygeus repair may foreshorten the vagina, it does not always occur.

22. **e. There may be posterior or caudal displacement of the vagina.** The caudal displacement of the vagina is thought to potentially contribute to the rate of anterior prolapse recurrence. By displacing the vaginal apex posteriorly, the procedure places the anterior compartment at risk for recurrent prolapse.

23. **b. Pudendal nerve.** The pudendal nerve courses around the ischial spine. Medial placement of the sutures 1.5 cm away from the ischial spine will help to avoid entrapment of the pudendal nerve. The other structures are farther away from the sacrospinous ligament and are less likely to be injured.

24. **c. The highest concentration of sacral nerves is by the ischial spine.** The highest concentration of sacral nerves is closest to the sacrum.

25. **e. Pain is musculoskeletal in origin.** The pain from sacrospinous ligament suspension either is gluteal or radiates down the leg posteriorly. It is neuropathic, and it occurs in 15% of patients. The pain may last 2 to 3 months in patients who have delayed absorbable sutures. Injection of the nerve with local anesthetic has been described to alleviate the pain.

26. **c. The dissection for the iliococcygeus suspension is as extensive as for the sacrospinous ligament fixation.** The dissection for the iliococcygeus suspension is not as extensive as that used to access the sacrospinous ligament. Advantages include using either the anterior or posterior approach, maintaining the vagina in a near-normal axis.

27. **d. Use of a biologic graft.** Permanent monofilament mesh has been shown to be superior to both cadaveric fascia lata graft (Culligan et al, 2005) and xenograft (Deprest et al, 2009). Secure fixation of the graft to both the sacral promontory and vaginal cuff, use of a monofilament mesh, and complete reduction of the enterocele with culdoplasty and tensioning so that the rectum is two fingerbreadths away from the mesh are key elements of the repair.

28. **e. a and d.** Severe bleeding can be encountered with shearing of the presacral and middle sacral veins. This may be avoided by placing sutures higher on the sacral promontory. Careful dissection is essential over the promontory. Sterile tacks may be used to stop the bleeding if encountered.

29. **c. The risk of the Moschowitz culdoplasty is ureteral obstruction due to angulation.** The Halban culdoplasty involves placing longitudinal sutures, and the Moschowitz culdoplasty involves placing purse-string sutures. The Moschowitz culdoplasty can result in ureteral angulation resulting in obstruction. A culdoplasty prevents enteroceles (not rectoceles) from forming. The end-to-end anastomosis sizer must be angled upward to see the cul-de-sac.

30. **d. Appropriate choice for those wishing to maintain sexual activity.** Both colpocleisis and partial colpocleisis are only considered for those patients who are not sexually active and do not wish to maintain the ability to be sexually active. Careful counseling is especially important with these procedures.

31. **a. Stress urinary incontinence.** Patients may give a history of stress urinary incontinence that improved over time as their pelvic organ prolapse worsened. Before undergoing colpocleisis, all women should be screened for occult stress urinary incontinence.

32. **c. Apical support from the cardinal uterosacral ligament.** Loss of apical support from the cardinal uterosacral ligament complex leads to uterine prolapse. Because the broad ligament also provides a small amount of support, failure to reconstitute the support from the cardinal uterosacral ligament complex at the time of hysterectomy does not lead to immediate apical prolapse.

33. **d. Grade II uterine prolapse or greater.** Endometriosis of unknown extent may make vaginal hysterectomy problematic. Obliteration of the cul-de-sac will preclude accessing the proper plane to identify the parametrium.

34. **e. b and d.** The key elements to prevent recurrent vaginal vault prolapse after vaginal hysterectomy is culdoplasty, which is a closure of the cul-de-sac. Attaching the pubocervical fascia to the rectovaginal fascia closes the cul-de-sac, thus preventing an enterocele. Attaching the vaginal apex to the cardinal uterosacral ligament complex reconstitutes the apical support.

35. **a. Levator plication.** Levator plication was associated with high rates of de novo postoperative dyspareunia. Therefore it has largely been abandoned.

36. **b. Constipation.** Constipation may be associated with dysmotility disorders of the rectum that do not improve with an anatomic repair. The symptoms most likely to improve are dyspareunia, the need for vaginal splinting, vaginal mass, and pressure.

37. **b. The presence of mesh turns a single compartment repair into a multicompartmental repair.** The mesh placed with vaginal kits often supports both the vaginal apex and the anterior and posterior compartments, making direct comparisons between kits and traditional repairs challenging. The kits utilizing trocars have complications that are unique to those techniques. The volume of mesh used is more than the amounts used in traditional repairs.

38. **b. Cardinal uterosacral ligament complex.** The systems utilize the other structures as fixation points or references.

39. **b. Recurrent prolapse.** When compared to native tissue repairs, recurrence rate are less with vaginal kits. Vaginal extrusion of mesh is not unique to the trocar kits. The other complications have been associated with kits involving trocars.

40. **e. Depend on the definition of failure used.** Failure rates depend on the definition of failure used. Weber's data from 2001 concluded a 40% failure rate; however, when it was reanalyzed in 2011 applying alternate failure criteria, the failure rate fell to 10% to 20%. Most modern series define anatomic failure as stage II or greater using the Pelvic Organ Prolapse Quantification (POP-Q) system, yet some patients with recurrent stage II prolapse remain asymptomatic and do not require further surgical correction.

CHAPTER REVIEW

1. The iliococcygeus and the coccygeus muscles fuse in the midline and attach to the coccyx forming a complex called the *levator plate* that supports the upper vagina and cervix.
2. The urethra is fused to the anterior vaginal wall for much of its length.
3. Vaginal support is provided by the endopelvic connective tissues.
4. The cardinal and uterosacral ligaments provide level I support of the uterus and upper vagina; the endopelvic and pubocervical fascia provide level II support of the mid-vagina while it attaches to the arcus tendineus fasciae pelvis; the distal vagina attaches to the levator ani muscles and perineal body to provide for level III support.
5. Pelvic organ prolapse is for the most part a quality-of-life issue.
6. Anterior compartment defects can be central, lateral, or both.
7. Anterior colporrhaphy and paravaginal repairs are both ineffective alone in the treatment of stress urinary incontinence. They do not suspend the vaginal apex.
8. Sacrospinous ligament fixation may result in posterior displacement of the vaginal apex and increase the risk of anterior compartment prolapse.
9. If either the bladder or rectum is injured during pelvic organ prolapse repair, mesh should not be used.
10. Twenty-nine percent of women require reoperation for failed incontinence and prolapse surgery.
11. Synthetic mesh grafts erode in 10% of patients in whom they are used for the repair.
12. Sacrospinalis ligament fixation is an effective method of correcting vaginal apical prolapse. It results in posterior displacement of the vaginal apex.
13. Abdominal sacrocolpopexy maximizes functional vaginal length without significant distortion of the anatomic vaginal axis.
14. Colpocleisis obliterates a portion of the vagina and may be used to prevent vaginal vault prolapse. It precludes functional sexual activity.
15. Cystoscopy after the administration of indigo carmine or methylene blue is recommended as a routine practice after anterior colporrhaphy.
16. All women with advanced-stage anterior compartment prolapse should be screened for occult stress urinary incontinence.
17. The pain from sacrospinous ligament suspension is either gluteal or radiates down the leg posteriorly. It is neuropathic, and it occurs in 15% of patients.

84 Slings: Autologous, Biologic, Synthetic, and Midurethral

Roger R. Dmochowski, David James Osborn, and W. Stuart Reynolds

QUESTIONS

1. The Integral Theory proposed by Petros and Ulmsten states that:
   a. urethral hypermobility is the primary cause of stress urinary incontinence.
   b. adequate function of the pubourethral ligaments, the suburethral vaginal hammock, and the pubococcygeus muscle helps to preserve continence.
   c. anchoring a sling to the rectus muscle allows it to respond to changes in intra-abdominal pressure.
   d. dynamic kinking of the urethra during stress preserves incontinence.
   e. synthetic mesh integrates into host tissue.

2. Which of the following statements about the preoperative assessment of a sling patient is TRUE?
   a. It is generally not necessary to perform a focused neurologic examination.
   b. Urgency is not associated with worse outcomes after sling surgeries.
   c. The American Urological Association (AUA) Guidelines state that a postvoid residual (PVR) volume should be checked on all patients.
   d. Cystoscopy should be performed in all patients to rule out bladder pathology.
   e. The abdominal leak-point pressure is traditionally defined by a pressure of less than 80 cm H_2O.

3. Which of the following statements regarding pubovaginal sling materials is TRUE?
   a. Harvesting a thin strip of fascia lata is associated with significant morbidity.
   b. The risk of perforation and exposure associated with synthetic slings is minimal.
   c. Harvesting a thin strip of autologous rectus fascia is not associated with herniation.
   d. Synthetic sling materials exhibit the least amount of degradation.
   e. Although concerning, disease transmission has never been documented with allograft materials.

4. An autologous pubovaginal sling (PVS) is indicated in all of the following conditions EXCEPT:
   a. urethral incompetence in a T12 spinal cord injury.
   b. low urethral resistance with decreased bladder compliance.
   c. urethral incompetence and large urethral diverticulum.
   d. proximal urethral loss secondary to long-standing indwelling Foley catheter.
   e. refractory stress urinary incontinence (SUI) after failed midurethral sling (MUS) and bulking agents.

5. Which of the statements about the normal female urethra and pelvic floor is TRUE?
   a. The female urethra is composed of four separate tissue layers, and the middle seromuscular layer is most important in enhancing the urethral sphincter mechanism during voiding.

   b. The Valsalva pressure of the bladder exceeds the resting closing pressure of the internal sphincter.
   c. The fast-twitch fibers of the external sphincter are responsible for sudden protection against incontinence, and slow-twitch fibers provide passive control through the involuntary guarding reflex.
   d. The levator ani, urethropelvic ligament, and round ligament provide needed support to the bladder neck and undersurface of the bladder.
   e. The PVS is placed at the bladder neck to provide adequate urethral coaptation at rest and to decrease urethral responsiveness to abdominal pressure.

6. Which of the following statements regarding materials for bladder neck pubovaginal slings is FALSE?
   a. The ideal material has minimal tissue reaction and complete biocompatibility.
   b. Stiffness and maximal load failure are the same between freeze-dried fascia lata and solvent-dehydrated and dermal grafts.
   c. The estimated risk of human immunodeficiency virus (HIV) transmission by an allograft sling is approximately 1 in 1,660,000.
   d. Porcine small intestinal submucosa has less tensile strength than cadaveric fascia lata.
   e. Synthetic materials are associated with high perforation rates during use for bladder neck PVS.

7. Before final tensioning of the rectus fascial autologous PVS:
   a. the vaginal incision should be closed and the weighted speculum removed.
   b. the abdominal skin incision should be closed.
   c. vaginal packing should be placed.
   d. the patient should be taken out of lithotomy position.
   e. a drain should be placed in the retropubic space.

8. In outcomes associated with PVS procedures, which of the following is/are TRUE?
   a. Reported cure rates after an autologous PVS procedure are 50% to 97%.
   b. Preoperative Valsalva leak point pressure is a reliable predictor of outcomes after sling surgery.
   c. Bladder neck PVS slings should be utilized for refractory or recurrent SUI but are associated with worse outcomes.
   d. In the Stress Incontinence Surgical Treatment Efficacy Trial (SiSTER) trial, cure rates and voiding symptoms were greater for the pubovaginal sling than for the Burch colposuspension.
   e. a and d

9. Which of the following statements about perforation and PVS material is TRUE?
   a. Synthetic slings perforate into the urinary tract 15 times more often than autologous, allograft, or xenograft slings.
   b. Urethral perforations are rarely associated with urinary retention and mixed urinary incontinence.
   c. Synthetic slings are less likely to be associated with vaginal exposure than autologous, allograft, and xenograft slings.

d. Perforation from synthetic slings requires removal of the entire sling from a vaginal and retropubic approach.

e. None of the above are true.

10. Which of the following statements is NOT associated with voiding dysfunction after a PVS procedure?

a. Obstruction, detrusor overactivity, or impaired detrusor contractility are all manifestations of voiding dysfunction for iatrogenic PVS obstruction.

b. Persistent urgency is more common than urinary retention in bladder outlet obstruction after a PVS procedure.

c. Fifty percent of affected patients have symptoms of overactive bladder, which can be avoided if sling lysis is performed within 2 weeks of PVS placement.

d. Urodynamic study is valuable in assessment and planning management.

e. There is up to a 20% recurrent SUI rate after urethrolysis.

11. Regarding the pathophysiology of incontinence:

a. hypermobility is the main underlying cause of SUI.

b. intrinsic sphincter deficiency (ISD) is rarely the primary cause of SUI.

c. ISD is the primary underlying cause of SUI for women, with hypermobility being a secondary finding.

d. the levator floor provides active compression to the proximal urethra.

e. the extrinsic urethral skeletal sphincter is the primary mechanism for urinary continence.

12. Obese patients who undergo MUS surgery:

a. clearly have a higher rate of sling-related complications.

b. should have been offered weight loss as an initial management option.

c. have a significantly higher risk of trocar injury at the time of sling placement.

d. have been consistently shown to have worse outcomes.

e. are at a greater risk for voiding dysfunction.

13. The MUS procedure incorporates all of the following EXCEPT:

a. insertion trocars used to transpose the implanted material into position.

b. the synthetic material used is a wide porosity mesh.

c. loose tension is placed on the sling material.

d. the sling is sutured to the underlying tissues for fixation purposes.

e. cystoscopy is a crucial component of the procedure.

14. Common presenting symptoms of voiding dysfunction after PVS surgery are:

a. urgency and frequency.

b. painful voiding and suprapubic pain.

c. incomplete emptying and straining.

d. associated with recurrent urinary tract infections.

e. all of the above.

15. In review of the efficacy outcomes obtained with mid-urethral procedures, which of the following is TRUE?

a. Mid-urethral slings are less effective than open colposuspension procedures.

b. Mid-urethral slings produce inferior results compared with laparoscopic colposuspensions.

c. Postoperative voiding dysfunction is more common with mid-urethra procedures than with other types of suspension procedures.

d. Mixed incontinence results are superior to those for pure SUI.

e. Five-year results demonstrate durability similar to 1-year results.

16. Which of the following is theorized to be TRUE regarding patients at risk for voiding dysfunction after PVS surgery?

a. Failure to relax the external striated sphincter is not associated with postoperative voiding dysfunction.

b. Patients who habitually void with abdominal straining will not have an increased risk of voiding dysfunction after PVS surgery.

c. Patients with pure stress urinary incontinence are more likely to have voiding dysfunction after PVS surgery.

d. Patients with subclinical impaired detrusor contractility are at increased risk for voiding dysfunction after PVS surgery.

e. Young patients are more at risk for voiding dysfunction after PVS surgery.

17. In elderly patients, mid-urethral slings:

a. are less effective than in younger patients.

b. are associated with rates of postoperative urgency higher than those in young patients.

c. are associated with satisfaction rates lower than those in young patients.

d. are associated with mixed incontinence resolution rates higher than those in young patients.

e. result in postoperative urinary retention occurring more frequently.

18. In a patient with voiding dysfunction after sling surgery:

a. it is generally appropriate to wait as long as 3 months after MUS surgery before considering surgical intervention.

b. it is generally appropriate to wait as long as 3 months after autologous PVS surgery before considering surgical intervention.

c. loosening a synthetic sling through traction with a cystoscope in the operating room is associated with little risk.

d. formal urethrolysis has been shown to be superior to sling incision.

e. intermittent catheterization is not advisable.

19. When mid-urethral slings are performed at the time of prolapse surgery:

a. risks of perforation, exposure, and infection are higher than in cases in which only a sling is performed.

b. concomitant hysterectomy has an adverse effect on incontinence outcome.

c. rates of urethrolysis for postoperative retention are higher.

d. occult incontinence is not adequately addressed.

e. rates of retention are slightly higher than in those undergoing a sling procedure only.

20. When mid-urethral slings are used as salvage procedures:

a. complication rates are higher than when mid-urethral slings are done primarily.

b. the technique needs to be altered when done as a primary procedure.

c. failure rates are unaffected by urethral hypermobility.

d. bladder perforation is less than in primary cases.

e. overall efficacy is similar to that of primary implantation.

21. Complications associated with mid-urethral slings include:

a. bladder perforation injury rates range as high as 5%.

b. voiding dysfunction ranges from 4% to 20%.

c. de novo urgency occurs in as many as 12% of patients.

d. wound healing is delayed in approximately 1%.

e. all of the above.

22. According to International Continence Society and International Urogynecological Association (IUGA) terminology pertaining to synthetic (prosthetic) mesh sling complications which of the following is TRUE?

a. The term *perforation* should be used when mesh is present within the urinary tract or bowel.

b. The term *exposure* should be used when mesh is present in the urinary tract or bowel.

c. The term *erosion* should be used when mesh is found in the urinary tract a year or more after surgery.

d. a and b

e. a and c

23. Material-related exposures and perforations associated with mid-urethral slings are:

a. decreased by the macroporous nature of the sling material.

b. unaffected by tension placed on the slings.

c. associated with vaginal exposures approximately 20% of the time.

d. associated with bladder perforation rates of 20%.

e. do not affect outcomes or satisfaction.

24. Which of the following statements about the anatomy of mid-urethral slings is TRUE?

a. The obturator nerve and vessels are less than 2 cm away from the transobturator sling at the level of the obturator foramen.

b. For retropubic slings, the dorsal nerve of the clitoris is typically <2 cm away from the sling.

c. The anatomic position of a single-incision sling is significantly affected by position of the legs.

d. A branch of the obturator artery that courses along the pubic bone is more likely to be injured with an in-to-out transobturator sling technique.

e. The periurethral fascia covering the posterior urethra is very thin.

25. Which of the following statements is FALSE regarding the treatment of patients with recurrent SUI with a MUS surgery?

a. Retropubic slings have been shown to have better outcomes than transobturator slings in patients with recurrent SUI in a few small series.

b. Repeat MUS surgery is significantly less effective at curing incontinence then primary MUS surgery.

c. A meta-analysis of MUS surgery for recurrent SUI found that retropubic MUS surgery was significantly better than transobturator MUS surgery.

d. Recurrent SUI after MUS surgery may be due to intrinsic sphincter deficiency

e. None of the above statements are false.

26. In regard to perforations associated with mid-urethral slings:

a. bladder perforations cannot be managed endoscopically in well-selected cases.

b. vaginal exposures cannot be managed conservatively.

c. exposures and perforations are not related to errant sling placement.

d. symptoms are not usually associated with exposure.

e. complete excision of exposed material should be performed.

27. In regard to the mechanics of mid-urethral slings, which of the following is TRUE?

a. Mid-urethral slings work primarily by compressing the urethra.

b. There is no evidence to support dynamics kinking of the urethra as a mechanism for continence for mid-urethral slings.

c. Placing a sling tight at the mid-urethra will help eliminate postoperative hypermobility.

d. It appears that a MUS works by impeding the movement of the posterior urethral wall.

e. Postoperative urethral hypermobility is associated with failure of the procedure.

28. Which of the following statements is TRUE?

a. Retropubic mid-urethral slings cure SUI better than transobturator mid-urethral slings.

b. The risk of urinary tract trocar injury is higher with retropubic mid-urethral slings than transobturator mid-urethral slings.

c. Postoperative voiding dysfunction is higher with transobturator mid-urethral slings than retropubic mid-urethral slings.

d. It is not necessary to perform cystoscopy after a transobturator MUS surgery.

e. It is not necessary to perform cystoscopy after a single-incision MUS surgery.

29. Voiding dysfunction associated with mid-urethral slings is:

a. not associated with changes in urodynamic parameters.

b. predictable based on unique preoperative voiding parameters such as flow rate.

c. managed by immediate sling release.

d. managed initially conservatively, but sling release should be contemplated when persistent voiding trials are not successful.

e. resolved by complete excision of the sling.

30. In regard to operative management for voiding dysfunction after MUS surgery:

a. single incision of the sling results in incontinence in the majority of patients.

b. it important to remove the entire sling.

c. similar to autologous pubovaginal slings, surgery should not be considered until at least 3 months after sling placement.

d. voiding dysfunction is usually transient.

e. loosening the sling in the operating room with a cystoscope is very safe option.

31. Complications associated with mid-urethral slings include:

a. superficial vaginal material exposure.

b. vascular perforation.

c. intestinal perforation.

d. significant hemorrhage requiring transfusion.

e. all of the above.

32. Which of the following statements is TRUE regarding sexual dysfunction after mid-urethral sling surgery?

a. Postoperative dyspareunia is not associated with MUS surgery.

b. Sling removal has been shown to improve dyspareunia.

c. It has been clearly shown that MUS surgery will improve the sexual function of a woman with incontinence.

d. A decrease in coital incontinence may improve sexual function.

e. b and d

33. Which of the following statements is TRUE regarding bleeding and hematomas after MUS surgery?

    a. The rate of undiagnosed hematomas is likely less than 5%.

    b. The majority of postoperative hematomas resolve without intervention.

    c. In the literature, the rate of severe bleeding is consistently less than 1%.

    d. The rate of hematomas and severe bleeding is lower after retropubic MUS surgery than transobturator MUS surgery.

    e. All of the above are true.

34. Regarding the transobturator technique, the:

    a. surgical placement of the tape requires insertion through the adductor longus tendon.

    b. tape never traverses the gracilis or adductor magnus brevis muscles.

    c. anterior branch of the obturator artery is located at the medial aspect of the obturator foramen.

    d. tape remains above the perineal membrane and outside the true pelvis and does not penetrate the levator ani group.

    e. dorsal nerve of the clitoris is in close juxtaposition to the tape.

35. The transobturator technique involves:

    a. either outside-in or inside-out approaches.

    b. no absolute requirement for cystoscopy.

    c. no risk of lower urinary tract injury.

    d. no risk of leg pain or dyspareunia.

    e. similar meshes in all available kits.

36. Reported outcomes with the transobturator MUS:

    a. appear to be relatively similar regardless of whether ISD is present preoperatively.

    b. include bladder, but not urethral, injury being reported.

    c. indicate that vaginal exposure is similar regardless of the type of tape used.

    d. show that voiding dysfunction is significantly less with this technique as compared with the retropubic approach.

    e. are not affected by the presence of urethral hypermobility.

37. Which of the following statements is TRUE regarding pain after MUS surgery?

    a. Groin pain is more commonly associated with the transobturator MUS surgical approach.

    b. When groin pain does occur, it persists longer after retropubic MUS surgery.

    c. Most groin pain resolves after 2 days.

    d. a and c

    e. a and b

38. Which of the following statements is TRUE regarding infection after MUS surgery?

    a. Severe infection is a common complication after MUS surgery.

    b. Randomized controlled trials demonstrate a vaginal wound infection rate of approximately 10%.

    c. There are no reports in the literature about delayed presentation of infection after MUS surgery.

    d. Obesity and diabetes are associated with fasciitis after pelvic surgery.

    e. All of the above are true.

39. Which of the following is FALSE regarding the surgical management of mesh perforation and exposure after MUS surgery?

    a. Observational treatment is not recommended for mesh perforation of the bladder.

    b. Endoscopic excision or ablation is an acceptable first step for patients with small areas of bladder perforation.

    c. A midline vaginal incision is acceptable for patients undergoing removal of mesh that has perforated into the urethra.

    d. Reconstruction should involve nonoverlapping suture lines and interposition of tissue such as a labial fat pad, greater omentum, or autologous fascial sling.

    e. In cases of mesh perforation of the urinary tract, the entire MUS needs to be removed.

40. Which of the following statements is TRUE regarding regulatory and legal issues related to sling mesh complications?

    a. The first MUS had to go through the premarket approval process, and then subsequent slings were approved through the 510(k) process.

    b. Mid-urethral slings can no longer use the 510(k) approval process.

    c. The FDA considers mesh complications to be "rare."

    d. In the legal profession, the § symbol does NOT stand for "section."

    e. Single-incision sling manufacturers are required to perform 522 postmarket surveillance studies.

ANSWERS

1. **b. Adequate function of the pubourethral ligaments, the suburethral vaginal hammock, and the pubococcygeus muscle helps to preserve continence.** They postulated that injury to any of these three components from surgery, parturition, aging, or hormonal deprivation could lead to impaired mid-urethral function and subsequent urinary incontinence.

2. **c. The American Urological Association (AUA) Guidelines state that a postvoid residual (PVR) volume should be checked on all patients.** Based on AUA guidelines, a urinalysis and measurement of PVR volume should be performed on all patients, but more extensive imaging is not part of the routine evaluation of urinary incontinence. However, in some patients abnormal findings in the history, physical examination, or urinalysis may warrant further imaging.

3. **d. Synthetic sling materials exhibit the least amount of degradation.** In 2008, Woodruff et al* examined explanted sling materials and determined that synthetic materials demonstrated the least amount of degradation. They also demonstrated the greatest amount of fibroblast and tissue ingrowth into the specimen.

4. **b. Low urethral resistance with decreased bladder compliance.** Decreased bladder compliance is of concern for upper tract deterioration. The addition of a PVS, by increasing bladder outlet resistance, would cause significant damage to the upper tracts. The compliance should be addressed before or concurrently to anti-incontinence measures. A PVS procedure is indicated for intrinsic sphincter deficiency (ISD) associated with urethral hypermobility, SUI presenting as concomitant cystoceles, SUI associated with urethral diverticulum, and SUI associated with urethral defects (e.g., urethrovaginal fistula) in which urethral reconstruction is required, and in women with SUI and associated neurogenic conditions.

5. **c. The fast-twitch fibers of the external sphincter are responsible for sudden protection against incontinence, and slow-twitch fibers provide passive control through the involuntary guarding reflex.** The female urethra is composed of four layers, with the middle muscular layer maintaining the resting urethral closure mechanism and the outer seromuscular layer augmenting this closing pressure. The levator ani, urethropelvic ligament, and pubocervical fascia provide support to the bladder neck and underside of the bladder. The round ligament provides support

---

*Sources referenced can be found in *Campbell-Walsh Urology, 11th Edition,* on the Expert Consult website.

to the uterus. A PVS is placed at the bladder neck to provide adequate urethral coaptation for increasing urethral responsiveness to abdominal pressure.

6. **b. Stiffness and maximal load failure are the same between freeze-dried fascia lata and solvent-dehydrated and dermal grafts.** Maximum load to failure, maximum load/graft width, and stiffness are significantly lower for the freeze-dried fascia lata group compared with the autologous, solvent-dehydrated, and dermal graft groups. The ideal graft material causes no tissue reaction, is completely biocompatible, leads to significant host fibroblast infiltration and neovascularization, and causes negligible perforation or exposure. The estimated risk of HIV transmission from an allograft is 1 in 1,667,600. The theoretical risk of developing Creutzfeldt-Jakob disease from a non-neural allograft is 1 in 3.5 million. Porcine small intestinal submucosa has less tensile strength than cadaveric fascia lata. Synthetic material is no longer used for bladder neck PVS because of the exceedingly high perforation rates.

7. **a. The vaginal incision should be closed and the weighted speculum removed.** A sling should never be tensioned before the weighted speculum or vaginal incision is closed. Tensioning before this step may result in failure of the procedure due to too much or too little tension. The abdominal incision is also closed after the sling is tensioned.

8. **e. a and d.** Cure rates reported in peer-reviewed literature for autologous PVS procedures are 46% to 97%. There are no risk factors that predict outcomes after PVS surgery for primary or recurrent SUI. The PVS is a valuable option for refractory and recurrent SUI and yields a cure rate of 86%. The SiSTER trial was a multicenter, randomized clinical trial (Albo et al, 2007) that found higher cure rates for the PVS procedure than the Burch colposuspension, but also more associated voiding symptoms (urinary tract infection, difficulty voiding, and postoperative urge incontinence, $P < .001$).

9. **a. Synthetic slings perforate into the urinary tract 15 times more often than autologous, allograft, or xenograft slings.** This includes sutures, bone anchors, and screws. Synthetic slings perforate 15 times more often into the urethra and are exposed 14 times more often into the vagina than autologous, allograft, and xenograft slings. Urethral perforation usually presents at a mean of 9 months as urinary retention, urgency, and mixed urinary incontinence.

10. **c. Fifty percent of affected patients have symptoms of overactive bladder, which can be avoided if sling lysis is performed within 2 weeks of PVS placement.** Transient urinary retention is common, and most patients return to spontaneous voiding within 10 days postoperatively. Obstructive symptoms may improve or resolve with time, which is the reason most physicians prefer waiting 3 months before considering surgical intervention. The incidence of voiding dysfunction after continence surgery varies from 2.5% to 35% and includes obstruction, detrusor overactivity, or impaired detrusor contractility. Persistent postoperative urgency incontinence and urgency present more commonly (8% to 25%) than frank retention. Although urodynamics do not preoperatively predict outcomes after anti-incontinence surgery or urethrolysis, it is useful in diagnosing and treating patients with obstruction after a PVS procedure. There is a 0% to 18% recurrent SUI rate after urethrolysis.

11. **c. ISD is the primary underlying cause of SUI for women, with hypermobility being a secondary finding.** Although urethral hypermobility is present in many women, most do not manifest incontinence and, therefore, ISD is considered to be the most important factor in women who experience urinary loss. The extrinsic urethral sphincter is not considered to be the primary mechanism for urinary continence in women. The ongoing debate regarding hypermobility and ISD is further compounded by the advent of midurethral slings, which clearly address hypermobility during stress events. Given the efficacy of midurethral slings, there has been some confusion regarding the role of hypermobility in promoting continence. However, most believe that the intrinsic urethral mechanism is of primary importance for urinary control.

12. **b. Should have been offered weight loss as an initial management option.** It has been consistently shown in the literature that obese patients with incontinence benefit from weight loss. The literature regarding improvement or cure of incontinence in patients with obesity compared with nonobese patients is mixed. Multiple authors have found a higher rate of bladder trocar injury in nonobese patients during MUS surgery.

13. **d. The sling is sutured to the underlying tissues for fixation purposes.** The tension-free vaginal tape (TVT) procedure incorporates several specific technical components. Insertion trocars are used in either a suprapubic or a vaginal approach to assist in implantation of the material in the retropubic area. It is now well known that type 1 synthetic meshes are best because of their wide porosity. In addition, this mesh should be monofilamentous. Most authorities recommend placement of loose tension only on the TVT, although some authorities now are placing greater tension on the TVT, with success being established in patients with lesser degrees of hypermobility. No suture fixation to the underlying periurethral fascia is necessary to anchor the sling. Cystoscopy is a vital component of this procedure to exclude urinary tract injury.

14. **e. All of the above.** The presentation of patients with voiding dysfunction is variable, and the symptoms range from complete urinary retention and urgency incontinence to the less obvious irritative symptoms. Obstruction may also present with recurrent urinary tract infections, prolonged suprapubic pain, and painful voiding, even if emptying is completed.

15. **e. Five-year results demonstrate durability similar to 1-year results.** Five-year (and now 7-year) longitudinal results have shown that midurethral slings have procedural durability in terms of efficacy. This efficacy is not substantially less than results obtained at 1 year. Randomized trials have demonstrated similar efficacy in patients undergoing either open colposuspensions or laparoscopic colposuspensions. Mid-urethral slings provide superior results compared with laparoscopic procedures. Although voiding dysfunction may be observed after any type of sling procedure, results suggest that midurethral slings are associated with less voiding dysfunction than either colposuspensions or bladder neck slings. Results with mixed incontinence are acceptable compared with other types of interventions for urinary incontinence but are less than those obtained in pure SUI.

16. **d. Patients with subclinical impaired detrusor contractility are at increased risk for voiding dysfunction after PVS surgery.** It has been shown that preoperative voiding dysfunction affects a patient's ability to empty after anti-incontinence surgery. Subclinical preoperative impaired detrusor contractility may manifest symptomatically with voiding dysfunction after PVS surgery. Dysfunctional voiding or failure of relaxation of the external urethral sphincter may also affect emptying after surgery. Also, a patient who habitually voids by abdominal straining may have difficulty emptying after incontinence surgery. Because of the variability of presenting symptoms following a pubovaginal sling, it is important to ascertain the predominant symptom with a thorough history.

17. **b. Are associated with rates of postoperative urgency that are higher than those in young patients.** Elderly patients experience higher rates of postoperative urgency associated with any sling material, and this is true for the mid-urethral sling as well. However, elderly patients have results similar to their younger peers, and therefore satisfaction rates are also similar to those of their younger peers. Mixed urinary incontinence resolution rates are similar to those of the younger population, and actual postoperative retention occurs to a similar degree as in younger patients, but postoperative voiding function may be slightly higher in the older population.

18. **b. It is generally appropriate to wait as long as 3 months after autologous PVS surgery before considering surgical intervention.** Obstruction following an autologous PVS usually improves or resolves with time, therefore, most physicians historically have preferred waiting 3 months before considering

surgical intervention after PVS (it may not be suitable to wait this long after midurethral slings). It is appropriate and effective to initially treat persistent voiding dysfunction conservatively. This includes temporary catheter drainage, clean intermittent catheterization, timed voiding, double voiding, biofeedback, pelvic floor muscle training, and anticholinergic therapy.

19. **d. Occult incontinence is not adequately addressed.** Midurethral slings performed at the time of prolapse surgery have now been shown to be safe and efficacious. Risks of perforation, exposure, and infection are no greater than when the midurethral sling is performed as a primary isolated procedure. Concomitant hysterectomy has been shown not to have an adverse effect on continence status associated with these procedures. In addition, rates of postoperative urethrolysis are no greater when the midurethral sling technology is combined with a prolapse correction. Rates of retention are also not appreciably higher in this population compared with those women undergoing isolated slings only.

20. **e. Overall efficacy is similar to that of primary implantation.** As salvage procedures, midurethral slings have overall efficacy similar to their use in primary implantation procedures. Complications should be no higher than when done as primary procedures. The technique remains the same, and no alteration is required. Success does appear to be reliant on hypermobility, and patients with less hypermobility would appear to have less overall functional success than those patients with greater hypermobility. Rates of bladder perforation may be somewhat higher in this population than in primary cases.

21. **e. All of the above.** Complications with midurethral slings are an important part of informed consent. Bladder perforation rates range as high as 5% and in some studies are somewhat higher. Voiding function rates vary from 4% to 20%, and this variance is largely related to definitional reasons based on literature evidence. De novo urgency occurs with postoperative voiding dysfunction in as many as 12% of patients, and wound healing can be affected in approximately 1% of patients; results represent dramatic improvement compared with historic dense weave meshes.

22. **d. a and b.** In 2010, the International Urogynecological Association (IUGA) and the International Continence Society (ICS) released a report clarifying and standardizing the terminology related to complications from insertion of synthetic and biological materials during female pelvic surgery. According to that report, synthetic mesh is termed a *prosthesis* and a biologic implant is termed a *graft*. Mesh located in the lower urinary tract is termed a *perforation* and extrusion of mesh through the skin or vagina is termed *exposure*.

23. **a. Decreased by the macroporous nature of the sling material.** Exposure and perforation associated with midurethral slings is clearly decreased by the use of macroporous monofilament sling material (type 1). Tension may have a role in increasing mesh-related complications even in macroporous slings. Vaginal exposure rates and bladder perforation rates are very low and do not exceed 5% to 10% with newer sling materials. When material complications do occur, however, they have an adverse impact on overall patient satisfaction.

24. **b. For retropubic slings, the dorsal nerve of the clitoris is typically <2 cm away from the sling.** The left and right dorsal nerves of the clitoris (DNC) run along the inferior surface of the ischiopubic rami and cross under the pubic bone approximately 1.4 cm from the midline. Therefore, when a placing a trocar it is important to stay at least 2 cm from the midline to avoid injuring the DNC.

25. **c. A meta-analysis of MUS surgery for recurrent SUI found that retropubic MUS surgery was significantly better than transobturator MUS surgery.** In 2013, Agur et al performed a meta-analysis of the 10 randomized, controlled trials that of midurethral slings that addressed recurrent SUI. The review included 350 women with a mean follow-up of 18.1 months. The authors found no significant difference in subjective cure rates in patients after retropubic versus transobturator MUS surgery.

26. **e. Complete excision of exposed material should be performed.** Management of exposures and perforations is complex and must be individualized. Primarily, all exposed material, whether it be vaginal or within the urinary tract, must be removed or in some manner covered. There have been successful reports of bladder management endoscopically, although this is contingent on absolute excision of all exposed material. Some authors have reported successful management of vaginal exposures with conservative use of topical estrogens and delayed primary closure as well as simple secondary intention healing. Exposures and perforations are clearly linked to technique, and errant sling placement has a high significance in creating perforations.

27. **d. It appears that a MUS works by impeding the movement of the posterior urethral wall.** Indeed, it appears that a midurethral sling works by impeding the movement of the posterior urethral wall above the sling, directing its motion in an anteroinferior or anterior direction. In addition, inward movement of the posterior urethral wall after placement of a midurethral sling results in urethral lumen narrowing (compression). This securing of the posterior wall of the urethra (with or without compression during stress maneuvers) is one theory of how midurethral slings achieve continence.

28. **b. The risk of urinary tract trocar injury is higher with retropubic midurethral slings than transobturator mid-urethral slings.** In the majority of published series comparing retropubic and transobturator midurethral slings, the rate of urinary tract trocar injury at the time of sling placement is higher with retropubic slings. However, there are numerous case reports of transobturator sling mesh perforating into the urinary tract. Therefore, cystoscopy should be performed after transobturator sling trocar passage.

29. **d. Managed initially conservatively, but sling release should be contemplated when persistent voiding trials are not successful.** Voiding dysfunction associated with midurethral slings is substantially less than with bladder neck slings but still occurs. Timing of intervention is dependent on surgeon experience but is trending toward earlier intervention. Most experts recommend a period of conservative management of a few days to 1 month. Persistent obstruction will require intervention. Urodynamic parameters are often affected in cases of persistent obstruction. Unfortunately, no preoperative factors are predictive of postoperative voiding dysfunction. Immediate release is not recommended because a short period of observation usually results in resolution of the voiding dysfunction. When sling release occurs, midline incision of the sling is all that is required; the entire sling does not need to be excised.

30. **d. Voiding dysfunction is usually transient.** Urinary obstruction after MUS surgery is usually transient and can be managed with short-term intermittent catheterization, although occasionally symptoms mandate sling release. Long-term retention after retropubic midurethral sling surgery is a rare complication. In these cases, removal or incision of the sling usually improves the patient's symptoms.

31. **e. All of the above.** Complications of technique include injury to surrounding structures and significant hemorrhage due to laceration of perivesical vessels. Intestinal and vascular complications can cause substantial morbidity and mortality.

32. **e. b and d.** The rate of de novo dyspareunia after MUS surgery is between 3% and 14.5%. Some authors attribute improved sexual function after MUS surgery to a significant decrease in coital incontinence. There is contradictory evidence in the literature that MUS surgery improves and worsens sexual function. There is evidence in the literature that sling removal can improve dyspareunia.

33. **b. The majority of postoperative hematomas resolve without intervention.** Tseng et al (2005) performed ultrasound on 62 women after MUS surgery and found that 8 (12.9%) patients had significant retropubic hematomas larger than 5 cm on the day after surgery. Repeat ultrasonographic examinations 1 month after surgery revealed all the hematomas except one had resolved.

In randomized controlled trials, the majority of bleeding complications occur in patients after retropubic MUS surgery.

34. **d. Tape remains above the perineal membrane and outside the true pelvis and does not penetrate the levator ani group.** The transobturator technique is unique because (when done correctly) it avoids entry into the true pelvis and the levator group. Errant sling placement through the adductor longus tendon can result in substantial pain. Smaller muscle groups, such as the magnus brevis and gracilis, are often traversed by this technique without substantial complications. The obturator vessels are lateral and superior to the area of insertion of the device. The dorsal nerve of the clitoris is separated from the trajectory of the device by at least 1 to 2 cm.

35. **a. Either outside-in or inside-out approaches.** The transobturator technique can be performed by insertion of the passing needles from either vaginal or obturator approaches. Associated risks of device use include leg pain, dyspareunia, and injury to surrounding structures. Cystoscopy is a useful safety adjunct and should be performed as an integral and necessary part of the transobturator MUS surgery. Different kits use different meshes, and not all meshes are similar. The kit to be used should be evaluated critically for this parameter.

36. **a. Appear to be relatively similar regardless of whether ISD is present preoperatively.** Transobturator MUS surgery outcomes are relatively similar to those seen with the retropubic slings, regardless of urethral function. Any lower urinary tract structure, including the ureter, can be injured by the transobturator trocar, including the urethra and bladder. Vaginal exposure is clearly related to mesh type. Voiding dysfunction is similar to retropubic techniques. Less urethral hypermobility probably militates against success rates with transobturator slings, such as those reported in women with higher degrees of urethral hypermobility.

37. **d. a and c.** Thigh and groin pain appear to be more commonly associated with the transobturator approach. In addition, it appears that groin pain persists longer after the transobturator midurethral slings. Most groin pain resolves after the second postoperative day.

38. **a. Obesity and diabetes are associated with fasciitis after pelvic surgery.** A review of necrotizing fasciitis in gynecologic surgery found that obesity (88%), hypertension (65%), and diabetes (47%) were all factors associated with the development of fasciitis after surgery. In their randomized controlled trial from 2002, Ward and Hilton found a 2% rate of vaginal wound infection after retropubic MUS surgery. In 2010, Richter et al found a 0.7% rate of vaginal wound infection in both the retropubic and transobturator MUS arms.

39. **c. A midline vaginal incision is acceptable for patients undergoing removal of mesh that has perforated into the urethra.** For slings that perforate into the urethra an inverted-U incision is best because this allows for exposure of the proximal urethra, bladder neck, and endopelvic fascia as well as providing a vaginal epithelial flap that avoids overlapping suture lines.

40. **e. Single-incision sling manufacturers are required to perform 522 postmarket surveillance studies.** In January 2012, the Food and Drug Administration (FDA) mandated that all manufacturers of synthetic prosthetic mesh and biologic graft materials marketed for pelvic organ prolapse repair and single-incision sling products perform 522 postmarket surveillance studies. Midurethral sling products (except single-incision slings) were excluded from this mandate because, in September 2011, an FDA advisory panel deemed existing midurethral sling products "safe and effective."

CHAPTER REVIEW

1. Urethral slings are the procedure of choice for the surgical correction of female SUI.
2. Slings should be placed at the bladder neck.
3. Slings are particularly helpful in treating ISD.
4. The majority of patients who require clean intermittent catheterization after PVS placement had a neurogenic bladder preoperatively.
5. Persistent urgency incontinence or urgency are more common presenting symptoms for bladder outlet obstruction after a sling placement than is frank retention.
6. Maximum urethral closure pressure occurs at the level of the midurethra.
7. Success of midurethral slings is less in patients with a fixed urethra and/or a low leak-point pressure.
8. Urethral mobility before midurethral sling procedures has been shown to be predictive of success; the more the proximal urethra moves during a Valsalva maneuver, the better the cure rate for incontinence.
9. For patients with persistently elevated residual urines and bothersome symptoms refractory to conservative management after a sling procedure, MUS release procedures consistently provide resolution of symptoms with maintenance of continence in the majority of patients.
10. Cystoscopy is an integral part of all urethral sling procedures to visualize any injury to the urethra or bladder.
11. Periurethral bulking agents have limited success in treating stress incontinence.
12. The use of autologous tissue for a sling has the lowest rate of erosion and infection.
13. The most common reason for patient dissatisfaction following sling surgery is the development of urgency symptoms and/or urgency incontinence.
14. Synthetic material is no longer used for bladder neck slings.
15. When synthetic mesh erodes into the urethra or bladder, the mesh must be removed.
16. Obese patients with incontinence benefit from weight loss.
17. When sling release is performed, a midline incision of the sling is all that is required; the entire sling does not need to be excised.

85 Complications Related to the Use of Mesh and Their Repair

Shlomo Raz and Lisa Rogo-Gupta

QUESTIONS

1. Which of the following statements is TRUE?
   a. Urinary obstruction always presents with elevated postvoid residuals.
   b. Mesh exposure is necessary to diagnose a patient with mesh complications.
   c. Vaginal estrogen sometimes resolves mesh exposure.
   d. If a patient does not have complications 3 months after mesh insertion, no further follow-up is needed.
   e. De novo lower urinary tract symptoms are never a sign of mesh complications.

2. Evaluation of a patient with possible mesh complications includes:
   a. history and review of medical records.
   b. history and physical examination, conversation with the original surgeon.
   c. history and physical examination, review of medical records.
   d. history and physical examination, diagnostic imaging, review of medical records.
   e. physical examination and diagnostic imaging.

3. Which of the following correctly identifies a possible surgical complication?
   a. Levator ani pain after mesh placed vaginally for rectocele repair
   b. Sacral pain and osteomyelitis after mesh placed vaginally for cystocele repair
   c. Rectal penetration after midurethral sling
   d. Rectus muscle pain after mesh placed vaginally for rectocele repair
   e. All of the above are correct

4. All of the following are appropriate diagnostic studies for the evaluation of mesh complications, EXCEPT:
   a. abdominal radiograph for mesh location.
   b. voiding cystourethrogram for urinary obstruction.
   c. computed tomographic (CT) scan for abdominal abscess.
   d. magnetic resonance imaging (MRI) for osteitis or osteomyelitis.
   e. translabial ultrasound for mesh location and size.

5. Mesh products may contain which of the following components?
   a. Zero to four arms
   b. Tined ends
   c. Postinsertion adjustment device
   d. Polypropylene material
   e. All of the above

6. All of the following are appropriate treatment options for patients with mesh complications, EXCEPT:
   a. partial mesh excision.
   b. complete mesh excision.
   c. medical management of complications.
   d. referral to another physician for a second opinion.
   e. routine annual follow-up.

7. Patients should be counseled regarding risks of some mesh placement procedures, including:
   a. mesh exposure (1% to 19%).
   b. buttock, groin, or pelvic pain (0% to 18%) and de novo dyspareunia (2% to 28%).
   c. mesh exposure (10%) and reoperation (8%).
   d. reoperation (1% to 22%).
   e. a, b, and d.

8. Which of the following is correct regarding outcomes of mesh removal?
   a. Surgical removal of mesh may improve pain in the majority of patients
   b. Risk of anterior prolapse recurrence after mesh removal is 60%.
   c. Risk of incontinence after sling removal ranges from 30% to 50%.
   d. a and c only
   e. a, b, and c

ANSWERS

1. **c. Vaginal estrogen sometimes resolves mesh exposure.** Answers a, b, and e suggest that complications always present similarly, which is incorrect. Answer d suggests that complications always present within 3 months following insertion, which is also incorrect. Complications may present in a variety of ways, and at any time.

2. **d. History and physical examination, diagnostic imaging, review of medical records.** History and physical examination are essential components of evaluation. Review of medical records and diagnostic imaging may also be useful in select patients.

3. **a. Levator ani pain after mesh placed vaginally for rectocele repair.** Levator ani, gluteal pain, and rectal penetration have been described after rectocele repairs performed with mesh augmentation. Sacral pain and osteomyelitis have been described after suspensions of the uterus, cervix, or vagina to the sacrum. Rectus muscle pain is typically described after midurethral sling placement.

4. **a. Abdominal radiograph for mesh location.** Abdominal radiograph is not commonly utilized for identification of mesh location. Answers b, c, d, and e all describe diagnostic studies that may be useful in select patients.

5. **e. All of the above.** The term "mesh products" is used to describe a multitude of products. Variation exists in product composition, fixation mechanism, shape, and additional features.

6. **e. Routine annual follow-up.** Patients with complications should be followed up closely for improvement, and answer e is appropriate for patients without complications.

7. **e. a, b, and d.** This describes the recommended counseling for patients undergoing mesh placement procedures.

8. **d. a and c only.** There is a 20% risk of recurrent anterior prolapse after mesh removal.

CHAPTER REVIEW

1. With the use of mesh in the vaginal area, there is a 10% erosion rate and up to a 28% incidence of dyspareunia.
2. Pain complications on occasion cannot be reversed, even with complete removal of the mesh.
3. Mesh exposure and dyspareunia may occur years later as vaginal atrophy occurs with aging.
4. There is a 30% to 50% risk of incontinence following sling excision, and a 20% incidence of anterior compartment prolapse.

QUESTIONS

1. Which of the following has been shown to be the ideal injectable agent?
   a. Coaptite (Bioform Medical, San Mateo, CA)
   b. Macroplastique (Cogentix Medical, Minnetonka, MN)
   c. Durasphere EXP
   d. Bulkamid (Contura International, Soeborg, Denmark)
   e. None of the above

2. Which of the following statements about the mechanism of action of injectables is most correct?
   a. It augments urethral mucosa.
   b. Its mechanism is not yet defined.
   c. It improves hermetic seal.
   d. It creates obstruction.
   e. It improves urethral coaptation.

3. Injectable agents are indicated for the treatment of stress urinary incontinence (SUI) due to intrinsic sphincter deficiency (ISD). Which of the following statements about urodynamics for ISD is TRUE?
   a. The diagnostic and predictive value of urethral pressure profilometry in characterizing ISD has been proved.
   b. The presence of hypermobility always raises the leak-point pressure (LPP), thus excluding ISD.
   c. ISD is not present if the LPP is >90 cm H_2O.
   d. Many studies have not confirmed the value of LPP in quantifying ISD.
   e. A low urethral pressure profile (UPP) characteristically predicts the presence of ISD.

4. Which of the following statements about the usefulness of cystoscopy before injection is TRUE?
   a. The relative degree of ISD versus hypermobility can be ascertained.
   b. Adverse urethral factors such as scarring or diverticula can be assessed.
   c. The amount of SUI can be assessed.
   d. Bladder neck hypermobility, which contraindicates injectables, can be measured.
   e. Cystoscopy should not be done before injectable agents.

5. Which of the following statements about injection techniques is TRUE?
   a. Both the periurethral and transurethral techniques have shown similar results.
   b. The transurethral technique can only be done with cystoscopic monitoring.
   c. The periurethral technique always requires a general anesthetic.
   d. The transurethral technique is more painful for patients.
   e. The periurethral approach is more commonly done.

6. Which of the following injectable agents requires the use of a ratcheted injection gun?
   a. Silicone microimplants (Macroplastique)
   b. Carbon-coated zirconium beads (Durasphere)
   c. Polyacrylamide hydrogel (Bulkamid)
   d. Calcium hydroxylapatite (Coaptite)
   e. Hyaluronic acid detranomer (Deflux) (Salix Pharmaceuticals, Raleigh, NC)

7. Which of the following statements regarding antibiotic prophylaxis for the use of injectable agents is TRUE?
   a. One week of a second-generation cephalosporin is required.
   b. Intravenous aminoglycoside must be given 1 hour pretreatment.
   c. A fluoroquinolone or trimethoprim-sulfamethoxazole for 24 hours or less can be recommended.
   d. A 3-day course of a fluoroquinolone has been shown in randomized studies of injectable agents to be most effective.
   e. Prophylactic antibiotics are not effective for prevention of urinary tract infection (UTI).

8. Which of the following statements about reinjections is TRUE?
   a. Reinjections never restore continence.
   b. Reinjections should always be done within 1 week.
   c. The site of reinjection should always be away from the previous injection site.
   d. Long-term reinjections are superior to short-term.
   e. The minimum timing for reinjections is variable and depends on the agent.

9. Which of the following methods of reporting injectable results may lead to an overestimate in success rate?
   a. Eliminating the failures from the denominator
   b. Reporting results after the first rather than the last treatment
   c. Accounting for missing data by imputing a value based on a previous result (last observation carried forward, LOCF)
   d. Use of a Kaplan-Meier curve to depict efficacy
   e. a, b, and c are correct

10. Which of the following is a rare complication of collagen injections for SUI?
    a. Urinary infection
    b. Urethrovaginal fistula
    c. Hematuria
    d. Urgency incontinence
    e. Retention

11. Which injectable agent was reported to migrate to pelvic lymph nodes seen in radiograph?
    a. Porcine collagen
    b. Silicone macroparticles
    c. Carbon-coated zirconium beads

d. Bovine collagen

e. Autologous fat

12. What is the minimum threshold for particle size that determines migration risk?

a. 20 μm

b. 40 μm

c. 60 μm

d. 80 μm

e. 100 μm

13. Which of the following complications were seen more frequently in the carbon-coated zirconium bead arm of collagen versus carbon-coated zirconium bead study?

a. Urgency and retention

b. Hematuria

c. Recurrent SUI

d. Mucosal prolapse

e. Particle migration

14. Which of the following agents showed a treatment benefit versus collagen in a randomized trial?

a. Zuidex (hyaluronic acid dextranomer) (Q-Med AB, Uppsala, Sweden)

b. Durasphere (carbon-coated zirconium bead)

c. Macroplastique (silicone microimplant)

d. Autologous fat

e. Coaptite (calcium hydroxylapatite)

15. Which of the following injectable agents failed to demonstrate noninferiority to collagen in a randomized clinical trial?

a. Teflon (Polytetrafluoroethylene paste) (DuPont, Wilmington, DE)

b. Zuidex (hyaluronic acid dextranomer with Implacer)

c. Autologous fat

d. Tegress (ethylene vinyl alcohol) (C.R. Bard, Covington, GA)

e. Bulkamid (polyacrylamide hydrogel)

16. Regarding the outcome of pelvic floor physiotherapy for post–radical prostatectomy incontinence, which statement is TRUE?

a. The treatment results are not seen until 18 months after surgery.

b. The outcome is not dependent on the postoperative starting time.

c. The results are equivalent to surgery.

d. At 12 months there is almost no difference compared with no treatment.

e. A combination of bulking agents and physiotherapy has been shown to be better than either alone.

17. Which statement about the outcome of injectable agents for postradical prostatectomy incontinence is TRUE?

a. Multiple treatment sessions are usually required.

b. The results are similar to those after artificial sphincter.

c. The combination of injectable agent and sling has been demonstrated to be superior to either modality alone.

d. Their noninvasive nature mandates their use in all patients.

e. Newer agents have been shown to be more effective than collagen.

18. Which of the following factors contribute to a poor response to injectable agent (collagen) following prostatectomy?

a. Prior radiation

b. Stricture

c. High-grade SUI

d. Low abdominal leak-point pressure (ALPP)

e. All of the above

19. Which of the following statements about results of silicone microimplants (Macroplastique) for post-prostatectomy incontinence are TRUE? (Select all that are true.)

a. Long-term deterioration of outcome is expected.

b. Noninferiority was demonstrated versus collagen.

c. Not as effective for more severe incontinence versus the artificial urinary sphincter (AUS).

d. Reinjections are not commonly required.

e. Patient satisfaction has been shown to be higher with the Macroplastique than Bulkamid

20. Which of the following is a recognized adverse factor for ProACT (Uromedica, Düsseldorf, Germany) balloon success?

a. Slowly rising prostate-specific antigen (PSA)

b. Prior radiation

c. Failed artificial sphincter

d. Detrusor overactivity

e. Urinary tract infection

ANSWERS

1. **e. None of the above.** The ideal injectable agent should be easily injectable and conserve its volume with time. It should also be biocompatible, nonantigenic, noncarcinogenic, nonmigratory, and cause little or no inflammatory reaction (Kershen and Atala, 1999)* or fibrotic ingrowth (Dmochowski and Appell, 2000). The components of the bulking agent should not separate or dissociate on injection, and if the agent contains microcrystalline or micropolymeric components, they should be reasonably uniform spheres of particle sizes greater than 110 μm that are nonfragile and adhere to host tissue (Dmochowski and Appell, 2000). If unsuccessful, it should not interfere with subsequent surgical intervention. To date, no substance has met all of these requirements.

2. **b. Mechanism not yet defined.** It is generally thought that these agents improve intrinsic sphincter function, although the exact mechanism has not been defined (Smith et al, 2009). Bulking agents such as collagen have been reported (McGuire and Appell, 1994; Monga et al, 1995) to augment urethral mucosa and improve coaptation and intrinsic sphincter function as evidenced by an increase in post-treatment abdominal leak pressure (Herschorn et al, 1992; Richardson et al, 1995; Winters and Appell, 1995). Bulking agents do not generally obstruct voiding after the initial post-treatment period (Monga et al, 1995).

3. **d. Many studies have not confirmed the value of LPP in quantifying ISD.** Because injectable agents are indicated for the ISD component of SUI, can urodynamic studies assess ISD? Two measures of urethral function have been used: maximum urethral closure pressure (MUCP) and abdominal leak-point pressure (ALPP). A MUCP of ≤20 cm H_2O has been suggested as an indicator of clinically significant urethral weakness, but there is controversy regarding the diagnostic and predictive value of urethral pressure profilometry in characterizing ISD (Weber, 2001). Similarly, an ALPP of ≤60 cm H_2O was identified as an indicator of severe ISD (McGuire et al, 1993), but many studies have not confirmed the test's value in quantifying the degree of ISD (Koelbl et al, 2009). Previously, ALPP measurements of initially ≤65 and then ≤100 cm H_2O were used as indicators of ISD to justify the use of injectable agents

*Sources referenced can be found in *Campbell-Walsh Urology, 11th Edition,* on the Expert Consult website.

(Appell and Winters, 2007). However, because ISD may be present in many patients with SUI with or without urethral hypermobility (Koelbl et al, 2009, 2013), the specific value of either the MUCP or ALPP may be of no importance in the clinical decision about the use of injectables. As with other patients with SUI who opt for interventional therapy, urodynamic studies may be helpful for the reasons mentioned earlier.

4. **b. Adverse urethral factors such as scarring or diverticula can be assessed.** Preinjection cystoscopy is helpful to make sure that there are no adverse factors or unexpected findings that may prevent or compromise the injection procedure, such as extensive urethral scarring from previous surgery, radiation, or trauma, foreign bodies, or urethral diverticula.

5. **a. Both the periurethral and transurethral techniques have shown similar results.** The periurethral and transurethral approaches for collagen were compared first by Faerber and colleagues (1998), who reported no significant difference in success rates and numbers of injections required in 24 patients with transurethral treatment versus 21 with a periurethral approach. However, significantly more collagen was required for the periurethral approach. Schulz and coworkers (2004) reported similar findings in 40 women randomly assigned to either technique. There was no difference in short-term success rate, but the 20 women assigned to the periurethral approach required more collagen than those assigned to the transurethral approach. Furthermore, the Cochrane review concluded that there are insufficient data to determine whether transurethral is superior to periurethral and whether midurethral offers any benefit versus bladder neck injection (Kirchin et al, 2012). The transurethral approach is now more commonly reported than the periurethral approach.

6. **a. Silicone microimplants (Macroplastique).** Because of its high viscosity, Macroplastique injections require the use of a ratcheted injection gun. The injection needle is 7 Fr with a 10-mm 18-G needle tip.

7. **c. A fluoroquinolone or trimethoprim-sulfamethoxazole for 24 hours or less can be recommended.** Although randomized trials have not been done, prophylactic antibiotics with a fluoroquinolone or trimethoprim-sulfamethoxazole (TMP-SMX) for 24 hours or less can be recommended (Wolf et al, 2008). An additional 2 to 3 days has also been suggested (Appell and Winters, 2007).

8. **e. The minimum timing for reinjections is variable and depends on the agent.** Although bovine glutaraldehyde cross-linked collagen (Contigen; C.R. Bard, Covington, GA) could be reinjected within 7 days, most clinicians waited 4 weeks or longer to assess response of the urethra and the need for reinjection (Appell and Winters, 2007). Silicone microimplant (Macroplastique) injections can be repeated after 12 weeks (Uroplasty). Carbon-coated zirconium beads (Durasphere) can be reinjected after a minimum of 7 days (Lightner et al, 2001) and calcium hydroxylapatite (Coaptite) after 1 month or less (Mayer et al, 2007). Polyacrylamide hydrogel (Bulkamid) has been reinjected at 1 to 2 months (Toozs-Hobson et al, 2012; Sokol et al, 2014).

9. **e. a, b, and c are correct.** A number of pitfalls in reporting of injectable studies can lead to inflated success rate. Because injectable agents can be repeated if the initial treatment fails, authors should specify whether that time point is after all treatments have been completed or whether it is from baseline. If durability is reported after all injections are administered, then an accurate picture of duration of efficacy can be conveyed. A Kaplan-Meier curve of efficacy has been useful in showing what happens to patients' continence outcome with time (Herschorn and Radomski, 1997; Lightner et al, 2001). Nevertheless some studies report duration of results from initial treatment (Richardson et al, 1995) or do not specify (Monga et al, 1995). This may overestimate success because failures are retreated and counted as successes within the follow-up period. Another pitfall is reporting success rates on cohorts of patients followed for the long term rather than on all patients treated

from the start (Stenberg et al, 2003). If the failed or lost-to-follow-up patients are not included in the denominator, the success rate will be higher.

Another problem encountered in clinical studies, especially longer-term studies, is accounting for missing data from patients who dropped out. One way of handling this is to impute or assign a value based on a previous result. A standard method is last observation carried forward (LOCF). Although this may solve the problem of missing data, it may bias the study in favor of a good outcome. For example, in the 2-year follow-up study of Bulkamid, Toozs-Hobson and coworkers (2012) reported a responder rate of 64% in 116 women. However, there were 135 women treated at the beginning of the study and only 86 were available for the 24-month follow-up. If one calculates the number of responders in the 86 evaluable patients using the 64% responder rate and then uses that number to calculate the percentage in the 135 patients, the success rate then becomes 41%, substantially less than that reported. In view of this potential bias, other more robust methods than LOCF are available to provide for missing data (Siddiqui et al, 2009).

10. **b. Urethrovaginal fistula.** Vesicovaginal fistula occurring after collagen injections for SUI in 2 women after cystectomy and neobladder was described by Pruthi and colleagues (2000). Carlin and Klutke (2000) reported a urethrovaginal fistula in a woman whose warfarin was not completely reversed. She had a postinjection hematoma and ultimately fistulized to the vagina.

11. **c. Carbon-coated zirconium beads.** Pannek and coworkers did report particle migration (2001). This was subsequently attributed the high pressure necessary to inject the viscous material with large particles, resulting in material displacement into vascular or lymphatic spaces (Appell et al, 2006). Durasphere EXP with smaller particles is less likely to lead to this.

12. **d. 80 μm.** The bead size of carbon-coated zirconium ranges from 212 to 500 μm, which is larger than the threshold for particle size migration of 80 μm (Malizia et al, 1984).

13. **a. Urgency and retention.** In the multicenter randomized trial of Durasphere versus collagen, the adverse event profiles were similar (Lightner et al, 2001). However, more women had significantly more post-treatment urgency and acute retention with Durasphere versus collagen, 24.7% and 16.9% versus 11.9% and 3.4%, respectively.

14. **c. Macroplastique (silicone microimplant).** Ghoniem and colleagues (2009) reported results of a North American multicenter randomized trial of Macroplastique versus collagen. After 1 year, 61.5% (75/122) with Macroplastique and 48% (60/125) with collagen had an improvement of at least 1 Stamey grade. This indicated that Macroplastique was noninferior to collagen (P < 0.001). The proportion of the patients who were dry was higher in the Macroplastique group at 36.9% versus 24.8% (P < 0.05). However, there were no significant differences in pad weight testing, quality-of-life scale, or adverse events.

15. **b. Zuidex (hyaluronic acid dextranomer with Implacer).** Lightner and colleagues (2009) reported 12-month outcomes of a North American prospective 2:1 randomized trial of Zuidex-Implacer versus collagen injected cystoscopically in 344 women. The study failed to demonstrate that Zuidex was noninferior to collagen. The proportion of women who achieved a 50% reduction in urinary leakage on provocation testing, the primary outcome, was achieved in 84% of collagen-treated women versus 65% of Zuidex-treated women. There was also a 15% incidence of pseudoabscess formation. This negative trial prompted the company to withdraw the Zuidex product.

16. **d. At 12 months there is almost no difference compared to no treatment.** Physiotherapy and pelvic floor rehabilitation have been shown to improve or enhance continence (decreased time to final continence level) in the postoperative period in two randomized studies, but only if such measures are instituted before or immediately after catheter removal (Van Kampen et al, 2000; Parekh et al, 2003). Maximum difference between physiotherapy and no treatment is achieved at

3 months, with almost no difference at 12 months. A randomized study in which randomization occurred 6 weeks after surgery showed no difference in continence at 6 months (Wille et al, 2003).

17. **a. Multiple treatment sessions are usually required.** Urethral bulking theoretically works by adding bulk and increasing coaptation at the level of the bladder neck and proximal urethra. Several agents have been used, including bovine collagen (Contigen), and silicone microparticles (Macroplastique). All agents share similar problems, including the need for multiple injections, deterioration of effect over time, and low cure rates.

18. **e.** Several authors have identified factors that negatively affect postprostatectomy incontinence treatment results, including extensive scarring or stricture formation, previous radiation, and high-grade stress incontinence and low ALPP (Aboseif et al, 1996; Sanchez-Ortiz et al, 1997; Smith et al, 1998; Cespedes et al, 1999).

19. **c. Not as effective for more severe incontinence versus the artificial urinary sphincter (AUS).** Imamoglu and colleagues (2005) demonstrated no difference in success with AUS versus Macroplastique in men with mild incontinence. However, in patients with more severe incontinence, the AUS was superior, with minimal improvement seen following transurethral Macroplastique.

20. **b. Prior radiation.** Reported risk factors for failure and complications were prior external beam radiotherapy (Lebret et al, 2008; Gregori et al, 2010) and severe preoperative incontinence (Gregori et al, 2010). Kocjanic and colleagues (2007) reported a continence rate of 67% in nonradiated patients compared to 36% in radiated patients.

CHAPTER REVIEW

1. Injection therapy is thought to improve intrinsic sphincter function by improving mucosal coaptation.
2. Injectable agents are indicated for the ISD component of SUI.
3. Detrusor overactivity should be treated before injection therapy because it may compromise the results. Sphincter and bladder dysfunction may coexist in a third of patients.
4. A maximum urethral closure pressure less than or equal to 20 cm H_2O or an abdominal leak point pressure less than or equal to 60 cm H_2O have been used to diagnose intrinsic sphincter deficiency; however, these parameters do not correlate with success after injection therapy.
5. The substance to be injected at the bladder neck or proximal urethra is injected immediately beneath the mucosa at the 3- and 9-o'clock position so as to coapt the mucosa.
6. The transurethral or paraurethral route of injection has similar results.
7. A catheter is not routinely used after injection except in patients who have retention; if that is the case, the catheter should be of small caliber.

8. Complications of injection therapy include urinary retention, urinary infection, detrusor overactivity, hematuria, incontinence, vaginal discomfort, vaginal wall erosion, and urethral mucosa prolapse.
9. On average, approximately one third of patients are cured at 18 months.
10. Autologous materials that have been used for bulking agents include chondrocytes, fibroblasts, fat, and umbilical cord stem cells. The results have been mixed.
11. Postprostatectomy, sphincter and bladder dysfunction may coexist in one third of patients.
12. Injectable agents are not effective in a scarred membranous urethra.
13. Factors that negatively affect postprostatectomy incontinence treatment results include extensive scarring or stricture formation, previous radiation, high-grade stress incontinence, and low ALPP.
14. Injectables have been used in continent diversions with variable success. Vesicovaginal fistula has been reported as a complication in these patients.

87 Additional Therapies for Storage and Emptying Failure

Timothy B. Boone and Julie N. Stewart

QUESTIONS

1. All of the following patients would be candidates for augmentation cystoplasty EXCEPT:
   a. a patient with a neurogenic bladder and poor bladder compliance who has failed anti-cholinergic medications and intravesical injections of botulinum toxin.
   b. a patient with a spinal cord injury and detrusor leak point pressures of greater than 40 cm H_2O and subsequent vesicoureteral reflux.
   c. a patient with refractory idiopathic detrusor overactivity.
   d. a patient with significant urinary frequency and a bladder capacity of less than 100 mL.
   e. a patient with rapidly progressing multiple sclerosis and bothersome neurogenic detrusor overactivity causing urinary leakage.

2. Of the following statements, which one is NOT a potential side effect of an ileocystoplasty?
   a. Hyperchloremic metabolic acidosis
   b. Bacterial colonization and increased risk of urinary tract infections
   c. Osteopenia
   d. Hypochloremic hyponatremic alkalosis
   e. Vitamin B_{12} deficiency

3. All of the following statements are TRUE regarding stimulated myoplasty for sphincteric deficiency EXCEPT:
   a. Muscle type conversion from fast-twitch to slow-twitch fibers through continuous electrical stimulation provides resting tone for urethral closure.
   b. The sartorius muscle is used as a free microsurgical flap.
   c. An autologous muscle transfer provides circumferential pressure on the urethra or bladder neck.
   d. The gracilis muscle is often utilized.
   e. Electrode leads are implanted in the muscle in a staged, second procedure.

4. Which of the following statements is FALSE regarding urethral compression devices in a male?
   a. Urethral pressure should be released at least twice per day.
   b. They should be removed while sleeping.
   c. Pressure-related injuries may occur in patients with altered cognition.
   d. The lowest pressure that relieves incontinence should be used.
   e. Patients with pure sphincteric incontinence will obtain the best results.

5. The Credé maneuver for emptying the bladder is relatively contraindicated in patients:
   a. with decreased outlet resistance.
   b. who are obese.
   c. with vesicoureteral reflux.
   d. with high-pressure detrusor overactivity.
   e. younger than the age of 2 years.

6. Incontinence-associated dermatitis (IAD) is associated with the following factors in the incontinent patient EXCEPT:
   a. It may be caused by infrequent pad changes.
   b. It is manifested by inflammation of the skin with redness and edema.
   c. It may lead to malignant lesions of the skin.
   d. It predominately occurs in skin folds.
   e. It promotes candidiasis and bacterial infections.

7. All of the following statements are TRUE regarding bladder outlet closure EXCEPT:
   a. Complete closure of the bladder neck is rarely necessary.
   b. The main indication is urethral destruction after prolonged catheter drainage.
   c. An obstructing sling or artificial urinary sphincter (AUS) is rarely feasible, if less than 1 cm of urethra exists.
   d. Reflex sphincteric activity may result in disruption of the bladder neck closure.
   e. The transvaginal approach has decreased the postoperative fistula rate.

8. Of the following statements, which one is FALSE regarding "trigger voiding" in spinal cord-injured patients?
   a. Trigger voiding can be induced by digital rectal stimulation.
   b. Reflex contractions can be generated by using somatic motor axons to innervate parasympathetic bladder ganglia cells.
   c. Rhythmic suprapubic manual pressure is usually the most effective method for trigger voiding.
   d. Trigger voiding induces a reflex decrease in outlet resistance in patients with detrusor-sphincter dyssynergia.
   e. Trigger voiding can be induced by squeezing the clitoris

9. Common complications associated with a continent catheterizable channel include all of the following EXCEPT:
   a. stomal stenosis.
   b. perforation of the catheterizable channel.
   c. incontinence from the stoma site.
   d. difficulty passing a catheter through the stoma due to stricture.
   e. stomal prolapse.

10. Which of the following statements is FALSE?
    a. Chronic indwelling urethral catheterization protects against poor bladder compliance and upper tract complications.
    b. Chronic indwelling urethral catheterization compared with clean intermittent catheterization (CIC) is associated with a higher incidence of urolithiasis.
    c. Asymptomatic bacteriuria is common in catheterized patients and does not usually require treatment.
    d. Periodic upper and lower tract evaluation is important in all patients managed with chronic indwelling catheters.
    e. There is still a role for anticholinergic medications in patients managing their bladders with a chronic indwelling catheter.

11. Clean intermittent catheterization is relatively contraindicated in patients with:

    a. a history of urethral stricture disease.

    b. bacteriuria.

    c. autonomic dysreflexia.

    d. decreased bladder compliance.

    e. a history of a bladder neck artificial urinary sphincter.

12. All of the following statements are TRUE regarding catheterization EXCEPT:

    a. there is no known association with intermittent catheterization and development of squamous cell carcinoma of the bladder.

    b. gross hematuria in a patient with a chronic indwelling catheter is likely related to infection or inflammation and does not require a thorough hematuria workup.

    c. urinary incontinence may worsen in patients with intrinsic sphincter deficiency who convert from an indwelling urethral to suprapubic catheter.

    d. there is a lower incidence of epididymitis in men who have chronic suprapubic catheters compared with urethral catheters.

    e. there is a low risk of developing squamous cell carcinoma of the bladder with chronic indwelling catheter use.

ANSWERS

1. **e. A patient with rapidly progressing multiple sclerosis and bothersome neurogenic detrusor overactivity causing urinary leakage.** A patient with a progressive neurologic disease, such as multiple sclerosis, may not have the ability to perform CIC in the future and an alternative treatment plan should be considered. Noncompliance with CIC puts the patient at risk for life-threatening spontaneous bladder perforation.

2. **d. Hypochloremic hyponatremic alkalosis.** All of the statements are potential side effects of an ileocystoplasty except hypochloremic hyponatremic alkalosis. This metabolic abnormality is associated with a gastrocystoplasty.

3. **b. The sartorius muscle is used as a free microsurgical flap.** The use of an autologous muscle transfer to form a neosphincter around the urethra has been reported in a few small clinical series. Case reports describe transposition of the gracilis muscle to the urethra or bladder neck by transection of the distal muscle at the tibial tuberosity with preservation of the proximal neurovascular pedicle. The gracilis muscle is wrapped around either the bladder neck or the bulbous urethra and attached to itself (bulbous urethra) or the back of the os pubis (bladder neck), ensuring circumferential pressure on the urethra with electrical stimulation of the myoplasty.

4. **a. Urethral pressure should be released at least twice per day.** These devices are primarily used to treat patients with pure sphincteric incontinence, most commonly postprostatectomy incontinence, because normal bladder capacity and storage pressures are a relative requirement. Compression devices should be unclamped regularly at 3- to 4-hour intervals, because prolonged or excessive compression can cause pressure-related injury to the penis. In addition, these devices should not be worn during an erection or while sleeping. Pressure-related injuries may also be more prevalent in patients with impaired sensation or cognition; therefore, penile clamp usage in this population should be considered a relative contraindication. Although these devices manage sphincteric incontinence relatively well, they are rarely used today because they are inconvenient, and many minimally invasive options for male sphincteric incontinence now exist. These devices remain useful for patients who cannot undergo surgical therapy because of medical conditions, and for patients who have severe leakage during the early postprostatectomy period while surgical treatment is contraindicated.

5. **c. With vesicoureteral reflux.** The Credé maneuver (manual compression of the bladder) is most effective in patients with decreased bladder tone who can generate an intravesical pressure greater than 50 cm H_2O and have decreased bladder outlet resistance. The Credé maneuver requires good hand control, is easier in a thin individual than an obese one, and is more easily performed in a child than in an adult. Voiding by Credé is unphysiologic, because active opening of the bladder neck does not occur, and increases in outlet resistance by a reflex mechanism may actually occur. If complete emptying does not occur, treatment to decrease outlet resistance can be contemplated, or an alternative method to empty the bladder should be used. Vesicoureteral reflux is a relative contraindication to external compression and straining maneuvers, especially in patients capable of generating a high intravesical pressure.

6. **c. It may lead to malignant lesions of the skin.** Prolonged exposure of the skin to a wet environment may lead to supersaturation and disruption of the skin's protective barriers, thus promoting skin maceration, dermatitis, and possibly infection. Incontinence-associated dermatitis (IAD) can be defined as inflammation of the surface of the skin with redness, edema, and, in some cases, bullae containing clear exudate. IAD predominately occurs in skin folds and may promote candidiasis or bacterial skin infections. IAD has not been associated with premalignant or malignant lesions of the skin.

7. **e. The transvaginal approach has decreased the postoperative fistula rate.** Complete closure of the bladder neck is rarely necessary, because a compressive bladder neck sling is more easily performed, is less morbid, and allows transurethral access if necessary. The main indication for bladder outlet closure is urethral destruction secondary to prolonged catheter drainage in neurogenic bladder patients. A case series using "tight" autologous pubovaginal sling and lower urinary tract reconstruction for urethras destroyed by long-term Foley catheter use reported excellent results with minimal incontinence. The authors concluded that at least 1 cm of normal urethra was required for proper functioning of the sling. The risk of complications, specifically a vesicovaginal fistula, is relatively common and can be difficult to repair. It is important to remember that a bladder neck closure is much more difficult than a simple closure of the bladder wall. The bladder neck is usually hyperactive in patients with neurologic disease, and every voiding reflex includes active opening and closing of the bladder neck, which forcibly attempts to destroy the bladder neck closure. To reduce this risk, postoperative suppression of the voiding reflex using prolonged continuous catheter drainage (3 weeks) and liberal use of anticholinergics is imperative. In addition, to reduce the risk of fistula, the repair must be watertight from the beginning, and this requires a precise mucosal closure using a running suture and multiple additional layers of muscle to reinforce the strength of the repair.

8. **d. Trigger voiding induces a reflex decrease in outlet resistance in patients with sphincter dyssynergia.** In some types of spinal cord injury or bladder dysfunction characterized by detrusor hyperreflexia, manual pressure may sometimes be used to initiate a reflexive bladder contraction—sometimes called "trigger voiding." The most effective method of initiating a reflex contraction is thought to be rhythmic suprapubic manual pressure, typically seven or eight compressions every 3 seconds. This rhythmic pressure is thought to produce a summation effect on the tension receptors in the bladder wall, resulting in an afferent neural discharge that activates the bladder reflex arc. Trigger voiding can also sometimes be induced by pulling the skin or hair of the pubis, scrotum, or thigh; squeezing the clitoris; or digital rectal stimulation. Surgical procedures to reduce outlet resistance should be considered, if significant obstruction or sphincter dyssynergia are present. In an animal model using neural rerouting, a detrusor contraction without striated sphincter dyssynergia could be initiated by scratching the skin or by

percutaneous electrical stimulation in the L7 dermatome. The pathway was found to be mediated by cholinergic transmission at both ganglionic and peripheral levels. The importance of this experimental model is that somatic motor axons were able to innervate parasympathetic bladder ganglion cells and therefore transfer somatic reflex activity to the lower urinary tract.

9. **b. Perforation of the catheterizable channel.** These catheterizable channels are not free of complications, and long-term issues with catheterization, incontinence and stomal stenosis can occur. A large retrospective study by Leslie et al (2011)* analyzed the long-term outcomes of 169 pediatric patients who had either undergone a Mitrofanoff appendicovesicostomy or a transverse ileal, or Monti, tube. The authors report a 39% revision rate (8% stricture, 4% prolapse, 10% incontinence, and 17% stomal stenosis at skin level). Perforation of the catheterizable channel has not been commonly reported as a complication.

10. **a. Chronic indwelling urethral catheterization protects against poor bladder compliance and upper tract complications.** The exact etiology of upper tract deterioration in patients with long-term indwelling catheters is unclear because the bladder should be well drained by a catheter; however, it is likely related to chronic "occult" or subclinical detrusor overactivity in the face of sphincteric dyssynergia providing a functional obstruction. Regardless of the etiology, it is clinically heralded by the development of poor detrusor compliance demonstrated on urodynamic studies.

11. **c. Autonomic dysreflexia.** CIC should be used cautiously in patients known to have autonomic dysreflexia because bladder filling and bladder overdistention can be triggers for autonomic dysreflexia.

12. **b. Gross hematuria in a patient with a chronic indwelling catheter is likely related to infection or inflammation and does not require a thorough hematuria workup.** The long-term risk of carcinoma in the spinal cord injury patient with a chronic catheter has been estimated to be 8% to 10%. This association has not been identified in patients performing intermittent catheterization. The development of gross hematuria in patients with a chronic indwelling catheter should prompt further evaluation, including upper tract imaging, urine cytology, cystoscopy, and consideration of bladder biopsy.

CHAPTER REVIEW

1. Indications for augmentation cystoplasty include poor bladder compliance, reduced capacity, and significant overactivity.
2. Chronic metabolic acidosis and osteopenia have been reported in patients over the long term who have had bladder augments with either ileum or colon.
3. Gastrocystoplasty is rarely used because of the development of bladder erosions, perforation, the hematuria dysuria syndrome, and adenocarcinoma in the gastric segment.
4. Bladder augmentation should only be considered in patients who have the capability for self intermittent catheterization.
5. In patients who use intermittent catheterization or in those with chronic indwelling catheters, the presence of asymptomatic bacteriuria does not require treatment. Continued prophylactic antibiotics are rarely indicated in this group as well.
6. Lapedes proposed that high intravesical pressures with bladder overdistention reduces bladder blood flow and makes the bladder susceptible to bacterial invasion and significant urinary tract infections.
7. CIC should be used cautiously in patients known to have autonomic dysreflexia.
8. The frequency of intermittent catheterization should be such that bladder volumes remain below 400 to 500 mL between catheterizations.
9. The advantage of a suprapubic cystostomy in males compared with continuous urethral catheterization is a lower incidence of epididymitis and urethral stricture disease, with preservation of sexual function.
10. When bladder neck incision is performed, it should occur at the 5- and 7-o'clock position and extend caudally just proximal to the verumontanum. This results in retrograde ejaculation approximately 30% to 50% of the time.
11. Sphincterotomy should be performed at the 12-o'clock position because this is the position least likely to cause significant hemorrhage.
12. Compression devices should be unclamped regularly at 3- to 4-hour intervals, because prolonged or excessive compression can cause pressure-related injury to the penis.
13. The Credé maneuver (manual compression of the bladder) is most effective in patients with decreased bladder tone who can generate an intravesical pressure greater than 50 cm H_2O and have decreased bladder outlet resistance. Vesicoureteral reflux is a relative contraindication to external compression.
14. Bladder neck closure is much more difficult than a simple closure of the bladder wall. The bladder neck is usually hyperactive in patients with neurologic disease, and every voiding reflex includes active opening and closing of the bladder neck, which forcibly attempts to destroy the bladder neck closure.
15. Catheterizable channels are not free of complications, and long-term issues with catheterization, incontinence and stomal stenosis can occur. There is a 39% revision rate (8% stricture, 4% prolapse, 10% incontinence, and 17% stomal stenosis at skin level).
16. The long-term risk of carcinoma in the spinal cord injury patient with a chronic catheter has been estimated to be 8% to 10%.

*Sources referenced can be found in *Campbell-Walsh Urology, 11th Edition,* on the Expert Consult website.

Aging and Geriatric Urology

Neil M. Resnick, Stasa D. Tadic, Subbarao V. Yalla, and W. Scott McDougal

QUESTIONS

1. With aging:
   a. renal function increases.
   b. bladder capacity declines.
   c. hepatic function remains relatively stable.
   d. pulmonary function declines.
   e. immunologic function remains stable.

2. Urinary tract infections (UTIs) in elderly women may best be decreased by:
   a. nitrofurantoin prophylaxis.
   b. systemic estrogen administration.
   c. cranberry juice.
   d. vaginal estrogen application.
   e. α-blocker therapy.

3. In demented elderly patients, incontinence:
   a. is inevitable.
   b. is virtually always due to detrusor hyperreflexia.
   c. is unlikely to respond to therapy.
   d. is multifactorial and often reversible.
   e. treatment should focus primarily on preventing skin breakdown.

4. Urinary incontinence (UI) in older people is usually:
   a. brought to a physician's attention by the patient.
   b. detected by the patient's primary physician.
   c. obvious to the urologist.
   d. detected by the physician but ignored.
   e. unknown to the patient's physician.

5. In older patients, involuntary bladder contractions:
   a. are rarely seen in asymptomatic patients.
   b. are primarily due to central nervous system (CNS) pathology.
   c. are almost always the cause of the patient's incontinence.
   d. are inevitable in demented patients.
   e. may not be the cause of the incontinence.

6. After the history and physical examination, evaluation of the incontinent older patient should include:
   a. cystoscopy.
   b. videourodynamics.
   c. postvoid residual assessment.
   d. urinary cytology.
   e. assessment of prostate size in a male.

7. Which of the following occurs as part of *normal* aging?
   a. Urinary incontinence
   b. A small increase in serum creatinine concentration
   c. Uninhibited detrusor contractions
   d. Increase in bladder capacity
   e. Urinary flow rate is unchanged

8. The cornerstone of treatment for persistent urgency incontinence is:
   a. behavioral therapy.
   b. flavoxate.
   c. oxybutynin.
   d. tolterodine.
   e. solifenacin.

9. Acute urinary retention in an older man:
   a. indicates the need for surgical decompression.
   b. is treated effectively with α-adrenergic blockers.
   c. can be seen with detrusor hyperactivity with impaired contractility (DHIC).
   d. is treated effectively with bethanechol.
   e. requires treatment of the underlying urinary tract abnormality.

10. Incontinence management products (e.g., garments/pads):
    a. are reimbursed by insurance companies.
    b. should include menstrual pads.
    c. generally cost less than a dollar per day.
    d. should be chosen according to the type of incontinence rather than its severity.
    e. should be tailored to the individual.

11. The voiding diary completed by an 83-year-old woman bothered by daytime incontinence discloses 800-mL output between 8:00 AM and 11:00 PM, and 1500 mL from 11:00 PM to 8:00 AM. The next step should be:
    a. to have her repeat it with a record of fluid intake.
    b. to take furosemide at 7:00 PM each evening to reduce nocturnal excretion.
    c. to use pressure-gradient stockings to minimize peripheral edema.
    d. to advise her to curtail fluid intake after dinner.
    e. none of the above.

12. Anticholinergic bladder relaxants may, ironically, actually exacerbate incontinence through all of the following mechanisms EXCEPT:
    a. causing/exacerbating confusion.
    b. causing/exacerbating impaired mobility.
    c. causing/exacerbating a dry mouth.
    d. causing/exacerbating subacute urinary retention.
    e. precipitating acute urinary retention.

13. A 78-year-old woman with dementia has responded modestly to donepezil (Aricept, a cholinesterase inhibitor) for the past year. The recent onset of urgency incontinence led her primary physician to prescribe tolterodine last month while awaiting your assessment. Her incontinence has responded well. The next appropriate step is to:
    a. discontinue tolterodine due to its interaction with donepezil.
    b. discontinue donepezil because her cognitive function is stable.

c. discontinue both drugs because she is stable and the urgency incontinence may reflect an adverse effect of the donepezil.

d. continue both drugs and monitor her for deterioration in cognitive function.

e. taper the tolterodine.

14. A 68-year-old obese woman with significant daily stress incontinence comes for a follow-up. Her bladder diary shows maximal voided volume of 125 mL during the daytime. Each of these measures is appropriate EXCEPT:

a. adjustment of fluid excretion and voiding intervals.

b. advising weight reduction.

c. teaching her postural maneuvers.

d. consideration of surgical correction.

e. pelvic floor muscle exercises.

15. A 72-year-old man has urinary urgency and postvoid residual (PVR) of 40 mL. He also has hypertension and aortic stenosis that has caused minimal symptoms. His friend suggested that he ask for terazosin because it helped him with similar symptoms. The most appropriate response is:

a. to prescribe terazosin and see him again in 4 weeks.

b. to prescribe alfuzosin instead, because it has a better side-effect profile.

c. to obtain medical consultation before prescribing the drug.

d. to perform urodynamic testing before deciding.

e. to prescribe an anticholinergic agent.

ANSWERS

1. **d. Pulmonary function declines.** Pulmonary surface area for oxygen diffusion decreases, which leads to alterations in the ventilation perfusion ratio. With aging, renal function and renal mass decline, bladder capacity remains relatively stable but elasticity and contractility decline, and hepatic and immunologic function decline.

2. **d. Vaginal estrogen application.** It has been proposed that vaginal estrogens promote the growth of lactobacillus and thereby lower vaginal pH, which helps reduce pathogen colonization. Systemic estrogens are generally not prescribed in the elderly and may in fact cause incontinence in this population. Nitrofurantoin should not be given during the long term in the elderly because it may reduce renal function and lead to pulmonary fibrosis. Cranberry juice has its advocates but has not been shown to be effective in randomized trials, and α-blocker therapy in the female would not be expected to have much of an effect on residual urine as the female has few alpha receptors at the bladder neck.

3. **d. Is multifactorial and often reversible.** Incontinence is never normal, even with dementia. Detrusor overactivity (DO) is the most common type of lower urinary tract dysfunction among demented incontinent nursing home residents, but it is also the most common dysfunction among their dry peers. Moreover, incontinence in 40% of these individuals is not associated with DO but with obstruction (in men), stress incontinence (in women), or a combination of an outlet and a detrusor problem, and the cause does not correlate with either the presence or severity of dementia. Thus it is no longer tenable to attribute incontinence a priori to DO. Because incontinence in the elderly is usually multifactorial, involving urinary tract as well as non–urinary tract contributions, it is often treatable. Even among nursing home patients, studies have documented more than a 50% reduction in incontinent episodes overall and full daytime continence in nearly 40% of residents. Particularly among demented individuals, nonurinary factors are prevalent and commonly include medication use, depression, fecal impaction, UTI, atrophic vaginitis, and disorders of fluid excretion.

It is important to prevent skin breakdown, but this should not be the primary approach to the incontinent nursing home resident.

4. **e. Unknown to the patient's physician.** Despite the fact that incontinence is so common and amenable to therapy, most patients do not mention it to a physician. Reasons include embarrassment, misperception that it is a normal part of aging, belief that it is untreatable, fear of complications associated with its evaluation and treatment, or misconception that only major surgery can cure it. Moreover, when patients do mention it, most physicians either dismiss it as a normal part of aging or merely check a urinalysis. With newer undergarments and pads that better absorb and deodorize, the doctor may be unaware of the problem unless he/she asks about it.

5. **e. May not be the cause of the incontinence.** It is important to realize that involuntary bladder contractions are found commonly in even continent, neurologically intact elderly; the prevalence ranges in various studies between 50% and 55%. This fact underscores the concept that such contractions are a risk factor for UI but not necessarily sufficient. Moreover, even when such contractions are the major contributor to UI, they may be due to a urethral abnormality. More than half of obstructed individuals and approximately 25% of those with stress incontinence have associated DO that usually remits with correction of the urethral abnormality alone. The proportion of elderly individuals in whom DO remits is likely lower, but clearly it is insufficient merely to identify involuntary contractions on cystometry and attribute the incontinence to them. To be considered the cause of the UI, such contractions must reproduce the patient's type of leakage, and urethral abnormalities must be excluded. This is particularly important because a bladder relaxant medication prescribed for DO that is actually due to obstruction may precipitate acute retention.

6. **c. Postvoid residual assessment.** Determining the PVR is essential in all incontinent older individuals, not only because retention can mimic other causes of UI, but also because knowledge of the PVR will affect therapy. For instance, an older woman with DO and PVR of 250 mL would be approached differently from a woman with DO and PVR of 5 mL. The rest of the diagnostic evaluation depends on the need for diagnostic certainty. However, if surgical correction is contemplated, or if the risk of empiric therapy exceeds the benefit, further testing is warranted. Cytology is indicated when bladder carcinoma is suspected and would be treated if found (i.e., not in a bedfast, demented patient). Cystoscopy has many indications, but it is not routinely required for evaluation of incontinence, nor is it alone sufficient to detect or exclude prostatic obstruction. Palpated prostate size correlates poorly with the presence of obstruction.

7. **c. Uninhibited detrusor contractions.** Incontinence is never part of normal aging. Even at age 90 years, at least half of people are continent. Although renal function declines in most older adults, there is no change in serum creatinine because of a concomitant and balanced decrease in muscle mass. Involuntary detrusor contractions are common in continent and even asymptomatic elderly, but are rarely seen during routine cystometry in younger people. Bladder capacity may decrease in the elderly, but there is no evidence for an increase. Flow rate declines, not only because obstruction becomes more likely in aging men, but also because detrusor contractility appears to decrease in both sexes.

8. **a. Behavioral therapy.** Behavioral therapy is the cornerstone of treatment for detrusor overactivity, although the type of therapy must be tailored to the individual. Bladder retraining attempts to restore a normal voiding pattern by progressively lengthening the voiding interval. Scheduled toileting aims to reduce incontinence by frequent voiding, which reduces total bladder volume and the chance of triggering involuntary bladder contractions. Prompted voiding works by regularly and frequently reminding cognitively impaired residents of the need to void. The role of medications is to supplement behavioral therapy, but only if needed. By reducing bladder irritability,

such agents allow the bladder to hold more urine before the spasm occurs. However, even when continence is restored by these drugs, detrusor overactivity is still generally demonstrable. Furthermore, if the drug increases residual urine more than total bladder capacity, it may paradoxically decrease functional capacity, allowing the persistent involuntary contraction to occur at more frequent intervals. Thus before deciding that drug therapy has failed, PVR should be remeasured. Except for flavoxate, each of the agents listed has been proved effective in randomized controlled trials that included a substantial number of elderly patients.

9. **c. Can be seen with detrusor hyperactivity with impaired contractility (DHIC).** The differential diagnosis for urinary retention extends beyond urethral obstruction, particularly in the elderly. Patients with underactive detrusor or detrusor hyperactivity with impaired contractility (DHIC) also may develop urinary retention. In addition, fecal impaction, pain (e.g., following hip replacement) and medications with urinary tract side effects (e.g., anticholinergics, sedating antihistamines, decongestants, and opiates) may induce acute urinary retention, particularly in patients with underlying bladder weakness or obstruction. Thus the bladder should be decompressed for at least a week while reversible causes are addressed; the larger the PVR, the longer should be the decompression. Decompression allows some restoration of detrusor strength, which also facilitates urodynamic testing should it be necessary. α-Adrenergic blockers are effective for men with symptoms of prostatism, but clinical trials excluded patients with significant urinary retention. Bethanechol, although originally designed to improve bladder emptying in unobstructed patients, has not proved effective for this purpose (and likely not for nonobstructed patients either). Decompression in some elderly patients can reduce but not eliminate residual urine; provided it does not cause symptoms or renal compromise, subclinical retention need not necessarily be treated in all elderly patients, even if obstruction is present.

10. **e. Should be tailored to the individual.** The cost of pads is rarely covered by insurance and can easily exceed $1/day. Menstrual pads, although often used for incontinence, are usually inappropriate. They are designed to absorb small amounts of slowly leaking viscid fluid rather than rapid gushes of urine. From among the numerous types of pads and garments, selection should be tailored to the individual's needs and comorbidity; the type of incontinence matters less than severity.

11. **e. None of the above.** The patient's altered pattern of fluid excretion may occur for a variety of reasons. The most common is accumulation of peripheral edema due to venous insufficiency, peripheral vascular disease, low albumin states (malnutrition, hepatic disease), congestive heart failure, or medications (e.g., nonsteroidal anti-inflammatory drugs [NSAIDs], dihydropyridine calcium channel blockers [e.g., nifedipine], or thiazolidinediones [e.g., rosiglitazone]). Each can be readily addressed. Before doing so, however, it is important to realize that the multiple pathologic conditions so often found in the elderly may be causal, contributory, a consequence, or unrelated to the condition for which the patient seeks help. In this individual, daytime leakage is the problem. Addressing the excess nocturnal excretion will not improve the daytime problem and, if it shifts the excess nocturnal excretion to the daytime (e.g., by use of pressure-gradient stockings), therapy may exacerbate the daytime leakage. If the nocturnal polyuria can be eliminated entirely (e.g., by substituting a drug that does not cause fluid retention), this should be done. If, however, therapy will only shift excretion to the daytime, one may elect not to treat if it is not dangerous (e.g., venous insufficiency). Evening furosemide risks inducing hypovolemia and increasing her risk of falls and fracture. Daytime predominance of incontinence suggests that she has stress incontinence, or DO associated with bladder neck incompetence that is exacerbated when she is upright. Once the cause is sorted out, the appropriate intervention can be prescribed,

but, in this individual, it should not include alteration of fluid intake: Her daytime output is too small to contribute to her daytime UI and, unless she is ingesting 2 L after dinner, her intake is also likely unrelated to her nocturnal polyuria. Moreover, the older kidney generally takes twice as long to respond to fluid restriction as the younger one; so, restricting fluid after dinner is apt to do little. This case highlights the need to tailor the evaluation and treatment to the patient rather than to a given abnormality.

12. **b. Causing/exacerbating impaired mobility.** All of the currently available bladder relaxant medications have anticholinergic properties and thus can cause anticholinergic side effects. Dry mouth (xerostomia) results from the anticholinergic effect on the salivary and parotid glands. Even the M_3-specific agents have this effect, because M_3 receptors are the predominant receptor in these glands as well as in the bladder. Because bladder relaxants generally do not abolish the involuntary detrusor contractions, the xerostomia-mediated increased fluid intake results in the bladder filling more frequently to the volume at which detrusor contractions may be triggered. Bladder relaxants often impair detrusor contractility and can lead to subacute retention. If the increase in PVR is more than the increase in total bladder capacity, the effective bladder capacity will decrease. In turn, this could allow involuntary contractions to occur at a lower effective volume; an increase in incontinence frequency can ensue.

13. **d. Continue both drugs and monitor her for deterioration in cognitive function.** Because cholinesterase inhibitors block the metabolism of acetylcholine, there is concern that they will provoke urgency incontinence, especially in older adults who already may have underlying age-related involuntary detrusor contractions that have not yet caused incontinence. However, despite prescription of these agents to millions of demented patients, there is little evidence that they cause incontinence. Moreover, because the benefits of these drugs for dementia are modest at best and are not seen in the majority of patients who use them, patients and families may decide that the benefit of the bladder relaxant outweighs the risk. Particularly in this patient, who has already benefited from tolterodine without notable cognitive deterioration, it is worth continuing therapy and monitoring her cognitive status.

14. **a. Adjustment of fluid excretion and voiding intervals.** Recent evidence suggests that weight loss will improve stress incontinence in obese women, and data support the use of postural maneuvers, pelvic floor muscle exercises, and surgical correction as well. Adjusting fluid excretion and voiding intervals can also be useful, especially for women with volume-dependent stress leakage. It can work particularly well for women with a threshold of at least 150 mL and best in those with a threshold greater than 250 mL. However, when the threshold is this low, the extent of fluid restriction required is usually not feasible and might even lead to dangerous dehydration.

15. **c. To obtain medical consultation before prescribing the drug.** Men with these lower urinary tract symptoms and a low PVR generally respond well to an α-adrenergic receptor blocker. However, many of these agents can reduce cardiac preload and thus impede adequate left ventricular filling and cardiac output, especially in individuals whose ventricular filling is already more difficult in the setting of left ventricular hypertrophy. The risk is exacerbated by the normal age-related decline that occurs in baroreflex sensitivity and further compounded in patients who take a β blocker and/or have aortic stenosis. Thus although the overall risks of orthostasis, falls, and fracture appear to be lower with the newer α-adrenergic agents, it would be prudent to obtain medical consultation before prescribing an α-blocker in this clinical setting. Anticholinergic therapy can be used in men with urgency and a low PVR but because of the risk of inducing a tachycardia in a man with aortic stenosis and thereby also reducing left ventricular filling—combined with the potential risk of inducing urinary retention—prescription of an anticholinergic should not be the next step.

CHAPTER REVIEW

1. Renal blood flow, renal mass, and functional reserve decrease with aging, which results in a 10-mL decrease in glomerular filtration rate (GFR) per decade.
2. Serum creatinine levels do not accurately reflect renal function in the elderly due to decreased muscle mass. The Cockcroft-Gault formula is more accurate than the Modification of Diet in Renal Disease equation for estimating GFR in the elderly population.
3. Antidiuretic hormone secretion decreases in older adults, resulting in increased nocturia.
4. With age, there is a decrease in cardiac output and stroke volume.
5. The majority of deaths in the perioperative period in geriatric patients are due to cardiovascular events; however, pulmonary problems are the major cause of prolonged hospitalization.
6. Hepatic function and immunologic function diminish with age.
7. With aging, there is a loss of muscle mass and an increase in body fat mass.
8. Bladder capacity does not change with age; however, bladder sensation, contractility, and ability to postpone voiding decline in both sexes with age.
9. Increased involuntary detrusor contractions and decreased bladder elasticity and compliance occur with aging. Indeed, detrusor overactivity is the most common type of lower urinary tract dysfunction in incontinent elderly of both sexes.
10. There is a decrease in striated muscle in the rhabdosphincter with age.
11. Urinary incontinence, UTIs, pelvic prolapse, and bladder outlet obstruction all increase with aging.
12. Stress incontinence in elderly women is usually associated with hypermobility and some degree of intrinsic sphincter deficiency.
13. A functional assessment is correlated with health care outcomes and includes: (1) activities of daily living, (2) mobility with a slow gate speed a strong predictor of mortality, and (3) cognition.
14. Cognitive changes are frequently seen following anesthesia in elderly patients.
15. There is no difference in mortality and morbidity between general and regional anesthesia in the elderly.
16. Major geriatric syndromes include frailty, falls, pressure ulcers, multiple medications, delirium, and urinary incontinence.
17. The frailty phenotype may include an unintentional weight loss in excess of 10 lb per year, reduced grip, slowing of the gait, decreased activity, and easy exhaustion with activity.
18. Elderly men on androgen deprivation therapy are at increased risks for fractures.
19. A number of medications should be used with caution or not used at all in the elderly. For example, Demerol and prolonged use of nitrofurantoin should not be given and caution should be exercised when prescribing antimuscarinics. Anticholinergic agents are one of the most common causes of delirium in the elderly, especially in those with preexisting cognitive or functional impairment.
20. Asymptomatic bacteriura in the elderly does not require treatment; it does not cause incontinence.
21. Peripheral edema may be mobilized when supine and cause nocturia.
22. Conservative measures used to treat excessive fluid output at night include compression stockings, changing the time diuretics are taken or administering a rapid acting diuretic in the late afternoon, and altering the diet.
23. Poststroke fecal and urinary incontinence are not uncommon.
24. Incontinence may be due to impaired mobility and/or cognition.
25. Timed voidings may be helpful in controlling incontinence.
26. An elevated postvoid residual is common in older adults.
27. Decreased fluid consumption may worsen urge incontinence due to the concentrated urine acting as an irritant on the detrusor.
28. Pelvic floor exercises, when done correctly, may be helpful in treating incontinence.
29. If a chronic indwelling catheter is required, a suprapubic tube is preferable to a urethral catheter.
30. α-Blockers are associated with the "floppy iris syndrome," and the ophthalmologist should be informed of their use prior to any ophthalmologic surgery.
31. An underactive bladder characterized by poor bladder emptying is not necessarily due to outlet obstruction and occurs in both men and women. Both structural and functional changes occur in the bladder. Currently there is no effective medication for this condition.
32. Sleep abnormalities may be responsible for nocturia and may worsen the severity of neurologic conditions which affect the bladder.
33. Nocturia once per night in the elderly is considered normal.
34. Nocturia is usually multifactorial in the elderly and thus is often not adequately addressed with a single treatment modality.
35. Hyponatremia is a significant risk factor when desmopressin is given to the elderly.
36. Fecal and urinary problems often coexist, and one may cause the other.
37. UTIs may present atypically in the elderly with symptoms of confusion, agitation, lethargy, and anorexia.
38. Vaginal estrogens are useful for reducing UTIs in elderly women.
39. Elder mistreatment screening is an important part of the urologic evaluation, just as child abuse screening is an important part of the pediatric urologic visit.

89 Urinary Tract Fistulae

Eric S. Rovner

QUESTIONS

1. The most common cause of vesicovaginal fistula in the nonindustrialized, developing world is:
   a. cesarean section.
   b. surgical trauma during abdominal hysterectomy.
   c. surgical trauma during vaginal hysterectomy.
   d. obstructed labor.
   e. none of the above.

2. The most common type of acquired urinary fistula is:
   a. vesicovaginal fistula.
   b. ureterovaginal fistula.
   c. colovesical fistula.
   d. rectourethral fistula.
   e. vesicouterine fistula.

3. Vesicovaginal fistulae (VVF) may occur as a result of:
   a. locally advanced vaginal cancer.
   b. incidentally noted and repaired iatrogenic cystotomy during hysterectomy.
   c. radiotherapy for cervical cancer.
   d. cystocele repair with bladder neck suspension.
   e. all of the above.

4. Intraoperative consultation is requested by a gynecologist for a possible urinary tract injury during a difficult abdominal hysterectomy. There is clear fluid noted in the pelvis. The gynecologist is particularly worried about postoperative VVF formation. All of the following statements are correct regarding counseling this gynecologist EXCEPT:
   a. The incidence of iatrogenic bladder injury during hysterectomy is approximately 0.5% to 1.0%.
   b. Approximately 0.1% to 0.2% of individuals undergoing hysterectomy develop a VVF.
   c. The risk of ureterovaginal fistula is greater than the risk of VVF in this setting.
   d. The absence of blue-stained fluid in the operative field following the administration of intravenous indigo carmine does not eliminate a possibility of a urinary tract injury.
   e. All of the above are true.

5. VVF due to obstructed labor are:
   a. the most common etiology of VVF in Nigeria.
   b. usually located at the vaginal apex.
   c. never associated with simultaneous rectovaginal fistula.
   d. typically found in multiparous women.
   e. usually smaller and simpler to repair than those associated with gynecologic surgery.

6. A 47-year-old woman presents with the new onset of constant urinary leakage 5 years after completing radiation therapy for locally advanced cervical carcinoma. All of the following may be considered part of the diagnostic evaluation EXCEPT:
   a. cystoscopy and possible biopsy.
   b. voiding cystourethrography (VCUG).
   c. computed tomographic (CT) scan of the abdomen and pelvis.
   d. urodynamics.
   e. ureteroscopy.

7. A 52-year-old woman with a history of an abdominal hysterectomy 2 months previously presents for the evaluation of a constant clear vaginal discharge since the surgery. Following oral intake of pyridium, her pads continue to have a clear watery discharge. The most likely diagnosis is:
   a. vesicovaginal fistula.
   b. ureterovaginal fistula.
   c. peritoneovaginal fistula.
   d. vesicouterine fistula.
   e. urethrovaginal fistula.

8. In the industrialized world, postsurgical VVF are associated with ureteral injury in approximately:
   a. 0.01% of cases.
   b. 0.1% of cases.
   c. 10% of cases.
   d. 25% of cases.
   e. 50% of cases.

9. A 68-year-old woman presents with a 1-week history of vaginal leakage 6 months after completion of radiation therapy for locally advanced cervical cancer. VCUG reveals a VVF. On physical examination the fistula is irregular and indurated, and approximately 3 mm in size. Cystoscopy reveals bullous edema surrounding the fistula, and biopsy of the fistula tract reveals only fibrosis without evidence of malignancy. There is no suggestion of recurrent malignancy on CT scan. She should be counseled that:
   a. the optimal timing for repair of this fistula may be in 5 to 6 months.
   b. the best chance to repair this fistula is with immediate surgical intervention.
   c. a vaginal approach is not indicated.
   d. the use of an adjuvant flap will not be necessary.
   e. the success rate for the repair of this fistula is similar to that of a nonradiated VVF.

10. The abdominal approach to VVF repair:
    a. is the preferred approach in all patients with VVF.
    b. has a higher success rate than the vaginal approach.

c. is suitable for the use of an omental interpositional flap.

d. is associated with less morbidity and a shorter hospital stay than the vaginal approach.

e. is more often associated with postoperative vaginal shortening and dyspareunia than the vaginal approach.

11. The vaginal approach to an uncomplicated VVF repair:

a. is most often bolstered with use of a gracilis flap.

b. may be accomplished with a three- or four-layer closure.

c. requires the use of nonabsorbable suture.

d. is not indicated for obstetric-related fistula.

e. is contraindicated if the fistula tract is within 2 cm of the ureter.

12. Principles of urinary fistula repair include all of the following EXCEPT:

a. excision of the fistula tract.

b. tension-free closure.

c. use of well-vascularized tissue flaps.

d. watertight closure.

e. adequate postoperative urinary drainage.

13. Level I evidence (one or more randomized control trials) exists to support which of the following statements?

a. Preoperative administration of topical estrogens improves tissue quality prior to the repair of VVF.

b. Preoperative administration of topical estrogens improves the success rate of transvaginal VVF repair.

c. Preoperative administration of broad-spectrum intravenous antibiotics improves the success rate of all types of VVF repair.

d. Suprapubic bladder drainage is superior to urethral (Foley) catheter drainage in preventing surgical failure following VVF repair.

e. None of the above.

14. Vaginal repair of VVF is contraindicated in:

a. multiparous women.

b. large fistulae.

c. radiation-induced fistulae.

d. fistulae located at the vaginal cuff.

e. none of the above.

15. Potential complications of repair for a VVF following abdominal hysterectomy include all of the following EXCEPT:

a. stress urinary incontinence.

b. dyspareunia.

c. recurrence of the fistula.

d. urinary urgency and frequency.

e. ureteral injury.

16. Advantages of the transabdominal approach to VVF repair as compared with the transvaginal repair include all of the following EXCEPT:

a. ease of mobilization of the omentum as an interpositional flap.

b. decreased rate of intraoperative ureteral injury.

c. preservation of vaginal depth.

d. easier access to the apical VVF in individuals with high narrow vaginal canals.

e. ability to perform an augmentation cystoplasty through the same incision.

17. Seventeen days following a transvaginal VVF repair, a cystogram is performed. The bladder is filled to 100 mL with contrast medium and several images are taken. There is no evidence of a fistula on the filling images; however, the patient was unable to void during the study. A postvoid film was not obtained. This study:

a. demonstrates successful repair of the VVF, and the catheter should be removed.

b. is nondiagnostic, because it was done too soon following repair.

c. is nondiagnostic, because there are no voiding images or postvoid images.

d. is nondiagnostic, because the bladder was not filled to an adequate volume.

e. should be terminated and cystoscopy performed to examine for a persistent fistula.

18. Before surgical mobilization, the blood supply to a potential Martius flap (fibrofatty labial flap) is through the:

a. inferior hemorrhoidal artery.

b. external pudendal artery.

c. uterine artery.

d. inferior epigastric artery.

e. gonadal artery.

19. An interpositional flap of the greater omentum during VVF repair:

a. may be able to reach the deep pelvis without any mobilization in some patients.

b. is most commonly based on the superior mesenteric artery.

c. is contraindicated in the setting of inflammation or infection.

d. should not be divided or incised vertically in the midline because this may compromise the blood supply.

e. is most commonly used during a transvaginal approach.

20. A 39-year-old woman presents with constant vaginal leakage for 1 month following an abdominal hysterectomy. She describes symptoms of stress incontinence before the hysterectomy. She has no urgency and is voiding normally. Physical examination demonstrates no obvious fistula tract at the vaginal cuff. Oral phenazopyridine is given, and the bladder is filled with 100 mL of saline mixed with indigo carmine. A gauze pad is packed from the apex of the vagina proximally to the introitus distally, and the patient is told to ambulate for 90 minutes. Upon the patient's return, the pad is removed and examined. The most proximal portion of the pad is stained yellow-orange, and the most distal portion is blue. This is most consistent with:

a. ureterovaginal fistula.

b. vesicovaginal fistula.

c. urethrovaginal fistula.

d. a and b.

e. a and c.

21. Ureterovaginal fistulae are:

a. not associated with transvaginal hysterectomy.

b. usually associated with normal voiding patterns.

c. best diagnosed on VCUG.

d. found more commonly following hysterectomy for malignancy than for benign indications.

e. usually located in the middle one third of the ureter.

22. Two weeks following an emergent cesarean section for fetal distress during labor, a 28-year-old woman reports constant leakage per vagina. Analysis of the collected fluid reveals it to have a high creatinine level consistent with urine. Physical examination,

including pelvic examination, reveals absolutely no abnormalities or surgical trauma to suggest a urinary fistula. There is no stress incontinence elicited on physical examination. Renal ultrasonography demonstrates no hydronephrosis, and the bladder is empty. The most likely diagnosis is:

a. occult vesicovaginal fistula.

b. occult ureterovaginal fistula.

c. urethrovaginal fistula.

d. vesicouterine fistula.

e. peritoneovaginal fistula.

23. Vesicouterine fistulae occur most commonly due to:

a. low-segment cesarean section.

b. vaginal delivery.

c. malignancy.

d. conization of the cervix.

e. myomectomy.

24. Potential options for therapy of vesicouterine fistula in a patient desiring long-term preservation of fertility include:

a. observation.

b. cystoscopy and fulguration of the fistula tract.

c. hormonal therapy.

d. surgical exploration and repair of the fistula with interpositional omental flap.

e. all of the above.

25. Two months following resection of a large urethral diverticulum extending proximally beyond the bladder neck, a patient complains of urinary leakage. All of the following may be the source of this patient's symptoms EXCEPT:

a. a urethrovaginal fistula.

b. a vesicovaginal fistula.

c. stress urinary incontinence.

d. a recurrent urethral diverticulum.

e. a vesicouterine fistula.

26. Urethrovaginal fistulae in the distal one third of the urethra:

a. are often asymptomatic.

b. are associated with significant bladder overactivity.

c. cannot be repaired using a vaginal flap technique.

d. can result in severe stress incontinence.

e. are usually the result of malignant infiltration.

27. The most common cause of a colovesical fistula is:

a. colon cancer.

b. bladder cancer.

c. prostate cancer.

d. Crohn disease.

e. diverticulitis.

28. CT scan findings suggestive of a colovesical fistula include:

a. intravesical mass, air in the bladder, and bladder wall thickening.

b. air in the bladder, bowel wall thickening adjacent to the bladder, and clear fluid in a bowel segment adjacent to the bladder.

c. air in the bladder, bladder wall thickening adjacent to a loop of thickened bowel wall, and the presence of colonic diverticula.

d. air in the colon, colonic mass adjacent to the bladder, and debris within the bladder.

e. air in the colon, bladder wall thickening, and an intravesical mass.

29. In the evaluation of a possible colovesical fistula, cystoscopy:

a. has high diagnostic accuracy in revealing the cause of the fistula.

b. has a high yield in identifying potential fistulae.

c. should not be performed due to the risk of sepsis.

d. is usually normal.

e. most commonly reveals a large connection to the bowel.

30. A 62-year-old man presents with pneumaturia and recurrent urinary tract infections. A cystoscopy is performed revealing a bullous lesion on the posterior bladder wall. Two hours later, a CT scan is performed revealing air in the bladder. In this patient, air in the bladder:

a. suggests colovesical fistula.

b. may be due to a bacterial infection.

c. may be due to instrumentation.

d. is a nonspecific finding.

e. all of the above.

31. The most common cause of a ureterocolic fistula is:

a. locally extensive colon cancer.

b. appendicitis with an associated abscess.

c. diverticulitis.

d. Crohn disease.

e. tuberculosis.

32. The incidence of rectal injury during radical retropubic prostatectomy is:

a. 0.1%.

b. 1.0%.

c. 5.0%.

d. 10%.

e. 20-fold higher in patients undergoing laparoscopic radical prostatectomy.

33. Rectourethral fistula (RUF) formation following brachytherapy for prostate cancer:

a. may require complex reconstructive surgery or urinary diversion for repair.

b. is located at the level of the prostate.

c. is associated with fecaluria.

d. may be associated with recurrent malignancy.

e. may relate to all of the above.

34. A 61-year-old otherwise healthy man returns to the office with symptoms of mild stress urinary incontinence and fecaluria 3 weeks following radical retropubic prostatectomy. A VCUG is performed and reveals a 1-mm fistula at the vesicourethral junction. The prostate-specific antigen (PSA) is undetectable, and the final pathology reveals organ-confined disease. This patient should be counseled that:

a. a York-Mason transsphincteric approach to this fistula is associated with a high risk of anal incontinence.

b. a trial of indwelling catheterization may result in resolution of the fistula.

c. immediate colostomy is indicated.

d. the stress incontinence will become more severe following repair of the fistula.

e. urinary and fecal diversion will be necessary to repair this fistula.

35. Pyelovascular fistulae:

a. are usually related to percutaneous procedures in the upper urinary tract.

b. are most often due to renal malignancy.

c. should be treated by removal of the nephrostomy tube.

d. usually occur following radiation therapy.

e. are usually fatal.

36. A 74-year-old woman with a history of colon cancer and external beam radiotherapy develops ureteral obstruction and a stent is placed. Three months later, she presents with severe anemia and ongoing bright red gross hematuria for several hours. On examination she is pale and tachycardic, with a thready pulse and a systolic blood pressure of 60. As resuscitation is initiated with fluids and blood transfusion, the next step in management is:

a. a CT scan of the abdomen and pelvis.

b. cystoscopy, removal of the stent, and retrograde pyelography.

c. immediate laparotomy and possible nephrectomy.

d. angiography.

e. a tagged red blood cell scan to lateralize the bleeding.

Imaging

1. See Figure 89-1. A 36-year-old woman presents with increased vaginal discharge 3 weeks after an abdominal hysterectomy. On the axial CT images in the delayed excretory phase, the most likely diagnosis is:

a. Vesicovaginal fistula.

b. Ureterovaginal fistula.

c. Colovesical fistula.

d. Ureteral duplication.

e. Vesicocutaneous fistula.

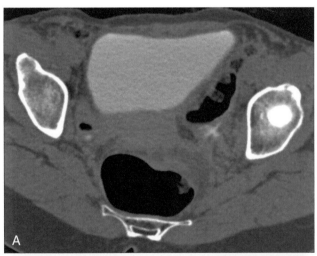

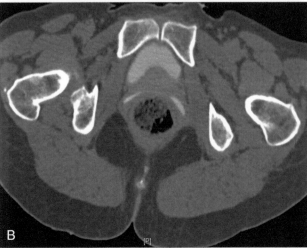

Figure 89-1.

ANSWERS

1. **d. Obstructed labor.** In the industrialized world, the most common cause of VVF is surgical trauma during gynecologic surgery, specifically hysterectomy. In the developing world, untreated obstructed labor results in ischemic necrosis of the anterior vaginal wall and underlying lower urinary tract and is the most common fistula in these geographic areas.

2. **a. Vesicovaginal fistula.** The vast majority of urinary fistulae involve the bladder and vagina in both the industrialized and nonindustrialized world. The other types of fistulae listed are much less common.

3. **e. All of the above.** Causes of VVF in the industrialized world include surgical trauma during hysterectomy, locally advanced gynecologic malignancy, anterior vaginal wall prolapse, anti-incontinence surgery, and pelvic radiotherapy. Intraoperative recognition and repair of bladder injury during hysterectomy should reduce the probability of VVF formation, but it does not eliminate the possibility.

4. **c. The risk of ureterovaginal fistula is greater than the risk of VVF in this setting.** The most common injury to the urinary tract during hysterectomy is a bladder laceration. Although ureteral injuries are not uncommon, they occur far less frequently than bladder injuries. Furthermore, ureterovaginal fistulae are much less common than VVF. The absence of blue-colored fluid in the pelvis does not exclude injury to the urinary tract. For example, a small bladder laceration may not be evident, especially if the bladder is decompressed with a Foley catheter.

5. **a. The most common etiology of VVF in Nigeria.** VVF in the developing world occur primarily due to obstructed labor. Typically, these occur in individuals who are young primigravidas with a narrow bony pelvis. These fistulae are usually large; located distally in the vagina, sometimes encompassing large segments of the trigone, posterior bladder wall, and bladder neck; and are often part of a larger complex of presenting signs and symptoms termed the "obstructed labor injury complex," which includes rectovaginal fistulae. Because of their size and extensive ischemia of the surrounding tissues, these fistulae are often difficult to repair.

6. **e. Ureteroscopy.** This individual does not have diagnosis of VVF, and therefore multiple considerations are present. Nevertheless, VVF is a strong possibility given the history of radiation therapy and pelvic malignancy. A VCUG can establish the presence of a fistula. Cystoscopy and biopsy of a fistula, if present, are mandatory to rule out recurrent malignancy. A CT scan of the abdomen and pelvis can evaluate for recurrent malignancy. Urodynamics may be helpful in evaluating for other types of incontinence, as well as assessing for bladder compliance and capacity in this individual, with a risk for impaired compliance due to radiation therapy. There is no indication for ureteroscopy in this individual.

7. **c. Peritoneovaginal fistula.** Clear fluid draining from the vagina following surgery should be properly characterized. A urinary fistula is a possible source; however, urinary incontinence (stress, urge, overflow, etc.) are strong considerations as well. A peritoneovaginal fistula is a rare complication of hysterectomy in which peritoneal fluid leaks through the vaginal cuff. The fluid may be collected and analyzed for creatinine level. A creatinine level similar to that found in serum excludes urinary fistula as the source of the fluid. In addition, if a pyridium pad test is negative (pads are wet but are not stained orange) then this is highly suggestive of a peritoneal vaginal cuff fistula.

8. **c. 10% of cases.** Approximately 10% to 12% of individuals with VVF are found to have an associated ureteral injury.

9. **a. The optimal timing for repair of this fistula may be in 5 to 6 months.** This patient has a VVF due to radiation therapy. It is recent in onset, suggesting that the fistula is immature and has a possibility of enlarging because the radiation injury has not yet completely demarcated. The optimal timing for repair of this fistula may be in 5 to 6 months. A reevaluation at that time will be needed to assess whether the VVF is now mature and

amenable to repair. Radiation-induced fistulae can be repaired vaginally, and adjuvant flaps are used to bolster the repair. The success rates for radiation-induced VVF are less than those associated with non-radiation-induced VVF, whether they are approached vaginally or abdominally.

10. c. Is suitable for the use of an omental interpositional flap. The choice of approach for VVF repair is generally individualized based on the patient's anatomy, clinical circumstances, and the experience of the operating surgeon. In experienced hands, success rates are similar between the two approaches. Advantages of the vaginal approach include a shorter hospital stay and less postoperative morbidity compared with the abdominal approach; however, vaginal shortening may be an issue with some types of vaginal VVF repairs, including the Latzko operation.

11. b. May be accomplished with a three- or four-layer closure. The vaginal approach to VVF repair uses a three- or four-layer closure. Absorbable suture is preferred to avoid complications related to foreign bodies in the urinary tract, including stone formation and infection. Gracilis flaps are rarely necessary as peritoneal flaps or Martius labial fat flaps are much more convenient and local. The vaginal approach is not contraindicated in obstetric fistula, or if the ureter is near the fistula tract.

12. a. Excision of the fistula tract. Although some authors have suggested that excision of the epithelialized portion of the fistula tract is beneficial, it is not required in all cases.

13. e. None of the above. There is no evidence-based medicine to support any of these statements. Although both topical estrogens and intravenous antibiotics are commonly used, this is on the basis of expert opinion. There is no preferred method for postoperative bladder drainage following VVF repair, although unobstructed drainage is critical in preventing disruption of the suture line.

14. e. None of the above. The transvaginal approach to VVF repair can be used in most patients with uncomplicated VVF. There are few absolute contraindications to the vaginal approach. Nulliparous individuals with VVF located at the vaginal cuff in a high narrow vagina can be challenging to repair vaginally due to anatomic considerations, but this approach is not contraindicated.

15. a. Stress urinary incontinence. Stress urinary incontinence may coexist with VVF; however, it is usually not related to the repair. One exception is the fistula located at the bladder neck or with involvement of the proximal urethra such as obstetric fistulae. These individuals may have new onset stress incontinence following repair due to destruction of the sphincter from the original injury.

16. b. Decreased rate of intraoperative ureteral injury. The transabdominal approach to VVF repair has several distinct advantages compared with the transvaginal approach. However, there are no studies to suggest that ureteral injury is less common using a transabdominal approach than a transvaginal approach.

17. c. Is nondiagnostic, because there are no voiding images or postvoid images. A postoperative cystogram should include voiding or postvoiding images to ensure that the VVF has been adequately repaired. Voiding may marginally increase the intravesical pressure, thereby providing opacification of some VVF that otherwise would be missed on simple filling cystograms. There is no standard filling volume for cystography. Generally, 2 to 3 weeks from surgery is an adequate time period for postoperative imaging. There is no indication for cystoscopy in this patient.

18. b. External pudendal artery. The blood supply to the Martius flap is provided from three sources: the internal and external pudendal arteries as well as the obturator artery. Generally, the small branches from the obturator artery, supplying the flap from a lateral direction, are sacrificed during mobilization. Furthermore, either the anterior (external pudendal) or posterior (internal pudendal) blood supply is divided in order to tunnel and then position the flap over the fistula.

19. a. May be able to reach the deep pelvis without any mobilization in some patients. The greater omentum has several favorable properties that support its use during transabdominal VVF repair. It is based on the right and left gastroepiploic arteries. Because of its rich blood supply and lymphatic properties, it can be a useful adjunctive measure in the setting of infection or inflammation. The blood supply enters the omentum perpendicular to its origin off the greater curvature of the stomach, enabling vertical incisions and mobilization into the deep pelvis. Wide mobilization may be necessary to permit the omentum to reach the deep pelvis in some cases; however, in many individuals the flap will reach into the deep pelvis without mobilization and without tension.

20. a. Ureterovaginal fistula. This patient has at least a ureterovaginal fistula, based on the yellow-orange staining at the proximal portion of the gauze pad. This would be consistent with the normal voiding pattern. The distal blue staining would be consistent with stress incontinence as noted by the patient preoperatively. Hysterectomy is not associated with formation of urethrovaginal fistula. Vesicovaginal fistula is less likely because the staining would tend to be green (a combination of blue and yellow) and located in the midportion of the pad. A VCUG would be most helpful in definitively ruling out a vesicovaginal fistula.

21. b. Usually associated with normal voiding patterns. Ureterovaginal fistulae involve the distal one third of the ureter. They most commonly occur in the setting of hysterectomy: Laparoscopic, abdominal, and vaginal hysterectomy may all result in ureterovaginal fistulae. Most ureterovaginal fistulae occur following hysterectomy for benign indications. Patients often do not complain of voiding dysfunction because the contralateral upper urinary tract provides filling of the bladder. VCUG is used primarily to exclude a concomitant VVF.

22. d. Vesicouterine fistula. The most common cause of vesicouterine fistula is low-segment cesarean section. The normal physical examination suggests a lack of surgical trauma to the vagina, which most likely excludes a vaginal fistula. In the postpartum period, urine from a vesicouterine fistula will leak out of the incompetent cervical os, resulting in constant urinary leakage. A VCUG will confirm the diagnosis.

23. a. Low-segment cesarean section. The vast majority of vesicouterine fistulae occur following low-segment cesarean section. Rarely, these may occur due to uterine rupture at the time of vaginal delivery.

24. e. All of the above. All of the listed options may preserve long-term fertility in patients with vesicouterine fistula. In those not desiring preservation of fertility, hysterectomy is indicated.

25. e. A vesicouterine fistula. It is very unlikely that a vesicouterine fistula can result from such a clinical circumstance. Stress incontinence, VVF, urethrovaginal fistula, and a recurrent diverticulum may all result in the described symptoms.

26. a. Are often asymptomatic. Distal urethrovaginal fistulae are often asymptomatic, because they originate beyond the sphincter. Vaginal voiding and pseudoincontinence may be present in some patients. A vaginal flap technique is an effective method of repair.

27. e. Diverticulitis. Diverticulitis is the most common cause of colovesical fistula in most series. Colon cancer is the second most common cause, followed by Crohn disease.

28. c. Air in the bladder, bladder wall thickening adjacent to a loop of thickened bowel wall, and the presence of colonic diverticula. The classic triad found on CT scan, which is suggestive of a colovesical fistula, includes: air in the bladder, bladder wall thickening adjacent to a loop of thickened bowel, and the presence of colonic diverticula.

29. b. Has a high yield in identifying potential fistulae. The finding of bullous edema during cystoscopy is nonspecific; however, in the appropriate clinical setting, this can be very suggestive of a colovesical fistula. Eighty percent to 100% of cases of colovesical fistulae have an abnormality noted on cystoscopy. Cystoscopy

and biopsy are useful to rule out a malignant fistula when this is a consideration.

30. **e. All of the above.** Air can be introduced into the bladder from instrumentation (i.e., cystoscopy or catheterization) or may be present due to infection with a gas-forming organism. Less commonly, air in the bladder results from a colovesical fistula.

31. **d. Crohn disease.** Most ureterocolic fistulae occur on the right side and occur in patients with Crohn disease. Left-sided fistulae in Crohn disease are much less common.

32. **b. 1.0%.** Most large series report a 1.0% to 1.5% incidence of rectal injury during radical retropubic prostatectomy. When recognized and repaired intraoperatively, very few of these injuries result in a rectourethral fistula. The incidence of rectal injury during laparoscopic radical prostatectomy, when performed by experienced surgeons, is similar to that reported in most open series.

33. **e. May relate to all of the above.** RUF commonly present with fecaluria, regardless of the etiology. RUF in the setting of prostatic malignancy should be biopsied to evaluate for the possibility of recurrent disease.

34. **b. A trial of indwelling catheterization may result in resolution of the fistula.** This is a small fistula and, as such, a trial of conservative therapy is warranted. Because this fistula is not associated with signs of local infection or sepsis, immediate colostomy is not indicated. A York-Mason operation is not associated with a high rate of anal incontinence. Furthermore, a single-stage approach may be attempted (without fecal diversion) in this uncomplicated fistula, if conservative measures fail. Finally, urinary incontinence may not worsen following surgical repair of the fistula.

35. **a. Are usually related to percutaneous procedures in the upper urinary tract.** Pyelovascular fistulae are most often related to interventional procedures in the upper urinary tract, especially percutaneous procedures. Renal neoplasms and radiation therapy are not usually causative of these fistulae. Initial treatment consists of tamponade of the bleeding vessel. If this is unsuccessful, angiographic embolization may be necessary.

36. **d. Angiography.** This individual is at high risk for a ureteroarterial fistula at the level of the stent. A CT scan and retrograde pyelography will both most likely be nondiagnostic. Removal of the stent could result in an increase in bleeding and be rapidly fatal. Angiography in the setting of active bleeding will provide both the diagnosis of a ureteroarterial fistula, if present, and a possible therapeutic intervention in the form of embolization or stent graft placement. Nephrectomy will not stop the acute hemorrhage. A red blood cell scan will be too time consuming, and although it may lateralize the side of the bleeding, it will delay a potentially lifesaving intervention.

Imaging

1. **b. Ureterovaginal fistula.** There is extraluminal contrast around the left distal pelvic ureter with contrast opacification of the vagina on the lower image. The bladder is normal in appearance with no contrast extravasation, making options a, c, and e incorrect. Ureteral duplication does not have this appearance.

CHAPTER REVIEW

1. Vesicovaginal fistulae may occur many years after completion of radiation therapy.
2. Clear vaginal discharge may not invariably represent a urinary fistula but may be a sign of a peritoneal vaginal fistula, lymphatic fistula, vaginitis, or fallopian tube fluid.
3. A fistula that does not heal following primary repair should be suspected of being associated with poor nutrition, a fungal infection, a malignancy, tuberculosis, distal obstruction, or the presence of a foreign body.
4. In the repair of fistulae, multiple layers should be used, and there should be no overlapping suture lines.
5. Long-term complications of vesicovaginal fistula repair include vaginal shortening and stenosis.
6. For an abdominal repair of a vesicovaginal fistula, it is essential to mobilize the bladder caudal to the fistula. Cholinergic agents are used liberally in the postoperative period following repair of a vesicovaginal fistula.
7. A Martius flap may be divided at either its superior or its inferior margin, because the vascular supply is provided at both ends of the graft.
8. A peritoneal flap is mobilized without opening the peritoneum, advancing it and securing it in a tension-free manner between the bladder and the vagina.
9. Following a ureteral injury, decompression of the upper tracks is essential.
10. Vesicouterine fistulae do not always present with urinary incontinence.
11. Soft tissue flaps are an important component of successful urethrovaginal fistula repair.
12. A recurrence of the malignancy should be ruled out in any fistula that develops following treatment of a primary malignancy with radiation therapy.
13. Vesicovaginal fistulae following hysterectomy are usually located on the anterior vaginal wall at the vaginal cuff.
14. Tissue interposition should be considered when repairing a fistula which failed primary closure, very large fistulae, and those occurring following radiation therapy.
15. The gracilis muscle, the rectus abdominis muscle, and a Martius pad are excellent flaps for tissue interposition.
16. An endovascular stent should be considered for ureterovascular (usually iliac) fistula repair.
17. Distal urethrovaginal fistulae are often asymptomatic because they originate beyond the sphincter.
18. Diverticulitis is the most common cause of colovesical fistula in most series. Colon cancer is the second most common cause, followed by Crohn disease.

90 Bladder and Female Urethral Diverticula

Eric S. Rovner

QUESTIONS

1. Congenital bladder diverticula are:
   a. usually multiple.
   b. strongly associated with bladder outlet obstruction.
   c. often found in smooth-walled bladders.
   d. located at the dome.
   e. usually less than 1 cm.

2. Acquired bladder diverticula are most commonly located:
   a. near the urethrovesical junction.
   b. adjacent to the ureter.
   c. at the dome.
   d. at the 10 o'clock and 2 o'clock position.
   e. posteriorly.

3. Videourodynamic evaluation in an adult female with a bladder diverticulum will likely reveal:
   a. impaired compliance.
   b. bladder outlet obstruction.
   c. intrinsic sphincter deficiency (ISD).
   d. low-pressure, low flow voiding.
   e. no abnormality.

4. Pathologic examination of a surgical bladder diverticulectomy specimen will likely reveal:
   a. absence of epithelium.
   b. premalignant or malignant changes.
   c. nephrogenic metaplasia.
   d. a poorly developed muscularis propria layer.
   e. trabeculation of the smooth muscle layer.

5. The most common malignant tumor associated with bladder diverticula is:
   a. urothelial.
   b. squamous cell.
   c. adenocarcinoma.
   d. sarcomatous.
   e. undifferentiated.

6. A 68-year-old man presents with hematuria. Cystoscopy reveals a 15-cm bladder diverticulum with a 3-mm papillary lesion at the base of the diverticulum. The next step is:
   a. biopsy of the papillary lesion.
   b. transurethral resection of the papillary lesion with deep muscle resection.
   c. urodynamics and transurethral prostatectomy (TURP) if bladder outlet obstruction is noted.
   d. bladder diverticulectomy.
   e. radical cystectomy and urinary diversion.

7. Acquired bladder diverticula are commonly found in association with:
   a. prostatic obstruction.
   b. calyceal diverticula.
   c. nephrogenic adenoma.
   d. infection of perivesical glands.
   e. erectile dysfunction (ED).

8. A 65-year-old man with bladder outlet obstruction and a 5-cm bladder diverticulum undergoes uneventful TURP. Postoperatively, the patient's symptoms are resolved, and a voiding cystourethrogram (VCUG) demonstrates satisfactory emptying of the bladder and the bladder diverticulum. The next step is:
   a. annual surveillance with cystoscopy and urine cytology.
   b. discharge from urologic care.
   c. transvesical bladder diverticulectomy.
   d. repeat urodynamics.
   e. computed tomographic (CT) cystogram.

9. Ten years following TURP, a 71-year-old man with congestive heart failure (CHF) and atrial fibrillation who is on Coumadin (warfarin sodium) has recurrent urinary tract infections (UTIs), and an American Urological Association (AUA) symptom score of 25. A videourodynamic study shows a 14-cm poorly emptying bladder diverticulum. The peak subtracted detrusor pressure (Pdet) during micturition is 15 cm H_2O with a Qmax of 3 mL/sec. Renal ultrasonography is normal. The next best step is:
   a. repeat TURP.
   b. clean intermittent self-catheterization (CIC).
   c. observation.
   d. bethanechol.
   e. CT urography.

10. Endoscopic examination of the lower urinary tract in the setting of bladder diverticula:
    a. is best performed with a rigid cystoscope.
    b. is associated with a high risk of perforation.
    c. should include examination of the entire interior of the diverticulum.
    d. is not indicated if an elective submucosal bladder diverticulectomy is planned.
    e. should always be performed with concomitant bilateral retrograde pyelograms (RPGs).

11. Bladder diverticula:
    a. often do not produce specific symptoms.
    b. can be associated with urinary tract infections.
    c. are commonly diagnosed incidentally during the evaluation of other symptoms or conditions.
    d. may be associated with persistent pyuria.
    e. All of the above.

12. Bladder diverticula associated with bladder outlet obstruction:
    a. are usually found in the absence of cellules and saccules.
    b. are associated with the universal finding of ipsilateral vesicoureteral reflux.
    c. cannot be imaged by CT.
    d. are associated with medial deviation of the pelvic ureter.
    e. are less likely to be associated with malignancy compared with congenital bladder diverticula.

13. Increased size of urethral diverticula at presentation correlates with:
    a. increased symptoms.
    b. risk of UTI.
    c. risk of recurrence postoperatively.
    d. risk of malignancy.
    e. risk of incontinence.

14. Common symptoms associated with urethral diverticula include all of the following EXCEPT:
    a. vaginal pruritus.
    b. dysuria.
    c. dyspareunia.
    d. postvoid dribbling.
    e. urinary urgency and frequency.

15. A 1.5-cm firm anterior vaginal wall mass is noted in a 35-year-old woman approximately 2 cm proximal to the urethral meatus at the level of the mid-urethra, without distorting the urethral meatus. It is nontender. Urine analysis is unremarkable. This mass may represent any of the following EXCEPT:
    a. vaginal wall cyst.
    b. Skene gland abscess.
    c. urethral diverticulum.
    d. vaginal leiomyoma.
    e. Gartner duct cyst.

16. The ostium of a urethral diverticulum is:
    a. most commonly found in the proximal one third of the urethra.
    b. most commonly found at the 10 o'clock and 2 o'clock position in the urethral lumen.
    c. usually seen on transvaginal ultrasound imaging.
    d. unable to be visualized with rigid cystoscopy.
    e. Usually located in the ventrolateral urethra.

17. Two weeks after removal of a 5-cm proximal urethral diverticulum extending beneath the trigone of the bladder, a 48-year-old woman returns to the office with complaints of urine staining her undergarments. Possible etiologies include:
    a. urethrovaginal fistula.
    b. ureterovaginal fistula.
    c. vesicovaginal fistula.
    d. stress urinary incontinence.
    e. all of the above.

18. During excision of the epithelial lining (sac) of a urethral diverticulum, a portion of the indwelling urethral catheter is seen at the base of the dissection. The next step is to:
    a. close the urethra and abort the procedure.
    b. perform buccal mucosal urethroplasty and abort the procedure.

c. complete the urethral diverticulectomy.
    d. vaginal inversion flap and closure of the urethra.
    e. close the urethra primarily, place a suprapubic tube, and harvest a Martius flap.

19. A VCUG is performed for evaluation of a possible urethral diverticulum (UD). The filling images are nondiagnostic. The radiologist calls you because the patient is unable to void under fluoroscopy in the radiology suite. The patient is taken off the imaging table and is able to void in the adjacent bathroom. The next step is:
    a. CT cystogram.
    b. transvaginal ultrasound.
    c. obtain postvoid images.
    d. endoluminal magnetic resonance imaging (MRI).
    e. positive pressure urethrography (PPU).

20. The most common malignancy found in urethral diverticula is:
    a. squamous.
    b. urothelial.
    c. adenocarcinoma.
    d. undifferentiated.
    e. sarcomatous.

21. Principles of surgical urethral diverticulectomy include all of the following EXCEPT:
    a. preservation or creation of urinary continence.
    b. excision of all identifiable periurethral fascia.
    c. identification of the ostium of the urethral diverticulum.
    d. closure of periurethral fascia following removal of the urethral diverticulum.
    e. watertight closure of the urethra.

22. The initial event implicated in the formation of most urethral diverticula is:
    a. congenital lack of fusion of the urethral crest.
    b. infection of vaginal cysts.
    c. traumatic vaginal delivery.
    d. infection of the periurethral glands.
    e. dysfunctional voiding.

23. In a patient with bothersome SUI and UD, anti-incontinence surgery is being considered. Of the choices listed below, the best concomitant surgical procedure to treat the SUI is:
    a. transobturator midurethral sling.
    b. retropubic midurethral sling.
    c. single-incision synthetic sling.
    d. autologous pubovaginal fascial sling.
    e. polypropylene bladder neck sling.

24. The ostia of UD are most commonly found at:
    a. 12 o'clock.
    b. 6 o'clock.
    c. 4 o'clock and 8 o'clock.
    d. 10 o'clock and 12 o'clock.
    e. none of the above.

Imaging

1. A 47-year-old woman presents with dribbling and recurrent urinary tract infections. See Figure 90-1.

   The most likely diagnosis on this axial and coronal T2-weighted MRI done with an endovaginal coil is:

   a. bladder prolapse.

   b. urethral diverticulum.

   c. bladder diverticulum.

   d. ureteral duplication.

   e. ectopic ureter.

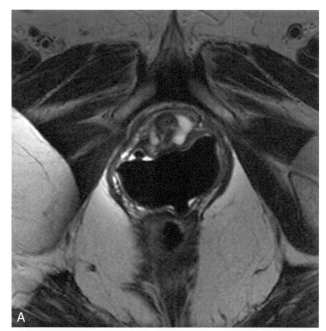

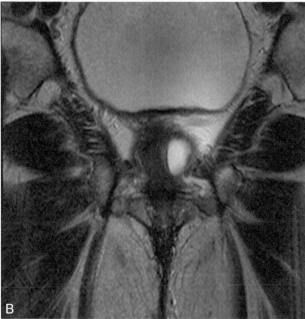

Figure 90-1.

ANSWERS

1. **c. Often found in smooth-walled bladders.** Unlike acquired bladder diverticula, congenital lesions are found in smooth walled bladders, and often adjacent to the ureteric orifice. Congenital bladder diverticula are usually solitary, often large, and not associated with bladder outlet obstruction. Congenital diverticula at the dome may be related to prune-belly syndrome, posterior urethral valves, or urachal anomalies.

2. **b. Adjacent to the ureter.** Similar to congenital bladder diverticula, acquired bladder diverticula are often located near the ureteric orifice. This area of the bladder is thought to be a location of relative anatomic weakness of the bladder wall, predisposing to the formation of bladder diverticula.

3. **b. Bladder outlet obstruction.** Bladder diverticula in adults are most commonly associated with some type of bladder outlet obstruction. In an adult female this may be due to prior anti-incontinence surgery (iatrogenic), dysfunctional voiding, neurogenic causes (e.g., detrusor external sphincter dyssynergia), or a variety of other conditions such as obstructing vaginal or urethral masses (e.g., malignancy).

4. **d. A poorly developed muscularis propria layer.** Though varying amounts of detrusor muscle fibers may be found on pathologic examination of surgical excised bladder diverticula, the muscularis propria layer is usually incomplete and the fibers are disorganized. Such a lack of a well-developed muscularis propria layer is a hallmark of a bladder diverticulum. Absence of an epithelial layer, nephrogenic metaplasia, and malignant changes are uncommonly reported in histological evaluation of bladder diverticula. Typically there is no trabeculation within the wall of a bladder diverticulum.

5. **a. Urothelial.** The most common malignant tumors seen within bladder diverticula are urothelial. The other types of tumors can be seen but are much less common.

6. **a. Biopsy of the papillary lesion.** A papillary lesion in a bladder diverticulum, similar to the rest of the urinary tract, may indicate a malignancy, but may also represent a benign lesion. Biopsy is warranted. Care should be taken to avoid perforation of the diverticulum wall during the biopsy as the wall lacks a muscularis propria layer. A 3-mm lesion can easily be biopsied without the use of a resectoscope. In the event that the biopsy demonstrates malignancy, perforation of the bladder wall risks malignant dissemination.

7. **a. Prostatic obstruction.** Acquired bladder diverticula are most commonly associated with bladder outlet obstruction (approximately 70%). They are also more common in males than in females, and the most common cause of bladder outlet obstruction in males is prostatic obstruction. There is no known association of bladder diverticula with calyceal diverticula, ED, nephrogenic adenoma or perivesical gland infection.

8. **a. Annual surveillance with cystoscopy and urine cytology.** Although the bladder diverticulum drains well, and the patient is asymptomatic, long term follow-up of bladder diverticula is warranted. The natural history of such lesions is unknown, and although the presumed etiology of malignant transformation is thought to be due to urinary stasis, this is unproved. Furthermore, it is possible that premalignant changes may have occurred during the time that the diverticulum was not draining well.

9. **b. Clean intermittent self-catheterization (CIC).** This patient is at high risk for major abdominal surgery. Removal of his diverticulum is likely to be a large surgical undertaking with substantial risk and is ill advised unless other conservative measures fail. Endoscopic treatment with TURP is also a risk due to anticoagulation. His detrusor pressure is low, suggesting that even an adequate outlet procedure (in this patient without definite evidence of obstruction) will not provide satisfactory emptying of the diverticulum. He has normal upper tracts but recurrent

UTIs, thus observation is not optimal. It is likely that his UTIs are due to urinary stasis in the diverticulum. CIC should adequately empty the diverticulum and reduce the risk of ongoing UTIs.

10. **c. Should include examination of the entire interior of the diverticulum.** Periodic endoscopic examination of bladder diverticula is warranted because of the risk of malignant transformation and early transmural involvement. The entire lining of the diverticulum should be examined. Rigid and flexible cystoscopes can be used. The upper urinary tract should be imaged. However, RPGs are not necessary unless otherwise indicated for another reason (e.g., a filling defect on urography).

11. **e. All of the above.** Bladder diverticula are most commonly recognized incidentally on evaluation for other signs and symptoms. There are no symptoms that are specific to bladder diverticula. Bladder diverticula are associated with UTIs and pyuria in some individuals.

12. **d. Are associated with medial deviation of the pelvic ureter.** Bladder diverticula found in association with lower urinary tract obstruction are commonly seen with saccules and cellules. Reflux is not a common finding with bladder acquired diverticula but may be present in some individuals, especially those with "Hutch" diverticula. Congenital bladder diverticula are not associated with malignancy. Medial deviation of the ureter can be seen on intravenous urography and CT with some large bladder diverticula due to the location of the diverticula relative to the ureter.

13. **c. Risk of recurrence postoperatively.** Although some urethral diverticula can be quite large, symptoms, malignancy risk, incontinence, and risk of UTI are not known to correlate with size. Large diverticula, including those extending in a "saddle bag" configuration, are more likely to recur.

14. **a. Vaginal pruritus.** Vaginal pruritus is not a symptom of urethral diverticula. Inflammatory and infectious conditions as well as lichen sclerosis (vulvar dystrophy) may cause vaginal pruritus. The other symptoms listed are often, although not invariably, individually or collectively associated with urethral diverticula. The classic triad of symptoms of urethral diverticula include the "3 D's"—dysuria, postvoid dribbling, and dyspareunia—although these are only uncommonly seen in the same patient.

15. **b. Skene gland abscess.** Skene gland abscess is usually associated with distortion of the urethral meatus due to its distal location. They are also often symptomatic with associated dyspareunia, and tenderness on physical examination. Vaginal wall cysts, vaginal leiomyoma, and Gartner duct cysts are firm anterior vaginal wall masses and are often nontender. Urethral diverticula in some cases may be asymptomatic and found incidentally in the evaluation of other conditions but do not result in distortion of the urethral meatus.

16. **e. Usually located in the ventrolateral urethra.** The ostium (opening) of a urethral diverticulum is most commonly found in the middle or distal third of the urethra, at the 4 o'clock and 8 o'clock positions. They are usually too small to be visualized by ultrasound but can often be seen with both rigid and flexible cystoscopy as a small opening in the urethral lumen ventrolaterally.

17. **e. All of the above.** Complications of urethral diverticulectomy include urinary fistula as well as stress incontinence. Large diverticula may extend beneath the trigone of the bladder, and excision of such lesions risks injury to the urethra, bladder, and ureters. De novo stress urinary incontinence (SUI) may occur following urethral diverticulectomy, which may be due to distortion or injury to the sphincter mechanism.

18. **c. Complete the urethral diverticulectomy.** Successful excision of a urethral diverticulum involves removal of the ostium that connects with the urethral lumen. This often results in direct visualization of the urethral catheter within the urethral lumen during surgery. The urethral defect is closed primarily with absorbable suture in a watertight fashion following completion of the removal of the sac. Additional procedures such as buccal mucosal urethroplasty, Martius flap, or vaginal flaps are not necessary to close the urethra.

19. **c. Obtain postvoid images.** In the absence of voiding images, many urethral diverticula will not be visualized during fluoroscopy, as there is no contrast in the urethra. This is a nondiagnostic but incomplete study. Postvoid images will often reveal retained contrast in the diverticulum. CT, ultrasound, MRI, and PPU are all potentially useful studies in the evaluation of diverticula, but every effort should be made to maximize the diagnostic potential of each radiographic imaging technique, and a postvoid image in this clinical scenario may provide useful diagnostic information.

20. **c. Adenocarcinoma.** The most common malignant tumor type found in urethral diverticula is adenocarcinoma. Although the other malignant tumors listed may be found, adenocarcinoma is the most common.

21. **b. Excision of all identifiable periurethral fascia.** Preservation of periurethral fascia is an important step in urethral diverticulectomy. This tissue is very important in reconstruction of the urethra to prevent fistula formation and close dead space. This tissue should not be excised.

22. **d. Infection of the periurethral glands.** Infection of the periurethral glands is felt to be the initial step in the formation of urethral diverticula. Such infection may lead to periurethral abscess formation and development of a cavity or space within the periurethral fascia that then becomes the anatomic location of a urethral diverticulum.

23. **d. Autologous pubovaginal fascial sling.** Stress urinary incontinence may accompany urethral diverticula. In symptomatic patients, concomitant repair can be considered. Urethral diverticula connect to the urethral lumen, and therefore the surgical excision of these lesions requires suture repair and closure of the ostium of the urethral diverticulum where it connects to the urethra. In such settings, the use of synthetic material for a sling is not advisable because of the risk of subsequent erosion of the synthetic material into the urethra. Autologous fascia is an excellent choice for a concomitant sling at the time of urethral diverticulectomy.

24. **c. 4 o'clock and 8 o'clock.** Urethral diverticula are thought to originate from infection of the periurethral glands. Such glands are located along the urethra and arborize laterally. They generally drain medially into the urethral lumen ventrolaterally at approximately the 4 o'clock and 8 o'clock positions of the middle and distal third of the urethra.

Imaging

1. **b. Urethral diverticulum.** The images demonstrate a fluid collection surrounding the urethra, compatible with a saddlebag urethral diverticulum. The coronal image clearly shows that the collection is separate from the bladder. (Options a and c are incorrect. An ectopic ureter would not have a saddlebag configuration.)

CHAPTER REVIEW

1. When the diverticulum encompasses the ureteral orifice in the setting of neurogenic bladder and vesicle ureteral reflux, it is termed a *Hutch diverticulum*.

2. Congenital diverticula generally occur lateral and posterior to the ureteral orifice and often are associated with vesicoureteral reflux.

3. Acquired bladder diverticula usually occur in the setting of obstruction or neurogenic vesicle dysfunction.

4. The major complications of diverticula include recurrent urinary tract infections, stones, carcinoma or premalignant change in the diverticulum, and upper tract deterioration as a consequence of obstruction or reflux.

5. Many diverticula are located adjacent to the ureter and may be very adherent to it. This has implications in surgical resection.

6. The urethropelvic ligament in the female is composed of two parts: (1) endopelvic fascia and (2) periurethral fascia. Within these two leaves of fascia lie the urethra, and this is the location of most urethral diverticula in woman.

7. The etiology of urethral diverticula in women has been attributed to recurrent urinary tract infection of periurethral glands with obstruction, suburethral abscess formation, and subsequent rupture of the infected gland into the urethra.

8. Skene glands do not communicate with the urethra.

9. Gartner duct cysts are located on the anterior lateral vaginal wall from cervix to introitus.

10. Urethral mucosa prolapse occurs in postmenopausal women and prepubertal girls.

11. A distinct layer of periurethral fascia should be preserved in managing excision of urethral diverticula for reconstruction.

12. When cancer occurs in a bladder diverticulum, the lack of a defined muscle wall makes biopsy and staging difficult because a deep biopsy may perforate, and without a deep biopsy proper staging may not be possible.

13. A urethra diverticulum may extend partially around the urethra, anterior to the urethra, or circumferentially around the urethra.

14. Stress incontinence occurs in approximately 10% of women after a repair of a urethra diverticulum.

15. Congenital bladder diverticula are usually solitary, often large, and not associated with bladder outlet obstruction.

16. The ostium (opening) of a urethral diverticulum is most commonly found in the middle or distal thirds of the urethra, at the 4 o'clock and 8 o'clock positions.

91

Surgical Procedures for Sphincteric Incontinence in the Male: The Artificial Urinary Sphincter and Perineal Sling Procedures

Hunter Wessells and Andrew Peterson

QUESTIONS

1. Which of the following is associated with a reduction in risk of artificial urinary sphincter (AUS) erosion?
   a. Transscrotal approach
   b. Proximal bulbar location
   c. Narrow back modification
   d. Inhibizone treatment
   e. Cuff placement over bulbospongiosus muscle

2. The most significant contraindication to AUS for sphincteric incontinence is:
   a. impaired cognitive function.
   b. pad weight test result >1000 mg/24 h.
   c. prior pelvic irradiation.
   d. detrusor overactivity.
   e. organic erectile dysfunction.

3. The most likely cause of gradual return of urinary incontinence (UI) 2 years after AUS is:
   a. mechanical failure.
   b. subcuff urethral atrophy.
   c. pressure-regulating balloon aneurysm.
   d. new onset detrusor overactivity.
   e. tubing kink.

4. A 54-year-old man with gravitational incontinence has a history of pelvic fracture urethral injury. Videourodynamics show mild detrusor overactivity and an open bladder neck. The best surgical treatment is:
   a. transurethral bulking agent.
   b. transobturator male sling.
   c. bone-anchored male sling.
   d. artificial urinary sphincter.
   e. catheterizable continent stoma.

5. In a man with a history of recurrent noninvasive bladder cancer and sphincteric urinary incontinence following transurethral resection of the prostate (TURP) with a pad weight of 230 g for 24 hours and leak-point pressure of 80 cm H_2O, the best solution for the incontinence is:
   a. bulbar AUS.
   b. bladder neck AUS.
   c. Cunningham clamp.
   d. transobturator male sling.
   e. cystectomy and urinary diversion.

6. During urethral dissection for implantation of a bulbar artificial urinary sphincter, a urethrotomy is made with the scissors. After repairing the urethral defect, the next step is:
   a. catheter drainage for 7 days and delayed replantation.
   b. placement of the cuff at a more distal location.
   c. transobturator sling placement.

   d. irrigation with antibiotic solution and transcorporeal cuff placement.
   e. tunica vaginalis flap coverage and bulbar cuff placement.

7. Efficacy of transobturator male sling post radical prostatectomy (RP) is reduced by prior:
   a. collagen injection.
   b. adjuvant radiation therapy.
   c. transurethral resection of the prostate.
   d. incision of bladder neck contracture.
   e. penile prosthesis.

8. The most likely urodynamic finding in men with incontinence after RP is:
   a. detrusor overactivity.
   b. impaired detrusor contractility.
   c. intrinsic sphincter deficiency.
   d. sensory urgency.
   e. detrusor hypocontractility.

9. A 59-year-old man develops a dense vesicourethral anastomotic stricture 2 years after bulbar AUS placement for post-RP UI. The best approach for treatment is:
   a. dilation with sounds.
   b. transurethral incision with Collins knife.
   c. laser incision with flexible ureteroscope.
   d. antegrade transurethral incision via suprapubic cystostomy.
   e. open cuff exploration with transurethral incision after cuff uncoupling.

10. A 43-year-old man with myelomeningocele has persistent incontinence after placement of a 4.0 cm bulbar artificial urinary sphincter. Urodynamics show Valsalva leak-point pressure (VLPP) of 55 cm H_2O and normal bladder capacity. The next step is:
    a. downsize the cuff to 3.5 cm.
    b. addition of tandem cuff.
    c. reposition cuff at the bladder neck.
    d. increase pressure-regulating balloon (PRB) to 71 to 80 cm H_2O.
    e. close bladder neck and create Mitrofanoff.

11. The most important technical difference in implantation of a bladder neck versus bulbar AUS is:
    a. cuff measurement.
    b. location of PRB.
    c. preperitoneal connections.
    d. choice of PRB.
    e. fluid volume in device.

12. The factors most likely to predict new overactive bladder symptoms after artificial urinary sphincter placement include:
    a. preoperative outlet procedure.
    b. VLPP less than 60 cm H_2O.

c. history of pelvic radiation.

d. cystometric capacity of 200 mL or less.

e. history of prior bladder neck contracture/stricture surgery.

13. All of the following factors are associated with an increased risk of cuff erosion of an AUS EXCEPT:

a. prior explanation for erosion.

b. prolonged catheterization.

c. prior transobturator sling surgery.

d. history of pelvic radiation.

e. history of hypertension.

14. In addition to a chief complaint and history of urinary leakage, prior to embarking on surgical therapy in the man with post-prostatectomy stress incontinence, the absolutely required evaluations include:

a. urodynamics.

b. voiding diary.

c. visual demonstration of stress incontinence with stress maneuvers.

d. pad weight test.

e. cystoscopy.

15. The most common pathogen involved in a primarily infected artificial sphincter is:

a. *Enterococcus*.

b. *Staphylococcus aureus*.

c. *Staphylococcus epidermidis*.

d. *Escherichia coli*.

e. *Candida*.

16. A 65-year-old male presents with stress incontinence after radical prostatectomy for Gleason 7 prostate cancer (pT3A). He has a history of adjuvant radiation therapy. He leaks urine with activity and when standing, has no urge component, and pad weight is 1200 mL per 24 hours. The most appropriate definitive therapy for his incontinence is:

a. quadratic male sling.

b. transobturator male sling.

c. AUS with bulbar placement.

d. AUS with transcorporeal placement.

e. urinary diversion.

ANSWERS

1. **c. Narrow back modification.** The narrow back modification was associated with a reduced risk of erosion. Transscrotal approach may not achieve as proximal a location of the cuff, but this is associated with potential risk of worse incontinence, not erosion. Inhibizone treatment has no literature to support its value in the prevention of erosion. Preservation of the bulbospongiosus muscle has not been shown to affect erosion rates.

2. **a. Impaired cognitive function.** Significant cognitive impairment puts a patient at risk for inability to safely use an AUS. Radiation therapy and prior urethral surgery are relative contraindications to sling surgery because of reduced efficacy, perhaps due to poor tissue coaptation or association with more severe incontinence. Although detrusor overactivity may reduce the efficacy of all devices, medical management can address many of these problems. Ischemic damage of the corpus spongiosum may increase risk of erosion, but in the absence of a traumatic arterial insufficiency to the entire pudendal bed, cavernosal blood flow would not be associated with outcomes of AUS.

3. **b. Subcuff urethral atrophy.** The narrow-backed AUS model 800 has improved mechanical reliability such that now atrophy is a more common cause of recurrent UI. New-onset detrusor overactivity is rare after AUS but may complicate any surgical treatment. The key is that slow onset of incontinence indicates atrophy, whereas sudden recurrence of incontinence indicates mechanical failure, fluid leak or erosion of the device.

4. **d. Artificial urinary sphincter.** This patient has a complex history with compromise of both rhabdosphincter and internal sphincter. Bulking agents are a consideration in cases of male urinary incontinence unrelated to radical prostatectomy, but the severity of incontinence makes this unrealistic. Thus, standard bulbar AUS is indicated. After urethral disruption due to pelvic fracture, neither transobturator nor bone-anchored slings are likely to reliably provide effective elevation, elongation, or compression because of distortion of the bony pelvic anatomy and high likelihood of rhabdosphincter damage. Continent diversion should be a last resort.

5. **d. Transobturator male sling.** The problem of urinary tract access is important to this case. Bulbar AUS will not allow appropriate instrumentation and transurethral resection of recurrent tumors. A male sling will allow passage of a 24-Fr resectoscope and is appropriate for this degree of incontinence. The other variables in this case indicate that this patient is an excellent candidate for a sling device with minimal to moderate urinary incontinence, high leak-point pressure, and no history of radiation. Urinary diversion is premature.

6. **a. Catheter drainage for 7 days and delayed replantation.** Urethral injury during any implant surgery places the patient at risk for device infection due to the presence of colonizing bacteria in the urethra. The risk of devastating device infection outweighs any benefit and thus the procedure should be aborted.

7. **b. Adjuvant radiation therapy.** Radiotherapy is associated with a lower success rate of bone anchored male slings and the transobturator male slings. The other listed conditions have not been associated with poor outcomes. Radiation tends to decrease the efficacy by approximately 50% in all patients undergoing transobturator male sling for stress incontinence.

8. **c. Intrinsic sphincter deficiency.** The sine qua non of UI post-RP is intrinsic sphincter deficiency. Detrusor dysfunction may be present in as many as 40% of these men, but is the primary cause of UI in less than 5%. Although detrusor overactivity may also be present, it is not a contraindication to moving forward with the treatment for sphincteric incontinence.

9. **c. Laser incision with flexible ureteroscope.** Dilation with sounds would be potentially risky to the cuff; bulbar cuffs do not allow the safe insertion of standard resectoscopes, making Collins knife incision impossible. The safest approach for an initial stricture would be laser incision through a smaller caliber endoscope such as a ureteroscope. Although exploration of the AUS cuff with uncoupling of the cuff will allow safe endoscopic management of strictures and tumors with resectoscopes, this should be reserved for cases not amenable to simple laser incision with small caliber and scopes. Antegrade incision is feasible but offers less control than the retrograde approach. Open surgical reconstruction should be reserved for refractory cases.

10. **a. Downsize the cuff to 3.5 cm.** This primary failure of AUS likely relates to incorrect sizing of the cuff. Although a tandem cuff or transcorporeal cuff could provide improved coaptation, in a 43-year-old man it is more appropriate to correct the cuff size than use up additional locations on the bulbar urethra. These will be necessary for future device replacements over time. Increasing the pressure in the PRB may also increase the risk of erosion. Long-term complications of bladder neck cuffs in men with normal vesicourethral junctions are low and the option of a bladder neck cuff placement should be considered before closing the bladder neck in an otherwise adequate bladder.

11. **d. Choice of PRB.** Bladder neck AUS require higher pressures to ensure coaptation. Cuff measurement and PRB location

require no modification; connections can be made intra-abdominally or in the subcutaneous space above the fascia; and usually the differences in fluid volume are nominal.

12. **d. Cystometric capacity of 200 mL or less.** The best indicators for patients who may develop overactive bladder after treatment of their outlet for sphincteric incontinence include a capacity of less than 200 mL on urodynamics or diary and the presence of symptomatic overactive bladder before surgical treatment for the incontinence. Patients with prior radiation therapy may develop urgency and frequency at a later time, but this is not a significant risk factor before proceeding with outlet procedures such as male slings or AUS. Leak-point pressure and prior procedures do not indicate a risk for development of overactive bladder.

13. **c. Prior transobturator sling surgery.** The placement of a transobturator sling before moving forward with an artificial urinary sphincter does not affect the outcomes of the artificial urinary sphincter. Prior erosions with the need for removal of the device, prolonged catheterization and instrumentation, and prior history of pelvic radiation, as well as hypertension and other comorbidities, do significantly affect the rates of subsequent erosion of these devices.

14. **c. Visual demonstration of stress incontinence with stress maneuvers.** Before embarking on the surgical management of stress incontinence, absolute requirements in the evaluation include a subjective history of urinary leakage with stress maneuvers, confirmation of leakage on physical exam, urinalysis to rule out infection, and evaluation of the postvoid residual. The inspection of pads soaked with urine is sufficient objective confirmation of leakage. Urodynamics may be helpful in cases where there may be mixed components of incontinence in addition to those cases with prior surgical interventions or other complex cases as indicated. The voiding diary is quite useful when evaluating stress versus urgency component but is still not absolutely required; cystoscopy is also helpful in evaluating the outlet but again is not absolutely required.

15. **c. *Staphylococcus epidermidis.*** Gram-positive bacterial infections are most commonly involved in infection of prosthetic devices in the genitourinary system (penile prosthesis and artificial urinary sphincter). Classically, *S. epidermidis* is most commonly involved on these devices. Although all of the other bacteria and fungal pathogens may also be involved, *S. epidermidis* is still most common.

16. **c. AUS with bulbar placement.** This patient's history of prior radiation therapy makes the transobturator sling outcome significantly worse. The radiation combined with very high volume of incontinence in a 24-hour period makes him an excellent candidate for the AUS. Although the device may not make him completely dry, it can significantly reduce the number of pads used per day and improve quality of life.

CHAPTER REVIEW

1. Endoscopic evaluation should precede surgical correction of urinary incontinence following radical prostatectomy or a TURP to evaluate the anatomy and eliminate bladder neck contracture; patients with suspected bladder outlet obstruction, significant bladder overactivity or impaired contractility should be evaluated with urodynamics.
2. An assessment of bladder capacity, compliance, and contractility is required before considering surgical correction of urinary incontinence.
3. Submucosal bulking agents are of limited efficacy in treating incontinence following radical prostatectomy.
4. After artificial sphincter placement, prolonged urinary retention requires suprapubic cystostomy drainage.
5. Determining the appropriate tension of the sling is the most critical portion of the operation.
6. Cuff atrophy requires downsizing, repositioning, tandem cuff placement, or transcorporeal surgery.
7. Incontinence after a TURP is rarely due to external sphincter injury.
8. Significant cognitive impairment puts a patient at risk for inability to safely use an AUS.
9. Radiation therapy and prior urethral surgery are relative contraindications to sling surgery
10. Moderate to severe incontinence is best treated with an AUS rather than a sling.
11. An absolute contraindication for surgical correction of incontinence is a decreased bladder compliance which would jeopardize renal function.
12. After AUS insertion a slow onset of incontinence indicates atrophy while the sudden recurrence of incontinence indicates mechanical failure, fluid leak, or erosion of the device.
13. Bulbar urethral placement of an AUS will not allow appropriate instrumentation and transurethral resection in patients with recurrent bladder tumors.
14. Detrusor overactivity, if present, is not a contraindication to the treatment for sphincteric incontinence.
15. Gram-positive bacterial infections are the most commonly involved in infection of prosthetic devices in the genitourinary system.

92 Tumors of the Bladder

David P. Wood, Jr.

QUESTIONS

1. What percentage of women will have squamous metaplasia of the bladder?
   a. 5%
   b. 15%
   c. 25%
   d. 40%
   e. 60%

2. Inverted papillomas are:
   a. a benign tumor of the bladder.
   b. a precursor to low-grade papillary cancer.
   c. chemotherapy resistant.
   d. an invasive tumor.
   e. best treated with antibiotics.

3. The incidence rate of urothelial cancer:
   a. has been decreasing recently because of less smoking.
   b. is higher in women than in men.
   c. is highest in developed countries.
   d. peaks in the fifth decade of life.
   e. is higher in Asia than Europe.

4. The mortality rate of urothelial cancer:
   a. is primarily related to lack of health care access.
   b. has been decreasing since 1990.
   c. is highest in underdeveloped countries.
   d. is proportionally higher in women than in men.
   e. is proportionally higher in white men than in African-American men.

5. What is the risk of a white male developing urothelial cancer in his lifetime?
   a. Less than 5%
   b. 20%
   c. 40%
   d. 60%
   e. 80%

6. The most common histologic bladder cancer cell type is:
   a. squamous.
   b. adeno.
   c. urothelial.
   d. small cell.
   e. leiomyosarcoma.

7. The mortality rate from bladder cancer is highest in:
   a. the United States.
   b. England.
   c. South America.
   d. China.
   e. Egypt.

8. Recent evidence suggests that physician practice may be related to bladder cancer deaths in the elderly. What percentage of deaths could be avoided?
   a. Less than 5%
   b. 30%
   c. 50%
   d. 70%
   e. 90%

9. Which gene is most commonly mutated in high-grade muscle invasive urothelial cancer?
   a. *Cyclin A*
   b. *TP53*
   c. *FGFR-3*
   d. *HRAS*
   e. *PTEN*

10. Which gene is most commonly mutated in carcinoma in situ (CIS)?
    a. *PI3K*
    b. *RB*
    c. *FGFR-3*
    d. *HRAS*
    e. *CD-44*

11. The chemotherapy proven to cause urothelial cancer is:
    a. doxorubicin.
    b. bleomycin.
    c. ifosfamide.
    d. etoposide.
    e. cyclophosphamide.

12. The increased risk of developing bladder cancer for a man who has a sister with bladder cancer is:
    a. twofold.
    b. 10-fold.
    c. 20-fold.
    d. 40-fold.
    e. 60-fold.

13. The risk of a family member developing bladder cancer if a first-degree relative has the disease is:
    a. related to secondhand smoke.
    b. higher in men.
    c. higher in smokers.
    d. related to inheritance of low-penetrance genes.
    e. most common in high-grade cancer.

14. The percent of patients presenting with non–muscle-invasive disease is:
    a. less than 5%.
    b. 20%.
    c. 40%.
    d. 60%.
    e. 80%.

15. A 30-year-old man has gross hematuria and cystoscopy reveals a papillary tumor. Transurethral resection of the tumor reveals a noninvasive 2-cm papillary low-malignant-potential urothelial tumor. Muscle is present in the resected specimen. All of the tumor is resected. The best treatment is:
    a. intravesical bacille Calmette-Guérin (BCG).
    b. repeat cystoscopy with random bladder biopsies.
    c. radical cystectomy because of the patient's young age.
    d. immediate mitomycin C intravesical therapy.
    e. observation.

16. The external agent most implicated in causing urothelial cancer is:
    a. β-naphthylamine.
    b. 4-aminobiphenyl.
    c. perchloroethylene.
    d. trichloroethylene.
    e. 4,4′-methylene bis(2-methylaniline).

17. If a woman stops smoking for 10 years after 30-pack-years of smoking, her risk of developing bladder cancer:
    a. is the same as if she still smoked.
    b. is the same as if she never smoked.
    c. is unrelated to the intensity of smoking.
    d. is very low because of her gender.
    e. gradually decreases with time.

18. Which food substance is associated with a low risk of urothelial cancer?
    a. Citrus
    b. Eggs
    c. Chicken
    d. Grapes
    e. Cherries

19. A man exposed to high doses of radiation (more than 500 mSv):
    a. has the same risk of urothelial cancer formation as a nuclear plant worker.
    b. will likely develop urothelial cancer within 5 years.
    c. is more likely to develop urothelial cancer if he is younger than 20 years.
    d. is 2 times more likely to develop urothelial cancer.
    e. should be quarantined for 3 months.

20. One of the main changes from the 1973 to 1998 World Health Organization urothelial classification system was that:
    a. there should be two grades of non-muscle-invasive bladder cancer.
    b. muscle-invasive disease should be segregated into inner and outer muscle involvement.
    c. perivesical fat involvement by tumors is stage T3.
    d. CIS can be low or high grade.
    e. Ta grade 1 tumors should be considered cancerous.

21. Genetic abnormalities associated with low-malignant potential Ta tumors include:
    a. fibroblast growth factor receptor-3 (FGFR-3).
    b. TP53.
    c. retinoblastoma (RB) gene.
    d. PTEN.
    e. loss of chromosome 17.

22. Urothelial cancer noninvasively involving the prostatic urethra:
    a. is stage T4a.
    b. is stage T4b.
    c. is not part of the 2010 tumor, node, metastasis staging system for bladder cancer.
    d. has a worse prognosis than perivesical fat involvement.
    e. should be treated with radical cystectomy.

23. A 40-year-old man has a T1 high-grade urothelial cancer on initial presentation. Muscle was present in the biopsy specimen. The next treatment is:
    a. BCG.
    b. repeat transurethral resection of a bladder tumor (TURBT).
    c. radical cystectomy.
    d. immediate mitomycin C instillation.
    e. neoadjuvant chemotherapy followed by radical cystectomy.

24. A 73-year-old man with a history of Ta bladder cancer is found to have a 0.5-cm papillary lesion in the prostatic urethra and undergoes extensive transurethral resection of the prostate, revealing high-grade noninvasive disease of the prostatic urethra without ductal or stromal involvement. The next best step is:
    a. perioperative mitomycin C.
    b. surveillance cystoscopy every 3 months.
    c. mitomycin C therapy.
    d. induction of and maintenance with BCG therapy.
    e. radical cystectomy.

25. A 62-year-old man undergoes a transurethral biopsy of a bladder tumor at the dome. Final pathology reveals muscle-invasive urothelial and small cell carcinoma. Metastatic workup is negative. The next step is:
    a. intravesical gemcitabine therapy.
    b. partial cystectomy.
    c. radical cystoprostatectomy.
    d. external beam radiotherapy.
    e. chemoradiation therapy.

26. When cisplatin-based chemotherapy is used, which of the following genetic mutations is associated with the worst prognosis?
    a. *FGFR-3* mutations
    b. *PTEN*
    c. *TP53*
    d. *RB*
    e. *PTEN, TP53,* and *RB*

27. Tumor suppressor genes are activated by:
    a. gene amplification.
    b. translocation.
    c. point mutations.
    d. DNA methylation.
    e. microsatellite instability.

28. The risk of urologic malignancy in a man with recurrent gross hematuria, but who had a previous negative evaluation, is:
    a. less than 5%.
    b. 20%.
    c. 40%.
    d. 60%.
    e. 80%.

29. Which of the following is not a high-risk factor in urothelial cancer formation in patients with microscopic hematuria?
    a. Age younger than 40 years
    b. Smoking
    c. History of pelvic radiation
    d. Urinary tract infections
    e. Previous urologic surgery

30. Commercially available fluorescence in situ hybridization kits test for abnormalities in which of the following chromosomes?
    a. 3, 7, 9, 17
    b. 2, 5, 8
    c. 4, 6, 9
    d. 1, 10, 12
    e. 13, 14, 16

31. Microsatellite analysis:
    a. detects telomeric repeats.
    b. amplifies DNA repeats in the genome.
    c. evaluates abnormalities on chromosome 9.
    d. detects DNA methylation.
    e. identifies hereditary urothelial cancer.

32. Smoking is responsible for what percent of bladder cancer in males?
    a. 5%
    b. 20%
    c. 40%
    d. 60%
    e. 80%

33. Which of the following is not sensitive to cisplatin chemotherapy?
    a. High-grade urothelial cancer
    b. Micropapillary cancer
    c. Squamous cell cancer

d. Adenocarcinoma
e. Small cell cancer

34. Nested variant of urothelial cancer can be confused with:
    a. cystitis cystica.
    b. micropapillary cancer.
    c. squamous cell cancer.
    d. small cell cancer.
    e. high-grade urothelial cancer.

35. The most common sarcoma involving the bladder is:
    a. angiosarcoma.
    b. chondrosarcoma.
    c. leiomyosarcoma.
    d. rhabdomyosarcoma.
    e. osteosarcoma.

36. Signet ring cell cancers:
    a. have a good prognosis.
    b. are sensitive to doxorubicin chemotherapy.
    c. usually present in advanced stage.
    d. are responsive to radiation therapy.
    e. are low-grade at initial presentation.

37. The risk of bladder cancer formation in a spinal cord-injured patient is:
    a. less than 5%.
    b. 20%.
    c. 40%.
    d. 60%.
    e. 80%.

38. For patients undergoing radical cystectomy for urothelial cancer, the risk of identifying prostatic urethral disease is:
    a. less than 5%.
    b. 20%.
    c. 40%.
    d. 60%.
    e. 80%.

39. Which of the following is NOT a risk factor for prostatic urethral cancer?
    a. Previous intravesical therapy
    b. CIS of the trigone
    c. CIS of the distal ureters
    d. Low-grade urothelial cancer
    e. Recurrent bladder tumors

Pathology

1. A 70-year-old man has microscopic hematuria. Cytology and computed tomography (CT) scan are negative. Cystoscopy reveals a raised 3-mm lesion on the trigone. The lesion is biopsied and is depicted in Figure 92-1A and B, and is reported as adenocarcinoma. The next step in management is:
    a. review the pathology slides with the pathologist.
    b. cystectomy.
    c. intravesical chemotherapy.
    d. bone scan.
    e. ask for special stains from pathology.

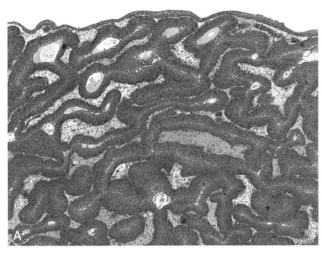

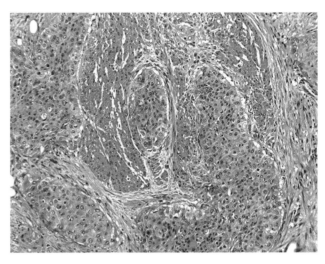

Figure 92-2. (From Bostwick DG, Cheng L. Urologic surgical pathology. 2nd ed. Edinburgh: Mosby; 2008.)

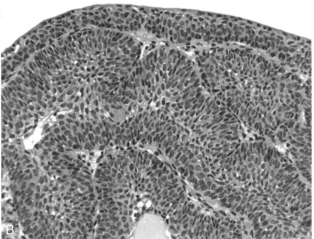

Figure 92-1. (From Bostwick DG, Cheng L. Urologic surgical pathology. 2nd ed. Edinburgh: Mosby; 2008.)

Imaging

1. See Figure 92-3. The depicted findings have an association with:
   a. bladder carcinoma.
   b. previous trauma.
   c. recurrent urinary tract infections.
   d. urolithiasis.
   e. ureteral spasm.

2. A 65-year-old man has gross hematuria. He has a history of tuberculosis. Cytology is suspicious, CT scan is normal, and cystoscopy reveals a papillary lesion cephalad to the trigone. The lesion is visually completely resected (Figure 92-2) and is reported as transitional cell carcinoma, grade 3. The next step in management is:
   a. intravesical BCG.
   b. immediate intravesical mitomycin C.
   c. repeat transurethral resection of bladder at the previous biopsied site.
   d. a cystectomy.
   e. ask the pathologist if there is muscularis propria in the specimen.

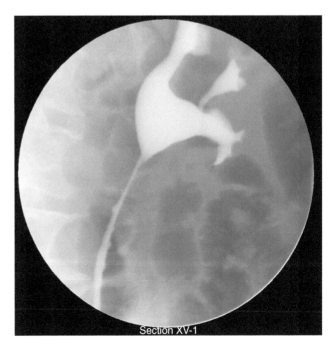

Figure 92-3.

2. Figure 92-4A is a delayed contrast-enhanced image through the pelvic ureters, and Figure 92-4B is an early contrast-enhanced image through the bladder. The next step in management is:

a. shockwave lithotripsy.

b. percutaneous nephrostolithotomy.

c. cystoscopy.

d. cystoscopy with ureteroscopy.

e. follow-up with imaging in 6 months.

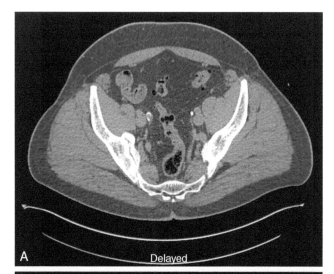

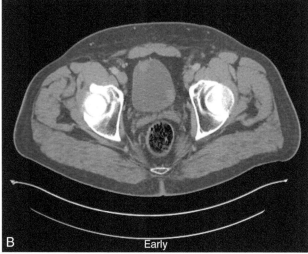

Figure 92-4.

ANSWERS

1. **d. 40%.** Approximately 40% of women and 5% of men have squamous metaplasia of the bladder that is usually related to infection, trauma, and surgery (Ozbey et al, 1999).* There are no racial differences, and squamous metaplasia is more common in women of childbearing age.

2. **a. A benign tumor of the bladder.** When diagnosed according to strictly defined criteria (e.g., lack of cytologic atypia), inverted papillomas behave in a benign fashion with only a 1% incidence of tumor recurrence (Sung et al, 2006; Kilciler et al, 2008). Occasionally, inverted papillomas are present with coexistent urothelial cancer elsewhere in the urinary system, occurring more commonly in the upper tract than the bladder (Asano et al,

---

*Sources referenced can be found in *Campbell-Walsh Urology, 11th Edition*, on the Expert Consult website.

2003). The use of fluorescence in situ hybridization to evaluate chromosomal changes can distinguish between an inverted papilloma and a urothelial cancer with an inverted growth pattern (Jones et al, 2007).

3. **c. Is highest in developed countries.** Sixty-three percent of all bladder cancer cases occur in developed countries, with 55% occurring in North America and Europe. There is a geographic difference in bladder cancer incidence rates across the world, with the highest rates in Southern and Eastern Europe, parts of Africa, Middle East, and North America, and the lowest in Asia and underdeveloped areas in Africa (Ferlay et al, 2007). The incidence of urothelial cancer peaks in the seventh decade of life.

4. **b. Has been decreasing since 1990.** The mortality rate of urothelial cancer has decreased by 5% since 1990, primarily because of smoking cessation, changes in environmental carcinogens, and healthier lifestyles (Jemal et al, 2008).

5. **a. Less than 5%.** A white male has a 3.7% chance of developing urothelial cancer in his lifetime, which is roughly 3 times the probability in white females or African-American males and more than 4.5 times the probability of an African-American female (Hayat et al, 2007; Jemal et al, 2008).

6. **c. Urothelial.** Histologically, 90% of bladder cancers are of urothelial origin, 5% squamous cell, and less than 2% adenocarcinoma or other variants (Lopez-Beltran, 2008). Urothelial carcinoma is the most common malignancy of the urinary tract and is the second most common cause of death among genitourinary tumors.

7. **e. Egypt.** The mortality rate from bladder cancer in Egypt is 3 times higher than in Europe and 8 times higher than in North America because squamous cell carcinoma is highly prevalent in Egypt (Parekh et al, 2002).

8. **b. 30%.** Mortality from bladder cancer is highest in elderly persons, particularly those past the age of 80, accounting for the third most common cause of cancer deaths in men over the age of 80 (Jemal et al, 2008). Whether this increase in mortality rate is related to tumor biology or changes in physician practice with the elderly is unclear. Recent evidence suggests that physician practice may be related to bladder cancer deaths in the elderly (Morris et al, 2009). These authors estimated that 31% of all bladder cancer deaths were avoidable, more commonly in noninvasive than invasive disease.

9. **b. *TP53*.** High-malignant potential, non–muscle-invasive bladder cancer is more likely associated with deletions of tumor suppressor genes such as *TP53* and *RB* (Chatterjee et al, 2004a; George et al, 2007; Sanchez-Carbayo et al, 2007).

10. **b. *RB*.** All CIS is high grade by definition. The genetic abnormalities associated with CIS include alterations to the *RB*, *TP53*, and *PTEN* genes (Cordon-Cardo et al, 2000; Lopez-Beltran et al, 2002; Cordon-Cardo, 2008).

11. **e. Cyclophosphamide.** The only chemotherapeutic agent that has been proven to cause bladder cancer is cyclophosphamide (Travis et al, 1995; Nilsson and Ullen, 2008). The risk of bladder cancer formation is linearly related to the duration and intensity of cyclophosphamide treatment, supporting a causative role. Phosphoramide mustard is the primary mutagenic metabolite that causes bladder cancer in patients exposed to cyclophosphamide.

12. **a. Twofold.** First-degree relatives of patients with bladder cancer have a twofold increased risk of developing urothelial cancer themselves, but high-risk urothelial cancer families are relatively rare (Aben et al, 2002; Murta-Nascimento et al, 2007; Kiemeney, 2008).

13. **d. Related to inheritance of low-penetrance genes.** The hereditary risk seems to be higher for women and nonsmokers, but it is not related to secondhand exposure to smoking in families. Most likely, there are a variety of low-penetrance genes that can be inherited to make a person more susceptible to carcinogenic exposure, thus increasing the risk of bladder cancer formation.

14. **e. 80%.** At initial presentation, 80% of urothelial tumors are non–muscle-invasive. There are multiple growth patterns of

urothelial cancer, including flat carcinoma in-situ (CIS), papillary tumors that can be low or high grade, and sessile tumors with a solid growth pattern. Non–muscle-invasive cancers can be very large because of lack of the genetic alterations required for invasion.

15. **d. Immediate mitomycin C intravesical therapy.** PUNLMP is a papillary growth with minimal cytological atypia that is more than seven cells thick and is generally solitary and located on the trigone (Holmang et al, 2001; Sauter et al, 2004). PUNLMP is composed of thin papillary stalks where the polarity of the cells is maintained and the nuclei are minimally enlarged. PUNLMP has a low proliferation rate and is not associated with invasion or metastases. Tumor recurrence is common, and thus perioperative treatment with mitomycin C is warranted.

16. **a. β-naphthylamine.** One of the first and most common chemical agents implicated in the formation of bladder cancer in dye and rubber workers is β-naphthylamine (Case and Hosker, 1954). Activation of aromatic amines allows DNA binding by enzymes that are selectively expressed in the population, making some subjects more susceptible to cancer formation, as described earlier related to the *NAT-2* and the *GSTM1* polymorphisms.

17. **e. Gradually decreases with time.** Smoking cessation does make a difference in urothelial cancer formation. Smokers who have stopped for 1 to 3 years have a 2.6 relative risk, and those who have stopped for more than 15 years have a 1.1 relative risk of bladder cancer formation (Wynder and Goldsmith, 1977; Smoke IAfRoCT, 2004).

18. **a. Citrus.** In general, a Mediterranean diet has the lowest urothelial cancer risk. In a case-controlled study, there were fewer cases of urothelial cancer in the group given a Mediterranean diet versus a standard Western diet, probably as a result of the increased ingestion of fruits and vegetables (de Lorgeril et al, 1998). Both fruits and vegetables, specifically citrus, apples, berries, tomatoes, carrots, and cruciferous vegetables, contain several active compounds that are important in detoxification.

19. **d. Is 2 times more likely to develop urothelial cancer.** There is a significant increased risk of dying from any cancer if a person is exposed to greater than 50 mSv. The relative risk of urothelial cancer formation is 1.63 in men and 1.74 in women. Interestingly, urothelial cancer formation after radiation is not age related, but the latency period is 15 to 30 years. However, there is no association with low-dose or industrial exposure of radiation therapy and bladder cancer formation. Importantly, urologic technicians and nuclear radiation workers do not have an increased risk of urothelial cancer formation.

20. **a. There should be two grades of non–muscle-invasive bladder cancer.** The two main changes were recognition that papillary Ta grade 1 urothelial cancers should not be considered cancers because of their indolent growth and lack of invasion, and the second was elimination of "grade 2" cancers that became a gray zone encompassing grade 1 and grade 3 cancers, causing interobserver variation.

21. **a. Fibroblast growth factor receptor-3 (*FGFR-3*).** Genetic abnormalities associated with low-grade cancer include deletion of 9q and alterations of *FGFR-3*, *HRAS*, and *PI3K* (Holmang et al, 2001; Cordon-Cardo, 2008). Low-grade carcinomas are immunoreactive for cytokeratin-20 and CD-44. The *TP53*, retinoblastoma *(RB)*, and *PTEN* genes and loss of chromosome 17 are all associated with high-grade cancer.

22. **c. Is not part of the 2010 tumor, node, metastasis staging system for bladder cancer.** Extension of the tumor into the prostatic urethra without stromal invasion is currently classified under the prostatic urethral section and does not carry an adverse prognosis for patients with known bladder cancer (Pagano et al, 1996).

23. **b. Repeat TURBT.** Because of this understaging, the American Urological Association (AUA) guidelines call for a repeat transurethral resection in patients with T1 tumors to assess for muscle-invasive disease even if muscle was present in the specimen (Hall et al, 2007).

24. **d. Induction of and maintenance with BCG therapy.** For patients with noninvasive prostatic urethral cancer, transurethral resection of the prostate with BCG therapy is appropriate (Palou et al, 2007). For patients with prostatic ductal disease, a complete TURP is warranted, plus BCG therapy. Although a radical cystectomy could be performed, a more conservative organ-sparing treatment is recommended.

25. **e. Chemoradiation therapy.** Small cell carcinoma of the bladder should be considered and treated as metastatic disease, even if there is no radiologic evidence of disease outside the bladder. Small cell carcinoma of the bladder accounts for much less than 1% of all primary bladder tumors. In general, small cell carcinoma of the bladder is very chemosensitive, and the primary mode of therapy is chemoradiation therapy.

26. **e. *PTEN*, *TP53*, and *RB*.** Overall genetic instability is the hallmark of invasive urothelial cancer, but, specifically, alterations of *TP53*, *RB*, and *PTEN* carry a very poor prognosis (Chatterjee et al, 2004a). *FGFR-3* mutations are associated with noninvasive bladder cancer.

27. **c. Point mutations.** Tumor suppressor genes are mainly activated by allelic deletion of one allele followed by point mutations of the remaining allele. Tumor suppressor genes are recessive or have a negative effect, resulting in unregulated cellular growth. Proto-oncogenes are generally activated by point mutations in the genetic code, gene amplification, and gene translocation. The activated proto-oncogenes become oncogenes that can cause cancer, and this is considered a positive or dominant growth effect (Lengauer et al, 1998; Wolff et al, 2005; Cordon-Cardo, 2008).

28. **a. Less than 5%.** Gross, painless hematuria is the primary symptom in 85% of patients with a newly diagnosed bladder tumor (Khadra et al, 2000; Alishahi et al, 2002; Edwards et al, 2006). The gross hematuria is usually intermittent and can be related to Valsalva maneuvers; therefore any episode of gross hematuria should be evaluated even if subsequent urinalysis is negative. Fifty percent of patients with gross hematuria will have a demonstrable cause, 20% will have a urological malignancy, and 12% will have a bladder tumor (Khadra et al, 2000). The risk of malignancy in patients with recurrent gross or microscopic hematuria that had a full, negative evaluation is near zero within the first 6 years (Khadra et al, 2000).

29. **a. Age younger than 40 years.** The guidelines recommend consideration for re-evaluation of low-risk individuals with microscopic hematuria, but repeat evaluation every 6 months with a urinalysis, cytology, and blood pressure (to detect renal disease) is recommended for high-risk patients. Age younger than 40 years is the only factor that is not associated with an increased risk of malignancy.

30. **a. 3, 7, 9, 17.** Fluorescence in situ hybridization (FISH) identifies fluorescently labeled DNA probes that bind to intranuclear chromosomes. The current commercially available probes evaluate aneuploidy for chromosomes 3, 7, 17, and homozygous loss of 9p 21 (Zwarthoff, 2008). The median sensitivity and specificity of FISH analysis is 79% and 70%, respectively (van Rhijn et al, 2005).

31. **b. Amplifies DNA repeats in the genome.** There are multiple markers available to identify short DNA repeats present throughout the chromosomes that are lost in some tumor cells. Microsatellite analysis amplifies these repeats in the genome that are highly polymorphic, and PCR amplification can detect tumor-associated loss of heterozygosity by comparing the peak ratio of the two alleles in tumor DNA in a urine sample with that ratio in a blood sample from the same individual (Steiner et al, 1997; Wang et al, 1997). The sensitivity and specificity of microsatellite analysis for the detection of urothelial carcinoma range from 72% to 97% and 80% to 100%, respectively (Steiner et al, 1997; Wang et al, 1997). Microsatellite analysis evaluates abnormalities on all chromosomes.

32. **c. 40%.** Smoking is responsible for 30% to 50% of all bladder cancers in males, and smokers have a twofold to sixfold greater risk for bladder cancer (Brennan et al, 2000; Boffetta, 2008). Smoking cessation will decrease the risk of eventual urothelial cancer formation in a linear fashion. After 15 years of not smoking, the risk of cancer formation is the same as for a person who

never smoked (Smoke IAfRoCT, 2004). The strong influence of smoking in bladder cancer formation prevents accurate determination of other less significant dietary, micronutrient, or lifestyle changes that may alter bladder cancer formation.

33. **b. Micropapillary cancer.** The most effective treatment for all stages of micropapillary urothelial carcinoma is surgical resection. Treatment with transurethral resection and BCG therapy is ineffective unless the tumor is completely resected (Kamat et al, 2007). Neoadjuvant chemotherapy does not appear effective in micropapillary urothelial carcinoma, similar to ovarian cancer (Bristow et al, 2002; Kamat et al, 2007). Neoadjuvant chemotherapy may actually worsen survival by delaying therapy when compared with immediate cystectomy. Cisplatin is effective against urothelial cancer and the associated variants of squamous cell, adenocarcinoma, and small cell cancer.

34. **a. Cystitis cystica.** The nested variant of urothelial cancer is a rare but aggressive cancer that has a male-to-female ratio of 6:1 and can be confused with benign lesions, such as Von Brunn nests that are in the lamina propria, cystitis cystica, and inverted papillomas (Holmang and Johansson, 2001). There is little nuclear atypia in nested variant urothelial carcinoma, but the tumor cells will often contain areas with large nuclei and mitotic figures. The mortality rate from nested variant urothelial carcinoma, despite aggressive therapy, is significant, with 70% dying of their disease within 3 years (Paik and Park, 1996).

35. **c. Leiomyosarcoma.** Leiomyosarcoma is the most common histologic subtype, followed by rhabdomyosarcoma and then, rarely, angiosarcomas, osteosarcomas, and carcinosarcomas. The male-to-female ratio is 2:1, and the average age at presentation is in the sixth decade of life. There are no clear agents that cause bladder sarcomas, although there is an association with pelvic radiation and systemic chemotherapy for other malignancies (Spiess et al, 2007). Importantly, bladder sarcomas are not smoking related.

36. **c. Usually present in advanced stage.** Primary signet ring cell carcinoma of the bladder is extremely rare, making up less than 1% of all epithelial bladder neoplasms (Morelli et al, 2006). Signet ring cell carcinoma can be of urachal origin and directly extend into the bladder. These tumors generally present as high-grade, high-stage tumors and have a uniformly poor prognosis. The primary treatment is radical cystectomy; however, in the majority of cases there are regional or distant metastases at the time of presentation, and the mean survival time is less than 20 months (Torenbeek et al, 1996). There are reports of elevated carcinoembryonic antigen (CEA) in patients with signet ring cell carcinoma. The prognostic significance of this elevated serum marker is unclear (Morelli et al, 2006). Understaging is very common in signet ring cell carcinoma, with peritoneal studding common at the time of surgical exploration.

37. **a. Less than 5%.** Spinal cord-injured patients are at risk for developing squamous cell carcinoma, most likely due to chronic catheter irritation and infection. Older studies have suggested a 2.5% to 10% incidence of squamous cell carcinoma in the spinal cord-injured population, with a mean delay of 17 years after the spinal cord injury (Kaufman et al, 1977). More recent analysis of the association of spinal cord-injury and bladder cancer formation has shown a remarkably lower risk of bladder cancer formation of 0.38%, most likely because of better catheter care (Bickel et al, 1991). This supports the concept that chronic infection and foreign bodies can lead to bladder cancer formation.

38. **c. 40%.** Prostatic urethral cancer is associated with urothelial cancer of the bladder in 90% of cases, primarily CIS, and most will have multifocal bladder tumors. However, the incidence of prostatic urethral disease in patients with primary urothelial cancer is only 3% (Rikken et al, 1987; Millan-Rodriguez et al, 2000). Secondary prostatic urethral involvement in patients with a history of urothelial cancer is approximately 15% at 5 years and 30% at 15 years, almost uniformly associated with extensive intravesical therapy (Herr and Donat, 1999). For patients undergoing radical cystectomy for urothelial cancer, the risk of identifying prostatic urethral disease is 40%.

39. **d. Low-grade urothelial cancer.** Risk factors for prostatic urethral involvement are CIS of the trigone, bladder neck, distal ureters, recurrent bladder tumors, and a history of intravesical chemotherapy (Wood et al, 1989b). Low-grade tumors rarely involve the prostatic urethra.

Pathology

1. **a. Review the pathology slides with the pathologist.** This is a classic inverted papilloma, and the inexperienced pathologist might mistake it for an adenocarcinoma. The location of the lesion would be unusual for adenocarcinoma, particularly in a patient with no risk factors, and should alert the clinician to review the slides with the pathologist.

2. **e. Ask the pathologist if there is muscularis propria in the specimen.** There are clear bundles of muscularis propria in the micrograph making the tumor at least a T2.

Imaging

1. **a. Bladder carcinoma.** Pseudodiverticulosis of the ureter is associated with bladder carcinoma in 30% of cases. This association has led many to recommend that patients with this diagnosis undergo surveillance of their bladder for the development of urothelial neoplasms. The etiology is unknown.

2. **d. Cystoscopy with ureteroscopy.** There are multiple enhancing masses in the fluid-filled urinary bladder on the early image. On the delayed image, the ureters are opacified with contrast, and there is a filling defect seen in the mildly dilated right ureter, suspicious for a synchronous ureteral lesion.

CHAPTER REVIEW

1. Inverted papillomas are associated with chronic inflammation.
2. Cystitis glandularis may be associated with pelvic lipomatosis.
3. Bladder cancers in adolescents and young adults generally are well differentiated and noninvasive.
4. The intensity and duration of smoking is linearly related to the risk of developing bladder cancer with no plateau; cessation of smoking reduces the risk.
5. There is a clear association between a healthy diet and a decreased risk of urothelial cancer.
6. There is no convincing evidence that alteration in fluid intake, alcohol consumption, ingestion of artificial sweeteners, or analgesic abuse increase the risk of bladder cancer; however, chronic irritation, bacterial infection, and radiation have all been associated with the development of bladder cancer.
7. Eighty percent of the time, low-grade, low-stage urothelial neoplasia (papillary urothelial neoplasia of low malignant potential) is associated with loss of chromosome 9.
8. Low-grade (stage 1), low-stage urothelial neoplasia is called papillary urothelial neoplasia of low malignant potential (PUNLMP); the terms low grade and high grade replace the old system of grades 2 and 3.
9. Prostatic urethral involvement by transitional cell carcinoma without invasion carries a relatively good prognosis; when it invades the prostatic stroma, the prognosis is less good, and when it directly invades the substance of the prostate from the bladder, the prognosis is poor.

10. Low-grade papillary lesions have a 60% recurrence rate but less than a 10% rate of progression to muscularis propria invasion, whereas high-grade lesions, particularly T1, may have a stage progression in as many as 50% of cases. Moreover, high-grade non-muscularis propria invasive tumors have an 80% incidence of recurrence.
11. Angiolymphatic invasion is a poor prognostic sign.
12. In muscularis propria invasive urothelial cancer, alterations in *TP53*, *RB*, and *PTEN* are poor prognostic indicators.
13. Genetic alterations in low-grade non-muscularis propria invasive disease include alterations in *FGFR-3* and deletions in chromosome 9.
14. Porphyrin-induced fluorescent cystoscopy and narrow-band imaging cystoscopy have been used to increase the sensitivity of cystoscopy.
15. To date, none of the urinary markers are sensitive or specific enough to replace cystoscopy for monitoring bladder cancer.
16. Sarcomas of the bladder, in decreasing order of frequency, include leiomyosarcoma, rhabdomyosarcoma, angiosarcoma, osteosarcoma, and carcinosarcoma.
17. *Schistosoma haematobium* is the causative agent of squamous cell carcinoma in endemic regions.
18. Altered growth patterns, such as micropapillary and nested patterns, carry a poor prognosis.
19. Normal bladder urothelium is less than 7 cell layers thick: papillary lesions are greater than 7 cell layers thick.
20. The incidence of urothelial cancer peaks in the seventh decade of life.
21. There is some evidence to indicate that BCG plus oral administration of vitamins A, B_6, C, E, and zinc result in a reduced risk of recurrent transitional cell carcinoma.
22. Histologically, 90% of bladder cancers are of urothelial origin, 5% squamous cell, and less than 2% adenocarcinoma or other variants.
23. All CIS is high grade by definition. The genetic abnormalities associated with CIS include alterations to the *RB*, *TP53*, and *PTEN* genes.
24. The only chemotherapeutic agent that has been proven to cause bladder cancer is cyclophosphamide.
25. First-degree relatives of patients with bladder cancer have a twofold increased risk of developing urothelial cancer themselves.
26. Urothelial cancer formation after radiation is not age related; the latency period is 15 to 30 years.
27. A repeat transurethral resection in patients with T1 tumors to assess for muscle-invasive disease should be performed, even if muscle was present in the original specimen.
28. Small cell carcinoma of the bladder is very chemosensitive.
29. The risk of malignancy in patients with recurrent gross or microscopic hematuria who had a full, negative evaluation is near zero within the first 6 years.
30. Neoadjuvant chemotherapy does not appear effective in micropapillary urothelial carcinoma.

93 Non–Muscle-Invasive Bladder Cancer (TA, T1, and CIS)

J. Stephen Jones

QUESTIONS

1. Postoperative intravesical chemotherapy (administered in the recovery room) is most appropriate for which of the following patients?
   a. Initial presentation of a solitary 3.0-cm, low-grade–appearing tumor on the posterior bladder wall
   b. Multifocal (n=4) low-grade, low-stage bladder tumor, all 4 to 10 mm in diameter
   c. 6.5-cm high-grade, broad-based tumor on lateral wall with deep resection
   d. a and b
   e. a, b, and c

2. Which of the following agents is contraindicated for postoperative intravesical chemotherapy (administered in the recovery room)?
   a. Thiotepa
   b. Bacille Calmette-Guérin (BCG)
   c. Mitomycin C
   d. Epirubicin
   e. b and c

3. Potential advantage(s) of tumor markers such as, BTA, stat NMP-22, and UroVysion (FISH) when compared with urinary cytology for monitoring patients with bladder cancer are improved:
   a. sensitivity.
   b. specificity.
   c. positive predictive value.
   d. a and c.
   e. a, b, and c.

4. Progression rates for low-grade Ta tumors range from:
   a. 0% to 3%.
   b. 3% to 10%.
   c. 10% to 17%.
   d. 17% to 25%.
   e. over 25%.

5. General anesthesia can be advantageous compared to spinal anesthesia when resecting a bladder tumor in which setting?
   a. Large, mobile papillary tumor
   b. Tumor in a posterior wall diverticulum
   c. Lateral location, at approximately 4 o'clock or 8 o'clock
   d. Extensive carcinoma in situ (CIS)
   e. Tumor at dome and along anterior bladder wall

6. A healthy 55-year-old man undergoes resection of a 2.0-cm bladder tumor in a posterior wall bladder diverticulum. Pathology demonstrates a pT1G3 bladder tumor with associated areas of carcinoma in situ (CIS). Muscularis mucosa is involved, but there is no definite muscularis propria in the specimen. Optimal management includes:
   a. repeat resection to stage the cancer.
   b. intravesical BCG therapy.
   c. partial cystectomy with excision of the diverticulum.
   d. radical cystectomy and neobladder urinary diversion.
   e. chemotherapy and radiation therapy.

7. The most important principle to follow when resecting tumor near or overlying a ureteral orifice is:
   a. stent frequently.
   b. avoid resection in most cases.
   c. avoid cautery in this area.
   d. resect at will—a stent or nephrostomy tube can be placed later.
   e. obtain an ultrasound preoperatively and place a nephrostomy tube if hydronephrosis is found.

8. A restaging transurethral resection of bladder tumor (TURBT) is indicated in which of the following situations?
   a. pT1, high grade tumor with no muscularis propria identified
   b. pTa, low grade tumor that is multifocal (n=5), for which resection appeared to be complete, but postoperative intravesical therapy was *not* administered
   c. pT1, high grade tumor with muscularis propria identified and negative
   d. a and c
   e. a, b, and c

9. The optimal laser for fulguration of bladder tumors is:
   a. CO_2.
   b. Neodymium-doped yttrium aluminium garnet (Nd:YAG).
   c. holmium.
   d. potassium titanyl phosphate (KTP).
   e. argon.

10. Intravesical mitomycin C chemotherapy for high-risk superficial bladder cancer:
    a. reduces the risk of progression.
    b. reduces the risk of recurrence.
    c. is preferred over BCG, particularly for CIS.
    d. is virtually free of side effects.
    e. is less expensive than BCG.

11. Contraindications to intravesical BCG therapy include which of the following:
    a. cirrhosis.
    b. history of tuberculosis (TB).
    c. total incontinence.
    d. immunosuppression.
    e. all of the above.

12. The combination of reduced-dose BCG and interferon-α for intravesical therapy is:
    a. more effective than BCG alone.
    b. more toxic than BCG alone.
    c. preferred first-line therapy for patients with multifocal CIS.

d. less expensive than BCG alone.

e. a reasonable option for BCG failures after one course of therapy.

13. Common side effects of thiotepa include:

a. irritative voiding symptoms and fever.

b. hematuria and irritative voiding symptoms.

c. bladder contraction and myelosuppression.

d. irritative voiding symptoms and myelosuppression.

e. flulike symptoms and fever.

14. Long-term (15 years) outcomes after intravesical BCG therapy for patients with high-risk non–muscle-invasive bladder cancer include the following:

a. approximately 50% progression rate.

b. approximately 25% alive and with bladder intact.

c. a high incidence of recurrence in extravesical sites (prostatic urothelium and upper tracts).

d. approximately 33% cancer-related mortality rates.

e. all of the above.

15. Understaging for patients with pT1 high-grade bladder cancer is approximately:

a. 5% to 10%.

b. 10% to 20%.

c. 20% to 30%.

d. 30% to 50%.

e. 50% to 70%.

16. A patient is diagnosed with a 1.0-cm pTa low-grade bladder cancer. Imaging of the upper tracts should be performed:

a. not indicated.

b. only at diagnosis.

c. at diagnosis and 5 years later.

d. at diagnosis and every other year thereafter.

e. at diagnosis and every year thereafter.

17. For patients with stage pTa low-grade bladder tumor and a negative cytology, random bladder biopsies:

a. are more likely to be positive in the prostatic fossa than the bladder.

b. must be done in a systematic manner.

c. should include sampling of the muscularis mucosa and preferably the muscularis propria, too.

d. are indicated at initial diagnosis and need not be repeated if negative.

e. are not indicated in most cases.

18. The risk of progression to muscle-invasive disease for patients with untreated CIS of the bladder is approximately:

a. 5% to 15%.

b. 15% to 25%.

c. 25% to 35%.

d. 35% to 45%.

e. higher than 45%.

19. Current consensus about p53 as a prognostic marker for bladder cancer is as follows:

a. established predictive factor for response to BCG therapy.

b. independent predictor of tumor progression for patients with pT1G3 disease.

c. stronger predictive value than grade for pTa tumors.

d. of no clinical value at present.

e. prospective validation required.

20. Which of the following disease entities is least common?

a. pTa low grade

b. pTa high grade

c. pT1 high grade

d. CIS of any form

e. pT2-3

21. The most important factor determining the long-term impact of BCG on progression is:

a. using a full dose with each instillation.

b. adding interferon.

c. maintenance therapy.

d. rolling side to side to ensure that BCG covers the entire urothelium.

e. washing the toilet with bleach after voiding each dose.

ANSWERS

1. **a. Initial presentation of a solitary 3.0 cm, low-grade–appearing tumor on the posterior bladder wall.** Postoperative intravesical chemotherapy should be considered for most cases of new, apparently low-grade non–muscle-invasive bladder cancer because it has been shown to reduce recurrence rates and improve outcomes for this disease. One major exception is the patient in whom an extensive resection has been performed or whenever there is a possible perforation. In these patients intravesical chemotherapy should be withheld due to concern about local extravasation and absorption. The benefit of postoperative intravesical chemotherapy is reduced in patients with recurrent or multiple tumors, and there is no clear benefit in patients with high-grade disease.

2. **b. Bacille Calmette-Guérin (BCG).** BCG should never be given in association with known trauma to the urinary tract, such as after transurethral resection of a bladder tumor (TURBT), due to concern over systemic absorption and sepsis. All of the other agents have shown efficacy in this setting with a favorable morbidity profile.

3. **a. Sensitivity.** Tumor markers such as BTA stat, NMP-22, and UroVysion (FISH) provide increased sensitivity, particularly for low-grade tumors. High specificity is the strength of urinary cytology. This approaches 90% to 100% in many series and has not been improved on with these other markers. Positive predictive value is highest for urinary cytology because the number of false positives is low. Put another way, if the cytology is positive, the patient usually has active disease.

4. **b. 3% to 10%.** Recurrence is common (50% to 70%) for patients with low-grade, pTa tumors, but progression to higher tumor stage is uncommon, occurring in about 5% to 10% of patients.

5. **c. Lateral location, at approximately 4 o'clock or 8 o'clock.** Resection along the lateral bladder wall posterolaterally places one in proximity to the obturator nerve, and this can lead to an obturator reflex. This can predispose to bladder wall perforation. In this situation, general anesthesia with complete paralysis is sometimes beneficial to allow the procedure to be performed in a safe and facile manner.

6. **d. Radical cystectomy and neobladder urinary diversion.** This patient should be strongly considered for radical cystectomy. Partial cystectomy is not a good option because of the presence of CIS, which indicates a high risk of field effect disease and subsequent recurrence. Deeper biopsies will risk perforation and would be unlikely to influence management. Understaging is

common with tumors in diverticuli, and high-grade invasive tumors like this are best managed with radical cystectomy to ensure local disease control and optimize outcomes on a long-term basis.

7. **c. Avoid cautery in this area.** A stent should be avoided if possible to prevent theoretical risk of reflux of tumor cells into the upper tracts. In most cases this area can be resected, and most ureters will remain unobstructed as long as the orifice is identified and cautery is not used in this area. Preoperative placement of a nephrostomy tube is often unnecessary as long as renal function is stable. Many patients with hydronephrosis will have invasive disease and will be undergoing urinary diversion in the near future, and this will relieve the obstruction. Hence, temporary nephrostomy tube placement is usually not required.

8. **d. a and c.** Patients with pT1 tumor for whom the muscularis propria was not identified are understaged about 50% of the time and a repeat resection is clearly indicated. Repeat resection of patients with pT1G3 tumor with muscularis propria present and negative are found to have residual or invasive disease 30% of the time. A repeat TURBT is thus indicated in both of these patient populations to accurately stage the tumor and to optimize patient management.

9. **b. Neodymium-doped yttrium aluminium garnet (Nd:YAG).** The Nd:YAG laser has the best properties (depth of penetration, intensity of energy for effective tumor ablation, etc.) for coagulation of bladder tumors and the greatest clinical experience demonstrating safety and efficacy in appropriately selected patients. CO_2 cannot be used in water and so is not an option at all.

10. **b. Reduces the risk of recurrence.** Mitomycin C (MMC) can reduce the risk of recurrence, but there is no convincing evidence that it can reduce progression rates, which is true for all forms of intravesical chemotherapy. Most comparative studies and meta-analyses suggest an advantage to BCG, particularly for CIS. MMC can lead to local bladder irritation and a number of other side effects, and is thus far from risk free.

11. **e. All of the above.** BGC is contraindicated in patients with liver disease (isoniazid cannot be given if they develop BCG sepsis), a personal history of TB, total incontinence (they cannot retain the BCG, so efficacy would be poor), and immunosuppression (BCG's mechanism of action is to stimulate an immune response). Other contraindications include disrupted urothelium, gross hematuria, or active or persistent symptomatic urinary tract infection (UTI).

12. **e. A reasonable option for BCG failures after one course of therapy.** BCG and interferon-α has shown activity in BCG failures and is one viable option for this challenging patient population. However, it is more expensive and there are no data to suggest that it is more effective than BCG alone. BCG remains the treatment of choice for CIS. BCG and interferon-α is well tolerated with a side-effect profile that is better on average than BCG alone, because most of the side effects are related to the BCG and its dose is reduced in this regimen.

13. **d. Irritative voiding symptoms and myelosuppression.** Irritative voiding symptoms are reported by 12% to 69% of patients receiving intravesical thiotepa. The low molecular weight of this agent (189 kD) predisposes to systemic absorption and myelosuppression. These are the two most common side effects of this agent.

14. **e. All of the above.** Data about long-term outcomes for patients with high-risk superficial bladder cancer treated with intravesical BCG therapy is derived primarily for the experience of Memorial Sloan Kettering (Cookson et al, 1997).* In this series, 50% of patient progressed, and one third died of cancer progression. Approximately one third developed disease in the prostatic fossa or upper tracts, and only 27% survived with an intact bladder. Such data should be considered when counseling patients about treatment options for high-risk disease.

15. **d. 30% to 50%.** The risk of understaging of a pT1 high-grade bladder tumor is approximately 30%, but it is even higher if there is no muscularis propria in the specimen. Altogether, the risk is about 30% to 50% in this high-risk patient population.

16. **a. Not indicated.** The incidence of upper tract tumor associated with pTaG1 bladder cancer is extremely low (0.3% to 2.3%), and current consensus is that upper-tract imaging is not indicated in this patient population (Oosterlinck et al, 2005). If hematuria is present, however, upper-tract imaging is indicated for its evaluation regardless of the finding of bladder tumor.

17. **e. Are not indicated in most cases.** The yield of random bladder biopsy in patients with low-grade, low-stage bladder tumors and a negative cytology is very low and is not indicated unless high-risk features are present.

18. **e. Higher than 45%.** Untreated CIS is very high risk (>50%) for progressing to muscle-invasive disease. Even patients with a complete response to intravesical BCG will experience progression in 30% to 40% of cases on longitudinal follow-up (Sylvester et al, 2005).

19. **e. Prospective validation required.** Almost all studies of p53 as a prognostic marker have been retrospective to date. Although promising, this marker will require prospective validation before it can be generally used for clinical decision making. However, the balance of available data has been promising, and the use of this marker for decision making in very challenging cases has been advocated by many in this field. Most studies suggest that p53 is not a good predictor of response to BCG therapy, and it is clearly not better than grade for predicting outcomes for pTa disease. Its ultimate role for predicting progression for pT1 high-grade tumors is not well defined at present.

20. **b. pTa high grade.** pTa low grade represents 50% to 70% of all non–muscle-invasive bladder tumors and is the most common of these entities. CIS is commonly associated with high-grade tumors and, overall, is found in approximately 10% to 20% of non-muscle-invasive bladder tumors. pT1 high grade is found in approximately 20% of patients with non–muscle-invasive bladder tumors. pT2-3 represents approximately 20% of all bladder cancer patients. pTa high grade is often misclassified, and in reality only represents approximately 5% to 10% of all non–muscle invasive tumors (Sylvester et al, 2005).

21. **c. Maintenance therapy.** Maintenance therapy is the only proven scenario demonstrating reduction of tumor progression. Dose reduction studies appear to support similar benefit for lower doses, which are usually better tolerated if side effects are identified with full dosing. Interferon is incrementally beneficial in certain circumstances. Options d and e are both without scientific basis, but are commonly recommended.

CHAPTER REVIEW

1. Low-grade Ta bladder cancer recurs at a rate of 50% to 70% and progresses in approximately 5%.
2. High-grade T1 lesions recur in more than 80% of cases and progress in 30% to 50%.
3. The most important risk factor for progression is grade.
4. A nodular or sessile appearance suggests deeper invasion.
5. Lymphovascular invasion increases the risk of muscularis propria invasion.
6. Hydronephrosis is often but not always associated with muscularis propria invasion.
7. Papillary low-grade tumors can often be removed with the resectoscope loop without the use of electrocautery.
8. A separate biopsy of the base of the tumor should be obtained after initial resection.
9. Tumors about the ureteral orifice should be resected with pure cutting current.
10. Mitomycin C is the most effective adjuvant intravesical therapy and, when used, should be administered within 6 hours of tumor resection. Postoperative intravesical chemotherapy should be considered for most cases of new, apparently low grade non–muscle-invasive bladder cancer because it has been shown to reduce recurrence rates and improve outcomes for this disease. It does not have a benefit in high-grade disease.
11. All chemotherapy should be withheld when there is an extensive resection or when there is a concern that a perforation may have occurred.
12. BCG should never be administered immediately following a tumor resection.
13. The mechanism of action of BCG is by initially binding to fibronectin and then the production of multiple cytokines.
14. After induction therapy, patients receiving maintenance BCG have a statistically significant decrease in recurrence rate compared with those receiving induction therapy alone.
15. BCG may delay the progression of high-risk bladder cancer; however, ultimately there may be no difference in long-term survival.
16. Quinolones should not be administered with BCG.
17. BCG plus interferon-α has a potential role regardless of prior BCG experience.
18. Risk factors for progression in patients with non–muscularis propria-invasive bladder cancer include high-grade tumors invading deeply into the lamina propria, lymphovascular invasion, associated diffuse CIS, bladder neck invasion, and disease that is refractory to initial therapy.
19. Although upper tract disease occurs in 0.8% to 4% of patients, when it does occur, the mortality rate is 40% to 70%.
20. Urothelial cancers are subdivided into papillary urothelial neoplasia of low malignant potential (old grade 1), low grade (old grade 2), and high grade (old grade 3).
21. Random biopsies in patients with normal-appearing urothelium is controversial; however, most agree that such biopsies are not indicated in those with low-risk disease.
22. BCG-refractory patients are at high risk for progression and should be considered for cystectomy.
23. For patients who have failed BCG, a second course results in 30% to 50% response rate.
24. Tumor recurrence on the initial 3-month surveillance cystoscopy and number of tumors on initial cystoscopy are strong predictors of recurrent disease.
25. Cytology is positive in one third of patients with low-grade disease and two thirds of patients with high-grade disease.
26. Megadose vitamins have shown promise in reducing recurrences of urothelial tumors.
27. BTA stat, NMP-22, and UroVysion (FISH) provide increased sensitivity, particularly for low-grade tumors. High specificity is the strength of urinary cytology. If the cytology is positive, the patient usually has disease.
28. BGC is contraindicated in patients with liver disease (isoniazid cannot be given if they develop BCG sepsis), a personal history of TB, total incontinence (they cannot retain the BCG, so efficacy would be poor), and immunosuppression (BCG's mechanism of action is to stimulate an immune response). Other contraindications include disrupted urothelium, gross hematuria, or active or persistent symptomatic UTI.
29. Long-term outcomes for a patients with high-risk superficial bladder cancer treated with intravesical BCG therapy is derived primarily from the experience of patients at Memorial Sloan Kettering. In their series 50% of patients progressed, and one third died of cancer progression. Approximately one third developed disease in the prostatic fossa or upper tracts, and 27% survived with an intact bladder.
30. Untreated diffuse CIS is very high risk for progressing to muscle invasive disease. Even patients with a complete response to intravesical BCG will experience progression in 30% to 40% of cases on longitudinal follow-up.

94 Management of Invasive and Metastatic Bladder Cancer

Thomas J. Guzzo and David J. Vaughn

QUESTIONS

1. Important components in the clinical staging of patients with muscle-invasive bladder cancer include:
   a. transurethral resection with adequate detrusor muscle in the specimen.
   b. bimanual examination under anesthesia.
   c. cross-sectional imaging of the abdomen and pelvis.
   d. laboratory studies including liver function tests.
   e. all of the above.

2. The most important pathologic predictor of outcome following radical cystectomy for muscle-invasive bladder cancer is:
   a. pT2a versus pT2b substaging.
   b. soft tissue margin status.
   c. nodal metastasis.
   d. ureteral margin status.
   e. prostatic urethral involvement.

3. All of the following have been reported to provide prognostic information with regard to pelvic lymphadenectomy EXCEPT:
   a. absolute number of lymph nodes removed.
   b. laterality of a single positive lymph node.
   c. lymph node density.
   d. extranodal extension.
   e. anatomic extent of the lymph node dissection.

4. A 52-year-old male with cT2N0Mx urothelial carcinoma is undergoing a radical cystoprostatectomy and planned orthotopic urinary diversion. What intraoperative finding would be an absolute contraindication to orthotopic diversion?
   a. Positive ureteral frozen section for carcinoma in situ (CIS)
   b. Positive apical urethral frozen section for urothelial carcinoma
   c. Suspicious lymphadenopathy
   d. Greater than 1.5-liter blood loss during the cystectomy
   e. None of the above

5. All of the following are true statements regarding neoadjuvant chemotherapy for muscle-invasive bladder cancer EXCEPT:
   a. Meta-analysis of available randomized trial data have reported an absolute 5% survival advantage for patients who receive neoadjuvant chemotherapy.
   b. Neoadjuvant chemotherapy is likely underutilized in the U.S.-based studies that use administrative data sets.
   c. Patients who are pT0 on final pathology following neoadjuvant chemotherapy have excellent oncologic outcomes.
   d. In patients in whom a cisplatin-based regimen is contraindicated, carboplatin-based chemotherapy provides similar oncologic efficacy.
   e. All of the above.

6. A 65-year-old woman with normal renal function undergoes upfront radical cystectomy, extended pelvic lymphadenectomy, and ileal conduit urinary diversion for bacille Calmette-Guérin-refractory bladder CIS. Final pathology is notable for T2N1M0 disease. The next step in management should be:
   a. enrollment in a clinical vaccine trial.
   b. adjuvant cisplatin-based chemotherapy.
   c. adjuvant pelvic external beam radiation therapy.
   d. combination chemotherapy/external beam radiation therapy.
   e. adjuvant carboplatin-based chemotherapy.

7. All of the following are contraindications to trimodal bladder preservation EXCEPT:
   a. a solitary, completely resected tumor.
   b. hydronephrosis.
   c. diffuse bladder CIS.
   d. T3 disease on cross-sectional imaging.
   e. multifocal tumors.

8. Predictors of a poor response to chemotherapy in patients with locally advanced or metastatic bladder cancer include:
   a. Karnofsky performance status below 80%.
   b. visceral metastasis.
   c. both a and b.
   d. neither a nor b.

9. Gemcitabine/cisplatin systemic therapy is often used in preference to MVAC (methotrexate, vinblastine, doxorubicin, and cisplatin) for patients with locally advanced and metastatic bladder cancer because of:
   a. studies demonstrating improved progression-free survival.
   b. studies demonstrating improved overall survival.
   c. better toxicity profile.
   d. oral administration compared with intravenous (IV) administration.
   e. cost.

10. An orthotopic neobladder in a woman undergoing anterior pelvic exenteration for muscle invasive bladder cancer is contraindicated in the setting of:
    a. age older than 75 years.
    b. nodal metastasis.
    c. recurrent urinary tract infection.
    d. a serum creatinine of 1.5.
    e. tumor invading the anterior vaginal wall.

ANSWERS

1. **e. All of the above.** Important components of staging patients with muscle-invasive bladder cancer include adequate transurethral resection, bimanual examination under anesthesia to assess local extent of disease, cross-sectional imaging, and serum laboratory values.

2. **c. Nodal metastasis.** Approximately 25% of patients with clinical T2 disease will have lymph node metastasis at the time of radical cystectomy. Lymph node status following surgery is a powerful predictor of long-term recurrence-free and overall

survival. Of patients with lymph node involvement, 70% to 80% will ultimately experience a recurrence following radical cystectomy.

3. **b. Laterality of a single positive lymph node.** Although some surgical series have demonstrated improved survival in patients with one positive lymph node compared with those with multiple positive nodes, the laterality of a single positive lymph node has no prognostic significance.

4. **b. Positive apical urethral frozen section for urothelial carcinoma.** The only contraindication to performing an orthotopic neobladder is a positive apical urethral margin and inability to achieve a negative margin of the retained urethra.

5. **d. In patients in whom a cisplatin-based regimen is contraindicated, carboplatin-based chemotherapy provides similar oncologic efficacy.** Although carboplatin is a reasonable choice for patients in whom cisplatin is contraindicated, it should not be considered a first-line therapy. Patients who cannot undergo neoadjuvant cisplatin-based chemotherapy should be considered for immediate cystectomy.

6. **b. Adjuvant cisplatin-based chemotherapy.** Adjuvant cisplatin-based combination chemotherapy should be considered. Randomized trials have thus far not been definitive in overall survival results on this subject. A meta-analysis suggests a 9% absolute benefit in overall survival, but the trials, often closed early or because of poor accrual, represent small numbers of patients, and not all of the patients in adjuvant chemotherapy trials are represented.

7. **a. A solitary, completely resected tumor.** Patients with solitary, completely resected tumors are ideal candidates for bladder preservation.

8. **c. Both a and b.** The Memorial Sloan Kettering Cancer Center group has published their data on 203 patients with unresectable or metastatic bladder cancer treated with MVAC (Bajorin et al, 1999). They found a Karnofsky performance status below 80% and visceral (lung, liver, bone) metastasis to be independent predictors of poor outcome. Median survival times for patients who had zero, one, or two risk factors were 33, 13.4, and 9.3 months, respectively.

9. **c. Better toxicity profile.** The toxicity of MVAC led to trials of alternative, less toxic chemotherapy regimens. Most notably, a phase III randomized trial comparing gemcitabine/cisplatin with MVAC was conducted in 405 patients (von der Maase et al, 2000, 2005).* There was no difference in response rates (49% vs. 46%), time to progression (7.4 vs. 7.4 months), and overall survival rates (13.8 vs. 14.8 months) between the two study arms. The updated study analysis confirmed equivalence of the two regimens (hazard ratio, 1.09, 95% confidence interval, 0.88-1.34; $P = .66$). The gemcitabine/cisplatin regimen was better tolerated, with only 37% of patients in that arm requiring dose modifications compared with 63% in the MVAC arm. Patients in the gemcitabine/cisplatin arm also experienced less grade 3/4 neutropenia, neutropenic fever, neutropenic sepsis, and mucositis. The toxicity-related death rate was also lower in the gemcitabine/cisplatin group (1% vs. 3%). Because of its equivalent efficacy and better tolerability, gemcitabine/cisplatin is the most widely used chemotherapeutic regimen for muscle-invasive and metastatic bladder cancer.

10. **e. Tumor invading the anterior vaginal wall.** The distal two thirds of the female urethra may serve as an adequate sphincter mechanism provided the risk of cancer in the retained urethra is low. Anterior vaginal wall involvement by a posterior-based bladder tumor or bladder neck or urethra involvement is a contraindication to urethra sparing and orthotopic bladder replacement because one cannot get an adequate distal vaginal margin and urethra margin (Stein et al, 1998). Age is not a contraindication as long as there is good pelvic support minimizing the risk of stress incontinence and the patient is capable of intermittent catheterization should the need arise. Nodal metastasis is associated with a 15% local recurrence rate with only a modest risk of invasion of the neobladder, and a thorough node dissection minimizes this risk (Lerner, 2009). Bilateral hydronephrosis, although indicating a deeply invasive cancer, is not a de facto contraindication (Stimson et al, 2010).

CHAPTER REVIEW

1. Among those with muscularis propria–invasive bladder cancer, 80% are seen with the disease at initial presentation.

2. Deaths due to bladder cancer invariably occur as a result of distant metastases present at the time of local regional therapy and usually occur within the first 2 years following treatment. Therefore muscularis propria–invasive bladder cancer should be considered a systemic disease.

3. The micropapillary variant is an aggressive disease and does not respond particularly well to chemotherapy.

4. T1 grade 3 bladder tumors should routinely be re-resected because understaging is not an uncommon event.

5. Fat can be observed in the bladder wall and should not be confused with perivesical fat.

6. Lymphatic and vascular invasion are risk factors for metastases.

7. Following chemotherapy, metastases may occur in unusual locations, such as the central nervous system.

8. The incidence of pelvic node metastases is directly related to the depth of invasion and the presence of lymphovascular invasion.

9. As many as 50% of patients with muscularis propria–invasive bladder cancer succumb to their disease.

10. Of the randomized trials evaluating neoadjuvant therapy, most have not shown a definite survival advantage; however, a meta-analysis has shown a small survival advantage for those receiving neoadjuvant chemotherapy. The evidence for adjuvant chemotherapy conferring a survival advantage is less convincing.

11. Appropriate candidates for bladder preservation (transurethral tumor resection, chemotherapy, and radiation therapy thereby preserving the bladder) are those who have a solitary T2 lesion of small diameter with no associated hydronephrosis and a visibly complete resection. The patient should have normal renal function.

12. As many as 15% of patients with muscularis propria invasive tumors have no residual disease following transurethral tumor resection.

13. Factors that affect outcome include stage, performance, status, lymphovascular invasion, age, gender, and histology.

---

*Sources referenced can be found in *Campbell-Walsh Urology, 11th Edition,* on the Expert Consult website.

14. Predictors of a poor prognosis include poor performance status and the presence of visceral metastases.

15. Treatment of neuroendocrine bladder tumors includes neoadjuvant chemotherapy and surgical resection; neuroendocrine tumors may be associated with a paraneoplastic syndrome (hypercortisolism and hypercalcemia).

16. There is a significant survival benefit to those who are rendered P0 at the time of radical cystectomy.

17. The highest concentration of prostatic ducts are located from the mid prostate to the veru at the 5 and 7 o'clock positions and are the locations where CIS of the prostatic urethra is most likely to be found (biopsy should be performed in this location).

18. In women, bladder neck biopsies are a good surrogate for urethral biopsies when an orthotopic bladder is being considered.

19. Skip metastases in nodal disease for bladder cancer is a rare event—this is not true of prostate cancer.

20. Ureteral margin status is a predictor of upper-tract recurrence.

21. Prostatic stromal invasion carries a high risk of recurrent disease.

22. Patients who are not good candidates for cisplatin chemotherapy are those with a poor performance status, a creatinine clearance less than 60 mL/min, hearing loss, peripheral neuropathy, and heart failure.

23. Although carboplatin is a reasonable choice for patients in whom cisplatin is contraindicated, it should not be considered a first-line therapy.

95 Transurethral and Open Surgery for Bladder Cancer

Neema Navai and Colin P.N. Dinney

QUESTIONS

1. The administration of neoadjuvant chemotherapy has improved survival in muscle-invasive bladder cancer from:
   a. 16 to 42 months.
   b. 23 to 54 months.
   c. 37 to 51 months.
   d. 46 to 77 months.
   e. 75 to 85 months.

2. Upper-tract imaging for urothelial carcinoma may include all of the following EXCEPT:
   a. renal ultrasound.
   b. computed tomography (CT) abdomen and pelvis.
   c. whole-body positron emission tomography (PET)/CT.
   d. magnetic resonance imaging (MRI) abdomen and pelvis.
   e. retrograde pyelogram.

3. MRI-based contrast agents are absolutely contraindicated at which glomerular filtration rate (GFR) level?
   a. <15 mL/min
   b. <20 mL/min
   c. <30 mL/min
   d. <35 mL/min
   e. <60 mL/min

4. The improvement in 5-year survival and median survival when more than 10 lymph nodes are removed is approximately:
   a. 15%, 24 months.
   b. 10%, 36 months.
   c. 20%, 24 months.
   d. 5%, 15 months.
   e. 15%, 15 months.

5. Which of the following statements is TRUE?
   a. Urethral recurrence following radical cystectomy is approximately 8% at 5 years.
   b. Even patients with a negative intraoperative urethral frozen section are at high risk for recurrence.
   c. The negative predictive value of urethral frozen section is poor.
   d. Orthotopic neobladder is protective against urethral recurrence and therefore a positive urethral margin is not a contraindication.
   e. Orthotopic neobladder can only be performed after nerve-sparing radical cystectomy.

6. Which of the following statements is FALSE regarding nerve-sparing radical cystectomy?
   a. A technique analogous to radical prostatectomy is used.
   b. Sexual function is similar for capsular-sparing and conventional nerve-sparing techniques.
   c. Age is a strong predictor of the return of erectile function.
   d. Nerve sparing does not increase local recurrence rates.
   e. Ejaculatory function can be maintained with subtotal prostate resection.

7. Anterior pelvic exenteration includes removal of the following EXCEPT:
   a. uterus.
   b. cervix.
   c. ovaries.
   d. urethra.
   e. vaginal introitus.

8. Partial cystectomy is appropriate in which of the following settings?
   a. 4-cm T2 lesion in the trigone
   b. 1-cm T2 lesion in the dome
   c. 3-cm T2 lesion in the dome with carcinoma in situ (CIS) in one location
   d. 1-cm T2 lesion with pelvic lymphadenopathy on imaging
   e. Carcinoma in situ (CIS) in two locations

9. Enhanced recovery includes all of the following EXCEPT:
   a. alvimopan.
   b. neostigmine.
   c. pharmacologic thromboembolism prophylaxis.
   d. nasogastric suction.
   e. early enteral feeding.

10. Thromboembolism prophylaxis is needed:
    a. immediately before incision.
    b. postprocedure for 1 day.
    c. postprocedure for 1 week.
    d. postprocedure for 1 month.
    e. both a and d.

ANSWERS

1. **d. 46 to 77 months.** In a seminal randomized trial, Grossman and colleagues compared the treatment of muscle-invasive bladder cancer with radical cystectomy alone or surgery followed by three cycles of MVAC chemotherapy (methotrexate, vinblastine, doxorubicin, and cisplatin). They demonstrated a significant improvement in survival (46 vs. 77 months) in the neoadjuvant chemotherapy arm. This study serves as the basis for current treatment paradigms in muscle-invasive bladder cancer (Grossman et al, 2003).*

2. **c. Whole-body positron emission tomography (PET)/CT.** Conventional staging evaluation for upper-tract urothelial carcinoma should include evaluation of both the kidney parenchyma and the urothelial lumen. Although PET/CT can be useful for a staging evaluation, the resolution of imaging within the urinary tract is limited by the excretion of contrast material and lack of granular resolution.

*Sources referenced can be found in *Campbell-Walsh Urology, 11th Edition,* on the Expert Consult website.

3. **c. <30 mL/min.** Although gadolinium contrast should be administered with caution in patients whose GFR is between 30 and 60 mL/min, it is absolutely contraindicated in those with GFR < 30 mL/min. This is due to the risk of nephrogenic systemic sclerosis.

4. **e. 15%, 15 months.** In a study of surgical factors that influence outcomes in bladder cancer treatment, Herr and colleagues found that a lymph node dissection inclusive of more than 10 nodes was associated with improvement in survival of 15 months (Herr et al, 2004).

5. **a. Urethral recurrence following radical cystectomy is approximately 8% at 5 years.** Factors that influence the risk of recurrence after radical cystectomy include orthotopic substitution with a positive urethral margin on frozen section analysis. This should be considered a contraindication for such a diversion. In addition, the negative predictive value is useful in the evaluation of urethral margins, and the risk of recurrence is only 8% at 5 years (Freeman et al, 1996).

6. **b. Sexual function is similar for capsular-sparing and conventional nerve-sparing techniques.** The rate of natural potency after radical cystectomy with conventional nerve sparing is lower than that of analogous prostatectomy series. Studies examining sexual function after subtotal resection (e.g., prostate sparing) have demonstrated improved results (Spitz et al, 1999); however, caution is advised because of the high risk of concurrent occult prostate cancer and potential for increased local recurrence.

7. **e. Vaginal introitus.** The vaginal introitus should be maintained for routine anterior exenteration. Satisfactory vaginal capacity can be maintained with both non–vaginal-sparing and vaginal-sparing approaches. In neither instance should a colpocleisis be performed as a matter of routine.

8. **b. 1-cm T2 lesion in the dome.** In the setting of muscle-invasive bladder cancer, partial cystectomy can be considered in very select patients. In those with small lesions and a lack of concurrent CIS, the results of partial cystectomy approach those of radical cystectomy (Kassouf et al, 2006; Capitanio et al, 2009).

9. **d. Nasogastric suction.** Postoperative nasogastric suction should be considered in patients with compromised airway protection; however, this has not been demonstrated to enhance recovery and need not be incorporated to facilitate return of bowel function postoperatively. Early enteral feeding, neostigmine, and alvimopan have all demonstrated efficacy in improving return of bowel function following abdominal surgery.

10. **e. Both a and d.** In addition to the administration of prophylaxis prior to incision, a reduction in postoperative thromboembolic events from 4.6 to 0.8% was observed in patients treated for 4 weeks following abdominal or pelvic surgery (Kakkar et al, 2010).

CHAPTER REVIEW

1. Before endoscopic treatment of bladder cancer, the patient should have upper-tract imaging.
2. Initial transurethral resection of a bladder tumor should routinely be performed to include muscle. There should be a 2-cm visibly negative margin on the surface.
3. Immediately following transurethral resection of bladder tumors, intravesical installation of epirubicin or mitomycin C modestly reduces recurrences but has little effect on progression.
4. Bacille Calmette-Guérin should never be instilled immediately following bladder tumor resection.
5. Before a cystectomy, the site of the abdominal stoma should be marked by an enterostomal therapist with the patient awake so that the proper location may be ascertained.
6. If prostate- or prostate capsule-sparing techniques are to be used in orthotopic bladder construction, preoperative evaluation to rule out occult cancer—either transitional cell or prostate adenocarcinoma—should be performed.
7. A radical cystectomy in the female includes complete removal of the urethra including the meatus.
8. Patients amenable to partial cystectomy should have a solitary lesion without associated CIS in which a 2-cm margin may be obtained, which is far enough away from the ureteral orifices and bladder neck that closure can be accomplished without compromising these structures.
9. Sixty-four percent of patients undergoing radical cystectomy have at least one perioperative complication in the first 3 months postoperative; 13% experience high-grade complications. The majority of complications are gastrointestinal.
10. The boundaries of a standard lymph node dissection are the genitofemoral nerve laterally, internal iliac artery medially, Cooper ligament caudally, and crossing of the ureter at the common iliac artery cranially.
11. The 90-day mortality rate for radical cystectomy is approximately 3%.
12. Routine administration of antibiotic prophylaxis in patients undergoing a transurethral resection of a bladder tumor is recommended and should be given 30 to 60 minutes before the procedure.
13. Transurethral resection of tumors on the lateral wall may initiate the obturator reflex and result in bladder perforation. This may be minimized by minimally distending the bladder, using bipolar cautery, and using general anesthesia with muscle paralysis.
14. Routine stenting of a resected ureteral orifice with cutting current is not necessary.
15. In preparation for a cystectomy and urinary diversion, mechanical and antibiotic bowel prep is controversial. The data to justify omitting this preparation come, for the most part, from the general surgical literature in which the bowel is not opened in the peritoneal cavity as it is in urology, particularly in continent diversions. Administration of intravenous antibiotic prophylaxis 30 to 60 minutes before the incision is recommended.
16. In women, the vagina should be prepped into the surgical field.
17. Care should be taken when using sealing instruments near the rectum because that organ may be injured by radiating heat.
18. Early enteral feeding, neostigmine, and alvimopan have all demonstrated efficacy in improving return of bowel function following abdominal surgery.

96 Robotic and Laparoscopic Bladder Surgery

Lee Richstone and Douglas S. Scherr

QUESTIONS

1. Laparoscopic ureteral reimplantation can be performed:
   a. with a cross-trigonal approach.
   b. with a Boari flap or bladder advancement flap.
   c. with a psoas hitch.
   d. via a traditional laparoscopic or robotic approach.
   e. all of the above.

2. All of the following are essential surgical aspects of the Boari flap or bladder advancement flap EXCEPT:
   a. an adequate-sized bladder must be present (200 to 300 mL).
   b. the contralateral vesical pedicle may be transected if necessary.
   c. the bladder flap should be slightly shorter than anticipated because bladder tissue can be easily stretched.
   d. a tension-free anastomosis is important.
   e. typically, a refluxing ureteral anastomosis is created.

3. Principles of open, laparoscopic, or robotic vesicovaginal fistula (VVF) repair include all of the following EXCEPT:
   a. good exposure of the fistulous tract.
   b. wide excision of the fibrous and scar tissue.
   c. tension-free repair of the vagina and bladder.
   d. interposition of a flap of peritoneum or omentum.
   e. adequate drainage.

4. Contraindications for laparoscopic enterocystoplasty include all of the following EXCEPT:
   a. diverticulosis.
   b. inflammatory bowel disease.
   c. renal failure.
   d. noncompliance.
   e. ulcerative colitis.

5. Which of the following statements is NOT correct regarding laparoscopic enterocystoplasty?
   a. Subtotal cystectomy is not always mandatory.
   b. Mesenteric pedicle of the selected bowel segment is wide and broad-based.
   c. Mesenteric window is closed.
   d. Reestablishment of bowel continuity is a critical step of the operation and may be performed extracorporeally for added security, if necessary.
   e. Bowel-to-bladder anastomosis is optimally performed with interrupted serosa-to-serosa sutures.

6. Partial cystectomy can be performed in all of the following circumstances EXCEPT:
   a. tumor at the bladder dome.
   b. tumor in the bladder diverticulum.
   c. solitary invasive bladder tumor located at a distance from the ureteric orifices.
   d. history of multiple tumors or carcinoma in situ (CIS).
   e. good bladder capacity.

7. Which of the following statements is TRUE regarding partial cystectomy?
   a. Thirty percent to 40% of patients with bladder cancer are candidates for a partial cystectomy.
   b. Five-year survival rates range from 80% to 90%.
   c. Laparoscopic partial cystectomy is now an established procedure.
   d. All of the above.
   e. None of the above.

8. Which of the following is a contraindication for laparoscopic radical cystectomy today?
   a. Multiple bladder tumors
   b. Nonbulky, invasive bladder cancer
   c. T4 disease
   d. Moderate obesity
   e. Open pelvic surgery

9. As regards radical cystectomy, all of the following have been performed laparoscopically EXCEPT:
   a. extended pelvic lymph node dissection.
   b. uterus- and vagina-sparing radical cystectomy.
   c. anterior pelvic exenteration in the female.
   d. orthotopic neobladder.
   e. Indiana pouch, constructed intracorporeally.

10. Anatomic boundaries of extended pelvic lymph node dissection include all of the following EXCEPT:
    a. external iliac artery (lateral).
    b. obturator nerve (posterior).
    c. aortic bifurcation area (proximal).
    d. internal inguinal ring (distal).
    e. bladder (medial).

11. Future directions for laparoscopic/robotic radical cystectomy are likely to include which of the following?
    a. Careful, prospective, long-term evaluation of oncologic and functional outcomes
    b. Evaluation of the potential advantages of intracorporeal bowel work
    c. Elimination of bowel through use of novel bladder substitutes
    d. International collaboration
    e. All of the above

ANSWERS

1. **e. All of the above.** All of the included answers are correct regarding laparoscopic ureteral reimplantation. Minimally invasive ureteral reimplant can be performed in a refluxing or nonrefluxing fashion, and with a cross-trigonal or tunneled approach if so desired. In cases with larger ureteral loss, a Boari flap or bladder advancement flap can be utilized, or a psoas hitch can be performed replicating open techniques. Finally, both a laparoscopic

and robotic approach to ureteral reimplantation has been described.

2. **c. The bladder flap should be slightly shorter than anticipated because bladder tissue can be easily stretched.** A tension-free anastomosis of the anterolateral bladder flap based on the ipsilateral vesical pedicle is critical. The bladder flap should be somewhat longer and wider than anticipated because the non-distended bladder shrinks in size, thus placing tension on the anastomosis. Ideally, a flap length-to-breadth ratio of 3:1 ensures good vascularity of its apex.

3. **b. Wide excision of the fibrous and scar tissue.** Wide circumferential excision of the fistula and associated scar tissue is not necessary and may not even be feasible. Only the fibrotic VVF tract and its edges need to be excised. Adequate mobilization of the anterior vaginal wall and posterior bladder wall is performed to achieve a tension-free repair. Care is taken not to compromise the ureteral orifices. An interposition graft of omentum is anchored between the vagina and the bladder with a stitch.

4. **a. Diverticulosis.** The presence of bowel pathology such as diverticulitis or ulcerative colitis requires the use of alternative, nondiseased bowel segments. Similar to open surgery, laparoscopic enterocystoplasty should not be performed in the presence of advanced renal or liver failure, inflammatory bowel disease, or short gut syndrome, or in a patient who is unable to perform or noncompliant in performing intermittent catheterization reliably. Diverticulosis is not a contraindication for performing enterocystoplasty.

5. **e. Bowel-to-bladder anastomosis is optimally performed with interrupted serosa-to-serosa sutures.** The technical principles of enterocystoplasty are identical between open surgical and laparoscopic techniques. Generous mobilization of the bladder allows creation of an adequate anteroposterior cystotomy. Subtotal cystectomy is necessary only in patients with severely symptomatic interstitial cystitis. An optimal segment of bowel based on a broad, well-vascularized mesenteric pedicle is selected that will reach the pelvis without tension. The bowel segment is isolated and bowel continuity reestablished by either intracorporeal or extracorporeal techniques, and the mesenteric window is closed. The isolated bowel segment is detubularized, and a bowel plate is created appropriately. A tension-free, watertight, full-thickness, circumferential, running anastomosis of the bowel segment to the bladder is created. Adequate urinary drainage is established.

6. **d. History of multiple tumors or carcinoma in situ (CIS).** Contraindications to partial cystectomy include multiple bladder tumors, tumors involving the bladder neck or posterior urethra or trigone, and concomitant CIS. History or current evidence of multifocal transitional cell carcinoma (TCC) with or without CIS is a contraindication for partial cystectomy. The ideal patient for partial cystectomy is one who has a solitary, organ-confined invasive bladder tumor located at the dome of a good-capacity bladder, without any concomitant multifocality or CIS.

7. **e. None of the above.** In large series of patients with bladder cancer, fewer than 10% of the patients are candidates for a partial cystectomy. In the properly selected patient, 5-year survival rate ranges from 50% to 70%. Laparoscopic partial cystectomy has only been performed in a few selected cases and is currently a controversial procedure.

8. **c. T4 disease.** Laparoscopic radical cystectomy is an emerging procedure performed at centers of laparoscopic expertise. At this writing, laparoscopic radical cystectomy should be offered to nonobese patients with nonbulky, organ-confined bladder cancer without pelvic lymphadenopathy on preoperative computed tomography (CT). Various conditions such as morbid obesity, prior radiotherapy, or pelvic surgery are relative contraindications because of the increase in laparoscopic technical complexity. Locally advanced T4 disease should not be approached laparoscopically.

9. **e. Indiana pouch, constructed intracorporeally.** Since the initial report of laparoscopic cystectomy in 1992 by Parra and colleagues, more than 300 laparoscopic radical cystectomies have been performed worldwide. In the female, laparoscopic anterior pelvic exenteration and uterus, fallopian tube, vagina-sparing radical cystectomy have been performed. In the male, conventional radical cystectomy and prostate-sparing radical cystectomy have been performed. Bilateral extended pelvic lymph node dissection with mean nodal yields of 21 lymph nodes has been reported. With regard to urinary drainage, ileal conduit, Mainz pouch, Indiana pouch (extracorporeally constructed), and orthotopic neobladder have all been performed laparoscopically. However, long-term follow-up outcomes are still lacking.

10. **a. External iliac artery (lateral).** Laterally, the dissection is extended up to the genitofemoral nerve. At the conclusion of an extended bilateral pelvic lymph node dissection, the external and internal iliac artery and vein, the common iliac artery, the obturator nerve, the pelvic side wall, and the perivesical area should be bilaterally devoid of lymphatic fatty tissue.

11. **e. All of the above.** Laparoscopic radical cystectomy is an evolving treatment modality with increasing experience being reported from multiple centers worldwide. With earlier detection of bladder cancer, careful application of laparoscopic techniques, and meticulous long-term follow-up, laparoscopic radical cystectomy is likely to emerge as a viable treatment option for the selected patient with bladder cancer.

CHAPTER REVIEW

1. Bladder surgery and the associated urinary diversion are associated with some of the highest rates of complications in urologic surgery.

2. Bladder diverticulectomy may be indicated in those of considerable size in which there is incomplete emptying, chronic or repeated urinary tract infection, bladder calculi, pain, or malignancy.

3. Any outlet obstruction must be addressed before the time of diverticulectomy.

4. In constructing a Boari flap, it is critical to ensure that the base of the flap is wide enough to provide for adequate vascularity. The base should be at least twice as wide at the apex as it is long to prevent contracture. Some recommend a 3:1 ratio.

5. Any patient considered for augmentation cystoplasty should be capable of self-intermittent catheterization.

6. In a partial cystectomy, a 2-cm margin should be outlined endoscopically with the electrocautery before opening the bladder because a decompressed bladder may distort the adequacy of the resection margin.

97 Use of Intestinal Segments in Urinary Diversion

Douglas M. Dahl

QUESTIONS

1. When a portion of stomach is to be used for augmentation, it should:
   a. always be based on the right gastroepiploic artery.
   b. include only the antrum.
   c. never extend to the pylorus.
   d. include a significant portion of the lesser curve.
   e. be mobilized with the omentum.

2. The ileum differs from the jejunum in that:
   a. it has a larger diameter.
   b. the mesentery is thinner.
   c. it has multiple arcades.
   d. the vessels in the mesentery are larger.
   e. the mesentery is longer.

3. When stomach is used for urinary diversion, the electrolyte abnormality that may occur is most commonly what type of metabolic alkalosis?
   a. Hyperchloremic
   b. Hypochloremic
   c. Hyperkalemic
   d. Hypernatremic
   e. Hypocalcemic

4. Postoperative bowel obstruction is most common when which of the following segments is used for diversion?
   a. Right colon
   b. Stomach
   c. Sigmoid
   d. Ileum
   e. Transverse colon

5. Mechanical bowel preparation results in a reduction in:
   a. bacterial counts per gram of enteric contents.
   b. bacterial count in the jejunum.
   c. total number of bacteria in the bowel.
   d. bacterial counts in the stomach.
   e. bacterial counts in the ileum.

6. Systemic antibiotics in elective surgery should be given:
   a. before the patient is anesthetized.
   b. before the skin incision is made.
   c. intraoperatively before closure commences.
   d. at any time in the perioperative period.
   e. postoperatively for 3 to 5 days.

7. The most common cause of a lethal bowel complication is:
   a. use of previously irradiated bowel.
   b. lack of mechanical bowel prep.
   c. lack of antibiotic bowel prep.
   d. placement of a drain adjacent to the anastomosis.
   e. failure to give preoperative antibiotics.

8. When stapled anastomoses are compared with sutured anastomoses, there is/are:
   a. fewer leaks.
   b. less compatibility with urine.
   c. reduced overall operative time.
   d. lesser incidence of bowel obstruction.
   e. earlier return of bowel function.

9. The use of a nasogastric tube in the postoperative period:
   a. hastens the return of intestinal motility.
   b. reduces the incidence of bowel leak.
   c. reduces postoperative vomiting.
   d. increases the risk of aspiration.
   e. reduces the incidence of anastomotic leak.

10. The abdominal stoma for a conduit should be:
    a. flush with the skin.
    b. placed through the belly of the rectus muscle.
    c. made as a loop to reduce parastomal hernia.
    d. made with the colon for the lowest complication rate.
    e. placed in the right lower quadrant.

11. The loop end ileostomy is best used in:
    a. the obese patient.
    b. the thin patient.
    c. when a stoma is revised.
    d. in female patients.
    e. in spinal cord injury patients.

12. Ureteral strictures occurring after an ileal conduit not associated with the ureteral intestinal anastomosis most frequently occur:
    a. at the ureteropelvic junction.
    b. in the right ureter several centimeters proximal to the ureteral intestinal anastomosis.
    c. on the left side where the ureter crosses the aorta.
    d. in the mid-ureter.
    e. in either ureter within several centimeters proximal to the anastomosis.

13. Renal deterioration after a conduit diversion with normal kidneys occurs in what percent of renal units?
    a. 20%
    b. 40%
    c. 50%
    d. 70%
    e. 80%

14. The most common cause of death in patients with ureterosig-moidostomies during the long term is:
    a. cancer.
    b. renal failure.
    c. acid base abnormalities.
    d. the primary disease.
    e. ammonium intoxication.

15. The minimal glomerular filtration rate (GFR) in mL/min necessary for a continent diversion is:
    a. 70.
    b. 60.
    c. 35.
    d. 25.
    e. 20.

16. The urinary diversion with the fewest intraoperative and immediate postoperative complications is:
    a. ileal conduit.
    b. colon conduit.
    c. Koch pouch.
    d. Indiana pouch.
    e. neobladder.

17. The jejunal conduit syndrome is manifested by:
    a. hyperchloremic metabolic acidosis.
    b. hypochloremic metabolic alkalosis.
    c. hyperkalemic, hyponatremic metabolic acidosis.
    d. hypokalemic, hyponatremic metabolic alkalosis.
    e. hyperkalemic metabolic alkalosis.

18. The primary advantage of a transverse colon conduit is:
    a. its ease of construction.
    b. the ability to perform a nonrefluxing anastomosis.
    c. less likely to be injured by radiation.
    d. reduced electrolyte problems.
    e. equidistant from each kidney, allowing for short ureteral length on both sides.

19. Total body potassium depletion is most common in:
    a. ureterosigmoidostomy.
    b. ileal conduit.
    c. colon conduit.
    d. sigmoid conduit.
    e. gastrocystoplasty.

20. In urinary intestinal diversion, serum creatinine may not be an accurate reflection of renal function because of:
    a. interfering substances.
    b. tubule secretion.
    c. tubule reabsorption.
    d. bowel reabsorption.
    e. decreased renal elimination.

21. Patients with urinary diversions who have a hyperchloremic metabolic acidosis with time:
    a. retain the ability to maintain the acidosis.
    b. lose the ability for electrolyte transport in the intestinal segments.

    c. compensate for the metabolic acidosis, thus eliminating risk.
    d. intermittently absorb ammonia when infection is present.
    e. tend to retain potassium.

22. Bone density abnormalities:
    a. are unlikely to occur with ileum.
    b. are most likely to occur with colon.
    c. are more common in patients with persistent hyperchloremic metabolic acidosis.
    d. are common in patients with total body potassium depletion.
    e. are unlikely to occur in patients with conduits.

23. Urinary intestinal diversion in children:
    a. increases the need for vitamin D.
    b. increases the need for calcium.
    c. limits linear growth.
    d. decreases epiphyseal growth.
    e. results in premature epiphyseal closure.

24. Cancer occurring in urinary intestinal diversion is most likely to occur in:
    a. augmentations.
    b. colon conduits.
    c. ileal conduits.
    d. ureterosigmoidostomies.
    e. sigmoid conduits.

25. Reconfiguring the bowel during the long term results in:
    a. decreased motor activity.
    b. increased volume.
    c. decreased metabolic complications.
    d. decreased absorption of solutes.
    e. increased absorption of solutes.

26. The syndrome of severe metabolic alkalosis in patients who have had a gastrocystoplasty is most likely to occur in patients who have:
    a. decreased aldosterone levels.
    b. jejunum interposed in the urinary tract.
    c. total body potassium depletion.
    d. elevated gastrin levels.
    e. decreased renin levels.

Imaging

1. See Figure 97-1. A 72-year-old man who had a cystectomy and ileal conduit urinary diversion for high-grade, T3 transitional cell carcinoma undergoes a loopogram (A) and a contrast-enhanced computed tomography (CT) scan (B). The most likely diagnosis is:
    a. normal studies.
    b. stricture at the left uretero-ileal anastomosis.
    c. recurrent urothelial tumor.
    d. technically poor-quality loopogram.
    e. abnormal reflux into the right ureter and collecting system.

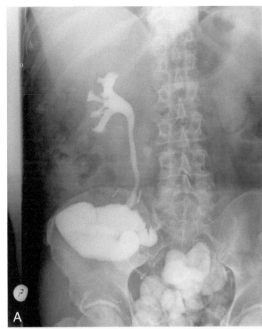

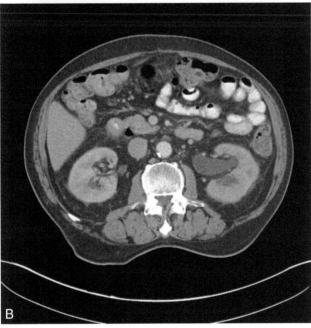

Figure 97-1.

ANSWERS

1. **c. Never extend to the pylorus.** When a wedge of fundus is used, it should not include a significant portion of the antrum and should never extend to the pylorus or all the way to the lesser curve of the stomach.

2. **c. It has multiple arcades.** The ileum, more distal in location, has a smaller diameter. It has multiple arterial arcades, and the vessels in the arcades are smaller than those in the jejunum.

3. **b. Hypochloremic.** Complications specific to the use of stomach include the hematuria-dysuria syndrome and uncontrollable metabolic alkalosis in some patients. When stomach is used, a hypochloremic, hypokalemic metabolic alkalosis may ensue.

4. **d. Ileum.** The incidence of postoperative bowel obstruction is 4% to 10%. Colon, stomach, and sigmoid obstruction result in a 4% incidence, less than that occurring with ileum.

5. **c. Total number of bacteria in the bowel.** The mechanical preparation reduces the amount of feces, whereas the antibiotic preparation reduces the bacterial count. A mechanical bowel preparation reduces the total number of bacteria but not their concentration.

6. **a. Before the patient is anesthetized.** Systemic antibiotics must be given before the operative event if they are to be effective.

7. **a. Use of previously irradiated bowel.** In one study of urinary intestinal diversion, 75% of the lethal complications that occurred in the postoperative period were related to the bowel. Eighty percent of these patients had received radiation before the intestinal surgery.

8. **b. Less compatibility with urine.** In general, anastomoses using reabsorbable sutures or reabsorbable staples are preferable for intestinal segments that are exposed to urine.

9. **c. Reduces postoperative vomiting.** In several studies there was no significant difference in major intestinal complications between those who had postoperative nasogastric tubes and those who did not; however, those who did not have gastric decompression showed a much greater incidence of abdominal distention, nausea, and vomiting.

10. **b. Placed through the belly of the rectus muscle.** All stomas should be placed through the belly of the rectus muscle and be located at the peak of the infraumbilical fat roll.

11. **a. The obese patient.** The loop end ileostomy is usually easier to perform than the ileal end stoma in the patient who is obese.

12. **c. On the left side where the ureter crosses the aorta.** Of importance is that ureteral strictures also occur away from the uretero-intestinal anastomosis. This stricture is most common in the left ureter and is usually found as the ureter crosses over the aorta beneath the inferior mesenteric artery.

13. **a. 20%.** Patients who are studied during the long term show a significant degree of renal deterioration. Indeed, 20% of renal units have shown significant anatomic deterioration.

14. **b. Renal failure.** The most common cause of death in patients who have had a ureterosigmoidostomy for more than 15 years is acquired renal disease (i.e., sepsis or renal failure).

15. **b. 60.** If the patient is able to achieve a urine pH of 5.8 or less, can establish a urine osmolality of 600 mOsm/kg or greater in response to water deprivation, has a GFR that exceeds 60 mL/min, and has minimal protein in the urine, he or she may be considered for a retentive diversion.

16. **a. Ileal conduit.** It is the simplest type of conduit diversion to perform and is associated with the fewest intraoperative and immediate postoperative complications.

17. **c. Hyperkalemic, hyponatremic metabolic acidosis.** The early and long-term complications are similar to those listed for ileal conduit except that the electrolyte abnormality that occurs is hyperkalemic, hyponatremic metabolic acidosis instead of the hyperchloremic metabolic acidosis of ileal diversion.

18. **c. Less likely to be injured by radiation.** The transverse colon is used when one wants to be sure that the segment of conduit used has not been irradiated in individuals who have received extensive pelvic irradiation.

19. **a. Ureterosigmoidostomy.** Hypokalemia and total body depletion of potassium may occur in patients with urinary intestinal diversion. This is more common in patients with ureterosigmoidostomies than it is in patients who have other types of urinary intestinal diversion.

20. **d. Bowel reabsorption.** Because urea and creatinine are reabsorbed by both the ileum and the colon, serum concentrations of urea and creatinine do not necessarily accurately reflect renal function.

21. **a. Retain the ability to maintain the acidosis.** The ability to establish a hyperchloremic metabolic acidosis appears to be retained by most segments of ileum and colon over time.

22. **c. Are more common in patients with persistent hyperchloremic metabolic acidosis.** Osteomalacia in urinary intestinal diversion may be due to persistent acidosis, vitamin D resistance, and excessive calcium loss by the kidney. It appears that the degree to which each of these contributes to the syndrome may vary from patient to patient.

23. **c. Limits linear growth.** There is considerable evidence to suggest that urinary intestinal diversion has a detrimental effect on growth and development.
24. **d. Ureterosigmoidostomies.** The highest incidence of cancer occurs when the transitional epithelium is juxtaposed to the colonic epithelium and both are bathed by feces.
25. **b. Increased volume.** Reconfiguring bowel usually increases the volume, but its effect on motor activity and wall tension over the long term is unclear at this time.
26. **d. Eelevated gastrin levels.** The syndrome of severe metabolic alkalosis is most likely to occur in patients with high resting gastrin levels who are dehydrated and fail to empty their pouch in a timely manner.

Imaging

1. **b. Stricture at the left uretero-ileal anastomosis.** The loopogram study is of good quality and demonstrates good opacification of the right ureter and collecting system, an expected finding (options d and e are incorrect). The lack of reflux into the left ureter and collecting system may be indicative of a stricture at the left uretero-ileal anastomosis, substantiated by the hydronephrotic left collecting system on the computed tomography (CT) image. Urothelial tumor recurrence is not a common cause for absence of reflux into the ureters on a loopogram (option c is less likely).

CHAPTER REVIEW

1. Perioperative care. The use of a preoperative mechanical bowel prep, oral antibiotic bowel prep, and postoperative nasogastric tube decompression in patients undergoing bowel surgery is controversial. Administering intravenous antibiotics 1 hour before the surgical incision is not controversial and is supported by many studies. Indeed, patients undergoing elective intestinal surgery in the studies that show no advantage to a mechanical and/or antibiotic bowel prep received preoperative intravenous antibiotics. It should be appreciated that these studies involve isolated anastomoses—not large segments of bowel that are opened, as is the case in urologic procedures.
2. Ureteral intestinal anastomotic strictures. Antirefluxing anastomoses have a 10% to 20% stricture rate; refluxing anastomoses have a 3% to 10% stricture rate. The Wallace ureteral intestinal anastomosis has the lowest stricture rate.
3. Renal function and urinary diversion. Serum creatinine and blood urea nitrogen do not accurately reflect renal function in patients with intestine in the urinary tract because these substances, when excreted by the kidney, are reabsorbed by the bowel. This is more likely to be a problem in continent diversions. A glomerular filtration rate (GFR) of at least 60 mL/min and an ability to acidify the urine are necessary prerequisites for a continent diversion.
4. The electrolyte abnormality that occurs when ileum or colon are used for the diversion is a hyperchloremic metabolic acidosis. These patients may have a potassium deficiency as well.
5. Significant perioperative infectious complications occur in approximately 10% of patients undergoing cystectomy and urinary diversion.
6. The most common cause of mortality in urologic procedures when the gut is used relates to complications involving the bowel.
7. Complications specific to the use of stomach include the hematuria-dysuria syndrome and uncontrollable metabolic alkalosis in some patients.
8. The incidence of postoperative bowel obstruction is 4% to 10%. Colon, stomach, and sigmoid obstruction result in a 4% incidence, less than that occurring with ileum.
9. The mechanical preparation reduces the amount of feces, whereas the antibiotic preparation reduces the bacterial count. A mechanical bowel preparation reduces the total number of bacteria but not their concentration.
10. If the patient is able to achieve a urine pH of 5.8 or less, can establish a urine osmolality of 600 mOsm/kg or greater in response to water deprivation, has a GFR that exceeds 60 mL/min, and has minimal protein in the urine, he or she may be considered for a retentive diversion.
11. Osteomalacia in urinary intestinal diversion may be due to persistent acidosis, vitamin D resistance, and excessive calcium loss by the kidney.
12. In patients with gastric tissue in the urinary tract (usually gastrocystoplasty), the syndrome of severe metabolic alkalosis is most likely to occur in those with high resting gastrin levels who are dehydrated and fail to empty their pouch in a timely manner.

98

Cutaneous Continent Urinary Diversion

James M. McKiernan, G. Joel DeCastro, and Mitchell C. Benson

QUESTIONS

1. A 45-year-old man had an ileal conduit diversion as a child for bladder exstrophy. He requests a continent diversion. Serum creatinine is 2 mg/dL. Loopogram shows bilaterally thin ureters with small kidneys. Which is the best procedure?
   a. Ureterosigmoidostomy
   b. T pouch using the ileal conduit
   c. Abandon continent diversion
   d. Penn pouch using the ileal conduit
   e. Indiana pouch

2. A 45-year-old man underwent ileal conduit urinary diversion as a child for bladder exstrophy. He presents requesting continent diversion. Serum creatinine is 2 mg/dL. Loopogram shows bilateral hydronephrosis and a pipestem conduit. What is the best course of action?
   a. Mainz II to avoid problems with dilated ureters
   b. T pouch abandoning the disease conduit
   c. No continent diversion
   d. Drain the upper tracts and reassess renal function
   e. Proceed to neobladder construction

3. A patient undergoing a cystectomy and planned continent cutaneous diversion has positive ureteral margin biopsies up to 2 cm above each iliac artery, at which point negative biopsies are obtained. What is the best course of action?
   a. Use the terminal ileum for ureteral implantation and a Mitrofanoff continence mechanism
   b. No continent diversion
   c. Mobilize the kidneys and stretch the ureters to the reservoir
   d. Use a T pouch with a long chimney
   e. Cutaneous ureterostomies

4. Preservation of the ileocecal valve can be maintained with which catheterizable pouch?
   a. T pouch or Kock pouch
   b. Le Bag
   c. Indiana pouch
   d. Mainz I or II
   e. Penn pouch

5. In which procedure to repair a nipple valve would resection of additional bowel be routinely required?
   a. Stones on exposed staples
   b. Nipple valve slippage
   c. Nipple valve atrophy
   d. Pinhole leak
   e. Anastomotic leak

6. A 10-year-old child has an ileal conduit for myelomeningocele. The conduit was replaced on two occasions for pipestem conduit development. The conduit is again affected by the same process. The patient's family wants a continent diversion. Which is the best procedure?
   a. Ureterosigmoidostomy
   b. Revise the conduit
   c. T pouch using the ileal conduit
   d. Penn pouch using the ileal conduit
   e. Indiana pouch using the ileal conduit

7. A patient with chronic active hepatitis and invasive bladder cancer associated with intravesical carcinoma in situ is scheduled for a cystoprostatectomy. The serum creatinine concentration is 1 mg/dL. Prostatic urethral biopsy shows mild atypia. What is the best diversion?
   a. T pouch
   b. Ileal conduit
   c. Right colon reservoir
   d. Mainz II
   e. Cutaneous ureterostomies

8. The highest reoperation rate in catheterizable pouches occurs with what type of sphincter?
   a. In situ appendix
   b. Imbricated terminal ileum
   c. Plicated terminal ileum
   d. Nipple valves
   e. Transposed appendix

9. Which of the Mitrofanoff sphincter deficiencies can be corrected surgically?
   a. Length of the appendix
   b. Absence of the appendix
   c. Stenosis of the appendix
   d. All of the above

10. Hematuria and skin breakdown may occur with what type of pouch?
    a. T
    b. Gastric
    c. Mainz
    d. Right colon
    e. All of the above

11. Preoperative colonoscopy is indicated in candidates for which reservoir procedures?
    a. Ileal
    b. Jejunal
    c. Rectal
    d. Gastric
    e. All of the above

12. What condition is more common in absorbable stapled ileal pouches?
    a. Urine leaks
    b. Valve failure
    c. Hydronephrosis
    d. Ischemic pouch contraction
    e. Ureteral stricture

13. Anastomotic transitional cell carcinoma develops in a patient who has undergone cystectomy and continent cutaneous urinary diversion. What is the best treatment?
    a. Distal ureterectomy and reimplantation
    b. Conversion to ileal conduit
    c. Ileal ureter interposition
    d. Nephroureterectomy
    e. Cutaneous ureterostomies

14. Drainage of mucus is most difficult with which sphincteric mechanism?
    a. Kock valve
    b. In situ appendix
    c. Imbricated ileum
    d. Plicated ileum
    e. Transposed appendix

15. Which continent cutaneous diversion allows for a refluxing ureteroenteric anastomosis?
    a. Mitrofanoff with implantation of the ureters into terminal ileum
    b. Mitrofanoff with implantation of the ureters into the colon
    c. T pouch
    d. Kock pouch
    e. Indiana pouch

16. Three years after radical cystectomy and construction of a Kock pouch, a patient presents with right lower quadrant discomfort and associated spurts of urinary leakage. The test most likely to diagnose the condition is:
    a. computed tomography (CT).
    b. intravenous pyelogram (IVP).
    c. urine culture and sensitivity.
    d. cystogram of pouch.
    e. urodynamics.

17. Three years after cystectomy and Kock pouch for bladder cancer, a patient presents with recurrent episodes of bilateral pyelonephritis. The test most likely to provide the correct diagnosis is:
    a. CT.
    b. IVP.
    c. urine culture and sensitivity.
    d. cystogram of the pouch.
    e. magnetic resonance imaging (MRI).

18. What is the most important feature in preventing nipple valve slippage?
    a. Absorbable staples
    b. Length of the intussusception
    c. Resecting adequate mesentery
    d. Attaching the nipple valve to the side wall of the reservoir
    e. Length of staple line

19. In a patient with pipestem conduit and bilateral hydronephrosis requesting conversion to continent urinary diversion, nephrostomy drainage results in clearance values of 40 mL/min on the right and 10 mL/min on the left. Serum creatinine is 1.8 mg/dL. The next step in management is:
    a. Mainz II to avoid problems with the dilated ureters.
    b. T pouch abandoning the disease conduit.
    c. no continent diversion.
    d. ureterosigmoidostomy.
    e. neobladder.

20. A patient with squamous cell cancer of the bladder desires cystectomy and continent diversion. He has lost 20 pounds in the month before surgery. The next step in management is:
    a. increase oral intake.
    b. conduct preoperative hyperalimentation.
    c. conduct postoperative hyperalimentation.
    d. proceed directly with surgery.
    e. count calories.

21. Preoperative evaluation with an oatmeal enema is required in which procedure?
    a. Right colon reservoir
    b. Mainz I pouch
    c. Mainz II procedure
    d. Le Bag pouch
    e. Indiana pouch

22. Follow-up urinary cytology and colonoscopy should be used in which type of continent diversion?
    a. Ureterosigmoidostomy
    b. Mainz II procedure
    c. Right colon reservoir
    d. All of the above

23. Nocturnal emptying of the patient's reservoir is required in which type of diversion?
    a. Ureterosigmoidostomy
    b. T pouch
    c. Right colon reservoir
    d. Penn pouch
    e. Ileal conduit

24. The appendix is sacrificed in patients undergoing which pouch construction?
    a. Indiana
    b. Le Bag
    c. Mainz I
    d. All of the above

25. Pouch stone development occurs most commonly with which pouch?
    a. T pouch
    b. Kock pouch
    c. Penn pouch
    d. Gastric-ileal composite pouch
    e. Le Bag

26. What is the typical catheter used for appendiceal sphincters?
    a. 22-French (Fr) straight-tipped
    b. 22-Fr coudé-tipped

c. 14-Fr straight-tipped

d. 14-Fr coudé-tipped

e. 20-Fr coudé-tipped

27. Urinary retention resulting from continent diversion occurs most commonly with what type of sphincter?

a. Appendiceal stoma

b. Benchekroun hydraulic valve

c. Nipple valve sphincter

d. Imbricated Indiana mechanism

28. Immediate postoperative initial pouch capacity is least in which pouch?

a. T or Kock ileal

b. Right colon

c. Gastric

d. Mainz I

e. Transverse colon

29. Elevated pouch pressures would potentially facilitate the continence mechanism seen with which valve or sphincter?

a. Benchekroun ileal valve

b. Kock valve

c. Appendiceal tunnel

d. Imbricated Indiana mechanism

e. All of the above

30. The long-term failure rate of continence mechanisms is greatest with which mechanism?

a. T pouch valve

b. Appendiceal tunnel

c. Benchekroun hydraulic valve

d. Imbricated terminal ileum

31. Absorbable staples in continent urinary diversion are best suited to what type of reservoir pouch?

a. Ileal

b. Right colon reservoir

c. Gastric-ileal composite

d. Gastric

e. None of the above

32. When creating a large intestinal reservoir from absorbable staples, why is bowel eversion necessary?

a. Because staples should not be used in reservoir construction

b. To inspect the inside of the reservoir

c. To avoid injury to the mesenteric blood supply

d. To allow application of the second row of staples

e. None of the above

33. Which of the following conditions make patients unsuitable candidates for continent urinary diversion?

a. Multiple sclerosis

b. Quadriplegia

c. Mental impairment

d. Severe physical impairment

e. All of the above

34. Which of the following sutures should NOT be used in the construction of a reservoir?

a. Chromic catgut

b. Plain catgut

c. Silk

d. Polyglycolic acid (Dexon)

e. Polyglactin (Vicryl)

35. Which of the following diversions place the patient at risk for the development of a late malignancy?

a. Ureterosigmoidostomy

b. T pouch

c. Mainz II

d. Indiana pouch

e. All of the above

36. Which of the following diversions places the patient at greatest risk for the development of a late malignancy?

a. Ureterosigmoidostomy

b. T pouch

c. Mainz II

d. Indiana reservoir

e. Le Bag

37. Continent urinary diversion has which of the following effects?

a. Results in a psychotic depression

b. Results in an improved psychosocial adjustment

c. Results in violent behavior

d. Bipolar behavior

e. None of the above

38. According to most randomized studies, which type of urinary diversion is associated with the highest reported quality of life?

a. Ureterosigmoidostomy

b. Continent ileal reservoir (Kock pouch)

c. Ileal conduit

d. Orthotopic neobladder

e. None—no conclusive studies have established higher satisfaction or quality of life with any one specific continent diversion

39. Which of the following is NOT true of continent urinary diversion?

a. It is the gold standard of urinary diversion.

b. It is a safe and reliable urinary diversion.

c. It is associated with an increased complication rate.

d. It is appropriate for selected individuals.

e. It requires stricter selection criteria than incontinent diversion.

40. Which of the following circumstances would contraindicate a rectal bladder?

a. Prior pelvic irradiation

b. Unilateral ureteral dilation

c. Bilateral ureteral dilation

d. Lax anal sphincter tone

e. All of the above

41. During the construction of a continent cutaneous urinary diversion, the surgeon should:

a. not be concerned about the continence mechanism because the mechanism will mold to the catheter.

b. not test the continence mechanism for ease of catheterization.

c. not be concerned about pouch integrity because the pouch will seal itself.

d. do none of the above.

e. do all of the above.

42. If the urine in a continent cutaneous reservoir is found to be infected, what should be done?
    a. Nothing needs to be done in the absence of symptoms.
    b. The urine should always be sterilized with appropriate antibiotics.
    c. The infection should be eradicated and prophylactic antibiotics prescribed.
    d. Administer an intravenous pyelogram to check for upper tract damage.
    e. Perform a pouch-o-gram.

43. The most appropriate and conservative care for pouch rupture is:
    a. broad-spectrum antibiotic therapy.
    b. careful radiologic imaging and antibiotic therapy.
    c. surgical exploration for repair of the rupture and broad-spectrum antibiotic therapy.
    d. pouch drainage and broad-spectrum antibiotic therapy.
    e. bilateral percutaneous nephrostomies.

44. The first pouch to use the Mitrofanoff principle was the:
    a. Mainz I.
    b. Penn.
    c. Kock.
    d. Indiana.
    e. Le Bag.

45. Which of the following represents the advantage of the gastric pouch?
    a. Electrolyte reabsorption is reduced.
    b. Absorptive malabsorption is avoided.
    c. Acid urine may reduce the risk of infection.
    d. All of the above
    e. None of the above

46. When converting from an ileal conduit to a continent diversion, the conduit should be:
    a. discarded because it is older and subject to higher complications.
    b. preserved for the ureteroileal anastomosis.
    c. incorporated into the continent diversion when possible.
    d. discarded because it is a potential nidus of infection.
    e. None of the above

47. Which of the following is TRUE of absorbable staples?
    a. Their use has been shown to shorten operative time.
    b. They are safe and reliable.
    c. Unlike nonabsorbable staples, they must not be overlapped.
    d. All of the above.
    e. None of the above.

ANSWERS

1. **c. Abandon continent diversion.** A creatinine level greater than 1.8 mg/dL indicates a level of renal function insufficient for continent diversion.
2. **d. Drain the upper tracts and reassess renal function.** The best course of action is to place ureteral cutaneous stents bilaterally (bypassing the pipestem segment) and reassess urinary function. In evaluating the hydronephrotic patient with impaired renal function for continent diversion, upper tract drainage is advised. If necessary, bilateral nephrostomy tubes can be used.

3. **a. Use the terminal ileum for ureteral implantation and a Mitrofanoff continence mechanism.** The best course of action is to perform a right colon reservoir with anastomosis of the ureters to the terminal ileum. The appendix or other pseudo-appendiceal (Mitrofanoff) mechanisms can be used for continence. The terminal ileum can accommodate short ureters.
4. **a. T pouch or Kock pouch.** Preservation of the ileocecal valve can be maintained with the T or Kock pouch. All other pouches use the right colon, so that the ileocecal valve is sacrificed.
5. **c. Nipple valve atrophy.** Nipple valve atrophy requires that a new nipple valve be made of additional bowel.
6. **b. Revise the conduit.** With significant small bowel compromise, as well as loss of the ileocecal valve in a neurogenic bladder patient, severe diarrhea may ensue.
7. **b. Ileal conduit.** The best approach is cystoprostatectomy and a conduit. Normal hepatic function is mandated in any patient undergoing continent diversion.
8. **d. Nipple valves.** The highest reoperation rate is associated with nipple valve sphincter failure.
9. **d. All of the above.** The caliber of Mitrofanoff mechanisms, the length of the appendix, stenosis, and even absence of the appendix can be resolved by surgical variations.
10. **b. Gastric.** Hematuria and cutaneous skin erosion may occur with a gastric pouch. With gastric reservoirs or composite reservoirs, the low pH of the urine may lead to hematuria and cutaneous breakdown.
11. **c. Rectal.** Preoperative colonoscopy is relatively indicated in candidates for any pouch. Any pouch using colon mandates preoperative colonic evaluation.
12. **d. Ischemic pouch contraction.** Because of the overlap of staple lines in absorbable stapled ileal pouches, ischemic pouch contraction may occur.
13. **a. Distal ureterectomy and reimplantation.** An additional segment of ileum can serve as a proximal limb to the reservoir. If nephrectomy is necessary, careful attention must be paid to the residual renal function.
14. **b. In situ appendix.** The small-diameter catheter used in draining appendiceal sphincter pouches allows for less effective mucus drainage.
15. **a. Mitrofanoff with implantation of the ureters into terminal ileum.** The implantation of the ureters into the terminal ileum may allow for reflux. The ileal cecal valve and the isoperistaltic ileal segment may either prevent or diminish reflux.
16. **c. Urine culture and sensitivity.** The most important diagnostic test is urine culture. The symptoms described are those of pouchitis. This is treated by appropriate antibiotic therapy.
17. **d. Cystogram of the pouch.** The proximal nipple valve may have failed, leading to reflux and pyelonephritis. This is tested by the pouch-o-gram.
18. **d. Attaching the nipple valve to the side wall of the reservoir.** This results in a relative lengthening of the valve rather than a foreshortening of the valve with pouch filling.
19. **c. No continent diversion.** In this case, although the serum creatinine level returns to 1.8 mg/dL, the clearance value measured is less than the 60 mL/min required for continent diversion. Continent diversion should be abandoned, and simple replacement of the conduit considered.
20. **b. Conduct preoperative hyperalimentation.** The 20-pound weight loss indicates a potential for nutritional depletion or metastatic disease. A careful search for metastatic disease should be undertaken. For the patient with nutritional depletion, preoperative hyperalimentation is suggested to be of value.
21. **c. Mainz II procedure.** Any procedure that relies on the intact anal sphincter for continence (i.e., the Mainz II pouch) requires an assessment of the sphincter before carrying out the operation. This can be assessed by an oatmeal enema, which mimics the constitution of a combination of the urinary and fecal streams.
22. **d. All of the above.** Follow-up urinary cytology and colonoscopy is mandatory with any procedure that combines urinary and fecal streams. Because of an increased risk of malignancy

even in the absence of admixture of urine and stool, all large intestinal pouches should be subjected to annual investigation by pouchoscopy and cytology.

23. **a. Ureterosigmoidostomy.** Nocturnal reservoir emptying may be required with any of the continent cutaneous reservoirs to prevent overdistention and possible rupture but is mandatory with ureterosigmoidostomy owing to the additional risk of fecal incontinence and metabolic acidosis.

24. **d. All of the above.** The appendix is sacrificed in patients undergoing Indiana, Le Bag, and Mainz I pouch reconstruction because it can serve as a nidus for infection and abscess formation.

25. **b. Kock pouch.** Pouch stone development occurs most commonly with the Kock pouch. Despite the exclusion of distal staples, the stapling techniques used to secure nipple valves will lead to a higher potential for stone development than in pouches not requiring nipple valves.

26. **d. 14-Fr coudé-tipped.** Larger catheters will not fit into the appendix. A straight catheter is more difficult to pass.

27. **c. Nipple valve sphincter.** Urinary retention occurs most commonly with nipple valve sphincters. If the chimney of the nipple valve is not near the surface of the abdomen, the catheter can be misdirected into folds of bowel rather than through the nipple valve.

28. **a. T or Kock ileal.** Immediate postoperative initial pouch capacity is least in ileal reservoirs (i.e., the T or Kock pouch). Small bowel pouches have initial capacities that are much lower than right colon pouches.

29. **a. Benchekroun ileal valve.** Because the Benchekroun ileal valve is hydraulic, higher pouch pressures would facilitate continence, whereas lower pouch pressures might lead to incontinence.

30. **c. Benchekroun hydraulic valve.** The long-term outcome of Benchekroun hydraulic ileal valve mechanisms is possibly the worst of all reported sphincteric mechanisms.

31. **b. Right colon reservoir.** The use of absorbable staples is best suited to large bowel pouches. With large bowel pouches there is no problem with staple lines causing subsequent bowel ischemia.

32. **d. To allow application of the second row of staples.** In an absorbable-stapled right colon pouch, bowel eversion is required to allow for the application of the second row of staples. Staple lines must not cross because this will prevent the bulky, absorbable staples from seating properly. The bowel is everted, a cut is made beyond the end of the staple line, and the next line of staples is applied.

33. **e. All of the above.** Patients with multiple sclerosis, quadriplegia, frailty, or mental impairment will at some point in their lives require the care of family members or visiting nurses, so they are poor candidates for any form of continent diversion.

34. **c. Silk.** All sutures used in the urinary tract should be absorbable.

35. **e. All of the above.** Late malignancy has been reported in all bowel segments exposed to the urinary stream, whether or not there is a commingling with feces.

36. **a. Ureterosigmoidostomy.** Although late malignancy has been reported in all bowel segments exposed to the urinary stream, whether or not there is a commingling with feces, the mixture of urothelium, urine, and feces poses the greatest risk.

37. **b. Results in an improved psychosocial adjustment.** Many studies from throughout the world have suggested an improved psychosocial adjustment of the patient undergoing continent urinary and fecal diversion compared with those patients with diversions requiring collecting appliances.

38. **e. None—no conclusive studies have established higher satisfaction or quality of life with any one specific continent diversion.** There are insufficient quality-of-life data from randomized studies comparing continent and incontinent urinary diversions to establish the superiority of any one technique.

39. **a. It is the gold standard of urinary diversion.** Ileal conduit should be considered the "gold standard" of urinary diversion.

40. **e. All of the above.** Dilated ureters, pelvic irradiation, and lax anal sphincteric tone are all contraindications to the procedure.

41. **d. Do none of the above.** The continence mechanism must be catheterized intraoperatively to ensure ease of catheter passage. This is an extremely important and crucial maneuver because the inability to catheterize is a serious complication that will often result in the need for reoperation.

42. **a. Nothing needs to be done in the absence of symptoms.** Most authors would suggest that bacteriuria in the absence of symptomatology does not warrant antibiotic treatment.

43. **c. Surgical exploration for repair of the rupture and broad-spectrum antibiotic therapy.** In general, these patients require immediate pouch decompression, radiologic pouch studies, and surgical exploration with pouch repair. If the amount of urinary extravasation is small and the patient does not have a surgical abdomen, catheter drainage and antibiotic administration may suffice in treating intraperitoneal rupture of a pouch. Patients managed with this conservative approach require careful monitoring.

44. **b. Penn.** The Penn pouch was the first continent diversion to use the Mitrofanoff principle, wherein the appendix served as the continence mechanism.

45. **d. All of the above.** Electrolyte reabsorption is greatly diminished, shortening of the absorptive bowel does not occur, and the acid urine may decrease the likelihood of reservoir colonization.

46. **c. Incorporated into the continent diversion when possible.** The authors prefer to use the conduit in some form whenever possible. The use of an existing bowel segment has the potential to diminish metabolic sequelae and may result in a lower complication rate.

47. **d. All of the above.** The use of absorbable staples has substantially reduced the time required to fashion bowel reservoirs and has demonstrated short-term and long-term reliability with respect to reservoir integrity and volume. They must not be overlapped because overlapping will prevent the proper close of the staple.

CHAPTER REVIEW

1. The ability to self-catheterize is essential in patients who are to be considered for a continent cutaneous diversion.
2. All patients should be prepared for the possibility of a traditional ileal conduit if intraoperative circumstances warrant it.
3. A patient should have a minimum creatinine clearance of 60 mL/min to undergo a continent urinary diversion.
4. Single J ureteral stents are used in all continent diversions. The stents are brought out through a separate abdominal stab wound, and a Malecot catheter should be placed into the reservoir and brought out through a separate stab wound as well.
5. In continent diversions, it is not clear at this time whether antirefluxing ureteral intestinal anastomoses are necessary to preserve the upper tracts; however, antirefluxing procedures are associated with a higher incidence of stricture over the long term.
6. Most patients are satisfied with the type of urinary diversion irrespective of whether it is continent or not.
7. It is often useful to secure the reservoir to the anterior abdominal wall to prevent the reservoir from migrating. This is conveniently done where the Malecot exits the reservoir onto the anterior abdominal wall.
8. Renal and hepatic function must be carefully evaluated before a continent diversion is performed. Significant abnormalities in either are a contraindication to continent diversion. The glomerular filtration rate should be 60 mL/min or greater.

9. Patients with rectal bladders are very prone to the complication of hyperchloremic acidosis and total body potassium depletion. These patients also have an increased incidence of rectal cancer.
10. The loss of the ileocecal valve in patients with neurologic or intestinal disorders subjects the patient to a significant risk of debilitating diarrhea.
11. Any procedure that relies on the intact anal sphincter for continence (i.e., the Mainz II pouch) requires an assessment of the sphincter before carrying out the operation. This can be assessed by an oatmeal enema.
12. Because of an increased risk of malignancy even in the absence of admixture of urine and stool, all large intestinal pouches should be subjected to annual investigation by pouchoscopy and cytology.
13. Nocturnal reservoir emptying may be required with any of the continent cutaneous reservoirs to prevent overdistention and possible rupture, but it is mandatory with ureterosigmoidostomy because of the additional risk of fecal incontinence and metabolic acidosis.
14. Small bowel pouches have initial capacities that are much lower than those of right colon pouches.
15. The use of absorbable staples is best suited to large bowel pouches. With large bowel pouches there is no problem with staple lines causing subsequent bowel ischemia.
16. Although late malignancy has been reported in all bowel segments exposed to the urinary stream, whether or not there is a commingling with feces, the juxtaposition of urothelium, urine, and feces poses the greatest risk.

99 Orthotopic Urinary Diversion

Eila C. Skinner and Siamak Daneshmand

QUESTIONS

1. Which of the following was the key finding that allowed application of orthotopic urinary diversion to women undergoing cystectomy?
   a. Confirmation that an intact bladder neck is required for continence
   b. Demonstration in cystectomy specimens that urethral involvement was rare in the absence of tumor at the bladder neck
   c. Understanding of the relationship between estrogen levels and continence in elderly women
   d. Studies showing that direct invasion into the uterus is relatively rare in women with invasive bladder cancer
   e. Quality-of-life studies showing that men with continent diversion had better quality of life than those with ileal conduit

2. The risk factor most predictive for urethra recurrence following cystectomy for urothelial carcinoma is:
   a. prostatic stromal invasion.
   b. node-positive disease.
   c. carcinoma in situ (CIS) in females.
   d. pathologic stage pT3b tumor at the trigone.
   e. history of multiple prior tumors.

3. An 80-year-old man with clinical cT2 bladder cancer lives alone but is active. His serum creatinine is 1.0 following neoadjuvant gemcitabine and cisplatin chemotherapy. He is interested in an orthotopic diversion. If he elects to have a continent diversion, the most important information to provide him so that postoperative expectations are met is:
   a. neoadjuvant chemotherapy increases the early complications of orthotopic diversion.
   b. older patients take longer to regain continence than younger patients.
   c. ileal conduit will be easier for him to take care of than a continent diversion.
   d. pyelonephritis is more common with continent diversion than ileal conduit.
   e. his risk of renal deterioration with continent diversion is higher than with ileal conduit.

4. Which of the following patients should NOT be offered an orthotopic neobladder?
   a. An 82-year-old healthy woman with recurrent cT1 and CIS following intravesical bacille Calmette-Guérin (BCG) and a prior vaginal hysterectomy
   b. A 53-year-old woman with an estimated glomerular filtration rate (eGFR) of 55 following neoadjuvant chemotherapy
   c. A 50-year-old man 2 years following low anterior colon resection with adjuvant chemotherapy and external beam radiation to the pelvis
   d. A 60-year-old woman with diabetes and hypertension
   e. A 58-year-old woman with palpable induration of the anterior vaginal apex

5. Which of these is a key requirement for construction of an orthotopic diversion?
   a. It should prevent vesicoureteral reflux to preserve renal function.
   b. It should be made of ileum or a combination of colon and ileum.
   c. The bowel used should be detubularized and fashioned into a spherical shape.
   d. It should be made with the smallest amount of bowel possible.
   e. The ureters should be anastomosed to an isoperistaltic segment of bowel.

6. Which of the following have been suggested to decrease the risk of urinary retention following ileal neobladder in women?
   a. Regular urethral dilation
   b. Tack the pouch to the anterior abdominal wall
   c. Biofeedback training in the early postoperative period
   d. Preservation of the uterus
   e. Construct a W pouch rather than a Studer type pouch

7. In performing a cystectomy and orthotopic ileal neobladder in a male, the most important step in preserving continence is to:
   a. construct a large-capacity reservoir.
   b. avoid excess dissection anterior to the urethra.
   c. perform a nerve-sparing procedure in all cases.
   d. avoid removal of the presacral lymph nodes.
   e. place a suprapubic catheter during the early postoperative period.

8. A 64-year-old man with recurrent CIS who strongly prefers an orthotopic or continent cutaneous diversion is found to have grossly node-positive disease at surgery. The next step is:
   a. close and refer for chemotherapy and radiation.
   b. complete the cystectomy but do an ileal conduit.
   c. complete the cystectomy but do a continent cutaneous diversion.
   d. complete the cystectomy and neobladder and refer for adjuvant chemotherapy.
   e. complete the cystectomy and neobladder and refer for adjuvant radiation therapy.

9. Before considering a continent orthotopic diversion, what evaluation is mandatory?
   a. Prostatic urethral biopsy
   b. Evaluation of renal function
   c. Colonoscopy to rule out colon polyps
   d. Biopsy of the bladder neck in a female
   e. Video-urodynamics to test the integrity of the external sphincter

10. The primary innervation of the rhabdosphincter that is responsible for continence in men and women following an orthotopic diversion is:
    a. parasympathetics from S2-S4.
    b. anterior branches of the sciatic nerve.

c. sympathetic nerves from the hypogastric plexus.

d. pudendal nerve.

e. femoral nerve.

11. Use of metallic surgical staples should be avoided in construction of a continent diversion because:

a. it is less secure than a hand-sewn closure.

b. they tend to be buried in the bowel mucosa.

c. the staples increases the risk of subsequent infection.

d. the staples become a nidus for stone formation.

e. they increase the risk of cancer developing in the segment.

12. A 71-year-old male is found on routine follow-up to have a pelvic recurrence 13 months after cystectomy and ileal neobladder. The mass is 2.5 cm in the obturator fossa, abutting the pouch. There is no hydronephrosis. He has good daytime continence but occasionally leaks at night. The next step is:

a. resection of the mass with removal of the pouch and conversion to an ileal conduit.

b. cystoscopy to look for invasion of the reservoir.

c. placement of a permanent suprapubic tube.

d. resection of the mass with preservation of the neobladder.

e. systemic chemotherapy with or without external beam radiation.

13. Asymptomatic bacteriuria in patients with orthotopic diversion:

a. carries a high risk of subsequent pyelonephritis.

b. leads to an increase in urethral recurrence.

c. does not generally require treatment.

d. is very rare in most reported series.

e. suggests probable outlet obstruction.

14. A 59-year-old man is 6 years out from a radical cystectomy and neobladder. He had excellent day and nighttime continence and no problems with infections, but recently has started to leak at night. The next step is:

a. video-urodynamics.

b. computed tomography (CT) scan looking for local recurrence.

c. check postvoid residual.

d. trial of long-term antibiotics.

e. magnetic resonance imaging (MRI) of the spine.

15. A 66-year-old male 2 years after a cystectomy and Hautmann ileal neobladder for pathologic stage T2N0M0 bladder cancer is found on routine CT scan to have a very distended neobladder and mild bilateral hydronephrosis. He has a postvoid residual of over 800 mL. Cystoscopy and digital rectal exam are normal. The next step is:

a. teach the patient intermittent catheterization.

b. dilate the urethra with van Buren sounds.

c. instruct the patient to credé while Valsava voiding.

d. convert the diversion to an ileal conduit.

e. decompress the neobladder with a catheter for 2 weeks and then resume regular voiding.

16. Quality-of-life studies of patients with orthotopic diversion:

a. are best done by the physician asking the patient about the function of his/her neobladder.

b. have generally shown that patients with continent diversions have a better quality of life than those with ileal conduits.

c. can be easily done with currently available questionnaires used for other populations.

d. have often been underpowered or affected by selection bias.

e. have shown that most patients with any urinary diversion have very poor quality of life.

17. A 70-year-old man who is 10 days postcystectomy and neobladder is readmitted with fever, and CT scan shows a large fluid collection near the reservoir that fills with contrast on delayed images. The catheter and ureteral stents are still in place. The next step is:

a. intravenous (IV) antibiotics and observation with frequent catheter irrigation.

b. exploration and repair of the pouch.

c. bilateral percutaneous nephrostomy tube placement.

d. percutaneous drainage of the fluid collection.

e. percutaneous placement of a suprapubic catheter.

18. A 53-year-old woman had an anterior exenteration and neobladder with omental flap interposition 3 months previously. She still has total incontinence day and night. The next step is:

a. reassurance and reinforce Kegel exercises.

b. refer for physical therapy for pelvic floor strengthening.

c. evaluate for possible vesicovaginal fistula.

d. prescribe extended-release oxybutynin.

e. fluorourodynamics.

19. A 70-year-old woman had a cystectomy and ileal neobladder diversion 5 years ago for pT2N0 urothelial cancer. CT scan is normal, and she has excellent continence and empties well with negative urine culture. The next step is:

a. refer her to her primary care physician for routine health maintenance.

b. continue annual CT abdomen and pelvis out to 10 years.

c. annual endoscopy of the pouch to screen for secondary malignancy.

d. annual cystogram and serum creatinine to evaluate for reflux nephropathy.

e. renal ultrasound and vitamin B_{12} level every 1 to 2 years.

20. Which of the following is NOT usually part of an Early Recovery After Surgery (ERAS) protocol applied to patients undergoing radical cystectomy?

a. Alvimopan BID beginning on the morning of surgery

b. Early feeding

c. No mechanical or antibiotic bowel prep

d. Continuous IV narcotics to optimize pain management

e. Early removal of nasogastric tubes

21. An otherwise healthy 90-year-old man had a cystectomy and ileal neobladder 15 years previously with a hemi-Kock pouch to the urethra. He presented with a creatinine of 4.0 and bilateral hydronephrosis on renal ultrasound that did not resolve with catheter drainage. The most likely cause of his problem is:

a. bilateral ureteral stones.

b. stenosis of the afferent nipple valve.

c. reflux nephropathy.

d. urinary retention.

e. cancer recurrence in the reservoir.

22. Which of the following is TRUE about robotic cystectomy with extracorporeal neobladder construction compared with standard open cystectomy?

a. Patients undergoing robot-assisted radical cystectomy have significantly fewer early and late complications.

b. Continence has been shown to be improved.

c. Long-term cancer control has been proven to be equivalent.

d. The surgery can be performed through a smaller incision.

e. Hospital stay has been shorter in the minimally invasive surgical series.

23. A 66-year-old man had a cystectomy and sigmoid neobladder 4 years previously and has good continence. He was noted on recent CT scan to have two 0.7-cm calcifications in the pouch. The next step is:

a. reassurance that the stones will probably pass.

b. shockwave lithotripsy.

c. metabolic stone evaluation.

d. begin intermittent catheterization.

e. cystoscopy and extraction of the stone.

24. A 49-year-old man had a cystectomy and neobladder 4 months previously. He has excellent continence in the daytime but still has accidents at night even though he gets up twice to empty. The next step is:

a. reassurance that the nighttime continence will likely improve with more time.

b. trial of extended release oxybutynin.

c. strict fluid restriction to no more than 1500 mL per day.

d. intermittent catheterization.

e. refer for physical therapy for pelvic floor strengthening.

ANSWERS

1. **b. Demonstration in cystectomy specimens that urethral involvement was rare in the absence of tumor at the bladder neck.** The two findings that paved the way for orthotopic diversion in women were retrospective pathologic studies showing that urethral involvement was rare in the absence of bladder neck involvement (in other words, "skip lesions" were rarely seen, suggesting oncologic safety) and studies showing that women could be continent without an intact bladder neck (previously thought to be required).

2. **a. Prostatic stromal invasion.** Two large studies have demonstrated conclusively that urethral recurrence in men is associated with prostatic stromal invasion in the cystectomy specimen.

3. **b. Older patients take longer to regain continence than younger patients.** Older men regain continence more slowly than younger men, but the majority of fit older men will ultimately have good control, especially in the daytime. Older men often have difficulty becoming independent in managing an ileal conduit, and in a man living alone a neobladder may actually be simpler.

4. **e. A 58-year-old woman with palpable induration of the anterior vaginal apex.** Women with palpable invasion of the anterior vaginal wall have a high risk of urethral tumor and should not undergo orthotopic diversion.

5. **c. The bowel used should be detubularized and fashioned into a spherical shape.** Orthotopic diversions can be made from small or large bowel. The key to obtaining a low-pressure reservoir with good volume is to detubularize the segment and reconfigure it into a spherical shape.

6. **d. Preservation of the uterus.** Late urinary retention ("hypercontinence") in women appears to be primarily due to posterior displacement of the pouch into the vagina resulting in a kinking at the urethral anastomosis. A number of maneuvers have been suggested such as sacrocolpopexy, but preservation of the uterus appears to be the most promising.

7. **b. Avoid excess dissection anterior to the urethra.** In preserving the urethra for an orthotopic bladder in males, one should be careful of the dorsal venous complex and avoid deep bites into the pelvic floor, especially anterior to the urethra where the rhabdosphincter is the most developed.

8. **d. Complete the cystectomy and neobladder and refer for adjuvant chemotherapy.** Patients with node-positive disease have a poor prognosis, but up to 30% may be long-term survivors, especially with adjuvant chemotherapy. Orthotopic diversion should not impact survival, and if a patient is highly motivated to avoid a stoma, this option can still be pursued.

9. **b. Evaluation of renal function.** In order to be considered a candidate for a continent diversion, a patient must have a glomerular filtration rate (GFR) in excess of 35 mL/min, and the kidneys must be capable of concentrating and acidifying the urine.

10. **d. Pudendal nerve.** The rhabdosphincter is innervated by the pudendal somatic nerve. The contribution to continence from the pelvic autonomic plexus is uncertain, although some nonrandomized studies suggest that preserving the neurovascular bundle posterolateral to the prostate may improve continence.

11. **d. The staples become a nidus for stone formation.** Metallic staples have a high association with subsequent stone formation, as was seen in the long-term experience with the hemi-Kock pouch. Recent efforts to perform intracorporeal neobladder using minimally invasive techniques have advocated using GIA staplers, but early results have suggested a high risk of stones.

12. **e. Systemic chemotherapy with or without external beam radiation.** Local recurrence of urothelial cancer will not usually impact the neobladder function. Rarely, direct invasion of the reservoir will cause bleeding or outlet obstruction. Prognosis is poor, and local resection is rarely successful in eradicating the tumor, so primary treatment should be systemic chemotherapy and possibly radiation (which can be safely applied around a neobladder).

13. **c. Does not generally require treatment.** In patients with orthotopic bladders, approximately one quarter have asymptomatic bacteriuria. After the initial 6 months it is rare for patients to have symptomatic infections or pyelonephritis, and bacteriuria does not require treatment.

14. **c. Check postvoid residual.** Patients who have a change in their continence after initial good function should be evaluated for possible urinary retention. This is often the first sign of incomplete emptying. Urodynamics are not necessary unless the pouch is made from colon, because ileal neobladders are very reliably low-pressure with good compliance.

15. **a. Teach the patient intermittent catheterization.** All patients who are considered for a continent diversion should be willing and able to perform self-catheterization. The likelihood of needing self-catheterization is lower in men than in women, with reported rates of 10% to 40% in most series.

16. **d. Have often been underpowered or affected by selection bias.** Quality-of-life surveys have not shown one type of urinary diversion to be superior over another, though the vast majority of studies have serious methodological flaws. Obviously, randomized studies in this area have been impossible. Most patients are reasonably well adapted socially, physically, and psychologically to their diversion. The key to this adaptation is appropriate and realistic preoperative education.

17. **d. Percutaneous drainage of the fluid collection.** If a patient has an undrained urine leak postoperatively, percutaneous drainage is the first step. Nephrostomy tubes can be placed if a large urine leak does not respond to percutaneous drainage with optimal catheter drainage. Open surgical repair should be avoided if possible because the complication rate is high and success in closing the leak in the face of acute postsurgical inflammation is low.

18. **c. Evaluate for possible vesicovaginal fistula.** A woman with persistent incontinence should be evaluated for a pouch vaginal fistula. This is most common when the anterior vaginal wall is removed with the specimen. It is best prevented by interposition of an omental pedicle but still can occur. Evaluation is easily performed with a speculum exam with methylene blue in the bladder.

19. **e. Renal ultrasound and vitamin B_{12} level every 1 to 2 years.** Long-term risks in diversion patients include late ureteral

stricture, stones, decreased bone density, and vitamin B_{12} deficiency. All of these can be silent, so long-term routine follow-up is required. Most primary care physicians are not familiar with this.

20. **d. Continuous IV narcotics to optimize pain management.** New ERAS protocols have resulted in shorter hospital stay. Avoidance of bowel prep and the use of the μ opioid inhibitor alvimopan have been proven effective in randomized trials.

21. **b. Stenosis of the afferent nipple valve.** Afferent nipple stenosis is a well-documented late complication of the classic hemi-Kock pouch with an intussuscepted nipple valve antireflux mechanism. Treatment includes nephrostomy tube placement and endoscopic incision of the valve mechanism.

22. **d. The surgery can be performed through a smaller incision.** A large series of patients undergoing robotic-assisted cystectomy with extracorporeal diversion showed no decrease in hospital stay or early or late complications compared with open series, and this was confirmed in one recent randomized trial from Memorial Sloan-Kettering. Oncologic efficacy appears to be similar, but long-term results are not yet available.

23. **e. Cystoscopy and extraction of the stone.** Stones can occur in all types of continent diversions. These stones should be removed endoscopically while they are still small.

24. **a. Reassurance that the nighttime continence will likely improve with more time.** Patients typically attain nighttime continence more slowly than daytime, with patients reporting improvement out to 1 to 2 years. Early on there is an obligate nocturnal diuresis from the pouch that aggravates this. If the patient has good daytime control, further efforts to strengthen the sphincter are unlikely to help the nighttime continence. There is no role for anticholinergics or urodynamics in this setting.

CHAPTER REVIEW

1. The volume of the reservoir generally increases over time. Reservoirs constructed from ileum generally have a greater increase in volume over time than pouches constructed with colon.

2. The risk factors in women that are most predictive of urethral cancer developing are vaginal wall invasion or bladder neck involvement of transitional cell carcinoma.

3. The majority of patients who have a urethral recurrence are symptomatic on presentation. A urinary cytology has a variable rate of yield but is generally low in this group of patients.

4. When orthotopic bladders are constructed in elderly patients, there is a slower time to achieve continence, an increased rate of stress incontinence, and an increased incidence of nighttime incontinence when compared with younger patients.

5. In order to consider a patient a candidate for a continent diversion, he or she must have a glomerular filtration rate (GFR) in excess of 60 mL/min, and the kidneys must be capable of concentrating and acidifying the urine. A minimum GFR of 35 mL/min is required for a conduit diversion if metabolic problems are to be manageable.

6. All patients who are considered for a continent diversion should be willing and able to perform self-catheterization, although for selected patients this may not be necessary.

7. In preserving the urethra for an orthotopic bladder in males, one should be careful of the dorsal venous complex, preserve the puboprostatic ligaments, and avoid deep bites into the pelvic floor. In females, the endopelvic fascia and levator muscles should be preserved.

8. In patients with orthotopic bladders, approximately one quarter have asymptomatic bacteriuria.

9. The need to perform an antireflux mechanism for the ureters in an orthotopic urinary diversion is unproved.

10. If there is any suggestion that a nerve-sparing technique might result in a positive surgical margin, the nerve should be sacrificed. This does not mean that the diversion cannot be successfully performed or that the patient will not be continent.

11. Nighttime incontinence occurs in approximately 25% to 75% of patients.

12. Urinary retention following orthotopic urinary diversion occurs in 10% to 25% of patients and is more common in women than in men.

13. It may take 3 to 6 months for daytime continence to develop in many patients. Nocturnal continence may take more than a year after surgery.

14. If a patient has an undrained urine leak postoperatively, percutaneous drainage and/or nephrostomy is preferable to open surgical repair because the latter is extremely difficult and the complication rate is high.

15. Obstruction from an antireflux valve may be clinically silent, and patients may present with hydronephrosis and/or renal failure.

16. A pouch vaginal fistula is a morbid complication in female patients and is most likely to occur when the anterior vagina is removed along with the bladder. It is best prevented by interposition of an omental pedicle.

17. Quality-of-life surveys have not shown one type of urinary diversion to be superior over another. Most patients are reasonably well adapted socially, physically, and psychologically to their diversion. The key to this adaptation is appropriate and realistic preoperative education.

18. Preserving the uterus and vagina and their supporting structures limits the risk of a vaginal fistula, improves sexual function, and may decrease urinary retention in women who undergo a continent diversion.

19. The absence of the guarding reflex and increased volume output at night due to secretion of fluid by the bowel and the physiologic diuresis that occurs in older patients in the supine position contributes to nighttime incontinence.

20. In women, one fourth will have daytime leakage, one third will have nighttime leakage, and two thirds will require self-catheterization at least once a day.

21. Women with palpable invasion of the anterior vaginal wall have a high risk of urethral tumor and should not undergo orthotopic diversion.

22. Long-term risks in diversion patients include late ureteral stricture, stones, decreased bone density, and vitamin B_{12} deficiency.

100 Minimally Invasive Urinary Diversion

Khurshid A. Guru

QUESTIONS

1. Regarding perioperative thromboprophylaxis treatment after robot-assisted radical cystectomy, which of the following is TRUE?
   a. Pneumatic compressions and leg stockings are adequate.
   b. Low-molecular-weight heparin can be used as a single dose before the operation.
   c. Low-molecular-weight heparin should be continued until 4 weeks after surgery.
   d. Both mechanical and pharmacologic prophylaxes are adequate for 48 hours perioperatively.
   e. No prophylaxis.

2. During robotic-assisted radical cystectomy and intracorporeal urinary diversion:
   a. use of a 30-degree up lens is advantageous for a deep female pelvis.
   b. a 0-degree lens can be used for the entire procedure.
   c. the camera port is inserted below the umbilicus.
   d. the camera can be easily switched to another robotic port.
   e. a five-port configuration is used.

3. Before embarking on intracorporeal urinary diversion, it is important to:
   a. perform a bowel segment washout.
   b. de-dock the robot and change the attachments to the ports.
   c. de-dock the robot and reduce the steep Trendelenburg position for both ileal conduit and neo bladder.
   d. de-dock the robot and reposition the port to a new configuration for urinary diversion.
   e. de-dock the robot and reduce the steep Trendelenburg position for neobladder only.

4. During robot-assisted intracorporeal urinary diversion, the benefit of the marionette stitch is to:
   a. identify the distal and proximal ends of the conduit.
   b. help in retaining orientation of the bowel.
   c. allow free movement of the bowel segment for creation of the conduit.
   d. prevent leakage of bowel contents during the creation of the conduit.
   e. allow free movement of the bowel segment and prevent inadvertent movements of the robotic instruments.

5. During creation of the neobladder, mobilization of the bowel to reach the urethra can be achieved by all of the following EXCEPT:
   a. reducing the Trendelenburg position.
   b. using a Penrose drain for gentle traction and stretching.
   c. mobilization of the urethra cephalad.
   d. incising the peritoneum over the mesentery.
   e. dissection of the ileum around the ileocecal junction.

6. Which of the following has been a major limitation of incorporating intracorporeal urinary diversion during robot-assisted radical cystectomy?
   a. Higher rates to open conversion
   b. Steep learning curve
   c. Limitation of instrument maneuverability
   d. Prolonged operative time
   e. Increased complication and readmission rates

7. Which of the following factors have NOT been credited for reducing complications of robot-assisted radical cystectomy?
   a. Reduced bowel manipulation
   b. Decreased insensible losses
   c. Increased blood loss
   d. Minimal need for analgesia
   e. Minimally invasive approach

8. The most common cause of complications after robot-assisted radical cystectomy and intracorporeal urinary diversion is:
   a. bleeding.
   b. sepsis.
   c. necrosis of the bowel segment.
   d. enteroenteric anastomotic leak.
   e. port site and para-stomal hernia.

ANSWERS

1. **c. Low-molecular-weight heparin should be continued until 4 weeks after surgery.** Based on 939 patients who underwent robot-assisted radical cystectomy, the incidence of hematologic and vascular complications was 10%. A survey of urologists who were aware of the American Urological Association (AUA) Best Practice Statement guidelines revealed that 51% were likely to use thromboprophylaxis (odds ratio, 1.4, confidence interval, 1.2-1.6). Eighteen percent of urologic oncologists and/or laparoscopic/robotic specialists and 34% of nonurologic oncologists and/or laparoscopic/robotic specialists avoided routine thromboprophylaxis in patients undergoing radical cystectomy. The former were more likely to use thromboprophylaxis ($P<.0001$) than other respondents. Urologists graduating after the year 2000 used thromboprophylaxis in high-risk patients undergoing radical cystectomy more often than did earlier graduates (79.2% vs. 63.4%, $P<.0001$). Based on the American College of Surgeons NSQIP (National Surgical Quality Improvement Program) database from 1307 patients who underwent radical cystectomy, the mean time to venous thromboembolism diagnosis was 15.2 days postoperatively; 55% of all venous thromboembolism events were diagnosed after patient discharge home. It is recommended to consider extended duration pharmacologic prophylaxis (4 weeks) in this high-risk surgical population.

2. **b. A 0-degree lens can be used for the entire procedure.** The majority of robot-assisted radical prostatectomy procedures use different lenses for the procedure. During robot-assisted radical

cystectomy, surgeons prefer a 0-degree lens. Special situations of a narrow, deep pelvis in association with obesity can require a 30-degree down lens for better visualization, especially for the proximal portion of the extended lymph node dissection.

3. **e. De-dock the robot and reduce the steep Trendelenburg position for neobladder only.** Traditionally, a steep Trendelenburg position has been used to avoid bowel in the operative field and also to get direct access to the deeper pelvis. Unfortunately, this works against intracorporeal neobladder, as urethral-neobladder anastomosis is difficult if the bowel tries to retract back into the abdominal cavity and is under tension. The ideal solution introduced by the Karolinska Institute group is reducing Trendelenburg and reversing the steps by performing the urethra-neobladder anastomosis during the initial part of the procedure.

4. **c. Allow free movement of the bowel segment for creation of the conduit.** Because of the multiple detailed steps required during intracorporeal urinary diversion in a narrow operative space, the marionette stitch helps in controlling the area of focus by acting as a retraction and exposing the correct surgical space to perform the right and left uretero-ileal anastomosis.

5. **c. Mobilization of the urethra cephalad.** Traditionally, a steep Trendelenburg position has been used to avoid bowel in the operative field and also to gain direct access to the deeper pelvis. Unfortunately this works against intra-corporeal neobladder because urethral-neobladder anastomosis is difficult if the bowel tries to retract back into the abdominal cavity and is in tension. Several options used to reduce tension and ease anastomosis include reducing Trendelenburg, performing the urethra-neobladder anastomosis at the beginning of the procedure, incising the peritoneum over the mesentery, dissection of the ileum around the ileocecal junction, and, finally, using temporary traction for stretching and holding the bowel in place for anastomosis.

6. **d. Prolonged operative time.** An initial goal of minimally invasive surgeons for bladder cancer was to ensure oncologic outcomes that included avoiding inadvertent entry into bladder or tumor, low soft tissue surgical margins, and a thorough extended lymph node dissection. Adequate literature has been published to ensure that all these surgical tenets are met in order to address complete intracorporeal surgery by performing diversion using robotic assistance. Attempts to perform intracorporeal urinary diversion have previously failed because of limitations of the instruments (observed in conventional laparoscopy), especially for reconstruction requiring prolonged operative time.

7. **c. Increased blood loss.** Based on 939 patients from the International Robotic Cystectomy Consortium (IRCC) several risk factors for development of any or high-grade complications were identified that included age, receipt of neoadjuvant chemotherapy, smoking history, and receipt of blood transfusion. During this study, the mortality rate at 90 days identified perioperative blood transfusion as a risk factor as well.

8. **b. Sepsis.** A study evaluated 935 patients in the IRCC database who had robot-assisted radical cystectomy and pelvic lymph node dissection with both intracorporeal (ileal conduit: 106; neobladder: 61), and extracorporeal urinary diversion (ileal conduit: 570; neobladder: 198). The 90-day complication rate was not significantly different between the two groups, but there was a trend favoring the intracorporeal group (41% vs. 49%, $P = .05$). Gastrointestinal complications and sepsis constituted the majority of the complications in all robot-assisted radical cystectomy series comparing intracorporeal and extracorporeal urinary diversion. Although both complications were significantly lower in the intracorporeal group, sepsis was the most common complication in that group.

CHAPTER REVIEW

1. Recovery following radical cystectomy and urinary diversion is primarily dependent on return of bowel function.
2. An absolute contraindication for a minimally invasive cystectomy is significant pulmonary disease.
3. Preoperative broad-spectrum antibiotics should be given 1 hour before the incision.
4. A preoperative antibiotic and/or mechanical bowel preparation is controversial provided an intravenous broad-spectrum antibiotic is given 1 hour before the skin incision.
5. Continuity of the bowel is re-established following the ureteral intestinal anastomosis.
6. Duplicate ureters should be identified before the procedure.
7. Maintaining proper orientation of the bowel is critical.
8. The 30-day complication rates for minimally invasive cystectomy are reported to be approximately 70%, with 37% being high grade (sepsis is the most common); reoperation rates in the first 30 days range between 15% and 20%.
9. Fifty-five percent of all thromboembolic events are diagnosed after the patient is discharged. The average time to diagnosis is 15 days.
10. Risk factors that are predictive of postoperative complications include age, prior chemotherapy, a history of smoking, and receipt of blood transfusions. Gastrointestinal complications and sepsis are the most common complications.

101 Genital and Lower Urinary Tract Trauma

Allen F. Morey and Lee C. Zhao

QUESTIONS

1. Which of the following is an absolute indication for open repair of blunt bladder rupture injury?
   a. Significant extraperitoneal bladder rupture with extravasation of contrast agent into the scrotum
   b. Significant extraperitoneal bladder rupture with gross hematuria
   c. Significant extraperitoneal bladder rupture that has not healed after 3 weeks of Foley catheter drainage
   d. Intraperitoneal bladder rupture
   e. Significant extraperitoneal bladder rupture associated with pelvic fracture requiring treatment by external fixation

2. Which of the following statements is TRUE regarding cystography for diagnosis of bladder injury?
   a. If the patient is already undergoing computed tomography (CT) for evaluation of associated injuries, CT cystography should be performed via antegrade filling of the bladder after intravenous administration of radiographic contrast material and clamping the Foley catheter.
   b. If plain film cystograms are obtained, the study is considered negative and complete if there is no extravasation of contrast agent seen on the filling film.
   c. CT cystography is best performed with undiluted contrast medium.
   d. An absolute indication for immediate cystography is the presence of pelvic fracture and microhematuria.
   e. None of the above.

3. Which of the following statements is TRUE about blunt bladder rupture injuries?
   a. They are present in 90% of patients presenting with pelvic fractures.
   b. They coexist with urethral disruption in 50% of cases.
   c. Extraperitoneal ruptures are always amenable to nonoperative treatment.
   d. High mortality rate is primarily related to nonurologic comorbidities.
   e. They are associated with microhematuria or no hematuria in 40% of cases.

4. The risk of complications from nonoperative treatment of extraperitoneal bladder rupture is increased by:
   a. associated orthopedic injury.
   b. associated vaginal injury.
   c. associated urethral injury.
   d. associated rectal injury.
   e. all of the above.

5. Three months after a urethral distraction injury, a patient is found to have a 2-cm obliterative posterior urethral defect. Which of the following is TRUE about the repair?
   a. One-stage, open, perineal anastomotic urethroplasty is preferred.
   b. Orthopedic hardware in the pubic symphysis area is a contraindication to open posterior urethroplasty.

   c. Buccal mucosa graft urethroplasty is recommended.
   d. Urethral stent placement is recommended.
   e. The patient is at high risk for incontinence after posterior urethral reconstruction surgery.

6. In a patient with a pelvic fracture from blunt trauma in whom no urine is returned after catheter placement, what is the best initial method to evaluate urethral injury?
   a. Retrograde urethrography
   b. CT of abdomen and pelvis
   c. Filiforms and followers
   d. Bladder ultrasonography
   e. None of the above

7. During exploration after a scrotal gunshot wound, 20% of the left testicular capsule is found to be disrupted. What should be done?
   a. Left orchiectomy
   b. Application of wet dressings and delayed testicular surgery
   c. Left testicular reconstruction with synthetic graft
   d. Closure of the scrotal laceration followed by ultrasonography
   e. Immediate primary repair of the left testis

8. A 23-year-old man is found to have an 80% transection of the proximal bulbar urethra after a gunshot wound with a 22-caliber pistol. A 1-cm urethral defect is visualized during cystoscopy. What is the most appropriate therapy?
   a. Buccal mucosa graft urethroplasty
   b. Spatulated, stented, tension-free, watertight repair of the urethra with absorbable sutures
   c. Suprapubic tube placement
   d. Urethral catheterization alone
   e. Perineal urethrostomy

9. Which of the following statements regarding penile fracture is FALSE?
   a. Most injuries occur ventrolaterally.
   b. Rupture of a superficial vein can sometimes mimic the presentation of a corporeal tear.
   c. Retrograde urethrography should be uniformly performed to assess for urethral injury.
   d. Patients with penile fracture who are treated nonoperatively are more likely to have longer hospital stays, a higher risk of infection, and penile curvature than those whose fracture is repaired surgically.
   e. Physical examination is usually sufficient in making the diagnosis or for deciding on surgical exploration.

10. The blood in a hematocele is contained in which of the following?
    a. Tunica albuginea
    b. Tunica vaginalis
    c. Dartos muscle
    d. Camper fascia
    e. Spermatic cord

11. Blunt scrotal trauma that results in testis rupture:
    a. is usually a bilateral process.
    b. is often diagnosed by the presence of intratesticular hypoechoic areas on ultrasonography.
    c. has a degree of hematoma that correlates with the extent of injury.
    d. requires conservative management that results in acceptable viability and function.
    e. is definitively diagnosed during physical examination alone in most cases.

12. Which of the following statements is TRUE regarding penile amputation injury?
    a. Microscopic reanastomosis of the corporeal arteries is recommended.
    b. The severed phallus should be placed directly on ice during transport.
    c. Microscopic dorsal vascular and neural reanastomosis is the best method of repair.
    d. Primary macroscopic reanastomosis invariably results in erectile dysfunction.
    e. Skin loss is rarely a problem after macroscopic repair.

13. What is the best option for coverage of acute penile skin loss?
    a. Foreskin flap for small distal lesions
    b. Meshed skin graft in a young child
    c. Wet-to-dry dressings
    d. Thigh flaps
    e. Burying the penile shaft in a scrotal skin tunnel

14. Which is FALSE about penile fracture?
    a. Penile fracture must be repaired immediately for the best outcomes.
    b. Ultrasonography can identify location of the corporal tear.
    c. Magnetic resonance imaging (MRI) can demonstrate disruption of the tunica albuginea.
    d. Rupture of the dorsal penile artery can have the same presentation as penile fracture.
    e. Bilateral corporal injury is more commonly associated with urethral injury.

15. Advantages of open suprapubic tube placement after posterior urethral disruption injuries include:
    a. inspection of bladder.
    b. an opportunity for controlled antegrade urethral realignment.
    c. allowance for large-bore catheter insertion.
    d. not jeopardizing continence or potency rates.
    e. all of the above.

Imaging

1. See Figure 101-1. This CT scan in a 22-year-old man involved in a motor vehicle accident indicates that the most likely diagnosis is:
   a. extraperitoneal bladder injury.
   b. intraperitoneal bladder injury.
   c. bladder contusion.
   d. combined intraperitoneal and extraperitoneal bladder injury.
   e. ureteral injury.

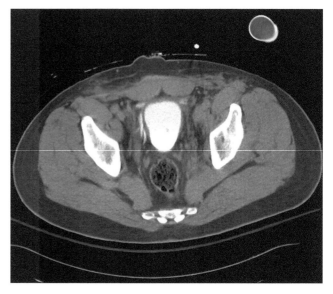

Figure 101-1.

ANSWERS

1. **d. Intraperitoneal bladder rupture.** When intraperitoneal bladder laceration occurs after blunt trauma, a large laceration of the bladder dome is usually produced that predisposes to urinary ascites and/or peritonitis if it is not repaired promptly.

2. **e. None of the above.** The CT cystogram must be performed via retrograde distention of the bladder with a diluted contrast medium. Most bladder lacerations are associated with gross hematuria, not microhematuria. A drainage film is required to complete a plain film cystogram.

3. **d. High mortality rate is primarily related to nonurologic comorbidities.** Bladder lacerations occur in approximately 10% of pelvic fractures and often occur in the context of multisystemic trauma.

4. **e. All of the above.** All of the listed concomitant injuries increase the risk of complications such as abscess, fistula, or incontinence.

5. **a. One-stage, open, perineal anastomotic urethroplasty is preferred.** Posterior urethral reconstruction including excision of the fibrotic segment with distal urethral mobilization and primary anastomosis is associated with the best long-term outcomes after urethral disruption. Incontinence occurs in less than 5% of patients.

6. **a. Retrograde urethrography.** Retrograde urethrography is the most reliable imaging study for urethral evaluation.

7. **e. Immediate primary repair of the left testis.** Immediate primary repair should be attempted in the setting of subtotal injury to an otherwise viable testis. Even extensive testicular injuries often can be safely salvaged, and tunica vaginalis grafts provide better outcomes than do synthetic grafts for complex repair.

8. **b. Spatulated, stented, tension-free, watertight repair of the urethra with absorbable sutures.** Immediate urethral repair with fine absorbable suture over a Foley catheter is associated with superior outcomes after penetrating injury. A proximal bulbar urethral pathologic process in a young man is uniquely amenable to primary anastomotic repair.

9. **c. Retrograde urethrography should be uniformly performed to assess for urethral injury.** Flexible cystoscopy performed at the time of surgical exploration is the simplest and most sensitive means to assess for urethral injury. Urethrography is of low yield in men with no hematuria, no blood at the meatus, and no voiding symptoms; intraoperative flexible cystoscopy is an appropriate alternative method of urethral evaluation.

10. **b. Tunica vaginalis.** Blood fills the space between the visceral and parietal layers of the tunica vaginalis.

11. **b. Is often diagnosed by the presence of intratesticular hypoechoic areas on ultrasonography.** Testicular rupture is often difficult to detect clinically. Ultrasound evaluation usually shows intratesticular heterogeneity as a sentinel finding; detection of a defect of the tunica albuginea is less common.

12. **c. Microscopic dorsal vascular and neural reanastomosis is the best method of repair.** Microvascular reanastomosis of the dorsal neurovascular structures is suggested as the preferred treatment modality whenever possible. Reanastomosis of the corporeal arteries is not recommended.

13. **a. Foreskin flap for small distal lesions.** Redundant foreskin provides excellent closure when ample viable tissue exists.

14. **a. Penile fracture must be repaired immediately or there is a decrement in erectile function.** Recent data has shown that a delay in surgery of as long as 7 days has no effect on the outcomes of penile fracture.

15. **e. All of the above.** Antegrade urethral realignment may simplify treatment of the defect, and a large-bore suprapubic catheter placed near the midline will promote subsequent identification of the prostatic apex during delayed reconstruction while preventing tube encrustation or obstruction.

Imaging

1. **a. Extraperitoneal bladder injury.** There is stranding in the soft tissues around the urinary bladder, and extraluminal contrast medium is seen in the space of Retzius anterior to the bladder, as well as in the right perivesical space. With intraperitoneal injuries, contrast medium would outline the bowel and not be confined to the perivesical space. Ureteral injuries are unusual with blunt abdominal trauma and would not have this appearance.

CHAPTER REVIEW

1. Penile fracture generally occurs at the base of the penis in a ventrolateral location where the tunica albuginea is thinnest.

2. If the location of the penile fracture is evident, a vertical ventral penile incision over the injury may be used. If the location of the injury is uncertain or there is an associated urethral injury, a distal circumcising incision should be made; if this incision is used in an uncircumcised patient, a limited circumcision should be performed before closure to prevent persistent edema of the foreskin.

3. Dog bites of the penis are treated with copious irrigation, debridement, and primary closure. Human bites should be irrigated, debrided, treated with antibiotics, and left open.

4. A fractured testis should be explored and repaired because the salvage rate is higher than when conservative nonoperative therapy is used.

5. Ninety percent of bladder ruptures are associated with pelvic fractures; 10% of pelvic fractures are associated with a bladder rupture.

6. Noncomplicated extraperitoneal bladder ruptures may be treated with urethral catheter drainage alone.

7. The bulbomembranous junction is more vulnerable to injury during pelvic fracture than is the prostatomembranous junction; thus, the external sphincter is often intact. In children, urethral disruptions generally occur at the bladder neck. In females, the urethral avulsion usually occurs proximally.

8. In females, urethral disruptions should be primarily repaired and vaginal lacerations should be closed.

9. Initial suprapubic cystostomy is the standard of care for major straddle injuries involving the urethra.

10. When intraperitoneal bladder laceration occurs after blunt trauma, a large laceration of the bladder dome is usually produced that predisposes to urinary ascites and/or peritonitis if it is not repaired promptly.

11. The CT cystogram must be performed via retrograde distention of the bladder with a dilute contrast medium. A drainage film is required to complete a plain film cystogram.

12. Flexible cystoscopy performed at the time of surgical exploration is the simplest and most sensitive means to assess for urethral injury.

13. In posterior urethral disruptions, urethral realignment, if done without dissection and expeditiously, may make a subsequent repair unnecessary or at the least realign the two ends, facilitating the repair.

102 Development, Molecular Biology, and Physiology of the Prostate

Ronald Rodriguez and Ashley Evan Ross

QUESTIONS

1. Which of the following is NOT considered a sex accessory tissue?
   a. Prostate gland
   b. Seminal vesicles
   c. Tunica albuginea
   d. Ampullae
   e. Bulbourethral gland

2. Which fetal hormone stimulates the development of the wolffian ducts?
   a. Estradiol
   b. Dihydrotestosterone (DHT)
   c. Estrone
   d. Testosterone
   e. Inhibin

3. Which one of the following statements about fetal development of the lower urogenital tract is FALSE?
   a. The urogenital sinus derives from the cloaca.
   b. The cloaca gets its name (L. "sewer") because it receives input from the gastrointestinal and urinary tracts.
   c. The seminal vesicles derive from the posterior portion of the wolffian ducts, whereas the prostate derives from the anterior portion.
   d. Sox9 is an early molecular marker of prostate development.
   e. The urogenital sinus is a primordial structure that contributes to bladder *and* prostate development.

4. Which fetal hormone is most important in stimulating the growth of the prostate during development?
   a. Estradiol
   b. DHT
   c. Estrone
   d. Testosterone
   e. Inhibin

5. Which one of the following statements is TRUE regarding the role of androgens in prostate development?
   a. Males will develop prostates in the presence of sufficiently high levels of androgens, but females will not.
   b. Females will develop prostates in the presence of sufficiently high levels of androgens, but males will not.
   c. Both males and females will develop prostates in the presence of sufficiently high levels of androgens.
   d. Prostate tissue rudiments with a normal androgen receptor in the epithelium but mutant androgen receptor in the mesenchyme will develop into normal prostates in the presence of sufficiently high levels of androgen.
   e. Prostate tissue rudiments with androgen receptor overexpression in the epithelium but mutant androgen receptor in the mesenchyme will develop into normal prostates in the absence of androgen.

6. Which α_1-adrenergic receptor subtype is linked to smooth muscle contraction in the prostate?
   a. α_D
   b. α_{1A}
   c. α_{1B}
   d. α_2
   e. α_{2B}

7. Which of the following is TRUE regarding testosterone?
   a. Testosterone is synthesized by the Sertoli cells of the testes.
   b. Testosterone is synthesized by the Leydig cells of the testes.
   c. Testosterone is a direct precursor of pregnenolone.
   d. 5α-Reductase is an enzyme that converts DHT into testosterone.
   e. Aromatase converts estrogens into testosterone.

8. Dehydroepiandrosterone (DHEA) has been suggested as a major source of testosterone within the plasma. What percentage of total testosterone has been determined to be derived from DHEA?
   a. 1%
   b. 2%
   c. 5%
   d. 15%
   e. 20%

9. To what is the majority of testosterone in the plasma bound?
   a. Insulin
   b. Cholesterol
   c. Prostaglandins
   d. TP53
   e. Sex hormone-binding globulin (SHBG)

10. Which 5α-reductase isoform predominates in the prostate gland?

    a. Type 1

    b. Type 2

    c. Type 3

    d. Type 4

    e. Type 5

11. What is the source of fructose in seminal plasma?

    a. Prostate gland

    b. Bulbourethral gland

    c. Vas deferens

    d. Seminal vesicles

    e. Basal cells

12. Compartmentalization of the androgen receptor from the cytosol to the nucleus is dependent on:

    a. dimerization.

    b. adenosine triphosphate (ATP).

    c. RAN-mediated transport.

    d. nuclear localization and nuclear export signals.

    e. all of the above.

13. Which feature of the androgen receptor polymorphisms is thought to impact on the overall activity of androgen target gene induction?

    a. Zinc finger motifs

    b. Poly CAG repeats

    c. Nuclear export signals

    d. Ligand binding domain

14. Which of the following is TRUE with regard to the effects of estrogens in prostate development?

    a. Estrogens are not required for the development of a prostate because ER-α and ER-β knockout mice have phenotypically normal prostates.

    b. ER-α regulates ductal formation.

    c. ER-β is required for prostates to allow sperm to mature to an active form.

    d. b and c

15. When the androgen receptor binds to an androgen response element, which of the following is (are) true?

    a. The dimerization of the receptor is always head to head, regardless of whether the sequence is a direct repeat or an inverted repeat.

    b. The dimerization occurs head to head for an inverted repeat and head to tail for a direct repeat.

    c. The dimerization of the androgen receptor occurs on the DNA template in a process that requires ATP and heat shock proteins.

    d. The androgen receptor can bind to a target androgen response element in either a head-to-head or a head-to-tail orientation, depending on the orientation of the structural gene.

ANSWERS

1. **c. Tunica albuginea.** Sex accessory tissues include the prostate gland, seminal vesicles, ampullae, and bulbourethral glands. They are believed to play a major, but unknown, role in the reproductive process.

2. **d. Testosterone.** The wolffian ducts develop into the seminal vesicles, epididymis, vas deferens, ampulla, and ejaculatory duct; the developmental growth of this group of glands is stimulated by fetal testosterone and not DHT.

3. **c. The seminal vesicles derive from the posterior portion of the wolffian ducts, whereas the prostate derives from the anterior portion.** The prostate develops from the urogenital sinus, not the wolffian duct.

4. **b. DHT.** The prostate first appears and starts its development from the urogenital sinus during the third month of fetal growth and development is directed primarily by DHT, not testosterone.

5. **c. Both males and females will develop prostates in the presence of sufficiently high levels of androgens.** If androgen (testosterone or DHT) levels are sufficiently high at the right time in fetal development, prostate development will proceed in the urogenital sinus regardless of whether the embryo is male or female. For prostate development to proceed, androgen receptor is required to be functional in the mesenchyme.

6. **b. α_{1A}.** Research work has demonstrated three subtypes of the α_1-adrenergic receptor (α_{1A}, α_{1B}, and α_{1D}), of which the α_{1A} receptor appears to be linked to contraction.

7. **b. Testosterone is synthesized by the Leydig cells of the testes.** Foremost among the hormones and growth factors that stimulate the prostate is the prohormone testosterone, which must be converted within the prostate into the active androgen DHT. Testosterone is synthesized in the Leydig cells of the testes from pregnenolone by a series of reversible reactions; however, once testosterone is reduced by 5α-reductase into DHT or to estrogens by aromatase, the process is irreversible. In other words, whereas testosterone can be converted into DHT and into estrogens, estrogens and DHT cannot be converted into testosterone.

8. **a. 1%.** Less than 1% of the total testosterone in the plasma is derived from DHEA.

9. **e. Sex hormone-binding globulin (SHBG).** The majority of testosterone bound to plasma protein is associated with SHBG.

10. **b. Type 2.** The type 2 isoform is mutated in 5α-reductase deficiency and is the dominant isoform present in the prostate gland.

11. **d. Seminal vesicles.** The source of fructose in human seminal plasma is the seminal vesicles. Patients with congenital absence of the seminal vesicles also have an associated absence of fructose in their ejaculates.

12. **e. All of the above.** After binding ligand, the androgen receptor dissociates from chaperonins, dimerizes, and then is transported to the nucleus via a nuclear localization motif, which activates Ran-dependent active transport, a process that is ATP dependent.

13. **b. Poly CAG repeats.** The shorter the length, the more actively the androgen receptor is thought to function.

14. **a. Estrogens are not required for the development of a prostate because ER-α and ER-β knockout mice have phenotypically normal prostates.**

15. **a. The dimerization of the receptor is always head to head, regardless of whether the sequence is a direct repeat or an inverted repeat.** Although most models predicted that inverted repeat and direct repeat androgen response elements would have dimers that bind with opposite polarity, this prediction was not observed in x-ray crystallography studies.

CHAPTER REVIEW

1. The seminal vesicles are extremely resistant to disease.
2. There are two major cellular components in the prostate: epithelial and stromal.
3. The stromal component consists of connective tissue, smooth muscle cells, and fibroblasts.
4. The epithelial component consists of basal cells, intermediate cells, and neuroendocrine cells.
5. The prostate contains a rich plexus of autonomic nerves.
6. Because of the diurnal variation of serum testosterone, to avoid inconsistency it should be measured in the morning.
7. The role of circulating adrenal androgens on prostate growth is minor.
8. Because the plasma half-life of testosterone is 10 to 20 minutes, patients who undergo bilateral orchiectomy are functionally castrate within 1 to 2 hours after surgery.
9. The androgen receptor is transported to the nucleus and then back to the cytoplasm; nuclear matrix is the major target for androgen and estrogen receptor binding in the nucleus.
10. The longer the CAG repeat in the androgen receptor, the lower its activity in activating target genes.
11. The source of prostaglandins, fructose, and semenogelin is the seminal vesicle.
12. The seminal vesicle contributes the most volume to the seminal fluid.
13. The source of citrate, zinc, spermine, and choline is the prostate.
14. Prostate-specific antigen is a serine protease and degrades semenogelin. Semenogelin gives rise to the coagulation of semen.
15. Complexed PSA is irreversibly bound to alpha1-antichymotrypsin and alpha2-macroglobulin.
16. Increases in human kallikrein 2, pro-PSA, and bound PSA are associated with prostate cancer.
17. Few drugs reach concentrations in the prostatic secretions that approach or surpass their concentrations in the serum. The exceptions include erythromycin, oleandomycin, sulfonamides, tetracycline, clindamycin, trimethoprim, and the fluoroquinolones.
18. Prostatic fluid is more acidic than is serum.
19. Acid phosphatase produced in the prostate may be elevated in prostate cancer; it is also produced in the bone and may be elevated in diseases that affect the bone such as Paget disease, osteoporosis, and bone metastases.
20. The wolffian ducts develop into the seminal vesicles, epididymis, vas deferens, ampulla, and ejaculatory duct; the developmental growth of this group of glands is stimulated by fetal testosterone and not DHT.
21. Testosterone is reduced by 5α-reductase into DHT or to estrogens by aromatase; the process is irreversible.

103 Benign Prostatic Hyperplasia: Etiology, Pathophysiology, Epidemiology, and Natural History

Claus G. Roehrborn

QUESTIONS

1. Which statement is correct regarding the role of androgenic hormones in the etiology of benign prostatic hyperplasia (BPH)?

   a. Testosterone and dihydrotestosterone are the sole causes of the hyperplasia taking place in the prostate after the age of 40 years.

   b. The total amount of androgen receptors in the prostate decreases with aging, leading to a lesser response to androgenic stimuli.

   c. Dihydrotestosterone is considered the more potent of the androgenic steroid hormones by a factor of approximately 10:1.

   d. Of the two 5α-reductase isoforms, type 1 is most commonly found in the prostate.

   e. Only testosterone produced in the testis and not in the adrenal gland enters into the prostate gland.

2. Regarding genetic and familial factors in the etiology of BPH, which statement is TRUE?

   a. There is no evidence that BPH is a familial disease.

   b. Any man who has undergone transurethral resection of the prostate (TURP) should alert his sons that their chances of requiring TURP is three times greater than age-matched controls.

   c. Cases of familial BPH tend to occur in men with smaller prostates than the sporadic cases of BPH.

   d. Approximately 50% of cases of BPH in men who undergo surgery when younger than the age of 60 years are estimated to be inheritable.

   e. The most likely inheritance pattern is autosomal recessive.

3. The prevalence of a disease is defined as the number of:

   a. diseased people per 100,000 population per year.

   b. existing cases per 100,000 population at a distinct target date.

   c. deaths per 100,000 population per year.

   d. deaths per number of diseased.

   e. cumulative cases of a disease over a specified time period.

4. Concerning the autopsy prevalence of BPH or stromoglandular hyperplasia of the prostate, which statement is correct?

   a. No adequate studies have been done to date.

   b. It is commonly found in men of all ages.

   c. It is very uncommon in men younger than 30 years.

   d. It is found in 100% of men beginning at the age of 40 years.

   e. International comparisons are impossible because of a lack of its definition.

5. Which of the following statements regarding the International Prostate Symptom Score (IPSS) is TRUE?

   a. Moderate symptom severity is defined as a score from 12 to 22 points.

   b. The IPSS score addresses voiding and storage symptoms as well as questions regarding incontinence.

   c. Quantitative symptom scores in BPH are not as important as are objective measures such as a flow rate recording.

   d. The IPSS score has been translated and validated in many languages.

   e. Physicians and nurses may fill out the IPSS score for their patients after consultation.

6. Which statement is TRUE regarding prostate volume?

   a. International studies show significant similarity in prostate volume in white, age-stratified men.

   b. Prostate volume assessment by digital rectal examination (DRE) is reproducible across examiners.

   c. Although there is a steady increase in total prostate volume with age, the transition zone volume increases only marginally.

   d. Magnetic resonance imaging (MRI) measurements are, in general, smaller compared with transrectal ultrasound measurements.

   e. DRE estimation of prostate volume is fairly accurate when done by an experienced urologist.

7. Concerning liver disease and BPH, which of the following statements is TRUE?

   a. Ethanol consumption increases circulating levels of estrogens.

   b. The risk of having surgery for BPH is increased in heavy drinkers.

   c. The intake of ethanol can decrease serum testosterone levels by a variety of mechanisms.

   d. Most autopsy studies find a higher prevalence of BPH in men with liver cirrhosis.

   e. In men with liver disease, histologic specimens of the prostate show a similar influence of estrogen such as seen in hormonally treated prostate cancer.

8. How do medications influence symptoms and flow rate?

   a. There is no documented influence of any medication on symptoms or flow rate.

   b. Antihistamines and bronchodilators significantly decrease urinary flow rates.

   c. Calcium channel blockers and β-adrenergic blockers reduce urinary flow rates significantly.

   d. Antidepressants, antihistamines, and bronchodilators increase the symptom score by several points.

   e. Anticholinergic agents decrease the peak urinary flow rate markedly.

9. Concerning correlations between baseline parameters, which statement is TRUE?

   a. A clinically useful correlation exists between prostate volume and serum prostate-specific antigen (PSA) level.

   b. Many studies have shown a significant correlation between the transition zone volume and symptom severity.

c. Correlation of symptoms, bother, interference, and quality of life are poor.

d. Urinary flow rate and prostate volume correlate highly with serum PSA level.

e. Serum PSA level shows a strong correlation with symptom frequency and bother.

10. Which statement is correct regarding the study of the natural history of BPH?

a. Placebo groups from treatment trials are useful because they do not have treatment biases.

b. A longitudinal population-based study has the fewest biases and is the most useful type of study.

c. Control groups from intervention or medical therapy trials reflect the natural history of the disease in unselected community-dwelling men.

d. Placebo groups have fewer selection biases compared with population-based studies.

e. No such studies have been conducted.

11. Regarding the magnitude of the placebo response and its perception, which of the following statements is TRUE?

a. Placebo response is not dependent on the baseline severity score.

b. Most patients report subjective improvement when the drop from baseline is 30%.

c. The higher the baseline score, the more of a drop is required for patients to subjectively feel improved.

d. Perception of improvement is independent of baseline score.

e. There are convincing data to demonstrate that the final score after treatment is more important than the baseline score or the drop from baseline.

12. Descriptive studies of the incidence rates of acute urinary retention (AUR) have demonstrated that:

a. depending on the population studied, incidence rates less than 5 to more than 130 cases/1000 man-years have been reported.

b. the incidence rates reported do not differ significantly between various studies and populations.

c. AUR has been poorly defined, and therefore no incidence rate can be calculated.

d. incidence rates of approximately 10/1000 man-years have been reported in all watchful waiting studies.

e. incidence rates of AUR have not been reported in the urologic literature, only prevalence rates.

13. What is the most significant finding regarding analytical epidemiology of AUR?

a. Serum PSA level is a more powerful predictor of AUR than is age.

b. Serum PSA level and prostate volume have limited ability to predict episodes of AUR.

c. Urinary flow rates in placebo control groups are strong predictors of AUR episodes.

d. Age has been found to be the most significant risk factor for AUR in population-based studies.

e. There is virtually no relationship between symptom frequency and bother and AUR episodes.

14. Which statement regarding surgery for BPH is TRUE?

a. The incidence rates of surgery are similar across wide geographic regions and ethnic backgrounds.

b. AUR is a harder and more objective end point compared to surgery.

c. Surgery is a less common end point compared with AUR.

d. Most patients with BPH eventually require surgery for their condition.

e. Surgery rates for BPH have remained stable since approximately 1990.

ANSWERS

1. **c. Dihydrotestosterone is considered the more potent of the androgenic steroid hormones by a factor of approximately 10:1.** The androgenic steroid hormones testosterone and dihydrotestosterone (DHT) have a permissive role in the development of BPH but are not the sole cause. The androgen receptor remains at high levels in the prostate in aging men and specifically in BPH tissues, maintaining responsiveness to androgenic stimuli. The most common of the two 5α-reductase isoforms in the benignly enlarged prostate gland is type 2.

2. **d. Approximately 50% of cases of BPH in men who undergo surgery when younger than the age of 60 years are estimated to be inheritable.** There is significant evidence to suggest that some cases of BPH are familial, with autosomal dominant being the most likely inheritance pattern. An increased risk for BPH surgery exists mostly for men who come to BPH surgery when younger than the age of 60 years, and men with familial cases of BPH have larger glands than men with sporadic cases.

3. **b. Existing cases per 100,000 population at a distinct target date.** When studying diseases by descriptive or analytical epidemiologic methods, it is important to have a good understanding of the definitions that apply. Most epidemiologic terms are expressed as rates, which are the number of cases for persons expressed over the population. The definitions that are of relevance are incidence rates, which are equal to the number of people/100,000 population/year getting a certain disease; prevalence, which is the number of existing cases of the disease of interest/100,000 at a distinct target date; mortality rate, which is the number of deaths/100,000 population/year; and fatality, which equals the number of deaths due to the disease/number of diseased people.

4. **c. It is very uncommon in men younger than the age of 30 years.** The autopsy prevalence of BPH has been studied as early as 1984 by Berry and colleagues.* Since then, many studies have been done on virtually all continents in many ethnic groups. It is astonishing that these studies find a very significant agreement in terms of the actual prevalence of histologic BPH or stromoglandular hyperplasia around the world. Stromoglandular hyperplasia or BPH is very uncommon in men younger than the age of 30 years, but then increases steadily in an almost linear manner. In fact, approximately 90% of men in their 80s have evidence of stromoglandular hyperplasia.

5. **d. The IPSS score has been translated and validated in many languages.** The IPSS symptom score is a seven-question, self-administered questionnaire that yields a total score ranging from 0 to 35 points. Men who score 0 to 7 points are classified as mildly symptomatic, those scoring from 8 to 19 points as moderately symptomatic, and those scoring from 20 to 35 points as severely symptomatic. The IPSS score addresses both voiding and storage, but not incontinence symptomatology. It is widely accepted that quantitative symptom scores are more important than, for example, urinary flow rate recordings. The IPSS score, the most widely utilized instrument, has been translated and culturally validated in many languages. Providers should abstain from filling in the questionnaire for their patients as it is validated as a self-reported symptom severity instrument.

6. **a. International studies show significant similarity in prostate volume in white, age-stratified men.** Prostate volume can

---

*Sources referenced can be found in *Campbell-Walsh Urology, 11th Edition*, on the Expert Consult website.

relatively easily be assessed by transrectal ultrasonography (TRUS). TRUS has been found to be a reliable measure that is reproducible across examiners, in contrast to digital rectal examination (DRE), which is only poorly reproducible. MRI is very expensive and it yields in general a larger volume compared with TRUS measurements. Of note is the fact that international studies show significant similarity in regard to total and transitional zone prostate volume in white, age-stratified men.

7. **c. The intake of ethanol can decrease serum testosterone levels by a variety of mechanisms.** It is known that alcohol intake may decrease plasma testosterone levels by reducing production of and increasing clearance of testosterone. However, despite this hypothetical reason for a lower incidence, an inverse relationship has been described. The age-adjusted multivariate relative risks for undergoing surgery for BPH in men drinking more than three or four glasses of alcohol per day is lower than in age-matched controls. Of course, this could be due to a bias against surgery in patients who are heavy drinkers and therefore in poor health. It is interesting to note, however, that in the majority of studies, namely, four of five, a lower prevalence of BPH is found in men with cirrhosis compared with those without cirrhosis.

8. **d. Antidepressants, antihistamines, and bronchodilators increase the symptom score by several points.** There is only one study that systematically assessed the effect of medications on urinary symptoms and flow rate. Cold medications containing α-sympathomimetics tend to exacerbate lower urinary tract symptoms by the expected effect on the smooth muscle of the bladder outlet. Data from the Olmsted County Study of Urinary Symptoms and Health Status Among Men show that daily use of antidepressants, antihistamines, or bronchodilators is associated with a 2- to 3-point increase in the symptom score. However, only the daily use of antidepressants is associated with a decrease in the age-adjusted urinary flow rate.

9. **a. A clinically useful correlation exists between prostate volume and serum PSA level.** In general there is an absence of useful baseline correlations between subjective and objective parameters such as symptoms, frequency, quality of life, and urinary flow rate measures of obstruction and prostate volume. However, symptom, bother, and interference with quality of life show excellent correlation with each other, and a clinically useful correlation exists between total and transition zone prostate volume and serum PSA in men with BPH.

10. **b. A longitudinal population-based study has the fewest biases and is the most useful type of study.** There are several ways to study the natural history of BPH. One can look at watchful waiting cohorts or placebo-controlled groups of medication trials, or study population-based groups of men longitudinally over time. The latter is clearly the best way of studying the natural history of the disease because it incurs the fewest biases.

However, it is also the most tedious and most expensive method. Placebo groups in medication trials clearly suffer from enrollment biases but do provide useful information.

11. **c. The higher the baseline score, the more of a drop is required for patients to subjectively feel improved.** The placebo response is partially a regression to the mean and partially an effect induced by the interaction between patient and doctor. The response is clearly dependent on the baseline severity score, with patients' higher scores having a larger decrease from baseline. The perception of subjective improvement has been shown to be dependent on the drop from baseline as well as on the baseline itself. For example, the higher the baseline score, the more of a drop from baseline is required for patients to have a subjective perception of improvement. Overall, a 3-point decrease is associated with a subjective perception of improvement.

12. **a. Depending on the population studied, incidence rates less than 5 to more than 130 cases/1000 man-years have been reported.** AUR has been studied during the past few years in population-based studies as well as in placebo-control groups from long-term treatment trials. The incidence rates differ significantly between different studies because of the inclusion and exclusion criteria and selection biases. Fortunately, AUR is a very clearly defined outcome and, thus, incidence rates can easily be calculated and compared.

13. **d. Age has been found to be the most significant risk factor for AUR in population-based studies.** In population-based studies such as the Olmsted County Study of Urinary Symptoms and Health Status Among Men, age is the most significant predictor of AUR. Data from placebo groups of long-term medical treatment trials demonstrate that serum PSA is the most powerful predictor of AUR together with prostate volume. Although this appears on the surface to be a contradiction, it can be relatively easily explained by the fact that in BPH treatment trials, elderly men with already an existing diagnosis of BPH are enrolled. Thus, age plays a lesser factor in terms of predicting AUR. In population-based studies in which men stratified by age are followed during long periods of time, age plays a more significant factor compared with PSA.

14. **b. AUR is a harder and more objective end point compared with surgery.** Incidence rates of surgery vary significantly across geographic regions and patients with different ethnic backgrounds. Depending on the interaction between patient and physician, the physician can convince the patient to undergo surgery or, based on the patient's comorbidities, talk him out of surgery. The same cannot be said for urinary retention. It is clear that a vast majority of patients do not require surgery in the course of their disease but, rather, can be treated effectively with reassurance alone or medication.

CHAPTER REVIEW

1. BPH is characterized by an increased number of epithelial and stromal cells, not an increase in their size.
2. Androgens are required for normal cell proliferation and differentiation and actively inhibit cell death.
3. Serum estrogen levels increase in men with age.
4. Early periurethral nodules are stromal; transition zone proliferation is glandular.
5. Prostatic stroma represents 40% of the gland. Smooth muscle is a prominent component of the stroma.
6. Autonomic system overactivity may contribute to lower urinary tract symptoms in men with BPH; the alpha 1a receptor is the most abundant form in the prostate.
7. Symptoms that use the AUA Symptom Index are classified as mild if the score is 0 to 7, moderate if it is 8 to 19, and severe if it is 20 to 35. A change of 3 points or more from time to time is subjectively discernible.
8. Men and women experience a decrease in maximum urinary flow rate as they age.
9. Bladder fibrosis is seen in both sexes with advancing age.
10. After spontaneous acute urinary retention (AUR), 15% of patients will have another episode and three fourths will undergo surgery; after precipitated AUR, 9% will have another episode and 26% will undergo surgery.
11. A significant portion of male lower urinary tract symptoms is related to age-related detrusor dysfunction and other conditions unrelated to the prostate.
12. DHT, the most potent androgen in the prostate, and androgen receptors remain high with age.
13. Androgen withdrawal results in apoptosis of prostate cells.
14. Estrogen receptors are found in the prostate and may play a role in BPH.
15. The size of the prostate does not correlate with the degree of obstruction.

16. Trabeculation is due to an increase in detrusor collagen.
17. A maximum flow rate less than 10 mL/sec in the male indicates a high probability of obstruction.
18. There is no relationship between vasectomy and BPH; however, there is a positive relationship between lack of physical activity, obesity, BMI, and LUTS/BPH.
19. Hydronephrosis is found in 7.6% of patients having surgery for BPH, one third of whom have renal insufficiency.
20. Some cases of BPH are familial, with autosomal dominant being the most likely inheritance pattern. Patients with familial BPH tend to have larger glands than those with sporadic BPH.
21. Cold medications containing α-sympathomimetics tend to exacerbate lower urinary tract symptoms by the expected effect on the smooth muscle of the bladder outlet.
22. A clinically useful correlation exists between total and transition zone prostate volume and serum PSA in men with BPH.

104 Evaluation and Nonsurgical Management of Benign Prostatic Hyperplasia

Thomas Anthony McNicholas, Mark J. Speakman, and Roger S. Kirby

QUESTIONS

1. Where does benign prostatic hyperplasia (BPH) originate? In the:
   a. transition zone.
   b. peripheral zone.
   c. periurethral glands.
   d. transition zone and periurethral zone.
   e. peripheral and periurethral zones.

2. A strong correlation exists between prostate volume and:
   a. serum prostate-specific antigen (PSA).
   b. American Urological Association (AUA) symptom score.
   c. peak urinary flow rate.
   d. postvoid residual.
   e. all of the above

3. Medications that may exacerbate lower urinary tract symptoms (LUTS) include:
   a. α-adrenergic antagonists.
   b. α-adrenergic agonists.
   c. β-adrenergic agonists.
   d. muscarinic agonists.
   e. phytotherapy.

4. What is the primary objective of the digital rectal examination (DRE) in evaluation of men with LUTS? To:
   a. estimate prostate volume.
   b. obtain prostatic secretions.
   c. identify prostate nodules.
   d. determine rectal tone.
   e. assess for prostatic tenderness.

5. In older men with LUTS, which test should be routinely performed to obtain the differential diagnosis?
   a. Urinalysis
   b. Peak flow rate
   c. Serum creatinine assay
   d. Renal ultrasonography
   e. Flexible cystoscopy

6. It is advisable in a man with LUTS/BPH and a slightly elevated creatinine level to perform:
   a. transurethral resection of the prostate (TURP).
   b. intravenous pyelogram.
   c. renal ultrasound.
   d. urodynamic study.
   e. flexible cystoscopy.

7. What percentage of men have histologically proven BPH with a serum PSA value of 4.0 ng/mL or greater?
   a. 5%
   b. 15%
   c. 30%
   d. 50%
   e. 80%

8. An AUA symptom score of 20 indicates severe:
   a. LUTS.
   b. BPH.
   c. bladder outlet obstruction.
   d. bladder dysfunction.
   e. overactive bladder (OAB).

9. An absolute indication for surgery (TURP or open prostatectomy) is:
   a. severe symptoms.
   b. postvoid residual (PVR) urine of 300 mL or more.
   c. single episodes of acute urinary retention.
   d. refractory gross hematuria secondary to BPH.
   e. Lack of response to an alpha blocker.

10. A low peak flow rate suggests:
    a. severe symptoms.
    b. bladder outlet obstruction.
    c. impaired detrusor contractility.
    d. b or c.
    e. detrusor overactivity.

11. What is the next step for a man with a PVR of 300 mL?
    a. Repeat the PVR assay
    b. Upper urinary tract imaging
    c. Urodynamic testing
    d. Cystoscopy
    e. TURP

12. The probability that a urodynamic study helps to decrease the failure rate of TURP in men with a peak flow rate of 15 mL/sec is approximately:
    a. 10%.
    b. 25%.
    c. 50%.
    d. 75%.
    e. 95%.

13. What is the percentage of men with LUTS who have uninhibited contraction?
    a. 10%
    b. 30%

c. 60%

d. 80%

e. 95%

14. What is the likelihood that uninhibited detrusor contractions (UDCs) in men with BPH will resolve after TURP?

a. Never

b. Unlikely

c. Likely

d. Always

15. The finding of bladder trabeculation suggests:

a. high-grade obstruction.

b. high successful rate after TURP.

c. high PVR.

d. chronic inflammation.

e. none of the above.

16. Imaging of the upper tract is indicated for:

a. prostate glands weighing more than 50 g.

b. urinalysis demonstrating hematuria.

c. bladder trabeculation.

d. severe LUTS.

e. PSA > 1.5 ng/mL.

17. An improvement in the AUA symptom score of 5 units correlates with which level of symptoms improved?

a. Marked

b. Moderate

c. Slight

d. None

18. Urodynamic testing reliably predicts response after:

a. TURP.

b. α-adrenergic blockers.

c. 5α-reductase inhibitors.

d. antimuscarinic therapy.

e. none of the above.

19. There is compelling evidence that PVR is:

a. related to symptom severity.

b. associated with the risk for urinary tract infection (UTI).

c. both a and b.

d. neither a nor b.

20. The definition of detrusor overactivity is bladder pressure greater than which level at a bladder volume of 300 mL or less?

a. 5 cm H_2O

b. 15 cm H_2O

c. 40 cm H_2O

d. 60 cm H_2O

21. The likelihood that a man with acute urinary retention will experience a subsequent episode of urinary retention within 1 week is approximately:

a. 20%.

b. 40%.

c. 60%.

d. 80%.

e. 100%.

22. The incidence of developing acute urinary retention is related to:

a. prostate size.

b. age.

c. severity of symptoms.

d. PSA level.

e. all of the above.

23. The best way to eliminate bias in a clinical study is to use:

a. honest investigators.

b. a placebo-controlled double-blind design.

c. randomization.

d. a large sample size.

e. cohort studies.

24. The larger the sample size, the:

a. less treatment effect required to achieve statistical significance.

b. better the study.

c. greater the treatment effect required to achieve statistical significance.

d. none of the above.

e. all of the above.

25. Which of the following is the attractive feature of medical therapy relative to TURP?

a. Fewer side effects

b. Reversible side effects

c. Less serious side effects

d. All of the above

e. Reduced long-term costs

26. During the past decade, the incidence of TURP in the United States has decreased by approximately:

a. 10%.

b. 50%.

c. 100%.

d. 200%.

27. Which of the following percentages of men older than 50 years have moderate or severe LUTS?

a. 2%

b. 5%

c. 30%

d. 50%

28. The ideal candidate for medical therapy should have which type of symptoms?

a. Severe

b. Moderate

c. Minimal

d. Bothersome

29. Smooth muscle accounts for what percentage of the area density of the prostate?

a. 5%

b. 10%

c. 20%

d. 40%

e. 60%

30. The tension of prostate smooth muscle is mediated by the:
    a. α_1 receptor.
    b. α_2 receptor.
    c. β_1 receptor.
    d. β_2 receptor.
    e. muscarinic cholinergic receptor.

31. What is the advantage of terazosin versus prazosin?
    a. Its longer half-life
    b. Its better absorption
    c. Its greater $\alpha1$-receptor selectivity
    d. None of the above.

32. Which α_1 receptor subtype mediates prostate smooth muscle tension?
    a. α_{1a}
    b. α_{1b}
    c. α_{1c}
    d. α_{1d}
    e. None of the above

33. The improvement in AUA symptom score after terazosin administration depends on baseline:
    a. age.
    b. prostate size.
    c. PVR.
    d. None of the above.

34. The mean treatment-related improvement in response to terazosin in AUA symptom score units is approximately:
    a. 2.
    b. 4.
    c. 6.
    d. 8.

35. The durability of the improvement in symptom scores and peak flow rates for α_1-adrenergic blockers has been reported to be up to how many months?
    a. 12
    b. 42
    c. 60
    d. 92

36. Which of the following α-adrenergic blockers does not lower blood pressure in men with uncontrolled hypertension?
    a. Terazosin
    b. Doxazosin
    c. Tamsulosin
    d. Prazosin

37. Retrograde ejaculation is most commonly seen with:
    a. terazosin.
    b. silodosin.
    c. finasteride.
    d. tamsulosin.
    e. alfuzosin.

38. Approximately what percentage of men have both BPH and hypertension?
    a. 5%
    b. 15%

c. 30%
d. 50%
e. 70%

39. What is the likely mechanism for dizziness after α_1-adrenergic blocker therapy?
    a. Vascular
    b. Central nervous system
    c. Carotid baroreceptor
    d. None of the above

40. The major advantage of tamsulosin 0.4 mg versus terazosin 10 mg is:
    a. greater efficiency.
    b. less retrograde ejaculation.
    c. no dose titration.
    d. greater lowering of blood pressure.

41. The embryologic development of the prostate is mediated primarily by:
    a. testosterone.
    b. dihydrotestosterone.
    c. androstenedione.
    d. estradiol.

42. Finasteride significantly decreases the long-term risk of:
    a. acute urinary retention.
    b. surgical intervention.
    c. symptom progression.
    d. all of the above.
    e. none of the above.

43. Finasteride is most effective at relieving hematuria in men with:
    a. prostatitis.
    b. enlarged prostate.
    c. transurethral prostatectomy.
    d. obstructing prostate.
    e. small prostates

44. Dutasteride:
    a. is a dual inhibitor of type 1 and type 2 5α-reductase.
    b. is more effective than finasteride.
    c. results in a 95% reduction in PSA after 6 months of therapy.
    d. is less likely than finasteride to result in loss of libido.
    e. is cheaper than finasteride.

45. The adverse event that limits the use of flutamide as a primary treatment of BPH is:
    a. breast tenderness.
    b. diarrhea.
    c. erectile dysfunction.
    d. loss of libido.

46. A potential advantage of cetrorelix, a gonadotropin-releasing hormone antagonist, for the treatment of BPH is:
    a. lower cost.
    b. ability to titrate the level of androgen suppression.
    c. ease of administration.
    d. rapid response.

47. A Veterans Affairs study demonstrated that terazosin is more effective than finasteride at rapidly relieving symptoms in men with:
    a. small prostates.
    b. intermediate-size prostates.
    c. large prostates.
    d. all of the above.

48. The Medical Therapy of Prostatic Symptoms (MTOPS) study confirmed that:
    a. α-adrenergic blockers and 5α-reductase inhibitors are equivalent in relieving symptoms.
    b. α-adrenergic blockers reduce the risk of acute urinary retention during 7 years of treatment.
    c. finasteride reduces the risk of adenocarcinoma of the prostate.
    d. a combination of an α-adrenergic blocker and a 5α-reductase inhibitor is the most effective way of preventing BPH progression.
    e. combination therapy was more effective than monotherapy after 6 months' treatment.

49. The Combination of Avodart and Tamsulosin (CombAT) Study showed that in men with larger prostates:
    a. the combination of dutasteride and tamsulosin was more effective than either agent alone.
    b. with time, the symptomatic response to dutasteride exceeded that to tamsulosin.
    c. both of the above.
    d. none of the above.
    e. tamsulosin did not affect ejaculation.

50. Combination therapy in LUTS/BPH using dutasteride and tamsulosin:
    a. should be continued long-term in all patients who respond.
    b. may be reduced to dutasteride alone after 6 months in all patients.
    c. may be reduced to dutasteride alone in 80% of patients with a baseline IPSS less than 20, after 6 months' treatment.
    d. may be reduced to dutasteride alone in all patients with a baseline IPSS less than 20, after 6 months' treatment.
    e. may be reduced to tamsulosin alone in in 80% of patients with a baseline IPSS less than 20, after 6 months' treatment.

51. The CombAT study showed that in men with a pretreatment PSA between 1.5 and 10 ng/mL:
    a. the combination of dutasteride and tamsulosin was more effective than either drug alone in improving symptoms.
    b. in men with larger prostates, although the tamsulosin effect was rapid, with time dutasteride was the more effective agent.
    c. combination therapy was significantly superior to tamsulosin but not dutasteride at reducing the RR of AUR or BPH-related surgery.
    d. none of the above.
    e. all of the above.

52. Antimuscarinic therapy is contraindicated in men with LUTS/BPH.
    a. Yes, in all such men.
    b. No, only in men with large and persistent residual urine volumes.

    c. No, not if combined with alpha blockers.
    d. Yes, if they have an enlarged prostate.
    e. No, OK in all men with OAB symptoms.

53. Men with significant obstruction, large residual urine volumes, and OAB who fail first line treatment with alpha blockers should be considered for:
    a. the addition of an antimuscarinic drug.
    b. surgical therapy.
    c. none of the above.
    d. the addition of phosphodiesterase 1 (PDE-1) inhibitors.
    e. psychotherapy.

54. Overactive bladder (OAB) symptoms in the male are:
    a. always secondary to bladder outflow obstruction (BOO).
    b. occur in all men with proven bladder outflow obstruction.
    c. should always be investigated with a filling/voiding cystometrogram.
    d. always secondary to benign prostatic enlargement (BPE).
    e. none of the above.

55. Studies of the use of antimuscarinic agents in men with LUTS and a significant storage component have shown that:
    a. the combination of tamsulosin and tolterodine showed a significant benefit over placebo in a patient's perception of benefit question.
    b. the number needed to treat was 5.
    c. trospium XR was safe and effective with significantly reduced frequency and urgency incontinence.
    d. fesoterodine added to an alpha blocker resulted in improvements in urinary frequency and bother.
    e. all of the above.

56. If a man with LUTs, stabilized on doxazosin, complains of erectile dysfunction, one should NOT give him:
    a. low-dose sildenafil.
    b. low-dose vardenafil.
    c. low-dose tadalafil.
    d. MUSE.
    e. a vacuum pump.

57. The amount spent on phytotherapy for the treatment of BPH is estimated to be:
    a. $10 million.
    b. $100 million.
    c. $1 billion.
    d. $10 billion.

58. The definitive mechanism of action for *Serenoa repens* is:
    a. inhibition of 5α-reductase.
    b. inhibition of cyclooxygenase.
    c. inhibition of lipoxygenase.
    d. inconclusive.

59. Potential future therapeutic avenues in BPH pharmacotherapy include:
    a. nitric oxide donors.
    b. α-adrenoceptor agonists.
    c. HMG coenzyme A inhibitors.
    d. endothelin antagonists.

ANSWERS

1. **d. Transition zone and periurethral zone.** The proliferative process originates in the transition zone and the periurethral glands.
2. **a. Serum prostate-specific antigen (PSA).** A strong correlation exists between serum PSA levels and prostate volume.
3. **b. α-adrenergic agonists.** Current prescription and over-the-counter medications should be examined to determine whether the patient is taking drugs that impair bladder contractility (anticholinergics) or that increase outflow resistance (α-sympathomimetics).
4. **c. Identify prostate nodules.** The DRE and neurologic examination are done to detect prostate or rectal malignancy, to evaluate anal sphincter tone, and to rule out any neurologic problems that may cause the presenting symptoms.
5. **a. Urinalysis.** In older men with BPH and a higher prevalence of serious urinary tract disorders, the benefits of an innocuous test such as urinalysis clearly outweigh the harm involved.
6. **c. Renal ultrasound.** An elevated serum creatinine level in a patient with BPH is an indication for imaging studies (ultrasonography) to evaluate the upper urinary tract.
7. **c. 30%.** Twenty-eight percent of men with histologically proven BPH have a serum PSA level greater than 4.0 ng/mL.
8. **a. LUTS.** The International Prostate Symptom Score (I-PSS), which is identical to the AUA Symptom Index, is recommended as the symptom scoring instrument to be used for the baseline assessment of symptom severity in men presenting with LUTS. When the I-PSS system is used, symptoms can be classified as mild (0 to 7), moderate (8 to 19), or severe (20 to 35). The I-PSS cannot be used to establish the diagnosis of BPH.
9. **d. Refractory gross hematuria secondary to BPH.** Surgery is recommended if the patient has refractory urinary retention (at least one failed attempt at catheter removal) or any of the following conditions, clearly secondary to BPH: recurrent urinary tract infection, recurrent gross hematuria, bladder stones, renal insufficiency, or large bladder diverticula.
10. **d. b or c.** One study found that flow rate recording cannot distinguish between bladder outlet obstruction and impaired detrusor contractility as the cause for a low Qmax.
11. **a. Repeat the PVR assay.** Residual urine volume measurement has significant intraindividual variability that limits its clinical usefulness.
12. **a. 10%.** One study recommended invasive urodynamic testing for patients with a Qmax higher than 15 mL/sec. For the population in their study, this would have resulted in an additional 9% of patients being excluded from surgery and a decrease in failure rate to 8.3%.
13. **c. 60%.** Overactive contractions are present in about 60% of men with LUTS and correlate strongly with irritative voiding symptoms.
14. **c. Likely.** UDCs resolve in most patients after surgery.
15. **e. None of the above.** Bladder trabeculation may predict a slightly higher failure rate in patients managed by watchful waiting but does not predict the success or failure of surgery.
16. **b. Urinalysis demonstrating hematuria.** Upper urinary tract imaging is not recommended for routine evaluation of men with LUTS unless they also have one or more of the following: hematuria; urinary tract infection; renal insufficiency (ultrasonography recommended); history of urolithiasis; and history of urinary tract surgery.
17. **b. Moderate.** The group mean changes in AUA Symptom Index for subjects rating their improvement as markedly, moderately, or slightly improved, unchanged, or worse were −8.8, −5.1, −3.0, −.7, and +2.7, respectively.
18. **e. None of the above.** Urodynamic testing does not predict symptom improvement after α-adrenergic blockade, transurethral microwave thermotherapy, or prostatectomy.
19. **d. Neither a nor b.** One study reported no correlation between the AUA symptom score and PVR volume. There are also no data documenting that the incidence of UTI is related to PVR volume.
20. **b. 15 cm H$_2$O.** The definition of detrusor instability is the development of a detrusor contraction exceeding 15 cm H$_2$O at a bladder volume less than or equal to 300 mL.
21. **d. 80%.** Of 59 Danish patients presenting to an emergency department with acute retention, 73% had recurrent urinary retention within 1 week after removal of the catheter.
22. **e. All of the above.** The incidence of acute urinary retention was related to age, severity of symptoms, and size of the prostate gland.
23. **b. A placebo-controlled double-blind design.** The only mechanism to ensure that the potential bias of the subject and the investigator does not influence the outcome is a randomized double-blind placebo-controlled design.
24. **a. Less treatment effect required to achieve statistical significance.** The larger the number of subjects enrolled in a study, the smaller the change required to achieve statistical significance.
25. **d. All of the above.** The attractive feature of medical therapy relative to prostatectomy is that clinically significant outcomes are obtained with fewer, less serious, and reversible side effects.
26. **b. 50%.** A 55% reduction in transurethral prostatectomy has occurred despite the progressively increasing number of men enrolled in the Medicare program.
27. **c. 30%.** Approximately 30% of American men older than 50 years of age have moderate to severe symptoms.
28. **d. Bothersome.** The ideal candidate for medical therapy should have symptoms that are bothersome and have a negative impact on the quality of life.
29. **d. 40%.** Smooth muscle is one of the dominant cellular constituents of BPH, accounting for 40% of the area density of the hyperplastic prostate.
30. **a. α$_1$ receptor.** The tension of prostate smooth muscle is mediated by the α$_1$ adrenergic receptors.
31. **a. Its longer half-life.** Terazosin and doxazosin are long-acting α-adrenergic blockers that have been shown to be safe and effective for the treatment of BPH.
32. **a. α$_{1a}$.** Prostate smooth muscle tension has been shown to be mediated by the α$_{1a}$ adrenergic receptors.
33. **d. None of the above.** The relationships between percent change in total symptom score and peak flow rate versus baseline age, prostate size, peak flow rate, PVR volume, and total symptom score were examined to identify clinical or urodynamic factors that predicted response to terazosin therapy. No significant association was observed between treatment effect and any of these baseline factors.
34. **b. 4.** The treatment-related improvement (terazosin minus placebo) in the AUA symptom score and urinary peak flow rate was 1.4 mL/sec and 3.9 symptom units, respectively.
35. **b. 42.** The initial improvements in symptom scores and peak flow rate in 450 subjects were maintained for up to 42 months.
36. **c. Tamsulosin.** The advantage of not lowering blood pressure in men who are hypertensive at baseline is controversial.
37. **d. Tamsulosin.** The treatment-related incidences of asthenia, dizziness, rhinitis, and abnormal ejaculation observed for 0.4 mg of tamsulosin were 2%, 5%, 3%, and 11%, respectively, and for 0.8 mg of tamsulosin were 3%, 8%, 9%, and 18%, respectively.
38. **c. 30%.** Approximately 30% of men treated for BPH have coexisting hypertension.
39. **b. Central nervous system.** The α$_1$-mediated dizziness and asthenia are likely due to effects at the level of the central nervous system.
40. **c. No dose titration.** The major advantage of 0.4 mg tamsulosin and slow-release alfuzosin is the lack of requirement for dose titration.
41. **b. Dihydrotestosterone.** The embryonic development of the prostate is dependent on the androgen dihydrotestosterone.
42. **d. All of the above.** The Proscar Long-Term Efficacy and Safety Study (PLESS) represents one of the longest duration multicenter randomized double-blind placebo-controlled studies reported in the literature on medical therapy for BPH. The unique findings of PLESS were related to incidences of both acute urinary retention

and surgical intervention for BPH. The risk reduction of acute urinary retention and BPH-related surgery was clinically relevant, especially in men with very large prostates.

43. **c. Transurethral prostatectomy.** These preliminary observations have been confirmed by a randomized, double-blind placebo-controlled study demonstrating that finasteride prevents recurrent gross hematuria secondary to BPH after prostatectomy.

44. **a.** Is a dual inhibitor of type 1 and type 2 5α-reductase. Unlike finasteride, which only inhibits the type 2 isoenzyme.

45. **a. Breast tenderness.** The incidences of breast tenderness and diarrhea in the flutamide group were 53% and 11%, respectively.

46. **b. Ability to titrate the level of androgen suppression.** A potential advantage of a gonadotropin-releasing hormone antagonist over the luteinizing hormone-releasing hormone agonists in the treatment of BPH is the ability to titrate the level of androgen suppression.

47. **d. All of the above.** In the study, the mean group differences between terazosin versus placebo and terazosin versus finasteride for all of the outcome measures other than prostate volume were highly statistically significant. Terazosin was more effective than finasteride in those subjects with large prostates.

48. **d.** A combination of an α-adrenergic blocker and a 5α-reductase inhibitor is the most effective way of preventing BPH progression. This was the key conclusion of the important MTOPS study that looked at finasteride versus doxazosin versus a combination of both and placebo in men with symptomatic BPH.

49. **c. Both of the above.**

50. **c. May be reduced to dutasteride alone in 80% of patients with a baseline IPSS less than 20, after 6 months' treatment.** As shown in the study by Barkin and colleagues (2003).*

51. **e. All of the above.**

52. **b. No, only in men with large and persistent residual urine volumes.** Antimuscarinics are only contraindicated if there is a large residual urine volume, as such men have a higher risk of retention.

53. **b. Surgical therapy.**

54. **e. None of the above.**

55. **e. All of the above.**

56. **c. Low-dose tadalafil.** The manufacturers of tadalafil recommend avoiding using it with doxazosin. However, care should be taken with the addition of any PDEI to men already optimized on an α-blocker, as there is an increased risk of symptomatic hypotension in all men being considered for this combination.

57. **c. $1 billion.** Use of these agents in the United States and throughout the world has escalated. It has been estimated that more than $1 billion was spent in the United States alone for these products.

58. **d. Inconclusive.** Although experimental data have suggested numerous possible mechanisms of actions for the phytotherapeutic agents, it is uncertain which, if any, of these proposed mechanisms is responsible for the clinical responses.

59. **d. Endothelin antagonists.** Although currently untested, endothelin antagonists represent a possible therapeutic avenue in BPH.

CHAPTER REVIEW

1. Patients with severe irritable symptoms and dysuria or microscopic hematuria should have a urine cytology.
2. Surgery is generally recommended for patients with refractory urinary retention, recurrent urinary tract infections, recurrent gross hematuria, bladder stones, renal insufficiency, and large bladder diverticula.
3. Flow rates are inaccurate if the voided volume is less than 150 mL. A peak flow rate (PFR) is better than an average flow rate.
4. Patients with a PFR greater than 15 mL/sec are less likely to have good treatment outcomes after prostatectomy. Patients with a flow rate less than 10 mL/sec have better surgical outcomes.
5. It takes at least a 3-point change in the IPSS for the patient to perceive a difference.
6. Conservative therapy to reduce the severity and bother of symptoms involves decreasing fluid intake, especially before bedtime, moderating alcohol and caffeine intake, and maintaining timed voiding schedules.
7. α-Adrenergic blockers may influence smooth muscle growth in the prostate. They may induce apoptosis.
8. α-Adrenergic blockers may induce the floppy iris syndrome, and patients should be warned of this if they are to have cataract surgery.
9. The maximal reduction in prostate volume requires 6 months after initiation of androgen suppressive therapy.
10. The rationale for aromatase inhibition is that estrogens may be involved in the pathogenesis of BPH.
11. Finasteride reduces prostate volume by approximately 20%. Maximum reduction in prostate volume following androgen deprivation occurs by 6 months.
12. Anticholinergic receptor blockers may be safely administered in patients with bladder outlet obstruction to reduce frequent voiding if they have PVR urine volumes less than 200 mL and do not report increasing hesitancy and show signs of increasing PVR urine volume when placed on such therapy.

13. Phosphodiesterase inhibitors have been known to improve IPSS scores. Phosphodiesterase inhibitors do not improve flow rate.
14. Concomitant use of α-adrenergic blockers and phosphodiesterase inhibitors may lead to hypotension.
15. Mortality increases sixfold in patients with renal insufficiency who are treated surgically for BPH.
16. PSA is of value in predicting the likelihood of response to 5α-reductase inhibitors and the risk of LUTS/BPH progression.
17. PSA is reduced by one-half in patients on 5α-reductase inhibitors.
18. The value of pressure flow studies and PVR in predicting the outcome of treatment is uncertain.
19. There is no convincing evidence in the aging male that an elevated PVR causes recurrent UTIs.
20. An elevated serum creatinine level in a patient with BPH is an indication for imaging studies (ultrasonography) to evaluate the upper urinary tract.
21. Overactive contractions are present in approximately 60% of men with LUTS and correlate strongly with irritative voiding symptoms.
22. Upper urinary tract imaging is not recommended for routine evaluation of men with LUTS unless they also have one or more of the following: hematuria; urinary tract infection; renal insufficiency (ultrasonography recommended); history of urolithiasis; and history of urinary tract surgery.
23. The definition of detrusor instability is the development of a detrusor contraction exceeding 15 cm H_2O at a bladder volume less than or equal to 300 mL.
24. Finasteride prevents recurrent gross hematuria secondary to BPH after prostatectomy.
25. A combination of an α-adrenergic blocker and a 5α-reductase inhibitor is the most effective way of preventing BPH progression.

*Sources referenced can be found in *Campbell-Walsh Urology, 11th Edition*, on the Expert Consult website.

105 Minimally Invasive and Endoscopic Management of Benign Prostatic Hyperplasia

Kevin T. McVary and Charles Welliver

QUESTIONS

1. In the last 30 years of benign prostatic hyperplasia (BPH) management, which of the following has been a general trend in endoscopic surgical treatment?
   a. With the widespread use of medical therapy for BPH, there has been a trend toward less use of surgical management.
   b. The advent of the bipolar resection system increased the overall percentage of endoscopic procedures done as transurethral resections of the prostate (TURPs).
   c. Socioeconomic factors involved in acceptance and use of laser technology have not been described.
   d. Younger men are more likely to undergo treatment for BPH than older men.
   e. Retreatment rates have not influenced the continued adoption of new endoscopic and minimally invasive treatments.

2. With regard to defining outcomes in BPH treatment, which of the following statements is NOT correct?
   a. Intent to treat analyses are commonly reported.
   b. Subjective symptoms (such as dysuria) can be influenced by observer reporting.
   c. Reports of long-term treatment efficacy are highly influenced by a loss of patients to follow-up and, possibly, reporting of responder data only.
   d. Comparisons across surgical techniques are often unfair because new technologies are frequently compared with a historic, and often inferior, data set.
   e. In a randomized controlled trial (RCT), comparison with TURP assumes that the surgeon performing the TURP has been sufficiently trained and can produce predictable results.

3. The minimum antibiotic coverage for treatment of BPH according to the American Urological Association (AUA) best practice statement is:
   a. ceftriaxone.
   b. ampicillin.
   c. fluoroquinolone.
   d. trimethoprim.
   e. acyclovir.

4. TURP should begin with resection of the:
   a. apical portion of the prostate.
   b. prostate floor.
   c. bladder neck.
   d. median lobe, if present.
   e. anterior portion of the prostate.

5. Transurethral resection (TUR) syndrome is caused by:
   a. absorption of fluid during procedures such as holmium laser enucleation of the prostate (HoLEP) and bipolar TURP.
   b. absorption of non–sodium-containing irrigating fluid, leading to an acute dilutional hyponatremia.
   c. irrigating fluid placed at a less than ideal height above the patient.
   d. a serum sodium of greater than 130 mEq/L.
   e. intraoperative ureteral injury.

6. Which of the following is TRUE of bipolar compared with monopolar TURP?
   a. In a meta-analysis of patients undergoing bipolar TURP, authors concluded that by treating 50 patients with bipolar TURP, one case of TUR syndrome could be prevented.
   b. A relative risk of 0.53 for blood transfusion with bipolar resection was found in meta-analysis.
   c. Improved visualization during bipolar TURP may also lead to a decrease in capsular perforations and operating time.
   d. Late complications such as bladder neck contracture and need for retreatment of BPH do not appear to be much different from those found with conventional TURP.
   e. All of the above.

7. Which of the following is TRUE about transurethral vaporization of the prostate (TUVP)?
   a. There is a large startup cost associated with the procedure due to the required purchase of new generators and equipment.
   b. Frequently leads to lower hemostasis related complications (transfusion, clot retention) compared to monopolar TURP
   c. Is available only as a monopolar technology
   d. Was first described in 2005
   e. It leads entirely to tissue vaporization.

8. Transurethral microwave therapy (TUMT) has been shown to:
   a. frequently cause erectile dysfunction.
   b. improve AUA Symptom Score (AUASS) by approximately 60% at 1 year.
   c. have comparable results in both the low energy and high energy platforms.
   d. increase density of nerve endings in the prostate.
   e. induce changes in prostate volume of greater than 50%.

9. Sham studies on urologic procedures for lower urinary tract symptoms (LUTS) due to BPH:
   a. frequently show statistically significant decreases in AUASS.
   b. are poorly tolerated by the patient.
   c. have significant side effects and should not be performed as part of research.
   d. have never shown a statistically significant improvement in objective measures such as peak urinary flow.
   e. have never been performed.

10. Which of the following is the most commonly reported complication/adverse event associated with TUMT?
    a. Blood transfusion
    b. Urinary tract infection
    c. Erectile dysfunction

d. Urethral stricture

e. Incontinence

11. Transurethral needle ablation (TUNA):

a. now universally regulates temperature based on impedance.

b. is required to be done in a hospital-based operating room with overnight admission.

c. should only be performed on prostates less than 50 mL in size.

d. has an equivalent need for retreatment for lower urinary tract symptoms (LUTS) due to BPH compared to TURP.

e. is not recommended in patients with metallic pelvic prostheses.

12. Which of the following is TRUE regarding transurethral incision of the prostate (TUIP)?

a. It commonly results in TUR syndrome.

b. It is generally only used in prostates larger than 60 mL.

c. It causes retrograde ejaculation in 80% of cases.

d. It results in removal of a large volume of prostate adenoma.

e. It may have a lower rate of ejaculatory dysfunction in patients when done unilaterally.

13. With regard to laser safety, which of the following statements is correct?

a. Eye protection is required for the surgeon only.

b. All windows or wall openings from the operating room (OR) must be covered.

c. Signs denoting that a laser is in use need only be displayed on the most commonly used door for that operating room.

d. Eye protection is required only when a video camera is not used during the case.

e. All laser energy is readily absorbed by air/irrigating fluid, making it safe to use in the OR.

14. Holmium laser resection of the prostate (HoLRP) differs from HoLEP in that HoLRP:

a. follows anatomic planes to remove the prostate in lobes.

b. requires the use of a morcellator.

c. preceded HoLEP chronologically and conceptually.

d. has been shown to be superior to TURP in recent meta-analyses.

e. uses a thulium laser.

15. Which of the following is TRUE of HoLEP?

a. Transient urinary retention is seen in more than 50% of patients.

b. A morcellator-related bladder injury has never been reported.

c. Bladder neck contracture may be more common in smaller prostate glands.

d. Overall complication rates increase significantly with increasing prostate size.

e. When observed, urinary incontinence is generally permanent.

16. Prostate vaporization:

a. ideally uses a wavelength that is readily absorbed by hemoglobin for improved hemostasis.

b. utilizes coagulation of tissue over ablation of tissue.

c. was ideally suited for the neodymium laser.

d. increases with decreasing laser wattage.

e. occurs frequently during TURP.

17. Patients on anticoagulation who undergo photoselective vaporization of the prostate (PVP) have an increased risk of:

a. erectile dysfunction.

b. blood transfusion.

c. TUR syndrome.

d. ejaculatory dysfunction.

e. time in the hospital after procedure.

18. The mechanism of action of prostate urethral lift is:

a. implantation of a radiation-eluting implant that causes tissue ablation with time.

b. primarily in compression of peripheral zone of the prostate.

c. primarily in compression of the transition zone of the prostate.

d. delayed tissue necrosis of the prostatic urothelium causing a decrease in local irritative symptoms.

e. implantation of a stent within the lumen of the urethra to relieve obstruction by the lateral lobes.

19. When using the prostate lift for treatment of LUTS due to BPH, implants are placed where in the prostate anatomically?

a. Anterolaterally

b. Posterolaterally

c. Anteriorly

d. Posteriorly

e. In the peripheral zone

20. Which statement is TRUE of prostate embolization?

a. The pelvic vasculature is generally straightforward, and the procedure is technically not challenging.

b. It is achieved by occluding the internal iliac vessels.

c. It is applicable to a wide variety of patients.

d. It incurs no radiation to the patient.

e. Bilaterally achieved embolization yields better results.

ANSWERS

1. **a. With the widespread use of medical therapy for BPH, there has been a trend toward less use of surgical management.** Although short periods of increase have been noted, the overwhelming trend in the past 30 years has been a decrease in endoscopic treatment of BPH, as shown in many Medicare database analyses. The market share of TURP has decreased, even with the common use of the bipolar technology. Payer data from Florida have displayed an irregular acceptance and use of lasers in BPH treatment depending on socioeconomic factors. Older men are more likely to display histologic findings of BPH and are more likely to undergo surgery for the disease; the widespread use of medications has also led to an overall more aged cohort seeking treatment after medical therapy is unsuccessful. Although initial acceptance of a new technology is common, frequently an unacceptable need for disease retreatment causes a technology to lose market share and fail.

2. **a. Intent to treat analyses are commonly reported.** The definition of outcomes and comparison of procedures in BPH treatment is fraught with many problems. Intent-to-treat analyses are exceedingly rare. Subjective symptoms (including comments on severity) are not frequently reported and are subject to both patient and observer reporting problems. Long-term reports may frequently skew toward patients who are responders to treatment, because patients who do not respond will either receive retreatment for disease (no longer included in data set) or seek treatment elsewhere and also be lost. Frequently, new technologies are compared with historic TURP data sets that use outdated equipment or techniques that are no longer in use and does not represent contemporary outcomes. Although RCTs generate a

high level of evidence, the outcomes from the control group are subject to the training of the surgeon in the control procedure and many not represent commonly found outcomes.

3. **c. Fluoroquinolone.** The minimum antibiotic coverage according to the AUA best practice statement would include the use of either a fluoroquinolone or trimethoprim-sulfamethoxazole (TMP-SMX). In patients with a positive urine culture or indwelling Foley catheter, additional or extended antibiotic coverage should be considered.

4. **d. Median lobe, if present.** Although many different plans for resection exist, resection of the median lobe (when present) is generally accepted as the first step.

5. **b. Absorption of non–sodium-containing irrigating fluid, leading to an acute dilutional hyponatremia.** Absorption of non–sodium-containing irrigating fluid into the prostatic venous system that is exposed during resection is the etiology of the disease. This risk appears to be unique to monopolar TURP; other BPH techniques (such as bipolar TURP, HoLEP, and laser vaporization) use isotonic/iso-osmolar irrigating fluid such as normal saline. The ideal height of irrigating fluid was determined to be 60 cm above the patient, as this balanced the benefits of visualization with systemic absorption. Heights above this level will lead to an increased systemic absorption. Generally, symptoms of TUR syndrome begin with a serum sodium of less than 120 mEq/L. Ureteral injury is not associated with TUR syndrome.

6. **e. All of the above.** All of the findings in a through d have been demonstrated in studies. The use of a sodium-containing iso-osmolar irrigating fluid has essentially eliminated the risk of TUR syndrome in bipolar TURP. The "cut and seal" action of the technology improves intraoperative hemostasis with better visualization, leading to less blood transfusion and quicker operating times. Differences in many late complications such as bladder neck contracture and need for retreatment have not been demonstrated in comparison to monopolar technology.

7. **b. Frequently leads to lower hemostasis related complications (transfusion, clot retention) compared to monopolar TURP.** Fewer bleeding-related complications have been demonstrated in TUVP studies when compared to monopolar TURP. The technology is available in both monopolar and bipolar technology, with the monopolar technique described in 1995 by Kaplan and Te. The leading edge of the electrode uses primarily vaporization with the lagging edge causing tissue coagulation, leading to the improved hemostasis seen in many studies.

8. **b. Improve AUA Symptom Score (AUASS) by approximately 60% at 1 year.** Although the precise mechanism of action of transurethral microwave therapy is still debatable, it likely works by either inducing nerve degeneration in the prostate or leading to morphologic changes (apoptosis and necrosis) in the tissue. The technique infrequently leads to erectile dysfunction, with modest changes in prostate volume frequently exhibited (25% at the most). The high-energy and heat shock platforms are an improvement versus the low-energy protocol with regard to clinical efficacy. Improvements in AUASS are 60% to 65% at 1 year and 45% at 3 years.

9. **a. Frequently show statistically significant decreases in AUASS.** Multiple sham studies have been performed as part of clinical trials on TUMT and prostate lift. Significant improvements in both AUASS and peak flow have been shown. Side effects of treatment are infrequent, and the sham procedures are well tolerated.

10. **b. Urinary tract infection.** Urinary tract infection is a fairly common finding after TUMT, likely because of the frequently seen transient urinary retention and prolonged catheterization. The rest of these complications occur in less than 10% of cases.

11. **e. Is not recommended in patients with metallic pelvic prostheses.** The TUNA system can now measure temperatures at the end of the thermocouples, and close regulation of tissue impedance is less critical than in the previous impedance-based systems. The procedure can be performed in an office-based setting, and hospital admission is not required. Prostate sizes of up to 70 mL can be treated. Retreatment rates for TUNA are higher than for TURP (Odds ratio (OR) = 7.4 in the meta-analysis by Bouza et al). TUNA is not recommended in patients with active urinary tract infection (UTI), metallic pelvic prosthesis (e.g., artificial hip), cardiac implants (defibrillator or pacemaker), or a high bladder neck.

12. **e. May have a lower rate of ejaculatory dysfunction in patients when done unilaterally.** The procedure is relatively short and does not cause TUR syndrome. The procedure is only appropriate for small prostate glands (generally less than 30 mL), and no prostate adenoma is removed. Retrograde ejaculation occurs in up to 37% of patients. Although this is controversial, most authors believe that the risk of retrograde ejaculation is lower if done unilaterally as opposed to bilaterally.

13. **b. All windows or wall openings from the operating room (OR) must be covered.** Eye protection is required for all classes of lasers used in urology currently. Eye protection should be utilized by the patient and all personnel in the room even if a video camera is used during the case. Signs should be placed on all entries to the OR. Any and all openings to the OR from which laser energy could escape should be covered to preclude injury to persons outside of the OR. Although holmium laser energy is absorbed in irrigating fluid, KTP/LBO laser energy is not readily absorbed in either fluid. Both of these lasers can damage the eye when outside the body as neither are readily absorbed/dispersed in air.

14. **c. Preceded HoLEP chronologically and conceptually.** Both technologies utilize a holmium laser for prostate incision. Answers a, b, and d are true of HoLEP and not HoLRP. HoLRP advanced to HoLEP when the use of a morcellator became commonplace and conceptually predates HoLEP.

15. **c. Bladder neck contracture may be more common in smaller prostate glands.** Even transient urinary retention is an uncommon finding after HoLEP because of the complete removal of the adenoma. Morcellator injuries to the bladder have been reported and can be catastrophic. Overall complication rates do not appear to increase with increasing gland size, although the study by Kuo et al, 2003* found that bladder neck contractures may be more common in smaller glands. Urinary incontinence can occur in up to 10% of cases but is almost always transient.

16. **a. Ideally uses a wavelength that is readily absorbed by hemoglobin for improved hemostasis.** Currently, the most commonly used prostate vaporization systems use a laser wavelength that is ideally absorbed by hemoglobin (532 nm), as this is felt to improve hemostasis during the vaporization. Ablation and vaporization are essentially interchangeable terms, and ablation/vaporization is vapored over coagulation. The bulk of tissue is vaporized, but a thin rim of coagulated tissue is left in the prostate for hemostasis. Although originally thought to be the ideal laser for the prostate, the neodymium:YAG laser originally fell out of favor because of the wavelength's partiality for tissue coagulation and not vaporization. Increasing laser wattage has increased vaporization rates, and TURP has minimal tissue vaporization as it removes the prostate through resection of prostate chips.

17. **e. Time in the hospital after procedure.** Patients who undergo PVP while on anticoagulation appear to be more likely to require longer times in the hospital. They also appear to require more continuous bladder irrigation and a longer time with a urethral catheter. Blood transfusions do not appear to be more frequent. TUR syndrome does not occur with PVP, as normal saline is used. Erectile dysfunction and ejaculatory dysfunction in patients on anticoagulation during PVP are not well studied.

18. **c. Primarily in compression of the transition zone of the prostate.** The prostate urethral lift system works by primarily compressing the transition zone of the prostate. The implants do no elute radiation or cause delayed tissue necrosis. The last answer describes prostate stents.

---

*Sources referenced can be found in *Campbell-Walsh Urology, 11th Edition,* on the Expert Consult website.

19. **a. Anterolaterally.** The implants in the prostate lift system are placed anterolaterally to avoid the neurovascular bundles (posterolateral) and the prostate veins (anterior). The implants work by primarily compressing the transition zone of the prostate and leading to an increased opening of the urethral lumen.
20. **e. Bilaterally achieved embolization yields better results.** The procedure is actually technically very challenging because of highly variable pelvic anatomy with small vessels feeding the prostate. Occlusion should be done a location much more distal than the internal iliac vessels. Radiation to the patient is considerable with the procedure. Because of strict inclusion criteria, patients frequently are deemed unacceptable for the procedure. When bilateral embolization is achieved, it appears that outcomes are improved.

CHAPTER REVIEW

1. Complications of urethral stent placement include hematuria, migration, infections, encrustation, epithelial hyperplasia, irritative urinary symptoms, and painful ejaculation.
2. With the use of TUNA, there is a 23% requirement for retreatment in 5 years. Thus long-term efficacy has not been clearly demonstrated.
3. Transurethral microwave therapy (TUMT) offers less morbidity than TURP but is not as effective in relieving outlet obstruction or improving symptoms.
4. A peak urinary flow rate of less than 15 mL/sec does not differentiate between outflow obstruction and detrusor impairment.
5. Venous bleeding after TURP can be controlled by filling the bladder with 100 mL of irrigating fluid and placing the catheter on traction for 5 to 10 minutes.
6. The TUR syndrome is secondary to dilutional hyponatremia (with volume overload) and may present as mental confusion, nausea, vomiting, hypertension, bradycardia, and visual disturbances. Iso-osmolar solutions such as glycine and sorbitol are just as likely to cause dilutional hyponatremia as water. The use of saline as the irrigant eliminates hyponatremia but not volume overload.
7. Intraoperative priapism is managed by injecting an α-adrenergic agent into the corpora.
8. Outcomes of a TURP are best for men who are most bothered by their symptoms.
9. TUIP is particularly effective for those with bladder neck occlusion, in patients with small prostates, and in those who are young.
10. Prostate-specific antigen (PSA) may be used as a surrogate for prostate volume.
11. 5α-Reductase inhibitors may successfully manage hematuria originating from the prostate.
12. Each centimeter above the normal 2.5-cm prostate urethral length equates to an additional 10 g in prostate weight.
13. Resection of the prostate apex is best performed at the termination of the procedure when hemostasis is adequate.
14. A routine TURP results in 800 to 1000 mL of fluid being absorbed into the systemic circulation.
15. After TURP, an improvement in symptoms occurs in 75% of patients; 16% require a reoperation in 7 years. Complications include bladder neck contracture in 2% (more common when small glands are resected), urethral stricture in 2% to 4%, and ejaculatory problems in the majority.
16. After TUMT, there is a 30% retreatment rate, and one third of patients remain obstructed on urodynamic assessment.
17. PVP can be performed safely in patients on anticoagulant medication.
18. When performing a TURP, resection of the median lobe (when present) is generally accepted as the first step.
19. The ideal height of irrigating fluid was determined to be 60 cm above the patient because this balanced the benefits of visualization with systemic absorption.
20. TUNA is not recommended in patients with active UTI, metallic pelvic prosthesis (e.g., artificial hip), cardiac implants (defibrillator or pacemaker), and a high bladder neck.
21. Eye protection is required for all classes of lasers used in urology currently.

106 Simple Prostatectomy: Open and Robot-Assisted Laparoscopic Approaches

Misop Han and Alan W. Partin

1. The major advantage of simple prostatectomy over transurethral resection of the prostate (TURP) in the management of prostatic adenoma includes:
   a. removal of the prostatic adenoma under direct vision.
   b. decreased risk of hypernatremia.
   c. shortened convalescence period.
   d. decreased perioperative hemorrhage.
   e. enhanced preservation of erectile function.
2. The suprapubic simple prostatectomy, in comparison to the retropubic simple prostatectomy, allows:
   a. direct visualization of the prostatic adenoma during enucleation.
   b. better visualization of the prostatic fossa after enucleation to obtain hemostasis.
   c. easier management of a large median lobe and/or bladder calculi.
   d. an extraperitoneal approach.
   e. possible management of concomitant ureteral calculi.
3. The suprapubic approach to the prostatectomy is ideal for the patient with a large prostatic adenoma and:
   a. multiple small bladder calculi.
   b. total prostate-stimulating antigen (PSA) greater than 10.0 ng/mL.
   c. erectile dysfunction.
   d. symptomatic bladder diverticulum.
   e. presence of dilated renal pelvis.
4. The most appropriate definitive treatment options for the patient with a 120-g prostatic adenoma and a symptomatic bladder diverticulum are:
   a. retropubic open prostatectomy with the fulguration of bladder diverticulum.
   b. long-acting α-adrenergic antagonist and prophylactic antibiotics.
   c. TURP followed by bladder diverticulectomy in 3 months.
   d. TURP and partial cystectomy.
   e. simple prostatectomy with bladder diverticulectomy.
5. The contraindications to simple prostatectomy include:
   a. multiple cores of Gleason 8 prostate cancer.
   b. bladder diverticulum.
   c. large bladder calculi secondary to obstruction.
   d. recurrent urinary tract infection.
   e. acute urinary retention.
6. Both retropubic and suprapubic simple prostatectomies:
   a. are performed in the space of Retzius.
   b. are ideal for patients with a large, obstructive prostatic adenoma and a concomitant, small bladder tumor.
   c. require no blood transfusion.
   d. cause no trauma to the urinary bladder.
   e. require control of the dorsal vein complex before the enucleation of an obstructive prostatic adenoma.
7. Compared with open simple prostatectomy, robot-assisted laparoscopic simple prostatectomy has:
   a. quicker operative time.
   b. longer hospital stay.
   c. decreased need for blood transfusion.
   d. shorter learning curve.
   e. decreased need for anesthesia.

ANSWERS

1. **a. Removal of the prostatic adenoma under direct vision.** When compared with TURP, simple prostatectomy offers the advantages of lower retreatment rate and more complete removal of the prostatic adenoma under direct vision and avoids the risk of dilutional hyponatremia (the TUR syndrome).
2. **c. Easier management of a large median lobe and/or bladder calculi.** The major advantage of suprapubic simple prostatectomy over the retropubic approach is that it allows direct visualization of the bladder neck and bladder mucosa. As a result, this operation is ideally suited for patients with a large median lobe protruding into the bladder or a clinically significant bladder diverticulum.
3. **d. Symptomatic bladder diverticulum.** Suprapubic simple prostatectomy is ideally suited for patients with a large median lobe protruding into the bladder, a clinically significant bladder diverticulum that requires repair, or large bladder calculi. It also may be preferable for obese men, in whom it is difficult to gain direct access to the prostatic pseudocapsule and dorsal vein complex.
4. **e. Simple prostatectomy with bladder diverticulectomy.** Combined suprapubic simple prostatectomy and bladder diverticulum is the best option for the patient with a massive benign prostatic hyperplasia (BPH) and a symptomatic bladder diverticulum because of easy access to both prostatic adenoma and bladder diverticulum. If the prostatectomy is performed without the diverticulectomy, incomplete emptying of the bladder diverticulum and subsequent, persistent infection may occur.
5. **a. Multiple cores of Gleason 8 prostate cancer.** Contraindications to simple prostatectomy include a small fibrous gland, the presence of significant prostate cancer, and previous prostatectomy or pelvic surgery that may obliterate access to the prostate gland.
6. **a. Are performed in the space of Retzius.** Both retropubic and suprapubic simple prostatectomies are performed in the space of Retzius. The dorsal vein complex does not have to be controlled before the enucleation of an obstructive prostatic adenoma during suprapubic simple prostatectomy.
7. **c. Decreased need for blood transfusion.** Compared with open simple prostatectomy, robot-assisted laparoscopic simple prostatectomy can be performed with smaller incisions with shorter hospital stay and decreased risk for perioperative hemorrhage and blood transfusion.

CHAPTER REVIEW

1. Of the indications for simple prostatectomy—(a) acute urinary retention, (b) recurrent or persistent urinary tract infections, (c) significant symptoms of bladder outlet obstruction not responsive to medical therapy, (d) persistent gross hematuria from the prostate, (e) pathologic changes of the kidneys secondary to prostatic obstruction, and (f) bladder calculi—the only absolute indication for prostatectomy is pathologic changes of the kidneys secondary to prostatic obstruction. All the others are relative indications because they may on occasion be corrected without the need for prostatectomy.

2. One should not consider doing a simple prostatectomy for glands of less than 75 g. If a simple prostatectomy is planned and it is discovered intraoperatively that the prostate is less than 50 g, it is prudent to abort the procedure and perform a transurethral resection of the prostate instead, because performing an open prostatectomy on small glands carries an extremely high complication rate.

3. Simple prostatectomy should be considered in patients who cannot be placed in the lithotomy position and who have a sufficiently large gland that can be enucleated. Small fibrous glands, the presence of prostate cancer, previous prostatectomy, and pelvic surgery are contraindications to open simple prostatectomy.

4. Although a cystoscopic examination is not indicated for routine evaluation of obstructive voiding symptoms, one must estimate the size of the prostate adenoma preoperatively to schedule the patient appropriately. Cystoscopy may be a crucial component of that estimation. Moreover, in patients who have hematuria or a urethral stricture, or in whom one needs to evaluate a known bladder calculus or diverticulum, cystoscopy is indicated.

5. More than 10% of patients undergoing simple prostatectomy will require one or more units of blood either intraoperatively or postoperatively.

6. The risks of simple prostatectomy include urinary incontinence, erectile dysfunction, retrograde ejaculation, urinary tract infections, bladder neck contracture, urethral stricture, and the need for a blood transfusion.

7. Nonurologic complications include pulmonary embolus, myocardial infarction, and stroke.

8. A chromic suture placed at the 5- and 7-o'clock positions at the level of the bladder neck in the prostatic fossa may be used to secure the major arterial supply to the prostate and aids in hemostasis. If the bladder neck appears obstructive, a wedge is excised dorsally and the bladder mucosa advanced into the prostatic fossa and secured with 4-0 chromic suture.

9. A method of controlling persistent hemorrhage from the prostatic fossa that cannot be controlled by the hemostatic sutures or fulguration may be accomplished with the Malament suture. A nylon suture is placed in a purse-string fashion around the bladder neck, brought out through the skin, and secured over the urethral catheter with the balloon inflated in the bladder, thus effectively tamponading the prostatic fossa. After several days the suture may be removed when hemostasis is adequate.

10. Following a suprapubic prostatectomy a Malecot suprapubic tube is placed. The proper flow of continuous irrigation is entering through the urethral catheter and exiting from the suprapubic tube.

11. Erectile dysfunction occurs in 5% and retrograde ejaculation in over 90%; 5% of patients develop bladder neck contractures.

12. A urethral catheter must be passed into the bladder before the skin incision is made.

13. The patient should be informed preoperatively that urgency and urge incontinence may occur for several months postoperatively.

14. Suprapubic simple prostatectomy is ideally suited for patients with a large median lobe protruding into the bladder, a clinically significant bladder diverticulum that requires repair, or large bladder calculi. It also may be preferable for obese men, in whom it is difficult to gain direct access to the prostatic pseudocapsule and dorsal vein complex.

107 Epidemiology, Etiology, and Prevention of Prostate Cancer

Eric A. Klein and Andrew J. Stephenson

QUESTIONS

1. Following the prostate-specific antigen (PSA) "cull effect," the incidence of prostate cancer in the United States:
   a. is decreasing.
   b. is stable.
   c. is increasing.
   d. increased initially, then decreased.
   e. is fluctuating.

2. In the United States, the highest prostate cancer incidence rates are seen in:
   a. whites.
   b. African Americans.
   c. Hispanic/Latinos.
   d. Asian Americans
   e. Native Americans.

3. Worldwide, prostate cancer:
   a. is the leading cancer diagnosis in men.
   b. is the leading cause of cancer-related mortality.
   c. incidence is highest in countries with the highest rates of screening.
   d. is entirely genetic in origin.
   e. has the lowest age-adjusted mortality rates per 100,000 men in North America.

4. With respect to two large randomized trials assessing the effect of PSA screening on prostate cancer mortality:
   a. overall incidence rates were higher in the European Randomized Study of Screening for Prostate Cancer (ERSPC) but overall mortality rates were higher in the Prostate, Lung, Colorectal, and Ovarian (PLCO) trial.
   b. the ERSPC showed no significant difference in survival between screened and unscreened men.
   c. the PLCO cancer screening trial demonstrated a 20% risk reduction in prostate cancer mortality in screened men compared to unscreened men.
   d. contamination of the control arm with PSA screening is a limitation of the PLCO cancer screening trial.
   e. both studies clearly show no benefit to PSA screening for prostate cancer.

5. Compared with a man with no family history of prostate cancer, the risk of developing prostate cancer in a man with one affected first-degree relative is:
   a. unchanged.
   b. 1.5 times higher.
   c. 2 to 3 times higher.
   d. 5 times higher.
   e. 100%.

6. Biologic functions of known prostate cancer susceptibility genes include:
   a. control of the inflammatory response.
   b. homeobox genes.
   c. DNA repair mechanisms.
   d. susceptibility to infection.
   e. all of the above.

7. Which of the following statements regarding gene fusions in prostate cancer are correct?
   a. The most frequent fusions are between the TMPRSS2 serine protease to members of the ETS family of oncogenic transcription factors.
   b. The *TMPRSS2-ERG* fusion gene is present in prostate stem cells.
   c. *TMPRSS2* expression has been shown to be induced by androgens.
   d. *TRMPSS2*-related gene fusions are highly specific for the presence of prostate cancer.
   e. All of the above.

8. All of the following statements regarding estrogens and prostate cancer are correct, EXCEPT:
   a. Estrogen's treatment effect is primarily related to a negative feedback on the hypothalamo-pituitary-gonadal axis.
   b. Estrogen's treatment effect is partly through a direct inhibitory effect of estrogens on prostate epithelial cell growth.
   c. Aromatase-knockout mice all develop prostate cancer in their lifetime.
   d. Stromal estrogen receptor (ER)α expression is silenced in early prostate cancers, and re-emerges with disease progression.
   e. Prostate epithelial ERβ may play an important role in initiation of prostate cancer.

9. Elevated serum levels of insulin-like growth factor (IGF) 1 have been associated with:
   a. higher serum PSA levels.
   b. lower body mass index.
   c. reduced intraprostatic inflammation.
   d. higher risk of developing prostate cancer.
   e. lower serum testosterone levels.

10. Evidence suggesting that vitamin D affects the risk of prostate cancer includes the fact that:
    a. men living in areas with less ultraviolet exposure have lower prostate cancer mortality rates.
    b. vitamin D levels are higher in older men.
    c. a calcium-poor diet predisposes men to prostate cancer.
    d. native Japanese, whose diet is rich in vitamin D derived from fish, have a high incidence of prostate cancer.
    e. polymorphisms conferring lower vitamin D receptor activity are associated with increased risk for prostate cancer.

11. High body mass index is associated with:
    a. protection against oxidative stress.
    b. higher circulating androgens.
    c. lower serum PSA levels.
    d. better cancer-specific survival after radical prostatectomy.
    e. lower free IGF-1.

12. Hypermethylation of the following genes may play a role in prostate cancer etiology:
    a. DNA repair genes (*GSTpi*, *GPX3*, and *GSTM1*).
    b. hormonal response genes (*ERαA*, *ERβ*, and *RARβ*).
    c. genes controlling the cell cycle (*CyclinD2* and *14-3-3σ*).
    d. tumor suppressor genes (*APC*, *RASSF1α*, *DKK3*, $p16^{INK4?-α}$, *E-cadherin*, and $p57^{WAF1}$).
    e. all of the above.

13. The existence of multiple prostate cancer susceptibility genes and chromosomal loci suggests:
    a. dominant inheritance pattern.
    b. common clinical features associated with all identified genes.
    c. genetic heterogeneity in the cause of prostate cancer.
    d. need for yearly screening in those with a family history.
    e. multifocal tumors in affected individuals.

14. Epigenetic mechanisms active in prostate cancer include:
    a. chromatin remodeling
    b. promoter hypomethylation and hypermethylation
    c. microRNAs that lead to gene silencing
    d. long noncoding RNAs
    e. all of the above.

15. Findings of the Selenium and Vitamin E Cancer Prevention Trial (SELECT) include:
    a. a significant reduction in the incidence of prostate cancer in the combination arm.
    b. a significant effect of selenium and vitamin E on reducing the risk of cardiovascular disease and nonprostate malignancies.
    c. a significant increased incidence of diabetes mellitus in the selenium arm.
    d. a reduction in prostate-cancer specific mortality.
    e. an increased risk of prostate cancer in those taking vitamin E alone.

16. The protective effect of lycopene against prostate cancer may best be achieved by consuming:
    a. cooked foods.
    b. pure form as oral capsules.
    c. pure form with other antioxidants.
    d. raw vegetables.
    e. fresh fruit.

17. In the Prostate Cancer Prevention Trial (PCPT), compared with placebo, finasteride use was associated with a higher incidence of:
    a. prostatitis.
    b. urinary tract infection.
    c. surgical intervention for lower urinary tract symptoms.
    d. sexual dysfunction.
    e. low-grade prostate cancer.

ANSWERS

1. **e. Is fluctuating.** According to Surveillance, Epidemiology, and End Results (SEER) estimates, the incidence of prostate cancer peaked in 1992, approximately 5 years after the introduction of PSA as a screening test, fell precipitously until 1995, increased slowly at a slope similar to that observed before the PSA era until 2001, and has fluctuated year-to-year since 2001, likely related to changing screening practices in the general population.

2. **b. African Americans.** African-American men have the highest reported incidence of prostate cancer in the world, with an incidence of 255.5 per 100,000 person-years and a relative incidence of 1.6 compared with white men in the United States (American Cancer Society). Although African Americans have experienced a greater decline in mortality than white men since the early 1990s, their death rates remain 2.4 times higher than whites. Many biologic, environmental, and social hypotheses have been advanced to explain these differences, ranging from postulated differences in genetic predisposition; differences in mechanisms of tumor initiation, promotion and/or progression; higher fat diets, higher serum testosterone levels, or higher body mass index; structural, financial, educational and cultural barriers to screening, early detection and aggressive therapy; and physician bias. There are currently no data that clearly indicate any of these hypotheses are the determinants of the observed differences in incidence or mortality, and it seems likely that the source of the disparity is multifactorial.

3. **c. Incidence is highest in countries with the highest rates of screening.** The age-standardized incidence rates per 100,000 men are highest in the highest income regions of the world where PSA screening is more commonly practiced, including North America (85.6), Australia–New Zealand (104.2), Western Europe (93.1), and Scandinavia (73.1), and lowest in Asia (7.2) and Northern Africa (8.1).

4. **d. Contamination of the control arm with PSA screening is a limitation of the PLCO cancer screening trial.** The trial has been criticized for high rates of prescreening (44% reported undergoing PSA testing before enrollment), poor compliance with prostate biopsy, and 52% contamination by ad hoc screening in the control arm. A follow-up study in which PLCO participants were questioned about PSA testing reported a 15% non-PSA testing rate in the control arm of PLCO, which is identical to the noncompliance with screening in the screening arm.

5. **c. 2 to 3 times higher.** In someone with a positive family history of prostate cancer, the relative risk increases according to the number of affected family members, their degree of relatedness, and the age at which they were affected (see Table 107-1).

6. **e. All of the above.** All of these biologic functions are represented in genes shown to predispose men with variant gene structure to prostate cancer.

7. **e. All of the above.** Gene fusions, once thought to be the exclusive domain of hematologic malignancies, are common in prostate cancer and are fundamental drivers of prostate cancer growth and progression. The most commonly observed fusion results from the fusion of the 5′ untranslated end of TMPRSS2 serine protease to members of the ETS family of oncogenic transcription factors, bringing the latter growth-promoting genes under androgen control. The most common fusion identified in localized prostate cancer involves TMPRSS2 fused to ERG (ETS-related gene, 21q22.3) in approximately 50% of patients

TABLE 107-1 Family History and Risk of Prostate Cancer

FAMILY HISTORY	RELATIVE RISK	95% CONFIDENCE INTERVAL
None	1	
Father affected	2.17	1.90-2.49
Brother affected	3.37	2.97-3.83
First-degree family member affected age < 65 years at diagnosis	3.34	2.64-4.23
>2 first-degree relatives affected	5.08	3.31-7.79
Second-degree relative affected	1.68	1.07-2.64

Data from meta-analysis assessing risk of prostate cancer for relatives of patients with prostate carcinoma (Zeegers MP, Jellema A, Ostrer H. Empiric risk of prostate carcinoma for relatives of patients with prostate carcinoma: a meta-analysis. Cancer 2003;97:1894–903).

(Kumar-Sinha et al, 2008).* The *TMPRSS2* gene is prostate specific and is expressed in both benign and malignant prostatic epithelium. *TRMPSS-related gene fusions are highly specific for the presence of prostate cancer.*

8. **c. Aromatase-knockout mice all develop prostate cancer in their lifetime.** Aromatase-knockout mice cannot produce 17β-estradiol locally in the prostate, and despite elevated testosterone and dihydrotestosterone they do not develop prostate cancer (McPherson et al, 2001). All of the other statements are correct.

9. **d. Higher risk of developing prostate cancer.** A recent combined analysis found a positive correlation between serum concentration of IGF-1 and subsequent prostate cancer risk. The odds ratio (OR) in the highest versus lowest quintile was 1.38 (95% confidence interval (CI) 1.19-1.60) (Roddam et al, 2008).

10. **e. Polymorphisms conferring lower vitamin D receptor activity are associated with increased risk for prostate cancer.** Interest in vitamin D as a determinant of prostate cancer risk comes from several epidemiologic observations: (1) men living in northern latitudes with less exposure to sunlight-derived ultraviolet (UV) have a higher mortality rate from prostate cancer; (2) prostate cancer occurs more frequently in older men, in whom vitamin D deficiency is more common both because of less UV exposure and age-related declines in the hydroxylases responsible for synthesis of active vitamin D; (3) African Americans, whose skin melanin blocks UV radiation and inhibits activation of vitamin D, have the highest worldwide incidence and mortality rates for prostate cancer; (4) dietary intake of dairy products rich in calcium, which depresses serum levels of vitamin D, are associated with a higher risk of prostate cancer; and (5) native Japanese, whose diet is rich in vitamin D derived from fish, have a low incidence of prostate cancer. Finally, polymorphisms resulting in vitamin D receptors with lower activity have been associated with increased risk for prostate cancer.

11. **c. Lower serum PSA levels.** Higher body mass index has been associated with increased biologic measures of oxidative stress, lower circulating androgen levels, lower serum PSA (perhaps as a consequence of lower circulating androgens), higher serum free IGF-1 levels, and worse cancer-specific survival after radical prostatectomy. Obese men have lower PSA levels and larger prostates, which together may lead to fewer biopsies and more sampling error, potentially contributing to an increased risk of high-grade disease.

12. **e. All of the above.** A variety of genes implicated in prostate cancer initiation and progression are affected by these processes, including hypermethylation of hormonal response genes

(*ERαA*, *ERβ*, and *RARβ*), genes controlling the cell cycle (*CyclinD2* and *14-3-3σ*), tumor cell invasion/tumor architecture genes (*CD44*), DNA repair genes (*GSTpi*, *GPX3*, and *GSTM1*), tumor suppressor genes (*APC*, *RASSF1α*, *DKK3*, $p16^{INK4?-\alpha}$, *E-cadherin*, and $p57^{WAF1}$), signal transduction genes (*EDNRB* and *SFRP1*), and inflammatory response genes (*PTGS/COX2*); hypomethylation of *CAGE*, *HPSE*, and *PLAU*; histone hypoacetylation of *CAR*, *CPA3*, *RARB*, and *VDR*; and histone methylation of *GSTP1* and *PSA*.

13. **c. Genetic heterogeneity in the cause of prostate cancer.** Current evidence suggests that most prostate cancer is polygenic in origin. GWAS studies have identified more than 70 risk alleles and chromosomal loci, many of which occur in noncoding areas of the genome.

14. **e. All of the above.** Epigenetic events affect gene expression without altering the actual sequence of DNA, and in prostate cancer all of the listed mechanisms are important.

15. **e. An increased risk of prostate cancer in those taking vitamin E alone.** SELECT demonstrated no beneficial effect of vitamin E or selenium on the risk of prostate cancer (alone or in combination). Hazard ratios (HR) for prostate cancer were 1.13 (99% CI: 0.95-1.13) for vitamin E, 1.04 (99% CI: 0.87-1.24) for selenium, and 1.05 (99% CI: 0.88-1.25) for selenium and vitamin E. A follow-up study that included an additional 54,464 person-years showed that dietary supplementation with vitamin E significantly increased the risk of prostate cancer among healthy men (HR 1.17; 95% CI: 1.004-1.36; $P = 0.008$).

16. **a. Cooked foods.** Lycopene is a red-orange carotenoid found primarily in tomatoes and tomato-derived products including tomato sauce, tomato paste, and ketchup, and other red fruits and vegetables. In an in vivo model in which male rats were treated with *N*-methyl-*N*-nitrosourea and testosterone to induce prostate cancer, a protective effect was observed for both calorie restriction and tomato powder but not pure lycopene. This observation suggests that tomato products contain compounds in addition to lycopene that modify prostate carcinogenesis and that reduced caloric consumption and a diet rich in tomato-based foods may be more beneficial than taking oral lycopene supplements in reducing the risk of prostate cancer.

17. **d. Sexual dysfunction.** The incidence of erectile dysfunction and other sexually related side effects was more frequent in the finasteride arm, whereas the incidence of prostatitis, urinary tract infection, benign prostatic hyperplasia, urinary retention, and surgical intervention for lower urinary tract symptoms or retention was lower.

CHAPTER REVIEW

1. The median age for diagnosis of prostate cancer is 68 years. Men with prostate cancer younger than 50 years account for 2% of all cases. The average age of death from prostate cancer is 77 years.
2. Prostate cancer is an indolent disease with a very low cause-specific death rate and will only impact life expectancy in a minority of men.
3. The risk of developing prostate cancer increases with the number of family members with prostate cancer, their degree of relatedness, and the age at which they were affected.
4. Approximately 15% of patients with prostate cancer have the familial or hereditary form.
5. Carriers of the HOXB13, BRCA1 and *BRCA2* genes have an increased risk for developing prostate cancer. BRCA2 related tumors are more aggressive.
6. Chronic inflammation and infections may play a role in the genesis of prostate cancer.
7. Estrogens may act as procarcinogens in the prostate.
8. The androgen receptor is biologically important in the development and progression of prostate cancer even after androgen deprivation therapy.
9. Finasteride improves the sensitivity of PSA and the digital rectal exam.
10. Several studies have shown that there is no increased risk for developing prostate cancer in those who have had a vasectomy.
11. The chemoprevention trials with 5 alpha reductase inhibitors showed a reduced risk of diagnosing prostate cancer by about 25%. While it is unclear in these trials whether there is an increased risk of developing high-grade tumors in those who

*Sources referenced can be found in *Campbell-Walsh Urology, 11th Edition*, on the Expert Consult website.

took 5 alpha reductase inhibitors for chemoprevention, several studies have shown no difference in overall mortality between patients who took 5 alpha reductase inhibitors and those who took a placebo.

12. African-American men have the highest reported incidence of prostate cancer in the world.

13. The most common gene fusion identified in localized prostate cancer involves *TMPRSS2* fused to *ERG* (ETS-related gene, 21q22.3) in approximately 50% of patients. The *TMPRSS2* gene is prostate specific, and is expressed in both benign and malignant prostatic epithelium. TRMPSS-related gene fusions are highly specific for the presence of prostate cancer.

14. Polymorphisms resulting in vitamin D receptors with lower activity have been associated with increased risk for prostate cancer.

15. Higher body mass index has been associated with increased biologic measures of oxidative stress, lower circulating androgen levels, lower serum PSA (perhaps as a consequence of lower circulating androgens), higher serum free IGF-1 levels, and worse cancer specific survival after radical prostatectomy.

16. There is no beneficial effect of vitamin E or selenium on altering the risk of prostate cancer (alone or in combination).

108 Prostate Cancer Tumor Markers

Todd M. Morgan, Ganesh S. Palapattu, Alan W. Partin, and John T. Wei

QUESTIONS

1. Serum prostate-specific antigen (PSA) levels are specific for the presence of prostate:
   a. disease.
   b. cancer.
   c. enlargement.
   d. inflammation.
   e. none of the above.

2. Most detectable PSA in sera is bound to:
   a. albumin.
   b. α_1-antichymotrypsin (ACT).
   c. α_2-macroglobulin.
   d. human kallikrein.
   e. none of the above.

3. TRUE or FALSE: As many as 75% of men presenting with elevated PSA levels are found not to have prostate cancer after transrectal ultrasonography (TRUS) biopsy.
   a. True
   b. False

4. Compared with prostatic tissue PSA levels, prostatic tissue levels of hK2 are:
   a. elevated in well-differentiated prostate cancer tissue.
   b. elevated in poorly differentiated prostate cancer tissue.
   c. depressed in well-differentiated prostate cancer tissue.
   d. depressed in poorly differentiated prostate cancer tissue.
   e. not measurable in prostatic cancer tissue.

5. The serum urine prostate cancer biomarker PCA-3 represents a:
   a. gene on chromosome 20q13.4.
   b. noncoding gene in the *TP53* cluster.
   c. noncoding mRNA with no known protein product.
   d. glycosylated protein of molecular weight 60 kD.
   e. high-molecular-weight nuclear matrix protein.

6. TRUE or FALSE: Evaluation of tissue from prostate cancer specimens has demonstrated higher mRNA expression levels compared with normal prostate tissue, suggesting that prostate cancer cells make more PSA than normal prostatic tissue.
   a. True
   b. False

7. A man with a PSA of 4 ng/mL while taking finasteride for 2 years stops this medication and begins taking saw palmetto. What should his PSA be on his next annual check-up?
   a. 2 ng/mL
   b. 4 ng/mL
   c. 6 ng/mL
   d. 8 ng/mL
   e. 10 ng/mL

8. Which of the following biomarkers has the greatest specificity for the presence of prostate cancer in patients with an elevated PSA?
   a. PCA3
   b. TMPRSS2:ERG
   c. fPSA
   d. phi
   e. 4Kscore

9. proPSA represents:
   a. the early form of the PSA protein in urine.
   b. PSA that has been autocleaved by another molecule several times.
   c. an early form of bound PSA found within the nucleus.
   d. an uncleaved free PSA molecule with a leader sequence.
   e. PSA that gets paid a high salary for hitting home runs.

10. Compared with men without prostate cancer, the fraction of free or unbound PSA in serum from men with prostate cancer:
    a. is equal.
    b. is lower.
    c. is greater.
    d. is undetectable by current assays.
    e. varies depending on which assay is used.

11. The value percentage of free PSA has been approved by the U.S. Food and Drug Administration (FDA) for use in improving:
    a. cancer detection in men with PSA levels less than 4 ng/mL.
    b. cancer detection in men with benign digital rectal examinations and PSA levels of 4 to 10 ng/mL.
    c. the determination of prognosis.
    d. cancer detection in men found to have atypical small acinar proliferation (ASAP).
    e. cancer detection in men with a family history of prostate cancer.

12. After starting finasteride, serum PSA should _____ and the percentage of free PSA should _____.
    a. increase, not change
    b. increase, increase
    c. decrease, not change
    d. decrease, decrease
    e. not change, not change

13. Immunohistochemical studies have demonstrated different expression patterns for hK2 and PSA in benign versus cancerous tissue and may be best described as:
    a. benign: intense PSA and minimal hK2 expression.
    b. cancer: intense PSA and minimal hK2 expression.
    c. benign: minimal PSA and hK2 expression.
    d. benign: intense PSA and hK2 expression.
    e. cancer: minimal PSA and hK2 expression.

14. In which of these regions may the methylation status affect gene expression and play a role in carcinogenesis?
    a. Stop codon
    b. Glycine-cytosine-rich regions
    c. Promoter region
    d. Thymine islands
    e. All of the above

15. The products of hypermethylated genes evaluated in prostate cancer development are:
    a. UROC28 and hepsin.
    b. GSTP1, APC, RARβ2, and RASSF1A.
    c. PCA3, PAC, ERG, and NMP 48.
    d. all of the above.

ANSWERS

1. **e. None of the above.** Although PSA is widely accepted as a prostate cancer tumor marker, it is organ specific and not disease specific. Unfortunately, there is an overlap in the serum PSA levels among men with cancer and benign disease. Thus elevated serum PSA levels may reflect alterations within the prostate secondary to tissue architectural changes, such as cancer, inflammation, or benign prostatic hyperplasia (BPH).

2. **b. α₁-antichymotrypsin.** The current clinically relevant immunodetectable complexed forms of PSA are bound to ACT and, to a lesser extent, to α_1-protease inhibitor (API). The sum of these and other presently unknown PSA complexes is represented by the term complexed PSA (cPSA). The major form of cPSA in serum, PSA bound to ACT, is found in greater serum concentrations in men with cancer than in men with benign disease.

3. **a. True.** Although as many as 30% of men seen with an elevated PSA level may be diagnosed after this invasive procedure, as many as 75% to 80% will not be found to have cancer.

4. **b. Elevated in poorly differentiated prostate cancer tissue.** Immunohistochemical studies reveal different tissue expression patterns for hK2 and PSA. In benign epithelium, PSA is intensely expressed compared with the minimal immunoreactivity of hK2. This is in contrast to cancerous tissue, in which more intense expression of hK2 is seen.

5. **c. Noncoding mRNA with no known protein product.** Using differential display and Northern blot analysis to compare normal and prostate cancer tissue, investigators identified the *PCA3* prostate-specific gene on chromosome 9q21-22. Study of this gene has determined that it may function as noncoding mRNA, because it has been found to be alternatively spliced, contains a high density of stop codons, and lacks an open reading frame.

6. **b. False.** Although prostate cancer cells do not necessarily make more PSA than normal prostate cells, elevated serum levels are likely a result of cancer progression and destabilization of the prostate histologic architecture (Stamey et al, 1987).* Studies have demonstrated that prostate cancer cells do not make more PSA but rather less PSA than normal prostatic tissue (Meng et al, 2002). Evaluation of tissue from prostate cancer specimens have demonstrated as much as 1.5-fold lower mRNA expression levels compared with normal prostate tissue (Meng et al, 2002).

7. **d. 8 ng/mL.** Finasteride (5 mg) and other 5α-reductase inhibitors for treatment of BPH have been shown to lower PSA levels by an average of 50% after 6 months of treatment (Guess et al, 1993). Thus one can multiply the PSA level by 2 to obtain the "expected" PSA level of a patient who has been on finasteride for 6 months or more. Although saw palmetto has not been shown to affect PSA levels, possible contamination of these unregulated supplements may include compounds that can alter PSA levels (i.e., PC-SPES, now off the market).

8. **b. *TMPRSS2:ERG.*** This gene fusion is one of the earliest events that occurs in prostate carcinogenesis and is therefore close to 100% specific for prostate cancer, when present. However, it is only present in approximately 50% of PSA-screened prostate cancers, and therefore its sensitivity is substantially lower.

9. **d. An uncleaved free PSA molecule with a leader sequence.** PSA originates with a 17–amino acid chain that is cleaved to yield a precursor inactive form of PSA termed proPSA (pPSA). The precursor form of PSA contains a 7–amino acid proleader peptide, in addition to the 237 constituent amino acids of mature PSA, and it is termed [-7]pPSA. Once released, the proleader amino acid chain is cleaved at the amino terminus by hK2, converting pPSA to its active 33-kD PSA form. In addition to hK2, pPSA may be activated to PSA by other prostate kallikreins, including hK4. Incomplete removal of the 7–amino acid leader chain has led to the identification of various other truncated or clipped forms of pPSA. These include pPSAs with 2-, 4-, and 5-leader amino acids ([-2]pPSA, [-4]pPSA, and [-5]pPSA). With cellular disruption, these inactive forms circulate as free PSA and may constitute the majority of the circulating free PSA in patients with prostate cancer.

10. **b. Is lower.** Although prostate cancer cells do not produce more PSA than benign prostate epithelium, the PSA produced from malignant cells appears to escape proteolytic processing. Thus men with prostate cancer have a greater fraction of serum PSA complexed to ACT and a lower percentage of total PSA that is free compared with men without prostate cancer (Christensson et al, 1993; Leinonen et al, 1993; Lilja et al, 1993; Stenman et al, 1994).

11. **b. Cancer detection in men with benign digital rectal examinations and PSA levels of 4 to 10 ng/mL.** Currently, the percentage of free PSA is FDA approved for use to aid PSA testing in men with benign digital rectal examinations and minimal PSA elevations, within the diagnostic gray zone of 4 to 10 ng/mL.

12. **c. Decrease, not change.** Free PSA and total PSA both decrease in men on finasteride. Because both decline, the percentage of free PSA is not altered significantly by this medication (Keetch et al, 1997; Panneck et al, 1998).

13. **a. Benign: intense PSA and minimal hK2 expression.** Immunohistochemical studies reveal different tissue expression patterns for hK2 and PSA. In benign epithelium, PSA is intensely expressed compared with the minimal immunoreactivity of hK2 (Tremblay et al, 1997; Darson et al, 1999). This is in contrast to cancerous tissue, in which more intense expression of hK2 is seen. Furthermore, hK2 immunohistochemically stains the different Gleason grades of prostate cancer differently than does PSA. This inverse staining relationship of hK2 is seen as intense staining in high-grade (Gleason primary grade 4 to 5) cancers and lymph node metastasis compared with minimal staining of low-grade (Gleason primary grade 1 to 3) cancers and even weaker association in benign tissue, in which PSA exhibits intense staining (Darson et al, 1997, 1999; Tremblay et al, 1997; Kwiatkowski et al, 1998).

14. **b. Glycine-cytosine-rich regions.** Segments within the gene promoter that are composed of glycine-cytosine-rich regions are termed *CpG islands.* Alterations in the methylation status of these regions may affect gene expression and have been shown to play a role in carcinogenesis (Jones et al, 2002). Furthermore, cumulative effects of environmental exposures, such as diet and stress, throughout one's life may impact DNA methylation status and thus contribute to risk of cancer development (Li et al, 2004).

15. **b. GSTP1, APC, RARβ2, and RASSF1A.** The products of hypermethylated genes that have been evaluated in prostate cancer development are glutathione S-transferase P1 (GSTP1), APC, RARβ2, and RAS-association domain family protein isoform A (RASSF1A).

*Sources referenced can be found in *Campbell-Walsh Urology, 11th Edition,* on the Expert Consult website.

CHAPTER REVIEW

1. Prostate-specific membrane antigen (PSMA), a transmembrane protein, has been identified in the central nervous system, intestine, and prostate.

2. PSA is a member of the human kallikrein gene family. PSA and human kallikrein-2 have been used in prostate cancer detection.

3. Ectopic expression of PSA occurs in breast tissue, adrenal, and renal carcinomas.

4. PSA is organ specific, not disease specific; its half-life is 2 to 3 days.

5. The most common cause of mortality in men with prostate cancer is cardiac disease.

6. Prostate cancer cells make less PSA than normal prostate tissue, gram for gram. Black individuals without prostate cancer have higher PSA values than white individuals. PSA expression is strongly influenced by androgens. Ejaculation can lead to a false increase in PSA. If it is elevated following an ejaculation, the PSA should be rechecked 48 hours following sexual abstinence.

7. Of serum PSA, 70% to 80% is bound to three proteins: α_2-macroglobulin, α_1-protease inhibitor, and α_1-antichymotrypsin. Patients with prostate cancer have a higher fraction of circulating PSA bound to these proteins, that is, they have a lower free PSA.

8. When PSA is released from the cell, a portion of an attached amino acid chain is cleaved, leaving a smaller amino acid chain attached, which inactivates its biologic activity. This molecule is termed *proPSA*. When this amino acid chain is cleaved from proPSA, PSA becomes active as a serum protease. ProPSA may be used to diagnose prostate cancer.

9. PCA-3 is a urine-based marker used in the diagnosis of prostate cancer. It has no known function. It is approved for use as a marker to suggest who should be rebiopsied in those who have had a previous negative biopsy for an elevated PSA.

10. Identifying circulating tumor cells has great promise for both diagnosis and staging of malignancies, including prostate cancer.

11. Prostate cancer susceptibility genes have been located on a number of chromosomes and are thought to increase the risk of developing prostate cancer.

12. Micro-RNAs are involved in the regulation of messenger RNAs and may serve as useful markers for detecting prostate cancer.

13. Metabolomics or the metabolic products of cancer cells have promise for detecting cancers in biopsy specimens.

14. Multi-marker models such as the PHI (prostate health index), which includes proPSA, free PSA, and total PSA, have the potential to improve the accuracy of predicting who will have a positive biopsy and who will have a negative biopsy.

15. Although prostate cancer cells do not necessarily make more PSA than normal prostate cells, elevated serum levels are likely a result of cancer progression and destabilization of the prostate histologic architecture.

16. Segments within the gene promoter that are composed of glycine-cytosine-rich regions are termed *CpG islands*. Alterations in the methylation status of these regions may affect gene expression and have been shown to play a role in carcinogenesis.

109 Prostate Biopsy: Techniques and Imaging

Leonard G. Gomella, Ethan J. Halpern, and Edouard J. Trabulsi

QUESTIONS

1. Prostatic corpora amylacea are calcifications:
   a. always associated with prostate infection.
   b. pathognomonic for acute prostatitis.
   c. most commonly seen between the transition and peripheral zone of the prostate.
   d. associated with hypoechoic lesions and prostate cancer.
   e. in the peripheral zone exclusively and are located in blood vessels.

2. Calcifications diffusely seen in the prostate on transrectal ultrasound are:
   a. called corpora amylacea.
   b. always considered abnormal and mandate biopsy.
   c. considered diagnostic for prostate cancer.
   d. are incidental findings usually due to advanced age.
   e. represent the walls of blood vessels.

3. Which of the following statements is TRUE about transrectal ultrasonography of the seminal vesicles?
   a. Masses in the seminal vesicles are the most common lesion seen on transrectal ultrasonography (TRUS) of the prostate.
   b. The seminal vesicles are usually asymmetrical and normally measure less than 2 cm in length in the adult.
   c. Most cystic masses in the seminal vesicle are malignant and related to prostate cancer.
   d. A solid mass in the seminal vesicle is always associated with malignancy
   e. Solid masses in the seminal vesicle can be caused by schistosomiasis in endemic regions.

4. Which of the following statements about the seminal vesicle (SV) when imaged by ultrasound is TRUE?
   a. The average seminal vesicle is approximately 4.5 to 5.5 cm in length.
   b. A unilaterally absent seminal vesicle suggests an undescended testicle on the ipsilateral side.
   c. Seminal vesicles are usually asymmetrical.
   d. The ejaculatory ducts run alongside the seminal vesicles and cannot be visualized on transrectal ultrasound.
   e. The seminal vesicles are difficult to image using standard TRUS probes.

5. Which of the following statements concerning ultrasonographic estimates of prostate size/volume is TRUE?
   a. Only one formula (prolate ellipse) is acceptable to determine prostate volume.
   b. There is a poor correlation between radical prostatectomy specimen weights and volume as measured by TRUS.
   c. The mature average prostate is between 20 and 25 g and remains relatively constant until about age 50, when the gland enlarges in many men.
   d. Prostate cancer is always associated with an increase in overall volume of the prostate.

   e. Planimetry with a stepping device should be used for routine prostate volume determinations.

6. A hypoechoic lesion of the prostate can be caused by all of the following EXCEPT:
   a. granulomatous prostatitis.
   b. transition zone, benign prostatic hyperplasia nodules.
   c. prostate cancer.
   d. hematologic malignancies.
   e. normal urethra.

7. Which of the following statements is TRUE about anesthesia for TRUS prostate biopsy?
   a. Intrarectal lidocaine gel is as effective as the injection of lidocaine.
   b. It is not necessary even with extended-core biopsies owing to the small size of the needle.
   c. It is best performed using direct injection of lidocaine into the prostate gland.
   d. It is typically performed using lidocaine, a long 22-gauge spinal needle, and the biopsy channel of the ultrasound probe.
   e. It is typically performed using digital guidance to ensure that the base of the prostate near the seminal vesicles is infiltrated.

8. When performing TRUS prostate biopsy:
   a. the left lateral decubitus position is most commonly used.
   b. the right lateral decubitus position is most commonly used.
   c. enemas should not be used before the procedure and may increase the risk of bleeding.
   d. intravenous antibiotic prophylaxis is necessary in all patients to prevent urosepsis.
   e. the dorsal lithotomy position with the use of stirrups increases the diagnostic accuracy of the prostate biopsies.

9. When performing TRUS prostate biopsy:
   a. only hypoechoic lesions should be sampled.
   b. sextant biopsy represents the standard of care for the diagnosis of prostate cancer today.
   c. the transition zone should be included in all initial biopsies, because of the high incidence of cancer in this area.
   d. a minimum of 12 systematic biopsies is now recommended.
   e. isoechoic lesions are rarely cancerous and should not be sampled unless they are calcified.

10. Which of the following statements is TRUE concerning TRUS appearance after treatment:
    a. With an ideal permanent implant, seeds should be distributed evenly throughout the gland with periurethral sparing.
    b. TRUS findings are accurate in determining residual cancer following external beam radiation.
    c. Androgen ablation will always reduce the size of the prostate by more than 50% regardless of baseline size.
    d. With prostate-specific antigen (PSA) recurrence following radical prostatectomy, the anastomosis should be biopsied.

e. Prostate volume decreases by over 50% at 6 months using agents such as finasteride.

11. Which of the following statements about antibiotic prophylaxis for TRUS biopsy is TRUE?

a. It eliminates the risk of any infection.

b. It reduces the risk of febrile urinary tract infection requiring hospitalization but does not prevent them.

c. It is not necessary if the probe is sterilized and an enema is given.

d. Epididymitis is the most common infection after TRUS biopsy even if antibiotics are used.

e. Bacteriuria is the only indication for antibiotics after TRUS prostate biopsy.

12. Hematospermia after TRUS biopsy:

a. usually requires hospitalization.

b. is eliminated with the routine use of antibiotics.

c. usually clears immediately after TRUS biopsy.

d. can persist for up to 4 to 6 weeks after TRUS biopsy.

e. is eliminated if the probe is held firmly against the prostate after the needle is passed.

13. Which of the following statements is TRUE in men with a negative prostate biopsy?

a. They can be assured that no cancer is present.

b. They will require repeated biopsy if one of the cores contains seminal vesicle.

c. Transurethral biopsy is the next step after an initial negative biopsy.

d. Additional biopsies demonstrate decreasing yield of detecting cancer, and the cancer tends to be of lower grade and stage.

e. They should undergo transperineal biopsy for all future biopsies because these have been shown to be the most accurate approach in large randomized European trials.

14. Risk factors for prostate biopsy related infection include all of the following EXCEPT:

a. recent antibiotic use.

b. diabetes mellitus.

c. prostate enlargement.

d. foreign travel.

e. White race.

15. Which of the following statements is TRUE concerning TRUS/magnetic resonance imaging (MRI) fusion biopsy?

a. It must be performed in an "in-bore MRI."

b. The MRI must be obtained within 24 hours of the prostate biopsy.

c. TRUS/MRI fusion biopsy relies on co-registration of the MRI and TRUS images at the time of biopsy.

d. It relies on a method known as "cognitive fusion."

e. Any MRI of the prostate can be used for the fusion biopsy.

16. Concerning prostate cancer on transrectal ultrasound, which statement is FALSE?

a. Thirty-nine percent of cancers are isoechoic.

b. 1% may be hyperechoic.

c. A hypoechoic lesion is malignant up to 57% of the time.

d. An irradiated prostate is diffusely hypoechoic.

e. Hypoechoic lesions are all high Gleason score and suggest extraprostatic disease.

Imaging

1. See Figure 109-1.

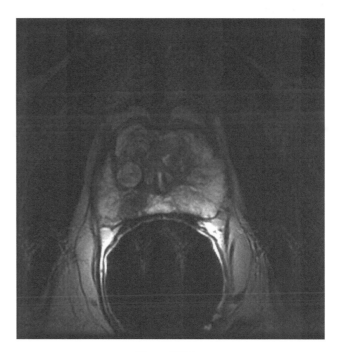

Figure 109-1.

A 62-year-old man with a PSA of 4.5 ng/dL has this axial T2-weighted endorectal coil MRI. The most likely diagnosis is:

a. extracapsular spread of prostate cancer.

b. cancer confined to the gland.

c. enlarged central gland due to benign prostatic hypertrophy.

d. neurovascular bundle involvement.

e. seminal vesicle involvement.

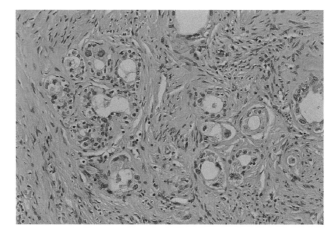

Figure 109-2. (From Bostwick DG, Cheng L. Urologic surgical pathology. 2nd ed. Edinburgh: Mosby; 2008.)

Pathology

1. A 52-year-old black male whose father died of prostate cancer has a PSA of 3 ng/mL for which he has a 12-core biopsy. The pathology on 8 of the cores is benign; however, 4 of the cores were read as normal seminal vesicle without prostate tissue, the pathology of which is depicted in Figure 109-2. The next step in management is:

a. inquire as to the presence of lipofuscin because it is not shown on this slide to confirm that it is seminal vesicle.

b. reassure the patient that the biopsy is benign.

c. ask the pathologist to stain for PSA to be sure this is not a poorly differentiated adenocarcinoma.

d. repeat the biopsy.

e. obtain a computed tomography (CT) scan to evaluate the seminal vesicles.

ANSWERS

1. **c. Most commonly seen between the transition and peripheral zone of the prostate.** Corpora amylacea develop in the surgical capsule between the transition and peripheral zones of the prostate.

2. **d. Are incidental findings usually due to advanced age.** Small, multiple diffuse calcifications are a normal result of age rather than a pathologic entity. Larger prostatic calculi associated with symptoms may be related to underlying infection or inflammation and require further evaluation

3. **e. Solid masses in the seminal vesicle can be caused by schistosomiasis in endemic regions.** Although cystic lesions of the seminal vesicle can be presumed to be benign, solid masses represent a small chance of malignancy. Schistosomiasis should be considered in the differential diagnosis of a solid seminal vesicle mass, especially in endemic regions (i.e., Nile river valley, South East Asia).

4. **a. The average seminal vesicle is approximately 4.5 to 5.5 cm in length.** The normal SV measures 4.5 to 5.5 cm in length and 2 cm in width, has a smooth, saccular appearance, and should be symmetrical.

5. **The mature average prostate is between 20 and 25 g and remains relatively constant until about age 50, when the gland enlarges in many men.** The prostate size increases at puberty. Many men develop symptomatic enlargement of the prostate that typically begins after age 50.

6. **d. Hematologic malignancies.** Many lesions can be hypoechoic, and many will prove to be malignant, reinforcing the need for biopsy of these lesions if seen. Many cancers, including hematologic malignancies of the prostate, are isoechoic.

7. **d.** It is typically performed using lidocaine, a long 22-gauge spinal needle, and the biopsy channel of the ultrasound probe. All recent studies indicate that infiltration of lidocaine around the neurovascular bundles increases tolerability of TRUS prostate biopsy.

8. **a. The left lateral decubitus position is most commonly used.** TRUS biopsy has become the gold standard to diagnose prostate cancer. It is most commonly performed with the patient in the left lateral decubitus position. Dorsal lithotomy may also be used in certain circumstances.

9. **d. A minimum of 12 systematic biopsies is now recommended.** Sextant biopsy revolutionized the utility of TRUS biopsy to diagnose prostate cancer. However, significant numbers of cancers were missed based on the analysis of radical prostatectomy specimens. Increasing to a minimum of 12 systematic biopsies has increased the diagnostic yield and is endorsed based on a recent white paper from the AUA (Bjurlin MA, Carter HB, Schellhammer P, et al. Optimization of initial prostate biopsy in clinical practice: sampling, labeling and specimen processing. J Urol 2013;189[6]:2039-46).

10. **a. With an ideal permanent implant, seeds should be distributed evenly throughout the gland with periurethral sparing.** Even distribution of seeds and urethral sparing is the hallmark of proper seed placement for interstitial brachytherapy.

11. **b. It reduces the risk of febrile urinary tract infection requiring hospitalization but does not prevent them.** Short-term use of prophylactic antibiotics can reduce the incidence of serious infections. Unfortunately, it does not completely eliminate the risk of infection.

12. **d. Can persist for up to 4 to 6 weeks after TRUS biopsy.** This can be a concerning side effect of prostate biopsy and is no clinical consequence. Patients should be counseled about the likelihood of hematospermia after TRUS biopsy.

13. **d. Additional biopsies demonstrate decreasing yield of detecting cancer, and the cancer tends to be of lower grade and stage.** Data from the large European screening study suggested that as the number of biopsy sessions increased to ultimately diagnose prostate cancer, the cancers diagnosed after several biopsy sessions were generally of lower grade and stage.

14. **e. White race.** Risk factors for prostate biopsy-related infection include non-White race, increased number of comorbidities, diabetes mellitus, prostate enlargement, foreign travel, and recent antibiotic use.

15. **c. TRUS/MRI fusion biopsy relies on co-registration of the MRI and TRUS images at the time of biopsy.** TRUS/MRI fusion requires a specific software platform. It combines the familiarity of real-time TRUS-guidance with detailed information from a diagnostic multiparametric MRI and superimposes both images via software image reconstruction. The reconstruction involves "image registration" or "image matching." A pre-biopsy MRI must identify target lesions suspicious for cancer based on imaging characteristics.

16. **e. Hypoechoic lesions are all high Gleason score and suggest extraprostatic disease.** There is a need to biopsy hypoechoic lesions, but these lesions are not pathognomonic for cancer as once thought and do not correlate with the aggressiveness of the disease as measured by Gleason score.

Imaging

1. **b. Cancer confined to the gland.** The small focus of prostate cancer is seen as a well demarcated low signal-intensity area in the right peripheral zone. The seminal vesicles are not included on this image and therefore cannot be accessed. The low signal-intensity capsule is well seen, bordering the tumor focus (options a and d are incorrect). Although there are a few enlarged nodules in the central gland, the gland itself is small in size (option c is incorrect).

Pathology

1. **d. Repeat the biopsy.** Although obtaining normal seminal vesicle on a prostate biopsy is not unusual, four cores is unusual and probably means that the systematic biopsy was not well directed. This patient is at high risk for prostate cancer in view of his race, family history, and elevated PSA for age. The biopsy needs to be repeated and done systematically by an experienced clinician.

CHAPTER REVIEW

1. There are five divisions of the prostate: (1) anterior fibromuscular stroma, (2) transition zone, (3) central zone, (4) periurethral zone, and (5) peripheral zone.

2. Calcifications may be seen along the surgical capsule, which is the junction between the transition zone and peripheral zone.

Multiple diffuse calcifications are often found incidentally and are not diagnostic of a specific entity.

3. A mass in the seminal vesicle that is cystic is usually benign, whereas a solid lesion has a small probability of being malignant. Schistosomiasis may cause solid lesions in the seminal vesicles.

4. Increasing the frequency of the ultrasound probe increases the resolution; decreasing the frequency increases the depth of penetration. It is important to eliminate an air interface between the ultrasound probe and the tissue being visualized.

5. A volume calculation of the prostate should always be performed and requires measurement of three dimensions: anteroposterior (AP) and sagittal. The former is performed at the mid-gland transversely and the latter just off the midline sagittally. Formulas used to calculate volume include those for an ellipse, a sphere, or a prolate (egg) shape. When a more accurate determination is required, multiple sections of the prostate must be measured using the technique of planimetry.

6. Thirty-nine percent of cancers are isoechoic; 1% are hyperechoic. A hypoechoic lesion contains cancer approximately 20% of the time.

7. All hypoechoic lesions should be biopsied; however, they may be caused by granulomatous prostatitis, infarct, or lymphoma in addition to cancer.

8. There is no PSA threshold at any age that can absolutely rule out cancer.

9. The preferred antibiotic prophylaxis for prostate biopsy is a fluoroquinolone given 2 hours prior to the procedure and for 48 hours following the procedure. For those at risk for endocarditis or those who have a prosthesis requiring additional coverage, intravenous ampicillin or vancomycin, if penicillin allergic, and gentamicin followed by fluoroquinolones is the appropriate prophylaxis.

10. Proper analgesia is performed by injection of 5 mL lidocaine bilaterally at the level of the seminal vesicles near the bladder base.

11. The best visualization of the biopsy path is in the sagittal plane.

12. Risk factors for prostate biopsy–related infection include non-White race, increased number of comorbidities, diabetes mellitus, prostate enlargement, foreign travel, and recent antibiotic use.

13. For individuals lacking a rectum, an ultrasound directed transperineal or CT-guided biopsy may be performed.

14. The benefit of a transperineal versus a transrectal biopsy approach is improved sampling of the prostatic apex and potential for less infectious complications.

15. A 12-core biopsy is standard on initial biopsy; increasing the number of cores to 18 to 20 at initial biopsy has minimal benefit.

16. Most suggest a self-administered enema be given before the biopsy.

17. The initial cancer detection rate for patients with a PSA between 4 and 10 µg/mL is 22%; subsequent biopsies for an elevated PSA result in a cancer detection rate of 10% on the second biopsy, 5% on the third, and 4% on the forth.

18. Isolated transition zone tumors without peripheral zone involvement occur less than 5% of the time.

19. For patients who have had multiple biopsies and no imaging abnormalities and who are suspect of harboring cancer, the two areas found most likely to be involved if cancer is present are the anterior zone and the apex. These areas may reliably be approached with a template biopsy or fusion biopsy.

20. Complications of prostate biopsy include febrile urinary tract infection, bacteremia, acute prostatitis, bleeding, hematospermia, acute urinary retention, and sepsis.

21. Newer imaging modalities allowing for the potential of targeted biopsy include Doppler to determine vessel density, determination of the elasticity of an area, endorectal MRI with dynamic contrast enhancement and diffusion weighting, and MRI spectroscopy.

22. Newer imaging modalities such as fusion biopsy, which couples the MRI image with the real-time ultrasound image, have the potential for allowing the clinician to target specific suspicious areas.

110 Pathology of Prostatic Neoplasia

Jonathan I. Epstein

QUESTIONS

1. All of the following statements are true about high-grade prostatic intraepithelial neoplasia (PIN), EXCEPT:
   a. glands are architecturally benign.
   b. if unifocal, PIN is not associated with an increased risk of cancer on rebiopsy.
   c. PIN shares some of the molecular findings with prostatic adenocarcinoma.
   d. PIN is the same as intraductal carcinoma.
   e. PIN does not by itself give rise to elevated serum prostate-specific antigen (PSA) levels.

2. Which of the following is TRUE about the pathologic staging of prostate adenocarcinoma?
   a. pT1c can be assigned to radical prostatectomy specimens.
   b. The difference between T1a and T1b is based on perineural and/or vascular invasion.
   c. pT2c by definition represents more advanced cancer than pt2a.
   d. pt2x refers to prostatectomy specimens with intraprostatic incision.
   e. Microscopic bladder neck muscle invasion is pT3b.

3. Which of the following is TRUE about prostate cancer tumor volume/location?
   a. Posterior/posterolateral in 85% of T1c cases
   b. Multifocal in 30% of cases
   c. Transition zone carcinomas extend out of the prostate at smaller volumes than peripheral zone cancers.
   d. Tumor volume in an independent predictor of prognosis, factoring in other pathological variables at radical prostatectomy.
   e. The number of involved chips distinguishes stages T1a and T1b.

4. All of the following are true about the Gleason grading system, EXCEPT:
   a. on needle biopsy, it sums the most common and highest patterns.
   b. on radical prostatectomy, it sums the most common and second most common patterns.
   c. it factors in cytology as well as glandular architecture.
   d. Gleason score 6 is for the most part the lowest score assigned on biopsy.
   e. Gleason score 6 cancers do not have the ability to metastasize.

5. Which of the following Gleason grade groupings is the most prognostically accurate?
   a. 2-4; 5; 6; 3 + 4; 4 + 3; 8-10
   b. 2-4; 5-6; 3 + 4; 4 + 3; 8, 9-10

   c. ≤6; 7; 8, 9-10
   d. ≤6, 3 + 4; 4 + 3; 8-10
   e. ≤6; 3 + 4; 4 + 3; 8; 9-10

6. All of the following findings at radical prostatectomy adversely affect prognosis, EXCEPT:
   a. tertiary grades.
   b. subdividing extra-prostatic extension into focal and non-focal.
   c. the extent of positive margins.
   d. perineural invasion.
   e. vascular invasion.

Pathology

1. See Figure 110-1.
   A 68-year-old man with an abnormal digital rectal exam (DRE) has a PSA of 4.2 ng/mL and has a needle biopsy of the prostate depicted in the figure. The tissue is stained with high-molecular-weight cytokeratin, and the pathologist reports the biopsy is consistent with benign prostatic hyperplasia (BPH). The next step is to:
   a. repeat the biopsy.
   b. ask the pathologist for additional molecular marker stains.
   c. follow up the patient with a PSA and DRE in 3 to 6 months.
   d. obtain endorectal magnetic resonance imaging (MRI).
   e. obtain a PCA3.

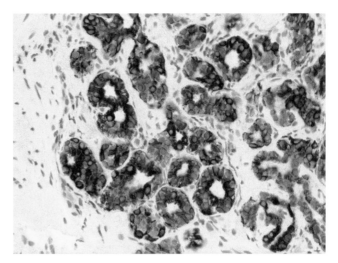

Figure 110-1. (From Bostwick DG, Cheng L. Urologic Surgical Pathology. 2nd ed. Edinburgh: Mosby; 2008.)

2. See Figure 110-2.

A 55-year-old man has a prostate biopsy depicted in the figure for a PSA of 4.5 and is reported as adenocarcinoma. The next step in management is:

a. ask the pathologist for a Gleason score and volume of cancer.
b. radical prostatectomy.
c. metastatic workup with abdominal computed tomography (CT) and bone scan.
d. endorectal MRI.
e. active observation.

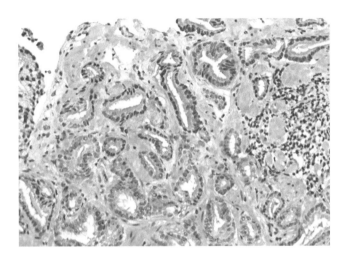

Figure 110-2. (From Bostwick DG, Cheng L. Urologic Surgical Pathology. 2nd ed. Edinburgh: Mosby; 2008.)

ANSWERS

1. **d. PIN is the same as intraductal carcinoma.** Intraductal carcinoma is morphologically worse than high-grade PIN and is typically associated with high-grade carcinoma. Whereas high-grade PIN is either just followed clinically or leads to a repeat biopsy, intraductal carcinoma is treated the same as high-grade invasive prostate adenocarcinoma.
2. **d. Pt2x refers to prostatectomy specimens with intraprostatic incision.** Pt2x means that the tumor is organ confined everywhere in the prostate except in the area of the positive margin where extraprostatic extension cannot be assessed because there is an intraprostatic incision and the edge of the prostate is not visualized in this area.
3. **a. Posterior/posterolateral in 85% of T1c cases.** Even though T1c tumors are nonpalpable, the majority are still in the posterior or posterolateral region.
4. **c. It factors in cytology as well as glandular architecture.** Gleason grading assesses only the architectural pattern.
5. **e. ≤6; 3+4; 4+3; 8; 9-10.** There is a progressive increase in adverse outcome in this sequence of Gleason scoring.
6. **d. Perineural invasion.** Perineural invasion in the radical prostatectomy specimen has no prognostic significance; however, there are conflicting data on whether it has any predictive value in biopsy specimens.

Pathology

1. **c. Follow up the patient with a PSA and DRE in 3 to 6 months.** The patient has BPH as demonstrated by the presence of a basal layer with the positive cytokeratin stain. Because of the abnormal DRE, close follow up is indicated.
2. **a. Ask the pathologist for a Gleason score and volume of cancer.** The figure demonstrates a straightforward Gleason 6 adenocarcinoma. The pathologist needs to report the Gleason score and the volume of cancer in the biopsy specimen in order for the physician to make an informed decision about management.

CHAPTER REVIEW

1. Prostatic intraepithelial neoplasia (PIN) is classified into low and high grade.
2. Low-grade PIN does not increase the risk of prostate cancer.
3. Rebiopsying patients with PIN is unnecessary unless there are multiple cores involved with high-grade PIN or there are other clinical indications.
4. Eighty-five percent of prostate adenocarcinomas are located in the peripheral zone, and 85% are multifocal.
5. Peripherally located cancers tend to extend outside the prostate through the perineural space. The presence of perineural invasion within the prostatectomy specimens does not worsen the prognosis. By contrast, vascular invasion increases the risk of metastatic disease.
6. Prostate cancer metastasizes, in descending order, to lymph nodes, bone, lung, bladder, liver, and adrenal glands.
7. Subdividing pathologic T2 disease has no prognostic significance.
8. Transition zone tumors require larger volumes than peripheral zone tumors for comparable rates of extraprostatic extension and/or distant metastases.
9. For needle biopsy specimens, the primary pattern (dominant pattern) and the highest grade (irrespective of volume) should be reported as the Gleason sum.
10. Adverse findings on needle biopsy generally accurately predict adverse findings in radical prostatectomy specimens. However, favorable findings on needle biopsy do not necessarily predict favorable findings in the radical prostatectomy specimen.
11. Benign glands are differentiated from malignant glands in that the former contain basal cells. These can be labeled, if necessary, with high-molecular-weight cytokeratin and TP63. Patients with atypical glands reported on biopsy specimens have a high likelihood of cancer on rebiopsy. Such findings should prompt a rebiopsy.
12. Adenosis (atypical adenomatous hyperplasia) is characteristically found in the transition zone, and although it may mimic carcinoma histologically, there is no increased risk for adenocarcinoma in patients with this diagnosis.
13. Only 25% of men with seminal vesicle invasion and few with lymph node metastases are biochemically free of disease following radical prostatectomy 10 years postoperatively.
14. Tumor volume correlates well with pathologic stage and Gleason grade in clinical T2 cancers; however, it is not an independent predictor of cancer progression once grade, stage, and margins are accounted for.
15. The prostate lacks a discrete histologic capsule.
16. Involvement of the seminal vesicles is almost always due to direct extension (T3b); it carries a poor prognosis.
17. Only 50% of men with positive margins progress following radical prostatectomy.
18. Endocrine therapy results in atrophic changes with squamous metaplasia in the prostate. Carcinomas in patients who have had endocrine therapy may appear artifactually higher in grade.
19. Primary urothelial carcinomas of the prostate show a propensity to infiltrate the bladder neck and surrounding tissue such that more than 50% of the patients are stage T3 or T4, and 20% have distant metastases at the time of presentation.
20. Intraductal carcinoma is morphologically worse than high-grade PIN and is typically associated with high grade carcinoma.

111 Diagnosis and Staging of Prostate Cancer

Stacy Loeb and James A. Eastham

QUESTIONS

1. Most immunodetectable prostate-specific antigen (PSA) in serum is bound to which of the following?

   a. Albumin

   b. α_1-Antichymotrypsin (ACT)

   c. α_2-Macroglobulin (MG)

   d. Human kallikrein

   e. Globulin

2. Serum PSA levels vary with which factor?

   a. Age

   b. Race

   c. Prostate volume

   d. ACT concentration

   e. Age, race, and prostate volume

3. Serum PSA elevations may occur with prostate:

   a. manipulation.

   b. cancer.

   c. enlargement.

   d. inflammation.

   e. All of the above.

4. Which of the following should be recommended for an elevated PSA?

   a. Repeat the measurement after cystoscopy.

   b. Give a 2-week course of fluoroquinolones, then repeat PSA.

   c. Give a 4 week course of doxycycline, then repeat PSA.

   d. Repeat the PSA measurement after a period of observation.

   e. All of the above.

5. Which of the following represent ways to adjust the PSA measurement?

   a. PSA density

   b. PSA velocity

   c. PSA transition zone density

   d. Percent free PSA

   e. All of the above

6. A 60-year-old man taking finasteride (Proscar) for 2 years with a PSA value of 4 ng/mL would most likely, if he were not taking finasteride, have which PSA value?

   a. 2 ng/mL

   b. 6 ng/mL

   c. 8 ng/mL

   d. 12 ng/mL

   e. 4 ng/mL

7. Which of the following tests has the highest positive predictive value for prostate cancer?

   a. PSA

   b. Digital rectal exam (DRE)

   c. Transrectal ultrasonography (TRUS)

   d. Combination of DRE and TRUS

   e. Human glandular kallikrein (hK2)

8. Which of the following statements about prostate cancer staging is FALSE?

   a. A goal of staging is to predict prognosis.

   b. Staging facilitates the selection of rational therapy on the basis of predicted extent of disease.

   c. Imaging can accurately identify all cases of pelvic lymph node metastases.

   d. PSA and DRE are components of the staging evaluation.

   e. Pelvic lymphadenectomy is the gold standard for the detection of pelvic lymph node metastases.

9. The currently available modalities for assessing disease extent in men with prostate cancer include:

   a. DRE.

   b. serum PSA.

   c. histologic grade.

   d. bone scan.

   e. all of the above.

10. Pathologic staging is superior to clinical staging because all of the following factors are confirmed in the final pathologic examination EXCEPT:

    a. PSA.

    b. surgical margin status.

    c. seminal vesicle involvement.

    d. tumor volume.

    e. capsular penetration.

11. What pathologic finding or findings at radical prostatectomy are highly predictive of the presence of occult metastatic disease?

    a. Positive surgical margins

    b. Seminal vesicle involvement

    c. Lymph node involvement

    d. Both b and c

    e. Both a and b

12. The finding of pathologic perineural invasion of cancer (PNI) on a prostate biopsy specimen suggests:

    a. organ-confined disease.

    b. low-grade disease at radical prostatectomy.

    c. a greater likelihood of capsular penetration.

    d. pelvic lymph node involvement.

    e. a bilateral nerve-sparing prostatectomy should not be considered.

13. As general guidelines regarding PSA levels and pathologic stage, which of the following statements is TRUE?

    a. Twenty-five percent of men with a PSA value less than 4 ng/mL have organ-confined disease.

    b. One hundred percent of men with a PSA value greater than 50 ng/mL have pelvic lymph node involvement.

    c. Ten percent of men with a PSA value greater than 10 ng/mL have extraprostatic extension.

    d. Serum PSA has no predictive value for staging.

    e. Seventy percent or more of men with a PSA value between 4 and 10 ng/mL have organ-confined disease.

14. With respect to the Gleason primary and secondary grade, all of the following statements are TRUE EXCEPT:

    a. Primary grade ranges from 1 to 5.

    b. Secondary grade ranges from 1 to 5.

    c. Secondary grade and primary grade are summed to provide a Gleason score (2 to 10).

    d. The primary grade represents the second-largest area of cancer on the biopsy specimen.

    e. The presence of a Gleason primary or secondary grade 4 or 5 on any biopsy specimen is predictive of poorer prognosis.

15. Which of the following variables are used to predict pathologic stage in the Partin tables?

    a. PSA

    b. Number of positive biopsy cores

    c. Gleason score

    d. Clinical stage

    e. a, c, and d are all correct.

Imaging

1. A 55-year-old man with a family history of prostate cancer had a 12-core prostate biopsy 1 year ago for a PSA of 2.6 ng/mL. Currently his PSA is 2.7 ng/mL and his DRE reveals a smooth soft minimally enlarged prostate with no nodules or firm areas. Prostate magnetic resonance imaging (MRI) with an endorectal coil is obtained and is depicted in Figure 111-1A: T2-weighted axial image of the prostate, Figure 111-1B: diffusion-weighted image of panel A; and Figure 111-1C: dynamic contrast enhancement image of 1A. The patient should be:

    a. reassured and scheduled for yearly PSA and rectal examination.

    b. sent back to his primary care physician for follow-up.

    c. scheduled for a directed prostate biopsy.

    d. scheduled for a saturation biopsy.

    e. followed with a PSA every 4 months and an MRI in a year.

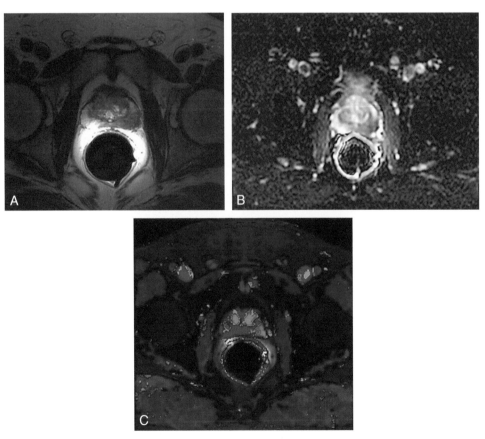

Figure 111-1. A, T2-weighted axial image of prostate MRI with endorectal coil. **B,** MRI image A, diffusion weighted. **C,** MRI image A with dynamic contrast enhancement.

ANSWERS

1. **b. α₁-Antichymotrypsin (ACT).** Most detectable PSA in sera (65% to 90%) is bound to ACT.

2. **e. Age, race, and prostate volume.** In the absence of prostate cancer, serum PSA levels vary with age, race, and prostate volume.

3. **e. All of the above.** Serum PSA elevations may occur as a result of disruption of the normal prostatic architecture that allows PSA to diffuse into the prostatic tissue and gain access to the circulation. This can occur in the setting of prostate disease (benign prostatic hyperplasia [BPH], prostatitis, and prostate cancer) and with prostate manipulation (prostate massage, prostate biopsy). The presence of prostate disease (prostate cancer, BPH, and prostatitis) is the most important factor affecting serum levels of PSA. PSA elevations may indicate the presence of prostate disease, but not all men with prostate disease have elevated PSA levels. Furthermore, PSA elevations are not specific for cancer.

4. **d. Repeat the PSA measurement after a period of observation.** The American Urological Association does not recommend giving empiric antibiotics for an elevated PSA. Manipulation of the urinary tract such as cystoscopy can lead to PSA elevations. Repeating an abnormal test after a period of observation is a good practice.

5. **e. All of the above.** Many different variations on the PSA test have been proposed to improve specificity. These include dividing by total prostate volume (PSA density) or volume of the transition zone (PSA transition zone density), examining changes over time (PSA velocity), and determining the proportion circulating in the free form (percent free PSA).

6. **c. 8 ng/mL.** Finasteride (a 5α-reductase inhibitor for treatment of BPH) at 5 mg has been shown to lower PSA levels by approximately 50% after 12 months of treatment. Thus one can multiply the PSA level by 2 to obtain the "true" PSA level of a patient who has been taking finasteride for 12 months or more. After 2 and 7 years of finasteride therapy, the PSA level should be multiplied by a factor of 2.3 and 2.5, respectively. Men who are to be treated with finasteride should have a baseline PSA measurement before initiation of treatment and should be followed with serial PSA measurements. If there is a rise in the PSA value when the patient is taking finasteride, these men should be suspected of having an occult prostate cancer.

7. **a. PSA.** PSA is the single test with the highest positive predictive value for cancer.

8. **c. Imaging can accurately identify all cases of pelvic lymph node metastases.** The goals in staging of prostate cancer are twofold: (1) to predict prognosis and (2) to rationally select therapy on the basis of predicted extent of disease.

9. **e. All of the above.** The currently available modalities for assessing disease extent in men with prostate cancer include DRE, serum tumor markers, histologic grade, radiographic imaging, and pelvic lymphadenectomy.

10. **a. PSA.** Pathologic staging is more useful than clinical staging in the prediction of prognosis because tumor volume, surgical margin status, extent of extracapsular spread, and involvement of seminal vesicles and pelvic lymph nodes can be determined.

11. **d. Both b and c.** The finding of seminal vesicle invasion or lymph node metastases on pathologic evaluation after radical prostatectomy is associated with a high risk of distant disease.

12. **c. A greater likelihood of capsular penetration.** PNI in a prostatectomy specimen has little independent prognostic staging value as initially reported by Byar and Mostofi (1972).* However, in biopsy cores, its presence is associated with a higher chance of non–organ-confined disease at prostatectomy. de la Taille and colleagues (1999) demonstrated that the presence of PNI on a biopsy specimen was closely associated with high PSA values, poorly differentiated tumor, and involvement of multiple cores with cancer, and thus a higher pathologic stage. Approximately 75% of men with PNI on a biopsy specimen will have capsular penetration on examination of the prostatectomy specimen.

13. **e. Seventy percent or more of men with a PSA value between 4 and 10 ng/mL have organ-confined disease.** As a general guideline, the majority of men (80%) who have prostate cancer with PSA values less than 4 ng/mL have pathologically organ-confined disease, two thirds of men with PSA levels between 4 and 10 ng/mL have organ-confined cancer, and more than 50% of men with PSA levels more than 10 ng/mL have disease beyond the prostate. Pelvic lymph node involvement is found in nearly 20% of men with PSA levels greater than 20 ng/mL and in most men (75%) with serum PSA levels greater than 50 ng/mL.

14. **d. The primary grade represents the second-largest area of cancer on the biopsy specimen.** The Gleason grading system is based on a low-power microscopic description of the architectural pattern of the cancer. A Gleason grade (or pattern) of 1 to 5 is assigned as a primary grade (the pattern occupying the greatest area of the specimen) and a secondary grade (the pattern occupying the second largest area of the specimen). A Gleason sum (2 to 10) is determined by adding the primary grade and the secondary grade. The presence of Gleason pattern 4 or greater (primary or secondary) or a Gleason sum of 7 or greater is predictive of a poorer prognosis.

15. **e. a, c, and d are all correct.** The "Partin tables" are probability tables for the determination of pathologic stage that are based on three parameters: preoperative clinical stage, serum PSA level, and Gleason sum. In the Partin tables, numbers within the nomogram represent the percent probability of having a given final pathologic stage based on logistic regression analyses for all three variables combined; dashes represent data categories in which insufficient data existed to calculate a probability. This information is useful in counseling men with newly diagnosed prostate cancer with respect to treatment alternatives and probability of complete eradication of tumor.

Imaging

1. **c. Scheduled for a directed prostate biopsy.** The T2-weighted image (Figure 111-1A) shows a well-demarcated low-signal-intensity area in the left peripheral zone with likely extracapsular extension. The diffusion-weighted image (**B**) shows restricted diffusion (dark area) in the same location as the abnormality seen in **A** and the dynamic contrast enhanced image (**C**) shows rapid uptake and loss of contrast (red area) in the same location of the abnormal left peripheral zone seen in **A**. These findings are highly suggestive of prostate cancer. The patient should have a directed biopsy to this area.

---

*Sources referenced can be found in *Campbell-Walsh Urology*, 11th Edition, on the Expert Consult website.

CHAPTER REVIEW

1. PSA levels are lower in hypogonadal men; statins may reduce PSA, whereas BPH, prostatitis, prostate manipulation, and prostate cancer increase serum levels of PSA.

2. PSA may be elevated within 24 hours following ejaculation; DRE does not result in a significant fluctuation of PSA.

3. Surgical therapy for BPH may reduce PSA.

4. A PSA velocity of more than 0.75 ng/mL/year in patients with levels between 4 and 10 prompts a concern for prostate cancer; a PSA density (PSAD) may also be used in this group for risk assessment.

5. A low noncomplexed PSA (free PSA) has a higher association with prostate cancer than does a high level of free PSA (>25%) in patients with PSAs between 4 and 10 ng/mL.

6. Prostate cancer screening was found in one study to reduce the rate of advanced disease at the time of diagnosis and reduce prostate specific mortality; however, in another prospective study there was no reduction in prostate specific mortality with screening. Moreover, it may increase morbidity due to increased unnecessary biopsies or treatment in some men.

7. There is some evidence that a PSA less than 1 ng/mL in patients aged 40 to 45 years may be used to inform the frequency of screening.

8. African Americans have higher PSA values than Whites.

9. A tertiary pattern of Gleason grade is reported if there is a small focus of a higher grade than the primary and secondary grades. The Gleason sum is a combination of the primary grade and the highest grade.

10. Bone scans are not appropriate for staging unless the PSA is greater than 20 ng/mL, the clinical stage is T3 or T4, or the patient has specific complaints referable to the bones.

11. MRI with diffusion-weighting and dynamic contrast enhancement has improved the specificity of MRI to predict cancer.

12. Specific criteria for who should have a pelvic lymphadenectomy as a preliminary staging procedure or combined with a radical prostatectomy have not been firmly established. At the very least, it probably should be done in patients with a Gleason score greater than 8, enlarged nodes on imaging, T3 disease on rectal exam, and/or a PSA greater than 20 ng/mL.

13. The majority of men (80%) who have prostate cancer with PSA values less than 4 ng/mL have pathologically organ-confined disease, two thirds of men with PSA levels between 4 and 10 ng/mL have organ-confined cancer, and more than 50% of men with PSA levels more than 10 ng/mL have disease beyond the prostate. Pelvic lymph node involvement is found in nearly 20% of men with PSA levels greater than 20 ng/mL and in most men (75%) with serum PSA levels greater than 50 ng/mL.

14. The "Partin tables" are probability tables for the determination of pathologic stage that are based on three parameters: preoperative clinical stage, serum PSA level, and Gleason sum.

112 Management of Localized Prostate Cancer

William J. Catalona and Misop Han

QUESTIONS

1. Prostate cancer is the cause of mortality in what percentage of U.S. men?
   a. 1%
   b. 3%
   c. 10%
   d. 16%
   e. 30%

2. An outcome comparison between different treatment modalities for localized prostate cancer is difficult because:
   a. most patients diagnosed with prostate cancer receive the same treatment.
   b. outcome measures are similar.
   c. the treatment outcomes in any patient series may be influenced by the malignant potential of the tumors as well as the treatment used.
   d. there are many effective treatments for clinically localized prostate cancer.
   e. randomized clinical trials eliminate selection bias.

3. Which statement is the best rationale for active surveillance protocols for localized prostate cancer?
   a. A prospective, randomized clinical trial demonstrated similar local cancer progression and metastasis rates for patients with clinically localized prostate cancer managed with deferred treatment and radical prostatectomy.
   b. In most active surveillance studies, only approximately 15% of patients develop objective evidence of tumor progression within 5 years.
   c. An accurate assessment of clinically insignificant or indolent cancers is determined by biopsy results.
   d. Active surveillance allows timely intervention as long as patients with localized prostate cancer are followed up semiannually with digital rectal examination and prostate-specific antigen (PSA) levels.
   e. The potential benefits of surgery do not outweigh potential complications in men with a life expectancy of less than 10 years and a low-grade prostate cancer.

4. What is an appropriate criterion used for recommending intervention during active surveillance for prostate cancer?
   a. PSA velocity less than 0.5 ng/mL/year
   b. More than 10% of a biopsy core involvement
   c. Previous cryotherapy of the prostate gland
   d. Gleason pattern 4 or 5 present
   e. Any positive repeat biopsy

5. What recent innovation has been most responsible for the wider use of radical prostatectomy?
   a. Discovery that the pudendal nerves are responsible for urinary continence
   b. Preservation of the external sphincter muscle that yields urinary continence rates in excess of 90%
   c. Frequent use of saturation biopsy under general anesthesia
   d. Magnification provided by robotic-assisted prostatectomy
   e. Elimination of pelvic lymphadenectomy in patients with low-risk tumor features

6. What features correctly characterize each of the following radical prostatectomy approaches?
   a. Perineal: more blood loss and a longer operative time than the retropubic approach
   b. Retropubic: higher risk for rectal injury and postoperative fecal incontinence
   c. Laparoscopic: lowest complication rate
   d. Laparoscopic: lowest positive surgical margin rate
   e. Robotic: less blood loss due to the pneumoperitoneum

7. What outcome do the Partin tables predict?
   a. Clinical stage
   b. Gleason score
   c. Pathologic stage
   d. Biochemical recurrence-free probability
   e. Cancer-specific survival probability

8. During the nerve-sparing portion of radical retropubic prostatectomy, the best approach is to:
   a. dissect the neurovascular bundles free of the posterolateral surface of the prostate gland.
   b. use bipolar electrocautery to transect the urethra.
   c. perform a retrograde dissection to identify the vas deferens.
   d. release the endopelvic fascia after the neurovascular bundle dissection.
   e. use a harmonic scalpel to release neurovascular bundles.

9. Which of the following is most closely associated with urinary continence recovery following radical retropubic prostatectomy?
   a. Preoperative renal function
   b. Pathologic tumor stage
   c. Performance of nerve-sparing surgery
   d. Patient age
   e. Bladder neck-sparing dissection

10. The return of erectile function following radical retropubic prostatectomy correlates best with:
    a. absence of preoperative hormonal therapy.
    b. absence of postoperative radiation therapy.
    c. absence of antihypertensive therapy.
    d. absence of a smoking history.
    e. nerve-sparing status.

11. Which statement is TRUE of "PSA bounce"?
    a. It is strongly associated with an intermittent androgen ablation therapy.
    b. It usually occurs within 2 years of radiation therapy.
    c. It should be treated immediately with combined androgen blockage therapy.
    d. It is more commonly associated with external beam radiation therapy.
    e. It does not exceed an increase of 2 ng/mL following radiation therapy.

12. What is the ASTRO (American Society of Therapeutic Radiation Oncology) definition for recurrence following radiation therapy?
    a. Three consecutive increases in PSA following radiation therapy, and back-dates the time of cancer progression to halfway between the second and third increase in PSA levels.
    b. Three consecutive increases in PSA following radiation therapy with at least one PSA bounce.
    c. Three PSA increases measured 12 months apart, and back-dates the time of cancer progression to halfway between the first and the second increase in PSA levels.
    d. Three consecutive PSA increases measured 6 months apart, and back-dates the time of cancer progression to halfway between the PSA nadir and the first rising PSA level.
    e. Three consecutive PSA increases of total 2 ng/mL after reaching a PSA nadir.

13. Which of the following criteria is a relative contraindication to external beam radiation therapy to the prostate?
    a. Previous radical retropubic prostatectomy
    b. Lower urinary tract symptoms
    c. Previous transurethral resection of prostate (TURP)
    d. Serum PSA less than 2 ng/mL
    e. History of hematospermia
14. Which of the following parameters is most predictive of favorable response to postoperative salvage radiation therapy?
    a. Preoperative PSA less than 10 ng/mL
    b. Extracapsular tumor extension
    c. PSA doubling time of more than 3 months
    d. Positive surgical margin
    e. Preradiation PSA greater than 2 ng/mL
15. Which of the following parameters is most associated with improved prostate cancer-specific survival with salvage radiotherapy for recurrence after surgery?
    a. PSA doubling time of less than 6 months
    b. Concurrent hormonal therapy
    c. Lymph node metastasis
    d. Initiation of salvage radiotherapy after PSA has risen above 2 ng/mL
    e. Previous robot-assisted laparoscopic prostatectomy

ANSWERS

1. **b. 3%.** About 1 in 7 men are diagnosed with prostate cancer during their lifetime. Because of effective treatment of some prostate cancers and the biological indolence relative to the life expectancy of others, only about 16% of men diagnosed with prostate cancer ultimately die of it. As a result, prostate cancer is the cause of death in about 3% of the U.S. male population

2. **c. The treatment outcomes in any patient series may be influenced by the malignant potential of the tumors as well as the treatment used.** Patients whose tumor has a low malignant potential are predetermined to fare better with most treatments. Therefore, the treatment outcomes in any patient series may be influenced by the malignant potential of the tumors and also by the treatment used. Accordingly, it is difficult to compare the results of different reports, because the patient populations usually are not strictly comparable.

3. **e. The potential benefits of surgery do not outweigh potential complications of surgery in men with a life expectancy of less than 10 years and a low-grade prostate cancer.** Traditionally, watchful waiting has been reserved for men with a life expectancy of less than 10 years and a low-grade (Gleason score 2 to 5) prostate cancer. However, active surveillance is now being studied in younger patients with low-volume, low- or intermediate- grade tumors to avoid or delay treatment that might not be immediately necessary.

4. **d. Gleason pattern 4 or 5 present.** During active surveillance, intervention is recommended if Gleason pattern 4 or 5 is present, more than two biopsy cores are involved, or more than 50% of a biopsy core is involved. Progression is more likely in patients who have cancer present on every biopsy procedure.

5. **b. Preservation of the external sphincter muscle that yields urinary continence rates in excess of 90%.** Recent innovations that have led to the wider use of radical prostatectomy include (1) the development of the anatomic radical retropubic prostatectomy, which allows the dissection to be performed with good visualization and preservation of the cavernosal nerves responsible for erectile function and preservation of the external sphincter muscle that yields urinary continence rates in excess of 90%; (2) the development of extended ultrasound-guided biopsy regimens, performed under local anesthesia as an office procedure; and (3) the widespread use of PSA testing, which has led to the great majority of patients being diagnosed with clinically localized disease.

6. **e. Robotic: less blood loss due to the pneumoperitoneum.** Remotely controlled, robot-assisted laparoscopic surgery recently has become popular because of its greater technical ease for the surgeon, especially for tying sutures and performing the vesicourethral anastomosis. Less blood loss due to the pneumoperitoneum is also an advantage over open surgical techniques.

7. **c. Pathologic stage.** Because imaging studies are not accurate for staging prostate cancer, preoperative clinical and pathologic parameters are used in the Partin tables to predict the pathologic stage, and thus identify patients most likely to benefit from the operation.

8. **a. Dissect the neurovascular bundles free of the posterolateral surface of the prostate gland.** Meticulous dissection is required to preserve the neurovascular bundles during the nerve-sparing radical retropubic prostatectomy. In performing nerve-sparing surgery, the neurovascular bundles are identified at the apex of the prostate, and the bundles are dissected free of the posterolateral surface of the prostate gland.

9. **d. Patient age.** The return of urinary continence following radical retropubic prostatectomy is strongly associated with patient age: more than 95% of men younger than 50 years are continent following surgery; 85% of men older than 70 years regain complete continence.

10. **e. Nerve-sparing status.** The return of erectile function following radical retropubic prostatectomy correlates with the age of the patient, preoperative potency status, extent of nerve-sparing surgery, and the era of surgery.

11. **b. It usually occurs within 2 years of radiation therapy.** Inflammation in the prostate gland can produce transient PSA elevation, called a PSA "bounce," following radiation therapy. PSA bounce usually occurs during the first 2 years after treatment and is less common with external beam therapy than with brachytherapy

12. **d. Three consecutive PSA increases measured 6 months apart, and back-dates the time of cancer progression to halfway between the PSA nadir and the first rising PSA level.** Until recently, the most frequent used definition for recurrence following radiation therapy was the American Society of Therapeutic Radiation Oncology (ASTRO) definition. It requires three consecutive PSA increases measured 6 months apart and back-dates the time of cancer progression to halfway between the PSA nadir and the first rising PSA level. Thus, it usually takes years to determine whether progression has occurred after radiotherapy.

    In recent years, the Phoenix definition was proposed to replace the ASTRO definition. It eliminates back-dating but requires the PSA level to rise by 2 ng/mL before treatment failure is declared. Thus, the time to recurrence is further prolonged after the PSA level begins to rise, and often it takes a considerably longer time for the PSA level to increase by 2 ng/mL. In some instances, adjuvant hormone therapy may be initiated before the PSA rises to 2 ng/mL. In practice, the Phoenix definition can yield results that are even more favorable than those obtained with the ASTRO definition.

13. **c. Previous transurethral resection of prostate (TURP).** A prior transurethral resection of the prostate is a relative contraindication to brachytherapy and external beam radiation therapy because the prostate does not hold the seeds well, and radiation after transurethral resection of the prostate is associated with an increased risk for urethral stricture. The presence of severe obstructive urinary symptoms is also a relative contraindication because of the risk for acute urinary retention, which is an even greater risk in patients treated with brachytherapy. Another relative contraindication is inflammatory bowel disease.

14. **d. Positive surgical margin.** Adjuvant radiotherapy is most likely to benefit patients with positive surgical margins or extracapsular tumor extension without seminal vesicle invasion or lymph node involvement. However, not all patients with extracapsular tumor extension or positive margins have tumor recurrence without radiotherapy, and most patients with highly adverse findings have treatment failure with distant metastases, despite adjuvant radiotherapy.

15. **a. PSA doubling time of less than 6 months.** Trock et al reported on a retrospective study of men with PSA failure after radical prostatectomy that is unique in that patients received either no treatment, salvage radiation therapy, or salvage radiation therapy with androgen-deprivation therapy. They reported that salvage radiation was associated with a threefold reduction in prostate cancer mortality, and although the addition of hormone therapy provided no additional decrease in the risk for mortality, the patients who received hormone therapy had higher-risk disease. Therefore, hormone therapy probably provided additional benefit for these high-risk patients. The benefit was strongest in those with the shortest PSA doubling times.

CHAPTER REVIEW

1. Approximately 81% of prostate cancer cases detected appear to be localized at the time of detection. Only 4% of patients present with metastatic disease at the time of diagnosis.

2. Patients who have greater than a 10-year life expectancy and may be considered for active surveillance should have low-volume disease, low- or intermediate-grade tumors (up to Gleason $3+4=7$), nonpalpable lesions, and PSAs that are below 10. Many would suggest that any Gleason grade of 4 or 5 on biopsy makes the patient ineligible for active observation.

3. Patients who are actively observed should routinely have an interval biopsy. Follow-up biopsies in which no cancer is detected significantly decrease the risk of progression in these patients. Intervention is recommended if Gleason pattern 4 or 5 is present, more than two biopsy cores are involved, or more than 50% of a biopsy core is involved. Progression is more likely in patients who have cancer present on every biopsy procedure.

4. Approximately 25% to 50% of patients who choose active observation develop objective evidence of tumor progression within 5 years.

5. The median time from PSA failure to the development of metastatic disease after radical prostatectomy is 8 years, and from the time of metastases to death is 5 years. Thus there is a total of 13 years following detectable PSA after radical prostatectomy before death due to prostate cancer usually occurs. Moreover, only one third of the patients with detectable PSAs will develop clinical metastases.

6. Neoadjuvant hormone therapy does not enhance the resectability of prostate cancer in those patients undergoing a radical prostatectomy.

7. Bone scan, computed tomography (CT) scan, and magnetic resonance imaging (MRI) are not indicated preoperatively in patients with a Gleason score less than 7, a PSA less than 10 ng/mL, nonpalpable disease, and lack of extensive involvement of the majority of the cores.

8. Possible overdiagnosis of insignificant cancer occurs in 6% to 20% of radical prostatectomy specimens.

9. Adverse prognostic factors following radical prostatectomy include non–organ-confined disease, lymphovascular invasion, seminal vesicle invasion, extracapsular tumor extension, positive surgical margins, and lymph node metastases.

10. In those instances of high-grade adenocarcinomas and neuroendocrine tumors that do not produce much PSA, recurrent disease may be diagnosed by palpation, thus indicating a role for digital rectal exam (DRE) in monitoring.

11. The most common late complications of radical prostatectomy are erectile dysfunction, urinary incontinence, inguinal hernia, and urethral stricture.

12. Intensity-modulated radiation therapy (IMRT) generally delivers in excess of 75 Gy.

13. Side effects of external beam radiation therapy include 5% to 10% persistent irritable bowel symptoms and 10% to 15% intermittent rectal bleeding. Approximately half of patients will be impotent.

14. Patients who have high-volume disease or high Gleason scores benefit from androgen-deprivation therapy before administering radiation therapy.

15. Brachytherapy with either iodine-125 or palladium-103 delivers 125 to 145 Gy to the prostate; it is seldom used in prostates which exceed 60 grams and those with high Gleason scores.

16. Not all patients with extracapsular tumor extension or positive surgical margins have a PSA failure. Those patients would not be expected to benefit from adjuvant radiation therapy.

17. There is no compelling evidence that an extensive pelvic lymphadenectomy is more beneficial than a standard lymphadenectomy when indicated.

18. In those who maintain erectile function following radical prostatectomy, the erection is generally less firm than it was preoperatively.

19. Only approximately one-third of patients who have a biochemical recurrence following radical prostatectomy will develop metastases.

20. Most patients with positive surgical margins are cured by the radical prostatectomy.

21. Following radiation therapy, inflammation in the prostate gland can produce transient PSA elevation, called a PSA "bounce." PSA bounce usually occurs during the first 2 years after treatment and is less common with external beam therapy than with brachytherapy.

22. Following radiation therapy, a meaningful elevation in PSA has several definitions: The ASTRO definition requires three consecutive PSA increases measured 6 months apart and back-dates the time of cancer progression to halfway between the PSA nadir and the first rising PSA level. The Phoenix definition was proposed to replace the ASTRO definition. It eliminates back-dating but requires the PSA level to rise by 2 ng/mL before treatment failure is declared. Thus it may take years to determine whether progression has occurred after radiotherapy.

23. A prior transurethral resection of the prostate is a relative contraindication to brachytherapy.

24. The role of adjuvant radiotherapy following radical prostatectomy is controversial because not all patients with extracapsular tumor extension or positive margins have tumor recurrence without radiotherapy, and most patients with highly adverse findings have treatment failure with distant metastases, despite adjuvant radiotherapy.

113 Active Surveillance of Prostate Cancer

Herbert Ballentine Carter and Marc Arnaldo Dall-Era

QUESTIONS

1. Watchful waiting is appropriate for men who:
   a. are 70 years of age or older.
   b. have impalpable cancer not visible on imaging studies.
   c. have a serum prostate-specific antigen (PSA) level less than 10 ng/mL.
   d. have a life expectancy approximately 10 years or less and well to moderately differentiated cancer.
   e. have no major comorbidities.

2. Which of the following is important for monitoring men on watchful waiting?
   a. Periodic PSA testing
   b. Serial transrectal ultrasound
   c. Repeat prostate biopsy
   d. Endorectal magnetic resonance imaging (MRI)
   e. None of the above

3. For men with well or moderately differentiated prostate cancer on watchful waiting, the 10-year cancer-specific mortality is approximately:
   a. 1%.
   b. 5%.
   c. 15%
   d. 30%.
   e. 50%.

4. For men with well-differentiated prostate cancer, the rate of metastases within the first 10 years of watchful waiting is approximately:
   a. 5%.
   b. 10%.
   c. 20%.
   d. 50%.
   e. 75%.

5. Compared with men treated by radical prostatectomy, men on watchful waiting have a higher risk of:
   a. bowel problems.
   b. obstructive voiding problems.
   c. metastases.
   d. death from prostate cancer.
   e. all of the above.

6. The best way to select men for active surveillance is:
   a. age at the time of cancer diagnosis.
   b. life expectancy.
   c. PSA level.
   d. results of imaging studies.
   e. assessment by multiple variables such as Epstein's risk assessment or nomogram.

7. During follow-up of men on active surveillance, how is digital rectal examination (DRE) most valuable?
   a. DRE is an indicator that a repeat biopsy is warranted.
   b. DRE is a means to assess prostate size as an indication for transurethral resection of the prostate.
   c. DRE is an indicator to order an imaging study such as transrectal ultrasound or endorectal MRI.
   d. DRE is a predictor of cancer progression.
   e. DRE has no apparent value in this setting.

ANSWERS

1. **d. Have a life expectancy approximately 10 years or less and well to moderately differentiated cancer.** Watchful waiting is a reasonable option in patients with a life expectancy of 10 years and clinically localized, well-differentiated, or moderately differentiated prostate cancer.

2. **e. None of the above.** Because the goal of watchful waiting is to limit morbidity and not to administer potentially curative treatment, PSA testing, repeat biopsy, and imaging studies are unimportant.

3. **c. 15%.** According to a study by Bill-Axelson and colleagues (2008),* men who were managed conservatively had a 14% cancer-specific mortality rate at 10 years after diagnosis.

4. **c. 20%.** Chodak and colleagues (1994) found that, for men with well-differentiated, clinical stage T1 to T2 cancer managed conservatively, the risk of metastasis at 10 years was 19%.

5. **e. All of the above.** In a randomized comparison of watchful waiting and radical prostatectomy in Sweden, men on watchful waiting experienced significantly more obstructive voiding complaints, bowel problems, metastases, and death from prostate cancer.

6. **e. Assessment by multiple variables such as Epstein's risk assessment or nomogram.** Models that incorporate multiple factors have proven to be better predictors of indolent prostate cancer than any single factor.

7. **a. DRE is an indicator that a repeat biopsy is warranted.** None of the current active surveillance studies has found DRE to be an independent predictor of cancer progression, although it can be useful in determining that a repeat biopsy should be taken.

*Sources referenced can be found in *Campbell-Walsh Urology, 10th Edition,* on the Expert Consult website.

CHAPTER REVIEW

1. Forty-two percent of American men 50 years or older who die of causes other than prostate cancer have prostate cancer at autopsy.

2. In the prostate cancer prevention trial it was found that 6.2% of men with a PSA less than 0.5 ng/mL and 25% of those with a PSA between 2.1 and 4 ng/mL had prostate cancer on biopsy.

3. It is generally accepted that organ-confined cancer less than 0.5 mL in volume with no Gleason grade 4 or 5 component is indolent and poses little if any risk to the patient.

4. Current estimates suggest that 20% to 40% of prostate cancers that are detected would never have been found in a subject's lifetime without screening—in other words, will never affect the patient's life.

5. The criteria generally used for selection of individuals for active observation include (a) no Gleason grade 4 or 5 in the biopsy; (b) no more than three cores positive, none of which is more than 50% involved (some suggest that there should be less than 3 mm of total involvement in the biopsy cores); (c) no palpable disease (controversial); and (d) a PSA less than 10 ng/mL with a PSA density less than 0.15 ng/mL per gram of tissue.

6. In most series of patients on active observation, approximately a third during a period of 5 years will receive definitive treatment.

7. PSA kinetics are extremely complex, so it is difficult to establish specific PSA criteria that predict progression.

8. A repeat biopsy is an integral part of all active observation protocols.

9. Indications for abandonment of active observation are an increased amount of cancer on repeat biopsy, an increased Gleason sum, a rapidly rising PSA, and patient anxiety.

10. Definitive therapy for disease progression in those on active observation appears to be effective in the majority of patients, although no long-term studies are available to firmly establish this.

11. Ten-year cancer-specific mortality for low-risk prostate cancer is approximately 3%.

12. Men with intermediate- and high-risk prostate cancer appear to benefit from treatment.

13. Approximately one third of patients will be upgraded on active surveillance during a 10-year period.

14. Endorectal MRI with diffusion weighting and contrast enhancement has a high negative predictive value and may be of help in selecting patients for active observation, although there are no prospective studies that would confirm this.

15. More extensive biopsies during the standard 12-core biopsy have not been shown to be helpful in patient selection for active observation.

114 Open Radical Prostatectomy

Edward M. Schaeffer, Alan W. Partin, and Herbert Lepor

QUESTIONS

1. What is the arterial blood supply to the prostate?
   a. The pudendal artery
   b. The superior vesical artery
   c. The inferior vesical artery
   d. The external iliac artery
   e. The obturator artery

2. What vessels are located in the neurovascular bundle?
   a. Capsular arteries and veins
   b. Pudendal artery and vein
   c. Hemorrhoidal artery and vein
   d. Santorini plexus
   e. Accessory pudendal artery

3. A radical prostatectomy may compromise the arterial blood supply to the penis by injuring the aberrant blood supply from which artery?
   a. The obturator artery
   b. The inferior vesical artery
   c. The superior vesical artery
   d. The penile artery
   e. All of the above

4. The main parasympathetic efferent innervation to the pelvic plexus arises from:
   a. S1.
   b. S2-S4.
   c. T11-L2.
   d. L3-S1.
   e. T5-T8.

5. What is the relationship of the neurovascular bundle to the prostatic fascia?
   a. Inside Denonvilliers fascia
   b. Outside the lateral pelvic fascia
   c. Inside the prostatic fascia
   d. Between the layers of the prostatic fascia and the levator fascia
   e. Both inside and outside the prostatic fascia

6. Why is there less blood loss during radical perineal prostatectomy?
   a. It is easier to ligate the dorsal vein complex through the perineal approach than through the retropubic approach.
   b. There is no need to divide the puboprostatic ligaments.
   c. The dorsal vein complex is not divided because the dissection occurs beneath the lateral fascia and anterior pelvic fascia.
   d. Because the perineum is elevated, there is lower venous pressure.
   e. The arterial supply to the prostate is ligated early.

7. Which anatomic structure is responsible for the maintenance of passive urinary control after radical prostatectomy?
   a. Bladder neck
   b. Levator ani musculature
   c. Preprostatic sphincter
   d. Striated urethral sphincter
   e. Bulbar urethra

8. What is the major nerve supply to the striated sphincter and levator ani?
   a. The neurovascular bundle
   b. The sympathetic fibers from T11 to L2
   c. The pudendal nerve
   d. The obturator nerve
   e. The accessory pudendal nerve

9. What is the posterior extent of the pelvic lymph node dissection?
   a. The hypogastric vein
   b. The obturator nerve
   c. The obturator vessels
   d. The sacral foramen
   e. The pelvic side wall musculature

10. In opening the endopelvic fascia, there are often small branches traveling from the prostate to the pelvic sidewall. These branches are tributaries from the:
    a. obturator artery.
    b. external iliac artery.
    c. inferior vesical artery.
    d. pudendal artery and veins.
    e. neurovascular bundle.

11. How extensively should the puboprostatic ligaments be divided?
    a. Superficially, with just enough incised to expose the junction between the anterior apex of the prostate and the dorsal vein complex
    b. Extensively, down to the pelvic floor, including the pubourethral component
    c. Not at all; the puboprostatic ligaments should be left intact
    d. Widely enough to permit a right angle to be placed around the dorsal vein complex
    e. Not at all; the puboprostatic ligaments do not need to be divided to perform a radical prostatectomy

12. When the dorsal vein complex is divided anteriorly, what is the most common major structure that can be damaged, and what is the most common adverse outcome?
    a. Aberrant pudendal arteries; impotence
    b. Neurovascular bundle; impotence
    c. Striated urethral sphincter; incontinence
    d. Levator ani musculature; incontinence
    e. Both a and b

13. What is the most common site for a positive surgical margin and when does this occur?

    a. Posterolateral; during release of the neurovascular bundle

    b. Posterior; when the prostate is dissected from the rectum

    c. Apex; during division of the striated urethral sphincter–dorsal vein complex

    d. Bladder neck; during separation of the prostate from the bladder

    e. Seminal vesicles

14. How should the back-bleeders from the dorsal vein complex on the anterior surface of the prostate be oversewn and why?

    a. The edges should be pulled together in the midline to avoid bleeding.

    b. Bunching sutures should be used to avoid excising too much striated sphincter.

    c. The edges should be oversewn in the shape of a V to avoid advancing the neurovascular bundles too far anteriorly on the prostate.

    d. They should be oversewn horizontally to avoid a positive surgical margin.

    e. Oversewing the proximal dorsal vein complex is not required.

15. After the dorsal vein complex has been ligated and the urethra has been divided, what posterior structure, other than the neurovascular bundles, attaches the prostate to the pelvic floor?

    a. Rectourethralis

    b. Denonvilliers fascia

    c. Rectal fascia

    d. Posterior portion of the striated sphincter complex

    e. Neurovascular bundles

16. What are the advantages of releasing the levator fascia higher at the apex (more than one answer may be correct)?

    a. More soft tissue on the prostate

    b. Less traction on the neurovascular bundles as they are released

    c. Preservation of anterior nerve fibers

    d. Less blood loss

    e. Better visualization of the location of the cancer

17. Once the apex of the prostate has been released, what is the best way to retract the prostate for exposure of the neurovascular bundle?

    a. Traction on the catheter, producing upward rotation of the apex of the prostate

    b. Use of a sponge stick to roll the prostate on its side

    c. Downward displacement of the prostate with a sponge stick

    d. Use of finger dissection to release the prostate posteriorly

    e. Dissection with the sucker

18. To avoid a positive surgical margin, what is the best way to release the neurovascular bundle?

    a. Right-angle dissection beginning on the posterior surface of the prostate and dissecting anterolaterally

    b. With sharp dissection, laterally dissecting toward the rectum

    c. With finger dissection to fracture the neurovascular bundle from the prostate

    d. With electrocautery to separate the neurovascular bundle from the prostate

    e. Elevation of the prostate with traction on the Foley catheter

19. What is the latest point at which a decision can be made regarding preservation or excision of the neurovascular bundle?

    a. When perineural invasion is identified on the needle biopsy specimen

    b. When the neurovascular bundle is being released from the prostate and fixation is identified

    c. When the prostate has been removed and tissue covering the posterolateral surface of the prostate is thought to be inadequate

    d. When the patient is found to have a positive biopsy result at the apex

    e. When the Partin tables indicate a greater than 50% chance of extraprostatic extension

20. Before the lateral pedicles are divided, what is the last major branch of the neurovascular bundle that must be identified and released?

    a. Apical branch

    b. Posterior branch

    c. Capsular branch

    d. Bladder neck branch

    e. Seminal branch

21. When the vesicourethral anastomosis sutures are being tied, if tension is found, what is the best way to release it?

    a. Creating an anterior bladder neck flap

    b. Placing the Foley catheter on traction postoperatively

    c. Releasing attachments of the bladder to the peritoneum

    d. Using vest sutures

    e. Releasing the urethra from the pelvic floor

22. If there is excessive bleeding from the dorsal vein complex while it is being divided, what should be done?

    a. Abandon the operation and close the incision.

    b. Ligate the hypogastric arteries.

    c. Inflate a Foley balloon and place traction on it.

    d. Divide the dorsal vein complex completely over the urethra and oversew the end.

    e. Deflate the Foley catheter.

23. If a rectal injury occurs during the operation, the most appropriate next step is:

    a. to create a loop colostomy.

    b. to create an end colostomy.

    c. to create a Hartman pouch.

    d. to ensure interposition of the omentum following repair of the injury.

    e. to repair the rectal injury in two layers.

24. In postoperative patients who require transfusions of blood for hypotension, the best approach is to:

    a. avoid re-exploration because it might damage the anastomosis.

    b. perform re-exploration.

    c. place the Foley catheter on traction.

    d. administer fresh frozen plasma.

    e. serially monitor the patient in an intensive care unit setting.

25. What is the best way to ensure good coaptation of the anastomotic mucosal surfaces to avoid a bladder neck contracture?

    a. Hold the catheter on traction while tying the sutures.

    b. Use a sponge stick in the perineum.

    c. Use a Babcock clamp to hold the bladder down.

d. Use vest sutures.

e. Evert the bladder mucosa.

26. What is the most common cause of incontinence after radical prostatectomy?

a. Intrinsic sphincter deficiency

b. Detrusor instability

c. Failure to reconstruct the bladder neck

d. Injury to the neurovascular bundles

e. Bladder neck contracture

27. Preservation of the seminal vesicles during radical prostatectomy has demonstrated:

a. improved erectile function in the majority of men.

b. no increase in biochemical recurrence.

c. improved early and late urinary control.

d. increased rate of pelvic abscess.

e. none of the above.

28. Preservation of the bladder neck during radical prostatectomy has demonstrated:

a. improved erectile function.

b. improved long-term urinary control.

c. decreased surgical margins.

d. improved anastomotic stricture rate.

e. none of the above.

29. What percentage of men who had bilateral sural nerve grafting demonstrated full erections sufficient for penetration?

a. 9%

b. 13%

c. 26%

d. 38%

e. 57%

30. Sural nerve grafts are placed:

a. end to end on the ipsilateral side from the tumor.

b. above the bladder neck and below the pubic arch.

c. in reverse to the natural position (proximal to distal and distal to proximal).

d. in a circle to enhance nerve growth factor release.

e. next to the prostatectomy specimen in the pelvis until it is time for anastomosis.

31. Which complication has changed dramatically with experience with salvage prostatectomy?

a. Overall urinary incontinence

b. Potency

c. Blood loss

d. Rectal injury

e. Stricture rate

32. Which of the following statements about perineal prostatectomy is FALSE?

a. The pathologic outcomes are similar to those of radical retropubic prostatectomy and proven over considerable time.

b. It has experienced a resurgence of interest as a result of its low morbidity and rapid convalescence.

c. It fell out of favor as the principal technique in the 1970s, secondary to high intraoperative blood loss.

d. Nerve-sparing techniques have been applied to the approach, allowing for postoperative potency.

e. Partin tables allow for relatively accurate predictions of pathologic stage, forfeiting the need for staging lymphadenectomy in many patients.

33. With regard to postoperative neurapraxia, which of the following statements is TRUE?

a. The literature supports that it is almost always transient.

b. It usually results in a motor deficit that is transient.

c. Most studies show that a self-limited neurapraxia occurs in approximately 25% of patients.

d. The same rates of neurapraxia tend to occur in retropubic prostatectomy as well.

e. This is a major source of morbidity and the reason many surgeons do not use this approach.

34. Which of the following statements with regard to rectal injury associated with perineal prostatectomy is FALSE?

a. If unrecognized, it may result in the occurrence of a rectocutaneous or urethrocutaneous fistula.

b. Despite the close proximity of the rectum in the initial dissection, the incidence is fairly low.

c. It can be avoided when an assistant places gentle downward pressure on the Lowsley tractor while the rectourethralis muscle is divided.

d. If repaired with a two-layer closure, most clinical sequelae are avoided.

e. After repair with a two-layer closure, the operation can continue without a problem.

35. When selecting a patient for radical perineal prostatectomy, which of the following must always be considered?

a. Gleason score of biopsy specimen

b. Preoperative serum prostatic-specific antigen (PSA)

c. Mild degenerative lumbar disk disease

d. a and b only

e. All of the above

36. Which of the following statements is TRUE regarding the radical perineal prostatectomy?

a. Patients who require lymph node sampling for staging purposes should undergo a radical retropubic prostatectomy because the radical perineal prostatectomy, when combined with a laparoscopic lymph node dissection, yields much higher morbidity and is not cost effective.

b. Patients with ankylosis of the hips or spine may not tolerate a radical perineal prostatectomy.

c. Patients with a prior history of renal transplant surgery with the allograft in the right iliac fossa are not candidates for a radical perineal prostatectomy.

d. Morbid obesity is becoming a common contraindication to a radical perineal prostatectomy.

e. None of the above.

37. Which of the following statements regarding blood loss during radical perineal prostatectomy is TRUE?

a. Because transfusion rates are low, a blood type and crossmatch are not recommended before starting the case.

b. Unlike a radical retropubic prostatectomy, the dorsal venous complex is not usually encountered and blood loss is significantly reduced.

c. Transfusion rate in most reports is approximately 15%.

d. The dorsal venous complex is ligated early, resulting in reduced blood loss.

e. Rates of transfusion are generally greater than those in the retropubic literature.

38. Which of the following statements concerning postoperative care is TRUE?

a. The diet is rapidly advanced to a regular diet.

b. Most patients are discharged from the hospital by postoperative day 2.

c. A rectal suppository is administered on a scheduled basis while in the hospital to minimize Foley catheter discomfort except in cases of intraoperative rectal injury.

d. a and b only

e. All of the above

39. Which of the following statements is TRUE with regard to potency outcomes of the radical perineal prostatectomy?

a. Using a nerve-sparing technique, potency is shown to return in up to 70% of men.

b. Older patients are as likely to be as potent as younger patients if a nerve-sparing technique is used.

c. Pharmacotherapy is demonstrated to improve postoperative potency status.

d. All of the above

e. a and c only

40. In a perineal prostatectomy, exposure of the urethra is facilitated by:

a. encircling the urethra with umbilical tape.

b. the Lowsley retractor.

c. division of the puboprostatic ligaments.

d. division of the dorsal venous complex.

e. retraction of the neurovascular bundles medially.

41. Which of the following statements concerning the technique of urethral anastomosis is TRUE?

a. The presence of the Lowsley retractor assists in identifying the membranous urethral stump for the initial placement of interrupted sutures.

b. A running suture technique is advocated for a watertight anastomosis.

c. The visualization of the anastomosis is difficult, one of the few disadvantages of the radical perineal prostatectomy.

d. The sutures are interrupted in a tennis-racquet fashion.

e. The indwelling Foley catheter is not passed until after the anterior vesicourethral anastomotic sutures are placed and tied down.

ANSWERS

1. **c. The inferior vesical artery.** The prostate receives arterial blood supply from the inferior vesical artery.

2. **a. Capsular arteries and veins.** The capsular branches run along the pelvic sidewall in the lateral pelvic fascia posterolateral to the prostate, providing branches that course ventrally and dorsally to supply the outer portion of the prostate. Histologically, the capsular arteries and veins are surrounded by an extensive network of nerves. These capsular vessels provide the macroscopic landmark that aids in the identification of the microscopic branches of the pelvic plexus that innervate the corpora cavernosa.

3. **e. All of the above.** The major arterial supply to the corpora cavernosa is derived from the internal pudendal artery. However, pudendal arteries can arise from the obturator, inferior vesical, and superior vesical arteries. Because these aberrant branches travel along the lower part of the bladder and anterolateral surface of the prostate, they are divided during radical prostatectomy. This may compromise arterial supply to the penis, especially in older patients with borderline penile blood flow.

4. **b. S2-S4.** The autonomic innervation of the pelvic organs and external genitalia arises from the pelvic plexus, which is formed by parasympathetic visceral efferent preganglionic fibers that arise from the sacral center (S2 to S4).

5. **d. Between the layers of the prostatic fascia and the levator fascia.** The neurovascular bundles are located in the lateral pelvic fascia between the prostatic and levator fasciae.

6. **c. The dorsal vein complex is not divided because the dissection occurs beneath the lateral fascia and anterior pelvic fascia.** In an effort to avoid injury to the dorsal vein of the penis and Santorini plexus during radical perineal prostatectomy, the lateral fascia and anterior pelvic fascia are reflected off the prostate. This accounts for the reduced blood loss associated with radical perineal prostatectomy.

7. **d. Striated urethral sphincter.** The striated sphincter contains fatigue-resistant, slow-twitch fibers that are responsible for passive urinary control.

8. **c. The pudendal nerve.** The pudendal nerve provides the major nerve supply to the striated sphincter and levator ani.

9. **a. The hypogastric vein.** The obturator artery and vein are skeletonized but are usually left undisturbed and are not ligated unless excessive bleeding occurs. The dissection then continues down to the pelvic floor, exposing the hypogastric veins.

10. **d. Pudendal artery and veins.** The incision in the endopelvic fascia is carefully extended in an anteromedial direction toward the puboprostatic ligaments. At this point, one often encounters small arterial and venous branches from the pudendal vessels, which perforate the pelvic musculature to supply the prostate. These vessels should be ligated with clips to avoid coagulation injury to the pudendal artery and nerve, which are located just deep to this muscle as they travel along the pubic ramus.

11. **a. Superficially, with just enough incised to expose the junction between the anterior apex of the prostate and the dorsal vein complex.** The dissection should continue down far enough to expose the juncture between the apex of the prostate and the anterior surface of the dorsal vein complex at the point where it will be divided. The pubourethral component of the complex must remain intact to preserve the anterior fixation of the striated urethral sphincter to the pubis.

12. **c. Striated urethral sphincter; incontinence.** The goal is to divide the complex with minimal blood loss while avoiding damage to the striated sphincter.

13. **c. Apex; during division of the striated urethral sphincter–dorsal vein complex.** The exact plane on the anterior surface of the prostate can be visualized, avoiding inadvertent entry into the anterior prostate and ensuring minimal excision of the striated sphincter musculature. This is the most common site for positive surgical margins because it can be difficult to identify the anterior apical surface of the prostate.

14. **c. The edges should be oversewn in the shape of a V to avoid advancing the neurovascular bundles too far anteriorly on the prostate.** To avoid back-bleeding from the anterior surface of the prostate, the edges of the proximal dorsal vein complex on the anterior surface of the prostate are sewn in the shape of a V with a running 2-0 absorbable suture. If one tries to pull these edges together in the midline, the neurovascular bundles can be advanced too far anteriorly on the prostate.

15. **d. Posterior portion of the striated sphincter complex.** The posterior band of urethra is now divided to expose the posterior portion of the striated urethral sphincter complex. The posterior sphincter complex is composed of skeletal muscle and fibrous tissue.

16. **b. Less traction on the neurovascular bundles as they are released, and c. Preservation of anterior nerve fibers.** The purpose of this technique is to speed up recovery of sexual function

by reducing traction on the branches of the nerves to the cavernous bodies and striated sphincter and/or avoiding inadvertent transection of the small branches that travel anteriorly. However, because there is less soft tissue at the apex, the risk of positive margins may be increased.

17. **b. Use of a sponge stick to roll the prostate on its side.** When the surgeon releases the neurovascular bundle, there should be no upward traction on the prostate. Rather, the prostate should be rolled from side to side.

18. **a. Right-angle dissection beginning on the posterior surface of the prostate and dissecting anterolaterally.** After the plane between the rectum and prostate in the midline has been developed, it is possible to release the neurovascular bundle from the prostate, beginning at the apex and moving toward the base, by using the sponge stick to roll the prostate over on its side. Beginning on the rectal surface, the bundle is released from the prostate by spreading a right angle gently. With use of this plane, Denonvilliers fascia and the prostatic fascia remain on the prostate; only the residual fragments of the levator fascia are released from the prostate laterally.

19. **c. When the prostate has been removed and tissue covering the posterolateral surface of the prostate is thought to be inadequate.** Clues that indicate that wide excision of the neurovascular bundle is necessary include inadequate tissue covering the posterolateral surface of the prostate once the prostate has been removed, leading to secondary wide excision of the neurovascular bundle. This last point is important to understand. The surgeon does not have to make the decision about whether to excise or preserve the neurovascular bundle until the prostate is removed, and, if there is not enough soft tissue covering the prostate, one can excise the neurovascular bundle then.

20. **b. Posterior branch.** The surgeon should look for a prominent arterial branch traveling from the neurovascular bundle over the seminal vesicles to supply the base of the prostate. This posterior vessel should be ligated on each side and divided. By this method, the neurovascular bundles are no longer tethered to the prostate and fall posteriorly.

21. **c. Releasing attachments of the bladder to the peritoneum.** The anterior suture is tied initially. There should be no tension. If there is, the bladder should be released from the peritoneum.

22. **d. Divide the dorsal vein complex completely over the urethra and oversew the end.** If there is troublesome bleeding from the dorsal vein complex at any point, the surgeon should completely divide the dorsal vein complex over the urethra and oversew the end. This is the single best means to control bleeding from the dorsal vein complex. Any maneuver short of this will only worsen the bleeding. To gain exposure for the prostatectomy, one must put traction on the prostate. If the dorsal vein is not completely divided, traction opens the partially transected veins and usually worsens the bleeding.

23. **d. To ensure interposition of the omentum following repair of the injury.** It is wise to interpose omentum between the rectal closure and the vesicourethral anastomosis to reduce the possibility of a rectourethral fistula.

24. **b. Perform re-exploration.** Our findings suggest that patients requiring acute transfusions for hypotension after radical prostatectomy should undergo exploration to evacuate the pelvic hematoma in an effort to decrease the likelihood of bladder neck contracture and incontinence.

25. **c. Use a Babcock clamp to hold the bladder down.** We have found that the use of a Babcock clamp to approximate the bladder neck and urethra while the anastomotic sutures are tied has virtually eliminated bladder neck contractures in our practice.

26. **a. Intrinsic sphincter deficiency.** After radical prostatectomy, incontinence is usually secondary to intrinsic sphincter deficiency.

27. **e. None of the above.** Sparing of the seminal vesicles has not improved incontinence, potency, or margin status, and there have been no reported cases of pelvic abscess.

28. **e. None of the above.** Sparing of the bladder neck has not improved incontinence, potency, margin status, or stricture rates.

29. **c. 26%.** The percentage of men who had bilateral sural nerve grafting and demonstrated full erections (sufficient for penetration) was 26%.

30. **c. In reverse to the natural position (proximal to distal and distal to proximal).** Sural nerve grafts are placed in reverse to the natural position (proximal to distal and distal to proximal).

31. **d. Rectal injury.** Only rectal injury rates have dramatically changed.

32. **c. It fell out of favor as the principal technique in the 1970s secondary to high intraoperative blood loss.** In the 1970s, the procedure fell out of favor because the importance of pelvic lymphadenectomy was understood for the purposes of staging. However, with the advent of Partin tables, surgeons could accurately predict the chances of lymph node involvement, obviating the need for staging lymphadenectomy. Furthermore, laparoscopic lymphadenectomy has gained favor and allows for radical perineal prostatectomy and lymph node dissection in one operative setting in patients in whom it is required. Pathologic outcomes are not significantly different for either procedure. It offers shorter hospital stays and lower costs than the retropubic prostatectomy. Blood loss is significantly lower than with the retropubic approach. A nerve-sparing technique can be accomplished through the perineal approach.

33. **a. The literature supports that it is almost always transient.** Sensory neurapraxia of the lower extremity is reported to occur in approximately 2% of radical perineal prostatectomy cases. However, one study did report an incidence of 25%. This is reported significantly more often than with retropubic prostatectomy. True motor deficits are rare. Because of the transient nature, this is not a major source of morbidity.

34. **c. It can be avoided when an assistant places gentle downward pressure on the Lowsley tractor while the rectourethralis muscle is divided.** Traction on the Lowsley tractor during division of the rectourethralis muscle tents the rectum upward and increases the likelihood of injury. Traction should not be placed until after the rectourethralis muscle is divided. When unrecognized, a fistula may ensue. Although one report showed an incidence of rectal injury in 11% of cases, most series recognize an incidence of 1% to 5%. When the injury is recognized and repaired at the time of occurrence, the operation can continue without a problem.

35. **d. a and b only.** The patient's Gleason score and PSA value help determine the likelihood of organ-confined disease and, thus, the candidacy for a radical perineal prostatectomy. A history of degenerative disk disease is not a contraindication to surgery.

36. **b. Patients with ankylosis of the hips or spine may not tolerate a radical perineal prostatectomy.** Because of the necessity for either an exaggerated lithotomy or a modified exaggerated lithotomy position, ankylosis of the hips or spine may be a contraindication to the procedure. Concomitant radical perineal prostatectomy and laparoscopic lymph node dissection results in little increased morbidity and remains cost effective when compared with radical retropubic prostatectomy. Patients with prior renal transplantation or morbid obesity are often better candidates for a perineal approach than for the retropubic approach.

37. **b. Unlike a radical retropubic prostatectomy, the dorsal venous complex is not usually encountered and blood loss is significantly reduced.** The dorsal venous complex is usually not encountered, resulting in relatively lower blood loss when compared with the retropubic approach. A blood type and antibody screen are performed in the days or hours before surgery, but a crossmatch is generally unnecessary. Transfusion rates are generally around 5%.

38. **d. a and b only.** Postoperatively, the diet is advanced rapidly as tolerated, patients ambulate early, and the overwhelming majority of patients are discharged by the second postoperative day.

However, rectal stimulation or manipulation is prohibited in the postoperative period.

39. **e. a and c only.** In a series by Weldon and colleagues (1997),* up to 70% of the patients were potent postoperatively. Furthermore, pharmacotherapy has been demonstrated to improve potency outcomes. However, older age has been demonstrated to be a risk factor for postoperative impotence.

40. **b. The Lowsley retractor.** The apex of the prostate and adjacent urethra can be palpated easily because of the presence of the Lowsley retractor.

41. **e. The indwelling Foley catheter is not passed until after the anterior vesicourethral anastomotic sutures are placed and tied down.** During placement of the anterior vesicourethral anastomotic sutures, a red rubber catheter is placed transurethrally and used to identify the membranous urethral stump and also provide traction on the urethra to assist in placement of the sutures. The red rubber catheter is then removed, and the indwelling Foley catheter is then placed retrograde into the bladder. Simple interrupted sutures are placed for the anastomosis. A tennis-racquet technique is used for bladder neck reconstruction if necessary.

CHAPTER REVIEW

1. The dorsal vein has three major branches: a superficial branch in the midline and two lateral branches that span over the lateral aspects of the prostate.
2. The prostate is covered with three distinct fascial layers: Denonvilliers fascia, prostatic fascia, and levator fascia.
3. Denonvilliers fascia is most prominent and dense near the base of the prostate and overlying the seminal vesicles and thins dramatically more caudad at its termination at the striated sphincter.
4. Laterally the prostatic fascia fuses with the levator fascia.
5. Following radical prostatectomy, 15% to 20% of men develop an inguinal hernia. It is usually an indirect inguinal hernia.
6. The final decision whether to preserve the neurovascular bundles is made at surgery.
7. Findings that would indicate a neurovascular bundle should be resected include palpable induration in the lateral pelvic fascia, a neurovascular bundle that appears fixed to the prostate, and insufficient tissue on the posterolateral aspect of the specimen.
8. Thermal energy should never be used on or near the neurovascular bundles.
9. Bladder neck contractures occur in less than 10% of patients.
10. Factors important for recovery of erectile function include patient age, preoperative potency status, and preservation of the neurovascular bundles.
11. Potency improves with time such that in one study 42% of patients were potent at 3 months and 73% at a year.
12. In a randomized study using sural nerve grafting to preserve potency in patients in whom a neurovascular bundle needed to be sacrificed, there was no difference in those grafted versus those who were not.
13. Salvage radical prostatectomy should only be considered in men who have unequivocally clinically localized prostate cancer.
14. Complications following salvage radical prostatectomy include 50% incontinence, 24% anastomotic stricture, and nearly universal erectile dysfunction, with approximately a 45% recurrence rate at 5 years.
15. Complete excision of the seminal vesicle during radical prostatectomy is recommended for cancer control.
16. Surgery should be deferred for 6 to 8 weeks after biopsy and 3 months after a transurethral resection of the prostate.
17. During pelvic lymphadenectomy, one should preserve the lymphatic tissue covering the external iliac artery, which drains the lower extremity.
18. Accessory pudendal arteries should be preserved.
19. The most common site of a positive margin occurs at the apex, followed by the posterior and the posterolateral prostate.
20. The bladder mucosa should be advanced so that the urethral vesicle anastomosis opposes mucosa to mucosa, is water tight, and is tension free.
21. If postoperative phosphodiesterase type 5 inhibitors are to be used, on demand is preferred to daily dosing.
22. Aberrant pudendal arteries may arise from the obturator, inferior vesical, and superior vesical arteries and should be preserved so as not to compromise the blood supply to the penis.
23. Wide excision of the neurovascular bundle should be considered when there is inadequate tissue covering the posterolateral surface of the prostate once the prostate has been removed. The surgeon does not have to make the decision about whether to excise or preserve the neurovascular bundle until the prostate is removed, and, if there is not enough soft tissue covering the prostate, one can excise the neurovascular bundle then.
24. If there is troublesome bleeding from the dorsal vein complex at any point, the surgeon should completely divide the dorsal vein complex over the urethra and oversew the end.
25. Patients requiring acute transfusions for hypotension after radical prostatectomy should undergo exploration to evacuate the pelvic hematoma in an effort to decrease the likelihood of bladder neck contracture and incontinence.
26. Rectal stimulation or manipulation is prohibited in the postoperative period.

---

*Sources referenced can be found in *Campbell-Walsh Urology, 11th Edition,* on the Expert Consult website.

115 Laparoscopic and Robotic-Assisted Radical Prostatectomy and Pelvic Lymphadenectomy

Li-Ming Su, Scott M. Gilbert, and Joseph A. Smith, Jr.

QUESTIONS

1. With laparoscopic/robotic prostatectomy, use of continuous (versus interrupted) sutures for the vesicourethral anastomosis:
   a. minimizes incontinence.
   b. has a high rate of bladder neck contracture.
   c. can be performed with the need for only a single knot.
   d. requires an indwelling catheter for at least 2 weeks.
   e. eliminates the need for a pelvic drain.

2. With laparoscopic/robotic radical prostatectomy, positive margin rates are not influenced by:
   a. surgical technique.
   b. patient selection.
   c. the method of pathologic analysis.
   d. transperitoneal versus extraperitoneal exposure.
   e. tumor grade and stage.

3. Compared with open surgical approaches, laparoscopic/robotic prostatectomy has been consistently shown to decrease:
   a. postoperative pain.
   b. urinary incontinence.
   c. bleeding.
   d. erectile dysfunction.
   e. positive margins.

4. Positive surgical margins with laparoscopic/robotic prostatectomy:
   a. decrease while technical experience is gained.
   b. are rare at the prostatic apex.
   c. occur only when extracapsular disease is present.
   d. are seen most commonly at the prostate base.
   e. can be avoided by using a robotic-assisted approach.

5. An advantage of extraperitoneal versus transperitoneal approach to laparoscopic/robotic prostatectomy is:
   a. faster operating room time.
   b. shorter hospitalization.
   c. increased working space.
   d. avoidance of bowel manipulation.
   e. fewer positive margins.

6. Laparoscopic pelvic lymph node dissection:
   a. is difficult to perform along with robotic radical prostatectomy.
   b. should always be performed transperitoneally.
   c. has an increased risk of thromboembolic complication compared with open approaches.
   d. should only be performed for tumors lower than or equal to Gleason grade 7.
   e. can allow lymph node removal comparable with open surgery.

7. Rectal injury with laparoscopic/robotic radical prostatectomy:
   a. is best avoided by antegrade release of the rectum from the posterior prostate.
   b. is usually from trocar placement.
   c. can be avoided by bluntly dividing Denonvilliers fascia.
   d. should be treated with an immediate diverting colostomy.
   e. is often unrecognized and heals spontaneously.

8. Bleeding during laparoscopic/robotic radical prostatectomy is usually minimal because:
   a. the plane of periprostatic tissue dissection is different than with open surgery.
   b. the dorsal vein complex does not have to be divided.
   c. the pneumoperitoneum tamponades venous bleeding.
   d. suturing is easier than with open surgery.
   e. the Trendelenburg position decreases venous pressure.

9. Robotic assistance with laparoscopy is most useful in:
   a. trocar insertion and removal.
   b. maintaining a steady insufflation pressure.
   c. decreasing operating room costs.
   d. facilitating suturing.
   e. eliminating the need for a table side assistant.

10. The neurovascular bundle lies within which two periprostatic fascial planes?
    a. Prostate capsule and prostatic fascia
    b. Prostate capsule and levator fascia
    c. Prostatic fascia and levator fascia
    d. Denonvilliers fascia and prostate capsule
    e. Denonvilliers fascia and endopelvic fascia

11. Antegrade laparoscopic dissection of the prostate results in less blood loss compared with the retrograde approach, due in part to:
    a. early division of the dorsal venous complex and prostatic pedicles.
    b. early division of the prostatic pedicles and late division of the dorsal venous complex.
    c. less tissue manipulation.
    d. better visualization.
    e. late division of the dorsal venous complex and prostatic pedicles.

12. The higher cost of laparoscopic/robotic-assisted as compared with open radical prostatectomy is mostly a consequence of:

    a. higher blood loss and transfusion rates.

    b. a higher complication rate.

    c. a longer operative time and disposable equipment.

    d. longer hospital stays.

    e. higher surgical and anesthesia charges.

13. As a consequence of the CO_2 pneumoperitoneum used during minimally invasive prostatectomy, the anesthesia team must be most aware of the potential for:

    a. bleeding and hypotension.

    b. hypoxia and acidosis.

    c. tachycardia and hypertension.

    d. bradycardia and hypotension.

    e. hypercarbia and oliguria.

14. Positive margins at the prostatic apex:

    a. are more common with the robotic-assisted technique compared with open surgery.

    b. can occur due to protrusion of the posterior prostatic apex beneath the urethra.

    c. can occur more commonly with retrograde versus antegrade dissection of the prostate.

    d. are less common in laparoscopic versus open surgery.

    e. are less common than at the prostatic base.

15. Men who are not candidates for laparoscopic/robotic-assisted laparoscopic radical prostatectomy include those with:

    a. palpable tumors.

    b. history of prior pelvic surgery.

    c. morbid obesity.

    d. uncorrectable bleeding diatheses.

    e. prior neoadjuvant hormonal therapy.

ANSWERS

1. **c. Can be performed with the need for only a single knot.** The vesicourethral anastomosis may be accomplished using either an interrupted closure or a running continuous suture with a single knot (van Velthoven et al, 2003).*

2. **d. Transperitoneal versus extraperitoneal exposure.** Comparison of margin status between high-volume centers with the operations performed by experienced surgeons has shown no definitive advantage for one surgical approach versus the other in achieving negative surgical margins (Brown et al, 2003; Khan and Partin, 2005).

3. **c. Bleeding.** Because most of the blood loss that occurs during radical prostatectomy is from venous sinuses, the tamponade effect from the pneumoperitoneum helps diminish ongoing blood loss during laparoscopic robotic prostatectomy (LRP)/robot-assisted laparoscopic prostatectomy (RALP). Blood loss of less than a few hundred milliliters is routinely reported (Guillonneau et al, 2001; Hoznek et al, 2002).

4. **a. Decrease while technical experience is gained.** In most series of LRP and RALP, positive margin percentages decrease while greater familiarity with the procedure is obtained (Ahlering et al, 2004b; Salomon et al, 2004; Rassweiler et al, 2005).

5. **d. Avoidance of bowel manipulation.** While the extraperitoneal technique avoids violation of the peritoneal envelope, bowel manipulation is avoided. It is for this reason that patients with extensive prior abdominal surgery can undergo successful laparoscopic and robotic prostatectomy by the extraperitoneal route.

6. **e. Can allow lymph node removal comparable with open surgery.** Pelvic lymphadenectomy can be performed by open or laparoscopic techniques with no significant difference in nodal yield.

7. **a. Is best avoided by antegrade release of the rectum from the posterior prostate.** Thorough dissection of the rectum off of the posterior prostate is critical to minimize the risk of rectal injury during subsequent steps such as division of the urethra and dissection of the prostatic apex. With LRP and RALP, sharp and complete incision of the posterior layer of Denonvilliers fascia is necessary after seminal vesicle dissection to allow adequate mobilization of the rectum.

8. **c. The pneumoperitoneum tamponades venous bleeding.** Because most of the blood loss that occurs during radical prostatectomy is from venous sinuses, the tamponade effect from the pneumoperitoneum helps diminish ongoing blood loss during LRP/RALP. Blood loss of less than a few hundred milliliters is routinely reported (Guillonneau et al, 2001; Hoznek et al, 2002).

9. **d. Facilitating suturing.** Most surgeons believe that the robotic technology significantly facilitates suturing (especially for the vesicourethral anastomosis) and other aspects of the surgical dissection (Dasgupta, 2005).

10. **c. Prostatic fascia and levator fascia.** The neurovascular bundle travels between two distinct fascial planes that surround the prostate, namely, the prostatic fascia and levator fascia.

11. **b. Early division of the prostatic pedicles and late division of the dorsal venous complex.** Because the dorsal venous complex is divided early in the operation and the prostatic pedicles late, there is potentially a greater risk of ongoing bleeding with the retrograde technique (Rassweiler et al, 2001). In contrast, during the antegrade neurovascular bundle dissection, the arterial blood supply to the prostate (via the prostatic pedicles) is divided early and the dorsal venous complex is divided near the end of the operation, thus reducing blood loss during the operation.

12. **c. A longer operative time and disposable equipment.** In the study by Link and colleagues (2004), the factors that most influenced overall cost in order of importance included operative time, length of hospital stay, and consumable items (e.g., disposable laparoscopic equipment and trocars).

13. **e. Hypercarbia and oliguria.** The anesthesiologist must be aware of the potential consequences of CO_2 insufflation and pneumoperitoneum including oliguria and hypercarbia.

14. **b. Can occur due to protrusion of the posterior prostatic apex beneath the urethra.** Before division of the posterior urethra, great care must be taken to inspect the contour of the posterior prostatic apex. In some patients, the posterior prostatic apex can protrude beneath the urethra, resulting in an iatrogenic positive margin if not identified.

15. **d. Uncorrectable bleeding diatheses.** Contraindications to minimally invasive laparoscopic prostatectomy include uncorrectable bleeding diatheses or the inability to undergo general anesthesia due to severe cardiopulmonary compromise.

---

*Sources referenced can be found in *Campbell-Walsh Urology, 11th Edition*, on the Expert Consult website.

CHAPTER REVIEW

1. Accessory pudendal arteries traveling longitudinally along the anteromedial aspect of the prostate should be preserved because they may be important in preserving blood flow for erectile function.
2. When dissecting at the tip of the seminal vesicles, care should be taken not to use electrocautery because damage to the cavernosal nerves that travel adjacent to this area may be incurred.
3. The apical dissection is the most common site of positive margins following radical prostatectomy. It is important to note that at the apex there may be an anterior and/or posterior overlying lip of prostate tissue that needs to be recognized and excised along with the specimen before transecting the urethra.
4. A transperitoneal approach is not totally protective against the formation of a lymphocele. Clips should be used if lymphatics are identified to reduce the incidence of lymphocele formation.
5. When a wide margin of tissue is desired posteriorly, Denonvilliers fascia should be incised and the dissection carried forward between Denonvilliers fascia and perirectal fat.
6. When the ureteral orifices are too close to the resected bladder neck, closure at the 5 o'clock and 7 o'clock positions with interrupted sutures will recess the orifices away for the vesicourethral anastomosis.
7. Complications specific to the pneumoperitoneum, steep Trendelenburg, and hyperextension include hypercarbia, acidosis, fluid overload, increased intraocular pressure, and femoral neurapraxia.

116 Radiation Therapy for Prostate Cancer

Anthony V. D'Amico, Paul L. Nguyen, Juanita M. Crook, Ronald C. Chen, Bridget F. Koontz, Neil Martin, W. Robert Lee, and Theodore L. DeWeese

QUESTIONS

1. When managed with radiation alone, patients with high-risk prostate cancer have a 5-year prostate-specific antigen (PSA) failure-free survival rate of approximately:

   a. 75%.

   b. 60%.

   c. 33%.

   d. 10%.

2. Which of the following represents unfavorable intermediate-risk disease?

   a. Gleason 3 + 4, PSA 9.5, cT2a

   b. Gleason 4 + 3, PSA 9.5, cT3a

   c. Gleason 4 + 4, PSA 9.5, cT1c

   d. Gleason 4 + 3, PSA 12.8, cT2a

3. A 58-year-old man presents with a T2b, Gleason 7 (4 + 3: 80% pattern 4, 2/6 sextants positive, 4/10 cores), PSA 7.8 ng/mL. He is treated with 6 months combined androgen deprivation therapy (ADT) + 78 Gy intensity-modulated radiation therapy (IMRT). Testosterone recovers 6 months following completion of IMRT. At 12 months, PSA is 0.8 ng/mL; at 18 months, 2.6 ng/mL; at 24 months, 3.2 ng/mL; and now at 30 months, following IMRT, PSA is 5.4 ng/mL. The best next step in management is:

   a. because the most likely explanation for the rising PSA is testosterone recovery, reassure the patient and continue to follow up.

   b. arrange biopsy for presumed local failure.

   c. because patient clearly has failed radiotherapy, advise radical local salvage.

   d. because patient's PSA doubling time and time to biochemical failure make him an unlikely candidate for local salvage because they are indicative of systemic failure, arrange systemic staging with or without multiparametric magnetic resonance imaging (MRI) of the prostate.

   e. The PSA kinetics are compatible with a benign increase or "bounce." Reassure the patient and continue to monitor.

4. A 53-year-old man presents with T2a, Gleason 7 (3 + 4: 20% pattern 4, 1/6 sextants positive, 2/10 cores), PSA 5.9 ng/mL. He is treated with iodine-125 permanent seed prostate brachytherapy. At 12 months, PSA has fallen to 1.2 ng/mL. At 15 months, PSA is 1.8 ng/mL; at 18 months, it is 3.2 ng/mL. He is sexually active and asymptomatic. Which is the best next step?

   a. Brachytherapy has failed. Start ADT.

   b. Brachytherapy has failed. Arrange radical local salvage.

   c. Brachytherapy has failed. Arrange biopsy before radical local salvage.

   d. Recognizing that this is classic timing for a benign PSA bounce, contact his radiation oncologist, review the dosimetry of the implant, and continue to monitor the PSA every 3 months, planning for eventual biopsy if the PSA has not started to decline again by 30 months.

   e. Given his time to nadir of 12 months and PSA doubling time of 4 months, explain to the patient that this is almost certainly distant failure and discuss timing of ADT.

5. In two large trials that randomized patients with high-risk and locally advanced prostate cancer to androgen deprivation therapy with versus without radiation therapy, the addition of radiation improved what outcome by an absolute of 8% to 10%?

   a. Biochemical recurrence-free survival

   b. Clinical recurrence-free survival

   c. Metastasis-free survival

   d. Disease-specific survival

   e. Overall survival

6. Modern radiation therapy for prostate cancer differs from the technology used in the 1980s to 1990s in what ways? Modern radiation uses:

   a. computed tomography (CT)-based treatment planning.

   b. intensity-modulated radiation delivery.

   c. image guidance.

   d. dose-escalated radiation.

   e. all of the above.

7. A randomized trial comparing 76 Gy in 38 fractions to 70.2 Gy in 26 fractions found:

   a. the shorter regimen improved 5-year biochemical failure and had comparable rectal and urinary toxicity.

   b. the shorter regimen improved 5-year biochemical failure and had higher late urinary toxicity.

   c. the shorter regimen improved 5-year biochemical failure and had higher late rectal toxicity.

   d. the shorter regimen did not improve 5-year biochemical failure and had higher late urinary toxicity in men with poor baseline urinary function.

   e. the shorter regimen did not improve 5-year biochemical failure and had higher late rectal toxicity.

8. In 2013, radium-223 was approved by the U.S. Food and Drug Administration (FDA) for use in the treatment of men with _____ because of a prolongation in _____.

   a. castrate-resistant metastatic prostate cancer, overall survival

   b. castrate-resistant metastatic prostate cancer, disease-free survival

   c. castrate-resistant nonmetastatic prostate cancer, overall survival

   d. castrate-resistant metastatic prostate cancer, PSA failure–free survival

   e. castrate-resistant nonmetastatic prostate cancer, PSA failure–free survival

Imaging

1. A voiding cystourethrogram on a 72-year-old man who presents with urinary tract infections 2 years after combination external beam radiation therapy and brachytherapy for prostate cancer is depicted in Figure 116-1. The most likely diagnosis is:

   1. brachytherapy seed migration.
   2. urethra rectal fistula.
   3. vesico sigmoid fistula.
   4. urethra cutaneous fistula.
   5. vesico rectal fistula.

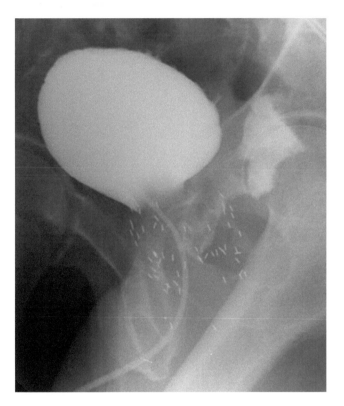

Figure 116-1.

ANSWERS

1. **c. 33%.** (D'Amico AV, Whittington R, Malkowicz S, et al. Biochemical outcome after radical prostatectomy, external beam radiation therapy, or interstitial radiation therapy for clinically localized prostate cancer. JAMA 1998;280:969–74.)
2. **d. Gleason 4+3, PSA 12.8, cT2a.** (Zumsteg ZS, Spratt DE, Pei I, et al. A new risk classification system for therapeutic decision making with intermediate-risk prostate cancer patients undergoing dose-escalated external-beam radiation therapy. Eur Urol 2013;S0302-2838(13)00257-1.)

3. **d. Because patient's PSA doubling time and time to biochemical failure make him an unlikely candidate for local salvage because they are indicative of systemic failure, arrange systemic staging with or without multiparametric magnetic resonance imaging (MRI) of the prostate.** This PSA increase is much too high to be due to testosterone recovery. Because this patient was treated with IMRT and not brachytherapy, this is not a benign increase. A 58-year-old man should not be denied potentially curative salvage, but his PSA kinetics are strongly suggestive of distant failure. Although ADT may well be the correct maneuver, systemic staging should be undertaken first. A post-treatment biopsy of the prostate should be interpretable 30 months after completion of treatment, but even if residual disease is demonstrated, this patient is at very high risk of also harboring systemic disease because of his PSA kinetics and should fully understand this before consenting to further local treatment.
4. **d. Recognizing that this is classic timing for a benign PSA bounce, contact his radiation oncologist, review the dosimetry of the implant, and continue to monitor the PSA every 3 months, planning for eventual biopsy if the PSA has not started to decline again by 30 months.** This is classic timing for a benign PSA bounce after brachytherapy monotherapy. Bounces are seen in 65% of men younger than 55 years, especially those who are sexually active, and can be quite dramatic, with kinetics characteristic of distant failure because of the early onset and rapid doubling. Reassurance, close monitoring, biopsy if the bounce has not resolved by 30 months, and systemic staging if the PSA approaches 10 ng/mL are appropriate.
5. **e. Overall survival.** In the NCIC/MRC trial of 1205 patients, the addition of radiation therapy significantly improved overall survival: 7-year survival 66% for ADT versus 74% ADT/RT ($P=.033$). In a Scandinavian trial (SPCG-7/SFUO-3) of 875 patients, radiation therapy decreased overall mortality: 10-year mortality was 39.4% for ADT versus 29.6% for ADT/RT ($P<.05$).
6. **e. All of the above.** CT-based treatment planning was developed in the 1990s, IMRT in the early 2000s, and image guidance more recently. Four randomized trials consistently demonstrated improved cancer control with "dose-escalated" radiation, which has changed the standard of care in prostate cancer radiation.
7. **d. The shorter regimen did not improve 5-year biochemical failure and had higher late urinary toxicity in men with poor baseline urinary function.** (Pollack A, Walker G, Buyyounouski MK, et al. Five year results of a randomized external beam radiotherapy hypofractionation trial for prostate cancer. Int J Radiat Oncol Biol Phys 2011;81(2):S1.)
8. **a. Castrate-resistant metastatic prostate cancer, overall survival.** (Parker C, Nilsson S, Heinrich D, et al.; ALSYMPCA Investigators. Alpha emitter radium-223 and survival in metastatic prostate cancer. N Engl J Med 2013;369(3):213–23.)

Imaging

1. **b. Urethra rectal fistula.** There is partial opacification of the irregular prostatic urethra with immediate filling of the rectum. The bladder is normal in appearance, making option e incorrect. The contrast is in the rectum, making a urethra cutaneous fistula and vesico sigmoid fistula incorrect. The seeds are located in the area one would expect following brachytherapy.

CHAPTER REVIEW

1. The advantage of brachytherapy is that there is a rapid falloff of dose within a few millimeters of the seed implant.
2. A pretreatment PSA velocity of greater than 2 ng/mL/yr is associated with an increased risk of biochemical failure following radiation therapy.
3. The ASTRO definition of failure following radiation therapy is three consecutive rises in PSA following the nadir. It is recommended that these determinations be obtained 3 to 4 months apart. The Phoenix definition of failure is a 2 ng/mL or more increase in PSA above the nadir.
4. A PSA nadir of less than 0.5 ng/mL is correlated with successful treatment.
5. PSA nadir is the strongest predictor of outcome.

6. Approximately 50% of potent men are impotent at 5 years following conformal external beam radiation therapy; 10% will have some rectal bleeding. Less common complications include urinary and fecal incontinence, hemorrhagic cystitis, and urethral stricture.

7. Conformal radiation therapy (CRT) uses a computerized algorithm to conform the dose of radiation to the contours of the prostate.

8. Intensity-modulated radiation therapy (IMRT) uses a set of radiation beams with changing intensities distributed across the field.

9. When IMRT is compared with CRT, lower doses are delivered to critical tissues such as rectum, bladder, and small bowel.

10. Heavy particle beams such as neutrons and protons exhibit a Bragg effect. This is manifested by a sharp falloff beyond the particle's tissue range, thus delivering little radiation beyond that point.

11. Iodine-125 has a half-life of approximately 60 days; palladium-103 has a half-life of 17 days.

12. Treatment of impending spinal cord compression due to prostate cancer consists of immediate ablation of androgens (most effectively accomplished by bilateral orchiectomy), steroids, and radiation therapy. Occasionally a decompression laminectomy is required emergently.

13. The dose delivered to the prostate with IMRT is 75 to 79 Gy; for brachytherapy with ^{125}I is 140 to 160 Gy; and for ^{103}Pd is 110 to 125 Gy.

14. Pretreatment risk stratification may be divided as follows: low risk—T1c-T2a, PSA less than 11 ng/mL and no Gleason score higher than 6; intermediate risk—T2b, PSA 11 to 20 ng/mL or Gleason score of 7; and high risk—T2c, PSA greater than 20 ng/mL or Gleason score greater than 7.

15. The percentage of positive biopsies and the PSA velocity have also been used for risk stratification.

16. Radiation causes significant changes in cell architecture that can make interpretation of biopsy specimens after radiation therapy difficult.

17. At present there does not appear to be any advantage of proton therapy over conventional photon IMRT.

18. Radium-223 used to treat metastatic prostate cancer to bone is an alpha particle emitter and as such there is less damage to hematopoietic marrow elements when compared with strontium-89.

19. A postradiation treatment biopsy of the prostate should be interpretable 30 months after completion of treatment.

117 Focal Therapy for Prostate Cancer

David C. Miller, Louis L. Pisters, and Arie S. Belldegrun

QUESTIONS

1. Technical innovations improving cryotherapy for prostate cancer include all EXCEPT the use of:
   a. transrectal ultrasound.
   b. urethral warming catheters.
   c. warming of neurovascular bundles.
   d. thermocouples placed in critical areas of the prostate.
   e. smaller-diameter cryoprobes allowing percutaneous insertion.

2. What is the most clinically important parameter of tissue ablation other than lowest temperature achieved by cryotherapy?
   a. The diameter of the cryoprobe
   b. The number of freeze/thaw cycles
   c. The velocity of tissue thawing
   d. The velocity of tissue freezing
   e. The duration of freezing

3. What is the characteristic appearance of frozen tissue on ultrasound?
   a. Mixed echogenicity
   b. Hyperechogenicity
   c. Anechogenicity
   d. Hypoechogenicity
   e. None of the above

4. Prostate cell death is likely to occur completely in a single freeze cycle when tissue temperature reaches:
   a. 20° C.
   b. 0° C.
   c. −20° C.
   d. −40° C.
   e. none of the above.

5. Failure after prostate cryotherapy may be defined as:
   a. failure to reach prostate-specific antigen (PSA) nadir by 2 months.
   b. PSA cutoff greater than 0.1 ng/mL.
   c. three consecutive elevations in PSA after nadir.
   d. PSA rise of 2 ng/mL above post-treatment nadir.
   e. c and d.

6. Two years after cryosurgery for clinical stage T2a, PSA 7, Gleason grade 3 + 4 cancer, a patient is found to have benign glands on a prostate biopsy specimen from the right apex. No malignancy is detected. The PSA level is detectable at 0.2 ng/mL. What is the next step in management?
   a. Repeat cryoablation of the left lobe
   b. Radiation therapy
   c. Surveillance
   d. Androgen deprivation
   e. Repeat biopsy

7. Which clinical parameter most accurately predicts cancer control after cryotherapy?
   a. PSA nadir less than 0.1 ng/mL
   b. Preoperative Gleason score less than 6
   c. Preoperative serum PSA level less than 15 ng/mL
   d. A prostate volume less than 40 mL
   e. Preoperative T stage

8. Potential advantages of primary cryotherapy for prostate cancer versus other local therapies include all EXCEPT:
   a. it is capable of destroying a biologically heterogeneous population of cancer cells, including cell populations that are resistant to radiation therapy and hormonal therapy.
   b. the freezing process can extend beyond the capsule of the prostate, potentially eradicating extracapsular disease.
   c. it is proven to be beneficial with adjuvant therapies.
   d. it can be repeated with minimal morbidity.
   e. it can treat high Gleason-score prostate cancer.

9. Salvage cryotherapy for radiorecurrent prostate cancer:
   a. will not reduce the PSA below 0.4 ng/mL.
   b. may be useful in the control of local spread in the face of distant metastases.
   c. has the same incidence of incontinence and fistula rates as primary cryotherapy.
   d. may be performed on all patients for whom irradiation fails.
   e. is unlikely to cure high-risk disease (PSA greater than 10 ng/nL and Gleason score greater than 7).

10. Clinical pretreatment factors associated with early treatment failure after salvage cryotherapy include:
    a. postradiation PSA greater than 10 ng/mL.
    b. recurrent cancer with Gleason score 9 or greater.
    c. postradiation PSA doubling time 16 months or less.
    d. all of the above.
    e. none of the above.

11. Two months after cryotherapy, a patient complains of urinary frequency and dysuria. Urinalysis reveals pyuria. What is the most likely diagnosis?
    a. Pelvic abscess
    b. Urethral sloughing
    c. Extravasation of urine
    d. Rectourethral fistula
    e. Bladder neck contracture

12. High-intensity focused ultrasound (HIFU) exerts what effect on prostate tissue?
    a. Tissue fragmentation with disruption of vascular architecture
    b. Coagulative necrosis
    c. Nuclear injury
    d. Cavitation
    e. Disruption of protein synthesis

13. The most common side effect of HIFU for localized prostate cancer is:

    a. impotence.

    b. urinary retention.

    c. bladder neck stricture.

    d. urethrorectal fistulae.

    e. incontinence.

ANSWERS

1. **c. Warming of neurovascular bundles.** Use of transrectal ultrasonography (TRUS) for real-time monitoring of the freezing process, use of a urethral warming catheter, use of thermocouples placed in critical areas of the prostate, and improved cryoprobes allowing percutaneous insertion are technical innovations that have all contributed to improving cryotherapy for prostate cancer.

2. **b. The number of freeze/thaw cycles.** In a clinical setting, the number of freezing cycles, the lowest temperature achieved, and the existence of any regional "heat sinks" may be more important factors relating to cancer destruction. Repeating a freeze/thaw cycle results in more extensive tissue damage compared with a single cycle.

3. **d. Hypoechogenicity.** Frozen tissue is significantly different from unfrozen tissue in sound impedance, resulting in strong echo reflection at the interface of frozen and normal tissue. The frozen area can be seen as a well-marginated hyperechoic rim with acoustic shadowing by ultrasonography. Sonography provides no information about the temperature distribution within the ice, nor does it show the extent of freezing at the lateral or anterior aspects of the prostate.

4. **d. $-40°$ C.** Complete cell death is unlikely to occur at temperatures higher than $-20°$ C, and temperatures lower than $-40°$ C are required to completely destroy cells.

5. **e. c and d.** There is no established definition of biochemical failure after cryotherapy, and different PSA cutoff levels of 0.3, 0.4, 0.5, and 1.0 ng/mL have been used in numerous studies. The American Society for Therapeutic Radiology and Oncology (ASTRO) definitions of failure based on three consecutive rises in the PSA level or PSA nadir plus 2 (Phoenix definition) have also been used.

6. **c. Surveillance.** Benign epithelium, often very focal, has been seen in as many as 71% of patients after cryotherapy. The significance of benign epithelium is unknown, and such findings may represent areas of the prostate not frozen to low temperatures, perhaps in the area of the urethral warmer.

7. **a. PSA nadir less than 0.1 ng/mL.** Biochemical failure is lowest among patients who achieve a PSA nadir less than 0.1 ng/mL. Biopsy failure is also lowest in patients with PSA nadirs less than 0.1 ng/mL.

8. **c. It is proven to be beneficial with adjuvant therapies.** Potential advantages that primary cryotherapy for prostate cancer offers versus other local therapies include the capability of destroying a biologically heterogeneous population of cancer cells including cell populations that are resistant to radiation therapy and hormonal therapy, extension of the freezing process beyond the capsule of the prostate, potentially eradicating extracapsular disease, repeat of treatment with minimal morbidity, and treatment of high-Gleason-score prostate cancer.

9. **e. Is unlikely to cure high-risk disease (PSA greater than 10 ng/mL and Gleason score greater than 7).** In patients who have experienced radiation therapy failure for prostate cancer, those with a PSA greater than 10 ng/mL and Gleason score of the recurrent cancer greater than 7 are unlikely to be successfully salvaged. The incidence of incontinence and fistulas is higher in salvage cryotherapy.

10. **d. All of the above.** Clinical factors associated with early treatment failure after salvage cryotherapy for radiorecurrent prostate cancer include a PSA level greater than 10 ng/mL, Gleason score greater than or equal to 9, and a postradiation PSA doubling time of 16 months or less.

11. **b. Urethral sloughing.** Tissue sloughing is manifested by irritative and obstructive voiding symptoms. Pyuria is noted as well. Urinary retention is not uncommon. This condition typically occurs 3 to 8 weeks after the procedure. Initial management consists of antibiotics.

12. **b. Coagulative necrosis.** Highly focused sound energy results in mechanical and thermal effects on tissue. In the case of HIFU, the primary mechanism of tissue ablation is by raising the temperature in the tissue above the level needed to create coagulative necrosis.

13. **b. Urinary retention.** HIFU results in acute swelling of the prostate gland, resulting in temporary urinary retention that usually lasts 1 to 2 weeks. This occurs in the majority of patients with the other complications listed occurring much less frequently.

CHAPTER REVIEW

1. The feasibility of focal therapy for a multifocal disease such as prostate cancer is based on the presumption that an index lesion is primarily responsible for disease progression and metastases.

2. The index lesion as the focus of disease progression and/or metastases is supported by: (1) a volume of tumor must be equal to or greater than 0.5 mL to be significant, (2) some studies indicate that a single lesion drives metastases and progression, (3) the presence of Gleason 4 or 5 and volume predict disease progression, and (4) tumors solely composed of Gleason 6 disease rarely progress.

3. The use of TRUS-guided biopsy to guide focal therapy is fraught with the following difficulties: it overdiagnoses clinically insignificant cancer; misses clinically significant cancers in 30% of cases—usually in the anterior or apical regions; it may underrepresent true cancer burden; and repeat biopsies do not give consistent results.

4. Clinically significant prostate cancer is usually defined as a volume equal to or greater than 0.5 mL and/or a Gleason score of 3 + 4 or greater.

5. On initial biopsy there is no significant difference between a 12-core and a 20-core TRUS biopsy.

6. Color Doppler, ultrasound elastography, and multiparametric magnetic resonance imaging (MRI) with T2 weighting, dynamic contrast enhancement, diffusion weighting, and spectroscopy are improved imaging techniques to detect cancer, but still have significant limitations in accurately predicting or eliminating disease.

7. MRI-TRUS fusion targeted biopsy appears to detect both more significant and insignificant cancers when compared to TRUS biopsy.

8. HIFU and cryosurgery are the two modalities most often employed in focal therapy.

9. The mechanism of injury for cryotherapy involves dehydration of the cell with rupture of the cell membrane, toxic concentration of cellular constituents, and vascular injury.

10. Cell destruction is determined by the cooling rate, warming rate, and lowest temperature achieved.

11. Slow thawing is more effective in tissue destruction than rapid thawing.

12. A minimum temperature of $-40°$ C and a double freeze/thaw cycle with urethral warming is recommended for cryotherapy.

13. Complications of cryotherapy include erectile dysfunction, which is common; long-term incontinence in 1% to 10% of patients; symptomatic urethral sloughing in 5% to 15% of patients; pelvic, rectal, or perineal pain; rectal urethral fistula; and osteitis pubis in a minority of patients.

14. HIFU provides an energy source 10,000 times stronger than diagnostic ultrasound, producing a focal area of heat with temperatures that can exceed 80° C.

15. Complications following HIFU therapy include transient urinary retention in almost all, prolonged urinary retention in 9%, urethral stricture in 3.6%, and rectourethral fistula in 1%.

16. TURP is not indicated for patients receiving focal HIFU.

17. Photodynamic therapy (with aminolevulinic acid), focal thermal therapy, radiofrequency ablation, and focal irreversible electroporation have been used for focal therapy but have few published data to evaluate their effectiveness.

18. Complications for focal therapies are dependent on the energy source but generally include urinary retention, urethral stricture, urinary incontinence, urinary tract infection, erectile dysfunction, and rectourethral fistula.

19. There are few long-term data to evaluate the predictive characteristics of postfocal therapy: biopsies, imaging, and PSA dynamics.

20. Cryotherapy, HIFU, brachytherapy, and radical prostatectomy have been used for salvage therapy following failed radiation therapy, all of which have significant post-therapy complications. For example, following salvage radical prostatectomy, the average disease-free rate at 5 years is 30% to 50%, with a 50% incontinence rate, a 20% urethral stricture rate, close to 100% impotence rate, and a 1% to 3% rectal injury rate. Similarly, cryotherapy has an average incontinence rate of 50%, a rectourethral fistula rate of 0% to 3%, 80% impotence rate, and perineal pain rate of 20%. Significant long-term cancer-free survival data are not available for the most part for the nonradical prostatectomy therapies.

118 Treatment of Locally Advanced Prostate Cancer

Maxwell V. Meng and Peter R. Carroll

QUESTIONS

1. Identification of patients with high-risk prostate cancer is best achieved by:
   a. transrectal ultrasonography.
   b. serum prostate-specific antigen (PSA).
   c. digital rectal examination.
   d. serum PSA, biopsy grade, clinical stage.
   e. PSA kinetics.

2. By using the Kattan postoperative nomogram, which of the following contributes most to the risk of biochemical recurrence after radical prostatectomy?
   a. Positive surgical margin
   b. Pretreatment serum PSA of 17 ng/mL
   c. Gleason 4 + 3 disease
   d. Established capsular penetration
   e. Seminal vesicle invasion

3. Neoadjuvant androgen deprivation (AD) before radical prostatectomy leads to:
   a. improved biochemical-free survival.
   b. improved overall survival.
   c. reduced positive surgical margins.
   d. reduced local recurrence.
   e. increased operative morbidity.

4. In men with locally advanced prostate cancer undergoing prostatectomy, clinical overstaging (i.e., pathologically organ confined disease) occurs in:
   a. less than 10%.
   b. 15% to 30%.
   c. 40% to 60%.
   d. 70% to 80%.
   e. more than 90%.

5. The use of high-dose antiandrogen monotherapy after prostatectomy in men with locally advanced disease:
   a. reduces disease progression.
   b. increases cardiac morbidity.
   c. does not have an impact on sexual function.
   d. improves overall survival.
   e. improves local disease control.

6. In men with locally advanced/high-risk prostate cancer, the most effective treatment among the following options is:
   a. brachytherapy + external-beam radiation therapy.
   b. neoadjuvant AD + external-beam radiation therapy.
   c. neoadjuvant AD + external-beam radiation therapy + adjuvant AD.

   d. concurrent AD plus external-beam radiation therapy.
   e. long-term AD alone.

7. Risk assessment schemes for prostate cancer are most accurate for patients with:
   a. low-risk disease.
   b. high-risk disease.
   c. the disease.
   d. metastatic disease.
   e. locally advanced cancers.

8. The current appropriate dose for adjuvant radiation therapy after radical prostatectomy is:
   a. less than 45 Gy.
   b. 45 to 50 Gy.
   c. 51 to 55 Gy.
   d. 56 to 60 Gy.
   e. greater than 60 Gy.

9. The use of AD in combination with radiation therapy for those with high-risk cancers is associated with all of the following EXCEPT:
   a. improved local control.
   b. improved biochemical-free survival.
   c. less gastrointestinal toxicity.
   d. worsened sexual function.
   e. more urinary frequency.

10. The benefits of early radiation therapy after radical prostatectomy in men with locally advanced disease are observed:
    a. for improved local control.
    b. for improved overall survival.
    c. in men with positive surgical margins.
    d. none of the above.
    e. all of the above.

Imaging

1. A 65-year-old man underwent a radical retropubic prostatectomy 4 years ago for a P3 N0 Gleason 8 adenocarcinoma of the prostate. Two years postoperatively, his PSA first became detectable and has slowly risen since then to its current value of 1.2 ng/mL. A computed tomography (CT) scan of the pelvis is obtained and is depicted in Figure 118-1. The most likely diagnosis is:
   a. retained seminal vesicle.
   b. enlarged lymph node.
   c. recurrence in the prostatectomy bed.
   d. rectal mass.
   e. rectal diverticulum.

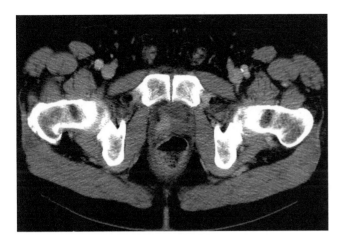

Figure 118-1. Computed tomography scan of pelvis.

ANSWERS

1. **d. Serum PSA, biopsy grade, clinical stage.** Although clinical stage, serum PSA, and Gleason score all individually predict pathologic stage and prognosis, the combination of these three variables increases the accuracy of this assessment.

2. **b. Pretreatment serum PSA of 17 ng/mL.** Despite the trend toward lower serum PSA at the time of diagnosis, PSA remains an important predictor of treatment failure, and greater elevations (greater than 8 ng/mL) of PSA contribute significantly to calculated biochemical recurrence.

3. **c. Reduced positive surgical margins.** The randomized and nonrandomized studies of neoadjuvant androgen deprivation in men with lower clinical stage (cT1-T2) clearly demonstrate a reduction in the rate of positive surgical margins; however, this advantage has not been observed in men with cT3c and has not translated into improved long-term PSA-free survival.

4. **b. 15% to 30%.** Recent data suggest that clinical overstaging occurs in approximately 27% of men with clinical stage T3 disease undergoing prostatectomy, consistent with the range in the literature of 7% to 26%.

5. **a. Reduces disease progression.** Bicalutamide at greater dose (150 mg) appears to have a positive effect in those men with locally advanced disease, with 43% reduction in disease progres-

sion and potential benefit of improved survival; however, it should be remembered that high-dose bicalutamide given to men with localized prostate cancer is associated with increased risk of death (hazard ratio: 1.23).

6. **c. Neoadjuvant AD+external-beam radiation therapy+adjuvant AD.** The accumulated data from multiple RTOG and EORTC trials suggests that improved outcomes are achieved with greater duration of administration of androgen deprivation in combination with external-beam radiation therapy, with apparent benefit of both neoadjuvant and adjuvant therapy.

7. **a. Low-risk disease.** Validation has confirmed the general accuracy of the available risk assessment tools, but there is a tendency to overestimate the risk of cancer recurrence in men with high-risk disease features.

8. **e. Greater than 60 Gy.** There is a trend to improve response to adjuvant radiation therapy and, most contemporary series report doses greater than 60 Gy, with potential threshold of either 61.2 or 64 Gy. Similarly, for primary radiation therapy, improved outcomes have been shown for higher doses (78 Gy or greater).

9. **c. Less gastrointestinal toxicity.** The longer application (longer than 6 to 9 months) of AD in conjunction with radiation therapy may be associated with increased rectal morbidity as well as sexual dysfunction.

10. **e. All of the above.** Data from European Organisation for Research and Treatment of Cancer (EORTC) 22911 and Southwest Oncology Group (SWOG) 8794 clearly demonstrate a benefit of adjuvant radiation therapy in men with pT3 disease, after radical prostatectomy, with respect to biochemical relapse-free, metastasis-free, and overall survival, as well as improved local control. The EORTC study suggests that patients who benefit the most are those with positive surgical margins.

Imaging

1. **c. Recurrence in the prostatectomy bed.** The pelvic CT scan demonstrates a mass in the prostatectomy bed on the right at the level of the urethra-vesicle anastomosis. Because the mass is anterior to the rectum, it is not likely to be a lymph node or seminal vesicle. In view of the radical prostatectomy specimen and the rising PSA, the mass is likely a prostate cancer recurrence in the prostatectomy bed.

CHAPTER REVIEW

1. At least 10% of men with newly diagnosed prostate cancer have locally advanced disease.
2. Risk assessment for locally advanced disease is best determined by a combination of PSA, T stage, cancer grade, and extent of cancer in the biopsy.
3. PSA recurrence following radical prostatectomy is influenced by Gleason score, extracapsular extension, seminal vesicle invasion, positive lymph nodes, and positive surgical margins.
4. Neoadjuvant androgen deprivation therapy before radical prostatectomy has no role.
5. Early androgen deprivation therapy appears to have a potential survival advantage in subsets of men with more aggressive disease. Unfortunately, side effects of the therapy may be a sequela.
6. The role of adjuvant radiation therapy following radical prostatectomy is controversial. A subset of patients apparently benefits from adjuvant radiation therapy. Unfortunately, all studies to date are flawed such that specific subsets of patients who will benefit have not been adequately defined.
7. Patients with seminal vesicle involvement or regional lymph node metastases are highly likely to develop progressive disease despite adjuvant local therapy.
8. EORTC trials suggest that improved outcomes are achieved with greater duration of administration of androgen deprivation in combination with external-beam radiation therapy for selected patients with high-grade disease.

119 Management of Biomedical Recurrence Following Definitive Therapy for Prostate Cancer

Eugene Kang Lee and J. Brantley Thrasher

QUESTIONS

1. What have the American Urological Association (AUA) and European Association of Urology (EUA) determined as the definition of prostate-specific antigen (PSA) failure following radical prostatectomy?
   a. Any level of detectable PSA following radical prostatectomy
   b. Two values of 0.1 ng/mL or higher
   c. 0.2 ng/mL
   d. 0.2 ng/mL with a confirmatory value
   e. 0.4 ng/mL with a confirmatory value

2. Which is NOT considered a high-risk feature following radical prostatectomy in determining the benefit of adjuvant radiation therapy?
   a. Positive surgical margin
   b. Positive pelvic lymph node
   c. Seminal vesicle invasion
   d. Extracapsular extension
   e. Pathologic T3 prostate cancer

3. Which imaging modality in PSA recurrence following radical prostatectomy has the highest sensitivity at the lowest PSA values?
   a. Radionucleotide bone scan
   b. Computed tomography (CT) of abdomen/pelvis
   c. Fluorodeoxyglucose–positron emission tomography (FDG-PET) scan
   d. Prostascint scan
   e. Multiparametric magnetic resonance imaging (MRI)

4. What is the minimum recommended dosage for salvage radiotherapy?
   a. 43 Gy
   b. 54 Gy
   c. 64 Gy
   d. 72 Gy
   e. 78 Gy

5. In Southwest Oncology Group (SWOG) 8794, which subset of patients did not benefit from adjuvant radiation therapy following radical prostatectomy?
   a. Positive surgical margins
   b. Seminal vesicle involvement
   c. Extracapsular extension
   d. None of the patients benefited from adjuvant radiation.
   e. All of the subgroups benefited from adjuvant radiation.

6. Which of the following factors was NOT a part of the "Phoenix" definition of PSA failure following definitive radiotherapy for prostate cancer?
   a. Can be used in patients receiving cryotherapy for prostate cancer

   b. Can be used in patients receiving concurrent androgen deprivation therapy
   c. PSA failure is defined as a rise of 2 ng/mL or more higher than the nadir PSA
   d. Date of failure is "at call"
   e. Biochemical outcomes should be 2 years short of the median follow-up for the group

7. Candidates for salvage prostatectomy following failed radiation therapy of the prostate should have all but which factor before treatment?
   a. Negative metastatic workup
   b. At least 10 years of life expectancy
   c. Biopsy-proven local recurrence
   d. Negative pelvic lymph node sampling
   e. PSA value less than 10 ng/mL

8. Which has the highest sensitivity in detecting recurrent local disease following radiation therapy for prostate cancer?
   a. Rectal exam
   b. Transrectal ultrasound
   c. MRI
   d. Prostascint scan
   e. PET scan

9. Which of these is NOT a commonly known side effect of androgen deprivation therapy (ADT)?
   a. Decreased bone mineral density
   b. Mania
   c. Hot flashes
   d. Fatigue
   e. Sexual side effects

10. The most important therapeutic consideration in selecting either local salvage therapy or systemic therapy for a patient with a rising PSA value after definitive local therapy is:
    a. patients with a rising PSA level after definitive local therapy should be started on hormonal therapy because they are destined to experience systemic relapse.
    b. patients with a rising PSA level should undergo salvage local procedures, such as radiation or cryotherapy or prostatectomy, before undergoing any systemic treatment.
    c. patients with a rising PSA level and no metastatic disease should be started on chemotherapy.
    d. patients with a rising PSA level should undergo neither systemic nor local treatments, because the only appropriate context in which to begin any intervention is when radiographic metastases have developed.
    e. patients with a rising PSA level should be risk stratified and treated with a modality of therapy that matches their risk of relapse, risk of developing local versus systemic disease, and risk of dying of other causes.

ANSWERS

1. **d. 0.2 ng/mL with a confirmatory value.** Throughout the radical prostatectomy literature, there have been more than 50 individual definitions for PSA failure. In 2007, the AUA Guidelines panel for localized prostate cancer released its recommendations for PSA failure following radical prostatectomy as 0.2 ng/mL with a confirmatory value greater than 0.2 ng/mL (Cookson et al, 2007).* Although higher values would result in greater specificity for disease recurrence and progression, the value of 0.2 ng/mL resulted in higher sensitivity and generalizability. The panel reported that in no way should this individual definition be used for determining the usage of adjuvant/salvage therapies and reiterated that this definition is not predictive of death outcomes.

2. **b. Positive pelvic lymph node.** It has been demonstrated in well-performed randomized clinical trials that patients with high-risk features following radical prostatectomy will benefit from adjuvant radiotherapy. SWOG 8794, European Organisation for Research and Treatment of Cancer (EORTC) 22911 and ARO 96-02 defined their patient population as those with extracapsular extension, positive seminal vesicles, and/or positive surgical margins (Bolla et al, 2005; Thompson IM et al, 2009, 2013; Thompson IM Jr et al, 2006; Wiegel et al, 2009).

3. **e. Multiparametric magnetic resonance imaging (MRI).** Traditional imaging techniques such as CT scan and bone scan demonstrate limited value at PSA values less than 10 ng/mL (Dotan et al, 2005; Okotie et al, 2004). Multiparametric MRI has shown reliability in identifying local recurrence even at low levels of PSA. In fact, MRI sensitivity may be as high as 86% at PSA values between 0.4 and 1.4 ng/mL and has also demonstrated an ability to perform better than PET-CT (Panebianco et al, 2012; Sciarra et al, 2008).

4. **c. 64 Gy.** In 1999, the American Society for Therapeutic Radiation Oncology (ASTRO) guidelines panel concluded that a minimum of 64 Gy should be used for salvage radiation following radical prostatectomy (Cox JD et al, 1999). This dosage was confirmed by the AUA guidelines in 2013 (Thompson IM et al, 2013). Modern reports suggest that salvage radiation dosages as high as 76 Gy may demonstrate effective biochemical recurrence-free survival with reasonable toxicities (De Meerleer et al, 2008; Ost, Lumen et al, 2011). It is hoped that studies such as SAKK 09/10 will clarify the role of dose escalation and identify an optimal therapeutic window for salvage radiation (http://clinicaltrials.gov/show/NCT01272050).

5. **e. All of the subgroups benefited from adjuvant radiation.** SWOG 8794 demonstrated the effectiveness of 60 to 64 Gy of adjuvant radiation following radical prostatectomy. Adjuvant radiation improved metastasis-free and overall survival. The study population included patients with high-risk features defined as extracapsular extension, seminal vesicle involvement, and positive surgical margins (Thompson IM et al, 2009; Thompson IM Jr et al, 2006).

6. **a. Can be used in patients receiving cryotherapy for prostate cancer.** In 2005, the "Phoenix definition" was created with the following criteria: rise of 2 ng/mL higher than the nadir PSA, failure was determined "at call," biochemical outcomes should be reported 2 years short of the median follow-up of the population, and could be used in patients who received concurrent ADT (Roach et al, 2006). The "Phoenix" definition was not meant to be used for other modalities of prostate cancer treatment.

7. **d. Negative pelvic lymph node sampling.** Although modern series of salvage prostatectomy demonstrate improved morbidity, patient selection is of the utmost importance (Heidenreich et al, 2010; Stephenson, Scardino et al, 2004). Patients who are candidates for salvage surgery must have at least 10 years of life expectancy, a negative metastatic workup, biopsy-proven local recurrence, and ideally a PSA value less than 10 ng/mL. A separate negative pelvic lymph node sampling is not imperative before undergoing salvage surgery, although sending lymph nodes for frozen section before prostatectomy would not be unreasonable.

8. **c. MRI.** Traditional imaging modalities have not demonstrated consistent ability to detect radiorecurrent prostate cancer. TRUS demonstrates sensitivities no better than digital rectal exam, and CT scans are not relevant at PSA values less than 20 ng/mL (Crook J et al, 1993). Alternatively, MRI with contrast enhancement, spectroscopy, and diffusion-weighted imaging has demonstrated improved sensitivity (Haider et al, 2008; Hara et al, 2012; Westphalen et al, 2010). In fact, diffusion-weighted imaging has demonstrated a sensitivity and specificity of 100% using a 22-core biopsy as a reference (Hara et al, 2012).

9. **b. Mania.** All other answers are commonly reported side effects of patients undergoing ADT.

10. **e. Patients with a rising PSA level should be risk stratified and treated with a modality of therapy that matches their risk of relapse, risk of developing local versus systemic disease, and risk of dying of other causes.** In the setting of biochemical recurrence following radical prostatectomy, patients' risks of metastasis and death are variable (Pound et al, 1999). Both metastasis-free and prostate-cancer survival depend on several factors such as Gleason score, PSA doubling time, and time from surgery to biochemical recurrence (Antonarakis et al, 2012; Freedland et al, 2005, 2006). All of these factors must be considered in salvage therapies. Clearly, patients with significant comorbidities and limited life expectancy are not good candidates for salvage local therapies, and this should be taken into consideration. The use of nomograms to help in decision-making processes is paramount.

CHAPTER REVIEW

1. After discontinued use of ablative hormonal therapy, testosterone levels generally return to baseline within 3 to 6 months; however, some patients can have extremely prolonged recovery periods, and some never recover. A follow-up serum testosterone must be obtained when evaluating a patient for treatment effect.

2. In the overwhelming majority of patients, biochemical relapse occurs far earlier than the development of radiographically observed metastases: In one study of radical prostatectomy patients, those in whom metastases developed on average were found to have them 8 years following the PSA recurrence, and in this group death due to prostate cancer occurred 5 years later.

3. Parameters often used in predicting the significance of a rising PSA level include pretreatment PSA level, grade of tumor, pathologic stage, time to relapse, and PSA doubling time (PSADT).

4. PSADT is often used to predict the time to the development of metastatic disease; however, it is unlikely that PSA kinetics follow the model of a single exponential equation. Therefore it is extremely difficult in many patients over a long period of time to characterize the PSADT.

5. The use of adjuvant androgen deprivation therapy because of a rising PSA value should take into account its effects on cognitive function, well-being, sexual health, cardiovascular risk, and the development of diabetes and osteoporosis, as well

---

*Sources referenced can be found in *Campbell-Walsh Urology, 11th Edition,* on the Expert Consult website.

as the likelihood that it would be effective in eradicating disease.

6. Patients who have demonstrable disease in the prostatic bed after radical prostatectomy should be considered for salvage radiation and/or hormonal therapy.

7. It is controversial whether an ultrasensitive PSA nadir is helpful in predicting clinical disease progression.

8. Several studies have suggested that patients with positive surgical margins benefit from adjuvant radiation therapy, and some studies suggest that those with T3a and T3b disease benefit as well; however, a significant number of these patients will never have a biochemical relapse without treatment.

9. Adjuvant radiation therapy may result in total urinary incontinence, radiation proctitis, radiation cystitis, and urethral stricture.

120 Hormone Therapy for Prostate Cancer

Joel B. Nelson

QUESTIONS

1. The effectiveness of estrogen as a hormone therapy for prostate cancer is primarily based on:
   a. direct cytotoxic effects of estrogen on prostate cancer cells.
   b. competitive binding of estrogen to the androgen receptor.
   c. inhibition of the conversion of cholesterol to pregnenolone.
   d. desensitizing luteinizing hormone–releasing hormone (LHRH) receptors in the anterior pituitary.
   e. negative feedback on luteinizing hormone (LH) secretion by the pituitary.

2. The expected response of a man to the administration of the nonsteroidal antiandrogens is:
   a. LH increases, testosterone decreases, estrogen decreases.
   b. LH increases, testosterone increases, estrogen decreases.
   c. LH increases, testosterone increases, estrogen increases.
   d. LH decreases, testosterone decreases, estrogen increases.
   e. LH decreases, testosterone increases, estrogen increases.

3. All of the following therapeutic approaches for androgen axis blockade are in current clinical use, EXCEPT:
   a. inhibition of androgen synthesis.
   b. blocking androgen action by binding to the androgen receptor in a competitive fashion.
   c. ablating the source of androgens.
   d. direct inhibition of androgen receptor–mediated pathways.
   e. inhibition of LHRH and LH release.

4. Nonsteroidal antiandrogens:
   a. do not act as agonists for prostate cancer cells when used in combination with LHRH agonists.
   b. allow long-term maintenance of erectile function and sexual activity at rates similar to men undergoing surgical castration.
   c. commonly induce gastrointestinal toxicity, manifest as constipation leading, on occasion, to fecal impaction.
   d. have pancreatic toxicity, ranging from reversible mild to fulminant, life-threatening suppurative pancreatitis; requires periodic monitoring of serum amylase and lipase.
   e. cause fluid retention and thromboembolism in the majority of patients.

5. Which of the following nonsteroidal antiandrogens is associated with interstitial pneumonitis and a delayed adaptation to darkness after exposure to bright illumination?
   a. Bicalutamide
   b. Flutamide
   c. Hydroxyflutamide
   d. Nilutamide
   e. Cyproterone acetate

6. Which of the following statements is TRUE concerning LHRH agonists?
   a. Based on a review of 24 trials, involving more than 6600 patients, survival after therapy with an LHRH agonist was significantly better than after surgical castration.
   b. Although depot preparations and osmotic pump devices allow dosing to extend from 28 days to 1 year, the most effective dosing regiment is daily.
   c. Current LHRH agonists are based on analogues of the native LHRH decapeptide by amino acid substitutions, particularly position 6 of the peptide.
   d. Widespread use of orally effective LHRH agonists has been limited by severe allergic reactions in some patients, even after previously uneventful treatment.
   e. The use of LHRH agonists is limited to combined androgen blockade.

7. Each of the following has been associated with a favorable initial response to androgen deprivation therapy, EXCEPT:
   a. the magnitude of the PSA decline.
   b. the rapidity of the PSA decline.
   c. the PSA doubling time before initiating androgen deprivation therapy (ADT).
   d. the Gleason score of the primary tumor.
   e. the maintenance of a detectable PSA.

8. Which of the following statements about the complications of ADT is TRUE?
   a. Most men undergoing ADT have normal bone mineral density before initiating therapy, and it usually takes at least a decade of treatment before the average man will develop osteopenia.
   b. Hot flashes occur in about one quarter of men on ADT but should always be treated because of the associated rare but life-threatening cardiovascular side effects.
   c. Erectile dysfunction after surgical castration or use of an LHRH is common but not inevitable: Although 1 in 5 men maintain some sexual activity, only 1 in 20 maintain high levels of sexual interest (libido).
   d. Because most men on ADT maintain lean muscle mass, the increase in weight is due to increases in adipose tissue.
   e. Gynecomastia and mastodynia are common with estrogenic compounds and antiandrogens but are effectively treated by external beam radiation after they occur.

9. Which of the following statements about the combination of 3 months of neoadjuvant ADT before radical prostatectomy is TRUE?
   a. Positive surgical margin rates are significantly reduced with ADT-treated patients.
   b. There is a significant reduction in biochemical (PSA) progression with ADT-treated patients.

c. The benefit of neoadjuvant ADT appears to be in men with locally advanced disease and/or those with high-grade disease.

d. Antiandrogen monotherapy has not shown a significant reduction of biochemical failure, but LHRH agonists have demonstrated this reduction.

e. Although the results of prospective randomized studies of this combination are mixed, the overall body of evidence supports the use of ADT in this setting.

10. Combined androgen blockade:

a. is designed to address the low levels of testicular androgens remaining after the use of LHRH agonists or antagonists.

b. typically uses an antiandrogens at the time of PSA rise after treatment with an LHRH agonist.

c. has not shown a survival advantage compared with an LHRH agonist alone.

d. significantly benefits men with minimally metastatic disease when used in combination with surgical castration.

e. using cyproterone acetate has a slightly worse outcome.

11. Compared with deferred ADT, early ADT instituted before the development of objective metastatic disease:

a. provides an overall survival advantage in all clinical disease states.

b. has an equivalent quality of life.

c. does not increase overall death rates.

d. does not prevent the emergence of castration-resistant prostate cancer.

e. should be offered to men with PSA recurrence after radical prostatectomy because of the rapid disease progression in this clinical setting.

12. In men with lymph-node metastatic prostate cancer discovered at the time of radical prostatectomy:

a. significant overall survival benefits of immediate ADT are limited to those with extrapelvic positive nodes.

b. a significant overall survival benefit of immediate ADT has been demonstrated in men who have also undergone subsequent radical prostatectomy.

c. a significant overall survival benefit of immediate ADT has been demonstrated in men who have not undergone subsequent radical prostatectomy.

d. b and c are correct

e. a, b, and c are correct

13. From a strictly financial point of view, which of the following forms of ADT is the least expensive?

a. Scrotal orchiectomy

b. LHRH agonist

c. Diethylstilbestrol (DES)

d. Antiandrogen monotherapy

e. LHRH antagonist

14. In a trial studying continuous ADT to intermittent ADT for men with rising PSA after radiation therapy:

a. prostate cancer–specific death was more common in the continuous ADT arm.

b. death unrelated to prostate cancer was more common in the intermittent ADT arm.

c. attrition from the intermittent arm was rare throughout the cycles.

d. duration of intermittent ADT progressively shortened over time.

e. quality of life was not improved in the intermittent arm.

15. There is general consensus that ADT should always be initiated in a hormonally intact patient in which of the following clinical settings?

a. Before radical prostatectomy with a clinical T2 tumor

b. In all clinical stages of men undergoing external beam radiation therapy

c. In those with clinically localized prostate cancer who do not want local treatment

d. In those with symptomatic metastatic disease

e. In those with high-grade prostatic intraepithelial neoplasia (PIN) on needle biopsy who refuse a subsequent biopsy

ANSWERS

1. **e. Negative feedback on luteinizing hormone (LH) secretion by the pituitary.** After the success of surgical castration in treating prostate cancer, the first central inhibition of the hypothalamic-pituitary-gonadal axis exploited the potent negative feedback of estrogen on LH secretion. Estradiol is a thousandfold more potent at suppressing LH and FSH secretion by the pituitary compared with testosterone. Although estrogen has some direct cytotoxic effects on prostate cancer cells, this is not its primary mode of action. All antiandrogens competitively bind to the androgen receptor. Aminoglutethimide inhibits the conversion of cholesterol to pregnenolone, an early step in steroidogenesis. The LHRH agonists desensitize LHRH receptors in the anterior pituitary.

2. **c. LH increases, testosterone increases, estrogen increases.** Unlike the steroidal antiandrogens, such as cyproterone acetate, which have central progestational inhibitory effects, the nonsteroidal antiandrogens simply block androgen receptors, including those in the hypothalamic-pituitary axis. Because those central androgen receptors no longer sense the normal negative feedback exerted by testosterone, both LH levels and—as the normal testicular response to increased LH—testosterone levels increase. Peripheral conversion of this excessive testosterone also increases estrogen levels, leading to gynecomastia and mastodynia associated with the nonsteroidal antiandrogens.

3. **d. Direct inhibition of androgen receptor–mediated pathways.** There are four therapeutic approaches for androgen axis blockade in current clinical use. All current forms of androgen deprivation therapy function by reducing the ability of androgen to activate the androgen receptor, whether through lowering levels of androgen or by blocking androgen–androgen receptor binding. Therefore, the androgen receptor is not directly affected by androgen deprivation therapy, leading many to hypothesize that hormone-refractory prostate cancer is a reactivation of androgen receptor–mediated pathways.

4. **b. Allow long-term maintenance of erectile function and sexual activity at rates similar to men undergoing surgical castration.** By blocking testosterone feedback centrally, the nonsteroidal antiandrogens cause LH and testosterone levels to increase, allowing antiandrogen activity without inducing hypogonadism and potency can be preserved. In clinical trials specifically examining erectile function and sexual activity in men on antiandrogen monotherapy, however, long-term preservation of those domains was 20% and not significantly different from that in men undergoing surgical castration. All antiandrogens can act agonistically on prostate cancer cells and, when used in combination with LHRH agonists, withdrawal of the antiandrogen can lead to declines in PSA and even objective responses. The common gastrointestinal toxicity is diarrhea, most often seen with flutamide. Liver toxicity, ranging from reversible hepatitis to fulminant hepatic failure, is associated with all nonsteroidal antiandrogens and requires periodic monitoring of liver function tests. The steroidal antiandrogen

cyproterone acetate is associated with fluid retention and thromboembolism.

5. **d. Nilutamide.** About one quarter of men on nilutamide therapy will note a delayed adaptation to darkness after exposure to bright illumination, and in approximately 1% of patients, nilutamide is also associated with interstitial pneumonitis, which can progress to pulmonary fibrosis. Hydroxyflutamide is the active metabolite of flutamide. Cyproterone acetate is a steroidal antiandrogen.

6. **d. Widespread use of orally effective LHRH agonists has been limited by severe allergic reactions in some patients, even after previously uneventful treatment.** The LHRH agonists exploit the desensitization of LHRH receptors in the anterior pituitary following chronic exposure to LHRH, thereby shutting down the production of LH and, ultimately, testosterone. Analogues of native LHRH increase their potency and half-lives. The initial flare in LH and testosterone may last 10 to 20 days, and co-administration of an antiandrogen is required for only 21 to 28 days. Survival after therapy with an LHRH agonist was equivalent to that for orchiectomy. The clinical utility of the first LHRH agonists was hampered by their short half-lives, requiring daily dosing. The LHRH antagonist abarelix has been associated with severe allergic reactions: All LHRH agonists are administered either IM or subcutaneously. LHRH can be used without combination with an antiandrogen.

7. **e. The maintenance of a detectable PSA.** The odds ratio of progressing to androgen-refractory progression at 24 months after starting ADT was 15-fold higher in those who did not achieve an undetectable PSA. The magnitude and rapidity of PSA decline, the pre-ADT PSA doubling time, and pretreatment testosterone levels are all associated with the ability to predict the response of to ADT. For each unit increase in Gleason score, the cumulative hazard of castration-resistant progression was nearly 70%.

8. **c. Erectile dysfunction after surgical castration or use of an LHRH is common but not inevitable: Although 1 in 5 men maintain some sexual activity, only 1 in 20 maintain high levels of sexual interest (libido).** The loss of sexual functioning is not inevitable with surgical or chemical castration, with up to 20% of men able to maintain some sexual activity. Libido is more severely compromised, with approximately 5% maintaining a high level of sexual interest. More than half of men undergoing ADT meet the bone mineral density criteria for osteopenia or osteoporosis; it is estimated osteopenia will develop in the average man within 4 years of initiating ADT. Hot flashes are among the most common side effects of ADT, affecting between 50% and 80% of patients. Hot flashes should be treated only in those who find them bothersome. Loss of muscle mass and increase in percent fat body mass are common in men undergoing ADT. Prophylactic radiation therapy (10 Gy) has been used to prevent or reduce gynecomastia and mastodynia, but it has no benefit once these side effects have already occurred.

9. **a. Positive surgical margin rates are significantly reduced with ADT-treated patients.** In both nonrandomized and randomized clinical trials, the pathological positive surgical margin rate is significantly reduced. In one study, the positive surgical margin rate fell from nearly 50% in hormonally intact patients to 15% in ADT-treated patients. Despite this improvement, there has not been a corresponding significant reduction in biochemical (PSA) progression in ADT-treatment patients, a finding in four separate prospective randomized studies. The benefit of ADT in men with locally advanced disease and/or high-grade disease has been in combination with external beam radiation therapy. There is no evidence that any form of 3-month neoadjuvant ADT before radical prostatectomy reduces biochemical failure rates.

10. **e. Using cyproterone acetate has a slightly worse outcome.** In studies of combined androgen blockade using the steroidal antiandrogen cyproterone acetate compared to LHRH agonists alone, the outcomes were slightly worse with the combination, suggesting increased non–prostate cancer deaths with this agent. Combined androgen blockade is designed to block the possible contribution of adrenal androgens to prostate cancer progression. Combined androgen blockade uses an antiandrogen along with an LHRH agonist: Addition of an antiandrogen at the time of PSA rise (evidence of hormone-refractory disease) is considered secondary hormonal manipulation. Several clinical trials have shown a slight but significant survival advantage for combined androgen blockade. A landmark randomized clinical trial comparing surgical castration alone with surgical castration combined with flutamide did not show a significant benefit in men with minimal metastatic disease.

11. **d. Does not prevent the emergence of castration-resistant prostate cancer.** The timing of the initiation of ADT has not prevented the development of castration-resistant prostate cancer. Although early ADT may provide an overall survival advantage in certain clinical disease states, in most studies there is no significant overall survival advantage. Indeed, in localized, low-risk prostate cancer, early ADT is associated with an increase in overall death rates. The natural history of disease progression after biochemical failure following radical prostatectomy is protracted: Median time to bone metastases is 10 years.

12. **b. A significant overall survival benefit of immediate ADT has been demonstrated in men who have also undergone subsequent radical prostatectomy.** A randomized prospective study of men with positive regional pelvic lymph nodes discovered at the time of radical prostatectomy showed an overall survival advantage to immediate ADT. In that study, all men also underwent the radical prostatectomy. A similar study, performed by the European Organisation for Research and Treatment of Cancer (EORTC) in men who did not undergo radical prostatectomy if positive nodes were discovered did not show a significant survival advantage to immediate ADT.

13. **c. Diethylstilbestrol (DES).** At a dose of 1 to 3 mg per day with no prophylactic breast irradiation, DES is the cheapest form of ADT. LHRH agonists would be cheaper than scrotal orchiectomy only if the patient lived a few months after the administration of ADT. Combined androgen blockade is the most expensive form of ADT.

14. **d. Duration of intermittent ADT progressively shortened over time.** The duration of intermittent ADT progressively shortened over time: the median interval of the "off cycle" was 20.1 months for the first interval, 13.2 months for the second cycle, 9.1 months for the third, and 4 to 5 months thereafter. Disease-specific death (prostate cancer and related treatments) was more common in the intermittent-therapy arm compared to the continuous-therapy, 120 versus 94, respectively; conversely, deaths unrelated to prostate cancer were more common in the continuous-therapy arm compared with the intermittent-therapy arm, 162 versus 148, respectively. Attrition from intermittent androgen deprivation progressively increased over time as patients either developed castration-resistant prostate cancer or died of another cause. Attrition occurred in only 5% of men in the first interval, whereas 68% had stopped intermittent therapy by the third interval. A secondary end point, improved quality of life in the intermittent-therapy arm, was associated with significantly better scores for hot flashes, desire for sexual activity, and urinary symptoms.

15. **d. In those with symptomatic metastatic disease.** In hormonally intact men with symptomatic metastatic prostate cancer, ADT is always indicated. There is no significant biochemical (PSA) disease-free advantage in men treated with neoadjuvant ADT. The benefits of ADT in combination with external beam radiation therapy are in men with locally advanced and/or high-grade disease. The use of ADT in men with low-risk, localized prostate cancer is associated with a significantly lower overall survival. There is no indication for ADT in the management of PIN.

CHAPTER REVIEW

1. Antiandrogens bind to the androgen receptor in a competitive fashion. They are either steroidal or nonsteroidal.
2. Steroidal antiandrogens suppress LH release. Thus the steroidal antiandrogens block the effects of testosterone on the receptor as well as lower testosterone through their progestational central inhibition effect. The nonsteroidal antiandrogens simply block androgen receptors
3. When performing an orchiectomy, double-ligating the transected segments of the cord with one being a transfixion suture is advised.
4. Initial exposure to LHRH agonists results in a flare of testosterone that may last for up to 20 days; the clinical effects of the flare may be blocked by the simultaneous administration of an antiandrogen. The two drugs should be administered together, and the antiandrogen therapy should be continued for 3 weeks.
5. After 4 years of androgen deprivation, the average man is osteopenic.
6. Hot flashes may be treated with megestrol, 20 mg twice daily.
7. Androgen deprivation therapy may result in bone loss, sexual dysfunction, hot flashes, decreased cognitive function, loss of muscle mass, increase in body fat, anemia, gynecomastia, diabetes, and increased cardiovascular mortality.
8. Twenty percent of individuals with metastatic prostate cancer die of non-prostate cancer causes.
9. Bilateral orchiectomy reduces testosterone by 90% within 24 hours.
10. The androgen receptor remains responsive to androgen even in the castration-resistant state; therefore, androgen deprivation therapy should be continued in the patient who has castration-resistant prostate cancer.
11. The steroid synthesis inhibitors aminoglutethimide, ketoconazole, and abiraterone require simultaneous glucocorticoid replacement. Aminoglutethimide requires mineral corticoid replacement as well, whereas abiraterone results in increased mineral corticoid production that may result in hypokalemia and hypertension.
12. Intermittent androgen deprivation therapy compared with continuous therapy is not superior and may be worse.
13. Many men with prostate cancer will never require androgen deprivation therapy because of the protracted course of the disease.
14. Estradiol is a thousandfold more potent at suppressing LH and follicle-stimulating hormone (FSH) secretion by the pituitary compared to testosterone.
15. Therapies that block the androgen receptor but do not lower testosterone, such as nonsteroidal antiandrogens, may produce excessive amounts of testosterone, which is peripherally converted to estrogens, leading to the gynecomastia and mastodynia.
16. All antiandrogens can act agonistically on prostate cancer cells and, when used in combination with LHRH agonists, withdrawal of the antiandrogen can lead to declines in PSA and even objective responses.
17. The LHRH agonists exploit the desensitization of LHRH receptors in the anterior pituitary following chronic exposure to LHRH, thereby shutting down the production of LH and, ultimately, testosterone.
18. Prophylactic radiation therapy (10 Gy) has been used to prevent or reduce gynecomastia and mastodynia, but it has no benefit once these side effects have already occurred. Once they are present, a simple mastectomy may be required in some men for cosmetic and symptomatic relief.
19. A clinical trial comparing surgical castration alone with surgical castration combined with flutamide did not show a significant benefit in men with minimal metastatic disease.
20. Although early ADT may provide an overall survival advantage in certain clinical disease states, in most studies there is no significant overall survival advantage. Indeed, in localized, low-risk prostate cancer, early ADT is associated with an increase in overall death rates.
21. The benefits of ADT in combination with external beam radiation therapy are limited to men with locally advanced and/or high-grade disease.

121 Treatment of Castration-Resistant Prostate Cancer

Emmanuel S. Antonarakis, Michael A. Carducci, and Mario A. Eisenberger

QUESTIONS

1. The term "castration-resistant disease" has replaced the older classification of "hormone-resistant disease" used to define all patients who demonstrate evidence of disease progression after initial androgen deprivation treatment because:

   a. androgen deprivation treatment focusing on medical/surgical castration is the initial systemic approach for patients with metastatic prostate cancer.

   b. in patients with castration-resistant disease, responses to subsequent androgen-receptor–targeted treatments continue to show a benefit.

   c. current data indicate that the androgen receptor continues to play a major role in the control of prostate cancer growth even when serum levels of testosterone are in the castrate range (less than 50 ng/dL).

   d. castration resistance does not equal hormone resistance.

   e. all of the above adequately describe the castration-resistant state.

2. Patients eventually stop benefiting from primary and secondary hormonal treatments and become refractory. Which of the following statement (s) INCORRECTLY defines the "castration-resistant" paradigm?

   a. Careful clinical monitoring of patients in clinical practice, including regular physical exams and sequential assessments of radiologic parameters and serum prostate-specific antigen (PSA) levels, facilitates early identification of patients who are becoming resistant to secondary hormonal manipulations.

   b. The definition of castration resistance is based on well-defined clinical and pathologic criteria such as Gleason score and extent of disease.

   c. Determination of castration resistance requires clinical evidence of disease progression to primary and secondary hormonal manipulations.

   d. The vast majority of patients treated with endocrine manipulations will develop evidence of disease progression and eventually require chemotherapy.

3. Docetaxel remains the standard first-line chemotherapy treatment for patients with metastatic castration-resistant prostate cancer considered candidates for this modality. Which of the following statement(s) is NOT true?

   a. Docetaxel infusion every 3 weeks (as many as 10 cycles) given in conjunction with daily oral prednisone is the standard schedule that has been shown to prolong survival and improve quality of life compared with mitoxantrone.

   b. Significant clinical benefits are seen in patients regardless of their age, functional status, and presence or absence of pain.

   c. Patients with metastatic castration-resistant disease who have favorable functional status (fully ambulatory, asymptomatic), no visceral involvement, and normal hemoglobin and serum lactate dehydrogenase (LDH) have survival outcomes frequently in excess of 2 years.

   d. Frequent toxicities associated with docetaxel treatment include fatigue, myelosuppression, modest neuropathy, lacrimation, and nail changes, among others. Routine evaluation before each cycle is indicated.

   e. Patients demonstrating rising serum PSAs during the first three cycles of treatment should be taken off treatment because it is not effective.

4. Cabazitaxel is another taxane approved for metastatic castration-resistant prostate cancer. In preclinical studies that used cancer cell lines and mouse xenograft models, cabazitaxel was shown to be active in docetaxel-sensitive tumors as well as those with primary or acquired docetaxel resistance. Which of the following statements adequately describes the clinical experience with this compound?

   a. Cabazitaxel was shown to prolong survival compared with mitoxantrone in patients previously treated with docetaxel.

   b. The toxicity pattern of cabazitaxel suggests a lower incidence of neuropathy, fatigue, lacrimation, and nail changes but has a higher incidence of neutropenic fever and diarrhea compared with docetaxel.

   c. Data on the TROPIC trial suggest that patients who fail to respond or develop early evidence of disease progression after docetaxel may benefit from cabazitaxel.

   d. Patients demonstrating disease progression after docetaxel can still survive longer than 1 year with cabazitaxel treatment.

   e. All of the above are correct.

5. After initial gonadal suppression, androgen receptor (AR) signaling is upregulated in castration-resistant disease and continues to play a major role in tumor growth. Which of the following statement(s) adequately describes AR-targeted treatments?

   a. CYP17 inhibitors target androgen synthesis both of adrenal and intracrine source and yield significant benefit in patients treated with first-line gonadal suppression who subsequently develop evidence of disease progression. This effect has been shown in patients with or without previous treatment with docetaxel.

   b. The side effects with abiraterone acetate include a mineralocorticoid excess state (efficiently prevented by a concomitant administration of prednisone), fatigue, abnormal liver function tests, possible cardiac toxicity, and potential drug interactions.

   c. Enzalutamide is a more recent nonsteroidal antiandrogen that differs from the first-generation compounds (flutamide, bicalutamide, and nilutamide) based on a greater AR affinity, AR nuclear translocation, and DNA binding. Most patients with castration-resistant disease benefit from treatment, which was shown to be significantly superior to placebo in prospective randomized trials.

   d. The benefits from CYP17 inhibitors (abiraterone) and AR antagonists (enzalutamide) are most likely more pronounced in patients who have not received prior docetaxel treatment.

   e. All of the above are correct.

6. Which of the following statements is correct regarding patients with widely metastatic prostate cancer who present with back pain?

   a. Administration of narcotic analgesics is the appropriate management, and if pain management becomes more challenging, patients should be referred to hospice.

b. All patients with known bone metastasis should be carefully assessed clinically for the possibility of epidural cord or nerve root compression. Administration of high-dose dexamethasone and early magnetic resonance imaging (MRI) should be used, and more definitive treatment with radiation or neurosurgical decompression should be considered.

c. Patients with back pain and stable skeletal radiographs should be treated with narcotic analgesics and corticosteroids. If improvement occurs, no further evaluation is necessary.

d. If the PSA is not rising and the workup with a bone scan and CT scans reveal stable disease, it can be assumed that cord compression or other complex neurologic involvement is unlikely.

e. Most current systemic treatments are effective for managing extensive bone metastasis even if there is evidence of nerve root or cord compression.

7. A small proportion of patients with advanced-stage disease develop a syndrome of rapid and dramatic development of severe symptoms (pain, obstruction, weight loss) and clinical evidence of rapidly growing disease with soft tissue and organ involvement. In these patients, typically serum PSA levels are either below detectable levels or grossly disproportionate to the other extent of disease parameters. Which statement is correct regarding this rare event in castration-resistant prostate cancer?

a. These patients usually benefit from hormonal therapy including all AR-targeted compounds

b. Serum PSA is low or undetectable and the PSA stains in tumor biopsies are usually negative. These tumors do not express androgen receptors.

c. A small proportion of patients demonstrate evidence of a rapidly progressing disease predominantly involving visceral sites, with low or no PSA expression. Biopsy is indicated because it will affect treatment decisions.

d. Patients with this clinical syndrome often demonstrate anaplastic tumors at biopsy, some with small-cell features, and most stain positive for neuroendocrine markers. Platinum-based chemotherapy has been show to offer some benefits for patients with the small-cell variety, whereas those with anaplastic tumors that are not of the small-cell subtype should be treated with taxane-based chemotherapy.

e. All statements are correct except a.

8. The radium-223 radiopharmaceutical was approved for the treatment of patients with metastatic castration-resistant disease. Which statement regarding ^{223}Ra is FALSE?

a. Radium-223 is an alpha-emitting radiopharmaceutical that has recently shown to be associated with a survival advantage compared to symptomatic/palliative care.

b. Alpha particles are approximately 7000 times heavier than beta particles, and as few as one or two hits can be sufficient to cause cell death, in comparison with hundreds or thousands of hits required from beta particles. In addition, alpha particles have a very short path length (less than 100 μm), which may spare surrounding healthy bone marrow, thereby limiting hematologic toxicities.

c. Radium-223 infusion has shown a very favorable toxicity spectrum with low hematological toxicity rates.

d. It is indicated for patients with bone metastasis, hemoglobin greater than 10 g/L and lymph-node metastasis smaller than 3 cm.

e. It was approved only for patients who have received prior docetaxel treatment.

9. Sipuleucel-T is a personalized vaccine derived from autologous CD54 + dendritic cells, the major class of antigen-presenting cells, which are apheresed from individuals and processed with a recombinant fusion protein made up of PAP and GM-CSF. Which statement is TRUE regarding this treatment?

a. Sipuleucel-T is approved for all patients with castration-resistant disease as long as they are symptomatic.

b. Sipuleucel-T treatment results in PSA declines and prolongation of progression-free survival, but no survival improvements.

c. Sipuleucel-T should be offered to patients with no evidence of metastasis as long as their disease is castration resistant.

d. Sipuleucel-T is a treatment option for patients with minimally or asymptomatic metastatic prostate cancer. Treatment is generally very safe. There is no evidence that sipuleucel-T treatment causes symptomatic relief, any clinically meaningful PSA declines, or delay in disease progression. The drug was approved based on a survival benefit compared to placebo.

ANSWERS

1. **e. All of the above adequately describe the castration-resistant state.**
2. **b. The definition of hormone resistance is based on well-defined clinical and pathologic criteria such as Gleason score and extent of disease.**
3. **e. Patients demonstrating rising serum PSAs during the first three cycles of treatment should be taken off treatment because it is not effective.**
4. **e. All of the above are correct.**
5. **e. All of the above are correct.**
6. **b. All patients with known bone metastasis should be carefully assessed clinically for the possibility of epidural cord or nerve root compression. Administration of high-dose dexamethasone and early magnetic resonance imaging (MRI) should be used, and more definitive treatment with radiation or neurosurgical decompression should be considered.**
7. **e. All statements are correct except a.**
8. **e. It was approved only for patients who have received prior docetaxel treatment.**
9. **d. Sipuleucel-T is a treatment option for patients with minimally or asymptomatic metastatic prostate cancer. Treatment is generally very safe. There is no evidence that sipuleucel-T treatment causes symptomatic relief, any clinically meaningful PSA declines, or delay in disease progression. The drug was approved based on a survival benefit compared to placebo.**

CHAPTER REVIEW

1. Androgen ablation induces apoptosis.
2. The androgen receptor may be stimulated by hormones other than androgens, including estrogens and progestins as well as growth factors and cytokines.
3. Patients with castration-resistant disease are not androgen independent and should be maintained on ablative hormonal therapy.
4. PSA doubling time (PSADT) may be used to predict bone scan progression and survival; a PSADT of less than 3 months is associated with a rapid clinical course.
5. When evaluating therapeutic agents, progression-free survival is a better end point than response rate.
6. PSA may or may not be affected by drugs that are efficacious, and therefore it is not a good marker to evaluate new drugs—perhaps circulating tumor cells will become a better marker.
7. Docetaxel is the first-line chemotherapeutic agent for metastatic castration-resistant prostate cancer.
8. Abiraterone inhibits enzymes involved in androgen synthesis. It does result in secondary mineralocorticoid excess with resultant hypertension and hypokalemia, and as such it is

commonly given with prednisone. Occasionally, when secondary mineralocorticoid excess causes significant abnormalities, a mineralocorticoid antagonist may be necessary.

9. Bone metastases in prostate cancer are usually blastic; hypercalcemia is rare.

10. Suspected spinal cord compression from prostate metastases may be diagnosed with a spinal MRI. Those with compression or impending compression, if they are not androgen suppressed, should have an immediate orchiectomy or be given aminoglutethimide or ketoconazole and high-dose corticosteroids. A decompression laminectomy and radiation therapy should be considered.

11. Bisphosphonates are used to limit skeletal events. Oral calcium supplements as well as vitamin D may be necessary.

12. Radiopharmaceuticals used to treat bone pain due to prostate metastases include the beta-emitters strontium-89 and samarium-153. These agents may cause severe myelotoxicity.

The alpha-emitter radium-223 shows promise in palliating bone pain without the myelosuppressive effects of the beta-emitters.

13. Rarely, patients with advanced prostate cancer may have a transformation of their tumor to a neuroendocrine/anaplastic variant. These tumors are endocrine resistant, frequently involve the viscera and brain, have little impact on PSA, and are treated with platinum-based chemotherapy.

14. After initial gonadal suppression, AR signaling is upregulated in castration-resistant disease and continues to play a major role in tumor growth.

15. Sipuleucel-T is a treatment option for patients with minimally or asymptomatic metastatic prostate cancer. Treatment is generally very safe. There is no evidence that sipuleucel-T treatment causes symptomatic relief, any clinically meaningful PSA declines, or delay in disease progression. The drug was approved based on a survival benefit compared with placebo.

122   Embryology of the Genitourinary Tract

John M. Park

QUESTIONS

1. The fetal kidneys develop from which of the following embryonic structures?
   a. Paraxial (somite) mesoderm
   b. Intermediate mesoderm
   c. Neural tube
   d. Lateral mesoderm

2. At what gestational time point does the metanephros development begin?
   a. 20th day
   b. 24th day
   c. 28th day
   d. 32nd day

3. Which of the following statements is TRUE of the metanephric development?
   a. It requires the reciprocal inductive interaction between Müllerian duct and metanephric mesenchyme.
   b. The calyces, pelvis, and ureter derive from the differentiation of the metanephric mesenchyme.
   c. Older, more differentiated nephrons are located at the periphery of the developing kidney, whereas newer, less differentiated nephrons are found near the juxtamedullary region.
   d. In humans, although renal maturation continues postnatally, nephrogenesis is completed by birth.

4. The fused lower pole of the horseshoe kidney is trapped by which of the following structures during the ascent?
   a. Inferior mesenteric artery
   b. Superior mesenteric artery
   c. Celiac artery
   d. Common iliac artery

5. The homozygous gene disruption (gene knockout) in which of the following molecules does NOT lead to a significant renal maldevelopment in mice?
   a. WT-1
   b. Pax-2
   c. GDNF
   d. p53

6. Which of the following statements is NOT TRUE of GDNF?
   a. It is a ligand for the RET receptor tyrosine kinase.
   b. GDNF gene knockout mice demonstrate an abnormal renal development.
   c. It is expressed in the metanephric mesenchyme but not in the ureteric bud.
   d. GDNF arrests the ureteric bud growth in vitro.

7. Which of the following statements is NOT TRUE of the renin-angiotensin system (RAS) during renal and ureteral development?
   a. The embryonic kidney is able to produce all components of the RAS.
   b. Both subtypes of angiotensin II receptor, AT_1 and AT2, are expressed in the developing metanephros.
   c. AT_1 gene knockout mice demonstrate a spectrum of congenital urinary tract abnormalities including ureteropelvic junction obstruction and vesicoureteral reflux.
   d. Infants born to mothers treated with angiotensin-converting enzyme inhibitors during pregnancy have increased rates of oligohydramnios, hypotension, and anuria.

8. The bladder trigone develops from which of the following structures?
   a. Mesonephric ducts
   b. Müllerian ducts
   c. Urogenital sinus
   d. Metanephric mesenchyme

9. The urachus involutes to become:
   a. verumontanum.
   b. the median umbilical ligament.
   c. appendix testicle.
   d. epoophoron.

10. Which of the following statements is NOT TRUE of bladder development?
    a. The bladder body is derived from the urogenital sinus while the trigone develops from the terminal portion of the mesonephric ducts.
    b. Bladder compliance seems to be low during early gestation, and it gradually increases thereafter.
    c. Epithelial-mesenchymal inductive interactions appear to be necessary for proper bladder development.
    d. Histologic evidence of smooth muscle differentiation begins near the bladder neck and proceeds toward the bladder dome.

11. The primordial germ cell migration and the formation of the genital ridges begin at which time point during gestation?
    a. Third week
    b. Fifth week

c. Seventh week

d. Ninth week

12. Which of the following statements is NOT TRUE of the paramesonephric (müllerian) ducts?

a. Both male and female embryos form paramesonephric (müllerian) ducts.

b. In male embryos, the paramesonephric ducts degenerate under the influence of the MIS (müllerian-inhibiting substance) produced by the Leydig cells.

c. In male embryos, the paramesonephric ducts become the appendix testis and the prostatic utricle.

d. In female embryos, the paramesonephric ducts form the female reproductive tract, including fallopian tubes, uterus, and upper vagina.

13. Which of the following structures in the male reproductive tract develops from the urogenital sinus?

a. Vas deferens

b. Seminal vesicles

c. Prostate

d. Appendix epididymis

14. Which of the following statements is NOT TRUE of normal prostate development?

a. It requires the conversion of testosterone into dihydrotestosterone by 5α-reductase.

b. It is dependent on epithelial-mesenchymal interactions under the influence of androgens.

c. It is first seen at the 10th to 12th week of gestation.

d. It requires the effects of MIS.

15. In female embryos, the remnants of the mesonephric ducts persist as the following structures EXCEPT:

a. epoophoron.

b. paroophoron.

c. hymen.

d. Gartner duct cysts.

16. Which of the following statements is NOT TRUE of the external genitalia development?

a. The appearance of the external genitalia is similar in male and female embryos until the 12th week.

b. The external genital appearance of males who are deficient in 5α-reductase is similar to that of females.

c. In males, the formation of distal glandular urethra may occur by the fusion of urethral folds proximally and the ingrowth of ectodermal cells distally.

d. In females, the urethral folds become the labia majora, and the labioscrotal folds become the labia minora.

17. The testicles descend to the level of internal inguinal ring by which time point during gestation?

a. Sixth week

b. Third month

c. Sixth month

d. Ninth month

18. Which of the following statements is NOT TRUE of the sex-determining region of the Y chromosome (SRY)?

a. Its expression triggers the primitive sex cord cells to differentiate into the Sertoli cells.

b. Approximately 25% of sex reversal conditions in humans are attributable to SRY mutations.

c. It is located on the short arm of the Y chromosome.

d. It causes the regression of mesonephric ducts.

ANSWERS

1. **b. Intermediate mesoderm.** Mammals develop three kidneys in the course of intrauterine life. The embryonic kidneys are, in order of their appearance, the pronephros, the mesonephros, and the metanephros. The first two kidneys regress in utero, and the third becomes the permanent kidney. In terms of embryology, all three kidneys develop from the intermediate mesoderm.

2. **c. 28th day.** The definitive kidney, metanephros, forms in the sacral region as a pair of new structures, called the ureteric buds, sprouts from the distal portion of the nephric duct and comes in contact with the blastema of metanephric mesenchyme at about the 28th day.

3. **d. In humans, although renal maturation continues postnatally, nephrogenesis is completed by birth.** It requires the inductive interaction between the ureteric bud and metanephric mesenchyme. The calyces, pelvis, and ureter derive from the ureteric bud. Older, more differentiated nephrons are located in the inner part of the kidney near the juxtamedullary region. In humans, although renal maturation continues to take place postnatally, nephrogenesis is completed before birth.

4. **a. Inferior mesenteric artery.** The inferior poles of the kidneys may fuse, forming a horseshoe kidney that crosses over the ventral side of the aorta. During ascent, the fused lower pole becomes trapped under the inferior mesenteric artery and thus does not reach its normal site.

5. **d. p53.** Mutant *WT-1* mice do not form ureteric buds, and in *Pax-2* gene knockout mice, no nephric ducts, müllerian ducts, ureteric buds, or metanephric mesenchyme form, and the animals die within 1 day of birth because of renal failure. Ureteric bud formation is impaired in GDNF (glial cell line–derived neurotrophic factor) knockout mice, but p53 gene knockout mice do not demonstrate significant renal developmental anomaly.

6. **d. GDNF arrests the ureteric bud growth in vitro.** GDNF promotes ureteric bud growth in vitro. Although the importance of RET in kidney development was clearly demonstrated, it is only recently that its ligand, GDNF, has been identified. GDNF is a secreted glycoprotein that possesses a cystine-knot motif. GDNF is expressed within the metanephric mesenchyme prior to ureteric bud invasion, and ureteric bud formation is impaired in GDNF knockout mice.

7. **c. AT$_1$ gene knockout mice demonstrate a spectrum of congenital urinary tract abnormalities, including ureteropelvic junction obstruction and vesicoureteral reflux.** AT$_2$ gene knockout mice demonstrate a spectrum of congenital urinary tract abnormalities, including ureteropelvic junction obstruction, multicystic dysplastic kidney, megaureter, vesicoureteral reflux, and renal hypoplasia.

8. **a. Mesonephric ducts.** The terminal portion of the mesonephric duct, called the common excretory ducts, becomes incorporated into the developing bladder and forms the trigone.

9. **b. The median umbilical ligament.** By the 12th week, the urachus involutes to become a fibrous cord, which becomes the median umbilical ligament.

10. **d. Histologic evidence of smooth muscle differentiation begins near the bladder neck and proceeds toward the bladder dome.** Between the 7th and 12th weeks, the surrounding connective tissues condense and smooth muscle fibers begin to appear, first at the region of the bladder dome and later proceeding toward the bladder neck.

11. **b. Fifth week.** During the fifth week, primordial germ cells migrate from the yolk sac along the dorsal mesentery to populate the mesenchyme of the posterior body wall near the 10th thoracic level. In both sexes, the arrival of primordial germ cells in the area of future gonads serves as the signal for the existing cells of the mesonephros and the adjacent coelomic epithelium to proliferate and form a pair of genital ridges just medial to the developing mesonephros.

12. **b. In male embryos, the paramesonephric ducts degenerate under the influence of the MIS (müllerian-inhibiting substance) produced by the Leydig cells.** A new pair of ducts, called

the paramesonephric (müllerian) ducts, begins to form just lateral to the mesonephric ducts in both male and female embryos. These ducts arise by the craniocaudal invagination of thickened coelomic epithelium, extending all the way from the third thoracic segment to the posterior wall of the developing urogenital sinus. The caudal tips of the paramesonephric ducts adhere to each other as they connect with the urogenital sinus between the openings of the right and left mesonephric ducts. The cranial ends of the paramesonephric ducts form funnel-shaped openings into the coelomic cavity (the future peritoneum). As developing Sertoli cells begin their differentiation in response to the SRY (sex-determining region of the Y chromosome), they begin to secrete MIS, which causes the paramesonephric (müllerian) ducts to regress rapidly between the 8th and 10th weeks. Small müllerian duct remnants can be detected in the developed male as a small tissue protrusion at the superior pole of the testicle, called the appendix testis, and as a posterior expansion of the prostatic urethra, called the prostatic utricle. In female embryos, MIS is absent, so the müllerian ducts do not regress and instead give rise to fallopian tubes, uterus, and vagina.

13. **c. Prostate.** Vas deferens, seminal vesicles, and appendix epididymis all develop from the mesonephric ducts. The prostate and bulbourethral glands develop from the urogenital sinus.

14. **d. It requires the hormonal effects of MIS.** The prostate gland begins to develop during the 10th to 12th week as a cluster of endodermal evaginations budding from the pelvic urethra (derived from the urogenital sinus). These presumptive prostatic outgrowths are induced by the surrounding mesenchyme, and this process depends on the conversion of testosterone into dihydrotestosterone by 5α-reductase. Similar to renal and bladder development, prostatic development depends on mesenchymal-epithelial interactions but under the influence of androgens. There is no evidence that MIS plays a direct role in prostate development.

15. **c. Hymen.** In the absence of MIS and androgens, the mesonephric (wolffian) ducts degenerate and the paramesonephric (müllerian) ducts give rise to the fallopian tubes, uterus, and upper two thirds of the vagina. The remnants of mesonephric ducts are found in the mesentery of the ovary as the epoophoron

and paroophoron, and near the vaginal introitus and anterolateral vaginal wall as Gartner duct cysts. The hymen develops from the endodermal membrane located at the junction between the vaginal plate and the definitive urogenital sinus, which is the future vestibule of the vagina.

16. **d. In females, the urethral folds become the labia majora, and the labioscrotal folds become the labia minora.** The early development of the external genital organ is similar in both sexes until 12th week. Early in the fifth week, a pair of swellings called cloacal folds develops on either side of the cloacal membrane. These folds meet just anterior to the cloacal membrane to form a midline swelling called the genital tubercle. During the cloacal division into the anterior urogenital sinus and the posterior anorectal canal, the portion of the cloacal folds flanking the opening of the urogenital sinus becomes the urogenital folds, and the portion flanking the opening of the anorectal canal becomes the anal folds. A new pair of swellings, called the labioscrotal folds, then appears on either side of the urogenital folds. In the absence of dihydrotestosterone, the primitive perineum does not lengthen, and the labioscrotal and urethral folds do not fuse across the midline in the female embryo. The phallus bends inferiorly, becoming the clitoris, and the definitive urogenital sinus becomes the vestibule of the vagina. The urethral folds become the labia minora, and the labioscrotal folds become the labia majora. The external genital organ develops in a similar manner in genetic males who are deficient in 5α-reductase and therefore lack dihydrotestosterone.

17. **b. Third month.** The testicle reaches the level of internal inguinal ring by the third month and passes through the inguinal canal to reach the scrotum between the seventh and ninth months.

18. **d. It causes the regression of mesonephric ducts.** When the Y-linked master regulatory gene, called *SRY*, is expressed in the male, the epithelial cells of the primitive sex cords differentiate into Sertoli cells, and this critical morphogenetic event triggers subsequent testicular development. Analysis of DNA narrowed the location of the SRY to a relatively small region within the short arm of the chromosome. It is now clear that only about 25% of sex reversals in humans can be attributed to disabling mutations of the SRY.

CHAPTER REVIEW

1. The glomerulus, proximal tubule, loop of Henle, and distal tubule are derived from the metanephric mesenchyme.
2. The remainder of the collecting system is formed from the ureteric bud.
3. The Weigert-Meyer rule states that the most lateral and cephalad ureteric orifice arises from the lower pole and may demonstrate reflux whereas the most medial and caudad orifice drains the upper pole and may be associated with a ureterocele.
4. Sertoli cells produce müllerian-inhibiting substance, which causes regression of the müllerian ducts.
5. Testosterone is secreted by the Leydig cells and stimulates the wolffian ducts to form the vas deferens and seminal vesicles.
6. The prostate and bulbourethral glands develop from the urogenital sinus.
7. Circulating androgens play a critical role in the development of the prostate.
8. When 5α-reductase is deficient, prostatic growth and development is severely compromised.
9. In the absence of müllerian-inhibiting substance and androgens, the wolffian ducts degenerate and the müllerian ducts give rise to the fallopian tubes, uterus, and upper two thirds of the vagina.
10. Boys with spina bifida have a 23% incidence of cryptorchidism.
11. If the *SRY* gene complex is translocated to an X chromosome, an XX female will have male characteristics.
12. The renin-angiotensin system is important for the normal development and growth of the kidney.
13. Circulating androgens and the conversion of testosterone to dihydrotestosterone (DHT) are critical to the normal development of the prostate and male external genitalia.
14. A defect in the WT1 gene may result in hypospadias, cryptorchidism, and ambiguous genitalia (disorders of sex development).
15. Defects in the androgen receptor result in abnormal masculinization of the external genitalia.
16. Abdominal pressure appears to be important for the transit of the testis through the inguinal canal and into the scrotum.
17. The embryonic kidneys are, in order of their appearance, the pronephros, the mesonephros, and the metanephros. The first two kidneys regress in utero, and the third becomes the permanent kidney.
18. Older, more differentiated nephrons are located in the inner part of the kidney near the juxtamedullary region.
19. Primordial germ cells migrate from the yolk sac along the dorsal mesentery to populate the mesenchyme of the posterior body wall near the 10th thoracic level.
20. Sertoli cells begin their differentiation in response to the SRY (sex-determining region of the Y chromosome); they begin to secrete MIS, which causes the paramesonephric (müllerian) ducts to regress.
21. Müllerian duct remnants in the male include the prostatic utricle and the appendix testis.

123 Renal Functional Development in Children

Victoria F. Norwood and Craig A. Peters

QUESTIONS

1. A 2-month-old infant born at 32 weeks gestation is expected to have:
   a. completed nephrogenesis but immature renal functional abilities.
   b. incomplete nephrogenesis and immature renal functional abilities.
   c. completed both nephrogenesis and renal functional maturation.
   d. functionally mature nephrons but ongoing formation of additional nephrons.
   e. no increased risk of chronic kidney disease (CKD) compared to an infant born at 38 weeks gestation.

2. A 2-week-old boy with bilateral moderate hydronephrosis who was born at 30 weeks gestation is found to have a serum creatinine of 0.7 mg/dL. This would suggest:
   a. significant renal dysfunction, possibly due to posterior urethral valves.
   b. maternal renal function.
   c. moderate renal dysfunction unrelated to his hydronephrosis.
   d. normal renal function without evidence of obstruction.
   e. likely hemolyzed specimen with inaccurate creatinine level.

3. A 4-year-old boy presents with swelling and decreased urine output. He has had eyelid edema on awakening for the past week. His blood pressure is 90/50 mm Hg, and he has marked eyelid edema, distended abdomen, and pitting edema of the legs and feet. Urinalysis showed a specific gravity of 1.030, pH 5, 3 + protein, and trace of blood. Serum studies show a sodium level of 131 mEq/L, blood urea nitrogen value of 30 mg/dL, creatinine level of 0.3 mg/dL, and albumin level of 1.6 g/dL. The appropriate next step in management is:
   a. quantitation of urinary protein excretion, renal ultrasound, and lipid panel.
   b. initiation of oral prednisone.
   c. workup for occult malignancy.
   d. quantitation of urinary protein excretion, renal ultrasound, lipid panel, and initiation of prednisone therapy.
   e. quantitative protein excretion, lipid panel, and prednisone therapy.

4. A 6-year-old, healthy girl undergoes a routine physical examination. Urinalysis reveals a specific gravity of 1.020, pH 6, trace protein, and moderate amount of blood on dipstick testing. The microscopic test shows 5 to 6 red blood cells per high-powered field. An inappropriate next step is:
   a. renal ultrasonography.
   b. random urine calcium and creatinine determinations.
   c. clean-catch urine culture.
   d. an empirical 10-day course of antibiotics.
   e. a repeat urinalysis in 2 weeks.

5. A urinalysis in an 8-year-old boy shows a specific gravity of 1.030, pH 5, trace protein, and moderate amount of blood.

He has a normal physical examination, including blood pressure of 96/56 mm Hg. On further history he was hospitalized 2 months ago with poststreptococcal glomerulonephritis. The most appropriate course of action is:
   a. cystoscopy.
   b. renal ultrasonography.
   c. a course of antibiotics after obtaining a urine culture.
   d. to reassure his family and obtain records from the outside institution.
   e. computed tomography (CT).

6. A 6-year-old boy is seen in the emergency department with the new onset of left-sided flank pain, gross hematuria, and vomiting. His blood pressure is 120/70 mm Hg, and the physical examination reveals right costovertebral angle tenderness. The urinalysis shows brown urine with a specific gravity of 1.030, pH 7, large amount of blood, and 2+ protein. The next step in diagnostic evaluation should NOT include:
   a. high-resolution CT of abdomen/pelvis without contrast.
   b. microscopic examination of the urine.
   c. cystoscopy.
   d. renal ultrasonography.
   e. serum electrolyte determination.

7. An 8-year-old is seen in the emergency room with 24 hours of severe left flank pain and nausea. Urinalysis shows a specific gravity of 1.024, pH of 6.3, and a serum creatinine of 0.4 mg/dl. He is afebrile and has had no surgery. The most appropriate next step is:
   a. no further imaging is needed.
   b. double-J ureteral stent placement.
   c. hospital admission and 4 days of antibiotics.
   d. abdominal ultrasound.
   e. CT urogram with and without contrast.

8. A 9-year-old girl presents after passing a 3-mm stone. On analysis, the stone is composed 100% of calcium oxalate. The next step is to:
   a. start a thiazide diuretic.
   b. obtain a 24-hour urine collection to test for calcium, creatinine, oxalate, and citrate.
   c. start potassium citrate.
   d. restrict dietary calcium.
   e. restrict dietary oxalate.

9. A 6-year-old boy is seen in the emergency department with new onset of headache and gross hematuria. He has no dysuria or fever but has vomited three times. He had a sore throat the week before, but it has resolved. His blood pressure is 140/90 mm Hg, and physical examination reveals a heart murmur. The urinalysis shows brown urine with a specific gravity of 1.030, pH 7, large amount of blood, and 2 + protein. The next step in the diagnostic evaluation should include all of the following EXCEPT:
   a. CT of the abdomen and pelvis.
   b. comprehensive metabolic panel.
   c. C3 determination.

d. antistreptolysin O titer.

e. microscopic examination of the urine.

10. A 3-year-old boy is seen in the emergency department with a respiratory problem and gross hematuria. He has no dysuria or abdominal pain but has fever, rhinorrhea, and cough. His blood pressure is 120/70 mm Hg, and physical examination shows rhinorrhea, mild pharyngeal erythema, and no peripheral edema or abdominal tenderness. The urinalysis shows brown urine with a specific gravity of 1.030, pH 7, large amount of blood, and 2+ protein. (His mother also has had hematuria in the past, and his maternal uncle is deaf and on hemodialysis.) The next step in diagnostic evaluation includes all of the following EXCEPT:

a. renal biopsy.

b. antistreptolysin O titer and C3.

c. comprehensive metabolic panel.

d. microscopic examination of the urine.

e. CT of the abdomen and pelvis.

11. **A 16-year-old boy with end-stage renal disease is managed with peritoneal dialysis (PD). He develops abdominal pain, vomiting, and a fever of 100.9° F. The next step in management is to:**

a. obtain blood and urine cultures.

b. start broad-spectrum antibiotics.

c. collect a specimen of dialysate for white blood cell count and culture.

d. change to hemodialysis.

e. administer intraperitoneal antibiotics.

12. During an evaluation for ongoing malaise and poor appetite, which followed initiation of treatment for otitis media four earlier, an 8-year-old boy is found to have a blood urea nitrogen level of 40 mg/dL and a creatinine of 1.4 mg/dL. His urinary sodium level is 13 mEq/L, fractional excretion of sodium (FE_{Na}) is 0.8%, and urinary osmolality is 410 mOsm/Kg. The most likely cause of his renal insufficiency is:

a. posterior urethral valves.

b. dehydration

c. interstitial nephritis.

d. hemolytic uremic syndrome.

e. previously unknown bilateral ureteropelvic junction obstruction.

13. A 9-year-old boy is found during routine examination to have a blood pressure of 120/90 mm Hg. The child was calm, and a properly sized blood pressure cuff was used for the measurement. The best next step in management is to:

a. repeat the measurement next week in the office.

b. obtain a fasting lipid profile.

c. perform renal ultrasonography.

d. obtain peripheral vein renin levels.

e. perform ambulatory blood pressure monitoring (ABPM).

14. An otherwise healthy 14-year-old boy is found to have 2+ protein on a urinalysis obtained as part of a sports physical for football. The most appropriate initial step in the evaluation should be:

a. referral to the first available pediatric urologist or nephrologist.

b. renal ultrasound, serum chemistries, and 24-hour urine protein quantitation.

c. initiation of oral prednisone.

d. spot protein and creatinine ratio on a first morning void following rest.

e. repeat urinalysis ASAP.

15. **A 5 year-old-boy with posterior urethral valves since birth has renal function that has slowly declined to a current creatinine of 1.7 mg/dl. His growth is impaired with height and weight less than the third percentile. The most appropriate management strategy is:**

a. referral to the nearest transplant program for initiation of transplant evaluation.

b. collaboration with a pediatric nephrologist about management of CKD.

c. repeat urodynamics in expectation of preemptive transplantation.

d. initiation of bicarbonate and growth hormone.

e. repeat valve ablation.

16. A 13-year-old boy presents with intermittent left flank pain and microscopic hematuria. Ultrasound shows bilateral renal calculi without evidence of obstruction. Urinalysis shows moderate RBCs, no WBCs, pH of 6.3, and hexagonal-shaped crystals. CT imaging demonstrates the calculi, which are found to have a Hounsfield density of 420 HU. The most appropriate initial therapy for this boy would be:

a. bilateral percutaneous nephrolithotomy.

b. bilateral ureteroscopic lithotomy.

c. urinary acidification and repeat imaging.

d. treatment with allopurinol.

e. treatment with dimercaptoproprionylglycine.

ANSWERS

1. **b. Incomplete nephrogenesis and immature renal functional abilities.** Nephrogenesis completes by 34 to 36 weeks postconception, whether in utero or ex-utero. Functional maturation continues for at least one year. Infants born prematurely most likely do not achieve their genetic endowment of normal nephrons and are at higher risk of developing CKD throughout life compared to infants born at term.

2. **d. Normal renal function without evidence of obstruction.** A serum creatinine of 0.7 mg/dl is within normal range for a premature infant. The moderate degree of hydronephrosis is unlikely to suggest obstruction severe enough to cause an elevated creatinine. While it is reasonable to rule out posterior urethral valves, the absence of dilated ureters would suggest it is of low likelihood.

3. **d. Quantitation of urinary protein excretion, renal ultrasound, lipid panel, and initiation of prednisone therapy.** The patient has hypoalbuminemia, edema, and proteinuria and most likely has nephrotic syndrome. In the absence of profound anasarca, the initial illness may be managed in the outpatient setting. Completion of diagnostic studies (quantitation of urinary protein, measurement of plasma lipids, and other studies as indicated), family education, and institution of a low-salt diet are followed by initiation of oral prednisone. A renal biopsy is not indicated if minimal change nephrotic syndrome is likely. Oral diuretics are not commonly prescribed unless careful observation is possible. Malignancy is very rarely associated with nephrotic syndrome in children. Renal ultrasonography only occasionally adds additional significant information but is usually performed at some point during the evaluation. Most children with primary nephrotic syndrome respond to corticosteroids within 14 days and have spontaneous diuresis with loss of edema and proteinuria.

4. **d. An empirical 10-day course of antibiotics.** Although asymptomatic hematuria may be caused by occult urinary tract infection, empirical treatment without culture is never the correct approach. Unfortunately this scenario happens far too frequently. It is reasonable to repeat the urinalysis before proceeding with diagnostic evaluation. If the hematuria persists, imaging

the kidneys and urinary tract and screening for hypercalciuria is a reasonable approach.

5. **d. To reassure his family and obtain records from the outside institution.** Given the previous history of postinfectious glomerulonephritis (in his case because of a preceding streptococcal infection), the most likely cause of microscopic hematuria is resolving nephritis. The microhematuria may persist for up to 1 year, while the proteinuria and macroscopic hematuria usually resolve within the 2-week acute phase. It would be helpful to confirm the diagnosis with review of medical records.

6. **c. Cystoscopy.** The clinical picture is that of a child presenting with a renal calculus. Cystoscopy is rarely indicated in the diagnostic evaluation, although it might be included during the treatment phase of nephrolithiasis in children. High-resolution CT without administration of a contrast agent is the test of choice, but one cannot argue that ultrasonography should be the first test. Examination of the urine is also a viable first step because children with nephritis occasionally complain of flank pain. Serum electrolytes would not be diagnostic of stone disease but could be helpful if vomiting has been significant.

7. **d. Abdominal ultrasound.** This clinical scenario is most consistent with acute presentation of a renal or ureteral stone. Ultrasound imaging to rule out hydronephrosis and to, often, reveal the stone is the best first step. Intervention for drainage is not indicated until appropriate analgesics have been initiated. CT imaging is unlikely to add further information and exposes the child to radiation.

8. **b. Obtain a 24-hour urine collection to test for calcium, creatinine, oxalate, and citrate.** A metabolic evaluation for the cause of calcium oxalate nephrolithiasis should be initiated because the differential diagnosis includes hyperoxaluria, hypercalciuria, renal tubular acidosis, or idiopathic calcium stones. In children, preventative treatment is rarely initiated without attempts to diagnose the underlying metabolic disturbance. Dietary calcium restriction below the recommended daily allowance is never a treatment for children with calcium stones with or without hypercalciuria.

9. **a. CT of the abdomen and pelvis.** With symptomatic hypertension and gross hematuria, one must entertain the possibility of acute glomerulonephritis. The prior history of pharyngitis is consistent with poststreptococcal-associated disease. Examination of the urine sediment for signs of glomerulonephritis (cellular casts) and documentation of renal function and electrolytes as well as elevated antistreptolysin O titer and decreased C3 are the usual steps taken to confirm the diagnosis. Hypertension is treated aggressively with salt restriction, loop diuretics, and antihypertensive agents. Resolution of the hypertension parallels resolution of the acute phase.

10. **e. CT of the abdomen and pelvis.** The presentation of gross hematuria during a respiratory infection is not characteristic of postinfectious glomerulonephritis because the onset of nephritis usually follows the infection. The positive family history is important because the onset of macroscopic hematuria during a respiratory infection is characteristic of two forms of chronic glomerulonephritis: (1) IgA nephropathy and (2) Alport hereditary nephritis. Imaging with ultrasound does not usually add to diagnostic accuracy but is often performed at some point, even if glomerulonephritis can be confirmed by microscopic examination of the urine. Patients with either IgA or hereditary nephritis would be expected to have normal C3. A renal biopsy is needed for diagnosis of IgA and is usually needed for diagnosis of hereditary nephritis, except in the case in which an affected relative has already undergone biopsy.

11. **c. Collect a specimen of dialysate for white blood cell count and culture.** Peritonitis is the most common complication of PD. Although the patient may undergo a full fever workup including urine and blood cultures as directed by the severity of the clinical presentation, the diagnosis of peritonitis is secured by collecting a sample of dialysate, which is often cloudy, and finding 100 WBCs/mm^3, of which 50% are neutrophils. Antibiotics will be administered after the cultures are collected. PD can continue while treating the peritonitis.

12. **b. Dehydration.** The biochemical analysis that was provided indicates a prerenal cause of acute renal injury. Prerenal azotemia may be present in the earliest phases of hemolytic uremic syndrome if volume depletion is present, but a diarrheal prodrome is expected. Posterior urethral valves, interstitial nephritis, and bilateral ureteropelvic junction obstruction are all associated with salt-wasting and impaired urinary concentrating ability.

13. **a. Repeat the measurement next week in the office.** This child's blood pressure is elevated, and measurement should be repeated and hypertension confirmed. ABPM could be considered but is recommended in children older than 10 years and is more practically performed after repeated office measurements. Therefore the blood pressure should be remeasured in the office. If hypertension is confirmed, the workup will include a complete metabolic panel, lipid profile, echocardiogram, and renal ultrasonography. Angiography and selective renin levels would be performed in the case of severe or recalcitrant hypertension.

14. **d. Spot protein and creatinine ratio on a first morning void following rest.** Low-grade proteinuria in an otherwise healthy teen, especially an athlete, is most likely either exercise-induced transient proteinuria or orthostatic proteinuria, both of which are benign. A first morning void, carefully collected to avoid contamination with urine from activities the day before (i.e., bladder was emptied prior to bed the night before) and quantitated by spot urine protein:creatinine ratio is the most efficient first step. If there is no significant protein on that sample (urine P:C <0.2) then no further workup or specialty referral is needed.

15. **b. Collaboration with a pediatric nephrologist about management of CKD.** Children with CKD from urologic disorder, even stage I with normal GFR, are best managed in a collaborative multi-specialty environment led by a team of urology and nephrology providers. Prevention, as opposed to treatment, of growth failure (as well as other sequelae of CKD) is imperative and generates the best possible foundation for successful renal transplantation and long-term outcome.

16. **e. Treatment with dimercaptoproprionylglycine.** The presence of bilateral low-density stones with crystalluria consistent with cystine in an adolescent is most likely that of cystinuria. While uric acid stones would be possible and urinary metabolic evaluation is appropriate, the most likely diagnosis is cystinuria. Initial surgical treatment would be appropriate for uncontrolled pain, obstruction or infection (Patel et al, 2014).*

CHAPTER REVIEW

1. Nephrogenesis is not complete until 36 weeks in utero; two-thirds of the nephrons develop in the third trimester.

2. At the time of birth, GFR is about 10% of the adult value. It is dependent upon gestational age and doubles in the first two weeks of life.

---

*Sources referenced can be found in *Campbell-Walsh Urology, 11th Edition,* on the Expert Consult website.

3. Serum creatinine at birth reflects maternal creatinine; by 1 to 3 months it should decrease to about 0.3 mg/dl.

4. Neonatal concentrating ability, the ability to excrete a large fluid load, the ability to conserve sodium, and the ability to excrete potassium and to acidify the urine are all limited in the newborn and take between six months and one year to approach the normal adult capabilities. These abnormalities are even more pronounced in the premature infant.

5. Normal fractional excretion of sodium for an infant is 1% to 3%; for an adult, it is less than 1%.

6. Normal serum bicarbonate in an infant is 15 to 18 mM/L due to the physiologic limitations for acidification.

7. Water makes up 80% of the body weight of the newborn.

8. Fetal urine output is required for normal alveolar development in utero.

9. Isotonic saline is usually used as the maintenance fluid in hospitalized children.

10. Isolated microscopic hematuria in children is usually benign; gross hematuria has a defined etiology in two-thirds of patients.

11. Hematuria in the presence of significant proteinuria indicates glomerular disease.

12. Hypercalciuria is one of the most common causes of recurrent or persistent microscopic hematuria.

13. Hypercalciuria may be diagnosed by a calcium: creatinine ratio greater than 0.2 mg or a 24-hour calcium excretion exceeding 0.4 mg/Kg.

14. Normal urinary protein excretion in a child is less than 100 mg/meter^2/day

15. The etiology of proteinuria may be divided into three categories: (1) an abnormality of glomerular permeability, (2) tubule dysfunction, and (3) excessive plasma protein concentrations.

16. Proteinuria is characterized as transient, orthostatic, or fixed.

17. Reflux nephropathy may result in proteinuria.

18. Fanconi syndrome is a generalized dysfunction of the proximal renal tubule.

19. Type 4 RTA is a distal RTA associated with hyperkalemia, defective NH4 metabolism, and aldosterone resistance. It is most commonly seen with obstructive uropathy or multicystic dysplasia.

20. Polydipsia, polyuria, and poor growth are common features of renal tubule disorders.

21. The most common cause of acquired nephrogenic diabetes insipidus is obstructive uropathy. Other causes include lithium and amphotericin administration.

22. Hypercalciuria is the most common cause of stones in children.

23. Metabolic causes of stone disease in children include: (1) type I RTA (calcium stones), (2) primary hyperoxaluria (calcium oxalate stones), (3) cystinuria (cystine stones), and (4) Lesch-Nyhan syndrome (uric acid stones).

24. Inflammatory bowel disease, prematurity, the use of lasix, the use of steroids, malignancy, and genetic abnormalities should be considered in the etiology of stone disease in children.

25. A significant cause of hypertension in children is obesity.

26. The most common cause of acute kidney injury in children is systemic illness or its treatment.

27. Acute kidney injury is an independent risk factor for mortality.

28. The etiology of end stage renal disease in children is renal cystic, hereditary, or congenital disorders in 36% of cases.

29. Uncorrected acidosis in children results in retardation of linear growth and decreased bone mineralization.

30. Preemptive transplantation prior to the initiation of dialysis is the goal for all children with CKD.

124 Perinatal Urology

Joseph G. Borer and Richard S. Lee

QUESTIONS

1. A 34-week-old female fetus has evidence of normal amniotic fluid and unilateral upper pole hydroureteronephrosis with no evidence of an intravesical ureterocele. What does this most likely represent?
   a. Vesicoureteral reflux (VUR)
   b. Ureteropelvic junction obstruction
   c. Obstructed ectopic ureter
   d. Cloacal malformation
   e. None of the above

2. Which of the following statements is TRUE?
   a. Intermittent or varying degrees of hydronephrosis or hydroureter is pathognomonic of VUR
   b. VUR cannot be definitively diagnosed on prenatal ultrasound.
   c. Increasing degrees of hydronephrosis increases the risk of VUR.
   d. Decreasing degrees of hydronephrosis decreases the risk of VUR.
   e. None are true.

3. A 37-week-old fetus with a previously normal-appearing ultrasound (US) has a newly diagnosed enlarged left kidney with loss of corticomedullary differentiation, echogenic streaks, branching hyperechoic vessels, and a calcified intramural inferior vena caval plaque. What is the most likely diagnosis?
   a. Renal artery thrombosis
   b. Renal vein thrombosis
   c. Congenital mesoblastic nephroma
   d. Autosomal recessive polycystic kidney disease (ARPKD)
   e. Wilms tumor

4. A 31-week-old male fetus has a thick-walled dilated bladder, dilated posterior urethra, unilateral severe hydroureteronephrosis, and late-onset oligohydramnios (after 29 weeks). There are no other US findings. Serial bladder taps have been performed, with the latest indices Na 90 (previous 115), Cl 100 (previous 120), Osm 190 (previous 225). As the consulting urologist, you would recommend:
   a. early delivery at 31 weeks.
   b. early delivery after 32 weeks.
   c. in utero urinary tract decompression with shunt.
   d. amnioinfusion with concomitant in utero shunt placement.
   e. observation with delivery at term.

5. In which scenario is in utero decompression by shunt reasonable?
   a. Single male fetus with decreasing amniotic fluid after 28 weeks
   b. Single male fetus with severe bilateral renal cystic disease at 24 weeks
   c. Female fetus with bilateral echogenic kidneys, decompressed bladder volume, and oligohydramnios
   d. Single male fetus with severe hydronephrosis and oligohydramnios at 21 weeks
   e. A twin male fetus with severe hydronephrosis and oligohydramnios at 21 weeks and a normal twin

6. To best distinguish between severe unilateral hydronephrosis and a multicystic dysplastic kidney (MCDK), which of the following combination best represents a MCDK?
   a. Minimal or absent renal parenchyma
   b. Absence of a central large cyst

   c. Appearance of multiple non-communicating cysts
   d. a, b, and c
   e. a and c

7. A 28-week-old fetus has bilaterally enlarged echogenic kidneys without renal cysts, hepatobiliary dilatation, and severe oligohydramnios. These findings suggest which diagnosis?
   a. ARPKD
   b. Posterior urethral valves
   c. Bilateral MCDK
   d. Autosomal dominant polycystic kidney disease (ADPKD)
   e. Bilateral multilocular cystic nephroma

8. A 2-month-old male infant with an antenatal history of left moderate to severe hydronephrosis has a postnatal ultrasound at 24 hours of life demonstrating mild hydronephrosis. A follow-up US at 2 months demonstrates left severe hydronephrosis. This can be explained by:
   a. intermittent changing hydronephrosis consistent with VUR.
   b. physiologic oliguria in the newborn.
   c. worsening obstruction.
   d. ureterocele disproportion.
   e. none of the above.

9. Prenatal imaging findings that are consistent with bladder exstrophy include all of the following EXCEPT:
   a. Absence of bladder filling documented on repetitive fetal imaging
   b. Volume of amniotic fluid appropriate for fetal gestational age
   c. Lower abdominal wall mass
   d. Spinal cord or spinal column abnormality
   e. Low-set umbilicus and inability to clearly visualize genitalia

10. Cloacal exstrophy is most likely in the differential diagnosis when fetal ultrasonography and/or magnetic resonance identify which of the following?
    a. Normal number, location, and anatomy of the kidneys
    b. Omphalocele
    c. Lower abdominal wall mass, absence of bladder filling on serial imaging, ectopic kidney, and spinal cord tethering
    d. 46,XY karyotype on amniocentesis and diminutive genitalia
    e. Renal agenesis and contralateral hydronephrosis

11. 46,XX karyotype, cystic pelvic mass, bilateral hydroureteronephrosis, and the presence of ascites in a fetus are findings and characteristics most consistent with which diagnosis?
    a. Cloacal exstrophy
    b. Cloaca
    c. Bladder exstrophy
    d. Imperforate anus
    e. Prune-belly syndrome

12. FALSE statement(s) regarding the identification of a solid renal mass on fetal imaging include which of the following?
    a. When possible, delivery should be planned at a pediatric tertiary care center to avoid a potentially life-threatening condition in early neonatal life.
    b. A solid renal mass identified in the fetus is most often consistent with a malignant tumor.
    c. Prenatal identification of a renal mass warrants careful immediate postnatal monitoring of the neonate.
    d. A solid renal mass in the fetus is a relatively common finding.
    e. Both b and d.

ANSWERS

1. **c. Obstructed ectopic ureter.** A duplication anomaly with upper pole hydroureteronephrosis is typically associated with a ureterocele, an ectopic ureterocele, or an ectopic ureter causing obstruction. A dilated ureter is typically identified.

2. **b. VUR cannot be definitively diagnosed on prenatal ultrasound.** Previous studies have demonstrated that the degree of hydronephrosis does not correlate with the incidence of VUR.

3. **b. Renal vein thrombosis.** The ultrasound appearance of the kidney during renal vein thrombosis can be renal enlargement, loss of the corticomedullary differentiation, echogenic streaks, lack of definition of renal sinus echoes, and loss of venous flow in the affected kidney evident on Doppler imaging.

4. **e. Observation with delivery at term.** Serial bladder sampling during 3 days has been used to help determine whether the fetus is a viable candidate. The serial nature of the procedure allows one to see the subsequent trend of urine osmolality and electrolyte composition as a reflection of fetal kidney response. This fetus has encouraging urine electrolytes and only unilateral hydroureteronephrosis.

5. **d. Single male fetus with severe hydronephrosis and oligohydramnios at 21 weeks.** In utero intervention is currently indicated when the fetus's life is at risk. In utero decompression by shunting is only indicated in instances of presumed bladder obstruction in the setting of oligohydramnios. In utero intervention in the case of a twin gestation may place the other fetus at risk and therefore is not recommended.

6. **d. a, b, and c.** The findings of multiple noncommunicating cysts, minimal or absent renal parenchyma, and the absence of a central large cyst are diagnostic of a multicystic dysplastic kidney.

7. **a. ARPKD.** Bilaterally enlarged echogenic kidneys without renal cystic disease, particularly if associated with hepatobiliary dilatation or oligohydramnios, suggest autosomal recessive polycystic kidney disease.

8. **b. Physiologic oliguria in the newborn.** It is important to keep in mind that a postnatal ultrasound examination performed within the first 48 hours of life may not yet demonstrate hydronephrosis or may underestimate the degree of hydronephrosis secondary to physiologic oliguria.

9. **d. Spinal cord or spinal column abnormality.** Ultrasound findings in a fetus with bladder exstrophy include nonvisualization of the fetal bladder, lower abdominal wall mass immediately inferior to a low-lying umbilicus, and diminutive genitalia. Other findings that may be evident to the experienced observer include normal kidneys in orthotopic position, normal vertebrae and spinal cord, abnormal symphyseal diastasis, and anteriorly displaced anus.

10. **c. Lower abdominal wall mass, absence of bladder filling on serial imaging, ectopic kidney, and spinal cord tethering.** The prenatal diagnosis of cloacal exstrophy should be suspected with findings of nonvisualization of the bladder in association with a low-lying umbilicus, lower abdominal wall mass—typically omphalocele—and kidney (number, location, and/or appearance) and lumbosacral spine abnormalities.

11. **b. Cloaca.** Persistent cloaca should be considered in any female fetus presenting with hydronephrosis and a large cystic mass arising from the pelvis.

12. **e. Both b and d.** Congenital mesoblastic nephroma is a rare benign congenital renal tumor and is the most common solid renal tumor in the neonatal period. Malignant tumors are rare. Delivery at a pediatric tertiary care center should be planned to avoid a potentially life-threatening condition in early neonatal life.

CHAPTER REVIEW

1. Oligohydramnios after 18 to 20 weeks may be the result of urinary tract obstruction or poor renal function.

2. Inability to identify the bladder on repeat prenatal ultrasound studies should suggest the diagnosis of exstrophy.

3. Dilatation of the posterior urethra (keyhole sign) suggests posterior urethral valves.

4. Neural tube defects are diagnosed prenatally by α-fetoprotein and screening with ultrasonography.

5. Adrenal hemorrhage may appear as eggshell calcifications in contrast to the fine stippled calcifications of neuroblastoma.

6. An indication that renal function is salvageable is suggested by a fetal urine specimen in which the urinary sodium value is less than 100 mEq/L, the chloride value is less than 110 mEq/L, and the osmolality is less than 200 mOsm/kg.

7. Postnatal ultrasonography performed within the first 48 hours of life may not demonstrate hydronephrosis owing to decreased urine formation.

8. A dimercaptosuccinic acid scan is recommended to confirm the diagnosis of multidysplastic kidney when the ultrasound findings are not classic to differentiate it from cystic nephroma.

9. The most common form of congenital adrenal hyperplasia (CAH) is 21-hydroxylase deficiency. Genital ambiguity in females can be minimized in CAH patients with prenatal treatment with dexamethasone.

10. Congenital mesoblastic nephroma is the most common solid renal tumor in the newborn. Wilms tumors are rare in the neonate.

11. Oligohydramnios in the second trimester is often associated with a lethal postnatal outcome due to pulmonary hypoplasia.

12. Bilateral hydronephrosis suggestive of bladder outlet obstruction should be evaluated promptly after birth. In boys the etiology is usually posterior urethral valves; in girls it usually is an obstructing ectopic ureterocele.

13. The ultrasound appearance of the kidney following renal vein thrombosis includes renal enlargement, loss of the corticomedullary differentiation, echogenic streaks, lack of definition of renal sinus echoes, and loss of venous flow in the affected kidney evident on Doppler imaging.

14. In utero decompression by shunting is indicated only in instances of presumed bladder obstruction in the setting of oligohydramnios.

15. The findings of multiple noncommunicating cysts, minimal or absent renal parenchyma, and the absence of a central large cyst are diagnostic of a multicystic dysplastic kidney.

16. In bladder exstrophy, usually the vertebrae and spinal cord are normal, and there is an abnormal symphyseal diastasis and anteriorly displaced anus. In cloacal exstrophy, lumbosacral spine abnormalities may occur.

125   Evaluation of the Pediatric Urology Patient

Thomas F. Kolon and Douglas A. Canning

QUESTIONS

1. Which one of the following patients does NOT need to be seen emergently?
   a. A newborn with hydronephrosis in a solitary kidney
   b. A 4-year-old boy with acute right scrotal pain
   c. A 12-year-old girl with microscopic hematuria found during a routine examination
   d. An 8-year-old boy with sickle-cell anemia and a 5-hour history of priapism
   e. A male newborn with a distended bladder, bilateral hydronephrosis, and respiratory insufficiency

2. Which of the following is a potential complication of neonatal circumcision?
   a. Wound infection
   b. Meatal stenosis
   c. Cicatrix
   d. Death
   e. All of the above

3. The pediatric kidney is particularly susceptible to trauma due to:
   a. relatively increased renal size.
   b. limited visceral adipose tissue.
   c. limited chest wall protection.
   d. increased mobility.
   e. all of the above.

4. What is the optimal timing of spinal ultrasonography during screening for occult spinal dysraphism?
   a. Before 6 months of age
   b. 6 months to 2 years of age
   c. At any age before puberty
   d. At any age
   e. Never. Ultrasound is not useful to screen for dysraphism.

5. What is the most commonly detected etiology for asymptomatic microscopic hematuria in children?
   a. Fibroepithelial polyp
   b. Hypercalciuria
   c. Poststreptococcal glomerulonephritis
   d. Uncomplicated urinary tract infection
   e. Hyperuricosuria

6. Findings associated with the Beckwith-Wiedemann syndrome include:
   a. macroglossia.
   b. hepatosplenomegaly.
   c. nephromegaly.
   d. macrosomia.
   e. all of the above.

7. A voiding cystourethrogram is essential in the diagnosis of which clinical conditions?
   a. Ureteropelvic junction obstruction
   b. Primary obstructive megaureter
   c. Posterior urethral valves
   d. Nephrolithiasis
   e. All of the above

8. When should a child with suspected congenital adrenal hyperplasia be tested?
   a. Before discharge from the nursery
   b. At the first well-baby visit
   c. Only if undergoing general anesthesia
   d. At puberty
   e. No testing is required

9. All of the following statements about the pediatric abdominal examination are true EXCEPT:
   a. renal pathology is the source of as many as two thirds of neonatal abdominal masses.
   b. abdominal distention at birth or shortly afterward suggests either obstruction or perforation of the gastrointestinal tract.
   c. the abdominal wall is normally strong, especially in infants with hydronephrosis.
   d. a solid flank mass may be due to renal venous thrombosis.
   e. in cloacal exstrophy, an omphalocele is superior to the cecal plate and lateral bladder halves with prolapsed ileum in the midline.

10. Which of the following statements is FALSE about cutaneous markers of occult spinal dysraphism?
    a. Forty percent of patients with atypical presacral dimples have associated occult spinal dysraphism.
    b. A combination of two or more congenital midline skin lesions is the strongest marker of occult spinal dysraphism.
    c. A presacral dimple less than 2.5 cm from the anal verge at birth may indicate spina bifida or cord tethering.
    d. Sacral hypertrichosis may be associated with spinal dysraphism.
    e. All of the above are true.

11. Sexual abuse can be associated with which of the following physical examination findings?
    a. Bruised vaginal mucosa in a prepubertal child
    b. Penile discharge
    c. A normal genital and perineal examination
    d. a and c
    e. a, b, and c

12. Urethral meatal stenosis in the infant occurs most commonly:
    a. as a result of birth trauma.
    b. after urinary tract infection.

c. after a voiding cystourethrogram (VCUG).

d. after healing of the inflamed, denuded glans after circumcision.

e. from penile adhesions.

13. In newborns with ambiguous genitalia, palpation of a gonad rules out which disorder of sexual development (DSD)?

a. Ovotesticular disorder

b. Mixed gonadal dysgenesis

c. Partial androgen insensitivity

d. Pure gonadal dysgenesis

e. Persistent müllerian duct syndrome

14. Secondary urinary incontinence is defined as:

a. diurnal and nocturnal enuresis.

b. incontinence associated with urinary tract infection.

c. urinary incontinence associated with constipation.

d. urinary incontinence after a dry interval greater than 6 months.

e. urinary incontinence associated with a neurologic condition.

15. A newborn should have a scrotal hydrocele surgically corrected in the neonatal period if:

a. it is large.

b. it is changing in volume.

c. it accompanies a symptomatic hernia.

d. a, b, and c.

e. b and c.

ANSWERS

1. **c. A 12-year-old girl with microscopic hematuria found during a routine examination.** In the absence of other symptoms, microscopic hematuria in children is not an emergency. Bilateral hydronephrosis or hydronephrosis in a solitary kidney both represent emergencies and should be evaluated as soon as possible. Acute scrotal pain should always be considered testicular torsion until proven otherwise. Boys with sickle cell anemia are at increased risk for priapism and should always be treated immediately to decrease the long-term sequelae associated with priapism.

2. **e. All of the above.** Wound infections, meatal stenosis, removal of too much/too little prepuce, cicatrix, and even death are all potential complications of neonatal circumcision.

3. **e. All of the above.** The pediatric kidney is particularly susceptible to trauma due to limited visceral adipose tissue, limited chest wall protection, relatively increased renal size, and increased mobility of the kidney.

4. **a. Before 6 months of age.** Ossification of the posterior elements after 6 months of age prevents an acoustic ultrasound window. After 6 months, spinal magnetic resonance imaging (MRI) is recommended when an occult spinal dysraphism is suspected.

5. **b. Hypercalciuria.** Most microscopic hematuria in children is transient and the source is not identified. The most commonly identified etiology of asymptomatic microhematuria in children is hypercalciuria.

6. **e. All of the above.** Beckwith-Wiedemann syndrome is caused by a mutation on chromosome 11p15.5. Clinical features include macroglossia, nephromegaly, organomegaly (hepatosplenomegaly), macrosomia (gigantism), and hemihypertrophy. Many of the affected infants have hypoglycemia in the first few days of life. Patients are at increased risk for specific tumors (e.g., adrenal carcinoma, Wilms tumor, hepatoblastoma, and rhabdomyosarcoma).

7. **c. Posterior urethral valves.** The diagnosis of posterior urethral valves requires visualization of the urethra during voiding. Bladder diverticula, a pronounced bladder neck, dilated posterior urethra, vesicoureteral reflux, and valve leaflets can all be associated with posterior urethral valves and are visible on voiding cystourethrogram. Ureteropelvic junction obstruction and primary obstructive megaureter are both obstructions above the level of the urethra and are usually evaluated with ultrasonography and a MAG3 renal scan or magnetic resonance urogram. Nephrolithiasis is typically evaluated using ultrasonography and computed tomography (CT) scan when necessary.

8. **a. Before discharge from the nursery.** Congenital adrenal hyperplasia may result in salt wasting; therefore, infants with ambiguous genitalia must be quickly evaluated and stabilized.

9. **c. The abdominal wall is normally strong, especially in infants with hydronephrosis.** Renal pathology accounts for approximately two thirds of abdominal masses found in the neonate. Solid masses include neuroblastoma, congenital mesoblastic nephroma, teratoma, and renal enlargement due to renal venous thrombosis. The abdominal wall is normally weak in premature infants and on occasion in those with hydronephrosis.

10. **c. A presacral dimple less than 2.5 cm from the anal verge at birth may indicate spina bifida or cord tethering.** The lower back should be examined for any evidence of cutaneous markers of occult spinal dysraphisms that may account for abnormal bladder function. In a series of 207 neonates with sacral and presacral cutaneous stigmata, 40% of patients with atypical dimples were found to have occult spinal dysraphism. An "atypical" presacral dimple is defined as a dimple that is off center, more than 2.5 cm from the anal verge at birth, or deeper than 0.5 cm. Sacral hair tuft (hypertrichosis) may also be associated with spinal dysraphism.

11. **e. a, b, and c.** Although penile discharge and bruised vaginal mucosa can reflect sexual abuse, the possibility of sexual abuse should not be dismissed in the absence of physical examination findings. Only 11% of girls evaluated in a sexual abuse clinic demonstrated suggestive physical examination findings.

12. **d. After healing of the inflamed, denuded glans after circumcision.** Meatal stenosis is not unusual after circumcision. It may result from contraction of the meatus after healing of the inflamed, denuded glans tissue that occurs after retraction of the foreskin or from damage to the frenular artery at the time of circumcision.

13. **d. Pure gonadal dysgenesis.** Particular attention to the symmetry of the examination is important if a disorder of sex development is thought to exist. A symmetrical gonadal examination (gonads palpable on each side or impalpable on both sides) suggests a global disorder, such as congenital adrenal hyperplasia or androgen insensitivity. When a gonad is palpable, female congenital adrenal hyperplasia (ovaries are not palpable) and pure gonadal dysgenesis (bilateral streak gonads are not palpable) are ruled out.

14. **d. Urinary incontinence after a dry interval greater than 6 months.** Although urinary incontinence can be associated with infection, constipation, and neurologic disease, secondary urinary incontinence is defined as occurring after a dry interval greater than 6 months.

15. **e. b and c.** A hydrocele that changes in volume suggests a patent processus vaginalis. These infants are at risk for an inguinal hernia. The processus vaginalis is less likely to close after birth. If a hernia has been symptomatic, it should be corrected in the newborn period. A large scrotal hydrocele may still resorb and get smaller with time—distinction must be made from an abdominoscrotal hydrocele.

CHAPTER REVIEW

1. The most common malignant abdominal tumor in infants is a neuroblastoma, followed by Wilms tumor.
2. Undescended testes are present in 30% of preterm neonates and 3% of full-term neonates; the testis will likely not descend after 6 months of age.
3. The most common prepubertal testicular/paratesticular tumor is teratoma, followed by rhabdomyosarcoma, epidermoid cyst, yolk sac tumor, and germ cell tumor, in that order.
4. Very few children hold the urine and not the stool. Conversely, children who retain stool nearly always retain urine.
5. Gross hematuria in the newborn is an emergency, because it may indicate renal venous thrombosis or renal artery thrombosis.
6. In general, blunt renal trauma is treated nonoperatively, except when there is a major vascular avulsion or extensive urinary extravasation.
7. In the newborn, the foreskin is adherent to the glans, and adhesions should not be separated unless a circumcision is performed.
8. A positive dip stick for blood requires a microscopic examination. Absence of red blood cells in the microscopic examination indicates hemoglobinuria or myoglobinuria.
9. Continuous leakage of urine in a girl should suggest ectopic ureter.
10. Infants younger than 6 months of age and uncircumcised male infants are at increased risk for urinary tract infections.
11. Patients with myelomeningoceles are at increased risk for latex allergy.
12. Most microscopic hematuria in children is transient and the source is not identified. The most commonly identified etiology of asymptomatic microhematuria in children is hypercalciuria.
13. Beckwith-Wiedemann syndrome is caused by a mutation on chromosome 11p15.5. Clinical features include macroglossia, nephromegaly, organomegaly (hepatosplenomegaly), macrosomia (gigantism), and hemihypertrophy. Many of the affected infants have hypoglycemia in the first few days of life. These individuals are at increased risk for adrenal carcinoma, Wilms tumor, hepatoblastoma, and rhabdomyosarcoma.
14. Renal pathology accounts for approximately two thirds of abdominal masses found in the neonate.
15. If a disorder of sex development is thought to exist, a symmetrical gonadal examination (gonads palpable on each side or impalpable on both sides) suggests a global disorder, such as congenital adrenal hyperplasia or androgen insensitivity. If the gonads are nonpalpable, congenital adrenal hyperplasia is likely.
16. A hydrocele that changes in volume suggests a patent processus vaginalis.

126 Pediatric Urogenital Imaging

Hans G. Pohl and Aaron D. Martin

QUESTIONS

1. Areas of renal scarring on dimercaptosuccinic acid (DMSA) scan have the following characteristic appearance:
   a. photon-intense lesion with normal reniform shape preserved.
   b. photon-deficient lesion without preservation of reniform shape.
   c. photon-deficient lesion with normal reniform shape preserved.
   d. photon-intense lesion without preservation of reniform shape.
   e. photon-deficient lesion located centrally.

2. A 6-year-old child with grade 4 hydronephrosis found on ultrasound after a urinary tract infection (UTI) is referred for evaluation. No stones are seen on the study, and there is no hyoureter. The following test should be performed:
   a. MAG-3 diuretic renography.
   b. computed tomographic (CT) urogram.
   c. intravenous pyelogram (IVP).
   d. retrograde pyelogram.
   e. repeat ultrasonography.

3. A 14-year-old presents to the emergency department at 1 AM with sudden-onset, severe left testicular pain, swelling, and nausea with one episode of emesis. He has been in pain for 7 hours at the time you evaluate him, and no imaging has yet been performed. The next step is:
   a. call for ultrasonography to come in to confirm torsion.
   b. reassure the patient this is likely epididymitis and give a trial of nonsteroidal anti-inflammatory drugs (NSAIDs).
   c. obtain urinalysis, treat empirically with antibiotics, and send home with narcotic pain meds.
   d. take him immediately for surgical exploration.
   e. obtain testicular scintigraphy to differentiate between torsion and an inflammatory process.

4. Technetium-99 m (^{99m}Tc)-dimercaptosuccinic acid is taken up by which renal cells?
   a. Thin segment loop of Henle
   b. Glomerulus
   c. Proximal tubule
   d. Distal tubule
   e. Collecting tubule

5. A 1-year-old boy is referred to your office for a right undescended testicle. The examination reveals a normal left descended testicle and a nonpalpable right testicle. The next step is:
   a. obtain a scrotal/pelvic ultrasound to determine the presence and/or location of the nonpalpable gonad.
   b. obtain pelvic magnetic resonance imaging (MRI) to determine the presence and/or location of the nonpalpable gonad.
   c. obtain testicular scintigraphy to determine the presence and/or location of the nonpalpable gonad.
   d. proceed to surgical exploration for cryptorchidism without further imaging.
   e. have the child return in 6 months for repeat examination and consider hormonal therapy to encourage spontaneous descent.

ANSWERS

1. **b. Photon-deficient lesion without preservation of reniform shape.** A scar on DMSA scan will create a defect in the reniform shape, whereas acute pyelonephritis will simply be a photon-deficient area with preserved reniform borders.

2. **a. MAG-3 diuretic renography.** This child's sonogram is concerning for ureteropelvic junction obstruction. MAG-3 diuretic renography will provide quantitative functional and descriptive anatomic information that cannot be ascertained in full by the other modalities.

3. **d. Take him immediately for surgical exploration.** Testicular torsion is a clinical diagnosis and does not require imaging unless the exam and symptoms are equivocal. Surgical therapy should not be delayed for imaging if the clinical picture is indicative for torsion.

4. **c. Proximal tubule.** DMSA is taken up and bound to the proximal tubules allowing for the best and most reliable imaging of the renal cortex. MAG-3 is filtered and also taken up by the proximal tubules but not bound, allowing rapid clearance to assess drainage of the collecting system.

5. **d. Proceed to surgical exploration for cryptorchidism without further imaging.** Per American Urological Association cryptorchidism guidelines, imaging rarely assists in decision making in these cases because of poor sensitivity and specificity, and therefore should not be obtained. Hormonal therapy has low response rates and little evidence of long-term efficacy. If the 6-month examination does not reveal spontaneous descent, it is recommended that an orchiopexy be performed within 1 year.

CHAPTER REVIEW

1. The benign nature of MRI exposure in the child has been questioned based on changes in gene expression that occur related to the magnetic field.
2. On renal ultrasound in the newborn, the renal cortex is slightly hypoechoic with discrete interfaces between cortex and medulla.
3. In cystic disease of the kidney, the cysts do not communicate, unlike the "cysts" (dilated calyces) in a hydronephrotic kidney, which do communicate.
4. Ultrasound for the evaluation of the routine cryptorchid testis is not indicated.
5. A DMSA scan that reveals an area of photon deficiency in the acute setting is consistent with acute pyelonephritis, whereas a

photopenic area that lasts more than 6 months is likely a renal scar. Also, a scar on DMSA will create a defect in the reniform shape, whereas acute pyelonephritis will simply be a photon-deficient area with preserved reniform borders.

6. Diuretic renography may be falsely positive due to dehydration or lack of bladder drainage; there are no established $T_{1/2}$ values in young children, and it is the character of the curve that suggests the diagnosis.

127 Infection and Inflammation of the Pediatric Genitourinary Tract

Christopher S. Cooper and Douglas W. Storm

QUESTIONS

1. The primary symptom in a 3-month-old that leads to the diagnosis of a pediatric urinary tract infection (UTI) is:
   a. diarrhea.
   b. frequency.
   c. fever.
   d. jaundice.
   e. foul-smelling urine.

2. Which of the following factors would not increase the probability of a UTI in a febrile girl?
   a. Age less than 12 months
   b. Temperature 39° C or higher
   c. African-American race
   d. Absence of other source of infection
   e. Recent previous UTI

3. A false-negative urinary nitrite test for UTI may be caused by all of the following EXCEPT:
   a. gram-positive bacterial UTI.
   b. urinary retention.
   c. dilute urine.
   d. yeast infection.
   e. frequent urination.

4. Which of the following tests has the highest sensitivity for UTI?
   a. Leukocyte esterase
   b. Urinary nitrite
   c. Urinary nitrate
   d. Serum procalcitonin
   e. Urine protein

5. Which of the following statements is FALSE regarding dimercaptosuccinic acid (DMSA) renal scan?
   a. The maximum sensitivity for detection of acute pyelonephritis is within 1 week from the onset of symptoms.
   b. Demonstration of irreversible renal damage and scar may require a renal scan at least one year after pyelonephritis.
   c. The risk of an abnormal scan increases with increased grades of vesicoureteral reflux (VUR).
   d. The estimated radiation dose is approximately 1 mSv.
   e. DMSA is bound to the glomerular basement membrane, providing excellent cortical imaging but slow excretion.

6. Which of the following statements regarding imaging is most likely to be broadly accepted?
   a. All children with febrile UTI require a voiding cystourethrogram (VCUG).
   b. All children with a febrile UTI require a renal ultrasound.
   c. All children with fever persisting longer than 48 hours after appropriate antibiotics require a renal and bladder ultrasound.
   d. All children with a febrile UTI require a DMSA.

   e. All children with fever persisting longer than 48 hours after appropriate antibiotics require a computed tomography (CT) scan.

7. The most common pediatric uropathogen is:
   a. *Escherichia coli.*
   b. *Klebsiella.*
   c. *Proteus.*
   d. *Enterobacter.*
   e. *Citrobacter.*

8. Ampicillin should be strongly considered for use with neonates because of the increased incidence of which uropathogen?
   a. *E. coli*
   b. *Klebsiella*
   c. *Pseudomonas*
   d. *Enterococcus*
   e. *Staphylococcus aureus*

9. Which of the following antibiotics would NOT be a good choice for a child with suspected pyelonephritis?
   a. Fluoroquinolones
   b. Trimethoprim
   c. Cephalosporin
   d. Nitrofurantoin
   e. Gentamicin

10. Which of the following antibiotics is contraindicated in children younger than 6 weeks?
    a. Trimethoprim-sulfamethoxazole
    b. Amoxicillin-clavulanate
    c. Cephalexin
    d. Piperacillin
    e. Tobramycin

11. Which of the following have been identified as risk factors for UTI?
    a. Constipation
    b. Bladder dysfunction
    c. High-grade VUR
    d. Female gender, older than 1 year
    e. All of the above

12. Which of the following is NOT true regarding renal scars?
    a. Increased incidence occurs with delayed treatment of a UTI
    b. May be indistinguishable on renal scan from renal dysplasia
    c. Most frequently seen in midportion of the kidney parenchyma
    d. Involve a loss of renal parenchymal tissue
    e. Have been associated with an increased risk of hypertension

13. Children with significant bilateral renal scars require:
    a. prophylactic antibiotics.
    b. renin-angiotensin antagonists.

c. dietary modification.

d. long-term assessment of proteinuria.

e. none of the above.

14. Which of the following statements regarding recurrent UTIs is FALSE?

   a. The risk of a recurrent UTI is higher in a boy with an initial UTI who is younger than 1 year than in one who is older than 1 year.

   b. 10% to 30% of children will develop at least one recurrent UTI.

   c. The recurrence rate is highest within the first 3-6 months following a UTI.

   d. The more frequent and more recurrent a child's UTIs, the more likely the child is to have subsequent UTIs.

   e. The risk of renal scars increases with recurrent UTIs.

15. In children aged 0 to 24 months who present with a fever, which of the following signs/symptoms are not useful in suspecting that they may have a UTI as the cause of their fever?

   a. Fever above 40° C

   b. Vomiting

   c. History of a previous UTI

   d. Suprapubic tenderness

   e. Uncircumcised penis

16. Which of the following statements is FALSE?

   a. Virulent bacteria that cause UTIs are otherwise known as *uropathogenic bacteria*.

   b. Virulent bacteria possess different adaptations and fitness factors that allow them to subvert or hijack host defenses and reside in an environment in which they would not normally preside.

   c. Virulent bacteria have mechanisms that allow the bacteria to initially attach to urogenital mucosal surfaces and then interact with these tissues by setting off cascades of signaling and other immunologic response events and subsequently invade the bladder.

   d. Commensal bacteria cannot cause UTIs.

   e. Commensal bacteria are defined as lacking the virulent traits that would allow a bacteria to subvert a host's immune defenses.

17. Which of the following is NOT considered a bacterial virulence trait?

   a. Properties that improve bacterial adherence

   b. Properties that allow bacterial nourishment in otherwise adverse environments

   c. Flagellar attachments that allow bacteria to move more quickly

   d. Properties that protect bacteria from the host's immune response

   e. Toxins that allow bacteria to invade host cells

18. Which of the following statements is FALSE?

   a. In children younger than 1 year, UTIs are more common in boys than girls.

   b. After 1 year, UTIs are more prevalent in females than males, except in elderly individuals.

   c. It has been estimated that 7% of girls and 2% of boys suffer a UTI by the age of 6 years.

   d. 3% to 5% of febrile children have a UTI.

   e. In sexually active teenagers, there is a female predominance of UTIs.

19. Which of the following is a TRUE statement?

   a. Circumcision reduces the rate of UTI development in the first 12 months of life by almost twentyfold.

   b. Circumcision reduces the rate of UTI development in the first 6 months of life by almost fivefold.

   c. Circumcision reduces the rate of UTI development in the first 6 months of life by almost tenfold.

   d. Circumcision reduces the rate of UTI development in the first 18 months of life by almost fivefold.

   e. Circumcision does not reduce the rate of UTI.

20. Which of the following statements is FALSE regarding the role that vesicoureteral reflux (VUR) plays in pediatric UTI development?

   a. VUR has been identified in 1% to 2% of all newborns.

   b. VUR is found in 25% to 40% of children after their first episode of UTI.

   c. In children who are found to have a DMSA-proven episode of pyelonephritis, 66% will be found to have VUR.

   d. Kidneys associated with higher grade VUR (grades III and IV) are twice as likely to have pyelonephritic changes on DMSA scan.

   e. Obtaining a voiding cystourethrogram (VCUG) in only those children with an abnormal DMSA scan may miss 15% to 30% of children with dilating VUR.

21. A 9-year-old female referred for treatment of multiple afebrile UTIs suffers from urinary urgency and is known to prolong using the toilet. She suffers from day and nighttime urinary incontinence. She also has a bowel movement only every few days that is typically hard and painful. She underwent a renal ultrasound that showed normal upper tracts and a thick-walled bladder. A VCUG was performed that showed Grade II left VUR and a spinning top urethra. Which of the following statements regarding treatment of this child is TRUE?

   a. The use of anticholinergics in this child would not help resolve her VUR.

   b. Biofeedback would be of no use in this patient because it has not been shown to improve VUR resolution and further UTI development.

   c. Treatment of her constipation may improve her day and nighttime urinary incontinence and help reduce the incidence of recurrent UTIs.

   d. The implementation of a timed voiding schedule would not be appropriate because this child requires urgent surgical therapy for treatment of her VUR to prevent further UTI development.

   e. Treatment of her dysfunctional elimination should not be considered because she has VUR.

22. Multiple studies demonstrate that _____ of individuals who intermittently catheterize develop chronic bacteria and/or pyuria and most are asymptomatic.

   a. 40% to 80%

   b. 50% to 90%

   c. 30% to 60%

   d. 10% to 25%

   e. 45% to 85%

23. Which of the following statements is FALSE?

   a. Catheter-associated UTI is the second most common nosocomial infection, accounting for more than 1 million cases each year in U.S. hospitals and nursing homes.

   b. The risk of UTI increases with the length of time that the catheter is in place.

c. Nosocomial UTIs typically necessitate one extra hospital day per patient and nearly 1 million extra hospital days annually.

d. The best way to avoid a catheter-related UTI and its related cost is the judicious use of urinary catheters and to remove urethral catheters in hospitalized patients as soon as they are no longer medically necessary.

e. In children, nosocomial UTIs account for 6% to 18% of nosocomial infections on pediatric hospital services.

24. A 9-year-old female presents with fevers, nausea, vomiting, and flank pain and is shown to have a culture-proven UTI. If she underwent a DMSA scan, how likely is it that the scan would show changes associated with pyelonephritis?

    a. 95% to 100%
    b. 50% to 66%
    c. 60% to 75%
    d. 70% to 85%
    e. 10% to 25%

25. Which of the following statements is FALSE regarding why bacteria within a biofilm may be difficult to eradicate with antibiotics?

    a. Antibiotics often fail to penetrate the full depth of a biofilm.
    b. Organisms within a biofilm often grow quickly, resulting in resistance to the antibiotics.
    c. Antimicrobial binding proteins are poorly expressed in these biofilm bacteria.
    d. Bacteria within a biofilm activate many genes that alter the cell envelope, the molecular targets, and the susceptibility to antimicrobial agents.
    e. Bacteria in a biofilm can survive in the presence of antimicrobial agents at a concentration 1000 to 1500 times higher than the concentration normally necessary to kill non–biofilm associated bacteria in the same species.

26. A girl who presents for a preschool physical is found to have more than 10^5 CFU/mL *E. coli* on a urine culture. She has never previously suffered a UTI and is asymptomatic. How should she be treated?

    a. Three-day course of antibiotics
    b. Urodynamics and kidney-ureter-bladder (KUB) radiography for evaluation of occult voiding dysfunction and constipation
    c. Renal ultrasound and VCUG
    d. No treatment or further evaluation is necessary.
    e. A catheterized urine specimen should be obtained to verify that this is truly a UTI.

27. Which of the following statements is FALSE?

    a. Recurrent urinary tract infections can be subdivided into unresolved bacteriuria, bacterial persistence, and reinfection.
    b. Unresolved bacteriuria is most commonly caused by inadequate bacterial therapy.
    c. Bacterial persistence and reinfection occur after sterile urine has been documented after previous UTI therapy.
    d. In cases of bacterial reinfection, typically a nidus causing the infection has not been eradicated.
    e. Asymptomatic bacteriuria (ASB) is defined as the presence of two consecutive urine specimens yielding positive cultures (more than 10^5 CFU/mL) of the same uropathogen in a patient who is free of any infectious symptoms.

28. Which of the following is TRUE regarding a renal abscess?

    a. Individuals presenting with a renal abscess commonly are more ill than patients with just pyelonephritis.
    b. In as many as 30% of renal abscess cases, the urine culture may be negative.

c. CT appears to be the most sensitive and specific imaging modality in making the diagnosis of a renal abscess.

d. Associated early CT findings include a poorly defined area of low attenuation or decreased enhancement or a striated, wedge-shaped zone of increased or decreased enhancement.

e. Ultrasound can detect an abscess as small as 2 cm and usually appears as a sonolucent area containing low-amplitude echoes.

29. Which of the following defines a UTI?

    a. If a suprapubic aspiration was performed, then recovery of any organisms defines a UTI.
    b. For catheterized specimens, recovery of at least 10,000 colony-forming units (CFU)/mL is required to define a UTI.
    c. 50,000 CFU/mL are required if the specimen was collected via a clean catch method.
    d. If a suprapubic aspiration was performed, then recovery of at least 10,000 CFU/mL organisms defines a UTI.
    e. No matter how the culture is collected, the presence of 10,000 CFU/mL defines a UTI.

ANSWERS

1. **c. Fever.** Although all of the choices may be symptoms of a UTI in infants and young patients, and UTI should be considered as a possible diagnosis, after the neonatal period, fever is usually the primary symptom that leads to the diagnosis of a pediatric UTI.

2. **c. African-American race.** The probability of a UTI in girls has been shown to be at least 1%, and 2% if they had two or more, or three or more, of the following risk factors, respectively: white race, age younger than 12 months, temperature at or above 39° C, fever lasting 2 days or more, or absence of another source of infection (Gorelick and Shaw, 2000).* In addition, children with a previous UTI are at increased risk for UTI. Children younger than 6 years with a documented UTI have been noted to have a 12% risk of recurrence per year in a community-based study (Conway et al, 2007).

3. **b. Urinary retention.** Urinary nitrite is reduced from dietary nitrates in the urine by gram-negative enteric bacteria. This conversion requires several hours to occur; thus, a first morning urine sample gives the best sensitivity with this test. Frequent urination, as is often the case in infants and small children, may not permit enough time for the urine in the bladder to undergo significant conversion of nitrates to nitrites and therefore result in a false-negative nitrite test more frequently than in older children (Mori et al, 2010). A dilute urine may also generate a false-negative test. Other reasons for a false-negative tests include infection with gram-positive organisms that do not reduce nitrates.

4. **a. Leukocyte esterase.** Leukocyte esterase has a relatively high sensitivity but low specificity. Urinary nitrite has a very high specificity. Urinary nitrite is formed by bacterial enzymatic reduction of urinary nitrate. Procalcitonin may be useful in identifying children with acute pyelonephritis.

5. **e. DMSA is bound to the glomerular basement membrane and providing excellent cortical imaging but slow excretion.** All other statements are true. DMSA is injected intravenously and taken up by the kidney, bound to the proximal renal tubular cells, and excreted very slowly in the urine, providing good and stable imaging of the renal cortex.

6. **c. All children with fever persisting longer than 48 hours after appropriate antibiotics require a renal and bladder ultrasound.** There is a lack of consensus among various guidelines around the world on what routine imaging, if any, is required

---

*Sources referenced can be found in *Campbell-Walsh Urology, 11th Edition*, on the Expert Consult website.

with a febrile UTI. However, significant clinical improvement including defervescence routinely takes at least 24 hours after beginning antibiotics (Hoberman et al, 1999). Ninety percent of children will have a normal body temperature within 48 hours of the start of therapy, but if the child is not improving after 48 hours, a renal and bladder ultrasound should be strongly considered.

7. **a. *Escherichia coli*.** *E. coli* remains the most common pediatric uropathogen (>80% of UTIs).

8. **d. *Enterococcus*.** Neonates and young infants should be covered for *Enterococcus* species when choosing empiric antibiotics, because the incidence of infections with this uropathogen is higher in early infancy than at a later age (Beetz and Westenfelder, 2011). *Enterococcus* is frequently sensitive to ampicillin and first-generation cephalosporins.

9. **d. Nitrofurantoin.** Nitrofurantoin has poor tissue penetration and should not be used for febrile UTI/pyelonephritis.

10. **a. Trimethoprim-sulfamethoxazole.** Trimethoprim-sulfamethoxazole is contraindicated in premature infants and newborns younger than 6 weeks. Sulfonamides may compete for bilirubin binding sites on albumin and cause neonatal hyperbilirubinemia and kernicterus, so TMP-SMX is avoided in the first 6 weeks of life.

11. **e. All of the above.** All of the listed options have been identified as risk factors. Boys in the first year of life have a higher incidence of UTIs than girls.

12. **c. Most frequently seen in midportion of the kidney parenchyma.** Pyelonephritic scarring occurs most commonly in the poles of the kidney and is associated with compound papillae (Hannerz et al, 1987).

13. **d. Long-term assessment of proteinuria.** Although certain children with significant bilateral renal scars may benefit from a, b, or c, on a routine basis, children with significant bilateral renal scars or reduction of renal function warrant long-term follow-up for assessment of hypertension, renal function, and proteinuria. Recent studies suggest that proteinuria not only may be a clinical feature of chronic kidney disease but may hasten its progression. The use of renin-angiotensin antagonists may slow the progression of chronic kidney disease in some of these patients (Wong et al, 2009).

14. **a. The risk of a recurrent UTI is higher in a boy with an initial UTI who is younger than 1 year than in one who is older than 1 year.** For boys younger than 1 year, 18% will develop a recurrent infection, usually within the next year. If the initial infection is in a boy older than 1 year, his risk of a reinfection increases to 32%. A similar trend is noted in girls younger than and older than 1 year of age, who have a recurrence risk of 26% and 40%, respectively (Winberg et al, 1974).

15. **b. Vomiting.** Vomiting has been shown to be nonspecific in predicting the presence of a UTI in patients aged 0 to 24 months of age. The remainder of the symptoms/signs are more specific for predicting the presence of a UTI.

16. **d. Commensal bacteria cannot cause UTIs.** Although virulent bacteria do account for the majority of UTIs, commensal bacteria may cause a small percentage of UTIs.

17. **c. Flagellar attachments that allow bacteria to move more quickly.** Flagella are considered a normal component of some bacteria and not necessarily a virulence trait. The remainder of the statements are true regarding virulence factors.

18. **b. After 1 year, UTIs are more prevalent in females than males, except in elderly individuals.** UTIs are more common in boys compared with girls younger than 1 year of age. After 1 year, UTIs are more common in females and remain so, even in elderly individuals.

19. **c. Circumcision reduces the rate of UTI development in the first 6 months of life by almost tenfold.** Although controversial, several studies have demonstrated that the risk of UTI appears to correlate with a period during the first 6 months of life when there is an increased amount of uropathogenic bacteria colonizing the prepuce, which appears to decrease and resolve by 5 years.

20. **c. In children who are found to have a DMSA-proven episode of pyelonephritis, 66% will be found to have VUR.** Although we continually question whether VUR may be present in a child who has suffered a pyelonephritic infection, it is important to remember that the majority of children who have suffered from pyelonephritis do not have VUR. Rushton et al (1992) found that in children suffering DMSA-proven pyelonephritis, only 37% are found to have vesicoureteral reflux.

21. **c. Treatment of her constipation may improve her day and nighttime urinary incontinence and help reduce the incidence of recurrent UTIs.** This child suffers from dysfunctional bowel and bladder issues that are known to contribute to UTI development and VUR. Treatment of her bladder issues with anticholinergics, biofeedback, and timed voiding would be appropriate, along with therapies to treat her constipation, even before considering surgical therapy. In fact, these conservative therapies often will eliminate the need for any surgery for VUR treatment.

22. **a. 40% to 80%.** Of individuals who intermittently catheterize, 40% to 80% develop chronic bacteriuria and/or pyuria. Most of these individuals are asymptomatic and do not require antibiotic prophylaxis or treatment.

23. **a. Catheter-associated UTI is the second most common nosocomial infection, accounting for more than 1 million cases each year in U.S. hospitals and nursing homes.** Catheter-associated UTIs are the most common nosocomial infection affecting children. The risk increases with the duration that the catheter is in place. The best way to avoid these infections is to use urinary catheters judiciously and to remove them from hospitalized patients as soon as they are no longer medically necessary.

24. **b. 50% to 66%.** We use signs and symptoms such as fever, flank pain, nausea, and vomiting to clinically define a pyelonephritic UTI. However, it is important to remember that acute changes on a DMSA scan at the time of a UTI are actually the gold standard for indicating that a child truly has pyelonephritis. When a patient presents with these pyelonephritic symptoms, a DMSA is positive only 50% to 66% of the time.

25. **b. Organisms within a biofilm often grow quickly, resulting in resistance to the antibiotics.** Bacteria within a biofilm have been found to grow at a slower than normal rate, making them more resistant to antibiotic therapy.

26. **d. No treatment or further evaluation is necessary.** Asymptomatic bacteriuria occurs in 0.8% of preschool girls and even fewer preschool boys. Children in this age group who are without VUR and/or other genitourinary abnormalities do not require antibiotics to clear their bacteria, as they do not appear to be at any risk for recurrent symptomatic infections, renal damage, or impaired renal growth.

27. **d. In cases of bacterial reinfection, typically a nidus causing the infection has not been eradicated.** Typically, a nidus causing a UTI has not been eradicated in cases of bacterial persistence, not bacterial reinfection.

28. **c. CT appears to be the most sensitive and specific imaging modality in making the diagnosis of a renal abscess.** Individuals presenting with a renal abscess often share symptoms similar to those of patients with pyelonephritis. In as many as 20% of renal abscess cases, the urine culture may be negative. Ultrasound can detect an abscess as small as 1 cm, which usually appears as a sonolucent area containing low-amplitude echoes. CT appears to be the most sensitive and specific imaging modality in making the diagnosis of a renal abscess.

29. **a. If a suprapubic aspiration was performed, then recovery of any organisms defines a UTI.** For catheterized specimens, recovery of at least 50,000 CFU/mL is required to define a UTI, and 100,000 CFU/mL are required if the specimen was collected via a clean catch method.

CHAPTER REVIEW

1. Urinary tract infections cause abnormally elevated renal pelvic pressures.
2. Clinical symptoms correlate poorly with bacterial localization in the urinary tract.
3. Microbial lipopolysaccharides trigger urothelial receptors (Toll-like receptors) to activate the innate local immune system, activating cytokines, chemokines, and neutrophils.
4. For children, when performing intermittent catheterization, neither sterile or single-use lubricated catheters nor antimicrobial prophylaxis is recommended.
5. In teenage females, sexually transmitted infections may progress to pelvic inflammatory disease, infertility, and chronic pelvic pain.
6. Suprapubic bladder aspiration is the most reliable method of determining whether a urinary tract infection is present.
7. Elevated C-reactive protein and procalcitonin have been associated with acute pyelonephritis.
8. Children with glucose-6-phosphate dehydrogenase deficiency should not be given nitrofurantoin.
9. Children with gross polynephritic nephropathy (reflux nephropathy) have a 10% to 20% risk of hypertension.
10. Significant proteinuria is a routine finding in patients with vesicoureteral reflux who have progressive deterioration of renal function.
11. Adenovirus is the most common cause of acute viral hemorrhagic cystitis in children.
12. Any catheter that has been left in place for more than 4 days will result in infected urine.
13. Mechanisms possessed by bacteria to promote their ability to cause a UTI include bacterial adhesion facilitated by pili, access to iron, production of hemolysin, capsular polysaccharides that interfere with the host's ability to detect antigen, and biofilms.
14. Age of first UTI, a mother with a history of UTI, and the presence of certain blood group antigens are risk factors for women for recurrent UTIs.
15. Bladder and bowel dysfunction (dysfunctional elimination syndrome) contribute to UTI. Correcting the dysfunction reduces the recurrence of UTI and improves VUR resolution.
16. Urethritis can be caused by *Neisseria gonorrhoeae*, *Chlamydia trachomatis*, and *Ureaplasma urealyticum*.
17. More than 5 to 10 white blood cells per high-power field is required for the diagnosis of UTI; a positive culture confirms the diagnosis.
18. A febrile UTI in a newborn or young infant requires hospitalization and parenteral antibiotics.
19. For a febrile UTI, antibiotics should be given for 7 to 14 days; for afebrile cystitis, a 2- to 4-day course is sufficient.
20. Renal dysplasia occurs with VUR and on DMSA scan may be mistaken for a renal scar.
21. Urinary nitrite is reduced from dietary nitrates in the urine by gram-negative enteric bacteria. This conversion requires several hours to occur; thus, a first morning urine gives the best sensitivity with the nitrite dipstick test. Frequent voiding may cause a false-negative test.
22. Neonates and young infants should be covered for *Enterococcus* species when choosing empiric antibiotics.
23. Boys in the first year of life have a higher incidence of UTIs than girls.
24. Pyelonephritic scarring occurs most commonly in the poles of the kidney and is associated with compound papillae.
25. Of individuals who intermittently catheterize, 40% to 80% develop chronic bacteruria and/or pyuria. Most of these individuals are asymptomatic and do not require antibiotic prophylaxis or treatment.
26. For catheterized specimens, recovery of at least 50,000 CFU/mL is required to define a UTI and 100,000 CFU/mL is required if the specimen was collected via a clean catch method.

128 Core Principles of Perioperative Management in Children

Carlos R. Estrada, Jr. and Lynne R. Ferrari

QUESTIONS

1. Prematurity and intrauterine growth restriction are defined as infants born before:
   a. 38 weeks and weighing less than 1500 g, respectively.
   b. 37 weeks and weighing less than 2500 g, respectively.
   c. 36 weeks and weighing less than 2500 g, respectively.
   d. 37 weeks and weighing less than 1500 g, respectively.
   e. 36 weeks and weighing less than 1500 g, respectively.

2. During the fetal stage of lung development, all branching resulting in the terminal bronchial airways occurs by:
   a. 12 weeks' gestation.
   b. 10 weeks' gestation.
   c. 16 weeks' gestation.
   d. 20 weeks' gestation.
   e. 24 weeks' gestation.

3. Compared with the adult heart, the neonatal and pediatric myocardium are:
   a. stiffer and less compliant.
   b. less stiff and less compliant.
   c. stiffer and more compliant.
   d. less stiff and more compliant.
   e. identical.

4. Following the relatively rapid rise in glomerular filtration rate (GFR) during the first few months of life, adult GFR is reached by:
   a. 3 to 4 years.
   b. 4 to 5 years.
   c. 6 months.
   d. 12 to 24 months.
   e. 10 years.

5. For a 7-month-old infant in the postoperative period who weighs 9 kg, the most appropriate maintenance fluid is:
   a. D5 1/4NS + 20 mEq/L KCl at 36 mL/hr.
   b. D5 1/2NS + 20 mEq/L KCl at 45 mL/hr.
   c. D5 1/2NS + 20 mEq/L KCl at 18 mL/hr.
   d. D5 1/4NS at 36 mL/hr.
   e. D5 1/2NS + 20 mEq/L KCl at 36 mL/hr.

6. The school-age child typically most fears:
   a. death.
   b. that they may not meet the expectations of adults.
   c. loss of control.
   d. injury.
   e. separation from their primary caregivers.

7. For a healthy child undergoing uncomplicated surgery, the risk of an adverse event is approximately:
   a. 1 in 10,000.
   b. 1 in 200.
   c. 1 in 2,000,000.

   d. 1 in 100,000.
   e. 1 in 200,000.

8. Routine diagnostic testing for surgery in a healthy 12-month-old child includes:
   a. a chest radiograph and complete blood count.
   b. a complete blood count, electrolytes, and prothrombin time (PT)/partial thromboplastin time (PTT).
   c. a chest radiograph, complete blood count, and PT/PTT.
   d. hemoglobin/hematocrit determination.
   e. no studies.

9. In preparation for surgery, children should fast from clear liquids:
   a. for 2 hours before surgery.
   b. for 3 hours before surgery.
   c. for 4 hours before surgery.
   d. for 6 hours before surgery.
   e. being nothing by mouth (NPO) after midnight.

10. For a child 6 years of age, assessment of postoperative pain is best done by:
    a. simply asking him or her about the pain.
    b. relying on appearance, because children cannot hide their pain well.
    c. using a visual analog scale.
    d. using a faces scale.
    e. asking the child's parents.

11. Poor and rapid metabolizers of codeine can be expected to:
    a. have good and poor pain relief, respectively.
    b. have little effect and have dangerously high plasma morphine levels, respectively.
    c. have dangerously high plasma morphine levels and little effect, respectively.
    d. have identical CYP2D6 enzyme genotypes.
    e. most likely be of North African and white descent, respectively.

12. Surgical antibiotic prophylaxis for a major class II operation is best:
    a. administered the night before surgery.
    b. administered following incision.
    c. administered immediately after surgery is complete.
    d. administered 1 hour before incision.
    e. not recommended/administered.

13. Blood volume in children can be most closely estimated as:
    a. 55 mL/kg.
    b. 25 to 50 mL/kg.
    c. 70 to 80 mL/kg.
    d. 100 mL/kg.
    e. 65 to 70 mL/kg.

14. Fever (greater than 38.5° C rectal temperature) in children within 24 hours of surgery is most likely due to:

    a. urinary tract infection.

    b. surgical-site infection.

    c. deep vein thrombosis.

    d. atelectasis.

    e. dehydration.

ANSWERS

1. **b. 37 Weeks and weighing less than 2500 g, respectively.** A baby born before 37 weeks' gestation is considered premature. The severity of prematurity may be indicated by the birth weight, although these two factors are not necessarily related. Infants weighing 2500 g or less at birth are considered low birth weight (LBW) in prematurity, but in an infant born full term, this weight would indicate intrauterine growth restriction (IUGR). This is an important distinction, because full-term neonates with IUGR usually have different problems than do premature infants.

2. **c. 16 Weeks' gestation.** Proper intrauterine growth and development are dependent on presence of normal amniotic fluid volume. Of particular relevance to urologists is lung development, which is dependent on amniotic fluid. The fetal stage of lung development begins at 7 weeks' gestation and proceeds to term. By the end of the 16th week of gestation, all lung branching occurs, resulting in the terminal bronchial airways. After this time, the only further growth that occurs is elongation and widening of existing airways.

3. **a. Stiffer and less compliant.** The neonatal and pediatric myocardium is stiffer and less compliant compared with the adult heart. This results in diminished preload capacity so that increases in end-diastolic ventricular volume and increases in right ventricular pressure result in decreased cardiac output at lower levels than in adult patients. In addition, infants and children have relatively higher resting heart rates. As a result, cardiac output in children is heart-rate dependent, because the stroke volume is relatively fixed. Decreases in heart rate in infants and children will result in decreases in cardiac output to a greater extent than a similar decrease in heart rate in an adult patient. A reduction of a child's heart rate to that of a typical adult would result in marked decrease in cardiac output.

4. **d. 12 to 24 months.** In utero, renovascular resistance is high, limiting renal blood flow. Immediately following birth, the distribution of renal cortical blood flow changes, with increased perfusion of the outer cortex and increased reactivity of the renal vascular bed. Consequently, the glomerular filtration rate (GFR) rises quickly despite renal blood flow remaining unchanged. In addition, water and electrolyte homeostasis is difficult to predict. GFR and tubular function double by 1 month of age (Kaskel),* and during the first 3 months of life, renovascular resistance continues to decrease, which results in further rises in GFR. Following this relatively rapid rise, GFR continues to increase more slowly toward adult levels, which are reached by 12 to 24 months of life. The maturation of renal tubular function lags behind the maturation of glomerular function, and therefore the neonate can concentrate urine to only approximately 50% of adult capability.

5. **e. D5 1/2 NS + 20 mEq/L KCl at 36 mL/hr.** The total requirements for maintenance fluids can be calculated by using the Holliday-Segar formula. After the fluid requirement is calculated, children usually receive either D5 1/4NS + 20 mEq/L KCl or D5 1/2NS + 20 mEq/L KCl. Children who are younger than 6 months old are generally given the solution with 1/4NS, because of their high water needs per kilogram. Children 6 months and older, however, should receive the solution with 1/2NS.

6. **b. That they may not meet the expectations of adults.** Age-appropriate treatment of children is essential to provide the best possible perioperative experience. Infants fear separation from their primary caregivers and exhibit stranger anxiety. Toddlers fear loss of control, so enabling a child to make choices, such as asking if the child has a color preference for his or her hospital gown, will diminish anxiety. Preschool-age children fear injury; they may fear, for example, that a blood draw may result in not enough blood being left in their bodies. The school-age child typically fears that he or she may not meet the expectations of adults. They are reluctant to ask questions for fear that they should already know the answer. Adolescents fear death and usually do not understand bodily functions.

7. **e. 1 in 200,000.** Most parents will state that they experience more anxiety about the anesthetic than the risks of the surgery. For a healthy child undergoing uncomplicated surgery, the risk of an adverse event is approximately 1 in 200,000. The risk of death under anesthesia is the most feared complication. This risk is 1 in 10,000 for all patients of any age undergoing any surgical procedure. However, the risk of death directly attributable to the anesthetic approaches zero, although the risk of cardiac arrests due to anesthesia remains approximately 4.5 in 10,000. The incidence of anesthetic-related complications and death is highest during the first year of life at 43:10,000, but this decreases dramatically during the second year of life to 5:10,000. Anesthetic risks increase by a factor of 6 during emergency procedures in all age groups.

8. **e. No studies.** Routine diagnostic testing in preparation for surgery is rarely indicated in healthy children, and studies that are ordered should be selected based on the general medical health of the patient and the procedure being performed. In general, measurement of hemoglobin/hematocrit in a healthy child undergoing elective surgery is unnecessary. A hemoglobin/hematocrit should be measured if significant blood loss is anticipated or if the child is younger than 6 months old or was born prematurely.

9. **a. For 2 hours before surgery.** It is no longer advisable or safe to restrict children to "NPO after midnight." The American Society of Anesthesiologists recommends fasting from clear fluids for 2 hours before anesthesia. Clear liquids consist of water, nonparticulate juices (e.g., apple, white grape), Pedialyte, and Popsicles. Fasting from breast milk for 4 hours and formula for 6 hours is recommended. The suggested fasting period for solid food is 6 hours for regular meals and 8 hours for fat-containing meals. However, individual institutions may have specific practice guidelines.

10. **d. Using a faces scale.** In general, children 8 years and older can reliably report pain on the visual analog scale used in adults. Children between the ages of 3 and 7 years can better report pain by using a faces scale that uses a series of drawings depicting increasing levels of distress.

11. **b. Have little effect and have dangerously high plasma morphine levels, respectively.** Codeine is a relatively weak opioid given its extremely low affinity for opioid receptors, and most of its analgesic effect is due to the 10% that is metabolized to morphine. The metabolism to morphine is predominantly by O-demethylation by the cytochrome P450 enzyme CYP2D6, which is known to show genetic polymorphism. Therefore, variations in CYP2D6 will result in variable abilities to metabolize codeine. In this way, individuals may be classified as poor metabolizers or ultrarapid metabolizers, depending on the phenotype of their CYP2D6 enzyme.

12. **d. Administered 1 hour before incision.** The timing of surgical antimicrobial prophylaxis is critically important, and the first dose should be given 30 minutes to 3 hours before incision to achieve bactericidal levels of the antibiotic at the site of incision.

13. **c. 70 to 80 mL/kg.** Blood volume in children varies with age, but can be estimated as 70 to 80 mL/kg.

*Sources referenced can be found in *Campbell-Walsh Urology, 11th Edition,* on the Expert Consult website.

14. **d. Atelectasis.** Postoperative fever is a very common early surgical problem, and its etiology is taught in the first days of medical school surgery clerkships as the four Ws: wind, wound, water, and walking. "Wind" refers to atelectasis, "wound" to a surgical-site infection (SSI), "water" to a urinary tract infection (UTI), and "walking" to fever caused by deep vein thrombosis (DVT) in the lower extremities. Fever, defined as greater than 38.5° C rectal temperature, is common within 24 hours of surgery and is usually caused by atelectasis.

CHAPTER REVIEW

1. Infants weighing 2500 g or less at birth are considered low birth weight (LBW) in prematurity, but in an infant born full term, this weight would indicate intrauterine growth restriction (IUGR). This is an important distinction, because full-term neonates with IUGR usually have different problems than premature infants.
2. Fluid requirements per 24 hours in children are calculated according to weight as follows: 1- to 10 kg, 100 mL/kg; 11 to 20 kg, +50 mL/kg; and greater than 20 kg, +25 mL/kg. Children who are less than 6 months old are generally given the solution with 1/4NS, because of their high water needs per kilogram. Children 6 months and older, however, should receive the solution as 1/2NS.
3. Lung development is dependent on an adequate amount of amniotic fluid.
4. A fetus with severe oligohydramnios may suffer pulmonary fibrosis.
5. Cardiac output in children is heart-rate dependent; the stroke volume is relatively fixed; infants have high heart rates, limiting their ability to increase cardiac output by increasing heart rate.
6. Neonates have an increased susceptibility to infection due to impaired T-lymphocyte function and deficiency of immunoglobulins.
7. The immune system does not become fully competent until approximately 8 years.
8. Anesthesia is most risky in the first year of life.
9. A family history of anesthesia-related events, liver problems, or malignant hyperthermia is part of the preoperative assessment.
10. Children should take clear liquids as long as 2 hours before anesthesia; solid foods should not be consumed for 8 hours prior to anesthesia.
11. In premature infants who undergo anesthesia, the major risk postoperatively is apnea; similarly, in full-term infants younger than 4 weeks of age, apnea is the major postoperative risk.
12. Children with spina bifida have a high incidence of latex sensitivity.
13. In response to planned surgery, infants fear separation, toddlers fear loss of control, preschool-age children fear injury, school-age children fear that they may not meet expectations of adults, and adolescents fear death.
14. A preoperative hematocrit should be obtained in children born prematurely and in those younger than 6 months.
15. It is unknown whether anesthesia is neurotoxic to the developing brain.
16. Children with ventriculoperitoneal (VP) shunts should be evaluated for a functional shunt preoperatively.
17. Children are at significant risk for hypothermia intraoperatively.
18. The maturation of renal tubular function lags behind the maturation of glomerular function, and therefore the neonate can concentrate urine to only approximately 50% of adult capability.
19. Codeine is a relatively weak opioid given its extremely low affinity for opioid receptors, and most of its analgesic effect is due to the 10% that is metabolized to morphine.

Principles of Laparoscopic and Robotic Surgery in Children

Pasquale Casale

QUESTIONS

1. The benefits of minimally invasive surgery (MIS) in children include all of the following EXCEPT:
   a. cosmesis.
   b. decreased convalescence.
   c. increased visualization.
   d. increased control of cancer margins.
   e. shorter hospital stay.

2. Strong contraindications to laparoscopic surgery in children include all of the following EXCEPT:
   a. von Willebrand disease.
   b. pulmonary hypertension.
   c. sepsis.
   d. malignancy.
   e. hemophilia.

3. In regard to comparing the adult patient with the pediatric patient:
   a. Half of the height in centimeters equals an eighth of the intra-abdominal space in liters.
   b. An eighth of the height in centimeters equals an eighth of the intra-abdominal space in liters.
   c. An eighth of the height in centimeters equals half of the intra-abdominal space in liters.
   d. Half of the height in centimeters equals half of the intra-abdominal space in liters.
   e. Half of the height in centimeters equals a fourth of the intra-abdominal space in liters.

4. Which of the following statements describes the difference between bipolar vessel sealing devices and ultrasonic shears?
   a. Bipolar devices provided a more secure seal up to 8-mm vessels; however, the ultrasonic devices had less thermal spread and used less surgical time.
   b. Bipolar devices provided a less secure seal up to 7-mm vessels; however, the ultrasonic devices had less thermal spread and used less surgical time.
   c. Bipolar devices provided a more secure seal up to 7-mm vessels; however, the ultrasonic devices had less thermal spread and used less surgical time.
   d. Bipolar devices provided a more secure seal up to 7-mm vessels; however, the ultrasonic devices had more thermal spread and used less surgical time.
   e. Bipolar devices provided a more secure seal up to 7-mm vessels; however, the ultrasonic devices had less thermal spread and used more surgical time.

5. Nitrous oxide gas has the following effect on laparoscopy:
   a. It is flammable.
   b. It increases hypercarbia.
   c. It decreases intracranial pressure.
   d. It increases bowel distention.
   e. It increases gastric emptying.

6. Insufflation of CO_2 has the following hemodynamic effects:
   a. The heart rate and mean arterial pressure increase, while the venous return and cardiac output decrease.
   b. The heart rate and mean arterial pressure decrease, while the venous return and cardiac output decrease.
   c. The heart rate and mean arterial pressure increase, while the venous return and cardiac output increase.
   d. The heart rate and mean arterial pressure decrease, while the venous return and cardiac output increase.
   e. The heart rate and mean arterial pressure stay constant, while the venous return and cardiac output decrease.

7. Renal effects of insufflation include all of the following EXCEPT:
   a. decreased glomerular filtration rate (GFR).
   b. decreased creatinine clearance.
   c. decreased renal blood flow.
   d. decreased urine output.
   e. decreased long-term renal reserve.

8. Hypercarbia causes all of the following EXCEPT:
   a. increased heart rate.
   b. vasodilation.
   c. increased cardiac contractility.
   d. increased intracranial pressure.
   e. pulmonary hypertension.

9. All of the following statements regarding the boundaries of the retroperitoneal space are true EXCEPT:
   a. posteriorly: the paraspinous, psoas, and quadratus lumborum muscles, which are anatomically fixed structures.
   b. laterally: the skin and subcutaneous fat.
   c. anteriorly: the mobile posterior parietal peritoneum and its contents.
   d. superiorly: the diaphragm.
   e. inferiorly: contiguous with the extraperitoneal portions of the pelvis.

10. If vascular entry of insufflation occurs:
    a. Nothing needs to be done because it is completely reversible.
    b. The patient should be placed in reverse Trendelenburg position with the right side up to trap the air embolus in the right atrium.
    c. The patient should be placed in Trendelenburg position with the right side up to trap the air embolus in the right atrium.
    d. The patient should be placed in reverse Trendelenburg position with the left side up to trap the air embolus in the right atrium.
    e. The patient should be placed in reverse Trendelenburg position with the left side up to trap the air embolus in the left atrium.

ANSWERS

1. **d. Increased control of cancer margins.** Laparoscopic surgery has gained widespread acceptance given the reliability and durability of outcomes. The proposed benefits of laparoscopic surgery versus the standard open approach include better cosmesis, increased magnification improving visualization, reduced postoperative pain, and shorter hospital stays. Its role in pediatric urologic oncology is in its infancy and limited data are available.

2. **d. Malignancy.** Contraindications to laparoscopy in infants, children, and adolescents are the same as for any other surgical procedure, except for evidence of limited pulmonary reserve, which may be considered a relative contraindication. If the patient is septic, in shock, or exhibits a coagulopathy, these should be corrected before MIS is contemplated. If surgery is deemed essential under these circumstances, then it probably should be performed by using open techniques.

3. **a. Half of the height in centimeters equals an eighth of the intra-abdominal space in liters.** Whereas an adult pneumoperitoneum will typically provide a 5- to 6-L working space, a 1-year-old boy will present a 1-L intra-abdominal space. A good rule of thumb is that half of the height in centimeters is equivalent to an eighth of the intra-abdominal space in liters.

4. **c. Bipolar devices provided a more secure seal up to 7-mm vessels; however, the ultrasonic devices had less thermal spread and used less surgical time.** Mischra performed a meta-analysis of the literature comparing these devices. The analysis found that bipolar devices provided a more secure seal up to 7-mm vessels; however, the ultrasonic devices had less thermal spread and used less surgical time. Based on the data, he concluded that it seemed to depend on the surgeon's experience to decide which energy source to use for each particular part of a specific procedure.

5. **d. It increases bowel distention.** Nitrous oxide gas increases bowel distention, potentially bringing the peritoneum closer to the area of dissection for retroperitoneal procedures and decreasing working space in transperitoneal procedures.

6. **a. The heart rate and mean arterial pressure increase, while the venous return and cardiac output decrease.** While gas is placed in the closed space of the operative field, the pressure rises and cardiovascular, pulmonary and renal effects occur. The heart rate and mean arterial pressure increase while the venous return and cardiac output decrease. These parameters are seen even when pressure is set at a standard working level of 10 mm Hg. Above a level of 15 mm Hg, more profound hemodynamic alterations are expected to occur, with further decrease in cardiac output.

7. **e. Decreased long-term renal reserve.** Renal effects occur secondary to gas insufflation, manifested by decreased glomerular filtration rate and urine output. Animal studies have shown that gas insufflation causes renal vein compression inducing decreased renal blood flow, decreased urine output and diminished creatinine clearance. These effects do not appear to cause renal damage in humans, however.

8. **e. Pulmonary hypertension.** The hemodynamic effects of hypercarbia are increased heart rate, vasodilation, increased cardiac contractility, and increased intracranial pressure. Although in healthy children there is little if any added cardiorespiratory risk from laparoscopic procedures, children with cardiopulmonary compromise require close and careful monitoring.

9. **b. Laterally: the skin and subcutaneous fat.** The boundaries of the retroperitoneal space are: (1) posteriorly and laterally: the paraspinous, psoas, and quadratus lumborum muscles, which are anatomically fixed structures; (2) anteriorly: the mobile posterior parietal peritoneum and its contents; (3) superiorly: the diaphragm; and (4) inferiorly: contiguous with the extraperitoneal portions of the pelvis.

10. **b. The patient should be placed in reverse Trendelenburg position with the right side up to trap the air embolus in the right atrium.** Vascular entry of insufflation can be catastrophic. If vascular entry is noted after insufflation has started, the patient should be placed in reverse Trendelenburg position with right side up to trap the air embolus in the right atrium. The air can then be retrieved with catheterization aided by transesophageal ultrasound.

CHAPTER REVIEW

1. Gastric distention following intubation should be immediately decompressed because of the rapid gastric emptying time in children—if this is not done, air may enter the small bowel, causing bowel distention.

2. The distance from the abdominal wall to vital structures may be very small in children; for example, the great vessels may be as little as 5 cm from the anterior abdominal wall.

3. Bipolar devices provide a more secure seal in vessels 7 mm or less when compared with ultrasonic devices; however, the latter have less thermal spread.

4. Nitrous oxide gas inhalation increases bowel distention,

5. Intraperitoneal gas insufflation causes renal vein compression, inducing decreased renal blood flow, decreased urine output, and diminished creatinine clearance.

6. If vascular entry is noted after insufflation has started, the patient should be placed in reverse Trendelenburg position with the right side up to trap the air embolus in the right atrium.

130   Anomalies of the Upper Urinary Tract

Ellen Shapiro and Shpetim Telegrafi

QUESTIONS

1. During a left inguinal herniorrhaphy, the vas was absent and a 3-mm golden-yellow nodule was found along the spermatic cord. This boy may also have:
   a. a left appendage epididymis.
   b. left renal agenesis.
   c. malpositioned left adrenal gland.
   d. absent left head of epididymis.
   e. absent left testis.

2. A 14-year-old girl with abdominal pain undergoes an abdominal and pelvic ultrasound. A solitary right kidney is seen. Her abdominal pain is most likely associated with:
   a. skeletal anomalies.
   b. a unicornuate uterus.
   c. imperforate hymen.
   d. a didelphic uterus.
   e. an absent left ovary.

3. A 27-year-old man has infertility. A pelvic ultrasound reveals a right pelvic kidney and a left orthotopic kidney. The most likely cause of his infertility is:
   a. absence of the right vas.
   b. history of bilateral cryptorchidism.
   a. absence of the mid and lower pole of the right epididymis
   b. dysplasia of the right testis.
   c. a subcoronal hypospadias.

4. The renal segment with the most variable blood supply is the:
   a. apex.
   b. upper.
   c. middle.
   d. lower.
   e. posterior.

5. A 29-year-old hypertensive woman was found to have a 2.7-cm renal artery aneurysm. Excision is recommended:
   a. if the aneurysm increases in size to 3 cm.
   b. when the woman is no longer of childbearing age.
   c. at this time.
   d. if there is no arteriovenous (AV) fistula.
   e. when the hypertension is well controlled.

6. A 5-year-old girl with a pelvic kidney has hydronephrosis most commonly due to:
   a. vesicoureteral reflux.
   b. malrotation.
   c. ureterovesical junction obstruction.
   d. ureteropelvic junction obstruction.
   e. ectopic ureter.

7. A newborn girl was noted prenatally to have coarctation of the aorta and horseshoe kidney. The next step is:
   a. voiding cystourethrogram.
   b. Magnetic resonance urography (MRU) with gadolinium.
   c. echocardiogram.
   d. obtain a karyotype.
   e. skeletal series.

8. Unilateral renal agenesis is commonly associated with:
   a. normal position of the splenic flexure.
   b. normal position of the adrenal gland.
   c. ipsilateral undescended testis.
   d. normal position of the hepatic flexure.
   e. rudimentary uterus.

9. Bilateral renal agenesis (BRA) is associated with mutations of:
   a. *GFRα1*.
   b. *GFDNF*.
   c. *RET*.
   d. *WNT*.
   e. *Pax2*.

10. Unilateral renal agenesis (URA) can be reliably diagnosed by finding:
    a. a single umbilical artery.
    b. preauricular skin tag(s).
    c. an imperforate hymen.
    d. absence of renal artery at L1-L2.
    e. specific radiographic evidence.

11. Male predominance of occurrence is most striking in:
    a. unilateral renal agenesis.
    b. bilateral renal agenesis.
    c. crossed fused ectopia.
    d. ectopic kidney.
    e. calyceal diverticulum.

12. The incidence of unilateral renal agenesis is:
    a. 1:2500.
    b. 1:4000.
    c. 1:1100.
    d. 1:5000.
    e. 1:500.

13. Unilateral renal agenesis and a unicornuate uterus will form when the embryological insult occurs at which gestational time?
    a. Before the fourth week
    b. At the start of the fourth week
    c. At the end of the fourth week
    d. At the start of the fifth week
    e. At the end of the fifth week

14. In autopsy studies, unilateral renal agenesis was found in association with:
    a. absence of the gonad.
    b. a normally developed ureter.
    c. an ectopic ureteral orifice.
    d. adrenal agenesis.
    e. absence of the head of the epididymis.

15. Most ectopic kidneys are clinically asymptomatic EXCEPT:
    a. pelvic kidneys.
    b. thoracic kidneys.
    c. kidneys with ectopic ureters.
    d. lumbar kidneys.
    e. abdominal kidneys.

16. The isthmus of a horseshoe kidney is located adjacent to which vertebrae?
    a. Th12 and L1
    b. L1 and L2
    c. L3 and L4
    d. L5 and S1
    e. S1 and S2

17. Between the sixth and ninth week, normal rotation of the kidney toward the midline to attain its orthotopic position involves:
    a. 60 degrees of lateral rotation.
    b. 90 degrees of lateral rotation.
    c. 180 degrees of lateral rotation.
    d. 90 degrees of medial rotation.
    e. 180 degrees of medial rotation.

18. Congenital renal arteriovenous fistulas are:
    a. usually congenital.
    b. cirsoid in configuration.
    c. symptomatic before the third decade.
    d. more common in males.
    e. usually located in the lower pole.

19. Bilateral megacalycosis:
    a. occurs more frequently in females.
    b. has an increased number of dilated calyces.
    c. is associated with ureteral dilation.
    d. is autosomal recessive in inheritance pattern.
    e. shows an obstructive pattern on renal scan.

ANSWERS

1. **b. Left renal agenesis.** The finding of a 3-mm golden-yellow nodule is indicative of ectopic adrenal. The adrenal develops just medial to the gonadal ridge. Their close proximity explains their location along the spermatic cord and their incidental identification at the time of herniorrhaphy or orchidopexy. Histologically, the nodules contain adrenal cortex but no medulla. In this case, the absent vas should raise a red flag for possible ipsilateral renal agenesis because the ureteral bud and vas are both derived from the wolffian duct. In one study, 79% of adult males with absence of the vas deferens have an absent ipsilateral kidney, with left-sided lesions predominating. The lower pole and mid-pole of the epididymis are wolffian duct derivatives. The head of the epididymis is derived from the mesonephric tubules, which link the mesonephric or wolffian duct with the gonad.

2. **d. A didelphic uterus.** Unilateral renal agenesis can be associated with didelphic uterus and obstruction of the ipsilateral vagina resulting in hematocolpos. This would likely explain this girl's abdominal pain.

3. **b. History of bilateral cryptorchidism.** This man's infertility is most likely due to a history of bilateral cryptorchidism. An ipsilateral absent vas, abnormal epididymis, or a unilateral dysplastic gonad would not lead to infertility because a normal contralateral testis would be expected to be present. Bilateral cryptorchidism has been associated with infertility.

4. **a. Apex.** The vessel to the apical segment has the greatest variation in origin; it arises from (1) the anterior division (43%), (2) the junction of the anterior and posterior divisions (23%), (3) the main-stem renal artery or aorta (23%), or (4) the posterior division of the main renal artery (10%).

5. **c. At this time.** Generally, excision is recommended if (1) the hypertension cannot be easily controlled; (2) incomplete ring-like calcification is present; (3) the aneurysm is larger than 2.5 cm; (4) the patient is female and of childbearing age, because rupture during pregnancy is a likely possibility; (5) the aneurysm increases in size on serial angiograms; or (6) an arteriovenous fistula is present.

6. **d. Ureteropelvic junction obstruction.** The renal pelvis is usually anterior (instead of medial) to the parenchyma because the kidney has incompletely rotated. As a result, 56% of ectopic kidneys have a hydronephrotic collecting system. Half of these cases are due to obstruction of the ureteropelvic or the ureterovesical junction (70% and 30%, respectively), 25% from reflux grade 3 or greater, and 25% from the malrotation alone.

7. **d. Obtain a karyotype.** Horseshoe kidney and coarctation of the aorta are seen in patients with Turner syndrome (45,XO). Therefore, a karyotype should be obtained. Other stigmata may include lymphedema, shield chest, low hairline, and webbed neck.

8. **b. Normal position of the adrenal gland.** Unilateral renal agenesis is commonly associated with an adrenal gland that is in a normal position, although it may be flattened. Regardless of sex, both gonads are usually normal. The most common müllerian duct anomalies are a true unicornuate uterus with complete absence of the ipsilateral horn and fallopian tube or a bicornuate uterus with rudimentary development of the horn on the affected side. A plain film of the abdomen (or other radiographic study such as magnetic resonance imaging) showing the gas pattern of the splenic flexure in the left renal fossa suggests left renal agenesis, ectopia, or crossed ectopia, whereas the gas pattern of the hepatic flexure positioned in the right renal fossa suggests congenital absence of the right kidney.

9. **c. RET.** The association between abnormal kidney development and mutations of *RET, GDNF,* and *GFRα1* in 29 stillborn fetuses with BRA or unilateral renal agenesis. Mutations in *RET* were found in 7 of 19 fetuses with BRA and 2 of 10 fetuses with URA. A mutation in *GDNF* was found in only 1 fetus with URA who also had mutations in RET. No *GFRα1* mutations were observed. These data suggest that congenital renal agenesis results from *RET* mutations that prevent or impede the embryonic development of *RET*-dependent structures.

10. **e. Specific radiographic evidence.** Unilateral renal agenesis can be diagnosed reliably with radiographic examinations including abdominal and pelvic ultrasound, dimercaptosuccinic acid (DMSA) scan, and/or magnetic resonance angiography (MRA).

11. **b. Bilateral renal agenesis.** Male predominance is most striking in bilateral renal agenesis, with almost 75% of affected individuals being male. For unilateral renal agenesis, there is a male-to-female ratio of 1.8:1. Crossed fused ectopia has a slight male predominance (3:2), whereas ectopic kidneys have no significant difference in incidence between the sexes.

12. **c. 1:1100.** The incidence of unilateral renal agenesis is 1:1100.
13. **a. Before the fourth week.** Unilateral renal agenesis and a unicornuate uterus will form when the embryological insult occurs before the fourth week. If the insult occurs early in the fourth week of gestation and affects both the wolffian duct and the ureteral bud, maldevelopment of the wolffian duct affects renal development, müllerian duct elongation, contact with the urogenital sinus, and subsequent fusion. Therefore, a didelphic uterus will form with obstruction of the horn and vagina on the side of the unilateral renal agenesis. If the insult occurs after the 4th week, the wolffian duct and müllerian duct elongation and differentiation proceed normally and only the ureteral bud and metanephric blastema are affected, thereby resulting in isolated unilateral renal agenesis.
14. **d. Adrenal agenesis.** In autopsy studies of unilateral renal agenesis, adrenal agenesis occurs in fewer than 10%, although the ipsilateral adrenal gland may be flattened or "lying down." The ureter is not normally developed, and the ipsilateral ureter is completely absent in approximately 60% of cases. The gonad is usually normal in both sexes. The head of the epididymis is normally formed because it is derived from the mesonephric tubules that link the mesonephric duct to the gonad.
15. **c. Kidneys with ectopic ureters.** Most ectopic kidneys are clinically asymptomatic except for the unusual cases of an ectopic kidney with an ectopic ureter.
16. **c. L3 and L4.** The isthmus of a horseshoe kidney is located adjacent to the L3 and L4 vertebrae.
17. **d. 90 degrees of medial rotation.** Between the sixth and ninth week, normal rotation of the kidney toward the midline to attain its orthotopic position involves 90 degrees of medial rotation.
18. **b. Cirsoid in configuration.** Fewer than 25% of all renal arteriovenous fistulas (AVFs) are congenital. They are identifiable by their cirsoid configuration and multiple communications between the main or segmental renal arteries and venous channels. Although congenital, they rarely present clinically before the third or fourth decade. Women are affected three times as often as men, and the right kidney is involved slightly more often than the left. The lesion is usually located in the upper pole (45% of cases), but not infrequently it may be found in the midportion (30%) or in the lower pole (25%) of the kidney.
19. **b. Has an increased number of dilated calyces.** Megacalycosis is defined as a nonobstructive enlargement of calyces resulting from malformation of the renal papillae. The calyces are generally dilated and malformed and may be increased in number. The renal pelvis is not dilated, nor is its wall thickened, and the ureteropelvic junction is normally funneled without evidence of obstruction. The ureter is usually normal. It occurs predominantly in males in a ratio of 6:1. Bilateral disease has been seen almost exclusively in males, whereas segmental unilateral involvement occurs only in females.

CHAPTER REVIEW

1. In bilateral renal agenesis, 40% of affected infants are stillborn. The ureters are almost always absent, and the bladder is either absent or hypoplastic. The adrenal glands, however, are usually in their normal anatomic position.
2. In patients with bilateral renal agenesis associated with oligohydramnios, Potter facies are pathognomonic of the process. Pulmonary hypoplasia is frequently present.
3. Ultrasound screening is recommended for parents and siblings of infants with unilateral or bilateral renal agenesis—there is a higher risk of renal agenesis in this population.
4. In unilateral renal agenesis, the ipsilateral ureter is completely absent in 60% of cases. Abnormalities of the contralateral ureter are not uncommon; reproductive tract anomalies in females are also common.
5. With unilateral renal agenesis, one quarter of the contralateral ureters reflux.
6. There is an association of genital anomalies with renal ectopia. The upper pole of the ectopic kidney usually joins with the lower pole of the normal kidney.
7. In all types of fusion anomalies, the ureter from each kidney is usually orthotopic.
8. The highest incidence of associated anomalies occurs with solitary renal ectopia. Associated anomalies in the male include cryptorchidism, and vaginal atresia or unilateral uterine anomalies in the female.
9. In a horseshoe kidney, the isthmus is bulky and consists of parenchymatous tissue with its own blood supply.
10. The blood supply to a horseshoe kidney is variable.
11. Ureteropelvic junction obstruction in horseshoe kidneys occurs one third of the time.
12. The incidence of Wilms tumors and renal pelvic tumors in horseshoe kidneys is higher than would be expected in the general population. There is no increased risk of renal cell carcinoma.
13. Renal arteries are end arteries and, as such, have no collaterals.
14. Arteriovenous fistulas may result in hypertension in 50% of cases, due to relative ischemia beyond the fistula. It is renin-mediated hypertension.
15. Infundibulopelvic stenosis is usually bilateral and is commonly associated with vesicoureteral reflux.
16. Maternal diabetes is associated with a threefold increased risk of renal agenesis and dysplasia.
17. Patients born with renal agenesis may have decreased renal reserve in the remaining kidney, which results in a significant risk for end-stage renal disease.
18. Of adult males with absence of the vas deferens, 79% have an absent ipsilateral kidney.
19. Excision of a renal artery aneurysm is recommended if (1) the hypertension cannot be easily controlled; (2) incomplete ringlike calcification is present; (3) the aneurysm is larger than 2.5 cm; (4) the patient is female and of childbearing age, because rupture during pregnancy is a likely possibility; (5) the aneurysm increases in size on serial angiograms; or (6) an arteriovenous fistula is present.

131 Renal Dysgenesis and Cystic Disease of the Kidney

John C. Pope IV

QUESTIONS

1. Which of the following is a correct match?
   a. von Hippel-Lindau disease and adenoma sebaceum
   b. Tuberous sclerosis and angiomyolipoma
   c. Autosomal dominant polycystic kidney disease (ADPKD) and salt-losing nephropathy
   d. Congenital nephrosis (Finnish type) and medullary cysts
   e. Autosomal recessive polycystic kidney disease (ARPKD) and colonic diverticulosis

2. The primary feature(s) associated with Ask-Upmark kidney (segmental hypoplasia) is/are:
   a. hypertension.
   b. renal artery intimal disease.
   c. found in young men and boys.
   d. b and c.
   e. a and c.

3. The development of acquired renal cystic disease (ARCD) is most related to which factor?
   a. Age of the patient
   b. Duration of renal failure
   c. Recent initiation of hemodialysis
   d. *Escherichia coli* infection
   e. Genetic defect on chromosome 16

4. Which statement(s) about ARPKD is/are TRUE?
   a. The most severe forms develop later in childhood or adolescence.
   b. No matter the severity of the renal disease, all patients will have liver involvement in the form of congenital hepatic fibrosis.
   c. In newborns, ultrasound findings include very enlarged kidneys with increased parenchymal echogenicity.
   d. a and b
   e. b and c

5. Which of the following statements accurately describes a fundamental process essential for the development of renal cysts?
   a. Proliferation of epithelial cells in segments of the renal collecting system
   b. Accumulation of fluid within an expanding segment of the glomerulus
   c. An imbalance of the secretory and absorptive properties in proliferating tubular epithelial cells
   d. Hypertrophy of the basement membrane within the ascending loop of Henle
   e. Glomerular outpouching resulting from elevated glomerular hydrostatic pressure

6. Which of the following statement(s) is/are correct about ADPKD?
   a. The genetic defect is located on the short arm of chromosome 16.
   b. Most affected infants have congenital hepatic fibrosis.
   c. Renal cysts are infrequently seen on ultrasonographic scans of affected patients before 30 years of age.
   d. Glomerular cysts are never found in the kidneys of newborns diagnosed with ADPKD.
   e. The incidence of renal cell carcinoma in ADPKD is twice that in the normal population.

7. The following are extrarenal manifestations of ADPKD EXCEPT:
   a. hepatic cysts.
   b. intracranial (berry) aneurysms.
   c. cerebellar hemangioblastomas.
   d. colonic diverticulosis.
   e. mitral valve prolapse.

8. Which of the following statements is FALSE regarding unilateral multicystic dysplastic kidneys?
   a. The majority of multicystic dysplastic kidneys become smaller or ultrasonographically undetectable with time.
   b. There is an absence of communication between cysts on ultrasonographic scans.
   c. Cysts are usually found in communication with each other when injected intracystically with contrast material.
   d. The sine qua non for diagnosis of a multicystic dysplastic kidney is the presence of primitive ducts.
   e. Multicystic dysplastic kidneys appear more often in females and more often on the right side.

9. Flank pain is one of the most common presenting symptoms of ADPKD in adult patients. This is often caused by:
   a. bleeding into a cyst.
   b. renal cell carcinoma.
   c. cyst rupture.
   d. b and c.
   e. a and c.

10. Which gene is associated with a multiple malformation syndrome and clear cell renal cell carcinoma?
    a. *PDK1*
    b. *PDK2*
    c. *TG737*
    d. *Wnt-2*
    e. *VHL*

11. A benign multilocular cyst is seen most often:
    a. in males younger than 4 years and in females older than 30 years.
    b. in females younger than 4 years and in males older than 30 years.
    c. in males between 4 and 30 years.
    d. equally in both sexes before 4 years and in females after 30 years.
    e. equally in both sexes before 4 years and in males after 30 years.

12. What is the primary distinguishing factor between juvenile nephronophthisis (NPH) and medullary cystic kidney disease (MCKD)?

    a. NPH presents with polyuria and polydipsia, whereas MCKD does not.

    b. NPH is an autosomal recessive disorder, whereas MCKD is an autosomal dominant disease.

    c. NPH is diagnosed histologically with severe interstitial fibrosis, whereas MCKD is diagnosed by the presence of glomerulosclerosis.

    d. Most patients with MCKD have extrarenal manifestations of the disease, whereas patients with NPH are usually affected only in the kidneys.

    e. In patients with NPH, renal failure occurs in the third to fourth decade, whereas in patients with MCKD, renal failure typically occurs in adolescence.

13. A patient with which of the following entities has the highest likelihood of having a renal cell carcinoma develop?

    a. ADPKD

    b. Tuberous sclerosis

    c. von Hippel-Lindau disease

    d. Acquired renal cystic disease

    e. Medullary sponge kidney

14. Which of the following is FALSE pertaining to MCDK?

    a. MCDK is one of the most common causes of an abdominal mass in the newborn.

    b. In patients with MCDK, the contralateral renal moiety is frequently affected by urologic disease.

    c. MCDK is often difficult to differentiate from severe ureteropelvic junction obstruction.

    d. Data from large series show that MCDK is associated with an increased risk for hypertension.

    e. Roughly 40% of MCDKs will spontaneously involute over time.

15. Which of the following would confirm the diagnosis of tuberous sclerosis?

    a. Renal angiomyolipoma and multiple renal cysts

    b. Hamartomatous rectal polyps and facial adenoma sebaceum

    c. Renal angiomyolipoma and cardiac rhabdomyoma

    d. Multiple renal cysts, hepatic fibrosis, and pheochromocytoma

    e. Mitral valve prolapse, renal angiolipoma, and gingival fibromas

16. The following are true of von Hippel-Lindau (VHL) disease EXCEPT:

    a. VHL disease is an autosomal dominant syndrome.

    b. VHL disease is caused by a mutation in the tumor suppressor gene, *VHL*, located on chromosome 3.

    c. epididymal cysts are not infrequent in patients with VHL disease.

    d. pheochromocytomas, cerebellar hemangioblastomas, and retinal angiomas are common extrarenal manifestations of VHL disease.

    e. renal cell carcinomas, the most common manifestation, are seen in the vast majority of patients.

17. Renal sinus cysts are most likely derived from:

    a. vascular elements.

    b. renal parenchyma.

    c. renal pelvis.

    d. lymphatic system.

    e. nephrogenic rests.

18. Most simple renal cysts identified in utero:

    a. represent the first sign of a multicystic kidney.

    b. represent the first sign of ARPKD.

    c. represent the first sign of ADPKD.

    d. represent a calyceal diverticulum.

    e. resolve before birth.

19. Approximately what percentage of individuals older than 60 years will have an identifiable renal cyst on computed tomography (CT)?

    a. 1% to 5%

    b. 10%

    c. 33%

    d. 75%

    e. 90%

20. Which of the following groups of antibiotics include the best choice for treating an infected renal cyst in a patient with ADPKD?

    a. Trimethoprim-sulfamethoxazole, chloramphenicol, fluoroquinolones

    b. Cephalosporins, trimethoprim-sulfamethoxazole, doxycycline

    c. Gentamicin, cephalosporins, vancomycin

    d. Fluoroquinolones, metronidazole (Flagyl), vancomycin

    e. Doxycycline, amoxicillin, gentamicin

21. All of the following are reasonable treatment strategies for patients with ADPKD EXCEPT:

    a. management of hypertension.

    b. avoidance of surgical treatment for large or multiple cysts in patients with chronic flank pain.

    c. surgical treatment of symptomatic urinary stone disease.

    d. use of lipophilic antibiotics for treatment of a suspected renal cyst infection.

    e. screening with magnetic resonance imaging (MRI) or CT for berry aneurysms in patients with a family history of subarachnoid hemorrhage.

22. In neonates with a unilateral multicystic kidney, what is the incidence of contralateral vesicoureteral reflux?

    a. 0% to 7%

    b. 18% to 43%

    c. 50% to 67%

    d. 75%

    e. 7% to 15%

23. What is the most likely cause of flank pain and hematuria in a 50-year-old patient with end-stage renal disease who has been undergoing dialysis for 5 years?

    a. Acute renal vein thrombosis

    b. Acute renal artery thrombosis

    c. Renal cell carcinoma

    d. ARCD

    e. Uric acid stones

24. Which group of three findings best describes the typical ultrasonographic image of a multicystic dysplastic kidney?

    a. The cysts are organized around a central large cyst; there is no identifiable renal sinus; and there are communications between the cysts.

    b. The cysts have a haphazard distribution; there is absence of a central or medial large cyst; and there are no obvious communications between the cysts.

    c. The cysts have a haphazard distribution; there is no obvious renal sinus; and there is a large central cyst.

    d. Connections exist between the cysts; a medial cyst is present; and a renal sinus is usually present.

    e. The cysts are organized at the periphery; the largest is the central one; and there is an identifiable renal sinus.

25. The Mayer-Rokitansky-Küster-Hauser syndrome refers to which group of associated findings?

    a. Wilms tumor, nephrotic syndrome, ambiguous genitalia

    b. Caudad ureteric budding, lateral orifice position, lower pole dysplasia

    c. Hypertension, vesicoureteral reflux, deep cortical depression over an area of the kidney with "thyroidization" of tubules

    d. Bilateral renal agenesis, respiratory failure, oligohydramnios

    e. Unilateral renal agenesis or renal ectopia, ipsilateral müllerian defects, vaginal agenesis

26. Which one of the following conditions is most representative of a neoplastic growth?

    a. Benign multilocular cyst

    b. Oligomeganephronia

    c. Multicystic dysplastic kidney

    d. Calyceal diverticulum

    e. Ask-Upmark kidney

27. Which of the following is the best match?

    a. ARPKD and congenital hepatic fibrosis

    b. Medullary sponge kidney and predominance of glomerular cysts

    c. Juvenile nephronophthisis and cortical cysts

    d. Ask-Upmark kidney and hypotension

    e. von Hippel-Lindau disease and adenoma sebaceum

28. Which of the following matches is correct?

    a. ARPKD and chromosome 2

    b. ADPKD and chromosomes 4 and 16

    c. Tuberous sclerosis and chromosomes 9 and 15

    d. von Hippel-Lindau disease and chromosome 4

    e. Juvenile nephronophthisis and chromosome 6

29. A renal cyst with increased number of septa and prominent calcification in a nonenhancing cyst wall does not require exploration. According to the Bosniak grading system, this cyst would be categorized as:

    a. I.

    b. II.

    c. II F.

    d. III.

    e. IV.

30. Ultrasonography in neonates with ARPKD reveals kidneys that are hyperechogenic or "bright" in appearance. This finding is due to:

    a. the presence of many small punctate calcifications within the renal papillae.

    b. dysplastic, diseased renal parenchyma.

    c. a vast increase in small fat deposits within the renal sinuses.

    d. the presence of numerous microcysts created by tightly compacted, dilated collecting ducts that result in innumerable ultrasonographic interfaces.

    e. the presence of renal hamartomas with increased cortical vascularity.

31. Ultrasound and/or CT criteria for the diagnosis of a simple renal cyst include all the following EXCEPT:

    a. sharp, thin, distinct smooth walls and margins.

    b. thickness of cyst wall less than or equal to 3 mm.

    c. acoustic enhancement behind cyst (ultrasound).

    d. spherical or ovoid shape.

    e. homogeneous with absence of internal echoes.

32. A 50-year-old man with known von Hippel-Lindau disease presents with a single episode of gross hematuria. CT scan reveals a 3-cm enhancing mass in the upper pole of each kidney. Metastatic evaluation is negative. He is otherwise healthy. Appropriate treatment at this point would be:

    a. bilateral radical nephrectomy with the placement of a peritoneal dialysis catheter.

    b. bilateral upper pole partial nephrectomy.

    c. right radical nephrectomy with left upper pole partial nephrectomy.

    d. observation with serial CT every 4 months.

    e. CT-guided needle biopsy of each lesion with surgical removal if diagnosis confirms renal cell carcinoma.

Pathology

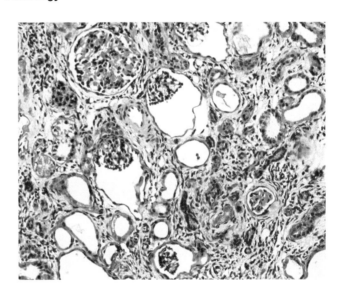

Figure 131-1. (From Bostwick DG, Cheng L. Urologic surgical pathology. 3rd ed. St. Louis: Elsevier; 2014.)

1. A 2-year-old boy has a right nephrectomy following an automobile accident for a shattered kidney with uncontrollable bleeding. The histology depicted in Figure 131-1 is reported as showing interstitial nephritis with cysts consistent with juvenile nephronophthisis. The next step in management is to:

    a. have the pathologist reexamine the specimen for evidence of nephrogenic rests.

    b. have the pathologist reexamine the specimen for an associated teratoma.

c. image the contralateral kidney for a renal mass.

d. image the liver for evidence of hepatic fibrosis.

e. inform the family that the child must be followed carefully for hypertension and decreased renal function.

ANSWERS

1. **b. Tuberous sclerosis and angiomyolipoma.** Angiomyolipomas occur in 40% to 80% of patients with tuberous sclerosis.

2. **a. Hypertension.** Hypertension and its sequelae (headache, hypertensive encephalopathy, retinopathy, etc.) are the hallmarks of Ask-Upmark kidney. Segmental vascular anomalies have been cited as a possible cause of the hypertension, but there is no evidence that renal artery intimal disease is associated. This disease is primarily found in young women and girls.

3. **b. Duration of renal failure.** At first, ARCD was thought to be confined to patients receiving hemodialysis. However, it shortly became apparent that the disorder is almost as common in patients receiving peritoneal dialysis and that it may develop in patients with chronic renal failure who are being managed medically without any type of dialysis. Thus ARCD appears to be a feature of end-stage kidney disease, rather than a response to dialysis.

4. **e. b and c.** The most severe form of ARPKD appears earliest in life, in the newborn period. All patients with ARPKD have liver involvement in the form of hepatic fibrosis and vary in the degree of biliary ectasia and periportal fibrosis. In both fetus and newborn, ultrasonography identifies bilateral, very enlarged, diffusely echogenic kidneys, especially when compared with the echogenicity of the liver. The increased echogenicity is due to the presence of numerous microcysts (created by tightly compacted, dilated collecting ducts) that result in innumerable interfaces. Compared with normal newborn kidneys, in ARPKD the pyramids are hyperechogenic because they blend in with the rest of the kidney, and the kidneys typically have a homogeneous appearance.

5. **c. An imbalance of the secretory and absorptive properties in proliferating tubular epithelial cells.** The fundamental processes that are essential for the development and progressive enlargement of renal cysts include (1) proliferation of epithelial cells in segments of renal tubule, (2) accumulation of fluid within the expanding tubule segment, and (3) disturbed organization and metabolism of the extracellular matrix. An imbalance of the secretory and absorptive properties in proliferating epithelial cells leads to a net accumulation of fluid in otherwise normal renal tubules. Recent evidence indicates that, beyond the loop of Henle, tubule cells have the capacity to secrete solutes and fluid on stimulation with $3',5'$-cyclic adenosine monophosphate (cAMP). This secretory flux operates in competition with the more powerful mechanism by which sodium (Na^+) is reabsorbed through apical epithelial Na^+ channels (ENaC). Under conditions in which Na^+ reabsorption is diminished, the net secretion of sodium chloride (NaCl) and fluid occurs.

6. **a. The genetic defect is located on the short arm of chromosome 16.** Infants with ARPKD have hepatic fibrosis, and infants with ADPKD rarely have hepatic fibrosis but commonly have cysts in the liver. Renal cysts are frequently seen in individuals on ultrasonography by the age of 20 years. Glomerular cysts are sometimes found in the kidneys of newborns diagnosed with ADPKD. The risk of renal cell carcinoma in patients with ADPKD is no higher than that in the general population.

7. **c. Cerebellar hemangioblastomas.** All are extrarenal manifestations of ADPKD except cerebellar hemangioblastomas, which are seen in patients with von Hippel-Lindau disease.

8. **e. Multicystic dysplastic kidneys appear more often in females and more often on the right side.** At any age, the condition is more likely to be found on the left side. Males are more likely to have unilateral multicystic dysplastic kidneys (2.4:1).

9. **a. Bleeding into a cyst.** Pain (flank and/or abdominal) is the most common presenting symptom in adults. This results from a number of possible factors: mass effect (cysts impinging on abdominal wall or neighboring organs), bleeding into the cysts, urinary tract infection (including infected cysts), and nephrolithiasis.

10. **e. VHL.** The gene associated with the transmission of von Hippel-Lindau disease is located on chromosome 3. In non–von Hippel-Lindau patients with sporadic clear cell renal cell carcinoma, 50% of cell lines are associated with a mutational form of the *VHL* gene.

11. **a. In males younger than 4 years and in females older than 30 years.** The great majority of patients present before the age of 4 years or after the age of 30 years. Five percent present between 4 and 30 years. The patient is 2 times as likely to be male if younger than 4 years and 8 times as likely to be female if older than 30 years.

12. **b. NPH is an autosomal recessive disorder, whereas MCKD is an autosomal dominant disease.** Although either condition can occur sporadically, juvenile nephronophthisis usually is inherited as an autosomal recessive trait, whereas medullary cystic disease usually is inherited in an autosomal dominant fashion. Juvenile nephronophthisis and medullary cystic disease both cause polydipsia and polyuria in more than 80% of cases, but not to the extent observed in patients with diabetes insipidus. Pathologically, NPH and MCKD are similar. Histologically, there is a characteristic triad present that includes (1) irregular thickening and disintegration of the tubular basement membrane, (2) marked tubular atrophy with cyst development, and (3) interstitial cell infiltration with fibrosis. Twenty percent of juvenile nephronophthisis families have extrarenal manifestations, whereas MCKD usually affects only the kidneys. Another important difference between the two entities is that renal failure develops in patients with NPH at a mean age of 13 years and almost always before 25 years. MCKD is a milder disease when it presents in early adulthood, but it will manifest in all patients by 50 years (Bernstein and Gardner, 1979).* End-stage renal disease (ESRD) in patients with MCKD most often develops in the third or fourth decade of life.

13. **c. von Hippel-Lindau disease.** Tuberous sclerosis and von Hippel-Lindau disease are associated with epithelial hyperplasia (and adenomas as well) and have an increased incidence of renal cell carcinoma (tuberous sclerosis, 2%, and von Hippel-Lindau disease, 35% to 38%).

14. **d. Data from large series show that MCDK is associated with an increased risk for hypertension.** All statements are true of MCDK, except that large series indicate MCDK is NOT associated with an increased risk of hypertension.

15. **c. Renal angiomyolipoma and cardiac rhabdomyoma.** Definitive diagnosis of tuberous sclerosis (TSC) is dependent on the presence of certain major and minor clinical features. The diagnosis of TSC requires two major features (renal angiomyolipoma, facial angiofibromas or forehead plaques, nontraumatic ungual or periungual fibroma, three or more hypomelanotic macules, shagreen patch, multiple retinal nodular hamartomas, cortical tuber, subependymal nodule, subependymal giant cell astrocytoma, cardiac rhabdomyoma, lymphangioleiomyomatosis) or one major plus two minor features (multiple renal cysts, nonrenal hamartoma, hamartomatous rectal polyps, retinal achromic patch, cerebral white matter radial migration tracts, bone cysts, gingival fibromas, "confetti" skin lesions, multiple enamel pits).

16. **e. Renal cell carcinomas, the most common manifestation, are seen in the vast majority of patients.** All statements are true of VHL disease except that renal cysts, NOT *renal cell carcinoma*, are the most common and often earliest manifestation as seen in 76% of patients.

17. **d. Lymphatic system.** The predominant type of renal sinus cyst appears to be one derived from the lymphatics.

---

*Sources refeenced can be found in *Campbell-Walsh Urology, 11th Edition*, on the Expert Consult website.

18. **e. Resolve before birth.** In 28 of 11,000 fetuses with renal cysts, 25 fetuses had the cysts resolve before birth. Of two cysts that remained postnatally, in one it was the first sign of a multicystic kidney.

19. **c. 33%.** In adults, the frequency of renal cyst occurrence increases with age. Using CT, one group demonstrated a 20% incidence of cysts by 40 years and approximately 33% incidence of cysts after 60 years.

20. **a. Trimethoprim-sulfamethoxazole, chloramphenicol, fluoroquinolones.** In the experience of one group of researchers, the only dependable antibiotics were those that were lipid soluble, namely, trimethoprim-sulfamethoxazole and chloramphenicol. Chloramphenicol produced better results. The fluoroquinolones, which are also lipid soluble, are proving useful. If a patient with suspected pyelonephritis does not respond to an antibiotic, and if the antibiotic used is not lipid soluble, one must consider whether the infection may be present in a noncommunicating cyst.

21. **b. Avoidance of surgical treatment for large or multiple cysts in patients with chronic flank pain.** All are reasonable treatment strategies for a patient with ADPKD, except that when conservative measures of chronic pain treatment fail, surgical management must be considered. Ultrasonography- or CT-guided cyst aspiration is a straightforward procedure and may be both diagnostic and therapeutic. Surgical unroofing of multiple or very large cysts can potentially alleviate symptoms of pain and can be performed either laparoscopically or through open flank or dorsal lumbotomy incisions. Surgical intervention appears to only improve symptomatology and does not appear to either accelerate the decline of renal function or preserve declining renal function.

22. **b. 18% to 43%.** Contralateral vesicoureteral reflux is seen even more often than contralateral ureteropelvic junction obstruction, being identified in 18% to 43% of infants.

23. **d. ARCD.** The most common presentation of ARCD is loin pain, hematuria, or both. Bleeding occurs in as many as 50% of patients.

24. **b. The cysts have a haphazard distribution; there is absence of a central or medial large cyst; and there are no obvious communications between the cysts.** Renal masses in infants most often represent either multicystic kidney disease or hydronephrosis, and it is important to distinguish the two, especially if the surgeon wishes to remove a nonfunctioning hydronephrotic kidney or repair a ureteropelvic junction obstruction while leaving a multicystic organ in situ. In newborns, ultrasonography is generally the first study performed. In a few cases, it is difficult to distinguish multicystic kidney disease from severe hydronephrosis. In general, however, the multicystic kidney has a haphazard distribution of cysts of various sizes without a larger central or medial cyst and without visible communications between the cysts. Frequently, very small cysts appear in between the large cysts. By comparison, in ureteropelvic junction obstruction, the cysts or calyces are organized around the periphery of the kidney, connections can usually be demonstrated between the peripheral cysts and a central or medial cyst that represents the renal pelvis, and there is an absence of small cysts between the larger cysts. When there is an identifiable renal sinus, the diagnosis is more likely to be hydronephrosis than multicystic kidney.

25. **e. Unilateral renal agenesis or renal ectopia, ipsilateral müllerian defects, vaginal agenesis.** The term *Mayer-Rokitansky-Küster-Hauser syndrome* refers to a group of associated findings that include unilateral renal agenesis or renal ectopia, ipsilateral müllerian defects, and vaginal agenesis. Drash syndrome includes Wilms tumor, nephrotic syndrome, and ambiguous genitalia; the findings of caudad ureteric budding, lateral orifice position, and lower pole dysplasia follow the bud theory; the grouping of hypertension, vesicoureteral reflux, and deep cortical depression over an area of the kidney with "thyroidization" of tubules defines the Ask-Upmark kidney; and the grouping of bilateral renal agenesis, respiratory failure, and oligohydramnios can lead the fetus to be born with Potter syndrome and Potter facies.

26. **a. Benign multilocular cyst.** For the benign multilocular cystic lesion, certain authors prefer the term *cystic nephroma*, because this term implies a benign but neoplastic lesion.

27. **a. ARPKD and congenital hepatic fibrosis.** All patients with ARPKD have varying degrees of congenital hepatic fibrosis.

28. **b. ADPKD and chromosomes 4 and 16.** For the genetic cystic disease ADPKD, the chromosomal defect is on chromosome 16 for *PKD1* and 4 for *PKD2*; *PKD3* has not been mapped. Autosomal recessive polycystic kidney disease involves chromosome 6; tuberous sclerosis involves chromosomes 9 and 16; von Hippel-Lindau disease involves chromosome 3; and juvenile nephronophthisis involves chromosome 2.

29. **c. II F.** The Bosniak classification has recently been updated to include category II F, as defined in the answer.

30. **d. The presence of numerous microcysts created by tightly compacted, dilated collecting ducts that result in innumerable ultrasonographic interfaces.** In both fetuses and newborns with ARPKD, ultrasonography identifies bilateral, very enlarged, diffusely echogenic kidneys, especially when compared with the echogenicity of the liver. The increased echogenicity is due to the presence of numerous microcysts (created by tightly compacted, dilated collecting ducts) that result in innumerable interfaces. Compared with normal newborn kidneys, in ARPKD the pyramids are hyperechogenic because they blend in with the rest of the kidney, and the kidneys typically have a homogeneous appearance.

31. **b. Thickness of cyst wall less than or equal to 3 mm.** One can safely make the diagnosis of a classic benign simple cyst by ultrasonography when the following criteria are met: (1) absence of internal echoes; (2) sharply defined, thin, distinct wall with a smooth and distinct margin; (3) good transmission of sound waves through the cyst with consequent acoustic enhancement behind the cyst; and (4) spherical or slightly ovoid shape. The CT criteria for a simple cyst are similar to those used in ultrasonography: (1) sharp, thin, distinct, smooth walls and margins; (2) spherical or ovoid shape; and (3) homogeneous content.

32. **b. Bilateral upper pole partial nephrectomy.** Because the tumors that characterize VHL disease are frequently multiple, bilateral, and recurrent, close surveillance and minimization of surgical procedures constitute the mainstay of treatment. For patients who have VHL disease and all patients who have hereditary cancer syndromes, the goal of treatment is cancer control, not cancer cure, and preservation of functional parenchyma to avoid the morbidity associated with renal loss. In patients who have VHL disease, surgical resection is performed with the understanding that microscopic disease probably is left behind. Currently, nephron-sparing surgery should be considered the standard of care for treating low-grade renal cell carcinoma in the setting of VHL disease. Patients with high-grade disease are still probably best served with bilateral nephrectomy. Although having the objective of sparing as much renal parenchyma as possible and preventing metastasis of the lesions already present, it is not curative surgery (Reed, 2009). Although this approach does not reduce the risk of recurrence, reported to be 75% to 85%, the 10-year disease-specific survival rates are quite high (81% to 94%) (Malek, 1987; Steinbach, 1995; Roupret, 2003; Ploussard, 2007). Classically, the survival rate after nephrectomy has been only 50%. Because most of these tumors are low grade, a nephron-sparing approach provides very good survival rates while avoiding the diminished quality of life that comes with bilateral nephrectomy and subsequent dialysis/transplantation. Laparoscopic and percutaneous image-guided ablative techniques, such as radiofrequency ablation and cryoablation, have also been used and are currently under investigation.

Pathology

1. **e. Inform the family that the child must be followed carefully for hypertension and decreased renal function.** The histology is classic for juvenile nephronophthisis showing chronic interstitial nephritis-fibrosis, atrophic tubules, and glomerular microcysts. It is usually inherited as an autosomal recessive. These patients have a high likelihood of developing hypertension and eventually chronic renal failure. They may also develop retinitis pigmentosa.

CHAPTER REVIEW

1. Potter facies is manifested by hypertelorism, prominent inner canthal folds, and a recessive chin.
2. Dysplasia is histologically manifested by embryonic, immature mesenchyme, and primitive renal components; it is often associated with ureteric bud abnormalities and/or urinary obstruction.
3. Renal hypoplasia is manifested by less than the normal number of calyces and nephrons with absence of dysplasia.
4. Oligomeganephronia is a reduced number of nephrons with hypertrophy of the remaining nephrons. Many patients with the disorder develop renal failure.
5. The Ask-Upmark kidney (segmental hypoplasia) is often associated with reflux and patients develop severe hypertension.
6. Autosomal dominant polycystic kidney disease is associated with cysts of the liver, pancreas, spleen and lungs, berry aneurysms, colonic diverticula, aortic aneurysms, and mitral valve prolapse. It usually becomes clinically manifest in the fourth and fifth decades.
7. Benign multilocular cyst and cystic nephroma fall into a spectrum of disease, with multilocular cyst on the one end being benign and, on the other end of the spectrum, cystic Wilms tumors being malignant. Multilocular cyst with nodules of Wilms tumor lies in the middle.
8. In the adult, there is a multilocular cystic renal cell carcinoma. Multilocular cystic lesions should therefore be removed.
9. One third of patients with medullary sponge kidneys have hypercalciuria.
10. Congenital bilateral absence of the vas is associated with cystic fibrosis; unilateral absence of the vas may be associated with ipsilateral absence of the kidney.
11. Von Hippel-Lindau syndrome is inherited as an autosomal dominant and is manifested by cerebellar and retinal hemangioblastomas; cysts of the pancreas, kidney, and epididymis; epididymal cystadenoma, pheochromocytoma, and clear cell renal cell carcinoma.
12. Multicystic dysplastic kidney has no identifiable normal renal parenchyma; it is not associated with an increased risk of either hypertension or malignancy.
13. Medullary sponge kidney has dilated collecting ducts and is associated with hypercalciuria, hypocitraturia, and renal calculi.
14. All patients with autosomal recessive polycystic kidney disease (ARPKD) have liver involvement in the form of hepatic fibrosis and varying degrees of biliary ectasia and periportal fibrosis.
15. Juvenile nephronophthisis usually is inherited as an autosomal recessive trait, whereas medullary cystic disease usually is inherited in an autosomal dominant fashion. Juvenile nephronophthisis and medullary cystic disease both cause polydipsia and polyuria, and pathologically they are similar.

132 Congenital Urinary Obstruction: Pathophysiology

Craig A. Peters

QUESTIONS

1. Congenital obstruction differs from acquired obstruction in that it:
   a. causes renal atrophy.
   b. induces interstitial fibrosis.
   c. alters renal homeostasis.
   d. affects tubular function.
   e. affects glomerular development.

2. Renal dysplasia associated with obstruction is characterized by:
   a. renal atrophy.
   b. glomerular cysts.
   c. fibromuscular collars.
   d. heterotopic bone formation.
   e. excess production of afferent arteriole renin.

3. After relief of a unilateral obstructing lesion, decreasing relative uptake on radionuclide renal imaging is most likely due to:
   a. glomerular hyperfiltration.
   b. asymmetrical renal growth.
   c. established renal tubular fibrosis.
   d. neural imbalance.
   e. compensatory hypertrophy.

4. In the obstructed kidney, epidermal growth factor (EGF) has been shown to:
   a. reduce renal apoptosis.
   b. reduce glomerular sclerosis.
   c. accelerate interstitial fibrosis.
   d. improve collecting duct function.
   e. reduce renin recruitment in the afferent arteriole.

5. Epithelial to mesenchymal transformation in the developing kidney is:
   a. a one-way process.
   b. the basis for glomerular sclerosis.
   c. integral to glomerular development.
   d. seen only in the setting of obstruction.
   e. reflected in the presence of α-smooth muscle actin.

6. Regulation of the extracellular matrix in the kidney:
   a. depends on normal expression of EGF.
   b. depends entirely on collagen synthesis.
   c. is not related to angiotensin expression.
   d. depends on balanced synthesis and degradation.
   e. is independent of transforming growth factor-β (TGF-β) activity.

7. The principal effects of congenital renal obstruction are:
   a. glomerulosclerosis, interstitial fibrosis, and atrophy.
   b. hypoplasia and increased epithelial-mesenchymal transformation.
   c. altered growth regulation, renal differentiation, and functional integration.
   d. glomerulosclerosis, renin downregulation, and tubular hypertrophy.
   e. increased growth, fibrosis, and tubular atrophy.

8. In the fetal kidney, angiotensin activity:
   a. is tightly regulated by EGF.
   b. acts predominantly through the AT-1 receptor.
   c. affects epithelial-mesenchymal transformations.
   d. is an important regulator of renal growth.
   e. is unaffected by renal obstruction.

9. Inflammatory changes in the congenitally obstructed kidney:
   a. are similar to those seen in postnatally obstructed kidneys.
   b. are mediated by the renin-angiotensin system.
   c. are minimal in the absence of overt infection.
   d. are the key element in glomerular damage.
   e. affect renal interstitial fibrosis.

ANSWERS

1. **e. Affects glomerular development.** Only congenital obstruction will change glomerular development, whereas acquired obstruction can produce all of the other changes indicated. Because it occurs during development, congenital obstruction can produce an altered developmental pattern, whereas acquired obstruction cannot change an already established pattern, only damage or distort it.

2. **c. Fibromuscular collars.** One of the histologic hallmarks of dysplasia is fibromuscular collars, so-called *primitive ducts* reflecting abnormal differentiation of the peritubular mesenchyme. Renal growth impairment is common with dysplasia; however, this is not atrophy but growth failure. Glomerular cysts are not characteristic of dysplasia. Heterotopic cartilage may be seen, but not bone. Excess renin expression may be seen in obstruction without dysplasia.

3. **b. Asymmetrical renal growth.** When renal function appears to decline after relief of obstruction, it is often due to different growth and functional development rates of the two kidneys, when the affected kidney cannot increase its absolute function as rapidly as the other intact kidney. This produces a progressive differential functional uptake on nuclear imaging that gives the impression of functional loss that is relative and not absolute.

4. **a. Reduce renal apoptosis.** Administration of EGF to the congenitally obstructed kidney can reduce renal apoptosis and reduce the effects of growth impairment. The other effects have not been reported.

5. **e. Reflected in the presence of α-smooth muscle actin.** Epithelial to mesenchymal transformations are an important part of renal development but have not been shown to be part of normal glomerular development. It is the presumed basis for the presence

of α-smooth muscle actin in the obstructed kidney. It is bidirectional.

6. **d. Depends on balanced synthesis and degradation.** Extracellular membrane (ECM) regulation is due to collagen synthesis rates as well as to the rate of ECM breakdown. The latter is determined by the balanced activities of the TIMPs and MMPs; these are regulated in part by TGF-β and the renin-angiotensin system.

7. **c. Altered growth regulation, renal differentiation, and functional integration.** The key patterns defining congenital renal obstruction are altered growth regulation, renal differentiation, and functional integration, although interstitial fibrosis, tubular hypotrophy, and increased epithelial-mesenchymal transformation are components of these changes.

8. **d. Is an important regulator of renal growth.** In the developing kidney, angiotensin is an important growth regulator, as well as mediator of fibrosis, and is altered significantly by obstruction. Fetal angiotensin acts predominantly through the AT2 receptor until late in gestation, when the AT1 receptor begins to exert a greater role.

9. **c. Are minimal in the absence of overt infection.** In contrast to acquired obstruction, congenital obstruction is not characterized by a significant inflammatory infiltrate, except when complicated by infection.

CHAPTER REVIEW

1. A damaged kidney does not have the functional reserve to maintain normal renal function over time as the child grows. Thus, with time, the creatinine concentration will rise in patients who have no functional reserve in their nephron mass.

2. Obstructive processes may produce dysplasia.

3. In some cases, congenitally obstructed kidneys are smaller. This is not a result of atrophy but of hypoplasia.

4. A critical determinant of dysplasia in the kidney is complete obstruction early in gestation.

5. A universal characteristic of obstruction is renal fibrosis with infiltration of the interstitium with extracellular matrix.

6. The frequency with which a post obstructed kidney has progressive deterioration in renal function is 20% to 40%; it does not have the renal reserve of a normal kidney and may have a reduced number and function of nephrons. This results in hyperfiltration resulting in glomerulosclerosis and a progressive decline in renal function.

7. Measures of urinary sodium, chloride, osmolality, and calcium correlate with fetal renal function. When these measures approach serum levels, irreversible damage is suggested.

8. The distinctness of the calyx is helpful in determining the functionality of the obstruction. Thus, no caliectasis suggests a mild to minimal degree of functional obstruction.

9. ^{99m}Tc-Mercaptoacetyltriglycine is generally used for diuretic renography. It is taken up and excreted by the renal tubules relatively rapidly with little glomerular filtration.

10. If the diuretic renogram shows a T1/2 greater than 20 minutes, the kidney is presumed to be obstructed; if it is less than 10 minutes it is presumed normal; if it is between 10 and 20 minutes, it is considered indeterminate.

11. Obstruction can be very harmful to the developing kidney, far beyond that seen in the mature kidney. The effects of obstruction may be not be reversible owing to alterations in structure and function in the developing kidney that do not occur in the mature kidney.

12. When obstruction results in a growth impairment, the results are fewer nephron units and delayed nephron maturation.

13. Angiotensin appears to be a key modulator of the inflammatory response in renal obstruction. It is also an important growth regulator, as well as mediator of fibrosis, and is altered significantly by obstruction.

14. Renal renin is increased in the obstructed kidney.

15. Inflammation with interstitial infiltration of lymphocytes is a common finding in postnatal acquired obstruction.

16. When renal function appears to decline after relief of obstruction, it is often due to differential growth and functional development rates of the two kidneys, when the affected kidney cannot increase its absolute function as rapidly as the contralateral intact kidney. This produces a progressive differential functional uptake on nuclear imaging that gives the impression of functional loss that is relative and not absolute.

17. In contrast to acquired obstruction, congenital obstruction is not characterized by a significant inflammatory infiltrate, except when complicated by infection.

133 Surgery of the Ureter in Children

L. Henning Olsen and Yazan F.H. Rawashdeh

QUESTIONS

1. Which of the following statements is NOT correct concerning laparoscopic pyeloplasty?
   a. It is discounted early as unacceptable due to degree of difficulty.
   b. It can be performed after a failed previous pyeloplasty.
   c. It has an overall higher success rate than endopyelotomy.
   d. It should be performed in patients of all ages.
   e. Many different techniques for laparoscopic approach have been described.

2. In regard to closure of trocar sites:
   a. closing fascial wounds larger than 3 mm is recommended.
   b. fascial closure devices facilitate closure in the obese patient.
   c. omentum is the most common herniated intra-abdominal structure.
   d. trocars should not be removed before the intra-abdominal pressure is close to normal.
   e. all of the above are true.

3. Which is NOT true for transperitoneal procedures?
   a. Sutures may be passed through the anterior abdominal wall.
   b. For lower abdominal procedures, infants are best positioned across the foot of the bed.
   c. Laxity of the infant abdominal wall can limit exposure due to compression.
   d. Cannula fixation is a common problem in pediatric laparoscopy.
   e. Visibility is usually a problem.

4. A recognized risk of laparoscopy in all infants is:
   a. use of monopolar cautery.
   b. ventilatory compromise.
   c. abdominal adhesions.
   d. decreased renal perfusion.
   e. compartmental syndrome.

5. Which of the following is a relative contraindication to retroperitoneoscopic surgery in the pediatric population?
   a. Abnormalities such as horseshoe kidneys
   b. Spinal deformity
   c. Previous abdominal surgery
   d. Weight
   e. Intestinal malrotation

6. Hypothermia during laparoscopy in all infants is caused by:
   a. insufflation of a large amount of CO_2 due to port leakage.
   b. high-frequency ventilation.
   c. room-temperature insufflation.
   d. evaporation.
   e. cold room temperature.

7. Regarding pediatric minimally invasive surgery in obese patients:
   a. suture can be placed from the skin at the entry site to the cannula to keep the cannula from sliding off if rapid desufflation is encountered.
   b. hitch stitches are helpful.
   c. an insufflation needle works well in most children, because the abdominal wall is thin.
   d. bladeless optical trocars or open access for the camera port might be helpful.
   e. higher insufflation pressures are needed.

8. Which of the following statements is TRUE regarding primary obstructive megaureters?
   a. It is caused by a dysfunctional juxtavesical segment that is unable to propagate urine at acceptable rates of flow.
   b. It most commonly occurs with neurogenic and non-neurogenic voiding dysfunction or infravesical obstructions such as posterior urethral valves.
   c. It may be due to acute infections, nephropathies, or other medical conditions, causing significant increases in urinary output that overwhelm maximal peristalsis.
   d. It is diagnosed when reflux, obstruction, and secondary causes of dilatation are ruled out.
   e. None of the above.

9. Which of the following statements is TRUE regarding secondary obstructive megaureters?
   a. It is caused by an aperistaltic juxtavesical segment that is unable to propagate urine at acceptable rates of flow.
   b. It most commonly occurs with neurogenic and non-neurogenic voiding dysfunction or infravesical obstructions such as posterior urethral valves.
   c. It may be due to acute infections, nephropathies, or other medical conditions causing significant increases in urinary output that overwhelm maximal peristalsis.
   d. It is diagnosed once reflux, obstruction, and secondary causes of dilatation are ruled out.
   e. None of the above.

10. Which of the following is TRUE regarding the surgical management of megaureters?
    a. Ureteral tailoring is usually necessary to achieve the proper length-to-diameter ratio required of successful reimplants.
    b. Plication or infolding is useful for the more severely dilated ureter.
    c. Excisional tapering is preferred for the moderately dilated ureter.
    d. Narrowing the ureter may theoretically lead to less effective peristalsis.
    e. Patients usually have such massively dilated and tortuous ureters that straightening with removal of excess length and proximal revision becomes necessary.

11. Which of the following is the most serious complication to ureteral tailoring?

   a. Gradual tapering can cause an abrupt change of the ureteral caliber and subsequent kinking.

   b. A too-short intravesical tunnel can cause vesicoureteral reflux.

   c. Compromise of the distal vasculature of the ureter with subsequent fibrosis

   d. Secondary stenosis of the ureteral orifice

   e. Bladder dysfunction after intravesical dissection

ANSWERS

1. **d. Should be performed in patients of all ages.** In newborns, access to the ureteropelvic junction (UPJ) requires only a very small incision.
2. **d. Trocars should not be removed before the intra-abdominal pressure is close to normal.** Lowering the pressure before removing the trocars will reveal that the hemostasis is under control and prevents intra-abdominal (bowel, omentum) content from entering the port holes.
3. **e. Visibility is usually a problem.** The peritoneal lining mirrors the light from the telescope, giving better visibility than in the retroperitoneal route.
4. **a. Use of monopolar cautery.** Monopolar cautery increases the risk of unrecognized lesions to intra-abdominal organs, particularly the bowel.
5. **a. Abnormalities such as horseshoe kidneys.** Access to the UPJ from the posterior aspect is extremely difficult in horseshoe kidneys.
6. **a. Insufflation of a large amount of CO_2 due to port leakage.** The large amount of gas exchange lowers the intra-abdominal temperature significantly.
7. **d. Bladeless optical trocars or open access for the camera port might be helpful.** Blind access to the peritoneal cavity imposes and inherent risk of organ damage.
8. **a. It is caused by a dysfunctional juxtavesical segment that is unable to propagate urine at acceptable rates of flow.** Obstruction results from the presence of an abnormal adynamic segment at the terminal end of the ureter near or at the ureterovesical junction (UVJ).
9. **b. It most commonly occurs with neurogenic and non-neurogenic voiding dysfunction or infravesical obstructions such as posterior urethral valves.** High bladder pressure might result in secondary reflux.
10. **a. Ureteral tailoring is usually necessary to achieve the proper length-to-diameter ratio required of successful reimplants.** Especially in small children, the reimplant can be otherwise impossible.
11. **c. Compromise of the distal vasculature of the ureter with subsequent fibrosis.** Fibrosis can lead to recurrent obstruction and require a redo. However, when performed with care, the risk of vascular compromise should be minimal.

CHAPTER REVIEW

1. Congenital UPJ obstruction is due to an abnormal development of the musculature of the UPJ.
2. UPJ obstruction occurs more commonly in boys and on the left side.
3. UPJ obstruction may be seen with vesicoureteral reflux.
4. Dismembered pyeloplasty for the repair of a UPJ is favored by many because of its broad applicability, the removal of the pathologic segment of ureter, and the ease with which a reduction pyeloplasty may be incorporated into the procedure.
5. Megaureters may be caused by an intrinsic abnormality of the distal ureter, reflux, or obstruction; they are classified as: (1) obstructing, (2) refluxing, (3) nonobstructing nonrefluxing, and (4) obstructed refluxing.
6. The majority of nonrefluxing, nonobstructed megaureters discovered in infancy will resolve spontaneously in the first few years of life; patients with a ureter diameter less than 10 mm are highly likely to never require surgery.
7. Acute management of an obstructed megaureter in the neonatal period may be by percutaneous nephrostomy; however, the nephrostomies are difficult to keep in place. A more manageable temporizing procedure may be accomplished by an end-cutaneous ureterostomy or refluxing vesicoureteral anastomosis.
8. Folding techniques for ureteral tailoring are not applicable in ureters greater than 1.75 cm in diameter.
9. Indications for surgical therapy in UPJ obstruction or megaureter are symptoms from the obstruction, a progressive decrease in renal function, and a sequential increase in renal pelvic diameter.
10. A concomitant reimplantation and dismembered pyeloplasty should be discouraged, as the ureteral blood supply may be compromised.
11. Ureteral polyps are most often found in the proximal third of the ureter.
12. During laparoscopy monopolar cautery increases the risk of unrecognized lesions to intra-abdominal organs, particularly the bowel.
13. Primary obstructive megaureter is thought to be caused by a dysfunctional juxtavesical segment that is unable to propagate urine at acceptable rates of flow.
14. Secondary obstructive megaureter most commonly occurs with neurogenic and non-neurogenic voiding dysfunction or infravesical obstructions such as posterior urethral valves.

134 Ectopic Ureter, Ureterocele, and Ureteral Anomalies

Craig A. Peters and Cathy Mendelsohn

QUESTIONS

1. All of the following are possible drainage sites for an ectopic ureter in a female except the:
   a. fallopian tube.
   b. uterus.
   c. ovary.
   d. vagina.
   e. urethra.

2. Inadequate interaction between the ureteral bud and metanephric blastema will most likely lead to which of the following conditions?
   a. Dysplasia
   b. Hydronephrosis
   c. Reflux
   d. Ureteral ectopia
   e. Multicystic dysplasia

3. The relationship between the upper and lower pole orifices in a complete ureteral duplication is best described by the upper pole:
   a. orifice being cephalad and lateral to the lower orifice.
   b. ureter joining the lower pole ureter just before entry into the bladder.
   c. orifice being caudal and medial to the lower pole orifice.
   d. orifice and lower pole orifice being located transversely side by side.
   e. ureter joining the bladder neck caudal to the lower pole orifice.

4. The most common site of drainage of an ectopic ureter in a male is:
   a. vas deferens.
   b. anterior urethra.
   c. seminal vesicle.
   d. posterior urethra.
   e. ampulla of the vas.

5. All of the following contribute to vesicoureteral reflux EXCEPT:
   a. lateral ureteral insertion.
   b. lax bladder neck.
   c. poorly developed trigone.
   d. gaping ureteral orifice.
   e. short intramural tunnel.

6. The voiding pattern most often seen in a girl with an ectopic ureter is:
   a. urge incontinence.
   b. stress incontinence.
   c. continuous incontinence.
   d. interrupted urinary stream.
   e. overflow incontinence.

7. Which of the following findings is most likely present on an ultrasound in a patient with an ectopic ureter in a duplicated system?
   a. Echogenic parenchyma of the lower pole of the kidney
   b. Medially displaced lower pole of the kidney
   c. Cystic structure in the bladder
   d. Tortuous lower pole ureter
   e. Cystic changes in the upper pole of the kidney

8. Ureteroceles can be associated with all of the following EXCEPT:
   a. smoking during pregnancy.
   b. vesicoureteral reflux.
   c. white race.
   d. female gender.
   e. duplicated kidneys.

9. All of the following can be caused by a ureterocele. Which is the LEAST likely?
   a. Bladder outlet obstruction
   b. Upper pole obstruction
   c. Lower pole reflux
   d. Urinary incontinence
   d. Contralateral reflux

10. A child known to have a ureterocele based on ultrasound imaging undergoes cystography, but no filling defect is noted. The most likely explanation is:
    a. ureterocele eversion.
    b. lower pole reflux.
    c. ureterocele effacement.
    d. ureterocele prolapse.
    e. ureterocele disproportion.

11. A girl undergoes open resection of a large ectopic ureterocele. After removal of the catheter, she has high postvoid residuals demonstrated on a sonogram. Which complication is most likely responsible?
    a. Persistent reflux
    b. Prolapsing residual ureterocele tissue
    c. Neurapraxia secondary to bladder retraction
    d. Excessive buttressing of deficient detrusor at the bladder neck
    e. Residual flap of the ureterocele in the urethra

12. What is the preferred method of endoscopic treatment of a ureterocele?
    a. Resection of the roof of the ureterocele
    b. Puncture of the ureterocele's urethral extension
    c. Puncture of the roof of the ureterocele
    d. Transverse incision at the base of the ureterocele
    e. Resection of the base of the ureterocele only

13. An adult is evaluated as a possible kidney donor. An excretory urogram demonstrates a round contrast agent-filled area at the bladder base with a thin radiolucent rim around it. What is the most likely diagnosis?

    a. Single-system kidney with a ureterocele

    b. Marked opacification delay of the kidney

    c. Radioopaque stone filing the ureterocele

    d. Extension of a ureterocele to the bladder neck and urethra

    e. Reflux

14. A white infant is found to have a smooth interlabial mass on the posterior aspect of the urethra. What would be the most appropriate initial management?

    a. Chemotherapy

    b. Puncture of the mass

    c. Topical estrogen cream

    d. Observation

    e. Resection of the mass

15. An 11-year-old child presents with flank pain and hematuria. There is left hydronephrosis to the ureteropelvic junction. There is no ureteral dilation. Diuretic renography shows symmetric uptake in both kidneys and a very delayed washout time with a half-life of 50 minutes. At the time of surgery, a retrograde pyelogram shows a proximal ureteral filling defect. The best course of action is:

    a. abandon the procedure and obtain computed tomography (CT) imaging with contrast.

    b. perform ureteroscopic biopsy.

    c. perform radical nephroureterectomy.

    d. perform ureteroscopic excision of the presumed fibroepithelial polyp.

    e. proceed with dismembered pyeloplasty and resect a fibroepithelial polyp.

16. An infant is seen with an intravesical ureterocele, no reflux, and an echogenic moderately dilated upper pole that has limited function. The washout curve of the upper pole moiety shows a $t_{1/2}$ of 10 minutes. The most appropriate treatment option would be:

    a. Observation with repeat ultrasound in 6 months

    b. Ureterocele excision and common sheath reimplantation

    c. Transureteral incision of the ureterocele

    d. Prophylactic antibiotics, observation, and repeat ultrasound in 4 months

    e. Upper pole partial nephrectomy

17. Which of the following statements regarding duplex kidneys is TRUE?

    a. Duplex kidneys are the same size as single-system kidneys.

    b. The upper pole moiety is the more likely of the two to have a ureteropelvic junction obstruction.

    c. The duplex kidney arises as a consequence of two separate ureteric buds.

    d. A duplex kidney results from two separate metanephric blastemal entities arising near the mesonephric duct.

    e. The lower pole ureter is less likely to have vesicoureteral reflux.

18. In a child with a functioning nondilated upper pole segment associated with an ectopic ureter, the most efficient therapeutic option(s) (more than one answer may be correct) would be:

    a. common sheath ureteral reimplantation.

    b. upper to lower ureteropyelostomy.

    c. upper to lower distal ureteroureterostomy.

    d. upper pole partial nephrectomy.

    e. upper pole ureteral reimplantation.

19. Initial endoscopic incision of a ureterocele offers the following advantages EXCEPT:

    a. early relief of bladder outlet obstruction.

    b. potential for definitive therapy.

    c. possible improvement in trigonal deficiency.

    d. potential for improved function of the affected renal segment.

    e. decompression of a dilated upper pole ureter.

20. What is the most common form of ureteral triplication?

    a. All three ureters joining to terminate in a single bladder orifice

    b. Three ureters joining to form two ureteral orifices

    c. Three ureters draining as three separate orifices

    d. One of the three ureters terminating ectopically, the other two draining orthotopically

    e. Two ureters draining into three orifices

21. Failure of atrophy of which vessel leads to the formation of a preureteral vena cava?

    a. Posterior cardinal vein

    b. Subcardinal vein

    c. Supracardinal vein

    d. Umbilical artery

    e. Inferior vitelline vein

22. Which of the following types of ureterocele is associated with the lowest incidence of secondary procedures after transurethral decompression?

    a. Ectopic ureterocele

    b. Ureterocele in a female patient

    c. Intravesical ureterocele

    d. Ureterocele associated with a duplicated system

    e. Cecoureterocele

23. After the perinatal period, what is the most common method of presentation of a ureterocele?

    a. Incontinence

    b. Abdominal mass

    c. Failure to thrive

    d. Stranguria

    e. Urinary tract infection

24. A patient with a suspected ectopic ureter due to incontinence has no hydronephrosis on an ultrasonographic study and apparent single systems bilaterally. Which of the following tests is a sensitive method of determining if there is an ectopic ureter and associated renal moiety?

    a. Diethylenetriaminepentaacetic acid (DTPA) renal scanning

    b. Magnetic resonance imaging (MRI) of the abdomen and pelvis

    c. Nuclear voiding cystourethrography

    d. Positron emission tomography

    e. Intravenous pyelography

ANSWERS

1. **c. Ovary.** An ectopic ureter may drain into any of the structures related to the Wolffian duct and can rupture into the adjoining fallopian tube, uterus, upper vagina, or the urethra.

2. **a. Dysplasia.** Clinical and experimental observations combine to support the commonly held notion that dysplasia is the product of inadequate ureteric bud-to-blastema interaction. The other conditions may include such an abnormal interaction but are not specifically the result of that interaction.

3. **c. Orifice being caudal and medial to the lower pole.** The upper pole orifice is caudal and medial to the lower pole orifice because of its later incorporation and migration into the trigonal structure. The lower pole orifice is more cranial and lateral to the caudad medial upper pole orifice.

4. **d. Posterior urethra.** In the male, the posterior urethra is the most common site of the termination of the ectopic ureter. All other sites except the anterior urethra are possible sites of ectopic ureteral insertion.

5. **b. Lax bladder neck.** It is owing to the combined effects of the lateral ureteral orifice position, the ureter's shortened submucosal course, the poorly developed trigone, and the abnormal morphology of the ureteral orifice that primary vesicoureteral reflux develops.

6. **c. Continuous incontinence.** Continuous incontinence in a girl with an otherwise normal voiding pattern after toilet training is the classic symptom of an ectopic ureteral orifice. This may not be obvious in a girl who has not yet been toilet trained, but can occasionally be seen as slow steady dribbling of urine on direct observation.

7. **d. Tortuous lower pole ureter.** The most obvious imaging sign on ultrasonography of an ectopic ureter is a tortuous dilated ureter due to distal obstruction. This is not always present, but when seen should direct further attention to the distal ureter and bladder to also assess for the presence of a ureterocele, which would appear as a cystic structure in the bladder. The upper pole may be dysplastic, but cystic changes are uncommon. The lower pole is usually normal, but may be hydronephrotic, yet uncommonly echogenic. The lower pole is displaced laterally, not medially.

8. **a. Smoking during pregnancy.** Ureteroceles occur most frequently in females (4:1 ratio) and almost exclusively in whites. Approximately 10% are bilateral. Eighty percent of all ureteroceles arise from the upper poles of duplicated systems, and approximately 50% will have associated vesicoureteral reflux.

9. **a. Bladder outlet obstruction.** Ultrasonographic study may show a dilated ureter emanating from a hydronephrotic upper pole. This finding should signal the examiner to image the bladder to determine whether a ureterocele is present. If the lower pole is associated with reflux, or if the ureterocele has caused delayed emptying from the ipsilateral lower pole, this lower pole may likewise be hydronephrotic. Similarly, the ureterocele may impinge on the contralateral ureteral orifice or obstruct the bladder neck and cause hydronephrosis in the opposite kidney, but the latter is uncommon. The upper pole parenchyma drained by the ureterocele will exhibit varying degrees of thickness and echogenicity. Increased echogenicity correlates with dysplastic changes. Reflux may also be seen in the contralateral system if the ureterocele is large enough to distort the trigone and the opposite ureteral submucosal tunnel. In one series, 28% of patients had reflux in the contralateral unit.

10. **c. Ureterocele effacement.** Voiding cystourethrography can usually demonstrate the size and laterality of the ureterocele as well as the presence or absence of vesicoureteral reflux. If early filling views are not obtained, the ureterocele may efface and the filling defect may not be visible. In some cases the ureterocele will evert and appear as a diverticulum.

11. **e. Residual flap of the ureterocele in the urethra.** The authors of one study emphasized the need for passing a large catheter antegrade through the bladder neck to ascertain that all mucosal lips that might act as obstructing valves have been removed. In some large ureteroceles, if repair of the maldeveloped trigone is not adequate, a posterior defect at the bladder neck can act as an obstructive valve during voiding.

12. **d. Transverse incision at the base of the ureterocele.** Our preferred method of incising the ureterocele is similar to that described by Rich and colleagues in 1990, a transverse incision

through the full thickness of the ureterocele wall using the cutting current. The incision should be made as distally on the ureterocele and as close to the bladder floor as possible to lessen the chance of postoperative reflux into the ureterocele.

13. **a. Single-system kidney with a ureterocele.** Excretory urography often demonstrates the characteristic cobra head (or spring-onion) deformity: an area of increased density similar to the head of a cobra with a halo or less dense shadow around it. The halo represents a filling defect, which is the ureterocele wall, and the oval density is contrast material excreted into the ureterocele from the functioning kidney.

14. **b. Puncture of the mass.** A ureterocele that extends through the bladder neck and the urethra and presents as a vaginal mass in girls is termed a prolapsing ureterocele. This mass can be distinguished from other interlabial masses (e.g., rhabdomyosarcoma, urethral prolapse, hydrometrocolpos, and periurethral cysts) by virtue of its appearance and location. The prolapsed ureterocele has a smooth round wall, as compared with the grapelike cluster that typifies rhabdomyosarcoma. The color may vary from pink to bright red to the necrotic shades of blue, purple, or brown. The ureterocele usually slides down the posterior wall of the urethra and, hence, the urethra can be demonstrated anterior to the mass and can be catheterized. The short-term goal is to decompress the ureterocele. The prolapsing ureterocele may be manually reduced back into the bladder; however, even if this is successful, the prolapse is likely to recur. Subsequent management is determined by further functional evaluation.

15. **e. Proceed with dismembered pyeloplasty and resect a fibroepithelial polyp.** This scenario most likely represents a fibroepithelial polyp of the ureteropelvic junction creating or associated with obstruction. The best approach is to proceed with the planned pyeloplasty and identify and resect the polyp thoroughly, followed by performing a conventional dismembered pyeloplasty. At times polyps may be multiple and complex, so this possibility should be looked for.

16. **d. Prophylactic antibiotics, observation, and repeat ultrasound in 4 months.** In the setting of no reflux and a draining upper pole associated with a ureterocele, the option of observation with prophylactic antibiotics has been seen to permit spontaneous resolution and no surgical intervention. Prophylactic antibiotics are recommended until resolution is demonstrated.

17. **c. The duplex kidney arises as a consequence of two separate ureteral buds.** Duplication anomalies arise as a consequence of two ureteral buds forming and inducing separate segments of the metanephric blastema. The duplex kidney may be completely normal, although it tends to be longer than normal, but if there is abnormal development, reflux and ureteropelvic junction obstruction occurs, most often in the lower pole, while ectopic ureteral insertion with or without a ureterocele is nearly always associated with the upper pole.

18. **b and c.** When the upper pole of a duplex system associated with an ectopic ureter demonstrates function, preservation is typically recommended. Two reasonable options exist for this, including proximal ureteropyelostomy which excises most of the usually dilated upper pole ureter, or distal ureteroureterostomy, which permits drainage without any manipulation of the perirenal tissues. There are no data to support one over the other, and both are reasonable options. There is no evidence to indicate that the so called *yo-yo phenomenon* of urine refluxing into more dilated segments of ureter is a clinically significant concern.

19. **c. Possible improvement in trigonal deficiency.** Transurethral puncture of a ureterocele offers all of the listed possible, but not certain, advantages, except to improve trigonal deficiency that can be associated with a severe ureterocele. This deficiency, which may lead to persisting reflux and bladder outlet obstruction, may require corrective surgery.

20. **a. All three ureters joining to terminate in a single bladder orifice.** In the classification used by most investigators, there are four varieties of triplicate ureter. In one variety, all three ureters unite

and drain through a single orifice. This appears to be the most common form encountered although all others have been reported.

21. **b. Subcardinal vein.** If the subcardinal vein in the lumbar portion fails to atrophy and becomes the primary right-sided vein, the ureter is trapped dorsal to it.

22. **c. Intravesical ureterocele.** Several studies have indicated that intravesical ureteroceles fared better than extravesical ureteroceles with regard to decompression, preservation of upper pole function, newly created reflux, and need for secondary procedures. Nonetheless, the clinical scenario will be the most important indicator of the appropriateness of endoscopic incision for a ureterocele in a particular patient.

23. **e. Urinary tract infection.** Many ureteroceles are still diagnosed clinically. The most common presentation is that of an infant who has a urinary tract infection or urosepsis. In the early perinatal period, prenatal identification of hydronephrosis is currently the most common means of diagnosis.

24. **b. Magnetic resonance imaging (MRI) of the abdomen and pelvis.** Occasionally, the renal parenchyma associated with an ectopic ureter is difficult to locate on ultrasound and may be identified only by alternative imaging studies. In such cases in which an ectopic ureter is strongly suspected because of incontinence yet no definite evidence of the upper pole renal segment is found, CT or MRI has demonstrated the small, poorly functioning upper pole segment.

CHAPTER REVIEW

1. An ectopic ureter in a duplex system inevitably drains the upper pole.
2. In females, the ectopic ureter may enter from the bladder neck to the perineum or into the vagina, uterus, or rectum.
3. In males, the ectopic ureter always enters the urogenital system above the external sphincter and may enter wolffian duct structures, such as the vas deferens, seminal vesicles, and ejaculatory duct.
4. The orifice of a cecoureterocele is within the bladder; however, the ureterocele may extend beyond the bladder neck into the urethra.
5. The ectopic ureter inserts into the wolffian duct structure and not directly into a müllerian structure. Therefore, in the female, for an ectopic ureter to enter the vagina, cervix, or uterus, it requires a rupture into those structures.
6. The Weigert-Meyer rule states that an ectopic ureter or ureterocele is associated with the upper pole and is located caudal and medial to the lower pole ureteral orifice.
7. A young boy presenting with epididymitis might have an ectopic ureter.
8. A toilet-trained girl with verified continuous urinary leakage should be evaluated for an ectopic ureter.
9. A ureterocele or ectopic ureter associated with a patulous bladder neck may be complicated by incontinence. Cecoureteroceles are at particular risk for this.
10. On endoscopy, ureteroceles vary in their appearance with bladder filling.
11. An obstructed ureterocele may be treated endoscopically by multiple punctures or by a transverse incision. Both techniques have similar rates of success in decompression. In a transurethral incision of the ureterocele, the incision is made transversely as close to the bladder floor as possible. This may prevent subsequent reflux.
12. In patients with an ectopic ureter who present with sepsis and have massive ureteral dilatation, a temporary end ureterostomy may be the best management.
13. When the upper pole of the kidney is removed for an ectopic ureter, the residual stump is rarely problematic.
14. The separation of duplex ureters distally in the intravesical dissection should be discouraged because it may injure the common blood supply.
15. Conditions that routinely affect the single-system kidney generally affect the lower pole of a duplex system, such as ureteropelvic junction obstruction and vesical ureteral reflux. Conditions that affect the upper pole are more likely due to abnormal ureteral formation, such as ectopia and ureterocele.
16. On a voiding cystourethrogram, if early filling views are not obtained, a ureterocele may efface and the filling defect may not be visible.
17. Fibroepithelial polyps most commonly occur at the ureteropelvic junction but may occur anywhere in the ureter.
18. Correction of the circumcaval ureter requires ureteral division and relocation ventral to the vena cava.
19. When the upper pole of a duplex system associated with an ectopic ureter demonstrates function, preservation of renal tissue is typically recommended. Two reasonable options exist for this, including proximal ureteropyelostomy, which excises most of the usually dilated upper pole ureter, or distal ureteroureterostomy, which permits drainage without any manipulation of the perirenal tissues. No data exist to support one versus the other, and both are reasonable options.

135 Surgical Management of Pediatric Stone Disease

Francis X. Schneck

QUESTIONS

1. Which component(s) of present-day Western diets is(are) thought to contribute to the increasing prevalence of nephrolithiasis in the pediatric population?
   a. Protein
   b. Potassium and magnesium
   c. Saturated fats and cholesterol
   d. Sodium and carbohydrates
   e. Calcium

2. A 5-year-old boy is seen in the office with complaints of intermittent right flank pain. There have been no episodes of nausea, vomiting, or fevers. He has 3+ blood on a urine dip. His physical exam reveals some mild right costovertebral angle (CVA) tenderness. Which imaging modality should be used first?
   a. Magnetic resonance imaging (MRI)
   b. Plain radiograph, kidney-ureter-bladder (KUB)
   c. Ultrasound
   d. Computed tomography (CT) scan
   e. Retrograde pyelogram

3. A 12-year-old girl is found to have a 5-mm left distal ureteral stone after an acute episode of left flank pain. She responded well to conservative therapy (intravenous [IV] hydration and pain medication) and her pain subsides. The next step in management is:
   a. given the size of the stone, it will most likely pass in 6 weeks.
   b. given the size of the stone, it will most likely not pass, and planning for an endourological procedure is advisable.
   c. given the size of the stone, it will most likely not pass, but a trial of oral therapies such as alpha-blockers and steroids may facilitate stone passage.
   d. given the size of the stone, it will most likely not pass, but a trial of oral therapy with a calcium channel blockers may facilitate stone passage.
   e. the stone has most likely passed, and no further interventions will be needed.

4. A 10-year-old male with spina bifida had an augment cystoplasty, bladder neck reconstruction, and bilateral Glenn-Anderson ureteral reimplantation for high-grade reflux at age 7 years. He was found to have a 1-cm renal pelvic stone. The therapy least likely to yield an efficacious (stone-free) result is:
   a. shockwave lithotripsy (SWL).
   b. ureteroscopy with laser lithotripsy.
   c. ureteral stenting and ureteroscopy with laser lithotripsy 6 weeks later.
   d. percutaneous nephrolithotomy (PCNL).
   e. open pyelolithotomy.

5. With regard to SWL in the treatment of pediatric nephrolithiasis, treatment failures are associated with:
   a. high stone burdens (i.e., 2-cm calcium oxalate monohydrate stone).
   b. sizeable infundibular length.
   c. an infundibulopelvic angle greater than 45 degrees.
   d. staghorn calculi.
   e. a, b, and c.

6. Complications that may occur during ureteroscopy while treating a ureteral stone include:
   a. hypothermia and hyponatremia.
   b. ureteral avulsion.
   c. hypertension.
   d. all of the above.
   e. a and b.

7. A 9-year-old female with cystinuria is found to have a right 2-cm renal pelvic stone. The best treatment option to treat her stone is:
   a. extracorporeal SWL (ESWL).
   b. ureteroscopy with laser lithotripsy and stone basketing.
   c. PCNL.
   d. medical therapy with potassium citrate and tiopronin.
   e. anatrophic nephrolithotomy.

8. The most common chemical composition of a bladder stone found in a child from a developing country would be:
   a. struvite.
   b. ammonium acid urate.
   c. uric acid.
   d. calcium oxalate monohydrate.
   e. calcium oxalate dehydrate.

ANSWERS

1. **d. Sodium and carbohydrates.** It has been speculated that diets rich in sodium and carbohydrates may be a contributing factor to the etiology of urolithiasis in this cohort of children.

2. **c. Ultrasound.** Ultrasound has a more limited role in the assessment of urolithiasis compared with CT but has the distinct advantage of no associated ionizing radiation. Therefore, ultrasound should be considered as a screening tool in the workup for nonemergent abdominal or flank pain.

3. **b. Given the size of the stone, it will most likely not pass, and planning for an endourological procedure is advisable.** In managing stone disease in the pediatric population, it is important to note that renal calculi smaller than 3 mm are likely to spontaneously pass, and stones 4 mm or larger in the distal ureter are likely to require endourologic treatment. This information should be relayed to caregivers and parents.

4. **a. Shockwave lithotripsy (SWL).** Recent data suggest that stone free rates in children with a history of urologic condition or urinary tract reconstruction are quite low (12.5%) and may be better served with ureterorenoscopy or PCNL.

5. **e. a, b, and c.** SWL failure and retreatment rates were associated with increased mean stone burden, increased infundibular length, and infundibulopelvic angle greater than 45 degrees. Staghorn calculi are uncommon in children and represent a management challenge. Although monotherapy success rates are low in adults, acceptable stone-free rates in children have been achieved with SWL.

6. **e. a and b.** Irrigating fluid, which may be used under pressure, should be isotonic and body temperature to avoid hypothermia and hyponatremia Other complications of ureteroscopy include unrecognized ureteral injury including mucosal flaps and tears, perforation, false passage, and partial to complete avulsion. Hypertension is not a recognized complication of ureteroscopy.

7. **c. PCNL.** This child would be best served with a PCNL because of the large stone burden. Although ureteroscopy is an option, multiple sessions would most likely be required. Cystine stones do not respond well to SWL. Medical therapy helps to prevent cystine stones, not treat them. Anatrophic nephrolithotomy is not an appropriate surgical treatment for this stone.

8. **b. Ammonium acid urate.** Bladder stones are more often found in children from developing countries and are thought to be related endemically to malnutrition. It is thought that diets low in animal protein and phosphorus (breast milk as opposed to cow's milk) in addition to vitamin A deficiency are contributory. Bladder stones from children in these developing countries are most often composed of ammonium acid urate. In contrast, among children from industrialized nations, bladder stones are most often found in those with spinal cord injuries or congenital abnormalities such as spina bifida. Very often these children have undergone augment cystoplasty and/or manage their bladders by clean intermittent catheterization.

CHAPTER REVIEW

1. Although reference ranges for 24-hour urine metabolites in children who form stones are not standardized, initial workup should include a 24-hour urine for creatinine, sodium, calcium, oxalate, uric acid, and citrate.

2. A metabolic abnormality is often present in pediatric stone formers; hypocitraturia is the most common abnormality.

3. An unenhanced helical CT scan is the imaging modality of choice in a patient with a suspected stone or in a known stone former; however, ultrasound should be used as a screen in a patient with nonemergent abdominal or flank pain to limit radiation exposure.

4. There has been a dramatic increase in pediatric nephrolithiasis, especially among white adolescent females.

5. Renal/ureteral calculi smaller than 3 mm are likely to spontaneously pass; calculi larger than 4 mm usually require endourologic management.

6. There is a theoretical risk that children treated with SWL will develop diabetes or hypertension.

7. Perioperative antibiotics are indicated for those patients requiring urologic instrumentation.

8. SWL has been the preferred treatment for proximal ureteral and renal calculi smaller than 15 mm.

9. Ureteral stenting after a procedure should be considered in patients with solitary kidneys, staghorn calculi, large ureteral calculi, prior obstruction, or abnormal anatomy. It may also be used to dilate the small ureter prior to ureteroscopy.

10. SWL has a poor success rate for stones with densities greater than 1000 Hounsfield units and those with previous urinary tract reconstruction.

11. Dilation of the pediatric ureter does not result in an unacceptable risk of the development of reflux or stricture.

12. Contraindications for ureteroscopic stone management include staghorn calculi, recurrent stone formers amenable to PCNL, and those with anatomic abnormalities precluding retrograde access.

13. Distal ureteral stones are best managed ureteroscopically.

14. Ureteroscopy should be performed under general anesthesia with the patient paralyzed. Isotonic body-temperature fluids should be used for the irrigant.

15. The most common complication of ureteroscopy is an unrecognized ureteral injury.

16. Indications for PCNL include a stone burden greater than 1.5 cm, lower pole calculi greater than 1.0 cm, calculi of cystine or struvite composition, and anatomic abnormalities making stone clearance difficult.

17. Spinal deformities may alter the anatomic location of the kidney, increasing the incidence of adjacent organ injury during percutaneous access.

18. Bladder stones in children in underdeveloped countries are due to malnutrition—a diet low in animal protein, phosphorus, and vitamin A—and usually consist of ammonium acid urate. In developed countries, bladder calculi are usually due to a neurogenic bladder or a reconstructed bladder.

19. Fifty percent of children with a reconstructed bladder will develop stones. Factors that play a role include stasis, bacterial colonization, retained mucus, or foreign body. The composition is usually struvite.

20. Percutaneous cystolithotripsy is the preferred method of managing bladder calculi in children.

136

Development and Assessment of Lower Urinary Tract Function in Children

Chung Kwong Yeung, Stephen Shei-Dei Yang, and Piet Hoebeke

QUESTIONS

1. Development of normal bladder function involves which of the following changes?
   a. Decrease in urine production and increase in bladder capacity
   b. Increase in urine production and increase in voiding frequency
   c. Increase in bladder capacity and decrease in voiding frequency
   d. Decrease in voided volume and increase in voiding frequency
   e. Increase in bladder capacity and no change in voided volume

2. Which of the following statements best describes urodynamic findings of maximum detrusor pressures with micturition (P_{det}max) in young infants with normal lower urinary tracts?
   a. There is no difference in P_{det}max compared with that in adults.
   b. Lower P_{det}max is observed in young infants compared with adults.
   c. Higher P_{det}max is observed in male infants only.
   d. Higher P_{det}max is observed in female infants only.
   e. Higher P_{det}max is observed in both male and female infants.

3. Which of the following statements on neurologic control of normal micturition is INCORRECT?
   a. Innervation of the bladder involves both the central somatic and the autonomic nervous system.
   b. Micturition is initiated with a full bladder by a simple spinal cord reflex.
   c. Micturition does not occur during sleep.
   d. Development of direct volitional control over the bladder-sphincter complex occurs.
   e. Neurologic control occurs at different levels of the central nervous system from spinal cord to brainstem.

4. The following is characteristic of children with urge syndrome:
   a. Vincent's curtsy sign.
   b. hold maneuver.
   c. urgency.
   d. small bladder capacity.
   e. all of the above.

5. Regarding normal parameters of lower urinary tract function, which statement is INCORRECT?
   a. Low bladder compliance (less than 20 mL H_2O) is frequently associated with neuropathic lower urinary tract dysfunction (LUTD) and may have detrimental effects on the upper tracts.
   b. The International Children's Continence Society (ICCS) views 6 years as the minimum age to adequately report lower urinary tract symptoms, and 5 years as the minimum age for functional bowel dysfunction.
   c. ICCS defines increased daytime urinary frequency as eight or more voids per day and decreased daytime urinary frequency as three or fewer voids per day.
   d. Bladder outlet obstruction can be suspected in cases with a Qmax less than 11.5 mL/sec (patients aged 4 to 6 years) or less than 15.0 mL/sec (patients aged 7 to 12 years).
   e. For children aged 4 to 6 years, repetitive postvoid residual (PVR) greater than 20 mL or greater than 10% bladder capacity (BC) can be regarded as elevated. For children aged 7 to 12 years, repetitive PVR greater than 10 mL or 6% BC can be defined as elevated.

6. A 7-year-old boy complains of daytime urinary urgency without daytime incontinence or nocturnal enuresis. Which of the following statements is INCORRECT?
   a. Urinalysis should be done to exclude urinary tract infection.
   b. Frequency-volume chart is necessary to document whether he has small voided volume throughout the day.
   c. Uroflowmetry may disclose a staccato flow pattern suggesting dysfunctional voiding.
   d. Postvoid residual urine may be normal or elevated.
   e. Anticholinergics will be the first-line treatment for him.

7. Regarding dysfunctional voiding, which statement is INCORRECT?
   a. Dysfunctional voiding is characterized by an intermittent and/or fluctuating flow rate due to intermittent contractions of the periurethral striated or levator ani muscles during voiding in neurologically normal children.
   b. A uroflow with electromyogram (EMG) or a videourodynamic study is required to document dysfunctional voiding.
   c. Staccato, interrupted, plateau, and even normal flow patterns can be observed in children with dysfunctional voiding.
   d. Dysfunctional voiding is frequently associated with urinary tract infection (UTI), vesicoureteral reflux, and various types of LUTS.
   e. Dysfunctional voiding is frequently observed in children after 1 year.

8. A 13-year-old boy complains of persistent nocturnal enuresis after medical treatment with antidiuretic hormone. Uroflowmetry disclosed voided volume = 250 ml, Qmax = 11.3 ml/s, plateau shaped curve. Postvoid residual urine was 10 ml. Which statement is incorrect?
   a. He may have congenital bladder outlet obstruction.
   b. If he had delayed bladder neck opening time (more than 4 seconds), he may have primary bladder neck dysfunction.
   c. Because he had a plateau-shaped uroflowmetry curve, discoordinated sphincter is unlikely.
   d. If image studies such as voiding cystography or videourodynamic study disclosed point stenosis at anterior urethra, an anterior urethral valve can be diagnosed.
   e. None of the above.

9. A 3-year-old girl is seen with febrile UTI and left grade 3 vesicoureteral reflux (VUR). She had an uroflowmetry of voided volume = 200 mL, Qmax = 22 mL/sec, and staccato flow pattern. Postvoid residual urine was 22 mL.

   a. She may have dysfunctional voiding.

   b. The predicted success rate of antireflux surgery is around 95%.

   c. Bladder overdistention may be the cause of staccato flow pattern.

   d. Fluid restriction and timed voiding may reverse this abnormal voiding pattern.

   e. Abnormal voiding posture may be the cause of staccato flow pattern.

ANSWERS

1. **c. Increase in bladder capacity and decrease in voiding frequency.** Development of normal bladder function involves an increase in bladder capacity in response to an increase in urine production. The voiding frequency decreases, whereas the voided volume of each micturition increases with age.

2. **e. Higher P_{det}max is observed in both male and female infants.** Urodynamic studies of infants with normal lower urinary tracts have documented significantly higher P_{det}max in both male and female infants compared with adults, although it was also noted that male infants had significantly higher P_{det}max compared with female infants.

3. **b. Micturition is initiated with a full bladder by a simple spinal cord reflex.** Studies have shown that even in full-term fetuses and newborns, micturition is modulated by higher centers.

4. **e. All of the above.** Detrusor overactivity during filling causes frequent attacks of sudden and imperative sensations of urge (urgency) which are often counteracted by voluntary contraction of the pelvic floor muscles in an attempt to compress the urethra (hold maneuver) exhibited as squatting (Vincent's curtsy+ sign). Children with urge syndrome have small bladder capacities for age.

5. **b. The International Children's Continence Society (ICCS) views 6 years as the minimum age to adequately report lower urinary tract symptoms, and 5 years as the minimum for functional bowel dysfunction.** ICCS defines 5 years of age as the minimum age to adequately report lower urinary tract symptoms (LUTS) and 4 years for functional bowel dysfunction.

6. **e. Anticholinergics will be the first-line treatment for him.** Based on the measurement of PVR, Thom et al. classified overactive bladder (OAB) as complete or incomplete emptying. Anticholinergics were recommended for OAB with complete emptying, and α-adrenergic antagonists for OAB with incomplete emptying (Thom, 2012).*

7. **e. Dysfunctional voiding is frequently observed in children after 1 year.** Dysfunctional voiding is frequently observed in infancy and subsides after 1 year of age.

8. **c. Because he had a plateau-shaped uroflowmetry curve, discoordinated sphincter is unlikely.** A discoordinated sphincter may occasionally present as a plateau-shaped curve.

9. **b. The predicted success rate of antireflux surgery is around 95%.** Operation for VUR associated with LUTD usually results in a lower success rate.

CHAPTER REVIEW

1. In infants and young children, the bladder is an abdominal organ and can readily be palpated when full.

2. Development of normal bladder function involves an increase in bladder capacity in response to an increase in urine production. The voiding frequency decreases, whereas the voided volume of each micturition increases with age.

3. Urodynamic studies of infants with normal lower urinary tracts have documented significantly higher P_{det}max in both male and female infants compared with adults, although it was also noted that male infants had significantly higher P_{det}max compared with female infants.

4. Immature detrusor sphincter coordination manifested as detrusor hypercontractility and interrupted voiding commonly occurs in the first 2 years of life and results in functional bladder outflow obstruction.

5. Even in newborns, micturition does not occur during sleep, suggesting modulation of micturition by higher centers.

6. The association of constipation with urologic pathology is referred to as the *dysfunctional elimination syndrome* (bladder bowel dysfunction). Abnormalities of bowel function are commonly present in young children with voiding dysfunction. These children tend to have more psychological difficulties, such as attention problems and oppositional behavior.

7. Giggle incontinence often results in complete emptying of the bladder.

8. In patients who develop acquired bladder sphincter dysfunction, a significant proportion also have bowel dysfunction.

9. There is a significant association of bladder dysfunction with nonresolution of high-grade vesicoureteral reflux.

10. In children, there is a poor correlation between maximal flow rate and outflow resistance. It is better to study the pattern of the flow curve.

11. In any evaluation of voiding dysfunction, abnormalities of the lower spine should be sought.

12. Nocturnal urine output in many enuretic children is in excess of bladder reservoir capacity during sleep.

13. Many enuretic children have a marked reduction in functional bladder capacity when compared with age-matched controls, and may have detrusor instability as well.

14. Normal voiding frequency by age is as follows: age 2 to 4 weeks: once per hour; age 2 to 3 years: 8 to 10 times per day; age 12 years: 4 to 6 times per day.

15. A positive family history may be present in many cases of non-neurologic LUTS in children.

16. All children with LUT dysfunction should have a screening ultrasound study, which should also include an assessment of residual urine.

17. Ultrasound measurement of bladder wall thickness is correlated with LUT dysfunction in children.

18. In general, a PVR greater than 20 mL is abnormal in children.

---

*Sources referenced can be found in *Campbell-Walsh Urology, 11th Edition*, on the Expert Consult website.

137 Vesicoureteral Reflux

Antoine E. Khoury and Darius J. Bägli

QUESTIONS

1. The estimated prevalence of vesicoureteral reflux in children with a urinary tract infection (UTI) is:
   a. 1%.
   b. 3%.
   c. 5%.
   d. 10%.
   e. 30%.

2. Which of the following statements regarding reflux is FALSE?
   a. Antenatally detected reflux is associated with a male preponderance.
   b. Antenatally detected reflux is usually low grade in boys when compared with that in girls.
   c. Antenatally detected reflux is usually bilateral in boys when compared with that in girls.
   d. When reflux is detected antenatally, renal impairment is frequently present at birth and is likely due to congenital dysplasia.
   e. The majority of reflux detected later in life occurs in females.

3. Which of the following statements regarding vesicoureteral reflux in regard to patient's race is TRUE?
   a. The incidence of vesicoureteral reflux is equal in children of all races.
   b. The disparity in the incidence of vesicoureteral reflux with respect to race becomes clearer in adulthood.
   c. The frequency of detected vesicoureteral reflux is lower in female children of African descent.
   d. African infants and white infants have a similar incidence of reflux, diagnosed on the basis of antenatal hydronephrosis.
   e. There is a clear understanding regarding the predisposition of reflux, because many of the studies have included patients from different countries around the world.

4. Which of the following statements is FALSE in regard to the diagnosis and treatment of sibling vesicoureteral reflux?
   a. On the basis of clinical judgment and the presence or absence of urinary tract infection (UTI), the patient's age should be taken into account in regard to the decision to proceed with diagnostic intervention to diagnose sibling reflux.
   b. It is reasonable to prescribe antibiotic prophylaxis while the decision to diagnose sibling reflux or not takes place.
   c. Once sibling reflux is diagnosed, the indications for correction are different from the indications for treating reflux in the general pediatric population diagnosed after UTI.
   d. Siblings who are younger than 5 years with normal imaging studies of the kidneys can be managed on the basis of clinical judgment, and it is not absolutely necessary to obtain a voiding cystogram.
   e. Siblings younger than 5 years who present with cortical renal defects have the most to lose by febrile UTIs in the presence of vesicoureteral reflux.

5. Primary reflux is a congenital anomaly of the ureterovesical junction with which of the following characteristics? A deficiency of the:
   a. longitudinal muscle of the extravesical ureter results in an inadequate valvular mechanism.
   b. longitudinal muscle of the intravesical ureter results in an inadequate valvular mechanism.
   c. circumferential muscle of the extravesical ureter results in an inadequate valvular mechanism.
   d. circumferential muscle of the intravesical ureter results in an inadequate valvular mechanism.
   e. longitudinal and circumferential muscles of the intravesical ureter results in an inadequate valvular mechanism.

6. What is the ratio of tunnel length to ureteral diameter found in normal children without reflux?
   a. 5:1
   b. 4:1
   c. 3:1
   d. 2:1
   e. 1:1

7. Which of the following statements is TRUE regarding children with non-neurogenic neurogenic bladders?
   a. Constriction of the urinary sphincter occurs during voiding in a voluntary form of detrusor-sphincter dyssynergia.
   b. Gradual bladder decompensation and myogenic failure result from incomplete emptying.
   c. Gradual bladder decompensation and myogenic failure result from increasing amounts of residual urine.
   d. All of the above.
   e. None of the above.

8. Which of the following statements is TRUE in regard to secondary vesicoureteral reflux?
   a. The most common cause of anatomic bladder obstruction in the pediatric population is posterior urethral valves, and vesicoureteral reflux is present in a great majority of these children.
   b. Anatomic obstruction of the bladder is a common cause of secondary vesicoureteral reflux in female patients.
   c. Patients with neurofunctional etiology for secondary vesicoureteral reflux benefit from immediate surgical intervention to try to correct vesicoureteral reflux.
   d. A sacral dimple or hairy patch on the lower back is not a significant finding in regard to evaluation and treatment of vesicoureteral reflux.
   e. The most common structural obstruction in male and female patients is the presence of a ureterocele at the bladder neck.

9. The complex anatomic relationships required of the ureterovesical junction may be gradually damaged by:
   a. decreases in bladder wall compliance.
   b. detrusor decompensation.
   c. incomplete emptying.

d. all of the above.

e. none of the above.

10. What does the initial management of functional causes of reflux involve?

a. Surgical treatment

b. Medical treatment

c. Observation only

d. All of the above

e. None of the above

11. Signs or symptoms of bladder dysfunction include:

a. dribbling.

b. urgency.

c. incontinence.

d. "curtsying" behavior in girls.

e. all of the above.

12. Treatment of bladder dysfunction and detrusor overactivity, regardless of its severity or cause, is directed at:

a. damping overactive detrusor contractions.

b. dilating the urethral sphincter.

c. lowering intravesical pressures.

d. all of the above.

e. a and c only.

13. There is a strong association between the presence of reflux in patients with neuropathic bladders and intravesical pressures of greater than:

a. 10 cm H_2O.

b. 20 cm H_2O.

c. 40 cm H_2O.

d. 60 cm H_2O.

e. 80 cm H_2O.

14. Bladder infections and their accompanying inflammation can also cause reflux by:

a. lessening compliance.

b. elevating intravesical pressures.

c. distorting and weakening the ureterovesical junction.

d. all of the above.

e. none of the above.

15. Which system provides the current standard for grading reflux on the basis of the appearance of contrast in the ureter and upper collecting system during voiding cystourethrography?

a. The Heikel and Parkkulainen System

b. The International Classification system

c. The Dwoskin and Perlmutter system

d. The National Classification System

e. The Dwoskin and Parkkulainen system

16. Which of the following is TRUE regarding accurately grading reflux with coexistent ipsilateral ureteropelvic junction (UPJ) obstruction?

a. It is not possible.

b. It is facilitated by obtaining a renal scan.

c. It is facilitated by obtaining an ultrasonographic scan.

d. It is facilitated by obtaining a computed tomographic (CT) urogram.

e. It is facilitated by obtaining a radionuclide cystogram.

17. Which of the following is TRUE regarding the presence of fever?

a. It may be an indicator of upper urinary tract involvement.

b. It may not always be a reliable sign of upper urinary tract involvement.

c. It increases the likelihood of discovering vesicoureteral reflux.

d. All of the above.

e. None of the above.

18. Complete evaluation including a voiding cystourethrogram (VCUG) and ultrasound are required for which of the following patients?

a. An uncircumcised male infant with a febrile illness and a positive urine culture obtained through a bagged specimen

b. A 3-year-old girl admitted to the hospital with pneumonia and found to have *Escherichia coli* on a urine culture without pyuria detected by microscopic analysis

c. A female patient with recurrent culture and urinalysis proven to have afebrile UTIs and later found to have scarring on a dimercaptosuccinic acid (DMSA) scan

d. Any child older than 5 years with documented UTIs

e. None of the above

19. Which of the following statements is TRUE regarding screening of older children who present with asymptomatic bacteriuria. They can be screened initially with:

a. ultrasonography.

b. cystography.

c. CT urogram.

d. renal scan.

e. nothing because they do not require any screening studies.

20. Which of the following is TRUE regarding cystography?

a. Cystography performed with a Foley catheter or while the patient is under anesthesia produces static studies that inaccurately screen for reflux or sometimes exaggerate its degree because of bladder overfilling.

b. Cystography performed in the presence of excessive hydration may mask low grades of reflux because diuresis can blunt the retrograde flow of urine.

c. Cystograms may show reflux only during active infections when cystitis weakens the ureterovesical junction with edema or by increasing intravesical pressures.

d. Cystograms obtained during active infections can overestimate the grade of reflux because the endotoxins produced by some gram-negative organisms can paralyze ureteral smooth muscle and exaggerate ureteral dilatation.

e. All of the above.

21. Which of the following statements is TRUE regarding radionuclide cystography?

a. It provides similar anatomic detail to that obtained with fluoroscopic cystography.

b. It is an accurate method for detecting and following reflux.

c. It is associated with more radiation exposure than is fluoroscopic cystography.

d. It is a less sensitive test than fluoroscopic cystography.

e. It provides more anatomic detail than fluoroscopic cystography.

22. Which of the following statements is TRUE regarding ultrasonography?

a. It is the diagnostic study of choice to initially evaluate the upper urinary tracts of patients with suspected or proven vesicoureteral reflux.

b. It can effectively rule out reflux.

c. It should be performed every 2 to 3 years in patients with reflux who are medically managed.

d. It is the study of choice for assessing renal function.

e. An ultrasonogram showing intermittent dilatation of the renal pelvis or ureter confirms the presence of reflux.

23. What is the best study for the detection of pyelonephritis and cortical renal scarring?

 a. Diethylenetriaminepentaacetic acid (DTPA) renal scan

 b. DMSA renal scan

 c. Mercaptoacetyltriglycine (MAG3) renal scan

 d. CT urogram

 e. Renal ultrasonographic scan

24. Which of the following is TRUE regarding urodynamic studies?

 a. They may be indicated in any child suspected of having a secondary cause for reflux (valves, neurogenic bladder, nonneurogenic neurogenic bladder, voiding dysfunction).

 b. They should be performed without the use of prophylactic antibiotics in children with secondary reflux.

 c. They help direct therapy in patients with secondary reflux.

 d. All of the above.

 e. Only a and c are true.

25. Which of the following is TRUE in regard to the evaluation of vesicoureteral reflux?

 a. Routine cystoscopy is indicated in the workup of patients with vesicoureteral reflux.

 b. The radiation doses with modern digital techniques have improved the anatomic detail, but the radiation dose with VCUG remains significantly higher than that of a radionuclide cystogram.

 c. Grading of reflux by VCUG and radionuclide cystogram is similar and comparable between the two imaging modalities.

 d. Ultrasonography provides an alternative means to evaluate the presence or absence of vesicoureteral reflux.

 e. Uroflowmetry is a valuable tool in the workup of a patient with vesicoureteral reflux.

26. Which of the following accurately describes what happens during ureteral development? A ureteral bud that:

 a. is medially (caudally) positioned from a normal takeoff at the trigone offers an embryologic explanation for primary reflux.

 b. is laterally (cranially) positioned from a normal takeoff at the trigone offers an embryologic explanation for primary reflux.

 c. fails to meet with the renal blastema offers an embryologic explanation for primary reflux.

 d. is laterally (cranially) positioned is often obstructed.

 e. fails to meet with the renal blastema is often obstructed.

27. In regard to the diagnosis of renal scars based on renal scintigraphy, which of the following is TRUE?

 a. An area of photopenia detected during an acute episode of pyelonephritis always represents renal scar.

 b. Photopenic areas may result from postinfection renal scarring and some renal dysplasia.

 c. Ultrasound is a sensitive and accurate diagnostic modality for renal scarring.

 d. Areas for photopenia detected during an acute episode of pyelonephritis that later resolve on a subsequent renal scan represent resolution of renal scarring.

 e. All of the above.

28. Which of the following is TRUE regarding hypertension?

 a. In children and young adults, it is most commonly caused by reflux nephropathy.

 b. It is not related to the grade of reflux or severity of scarring.

 c. It is not associated with abnormalities of Na^+,K^+-ATPase activity.

 d. All of the above.

 e. None of the above.

29. Which of the following factors might contribute to the effects of reflux on renal growth?

 a. The congenital dysmorphism often associated with, but not caused by, reflux?

 b. The number and type of urinary infections and their resultant nephropathy

 c. The quality of the contralateral kidney and its implications for compensatory hypertrophy

 d. The grade of reflux in the affected kidney

 e. All of the above

30. Which of the following statements is FALSE in regard to bladder and bowel dysfunction (BBD) and vesicoureteral reflux (VUR)?

 a. BBD lowers VUR resolution rates.

 b. BBD is associated with higher recurrence rates of VUR after successful endoscopic correction.

 c. BBD reduces the success rate of endoscopic implantation of dextranomer/hyaluronic copolymer (Dx/HA) and open surgical correction of VUR.

 d. BBD is associated with higher breakthrough infection rates.

 e. BBD is associated with increased incidence of UTI after surgery.

31. The anatomy of patients with ureteral duplication typically follows the Weigert-Meyer rule, in which the upper pole ureter enters the bladder:

 a. distally and medially, and the lower pole ureter enters the bladder proximally and laterally.

 b. proximally and medially, and the lower pole ureter enters the bladder distally and laterally.

 c. distally and laterally, and the lower pole ureter enters the bladder proximally and medially.

 d. proximally and laterally, and the lower pole ureter enters the bladder distally and medially.

 e. superior to the lower pole ureter.

32. Which of the following is not found to be associated with higher success rate of endoscopic correction of VUR?

 a. Volume of Dx/HA used

 b. Surgeon experience

 c. Volcano-shaped mound with no hydrodistention

 d. Negative intraoperative cystogram

 e. Utilization of the double hydrodistention-implantation technique

33. Which of the following accurately describes the state of the bladder during pregnancy?

 a. Urine volume decreases in the upper collecting system while the physiologic dilatation of pregnancy evolves.

 b. Bladder tone increases because of edema and hyperemia.

 c. Bladder changes predispose the patient to bacteriuria.

 d. All of the above.

 e. None of the above.

34. During pregnancy, the presence of vesicoureteral reflux in a system already prone to bacteriuria may lead to increased morbidity. What is an additional risk factor?
    a. Renal scarring
    b. Tendency toward urinary infections
    c. Hypertension
    d. Renal insufficiency
    e. All of the above

35. Which of the following statements is considered to be FALSE regarding reflux management?
    a. Spontaneous resolution of vesicoureteral reflux is common.
    b. Higher grades of vesicoureteral reflux are less likely to resolve than lower grades.
    c. Reflux of sterile urine is a benign process that does not lead to significant renal damage.
    d. The 2014 *New England Journal of Medicine* Randomized Intervention for Children with Vesicoureteral Reflux (RIVUR) study reported a 0.5% incidence of adverse reaction to prophylactic antibiotics and a 2% incidence of adverse reaction to the placebo.
    e. All of the above.

36. Regarding surgical correction of vesicoureteral reflux, which of the following is currently accepted?
    a. Extravesical ureteral reimplantation
    b. Intravesical ureteral reimplantation
    c. Endoscopic injection of bulking agent
    d. All of the above
    e. None of the above

37. Common to each type of open surgical repair for reflux is the creation of:
    a. a valvular mechanism that enables ureteral compression with bladder filling and contraction.
    b. a mucosal tunnel for reimplantation having adequate muscular backing.
    c. a tunnel length of three times the ureteral diameter.
    d. all of the above.
    e. none of the above.

38. Complete ureteral duplications with reflux can be best managed surgically by:
    a. separating the ureters and reimplanting them separately.
    b. a common sheath repair in which both ureters are mobilized with one mucosal cuff.
    c. performing an upper to lower ureteroureterostomy and reimplanting the lower ureter.
    d. performing a lower to upper ureteroureterostomy and reimplanting the upper ureter.
    e. none of the above.

39. Early postoperative obstruction can occur after a ureteral reimplant due to:
    a. edema.
    b. subtrigonal bleeding.
    c. twist or angulation of the ureter.
    d. blood clots.
    e. all of the above.

40. If early postoperative obstruction occurs after a ureteral reimplant, the next step is:
    a. immediate nephrostomy tube placement.
    b. immediate placement of a ureteral stent.

c. initial observation and diversion for unabating symptoms.
d. placement of both a nephrostomy tube and a ureteral stent.
e. reoperation.

41. Which of the following is TRUE regarding persistent reflux after ureteral reimplantation?
    a. It may be due to unrecognized secondary causes of reflux such as neuropathic bladder and severe voiding dysfunction.
    b. It seldom results from a failure to provide adequate muscular backing for the ureter within its tunnel.
    c. It may be repaired surgically by using minor submucosal advancements.
    d. All of the above.
    e. None of the above.

42. Which of the following is TRUE regarding the treatment of vesicoureteral reflux?
    a. Since the widespread acceptance of endoscopic treatment, the indications for surgical correction differ between the open endoscopic and laparoscopic approaches.
    b. Long-term follow-up data support the durability of endoscopic injection therapy.
    c. All injection materials provide a similar success rate and are just as easily injected under similar circumstances.
    d. The accuracy of the needle entry point during endoscopic injection, as well as the needle placement, are important components for the success of the surgical procedure.
    e. The learning curve for endoscopic injection is similar to the learning curve for open surgical reimplantation.

43. Which of the following is TRUE regarding the laparoscopic approach for ureteral reimplantation?
    a. The advantages of this approach versus open surgery include smaller incisions, less discomfort, and quicker convalescence.
    b. As with other laparoscopic procedures, experience is essential to the success of this approach.
    c. Costs may be increased because of lengthier surgery and the expense of disposable equipment.
    d. All of the above.
    e. None of the above.

44. After discontinuation of continuous antibiotic prophylaxis (CAP) in toilet-trained children: who is likely to develop recurrent UTI?
    a. Patients with higher grades of VUR
    b. Uncircumcised male children
    c. Children with BBD
    d. All of the above
    e. a and c only

45. Which patients were more likely to have febrile or symptomatic recurrences in the RIVUR Trial?
    a. Children with grade III or IV reflux at baseline
    b. Patients presenting with febrile index infection
    c. The presence of BBD at baseline
    d. All of the above
    e. a and c only

46. The 2011 American Academy of Pediatrics guidelines for management of the initial UTI in febrile infants and children age 2 to 24 months recommend obtaining:
    a. A renal and bladder ultrasound and a VCUG during the febrile episode
    b. A renal and bladder ultrasound and a VCUG 3 weeks after the febrile episode has resolved

c. A DMSA renal scan and, if positive, a VCUG

d. A renal and bladder ultrasound after confirmation of UTI by a properly collected urine specimen for culture and analysis

e. Wait for the second infection before performing any radiological testing

ANSWERS

1. **e. 30%.** A meta-analysis of studies of children undergoing cystography for various indications has indicated that the prevalence of vesicoureteral reflux is estimated to be 30% for children with UTIs and approximately 17% in children without infection.

2. **b. Antenatally detected reflux is usually low grade in boys when compared with that in girls.** The reflux is usually high grade and bilateral in boys when compared with reflux in girls.

3. **c. The frequency of detected vesicoureteral reflux is lower in female children of African descent.** One of the clear differences that has been established with several studies is the relative tenfold lower frequency of vesicoureteral reflux in female children of African descent.

4. **c. Once sibling reflux is diagnosed, the indications for correction are different from the indications for treating reflux in the general pediatric population diagnosed after UTI.** By taking into account the imaging of the kidneys first, as well as the patient's age and history of UTI, a rational top-down approach to sibling reflux screening emerges. In any sibling, however, in whom reflux is diagnosed, the indications for treatment remain the same as for general reflux in the pediatric population.

5. **b. Longitudinal muscle of the intravesical ureter results in an inadequate valvular mechanism.** Primary reflux is a congenital anomaly of the ureterovesical junction in which a deficiency of the longitudinal muscle of the intravesical ureter results in an inadequate valvular mechanism.

6. **a. 5:1.** In Paquin's novel study, a 5:1 tunnel length–ureteral diameter ratio was found in normal children without reflux.

7. **d. All of the above.** On the far end of this spectrum are children with non-neurogenic neurogenic bladders. Here, constriction of the urinary sphincter occurs during voiding in a voluntary form of detrusor-sphincter dyssynergia. Gradual bladder decompensation and myogenic failure result from incomplete emptying and increasing amounts of residual urine.

8. **a. The most common cause of anatomic bladder obstruction in the pediatric population is posterior urethral valves, and vesicoureteral reflux is present in a great majority of these children.** This diagnosis is obviously limited to male patients; consequently, female patients have a lower incidence of anatomic bladder obstruction. The most common structural obstruction in female patients is the presence of a ureterocele that prolapses and obstructs the bladder neck. Between 48% and 70% of patients with posterior urethral valves have vesicoureteral reflux, and relief of obstruction appears to be responsible for resolution of the reflux in a good number of those patients. The presence of a neurologic disorder should prompt the clinician to treat based on the primary etiology as opposed to proceeding with immediate surgical correction. One important aspect of the physical examination in children who present with vesicoureteral reflux is detection of potential occult spinal dysraphism, and this includes a thorough physical examination looking for sacral dimples, hairy patches, or gluteal cleft abnormalities.

9. **d. All of the above.** Decreases in bladder wall compliance, detrusor decompensation, and incomplete emptying gradually damage the complex anatomic relationships required of the ureterovesical junction.

10. **b. Medical treatment.** The initial management of functional causes of reflux is medical. It is imperative that clinicians inquire about, and determine, the voiding patterns of children with reflux.

11. **e. All of the above.** In addition to a careful physical examination, signs or symptoms of bladder dysfunction include dribbling, urgency, and incontinence. Girls often exhibit curtsying behavior, and boys will squeeze the penis in an attempt to suppress bladder contractions.

12. **e. a and c only.** Treatment of bladder dysfunction and detrusor overactivity, regardless of its severity or cause, is directed at dampening overactive detrusor contractions and lowering intravesical pressures.

13. **c. 40 cm H_2O.** There is a strong association between intravesical pressures of greater than 40 cm H_2O and the presence of reflux in patients with myelodysplasia and neuropathic bladders.

14. **d. All of the above.** Bladder infections (UTIs) and their accompanying inflammation can also cause reflux by lessening compliance, elevating intravesical pressures, and distorting and weakening the ureterovesical junction.

15. **b. The International Classification System.** The Heikel and Parkkulainen system gained popularity in Europe a few years before the Dwoskin and Perlmutter system became widely accepted in the United States. The International Classification System, devised in 1981 by the International Reflux Study, represents a melding of the two. It provides the current standard for grading reflux on the basis of the appearance of contrast in the ureter and upper collecting system during voiding cystourethrography.

16. **a. It is not possible.** Accurately grading reflux is impossible with coexistent ipsilateral obstruction.

17. **d. All of the above.** The presence of fever may be an indicator of upper urinary tract involvement but is not always a reliable sign. However, if fever (and presumably pyelonephritis) is present, the likelihood of discovering vesicoureteral reflux is significantly increased.

18. **c. A female patient with recurrent culture and urinalysis proven to have afebrile UTIs and later found to have scarring on a dimercaptosuccinic acid (DMSA) scan.** The presence of culture-proven UTIs in the setting of an abnormal renal scan should raise the question of vesicoureteral reflux, and it is reasonable to proceed with a VCUG and ultrasound in those patients. The other clinical scenarios include a patient without pyuria and a clear alternative source for her fever, as well as an infant diagnosed with UTI with a specimen obtained through a bagged collection. In those children the diagnosis of UTI should be questioned before proceeding with evaluation through cystogram and renal ultrasonography. Patients older than 5 years should not undergo immediate VCUG just on the basis of the presence of a UTI.

19. **a. Ultrasonography.** Older children who present with asymptomatic bacteriuria or UTIs that manifest solely with lower tract symptoms can be screened initially with ultrasonography alone, reserving cystography for those with abnormal upper tracts or recalcitrant infections.

20. **e. All of the above.** Excessive hydration may mask low grades of reflux because diuresis can blunt the retrograde flow of urine. Some reflux is demonstrated only during active infections when cystitis weakens the ureterovesical junction with edema or by increasing intravesical pressures. In addition, cystograms obtained during active infections can overestimate the grade of reflux because the endotoxins produced by some gram-negative organisms can paralyze ureteral smooth muscle and exaggerate ureteral dilatation.

21. **b. It is an accurate method for detecting and following reflux.** Nuclear cystography is the scintigraphic equivalent of conventional cystography. Although the technique does not provide the anatomic detail of fluoroscopic studies, it is an accurate method for detecting and following reflux.

22. **a. It is the diagnostic study of choice to initially evaluate the upper urinary tracts of patients with suspected or proven vesicoureteral reflux.** Ultrasonography is the diagnostic study of choice to initially evaluate the upper urinary tracts of patients with suspected or proven vesicoureteral reflux. However, the

appearance of the kidneys on ultrasound does not correlate with the absence or presence of reflux, or with its grade.

23. **b. DMSA renal scan.** Renal scintigraphy with technetium-99 m–labeled DMSA is the best study for detection of pyelonephritis and the cortical renal scarring that sometimes results.

24. **e. Only a and c are true.** Urodynamic studies may be indicated in any child suspected of having a secondary cause for reflux (e.g., valves, neurogenic bladder, non-neurogenic neurogenic bladder, voiding dysfunction), and they help direct therapy.

25. **e. Uroflowmetry is a valuable tool in the workup of a patient with vesicoureteral reflux.** Evaluation of the lower urinary tract cannot solely rely on imaging studies because reflux is considered to be a dynamic phenomenon. Uroflowmetry provides valuable information in the clinical assessment of these patients. Modern management of reflux does not include the routine evaluation through cystoscopy. The radionuclide cystogram has historically been described as a technique that requires a significantly lower dose of radiation than a regular VCUG, but the advances with modern digital techniques have significantly narrowed the difference between these two imaging modalities. Unfortunately, ultrasound cannot reliably detect the presence or absence of vesicoureteral reflux.

26. **b. Is laterally (cranially) positioned from a normal takeoff at the trigone offers an embryologic explanation for primary reflux.** As Mackie and Stevens have suggested, a ureteral bud that is laterally (cranially) positioned from a normal takeoff at the trigone offers an embryologic explanation for primary reflux, whereas those inferiorly (caudally) positioned are often obstructed.

27. **b. Photopenic areas may result from postinfection renal scarring and some renal dysplasia.** Vesicoureteral reflux, particularly reflux of higher grades, may result in renal dysplasia, which often appears scintigraphically identical to postinfection pyelonephritic scars. During an episode of active pyelonephritis, the renal scan may show an area of photopenia that later, if it persists, represents renal scarring secondary to the infection. Neither renal scan nor ultrasonography can differentiate accurately between renal dysplasia and renal scarring.

28. **a. In children and young adults it is most commonly caused by reflux nephropathy.** Reflux nephropathy is the most common cause of severe hypertension in children and young adults, although the actual incidence is unknown.

29. **e. All of the above.** Factors that might contribute to the effects of reflux on renal growth include the congenital dysmorphism often associated with (30% of cases), but not caused by, reflux; the number and type of urinary infections and their resultant nephropathy; the quality of the contralateral kidney and its implications for compensatory hypertrophy; and the grade of reflux in the affected kidney.

30. **c. BBD reduces the success rate of endoscopic implantation of dextranomer/hyaluronic copolymer (Dx/HA) and open surgical correction of VUR.** However, BBD is associated with increased incidence of UTI after surgery.

31. **a. Distally and medially, and the lower pole ureter enters the bladder proximally and laterally.** The anatomy of patients with ureteral duplication typically follows the Weigert-Meyer rule wherein the upper pole ureter enters the bladder distally and medially and the lower pole ureter enters the bladder proximally and laterally.

32. **d. Negative intraoperative cystogram.**

33. **c. Bladder changes predispose the patient to bacteriuria.** Bladder tone decreases because of edema and hyperemia, which are changes that predispose the patient to bacteriuria. In addition, urine volume increases in the upper collecting system as the physiologic dilatation of pregnancy evolves.

34. **e. All of the above.** It seems logical to assume that during pregnancy, the presence of vesicoureteral reflux in a system already prone to bacteriuria would lead to increased morbidity. Maternal history also becomes a factor if past reflux, renal scarring, and a tendency to get urinary infections are included. Women with

hypertension and an element of renal failure are particularly at risk.

35. **d. The 2014 *New England Journal of Medicine* RIVUR study reported a 0.5% incidence of adverse reaction to prophylactic antibiotics and a 2% incidence of adverse reaction to the placebo.** Adverse reactions to antibiotics were reported in 2% of *both* the antibiotic prophylaxis and placebo groups.

36. **d. All of the above.** Extravesical and intravesical ureteral reimplantation are all options for treatment of vesicoureteral reflux. In the past decade there has been widespread enthusiasm for endoscopic treatment, and different bulking agents have been used to correct vesicoureteral reflux by using minimally invasive techniques.

37. **a. A valvular mechanism that enables ureteral compression with bladder filling and contraction.** Common to each technique is the creation of a valvular mechanism that enables ureteral compression with bladder filling and contraction, thus reenacting normal anatomy and function. A successful ureteroneocystostomy provides a submucosal tunnel for reimplantation having sufficient length and adequate muscular backing. A tunnel length of five times the ureteral diameter is cited as necessary for eliminating reflux.

38. **b. A common sheath repair in which both ureters are mobilized with one mucosal cuff.** Approximately 10% of children undergoing antireflux surgery have an element of ureteral duplication. The most common configuration is a complete duplication that results in two separate orifices. This is best managed by preserving a cuff of bladder mucosa that encompasses both orifices. Because the pair typically share blood supply along their adjoining wall, mobilization as one unit with a "common sheath" preserves vascularity and minimizes trauma.

39. **e. All of the above.** Early after surgery, various degrees of obstruction can be expected of the reimplanted ureter. Edema, subtrigonal bleeding, and bladder spasms all possibly contribute. Mucus plugs and blood clots are other causes. Most postoperative obstructions are mild and asymptomatic and resolve spontaneously. More significant obstructions are usually symptomatic. Affected children typically present 1 to 2 weeks after surgery with acute abdominal pain, nausea, and vomiting.

40. **c. Initial observation and diversion for unabating symptoms.** The large majority of perioperative obstructions subside spontaneously, but placement of a nephrostomy tube or ureteral stent sometimes becomes necessary for unabating symptoms.

41. **a. It may be due to unrecognized secondary causes of reflux such as neuropathic bladder and severe voiding dysfunction.** Other than technical errors, failure to identify and treat secondary causes of reflux is a common cause of the reappearance of reflux. Foremost among these secondary causes are unrecognized neuropathic bladder and severe voiding dysfunction.

42. **d. The accuracy of the needle entry point during endoscopic injection, as well as the needle placement, are important components for the success of the surgical procedure.** The learning curve for endoscopic injection is believed to be different from that of open surgical reimplantation, but studies have not been carried out comparing these two surgical approaches for correction of vesicoureteral reflux. Treatment is currently based on the same indications, and these indications do not differ between the different types of intervention.

43. **d. All of the above.** The advantages of this approach versus open surgery include smaller incisions, less discomfort, brief hospitalizations (although many centers now perform open reimplants on an outpatient basis), and quicker convalescence. As with other laparoscopic procedures, a learning curve needs to be climbed and experience is essential to the success of this approach. Laparoscopic reimplantation requires a team with at least two surgeons; the repair is converted from an extraperitoneal to an intraperitoneal approach; operative time is longer than with open techniques (although with experience it is now becoming gradually shorter); and cost is increased because of lengthier surgery and the expense of disposable equipment.

44. **e. a and c only.** Uncircumcised male children older than 1 year do not appear to be at higher risk for development of recurrent UTI after discontinuation of CAP.
45. **d. All of the above.** Children with grade III or IV reflux at baseline, patients presenting with febrile index infection and the presence of BBD at baseline were considered event modifiers in the RIVUR trial and appear to benefit from CAP.
46. **d. A renal and bladder ultrasound after confirmation of UTI by a properly collected urine specimen for culture and analysis.** A VCUG is recommended only if the renal and bladder ultrasound is abnormal or if the child develops a second infection.

CHAPTER REVIEW

1. In patients with reflux, approximately one third of their siblings will have reflux.
2. Reflux that is inherited is thought to be due to an autosomal dominant pattern.
3. There is a frequent association of constipation and encopresis with reflux and UTIs.
4. If both the ureteropelvic junction (UPJ) and ureterovesical junction (UVJ) require operative repair, the UPJ should be repaired first.
5. There is an association of renal maldevelopment with high grades of reflux.
6. The cardinal renal anomalies associated with reflux are multicystic dysplastic kidney and renal agenesis.
7. Women with UTIs and reflux who have undergone a reimplantation will still be at significant risk for UTIs during pregnancy and should be monitored.
8. Almost 80% of low-grade and half of grade III reflux will resolve spontaneously.
9. Sterile reflux is benign.
10. Cohen's cross-trigonal technique of ureteral reimplantation is particularly well suited for small bladders and thick-walled bladders.
11. There is a 10% to 15% incidence of contralateral reflux after unilateral reflux is repaired.
12. Prophylactic bilateral reimplantation for unilateral reflux is not indicated.
13. Reflux is unlikely to be of any clinical significance in the absence of infection in a patient with normal bladder function.
14. The greatest risk for postinfection renal scarring is in the first year of life.
15. Reflux associated with a paraureteral diverticulum resolves at a similar rate to primary reflux.
16. There is a tenfold lower frequency of vesicoureteral reflux in female children of African descent.
17. The endoscopic repair of reflux is less invasive and less durable than the open surgical repair.
18. A 5:1 tunnel length–ureteral diameter ratio should be achieved in antireflux surgery for best results.
19. Bladder infections (UTIs) and their accompanying inflammation can also cause reflux by lessening compliance, elevating intravesical pressures, and distorting and weakening the ureterovesical junction.
20. Modern management of reflux does not include routine evaluation through cystoscopy.
21. Vesicoureteral reflux, particularly reflux of higher grades, may be associated with renal dysplasia, which often appears scintigraphically identical to postinfection pyelonephritic scars.
22. Reflux nephropathy is the most common cause of severe hypertension in children and young adults.
23. In a duplex system where one ureter refluxes and surgical reconstruction is indicated, both ureters should have a common sheath reimplantation because the paired ureters typically share blood supply along their adjoining wall, and mobilization as one unit with a "common sheath" preserves vascularity and minimizes trauma.
24. Failure to identify and treat secondary causes of reflux is a common cause of the reappearance of reflux following correction. Foremost among these secondary causes are unrecognized neuropathic bladder and severe voiding dysfunction.

138 Bladder Anomalies in Children

Dominic Frimberger and Bradley P. Kropp

QUESTIONS

1. At which point in time is fetal urine production sufficient so that at least 50% of bladders can be detected by ultrasound?
   a. 8 weeks
   b. 10 weeks
   c. 12 weeks
   d. 14 weeks
   e. 16 weeks

2. How can obstructive and nonobstructive bladder dilatation be distinguished on prenatal ultrasound?
   a. Thickness of the bladder
   b. Degree of ureteral dilation
   c. Presence of oligohydramnios
   d. Dilated bladder neck
   e. Size of the bladder

3. How is the presence of vesicoureteral reflux in congenital megacystis explained?
   a. High-pressure bladder
   b. Ectopic insertion of the ureteral orifice into the trigone
   c. Bladder dilation from continuous recycling of refluxing urine
   d. Obstruction of the bladder outlet
   e. High urine output

4. Which of the following is NOT considered a urachal anomaly?
   a. Patent urachus
   b. Umbilical-urachus sinus
   c. Urachal cyst
   d. Vesicourachal diverticulum
   e. Urethral-urachus fistula

5. Which other embryologic remnant must be differentiated from a patent urachus?
   a. Patent omphalomesenteric duct
   b. Choledochal cyst
   c. Meckel diverticulum
   d. Ureteral duplication
   e. Congenital bladder diverticulum

6. Which of the following congenital syndromes are NOT associated with bladder diverticula?
   a. Ehlers-Danlos
   b. Elfin facies
   c. Menkes syndrome
   d. Sutcliffe-Sandifer syndrome
   e. c and d

7. Which theories explain the development of duplicated bladders?
   a. Complete duplication of the bladder and hindgut is thought to occur due to partial twinning of the tail portion of the embryo.
   b. The development of a sagittal fissure on the cloacal plate occurs when the urorectal septum separates the urogenital from the digestive sinus.
   c. Failure of the lateral mesenchymal tissue to migrate
   d. Early rupture of the cloacal membrane
   e. a and b

ANSWERS

1. **b. 10 weeks.** The bladder can be visualized in approximately 50% of cases in the fetal pelvis at the tenth week of gestation, concurrent with the onset of urine production (Green and Hobbins, 1998).* The detection rate increases with fetal age to 78% at 11 weeks, 88% at 12 weeks, and almost 100% at 13 weeks.

2. **c. Presence of oligohydramnios.** It is very difficult to distinguish in utero whether the dilatation is due to obstruction or not. Obstructed cases present with moderate to severe oligohydramnios and a marked increase in renal echogenicity, whereas nonobstructed bladders tend to have normal amniotic fluid levels and regular renal echogenicity (Kaefer et al, 1997).

3. **c. Bladder dilation from continuous recycling of refluxing urine.** The observed reflux is not an after effect of obstruction, but rather the cause of the bladder dilatation from continuous recycling of the urine between the upper tract and bladder.

4. **e. Urethral-urachus fistula.** Four different urachal anomalies have been described: patent urachus, umbilical-urachus sinus, urachal cyst, and vesicourachal diverticulum. There is no such thing as a urethral-urachus fistula.

5. **a. Patent omphalomesenteric duct.**

6. **d. Sutcliffe-Sandifer syndrome.** Congenital diverticula are often found in children with generalized connective tissue diseases such as Ehlers-Danlos, elfin facies, or Menkes syndrome (Levard et al, 1989; Rabbitt et al, 1979; Daly and Rabinovitch, 1981). Sutcliffe-Sandifer syndrome is associated with gastroesophageal reflux.

7. **e. a and b.** Complete duplication of the bladder and hindgut is thought to occur due to partial twinning of the tail portion of the embryo (Ravitch and Scott, 1953). It also is suggested that the development of a sagittal fissure on the cloacal plate occurs when the urorectal septum separates the urogenital from the digestive sinus (Bellagha et al, 1993).

---

*Sources referenced can be found in *Campbell-Walsh Urology, 11th Edition,* on the Expert Consult website.

CHAPTER REVIEW

1. The fetal bladder empties every 15 to 20 minutes, so if it is not visualized, repeat ultrasound 15 to 20 minutes later should be performed.
2. When obstruction is the cause of a dilated bladder in the fetus, the mother usually has oligohydramnios.
3. Congenital megacystis is defined as a dilated, thin-walled bladder with a wide and poorly developed trigone. These bladders generally have wide-gaping ureteral orifices that are displaced laterally, causing massive reflux. Correcting the reflux often restores normal voiding dynamics.
4. Urachal remnants often undergo spontaneous resolution if discovered in patients younger than 6 months. An infected urachal remnant should be initially drained and treated with antibiotics; once the infection has subsided, an excision should be performed.
5. A urachal sinus must be differentiated from a persistent omphalomesenteric duct. The latter presents as a Meckel diverticulum connected to the umbilicus.
6. Urachal cysts do not communicate with either the bladder or umbilicus.
7. Portions of a bladder can be contained within a hernia sac.
8. Dilation of the fetal bladder due to obstruction is usually secondary to a urethral stricture, urethral valves, or urethral atresia. Extrinsic masses may also obstruct the bladder outlet.
9. Nonobstructed bladder dilation may be seen in prune-belly syndrome and neurogenic bladder.
10. Patients with bladder duplication often have associated genital anomalies and may have gastrointestinal anomalies.
11. Four different urachal anomalies have been described: patent urachus, umbilical-urachus sinus, urachal cyst, and vesicourachal diverticulum.
12. Congenital bladder diverticula are often found in children with generalized connective tissue diseases.

139 Exstrophy-Epispadias Complex

John P. Gearhart and Ranjiv Mathews

QUESTIONS

1. What is the live birth incidence of classic bladder exstrophy?
   a. 1 in 100,000
   b. 1 in 60,000
   c. 1 in 50,000
   d. 1 in 70,000
   e. 1 in 90,000

2. What is the live birth risk of bladder exstrophy in the offspring of individuals with bladder exstrophy and epispadias?
   a. 1 in 70
   b. 1 in 300
   c. 1 in 500
   d. 1 in 700
   e. 1 in 450

3. The main theory of embryologic maldevelopment in exstrophy is that of abnormal:
   a. underdevelopment of the cloacal membrane, preventing medial migration of the mesoderm tissue and proper lower abdominal wall development.
   b. overdevelopment of the cloacal membrane, preventing medial migration of the mesodermal tissue and proper lower abdominal wall development.
   c. infiltration of ectoderm into the cloacal membrane.
   d. infiltration of mesoderm into the cloacal membrane.
   e. invasion of endoderm into the cloacal membrane.

4. In evaluation of the skeletal defects of bladder exstrophy, Sponseller and colleagues (1995)* found that with classic bladder exstrophy, there are changes in the orientation of the pelvic bones. These include:
   a. external rotation of the posterior aspect of the pelvis of 12 degrees on each side.
   b. retroversion of the acetabulum.
   c. an 18-degree rotation of the anterior pelvis.
   d. a 30% shortening of the pubic rami in addition to a significant pubic symphyseal diastasis.
   e. All of the above.

5. Which of the following statements is TRUE regarding hernias in children with exstrophy?
   a. Identification at the time of initial closure is not possible.
   b. They are usually unilateral.
   c. They are noted in 80% of boys and 10% of girls.
   d. The orientation of the pelvic bones makes them infrequent.
   e. A patent processus vaginalis is rarely noted.

6. Which of the following statements is TRUE regarding the male genital defect in exstrophy?
   a. The posterior length of the corporeal bodies was 30% shorter than in healthy controls.
   b. The diameter of the posterior corporeal segments was less than in healthy controls.
   c. The shortening of the penis was due entirely to the pubic diastasis.
   d. The anterior corporeal segments are 50% shorter than those of healthy control participants.
   e. The angle between the corpora cavernosa is markedly reduced in boys with exstrophy.

7. Which of the following statements best describes findings regarding the prostate in exstrophy?
   a. Volume weight and the cross-sectional area appeared healthy compared with published results from control subjects.
   b. The prostate extended circumferentially around the urethra in all patients with exstrophy.
   c. Free prostate-specific antigen (PSA) values were greater than in healthy controls, indicating recurrent injury from infection.
   d. The vas deferens and seminal vesicles were abnormal due to the effect of the exstrophic bladder.
   e. Total PSA values were not measurable in men with exstrophy.

8. Which of the following accurately describes the vagina in the female patient with bladder exstrophy?
   a. Shorter than normal and of smaller caliber
   b. Vaginal orifice displaced posteriorly because of the anterior exstrophic bladder
   c. Shorter than normal but of normal caliber
   d. Longer than normal and of wider caliber
   e. Cervix enters the posterior vaginal wall

9. Findings regarding the structure and innervation of the exstrophic bladder include:
   a. density and binding affinity of the muscarinic receptors that were similar to norms.
   b. a decreased ratio of collagen to muscle in the exstrophic bladder.
   c. increased myelinated nerve profiles, indicating a later developmental stage.
   d. a threefold increase in the amount of type I collagen.
   e. study of vasoactive intestinal polypeptide, protein gene product 9.5, and calcitonin gene–related peptide that indicated the presence of dysinnervation.

10. Which of the following statements best describes bladder function in patients with bladder exstrophy?
    a. In patients who are continent after reconstruction, normal cystometrograms are noted in 10% to 25%.
    b. Eighty percent of patients had compliant and stable bladders before bladder neck reconstruction.

---

*Sources referenced can be found in *Campbell-Walsh Urology, 11th Edition,* on the Expert Consult website.

c. Involuntary contractions were noted infrequently after bladder neck reconstruction.

d. After bladder neck reconstruction, 90% maintained normal bladder compliance.

e. After successful closure, ultrastructure remains abnormal in the majority.

11. The characteristic prenatal appearance of bladder exstrophy includes which of the following?

a. Absence of bladder filling

b. Low-set umbilicus

c. Widening of the pubic ramus

d. Diminutive genitalia

e. All of the above

12. Newborn patient selection for immediate reconstruction is based on:

a. examination of the bladder in the nursery without anesthesia.

b. complete lack of any surface defects on examination.

c. indentation of the bladder under anesthesia or outward bulging when the child cries.

d. size of the phallus at birth.

e. extent of the pubic diastasis.

13. Fundamental steps in the modern staged reconstruction of bladder exstrophy include all of the following EXCEPT:

a. early bladder, posterior urethral, and abdominal wall closure.

b. early epispadias repair around age 1 year.

c. conversion of the bladder exstrophy to complete epispadias.

d. bladder neck reconstruction before the epispadias repair to provide early continence.

e. ureteral reimplantation at the time of bladder neck reconstruction.

14. What is the best treatment option at the time of birth in a child whose bladder template is judged to be too small to undergo closure?

a. Excision of the bladder with a nonrefluxing colon conduit

b. Immediate closure with epispadias repair to provide resistance and allow the bladder to grow

c. Delaying closure by 4 to 6 months with reassessment to see if the bladder will grow

d. Bladder closure, augmentation, ureteral reimplantation, and a continence procedure

e. Improve the potential for successful closure with an osteotomy

15. Combined osteotomy was developed for all of the following reasons EXCEPT:

a. the approach allows placement of an external fixator device.

b. superior cosmesis provided by this approach.

c. the need to turn a patient to perform an osteotomy.

d. better ease of pubic approximation.

e. reduced risk of malunion of the iliac wing and reduction of blood loss.

16. Complications that are associated with osteotomy and immobilization techniques include all of the following EXCEPT:

a. skin ulceration associated with use of mummy wrapping.

b. failure of the bladder and abdominal wall closure associated with the use of spica casting.

c. high rates of failure of reconstruction associated with the use of osteotomy and external fixation.

d. transient femoral nerve palsy with the use of osteotomy.

e. delayed union of the iliac wings after use of posterior osteotomy.

17. Other options have been described for reconstruction in bladder exstrophy. Which of the following statements is TRUE regarding the other described approaches?

a. The Warsaw approach includes bladder neck reconstruction at the time of initial bladder closure.

b. The Erlangen approach includes all of the features of reconstruction of the exstrophy in a single procedure.

c. The Seattle approach (CPRE) includes bladder neck reconstruction as part of the complete reconstruction of exstrophy.

d. Combined bladder closure and epispadias repair are performed in cases of primary exstrophy repair at birth.

e. The Warsaw approach uses the Young repair as the preferred method for epispadias reconstruction.

18. After initial primary bladder closure in the newborn, what should be done if recurrent urinary tract infections occur?

a. Voiding cystourethrogram

b. Bladder computed tomography (CT)

c. Ureteral reimplantation

d. Prophylaxis modified

e. Cystoscopy

19. After successful bladder closure, management should include all the following EXCEPT:

a. calibration of the urethral outlet 4 weeks after closure to ensure free drainage.

b. ultrasound evaluation of the kidneys and bladder.

c. intermittent antibiotics for urinary tract infections.

d. complete bladder drainage by suprapubic tube clamping.

e. yearly cystoscopic evaluation.

20. In a patient with bladder exstrophy who undergoes more than one closure of the bladder and urethral defect, what is the chance of having adequate bladder capacity for later bladder neck reconstruction?

a. 60%

b. 70%

c. 20%

d. 30%

e. 10%

21. The key concepts in the reconstruction of epispadias include all of the following EXCEPT:

a. correction of ventral chordee.

b. urethral reconstruction.

c. glans reconstruction.

d. penile skin coverage.

e. penile lengthening.

22. Information gleaned from most major series of bladder neck reconstruction indicates that the most important factor to predict success and eventual continence after bladder neck reconstruction is:

a. age of the child.

b. number of prior bladder infections.

c. number of attempts at bladder closure.

d. bladder capacity.

e. vesicoureteral reflux.

23. After bladder neck reconstruction, within what time period do the majority of patients achieve daytime continence?
    a. 2 years
    b. 1 year
    c. 2 months
    d. 6 months
    e. 4 years

24. After a failed bladder closure in the newborn period, an appropriate time period should elapse before attempting a secondary repair. What should this time period be?
    a. 2 months
    b. 18 months
    c. 2 years
    d. 6 months
    e. 15 months

25. All of the following statements are TRUE regarding the results of modern staged reconstruction of exstrophy EXCEPT:
    a. The onset of eventual continence and continence rates were unchanged in those who had initial successful closure.
    b. The modified Cantwell-Ransley repair has replaced the Young technique because there is less urethral tortuosity and lower fistula rates.
    c. Incidence of fistula formation was 12% at 3 months after epispadias repair.
    d. Continence is more likely in those patients undergoing initial closure before 72 hours of age or those who have closure after 72 hours of age with osteotomy.
    e. Continence rates are higher in those who have capacities of 85 mL or more at the time of bladder neck reconstruction.

26. Which of the following statements is TRUE regarding exstrophy failures?
    a. After successful secondary closure, 90% of patients develop dryness and voided continence.
    b. Dehiscence after complete primary repair may be associated with corporeal, urethral, and other major soft tissue loss.
    c. Bladder prolapse can be managed with minimal outlet procedures because this is considered a mild failure.
    d. Because the results of reclosure are poor, immediate resection of the bladder plate followed by neobladder construction is the preferred management.
    e. Posterior urethral stricture is usually a late complication occurring 4 to 6 years after initial closure.

27. Bladder neck reconstruction is designated as a failure if a 3-hour dry interval is not achieved within 2 years after surgery. Management of such failure is with the use of:
    a. collagen, which can lead to dryness.
    b. artificial urinary sphincter small bladder capacities.
    c. bladder neck transection, augmentation cystoplasty, and continent diversion.
    d. repeat bladder neck reconstruction in relatively tight bladder necks.
    e. repeat bladder neck reconstruction in bladder instability.

28. The risks of ureterosigmoidostomy in the exstrophy population include:
    a. pyelonephritis and hyperchloremic acidosis.
    b. pyelonephritis, hyponatremia, and rectal incontinence.
    c. low incidence for eventual development of cancer.
    d. poor outcomes with upper tract deterioration.
    e. prolapse of the abdominal stoma.

29. What is the live birth incidence of cloacal exstrophy?
    a. 1 in 400,000
    b. 1 in 20,000
    c. 1 in 750,000
    d. 1 in 1,000,000
    e. 1 in 500,000

30. Neurospinal abnormalities are noted in the majority of patients with cloacal exstrophy. All of the following statements are true EXCEPT:
    a. Thoracic defects may be noted in 10% of patients.
    b. The embryologic basis for the neurospinal defect has been identified as failure of neural tube closure.
    c. Autonomic bladder innervation is derived from a more medial location.
    d. Innervation of the duplicated corporeal bodies arises from the sacral plexus and courses medial to the hemibladders.
    e. Functional defects can include minimal lower extremity function.

31. Cloacal exstrophy is a multisystem abnormality. Which of the following is TRUE regarding cloacal exstrophy?
    a. The bones in a child with cloacal exstrophy were microscopically, markedly different from healthy controls.
    b. In the presence of a normal bowel length, there is low probability for the development of short-gut syndrome.
    c. The most common müllerian anomaly noted was partial uterine duplication.
    d. Cardiovascular and pulmonary anomalies are frequently noted.
    e. The most common upper urinary tract anomaly noted was multicystic dysplastic kidney.

32. What is the incidence of omphalocele associated with cloacal exstrophy?
    a. 40%
    b. 70%
    c. 95%
    d. 20%
    e. 60%

33. In the patient with cloacal exstrophy, hindgut remnants should be preserved to:
    a. enlarge the bladder.
    b. permit vaginal reconstruction.
    c. allow either bladder augmentation or vaginal reconstruction.
    d. provide additional length of bowel for fluid absorption.
    e. allow later anal pull-through surgery.

34. Gender assignment continues to remain a controversial aspect of cloacal exstrophy management. Current research indicates that:
    a. Psychosexual evaluation indicates that patients have marked female shift in development.
    b. Patients have feminine childhood behavior but developed masculine gender identity.
    c. Histology of the testis at birth is abnormal, and therefore removal has been recommended.
    d. Most recommend that gender be assigned on the basis of the ability for functional reconstruction rather than on karyotype.
    e. A functional and cosmetically acceptable phallus can now be constructed.

35. What is the live birth incidence of male epispadias?
    a. 1 in 150,000
    b. 1 in 200,000
    c. 1 in 400,000
    d. 1 in 117,000
    e. 1 in 250,000

36. What is the incidence of reflux in patients with complete epispadias?
    a. 10% to 20%
    b. 90%
    c. 70%
    d. 50%
    e. 30% to 40%

37. In the complete epispadias group, what is the predominant indicator of eventual continence?
    a. Length of the urethral groove
    b. Lack of spinal abnormalities
    c. Bladder capacity at the time of bladder neck reconstruction
    d. Age at bladder neck reconstruction
    e. Age at epispadias repair and degree of resistance provided

38. Many variations in anatomy have been reported in the exstrophy-epispadias complex. All of the following are true regarding exstrophy variants EXCEPT:
    a. The presence of musculoskeletal defects characteristic of the complex, with a normal urinary tract, is termed *pseudoexstrophy*.
    b. The bladder is completely exstrophied in the superior vesical fissure variant.
    c. With "covered" exstrophy, an isolated ectopic bowel segment has been frequently noted.
    d. An isolated segment of bladder is left on the abdominal wall, with a complete urinary tract within the bladder in duplicate exstrophy.
    e. A common embryologic origin has been postulated for developments of all of the variants.

39. Sexual function and libido in male and female exstrophy patients are:
    a. normal in males, abnormal in females.
    b. normal only in males.
    c. normal in both males and females.
    d. normal only in females.
    e. abnormal in both males and females.

40. What is the most common complication after pregnancy in female exstrophy patients?
    a. Premature labor
    b. Rectal prolapse
    c. Preeclampsia
    d. Cervical and uterine prolapse
    e. Oligohydramnios

41. Psychological studies of male and female children with bladder exstrophy find that:
    a. all have clinical psychopathology.
    b. they do not have clinical psychopathology.
    c. most have significant depression due to the condition.
    d. many children have gender dysphoria.
    e. half of males and half of females have clinical psychopathology.

42. Single-stage reconstruction by using the complete primary exstrophy repair technique offers several advantages versus staged reconstruction EXCEPT:
    a. the possibility to correct the penile, bladder, and bladder neck abnormalities of bladder exstrophy with one operation.
    b. the ability to achieve urinary continence without bladder neck reconstruction.
    c. correction of vesicoureteral reflux at the time of surgery.
    d. lower complication rates than previous attempts at single-stage reconstruction.
    e. initiation of bladder cycling early in life.

43. Single-stage reconstruction by using the complete primary exstrophy repair technique relies on which of the following to achieve continence?
    a. Reestablishment of normal anatomic relationships
    b. Bladder neck reconstruction at the time of primary surgery
    c. Osteotomy at the time of single-stage reconstruction
    d. Simultaneous epispadias repair
    e. None of the above

44. The following postoperative factors have been shown to increase the success of reconstruction for bladder exstrophy EXCEPT:
    a. immobilization with external fixators, Buck traction, a spica cast, or a mummy wrap.
    b. antibiotic therapy.
    c. prolonged nil per os (NPO) status to avoid abdominal distention.
    d. urinary diversion through ureteral stenting and suprapubic urinary drainage.
    e. adequate nutritional support.

45. Single-stage reconstruction by using the complete primary exstrophy repair technique can be safely performed because:
    a. the neurovascular bundles of the corporeal bodies lie laterally rather than dorsally on the corporeal bodies.
    b. the cavernosal bodies and urethral wedge are not actually separated from each other in this technique.
    c. the blood supply to the corporeal bodies and that to the urethral wedge are independent of each other.
    d. the blood supply is quickly reestablished once the components are "reassembled."
    e. the distal vascular communications between the corpora and urethral wedge are preserved.

46. The proximal limit(s) of dissection by using the complete primary exstrophy repair technique is/are:
    a. the intersymphyseal band.
    b. the muscles of the pelvic floor.
    c. the rectum.
    d. the corpora spongiosa.
    e. the endopelvic fascia.

47. Factors that mitigate against use of a single-stage reconstruction technique for cloacal exstrophy include the presence of:
    a. a large omphalocele.
    b. a wide pubic diastasis.
    c. a concomitant myelomeningocele.
    d. a small bladder plate.
    e. all of the above.

48. Complications of the complete primary exstrophy repair technique include:

    a. myogenic bladder failure.

    b. testicular atrophy.

    c. urethrocutaneous fistula.

    d. hip dislocation.

    e. epispadias.

ANSWERS

1. **c. 1 in 50,000.** The incidence of bladder exstrophy has been estimated as between 1 in 10,000 and 1 in 50,000 live births.

2. **a. 1 in 70.** Shapiro determined that the risk of bladder exstrophy in the offspring of individuals with bladder exstrophy and epispadias is 1 in 70 live births, a 500-fold greater incidence than in the general population.

3. **b. Overdevelopment of the cloacal membrane, preventing medial migration of the mesodermal tissue and proper lower abdominal wall development.** The theory of embryonic maldevelopment in exstrophy held by Marshall and Muecke is that the basic defect is an abnormal overdevelopment of the cloacal membrane, preventing medial migration of the mesenchymal tissue and proper lower abdominal wall development.

4. **e. All of the above.** Sponseller and colleagues found that patients with classic bladder exstrophy have a mean external rotation of the posterior aspect of the pelvis of 12 degrees on each side, retroversion of the acetabulum, and a mean 18-degree external rotation of the anterior pelvis, along with 30% shortening of the pubic rami.

5. **c. They are noted in 80% of boys and 10% of girls.** Connelly and colleagues, in a review of 181 children with bladder exstrophy, reported inguinal hernias in 81.8% of boys and 10.5% of girls.

6. **d. The anterior corporeal segments are 50% shorter than those of healthy control participants.** With the use of magnetic resonance imaging (MRI) to examine adult men with bladder exstrophy and comparison of this result with that from age- and race-matched control participants, it was found that the anterior corporeal length in male patients with bladder exstrophy is almost 50% shorter than that of healthy control participants.

7. **a. Volume weight and the cross-sectional area appeared normal compared with published results from control participants.** The volume, weight, and maximum cross-sectional area of the prostate appeared normal compared with published results from control subjects.

8. **c. Shorter than normal but of normal caliber.** The vagina is shorter than normal, hardly greater than 6 cm in depth, but of normal caliber.

9. **a. Density and binding affinity of the muscarinic receptors that were similar to norms.** Muscarinic cholinergic receptor density and binding affinity were measured in control participants and in patients with classic bladder exstrophy. The density of the muscarinic cholinergic receptors in both the control and exstrophy groups was similar, as was the binding affinity of the muscarinic receptor. Therefore it was thought by the authors that the neurophysiologic composition of the exstrophied bladder is not grossly altered during its anomalous development.

10. **b. Eighty percent of patients had compliant and stable bladders before bladder neck reconstruction.** Diamond and colleagues (1999), looking at 30 patients with bladder exstrophy at various stages of reconstruction, found that 80% of patients had compliant and stable bladders before bladder neck reconstruction.

11. **e. All of the above.** In a review of 25 prenatal ultrasonographic examinations with the resulting birth of a newborn with classic bladder exstrophy, several observations were made: (1) absence of bladder filling; (2) a low-set umbilicus; (3) widening pubis ramus; (4) diminutive genitalia; and (5) a lower abdominal mass that increases in size while the pregnancy progresses and as the intra-abdominal viscera increase in size.

12. **c. Indentation of the bladder under anesthesia or outward bulging when the child cries.** In minor grades of exstrophy that approach the condition of complete epispadias with incontinence, the bladder may be small yet may demonstrate acceptable capacity, either by bulging when the baby cries or by indenting easily when touched by a sterile gloved finger in the operating room with the child under anesthesia.

13. **d. Bladder neck reconstruction before the epispadias repair to provide early continence.** The most significant changes in the management of bladder exstrophy have been (1) early bladder, posterior urethral, and abdominal wall closure, usually with osteotomy; (2) early epispadias repair; (3) reconstruction of a continent bladder neck and reimplantation of the ureters; and, most importantly, (4) definition of strict criteria for the selection of patients suitable for this approach. Bladder neck repair usually occurs when the child is 4 to 5 years, has an adequate bladder capacity, and, most important, is ready to participate in a postoperative voiding program.

14. **c. Delaying closure by 4 to 6 months with reassessment to see if the bladder will grow.** Ideally, waiting for the bladder template to grow for 4 to 6 months in the child with a small bladder is not as risky as submitting a small bladder template to closure in an inappropriate setting, resulting in dehiscence and allowing the fate of the bladder to be sealed at that point.

15. **c. The need to turn a patient to perform an osteotomy.** Combined osteotomy was developed for three reasons: (1) osteotomy is performed with the patient in the supine position, as is the urologic repair, thereby avoiding the need to turn the patient; (2) the anterior approach to this osteotomy allows placement of an external fixator device and intrafragmentary pins under direct vision; and (3) the cosmetic appearance of this osteotomy is superior to that of the posterior iliac approach.

16. **c. High rates of failure of reconstruction associated with the use of osteotomy and external fixation.** Successful closure was noted in 97% of those immobilized with an external fixator and modified Buck traction.

17. **b. The Erlangen approach includes all of the features of reconstruction of the exstrophy in a single procedure.** This method is truly a "complete repair" because it accomplishes all of the facets of exstrophy reconstruction in a single procedure. Surgical repair is, however, performed at 8 to 10 weeks of age when the infant is larger and has had the opportunity to be medically stabilized.

18. **e. Cystoscopy.** An important caveat is that if there are recurrent urinary tract infections or if the bladder is distended on an ultrasonographic study, cystoscopy should be performed and the posterior urethra should be carefully examined anteriorly for erosion of the intrapubic stitch, which may be the cause of the recurrent infections.

19. **c. Intermittent antibiotics for urinary tract infections.** Before removal of the suprapubic tube, 4 weeks after surgery, the bladder outlet is calibrated by a urethral catheter or a urethral sound to ensure free drainage. A complete ultrasound examination is obtained to ascertain the status of the renal pelves and ureters, and appropriate urinary antibiotics are administered because all patients will have reflux postclosure. Residual urine is estimated by clamping the suprapubic tube, and specimens for culture are obtained before the patient leaves the hospital and at subsequent intervals to detect infection and ensure that the bladder is empty.

20. **a. 60%.** In one study, if a patient underwent two closures, the chance of having an adequate bladder capacity for bladder neck reconstruction was 60%.

21. **a. Correction of ventral chordee.** Regardless of the surgical technique chosen for reconstruction of the penis in bladder exstrophy, four key concerns must be addressed to ensure a functional and cosmetically pleasing penis: (1) correction of dorsal chordee, (2) urethral reconstruction, (3) glandular reconstruction, and (4) penile skin closure.

22. **d. Bladder capacity.** The most important long-term factor gleaned from a review of all these series is the fact that bladder capacity at the time of bladder neck reconstruction is an important determinant of eventual success.

23. **b. 1 year.** The vast majority of patients achieve daytime continence in the first year after bladder neck reconstruction.

24. **d. 6 months.** Dehiscence, which may be precipitated by incomplete mobilization of the pelvic diaphragm, and inadequate pelvic immobilization postoperatively, wound infection, abdominal distention, or urinary tube malfunction, necessitates a 6-month recovery period before a second attempt at closure.

25. **a. The onset of eventual continence and continence rates were unchanged in those who had initial successful closure.** The importance of a successful initial closure is emphasized by Oesterling and Jeffs (1987) and by Husmann and colleagues (1989), who found that the onset of eventual continence was quicker and the continence rate higher in those who underwent a successful initial closure with or without osteotomy.

26. **b. Dehiscence after complete primary repair may be associated with corporeal, urethral, and other major soft tissue loss.** Dehiscence and prolapse have also been reported after the "complete repair" and may be associated with glandular, corporeal, urethral plate, and other major soft tissue loss.

27. **c. Bladder neck transection, augmentation cystoplasty, and continent diversion.** A majority of bladder neck failures require eventual augmentation or continent diversion. The artificial urinary sphincter has been used with some success in patients who have a good bladder capacity. However, in most of these failures the bladder capacity is small and augmentation will be required. At the time of reoperative surgery, either the bladder neck is transected proximal to the prostate with a Mitrofanoff substitution, or a continence procedure such as an artificial sphincter or collagen injection, or both, is performed. In our extensive experience with failed bladder neck reconstructions, most of the patients have had several surgeries and need to be dry. In such cases the most suitable alternative is bladder neck transection, augmentation, and a continent urinary stoma (Gearhart et al, 1995b; Hensle et al, 1995).

28. **a. Pyelonephritis and hyperchloremic acidosis.** However, this form of diversion should not be offered until one is certain that anal continence is normal and after the family has been made aware of the potential serious complications including pyelonephritis, hyperchloremic acidosis, rectal incontinence, ureteral obstruction, and delayed development of malignancy.

29. **a. 1 in 400,000.** Fortunately, cloacal exstrophy is exceedingly rare, occurring in 1 in 200,000 to 400,000 live births.

30. **b. The embryologic basis for the neurospinal defect has been identified as failure of neural tube closure.** The embryologic basis for the neurospinal defects associated with cloacal exstrophy has been postulated to be secondary to problems with the disruption of the tissue of the dorsal mesenchyme rather than failure of neural tube closure (McLaughlin et al, 1995). Alternatively, it has been suggested that the defects that lead to the formation of cloacal exstrophy may lead to the developing spinal cord and vertebrae being pulled apart (Cohen, 1991).

31. **c. The most common müllerian anomaly noted was partial uterine duplication.** The most commonly reported müllerian anomaly was uterine duplication, seen in 95% of patients (Diamond, 1990). The vast majority of these patients had partial uterine duplication, predominantly a bicornate uterus.

32. **c. 95%.** In Diamond's series, the incidence of omphalocele was 88%, with a majority of all series reporting 95% or greater.

33. **d. Provide additional length of bowel for fluid absorption.** With the recognition of the metabolic changes in patients with ileostomy, an attempt is always made to use the hindgut remnant to provide additional length of bowel for fluid absorption.

34. **e. A functional and cosmetically acceptable phallus can now be constructed.** Most authors recommend assigning gender that is consistent with karyotypic makeup of the individual if at all possible. This policy can be supported by a report indicating that the histology of the testis at birth is normal (Mathews et al, 1999a). Furthermore, with evolution of techniques for phallic reconstruction, a functional and cosmetically acceptable phallus can now be constructed (Husmann et al, 1989).

35. **d. 1 in 117,000.** Male epispadias is a rare anomaly, with a reported incidence of 1 in 117,000 males.

36. **e. 30% to 40%.** The ureterovesical junction is inherently deficient in complete epispadias, and reflux has been reported between 30% and 40% in a number of series.

37. **c. Bladder capacity at the time of bladder neck reconstruction.** In the epispadias group, much as in the exstrophy group, bladder capacity is the predominant indicator of eventual continence.

38. **b. The bladder is completely exstrophied in the superior vesical fissure variant.** In the superior vesical fissure variant of the exstrophy complex, the musculature and skeletal defects are exactly the same as those in classic exstrophy; however, the persistent cloacal membrane ruptures only at the uppermost portion, and a superior vesical fistula that actually resembles a vesicostomy results. Bladder extrusion is minimal and is present only over the normal umbilicus.

39. **c. Normal in both males and females.** Sexual function and libido in exstrophy patients are normal.

40. **d. Cervical and uterine prolapse.** The main complication after pregnancy was cervical and uterine prolapse, which occurred frequently.

41. **b. They do not have clinical psychopathology.** The conclusions of this long-term study were that children with exstrophy do not have clinical psychopathology.

42. **c. Correction of vesicoureteral reflux at the time of surgery.** In most applications of the primary exstrophy repair technique, correction of vesicoureteral reflux is not performed, although some have reported performing ureteral reimplantation. All of the other elements are considered advantages of the primary repair.

43. **a. Reestablishment of normal anatomic relationships.** The fundamental basis of the primary repair technique is to reposition the bladder neck and urethral complex into the normal pelvic position more posteriorly than at birth. This permits more normal function of the pelvic floor in maintenance of continence. The other factors do not contribute as significantly to continence.

44. **c. Prolonged nil per os (NPO) status to avoid abdominal distention.** It is not necessary to maintain an NPO status after primary repair because this will compromise nutrition. If an ileus develops, appropriate decompression and management are necessary because abdominal distention strains the repair. All other factors contribute to a successful outcome.

45. **c. The blood supply to the corporeal bodies and that to the urethral wedge are independent of each other.** Because the three elements of the penis, the two corpora and the urethral wedge, are fully separated in the penile disassembly, their vasculature must be proximal, which it is; this is the reason this method is successful. Nevertheless, preservation of these proximal vascular supplies is essential.

46. **b. The muscles of the pelvic floor.** The limit of dissection along the penile structures is the pelvic floor, which is then split to permit repositioning of the bladder neck complex posteriorly.

47. **e. All of the above.** All of these factors would indicate that an attempt to perform a primary repair would be at high risk for failure, predominantly by dehiscence. Several of these factors may be present at one time.

48. **c. Urethrocutaneous fistula.** The most common complication after primary repair is development of a urethrocutaneous fistula on the ventrum of the penis. Other complications can include corporeal devascularization, hydronephrosis, and hypospadias.

CHAPTER REVIEW

1. The male-to-female ratio for exstrophy is 2.3:1.
2. The risk of bladder exstrophy in family members is increased.
3. Rectal prolapse frequently occurs in untreated exstrophy patients who have widely separated symphyses. It disappears after exstrophy closure.
4. If rectal prolapse occurs after closure, bladder outlet obstruction should be suspected.
5. The autonomic nerves are displaced laterally in patients with exstrophy.
6. Reflux occurs in 100% of patients with exstrophy; inguinal hernias are common.
7. An ectopic isolated bowel segment may be present in the lower abdominal wall.
8. Osteotomy is rarely performed in newborns unless the diastasis is greater than 4 cm.
9. The most reliable predictors of urinary continence are the size of the bladder template at birth and successful primary closure.
10. Approximately 75% of patients with exstrophy are continent after repair. Continence is defined as 3 hours of dryness.
11. Cloacal exstrophy consists of exstrophy of the bladder; complete phallic separation; wide diastasis of the pubis; exstrophy of the terminal ileum, which lies between the two halves of the bladder; rudimentary hindgut; imperforate anus; omphalocele; and not infrequently associated spinal defects. Spinal defects are not common in patients who only have exstrophy.
12. In adolescents and adults with exstrophy, concerns in the male are length, appearance, and deviation of the penis. In the female, concerns are the appearance of the external genitalia, adequacy of the vaginal opening, and uterine prolapse.
13. Women with exstrophy have delivered children; however, a frequent complication after pregnancy is cervical and uterine prolapse.
14. Closure of exstrophy: (1) reshapes the pelvis, (2) redistributes the levator group, and (3) smooths the contour of the pelvic floor.
15. At birth the exstrophy patient should have the umbilical cord secured with silk rather than an umbilical clamp to prevent trauma to the exposed bladder, and the bladder should be covered with a nonadherent film to minimize trauma and prevent desiccation of the bladder mucosa.
16. Bladder spasms must be controlled in the postoperative period following closure of the exstrophy.
17. Patients with epispadias may have associated vesicoureteral reflux and inguinal hernias, although the incidence is not as high as it is in bladder exstrophy.
18. The factor most likely to cause long-term disability in the reconstructed cloacal exstrophy patient is the associated neurologic deficit.
19. The basic defect in exstrophy is an abnormal overdevelopment of the cloacal membrane, preventing medial migration of the mesenchymal tissue and proper lower abdominal wall development.
20. Anterior corporeal length in male patients with bladder exstrophy is almost 50% shorter than that of healthy control participants.
21. Bladder neck repair usually occurs when the child is 4 to 5 years, has an adequate bladder capacity, and, most important, is ready to participate in a postoperative voiding program.
22. In a closed exstrophy patient, recurrent urinary tract infections should prompt evaluation for erosion of the anterior pubic stitch into the bladder or urethra.
23. A majority of bladder neck failures require eventual augmentation or continent diversion.
24. At birth ,most recommend assigning gender that is consistent with karyotypic makeup of the individual if at all possible.

140 Prune-Belly Syndrome

Anthony A. Caldamone and Francisco Tibor Dénes

QUESTIONS

1. Common findings in the prune-belly syndrome include all of the following EXCEPT:
   a. deficiency of abdominal wall musculature.
   b. urinary tract dilatation.
   c. palpable undescended testes.
   d. urachal pseudodiverticulum.
   e. vesicoureteral reflux.

2. Which of the following statements regarding the prognosis of patients with prune-belly syndrome is FALSE?
   a. The patient will likely be infertile.
   b. A substantial risk of renal failure exists.
   c. Testicular descent will not occur spontaneously.
   d. The male "pseudo-prune" phenotype is protected from renal failure.
   e. Chronic constipation and ineffective cough may result from abdominal wall laxity.

3. Complications involving which of the following organ systems are most likely to threaten the early survival of an infant with prune-belly syndrome?
   a. Cardiac
   b. Renal
   c. Pulmonary
   d. Gastrointestinal
   e. Endocrine

4. Ureteral dysfunction in prune-belly syndrome is related to all of the following EXCEPT:
   a. ureteral dilatation with failure of luminal coaptation during peristalsis.
   b. reduced smooth muscle tissue.
   c. failure of propagation of an electrical conduction due to increased fibrous connective tissue.
   d. more severe proximal ureteral dysfunction with failure to conduct a urinary bolus from the renal pelvis.
   e. abnormal myofilament content in smooth muscle cells.

5. Urodynamic bladder evaluation in prune-belly syndrome is primarily characterized by bladder enlargement with:
   a. elevated voiding pressures and detrusor-sphincter dyssynergia.
   b. high-amplitude uninhibited contractions.
   c. poorly contractile detrusor or myogenic failure.
   d. poor compliance.
   e. absent sensation.

6. The classic findings on prenatal ultrasound on prune-belly syndrome include all of the following EXCEPT:
   a. ambiguous genitalia.
   b. hydroureteronephrosis.
   c. distended bladder.
   d. early fetal ascites.
   e. irregular abdominal wall circumferences.

7. A management strategy of observation in the prune-belly syndrome is strongly supported by which finding?
   a. That spontaneous improvement in dilatation of the urinary tract generally occurs after puberty
   b. That vesicoureteral reflux occurs at low pressures and does not represent a threat to renal parenchyma
   c. That the risk of obstruction after ureteral reimplantation always outweighs the benefit
   d. That operative risks in this patient population are excessive
   e. None of the above

8. Which statement is most accurate when considering management of the lower urinary tract in the patient with prune-belly syndrome?
   a. Reduction cystoplasty is indicated when bladder capacity becomes greater than expected for age.
   b. Internal urethrotomy improves postvoid residual urine volumes without risk of incontinence.
   c. Reduction cystoplasty permanently improves bladder dynamics.
   d. Internal urethrotomy should be specifically based on pressure-flow studies.
   e. Routine intermittent catheterization should be used to improve postvoid residual urine volumes in all patients.

9. Which statement regarding orchiopexy in the patient with prune-belly syndrome is TRUE?
   a. It requires a microvascular testicular autotransplantation because of the high intra-abdominal position.
   b. It maintains endocrine function but has no potential to preserve spermatogenesis.
   c. It can be best accomplished by transperitoneal mobilization before 1 year of age.
   d. It should never involve use of the Fowler-Stephens technique because of unreliability of the collateral testicular blood supply.
   e. It is performed if spontaneous descent fails to occur by 2 years of age.

10. The most appropriate indication for prenatal intervention in suspected prune-belly syndrome is:
    a. oligohydramnios.
    b. urinary ascites.
    c. urethral atresia and progressive oligohydramnios.
    d. pulmonary hypoplasia.
    e. distended bladder.

11. The most appropriate initial management of the newborn with prune-belly syndrome includes:
    a. percutaneous drainage of the upper urinary tract after stabilization.
    b. stabilization and then vesicostomy if anesthetic risk permits.

c. stabilization and then bilateral cutaneous ureterostomy if anesthetic risk permits.

d. evaluation of pulmonary status and voiding cystourethrogram to rule out posterior urethral valves and reflux.

e. evaluation of pulmonary status, renal ultrasonographic study, and prophylactic antibiotics.

12. The prostatic urethra in prune-belly syndrome:

a. is dilated and associated with bladder neck hypertrophy on a voiding cystogram.

b. is sometimes associated with congenital urethral obstruction resulting in megalourethra.

c. is associated with a hypoplastic prostate with decreased epithelium and increased smooth muscle.

d. results in retrograde ejaculation.

e. is characterized by none of the above.

ANSWERS

1. **c. Palpable undescended testes.** Bilateral cryptorchidism is a central feature of the syndrome, and in most patients both testes are intra-abdominal, overlying the ureters at the pelvic brim near the sacroiliac level.

2. **d. The male "pseudo-prune" phenotype is protected from renal failure.** Although it is exceptionally rare to encounter a normal urinary tract in association with the characteristic abdominal wall defect in a male, the converse is not unusual. Some patients (with pseudo-prune-belly syndrome) with a normal or relatively normal abdominal wall exhibit many or all of the internal urologic features. These features may include dysplastic or dysmorphic kidneys or dilated and tortuous ureters. One report noted eight boys with relatively mild external features of the syndrome, five of whom progressed to renal failure, evidence that these children remain vulnerable to renal deterioration.

3. **c. Pulmonary.** The most urgent matters are actually those concerned with cardiopulmonary function. Pulmonary complications including pulmonary hypoplasia, pneumomediastinum, pneumothorax, and cardiac abnormalities must be excluded.

4. **d. More severe proximal ureteral dysfunction with failure to conduct a urinary bolus from the renal pelvis.** The proximal ureter usually displays a more normal appearance, an important feature when considering corrective surgery.

5. **c. Poorly contractile detrusor or myogenic failure.** Usually, the cystometrogram reveals excellent detrusor compliance; the end-filling pressure assumes a normal value; and the bladder functions well as a reservoir. However, bladder sensation during filling is shifted to the right with a delayed first sensation to void, and bladder capacity may be more than double the normal volume. Less consistent and less favorable results are seen with the voiding profile. The compressor capabilities of the detrusor are diminished by the frequent presence of vesicoureteral reflux and reduced detrusor contractility.

6. **a. Ambiguous genitalia.** The findings on prenatal ultrasound in prune-belly syndrome may not be diagnosed in all cases but would include hydronephrosis, an enlarged bladder, ascites presenting in the second trimester, and irregular abdominal wall circumference. Although external genital anomalies such as bilaterally undescended testes and megalourethra occur with prune-belly syndrome, these would not be detected on prenatal ultrasound as abnormalities of external genital development.

7. **e. None of the above.** The obvious implication of different studies was that a more aggressive approach was necessary to improve the fate of the infant with prune-belly syndrome. With the recognition that infection and progressive renal insufficiency are the factors that most often pose the greatest threat to quality of life and survival, surgical reconstruction to normalize the anatomy and function of the genitourinary tract was advocated. Early retailoring of the urinary system to reduce stasis and eliminate reflux or obstruction has included ureteral shortening, tapering and vesicoureteral reimplantation, and reduction cystoplasty. Reconstruction is best delayed until the child is approximately 3 months old, to allow for pulmonary maturation. This approach has been successful in achieving anatomic and functional improvement.

8. **d. Internal urethrotomy should be specifically based on pressure-flow studies.** Some initial improvement in voiding dynamics can be achieved by aggressive bladder remodeling. However, with long-term follow-up, there has been no evidence that this improvement is maintained, and excessive bladder volumes tend to recur with time. Internal urethrotomy is indicated in the rare patient with true anatomic urethral obstruction or in patients with urodynamic evidence of urethral obstruction by pressure-flow studies.

9. **c. It can be best accomplished by transperitoneal mobilization before 1 year of age.** Orchiopexy in all patients is now generally performed during infancy in an effort to maintain the germ cell population and protect spermatogenesis. In the neonate and in patients as old as 6 months, transabdominal complete mobilization of the spermatic cord almost always allows the testis to be positioned in the dependent portion of the scrotum without dividing the vascular portion of the spermatic cord. The Fowler-Stephens technique for performing orchiopexy in patients with intra-abdominal testes has become part of the standard urologic armamentarium.

10. **c. Urethral atresia and progressive oligohydramnios.** Because most hydronephrosis in prune-belly syndrome is well tolerated, its presence alone is not an indication for intervention. Similarly, oligohydramnios, pulmonary hypoplasia, distended bladder, and urinary ascites do not independently warrant prenatal intervention. The only situation with prune-belly syndrome that is potentially reversible is the pulmonary hypoplasia that is seen from urethral atresia and due to progressive oligohydramnios. Oligohydramnios that occurs early in the second trimester is generally indicative of severe renal dysplasia.

11. **e. Evaluation of pulmonary status, renal ultrasonographic study, and prophylactic antibiotics.** The most urgent matters are those concerned with cardiopulmonary function. After stabilization, urologic evaluation proceeds with physical examination and ultrasonography. Imaging requiring catheterization and the potential for introduction of bacteria should be avoided unless the results are necessary for immediate clinical decision making. Attention to sterile technique is crucial if invasive studies are performed. Once introduced, infection in a static system may be difficult to eradicate.

12. **d. Results in retrograde ejaculation.** The characteristically wide bladder neck merges with a grossly dilated prostatic urethra, so the junction is nearly imperceptible both radiographically and by gross inspection. The prostatic urethra does, however, taper to a relatively narrow membranous urethra at the urogenital diaphragm. Retrograde ejaculation is common.

CHAPTER REVIEW

1. The three major findings in prune-belly syndrome are (1) deficiency of abdominal musculature, (2) bilateral intra-abdominal testes, and (3) anomalous urinary tract usually composed of varying degrees of hydronephrosis, renal dysplasia, tortuous ureters, enlarged bladder, and dilated prostatic urethra.

2. The single most important determinant of renal function is the degree of renal dysplasia.

3. The majority (95%) of those with prune-belly syndrome are males.

4. The ureters lack smooth muscle cells and have an increased amount of fibrous connective tissue; the most normal portion of the ureter with the greatest amount of smooth muscle is in the proximal segment. This is the segment that should be preserved for reconstruction.

5. The bladder is usually massively dilated.

6. The vas and seminal vesicles are often atretic.

7. The fusiform type of megalourethra involves deficiencies of the corpus cavernosum and corpus spongiosum, whereas the scaphoid variety involves a deficiency of corpus spongiosum only.

8. The deficiency in the abdominal wall musculature is usually medial and inferior.

9. The disease is generally classified into three categories according to severity: category I, patients with marked oligohydramnios with renal dysplasia and pulmonary hypoplasia; category II, moderate renal insufficiency; and category III, mild manifestations in which renal function is well maintained.

10. Infection and progressive renal insufficiency are the greatest threat to long-term survival.

11. Abdominal wall reconstruction has been demonstrated to improve bladder emptying and result in a more effective cough and improved defecation.

12. Circumcision in the neonatal period is advisable if there is no structural deformity of the penis.

13. Upper track reconstruction is clearly indicated in patients with evidence of decreasing renal function in the presence of hydronephrosis, recurrent urinary tract infections, and progression of the hydronephrosis.

14. Patients with pseudo-prune-belly syndrome with a normal or relatively normal abdominal wall exhibit many or all of the internal urologic features of prune-belly syndrome. These features may include dysplastic or dysmorphic kidneys or dilated and tortuous ureters.

15. In the neonate and in patients up to at least 6 months of age, transabdominal complete mobilization of the spermatic cord almost always allows the testis to be positioned in the dependent portion of the scrotum without dividing the vascular portion of the spermatic cord.

141 Posterior Urethral Valves and Urethral Anomalies

Aseem Ravindra Shukla

QUESTIONS

1. A newborn infant with a history of antenatal hydronephrosis and oligohydramnios is evaluated with a renal/bladder ultrasound and voiding cystourethrogram. All of the following are characteristic findings of posterior urethral valves EXCEPT:

   a. hypertrophy and apparent elevation of the bladder neck.

   b. multiple bladder diverticula.

   c. bladder perforation with small amount of urinary extravasation causing ascites.

   d. rupture of an upper pole calyceal fornix causing distortion of the renal capsule.

   e. all of the above.

2. A 6-month-old child with a history of posterior urethral valves has a serum creatinine of 1.4 mg/dL. He has a dilated, thick-walled bladder and hydroureteronephrosis on sonography and evidence of dilating vesicoureteral reflux with no remnant valves on voiding cystourethrography. Which of the following BEST explains the renal impairment noted in this child?

   a. Increased intravesical storage pressures transmitted to the ureter, renal pelvis, and glomerular units causing architectural and functional changes

   b. High-grade vesicoureteral reflux

   c. Repeated afebrile urinary tract infections

   d. Family history

   e. Likely misdiagnosis of hydronephrosis for concurrent autosomal dominant polycystic kidney disease

3. A newborn diagnosed with posterior urethral valves is noted on voiding cystourethrogram (VCUG) to have unilateral high-grade vesicoureteral reflux into the right kidney that has no measurable renal function on nuclear renography. The left kidney displays normal uptake and excretion of nuclear tracer. Which of the following best characterizes this boy's renal status?

   a. Better long-term renal function due to protective effect of reflux into dysplastic right kidney

   b. No better or worse long-term renal function requiring close observation

   c. High risk of febrile urinary tract infections will require early nephroureterectomy of nonfunctioning renal unit

   d. Plan early right ureteral reimplantation reduce risk of pyelonephritis

   e. None of the above

4. All of the following findings on antenatal imaging should raise suspicion of posterior urethral valves EXCEPT:

   a. thickened bladder wall.

   b. bilateral pelvicaliectasis with ureterectasis.

   c. oligohydramnios.

   d. ambiguous genitalia.

   e. dilated posterior urethra (keyhole sign).

5. The most common cause of early neonatal mortality in a baby affected by posterior urethral valves is:

   a. urinary sepsis.

   b. end-stage renal disease not amenable to dialysis.

   c. pulmonary hypoplasia.

   d. urinary ascites due to calyx forniceal rupture.

   e. necrotizing enterocolitis.

6. A 3-year-old boy presents with urinary incontinence, stranguria, and occasional afebrile urinary tract infections. A renal ultrasound reveals moderate bilateral hydroureteronephrosis. The best next step in management is:

   a. a repeat renal ultrasound in 6 months.

   b. treatment of dysfunctional elimination syndrome with timed voiding and laxative.

   c. begin an alpha receptor blocker.

   d. Botox injection to the external urethral sphincter.

   e. voiding cystourethrogram.

7. Fetal intervention for obstructive uropathy secondary to posterior urethral valves has been shown to:

   a. diminish the incidence of end-stage renal disease.

   b. be associated with a high rate of fetal demise.

   c. lead to improved pulmonary function in the neonate.

   d. be most effective when accomplished by open fetal surgery.

   e. be associated with neonatal respiratory failure.

8. A premature neonate with a weight of 2500 g with impaired renal function and bilateral hydroureteronephrosis (right greater than left) is diagnosed with posterior urethral valves. After 1 week of bladder catheterization, a plan is made to proceed to the operating room for valve ablation. Cystoscopy is precluded by the small genitalia. Which of the following is the preferred initial surgical option?

   a. Creation of a vesicostomy

   b. Bilateral proximal loop ureterostomy

   c. Cystotomy with antegrade valve ablation

   d. Suprapubic tube placement until child is old enough for valve ablation

   e. Bilateral percutaneous nephroureteral stent placement

9. A 4-year-old boy with a history of ablation of posterior urethral valves in infancy is volitionally voiding with no incontinence, stable renal function, and no urinary tract infections. He has high-grade vesicoureteric reflux on the left side with stable hydroureteronephrosis that has not changed since infancy. What is the best management for this child?

   a. Cross trigonal ureteral reimplantation

   b. Vesicostomy

   c. Conservative management with timed voiding and anticholinergic therapy

   d. Cystoscopy with subureteral injection of Deflux

   e. Both a and d are correct

10. In cases of posterior urethral valves, the bladder transitions through three contractility patterns in childhood. Which is the correct order for the changes in bladder contractility?

    a. Detrusor hyperreflexia with high intravesical pressure; improved compliance with reduced intravesical pressures; high-capacity bladder and hypocontractility

    b. High-capacity bladder and hypocontractility; detrusor hyperreflexia with high intravesical pressure; improved compliance with reduced intravesical pressures

    c. Improved compliance with reduced intravesical pressures; high-capacity bladder and hypocontractility; detrusor hyperreflexia with high intravesical pressure

    d. High-capacity bladder and hypocontractility; improved compliance with reduced intravesical pressures; detrusor hyperreflexia with high intravesical pressure

    e. Detrusor hyperreflexia with high intravesical pressure; high-capacity bladder and hypocontractility; improved compliance with reduced intravesical pressures

11. All of the following are associated with the development of the valve bladder syndrome EXCEPT:

    a. high voiding pressures.

    b. incomplete bladder emptying with high postvoid residuals.

    c. renal tubular and glomerular impairment.

    d. previous history of vesicostomy.

    e. bilateral hydroureteronephrosis.

12. A child with a history of posterior urethral valve ablation suffers renal impairment and, ultimately, progresses to end stage renal disease. All of the factors below likely characterized his clinical course, EXCEPT:

    a. nadir creatinine at 1 year of life.

    b. renal dysplasia with or without vesicoureteral reflux.

    c. recurrent urinary tract infections.

    d. valve bladder syndrome.

    e. all of the above.

13. A 13-year-old boy with a history of posterior urethral valves progresses to end-stage renal disease and is a candidate for renal transplant. Of the complications listed, which one may be most likely to occur in a child with a history of posterior urethral valves?

    a. Acute graft rejection

    b. Vesicoureteral reflux

    c. Chronic graft rejection

    d. Ureteral obstruction at site of ureteroneocystotomy

    e. All of the above

ANSWERS

1. **c. Bladder perforation with small amount of urinary extravasation causing ascites.** Fetal and neonatal lower urinary tract obstruction due to posterior urethral valves may transmit enough pressure to the upper urinary tract to cause a rupture of a calyceal fornix, causing urine to be trapped within the renal capsule or causing ascites, in rare cases. However, bladder perforation is not a characteristic of posterior urethral valves, because the process actually leads to significant bladder wall hypertrophy.

2. **a. Increased intravesical storage pressures transmitted to the ureter, renal pelvis, and glomerular units causing architectural and functional changes.** Sustained increases in intravesical storage pressure during prolonged time intervals transmit these pressures to the ureter, renal pelvis, and ultimately, glomerular units.

Of the options provided, this is the most likely etiology of renal insufficiency in this child.

3. **b. No better or worse long-term renal function requiring close observation.** Contrary to previous assumptions, the so-called *vesicoureteric reflux and dysplasia* (VURD) syndrome is not a renal protective phenomenon. These children often have evidence of renal dysplasia detectable in the solitary functioning kidney increasing the likelihood of significant long-term renal impairment.

4. **d. Ambiguous genitalia.** All of the aforementioned findings are characteristic findings of posterior urethral valves on antenatal imaging, except ambiguous genitalia. Posterior urethral valves are not associated with external genital anomalies.

5. **c. Pulmonary hypoplasia.** Although the focus in posterior urethral valves is too often on the lower urinary tract and kidneys, the most profound complication and cause of perinatal mortality in infants affected by severe lower urinary tract obstruction remains pulmonary hypoplasia.

6. **e. Voiding cystourethrogram.** Despite the ubiquity of antenatal imaging today, delayed presentation of posterior urethral valves after 6 months of age is not uncommon. A high index of suspicion for posterior urethral valves must be assumed when a boy presents with lower urinary tract symptoms, especially recurrent urinary tract infections, but also overflow incontinence, gross hematuria, renal dysfunction, and, less commonly, ejaculatory dysfunction.

7. **c. Lead to improved pulmonary function in the neonate.** Fetal intervention for posterior urethral valves has not been shown to lower the incidence of end-stage renal disease but, in properly selected cases, it can offer the benefit of improved neonatal pulmonary function. Neonates with severe obstructive uropathy die of respiratory failure due to a noncompliant and hypoplastic lung.

8. **a. Creation of a vesicostomy.** In the low-birth-weight infant with renal impairment whose urethra will not accommodate an infant cystoscope, a vesicostomy is the ideal first option. The vesicostomy allows decompression of the obstructed system, allows continued bladder cycling, and is easily managed with diapers. Upper tract diversion is a reasonable option, but it does require bilateral incisions and also a complex follow-up surgery that can risk injury to the developing ureters.

9. **c. Conservative management with timed voiding and anticholinergic therapy.** Vesicoureteral reflux in children with posterior urethral valves is a common finding and should be understood to be a consequence of neonatal obstruction and the secondarily elevated bladder pressures. Management of this child should be centered on the lower urinary tract with attention to timed voiding, double voiding, and anticholinergics as necessary. Ureteral reimplantation is an option in atypical cases where urinary tract infections continue despite maximal bladder therapy.

10. **a. Detrusor hyperreflexia with high intravesical pressure; improved compliance with reduced intravesical pressures; high-capacity bladder and hypocontractility.** The bladder evolves through three distinct contractility patterns through childhood: (1) detrusor hyperreflexia in infancy and early childhood; (2) decreasing intravesical pressures and improved compliance bladder in childhood; and (3) increased capacity bladder with hypocontractility and atony in adolescence.

11. **d. Previous history of vesicostomy.** The theory of the valve bladder syndrome holds that although the bladder initially compensates for outlet obstruction by generating high voiding pressures, it begins to experience higher volumes of urine due to increasing urine production as the child grows. The polyuria due to nephrogenic diabetes insipidus secondary to evolving renal impairment augments the urine volumes entering a bladder that is increasingly unable to empty completely. As the postvoid residuals increase, the bladder no longer enjoys periods of complete relaxation, and the detrusor fibers are continuously in a state of partial or complete stretch, beginning a cascade of

gene expression and phenotypic changes that further impair contractility of the bladder. Creation of a vesicostomy has no impact on impairing bladder contractility.

12. **e. All of the above.** Risk factors known to affect the prognosis of an infant diagnosed with posterior urethral valves include age at diagnosis, renal dysplasia with or without vesicoureteral reflux, nadir creatinine at 1 year of life, recurrent urinary tract infections, and bladder dysfunction.

13. **d. Ureteral obstruction at site of ureteroneocystotomy.** The thickened bladder wall of patients with posterior urethral valves (PUV) may contribute to the significantly increased incidence of ureteral obstruction on univariate and multivariate analysis compared with a non-PUV transplant cohort, but recent studies saw no risk of increased graft loss or patient death despite ureteral obstruction, stenting or dilation.

CHAPTER REVIEW

1. Type I valves are the most common. These valves originate at the verumontanum and course distally.
2. Type II folds, which course from the verumontanum to the bladder neck, are no longer considered valves.
3. A type III valve is a membrane lying transversely across the urethra.
4. In patients with PUV, the bladder neck is elevated and hypertrophied. Renal dysfunction, reflux, and worsening hydronephrosis are due to bladder dysfunction.
5. Virtually all valve patients have hydroureteronephrosis.
6. Patients with posterior urethral valves fail to concentrate and acidify urine throughout childhood and adulthood.
7. Patients with urinary ascites have a poor prognosis.
8. The keyhole sign as seen on ultrasound or VCUG represents a dilated bladder and a dilated prostatic urethra, with a hypertrophied bladder neck in between.
9. Vesicoureteral reflux is present at birth in 50% of patients with posterior urethral valves.
10. The goal in treating posterior urethral valves cystoscopically is to incise them, not remove them.
11. It is imperative to document that the valve remnants are no longer obstructive following therapy.
12. If upper tract drainage is required, a low loop ureterostomy is preferred because it provides adequate drainage, can be placed beneath the diaper, and offers the least difficult reconstruction.
13. High-grade reflux is often associated with severe renal dysplasia.
14. The valve bladder may lead to deterioration of the upper tracts and incontinence during the patient's life.
15. The majority of patients with valve bladder have delayed daytime and nighttime continence.
16. The independent risk factors for predicting end-stage renal disease in patients with posterior urethral valves are the nadir serum creatinine and severe bladder dysfunction; renal impairment is due to renal dysplasia and obstructive uropathy .
17. Circumcision should be strongly considered in the neonatal period in patients with PUV to limit urinary tract infections.
18. Ablation of valves or vesicostomy will resolve reflux in 25% to 40% of patients.
19. PUV patients have polyuria due to impaired concentrating ability of the kidney.
20. The life time prevalence of end-stage renal disease in patients with PUV is 20% to 50%.
21. In patients with PUV at 1 year of life, a creatinine of less than 0.8 mg/dL portends a low risk for end-stage renal disease, whereas a creatinine of greater than 1.2 mg/dL suggests a high risk.
22. Anterior urethral valves often occur in the form of a diverticulum.
23. The treatment of congenital urethral strictures in the neonate is vesicostomy because the strictures are generally too long and dense to incise.
24. In urethral duplication, the ventral urethra is usually the functional urethra.
25. The most profound complication and cause of perinatal mortality in infants affected by severe lower urinary tract obstruction remains pulmonary hypoplasia.
26. Fetal intervention for posterior urethral valves has not been shown to lower the incidence of end-stage renal disease, but in properly selected cases, it can offer the benefit of improved neonatal pulmonary function.
27. In patients with posterior urethral valves, the bladder evolves through three distinct contractility patterns through childhood: (1) detrusor hyperreflexia in infancy and early childhood; (2) decreasing intravesical pressures and improved bladder compliance in childhood; and (3) increased capacity of the bladder with hypocontractility and atony in adolescence.
28. In the valve bladder, the polyuria due to nephrogenic diabetes insipidus secondary to evolving renal impairment augments the urine volumes entering the bladder, which is increasingly unable to empty completely.

142 Neuromuscular Dysfunction of the Lower Urinary Tract in Children

Dawn Lee MacLellan and Stuart B. Bauer

QUESTIONS

1. Which of the following is an acquired form of neuromuscular dysfunction of the lower urinary tract?
   a. Myelomeningocele
   b. Cerebral palsy
   c. Lipomeningocele
   d. Sacral agenesis
   e. Anorectal malformation

2. What is the primary goal in management of neuromuscular dysfunction of the lower urinary tract?
   a. Achievement of urinary continence
   b. Achievement of fecal continence
   c. Preservation of renal function
   d. Facilitation of sexual function
   e. Avoidance of urinary tract infection

3. The International Children's Continence Society (ICCS) recommends more frequent evaluation of children during periods of high rates of somatic growth when spinal cord tethering is more likely. These two development periods are:
   a. Newborn to toddler AND toddler to adolescent
   b. Newborn to toddler AND adolescent to adult
   c. Newborn to toddler AND adulthood
   d. Toddler to adolescent AND adolescent to adult
   e. Toddler to adolescent AND adulthood

4. The International Children's Continence Society's indications for repeat investigations before the routinely scheduled follow-up for neuromuscular dysfunction of the lower urinary tract do NOT include:
   a. urinary tract infections.
   b. development or worsening of hydronephrosis.
   c. worsening continence.
   d. change in lower extremity function.
   e. improved continence.

5. Which of the following may compromise bladder emptying in neuromuscular dysfunction of the lower urinary tract?
   a. Low capacity
   b. Low compliance
   c. Detrusor overactivity
   d. Detrusor sphincter dyssynergia
   e. Low outlet resistance

6. Initial minimally invasive treatment options to address inadequate bladder storage in neuromuscular dysfunction in children usually involve:
   a. overnight indwelling catheter drainage.
   b. antimuscarinics and clean intermittent catheterization.
   c. percutaneous cystostomy tube.
   d. endoscopic injection of botulinum toxin.
   e. robotic assisted augmentation cystoplasty.

7. The use of antimuscarinics for the treatment of detrusor overactivity in children does NOT result in the following:
   a. increased bladder capacity.
   b. decreased number of bladder contractions.
   c. decreased number of incontinence episodes.
   d. decreased number of catheterizations.
   e. decreased volume to first bladder contraction.

8. A possible predictor of poor clinical response to intravesical injection of botulinum toxin injection is preexisting:
   a. low maximum cystometric capacity.
   b. detrusor overactivity.
   c. more than five episodes of incontinence per day.
   d. poor detrusor compliance.
   e. previous botulinum toxin injections.

9. Which of the following increases the risk of developing lower urinary tract stones in children with bladder augmentation?
   a. Use of the ileal segment
   b. Routine bladder irrigation with water or saline
   c. Use of an antimuscarinic
   d. Catheterization of the urethra, rather than an abdominal stoma
   e. A mobile patient

10. The presentation of bladder malignancy in those with a history of bladder augmentation does NOT include:
    a. Presenting with advanced disease.
    b. Presenting at an older age than is typical for bladder malignancies.
    c. Presenting with atypical symptoms, such as vague abdominal pain, urosepsis or increased frequency of urinary tract infection (UTI), difficult catheterization, and renal failure.
    d. Presenting with a time lag of a minimum of 10 years after a bladder augmentation.
    e. Presenting with atypical signs, such as new hydronephrosis and bladder wall thickening.

11. Which of the following is the preferred approach to increase bladder capacity in children with neuromuscular dysfunction of the lower urinary tract?
    a. Autoaugmentation
    b. Enteric augmentation with a gastric segment
    c. Tissue-engineered bladder substitute
    d. Enteric augmentation with an ileal segment
    e. Enteric augmentation with an ileal-cecal segment

12. Worsening of bladder function after isolated bladder neck procedures including implantation of an artificial urinary sphincter or bladder neck fascial sling is more common in those with:

    a. preexisting detrusor overactivity and poor compliance.

    b. preexisting low maximum cystometric capacity.

    c. surgery in the postpubertal period.

    d. detrusor sphincter dyssynergia.

    e. history of prior bladder neck outlet procedures.

13. Which of the following is NOT an acceptable method of managing high-grade vesicoureteral reflux in children with neuromuscular dysfunction of the lower urinary tract?

    a. Clean intermittent catheterization

    b. Antimuscarinics

    c. Antibiotic prophylaxis

    d. Ureteral re-implantation

    e. Bladder emptying by the Credé maneuver

14. Prenatal surgery for children with myelomeningocele compared with standard postnatal closure has been noted to result in:

    a. an increased risk of fetal death and need for cerebrospinal fluid shunting.

    b. worsening of mental development and motor function at 30 months.

    c. fewer pregnancy complications.

    d. a lower risk of preterm labor.

    e. no improvement in bladder function.

15. Indications for the initiation of clean intermittent catheterization in the newborn with myelomeningocele do NOT include:

    a. postvoid residual urine measurement of 3 mL after the Credé maneuver.

    b. postvoid residual urine measurement of 10 mL after spontaneous voiding.

    c. the presence of detrusor sphincter dyssynergia on urodynamic studies.

    d. the presence of hydronephrosis and high-grade vesicoureteral reflux with poor bladder emptying.

    e. poor bladder compliance with bladder filling pressures greater than 40 cm H_2O.

16. The highest risk for the development of urinary tract deterioration in children with myelodysplasia is in those with initial urodynamic findings of:

    a. detrusor sphincter synergy.

    b. detrusor sphincter dyssynergy.

    c. complete denervation.

    d. low maximum cystometric capacity.

    e. detrusor overactivity.

17. The gold standard for measuring renal function in children with myelodysplasia is:

    a. serum creatinine.

    b. glomerular filtration rate as estimated by the Schwarz formula.

    c. glomerular filtration rate as estimated by the Modification of Diet in Renal Disease (MDRD) equation.

    d. serum cystatin C.

    e. nuclear renography.

18. Sexual function and satisfaction in men with myelomeningocele is better with the following condition:

    a. living with their parents.

    b. severe incontinence.

19. (continued)

    c. a sacral-level lesion of the neural tube defect.

    d. a thoracic-level lesion of the neural tube defect.

    e. the presence of hydrocephalus.

19. The most common finding associated with an occult neural tube defect is:

    a. a cutaneous abnormality overlying the lower spine.

    b. high-arched feet.

    c. claw or hammer toes.

    d. abnormal gait.

    e. absent perineal sensation.

20. In a 1-year-old child, definitive diagnosis of an occult neural tube defect is best made by:

    a. Spinal ultrasound.

    b. Urodynamic studies demonstrating findings consistent with neurogenic bladder dysfunction.

    c. Magnetic resonance imaging of the spine.

    d. Documentation of resolution of abnormal urodynamic findings after a detethering procedure.

    e. Abnormal electromyography of the external urinary sphincter.

21. Which of the following is UNLIKELY to be noted in a child with neuromuscular dysfunction of the lower urinary tract secondary to sacral agenesis?

    a. Urinary incontinence

    b. A maternal history of diabetes mellitus or gestational diabetes

    c. Flattened buttocks and a short, low gluteal cleft

    d. Absent perineal sensation

    e. Vesicoureteral reflux and recurrent urinary tract infections

22. Urodynamic studies of children with an anorectal malformation should be performed in all of the following circumstances EXCEPT:

    a. a bony malformation of the spine or a spinal cord defect.

    b. hydronephrosis.

    c. vesicoureteral reflux.

    d. urinary or fecal incontinence.

    e. a low insertion of the fistulous site.

23. Which of the following statements concerning bladder function in children with cerebral palsy is TRUE?

    a. They achieve nighttime urinary continence first.

    b. They achieve urinary continence at the same age as their age-adjusted peers.

    c. Lower urinary tract symptoms are more common in younger children.

    d. The most common urinary tract symptom is monosymptomatic nocturnal enuresis.

    e. Clinical symptoms of recurrent UTI and detrusor sphincter dyssynergia (retention, interrupted stream, and hesitancy) are associated with upper urinary tract deterioration.

24. The most common presenting urinary symptom in children with transverse myelitis is:

    a. urinary incontinence.

    b. urinary tract infection.

    c. urinary retention.

    d. urinary frequency.

    e. urinary urgency.

ANSWERS

1. **b. Cerebral palsy.** Cerebral palsy is the only acquired disease process in the list. The remainder are congenital.
2. **c. Preservation of renal function.** Although the other listed goals have important clinical and social implications, preservation of renal function is the primary goal of treatment. Achievement of urinary/fecal continence, sexual function, and avoidance of urinary tract infection are secondary goals of treatment.
3. **b. Newborn to toddler AND adolescent to adult.** The correct combination of growth periods in which the rate of somatic growth is highest is in the newborn to toddler and adolescent to adult age group. This recommendation is due to the fact that the highest rate of spinal cord tethering, and thus change in bladder/bowel function, is during periods of highest somatic growth.
4. **e. Improved continence.** Urinary tract infections, hydronephrosis, worsening continence, and a change in lower extremity function are more likely to indicate a significant change in bladder function than improved continence.
5. **d. Detrusor sphincter dyssynergia.** Detrusor sphincter dyssynergia is the only entity listed that may compromise bladder emptying. All other listed options would facilitate or encourage early bladder emptying.
6. **b. Antimuscarinics and clean intermittent catheterization.** The beneficial effects of early initiation of antimuscarinics and clean intermittent catheterization are well established. The other listed options would be considered to be more invasive or less established methods of intervention.
7. **e. Decreased volume to first bladder contraction.** Antimuscarinics in children result in increased bladder capacity, fewer bladder contractions, less incontinence, and fewer catheterizations. The question is worded negatively, so answer e is correct, because antimuscarinics would be expected to increase the volume to first bladder contraction, rather than decrease it.
8. **d. Poor detrusor compliance.** Kask et al (2013)* demonstrated that preexisting poor detrusor compliance predicts a poor clinical response to intravesical injection of botulinum toxin. One could postulate that the histologic changes that are present after the development of poor detrusor compliance are not amenable to the effects of botulinum toxin.
9. **a. Use of the ileal segment.** The use of an ileal segment has been shown to increase the risk of lower urinary tract stones. Catheterization through the urethra, rather than via an abdominal stoma, is associated with fewer lower urinary tract stones, presumably because of better drainage. A mobile patient and routine bladder irrigation decrease the risk of stones. The use of an antimuscarinic should not affect stone formation.
10. **b. Presenting at an older age than is typical for bladder malignancies.** Those with bladder augmentation present at a younger age, with atypical symptoms and advanced disease, usually with a minimum 10-year lag time between augmentation and presentation of bladder malignancy.
11. **d. Enteric augmentation with an ileal segment.** Lack of improvement in urodynamic and clinical symptoms, along with a high failure rate, makes autoaugmentation an undesirable option. Gastric segments are associated with more symptomatic side effects (such as hematuria dysuria syndrome) and metabolic complications than ileal segments. It is recommended to avoid the ileal-cecal segment in children with neural tube defects because it may aggravate bowel dysfunction. Phase II studies of tissue-engineered bladder revealed no improvement in urodynamic parameters and serious adverse events. Thus, the ileal segment is the most desirable for enteric augmentation.

12. **a. Preexisting detrusor overactivity and poor compliance.** Isolated bladder neck procedures, such as artificial urinary sphincter and bladder neck repairs, have been noted to lead to worsening of bladder function in as many as 30% of patients, especially those with preexisting detrusor overactivity and poor compliance. The remaining answers have not been associated with worsening of bladder function after isolated bladder neck procedures.
13. **e. Bladder emptying by the Credé maneuver.** Children with a reactive external urinary sphincter will have a reflex response of increased external urethral tone in response to the Credé maneuver, which can aggravate reflux and thus is contraindicated in this group. The other listed options are all reasonable methods of managing vesicoureteral reflux in those with neuromuscular dysfunction of the lower urinary tract.
14. **e. No improvement in bladder function.** Prenatal surgery for children with myelomeningocele compared with standard postnatal closure has been noted to decrease the need for cerebrospinal fluid shunting, improve neuromotor function, and increase pregnancy complications and the risk for preterm labor. The correct answer is there is no improvement in lower urinary tract function with prenatal versus postnatal closure.
15. **a. Postvoid residual urine measurement of 3 mL after the Credé maneuver.** A postvoid residual urine measurement of 3 mL after the Credé maneuver is within normal limits and does not require the initiation of clean intermittent catheterization (CIC). All other possible answers are indications for the initiation of CIC.
16. **b. Detrusor sphincter dyssynergy.** Within the first 3 years of life, more than 70% of children with detrusor sphincter dyssynergy will have urinary tract deterioration, whereas less than one quarter of those with synergy or complete denervation will have deterioration. Low maximum cystometric capacity and detrusor overactivity have not been associated with upper tract deterioration.
17. **e. Nuclear renography.** Although all possible answers are means of measuring renal function in children with myelodysplasia, nuclear renography is considered to be the gold standard.
18. **c. A sacral-level lesion of the neural tube defect.** Lesions above the sacral spinal cord, hydrocephalus, incontinence, and living with parents are associated with less sexual function and satisfaction compared with men with a sacral-level lesion.
19. **a. A cutaneous abnormality overlying the lower spine.** A cutaneous abnormality overlying the spine, such as a skin dimple, tuft of hair, skin tag, lipoma, vascular malformation, or asymmetric gluteal cleft, is noted in 90% of those with occult neural tube defect. The other listed answers are also noted in this entity, but their occurrence is much less frequent.
20. **c. Magnetic resonance imaging of the spine.** Spinal ultrasound may be used before ossification of vertebral bones (3 months of age). After this time, magnetic resonance imaging of the spine is required for definitive diagnosis of an occult neural tube defect.
21. **d. Absent perineal sensation.** Children with sacral agenesis have normal perineal sensation, thus d is incorrect. The remaining answers may be found in patients with sacral agenesis.
22. **e. A low insertion of the fistulous site.** Urodynamic evaluation in those with anorectal malformation is indicated if there is suggestion of possible spinal cord tethering (bony malformation of the spine or spinal cord defect) or signs and/or symptoms that might indicate a neurogenic defect such as hydronephrosis, vesicoureteral reflux, or urinary/fecal incontinence. Although spinal cord defects may be present in as many as a third of those with a low insertion of the fistula site, a low insertion site itself is not an indication for urodynamic study.
23. **e. Clinical symptoms of recurrent UTI and detrusor sphincter dyssynergia (retention, interrupted stream, and hesitancy) are associated with upper urinary tract deterioration.** Children with cerebral palsy usually achieve daytime dryness first, at an older age than their age-adjusted peers. Lower urinary tract symptoms become more prevalent in children with cerebral

*Sources referenced can be found in *Campbell-Walsh Urology, 11th Edition,* on the Expert Consult website.

palsy while they age. The most common symptom in these children is incontinence. Clinical symptoms of recurrent UTI and detrusor sphincter dyssynergia are associated with upper urinary tract deterioration and may warrant investigation with renal/bladder ultrasound and urodynamic studies.

24. **c. Urinary retention.** The most common presenting urinary symptom of transverse myelitis is urinary retention. Ninety-five percent of children in the acute phase of the disease will have urinary retention.

CHAPTER REVIEW

1. During urodynamics, bladder filling should occur at a rate of the calculated bladder capacity divided by 10 per minute.
2. Normal voiding pressure in boys is 55 to 80 cm H_2O, and in girls it is 30 to 65 cm H_2O.
3. In the myelomeningocele patient, the bony vertebral level provides little or no clue as to the neurologic level.
4. Upper motor neuron lesions result in an overactive detrusor, exaggerated sacral reflexes, detrusor sphincter dyssynergia, a thickened bladder wall, and a closed bladder neck.
5. Lower motor neuron lesions result in a noncontractile detrusor, denervation of the external sphincter, diminished or absent sacral reflexes, and a small smooth-walled bladder with an open bladder neck.
6. Assessment of the neonate with myelomeningocele involves renal ultrasonography and measurement of the postvoid residual urine.
7. Resting bladder pressure should be maintained below 30 cm H_2O. Resting pressures above 40 cm H_2O result in upper tract deterioration.
8. The neurologic lesion in myelodysplasia is a dynamic process and changes throughout childhood.
9. Bowel incontinence is frequently unpredictable and not associated with the attainment of urinary continence in myelodysplasia patients.
10. Sacral agenesis may result in bladder dysfunction not detected at birth and is usually brought to the physician's attention when the child fails at toilet training.
11. Sacral agenesis may manifest as either an upper or lower motor neuron lesion.
12. In patients with cerebral palsy, the presence of incontinence is usually related to the physical impairment.
13. In traumatic injuries of the spine, patients with upper thoracic and cervical lesions are likely to exhibit autonomic dysreflexia.
14. Women with low levels of folic acid or impairment of folic acid–mediated pathways are at increased risk for having a child with a neural tube defect.
15. Findings on initial urodynamic assessment warranting further investigation with a voiding cystourethrogram include detrusor overactivity, poor compliance, disorders of sex development, and elevated voiding pressure; moreover, reflux in myelodysplastic children is invariably associated with one of these abnormalities.
16. There are three categories of findings on urodynamics in myelodysplastic children: synergy, dyssynergia, and complete denervation.
17. Serum creatinine in myelodysplastic children is a poor predictor of renal function; serum cystatin C may be a better predictor.
18. In patients with neural tube defects, early intervention with CIC and antimuscarinics decreases UTIs, vesicoureteral reflux, upper tract deterioration, and the incidence of end-stage renal disease.
19. Puberty occurs as much as 2 years earlier in girls with myelodysplasia.
20. Indications for augmentation cystoplasty in patients with neural tube defects include poor bladder compliance, small capacity, and overactive detrusor.
21. Autoaugmentation is not effective in patients with myelodysplasia.
22. Occult spinal dysraphism in the newborn period may be suggested by a sacral defect or a cutaneous abnormality over the sacrum such as a skin dimple, tuft of hair, skin tag, lipoma, vascular malformation, or asymmetric gluteal cleft. Early detection and intervention addressing bladder dysfunction markedly improves renal and bladder outcomes.
23. Children of diabetic mothers are at increased risk for sacral agenesis.
24. In patients with anorectal malformations, a neurogenic bladder is usually associated with a spinal cord abnormality.
25. Children with cerebral palsy often achieve continence, although at a later date than their age matched peers.
26. The highest rate of spinal cord tethering, and thus a change in bladder/bowel function, is during periods of highest somatic growth.
27. Gastric segments used for augmentation cystoplasty are associated with more symptomatic side effects (such as hematuria dysuria syndrome) and metabolic complications than ileal segments. It is recommended to avoid the ileal-cecal segment in children with neural tube defects because it may aggravate bowel dysfunction.
28. Prenatal surgery for children with myelomeningocele compared with standard postnatal closure has been noted to decrease the need for cerebrospinal fluid shunting, improve neuromotor function, and increase pregnancy complications and the risk for preterm labor.
29. Within the first 3 years of life, more than 70% of children with detrusor sphincter dyssynergy will have urinary tract deterioration, whereas less than one quarter of those with synergy or complete denervation will have deterioration.

143 Functional Disorders of the Lower Urinary Tract in Children

Paul F. Austin and Gino J. Vricella

QUESTIONS

1. A 9-year-old female presents to the office with a chief complaint of daytime urinary incontinence. She denies dysuria, hematuria, or enuresis. She has never had a urinary tract infection (UTI) and there is no history of hydronephrosis. Her mother states that toilet-training occurred at 2 years of age and was "easy." A clean-catch urinalysis has been obtained by her pediatrician and is completely normal. When characterizing the incontinence, she states that she completely soaks her clothes, necessitating a change in wardrobe. She denies urgency or frequency and otherwise voids every 2 to 3 hours during the day. She states that the episodes are often associated with laughing at a funny joke or movie. She denies any issues with constipation. Assuming physical examination and voiding diary are normal, which of the following would be a reasonable first-line treatment strategy?

   a. Acupuncture
   b. Biofeedback
   c. Hypnosis
   d. Imipramine
   e. Oxybutynin

2. A 4-year-old female presents to the office with a chief complaint of labial adhesions, dysuria, daytime urinary incontinence, and recurrent UTIs. Her mother states that toilet-training was completed at 20 months and that there were no issues with this. Based on history and completed voiding diary, her elimination pattern is normal. Her mother states that during the past 3 months, however, she has noted that her underpants are damp and that this is often noted within a few minutes of the child having voided. They deny any urgency or frequency. She recently has been complaining of severe dysuria with two urinalyses (UAs) in the past 4 weeks demonstrating 5 to 10 white blood cells per high-power field (WBCs/hpf). Urine cultures have all been negative, and antibiotics have not helped with symptomatology. Physical examination reveals superficial labial adhesions with moderately erythematous external genitalia. Noninvasive urodynamics with pelvic ultrasound and uroflowmetry reveal a bell-shaped curve and an empty bladder with normal wall thickness. There is a small amount of fluid noted in the vagina. While the child climbs down off of the examining room table, there is involuntary leakage of urine. Repeat pelvic ultrasound reveals that the vaginal vault is empty. What is the most likely diagnosis?

   a. Bladder-bowel dysfunction
   b. Dysfunctional voiding
   c. Urge urinary incontinence
   d. Vaginal reflux
   e. Vesicoureteral reflux (VUR)

3. An 8-year-old male is brought in by his grandmother, who recently obtained guardianship due to parental divorce and the biological mother's recent untimely death. She states that his teachers have been complaining that for the last 4 months he spends most of his time in the restroom, asking to use the bathroom approximately every 15 minutes. He has had some occasional dysuria, but no hematuria or fevers. They deny any UTIs or daytime urinary incontinence. He has occasional constipation, but this is readily corrected with fruit juice and he generally has one soft, smooth bowel movement daily. He is generally able

to sleep through the night without having to wake to void, and they deny enuresis. The element in the history that will most often be able to distinguish pollakiuria from overactive bladder (OAB) is:

   a. a recent life event.
   b. male versus female gender.
   c. no history of UTIs.
   d. no urinary incontinence.
   e. the child does not wake to void.

4. Lower urinary tract dysfunction is associated with which of the following?

   a. Constipation
   b. Neuropsychiatric issues
   c. UTIs
   d. VUR
   e. All of the above

5. The purported mechanism of action for botulinum toxin in the treatment of children and adolescents with dysfunctional voiding is:

   a. reducing the frequency and intensity of uninhibited detrusor contractions during the filling phase of the bladder.
   b. smooth muscle relaxation at the bladder neck.
   c. paralysis of striated muscle of the external sphincter.
   d. stabilization of the motor end plate, inhibiting spinal cord feedback loops.
   e. none of the above.

6. A 4-year-old girl presents to your office with an 8-month history of recurrent UTIs, daytime urinary incontinence, urgency, dysuria and enuresis. Mother states that she refuses to wear pull-ups and will soak through underwear and clothes 1 to 2 times per week. She is also wet 7 out of 7 nights per week. Mother states that she will often "wait until the last minute" to void and is afraid of the toilets at school and so will often not void until she gets home. Mother does not think that daughter is constipated, but upon further questioning, she often has hard, large stools and will have a bowel movement once or twice a week. Urine cultures from her pediatrician's office reveal pansensitive *Escherichia coli* on three separate occasions in the last 2 months. A renal/bladder ultrasound demonstrates normal upper urinary tracts and a voiding cystourethrogram (VCUG) shows bilateral grade 2 VUR. Urinalysis in the office is negative. The best next step after the administration of antibiotic prophylaxis is:

   a. anticholinergics.
   b. bilateral Deflux (Salix Pharmaceuticals, Raleigh, NC) injection.
   c. bilateral ureteral reimplantation.
   d. biofeedback.
   e. voiding diary.

7. Which of the following organ systems is implicated in the pathogenesis of enuresis?

   a. Bladder
   b. Brain

c. Kidney

d. All of the above

e. None of the above

8. An 8-year-old male presents to your office with his parents for consultation regarding treatment for primary nocturnal enuresis. Behavioral modification, desmopressin, and the enuresis alarm have failed. Which of the following parameters is the best predictor of response to treatment with desmopressin?

a. Age of child

b. Bladder capacity

c. Motivation of family

d. Nocturnal polyuria

e. Poor arousal

ANSWERS

1. **b. Biofeedback.** Giggle incontinence (enuresis risoria) is an uncommon form of daytime incontinence and is classically seen in school-aged females. Typically, there is moderate to large amounts of urinary leakage triggered by laughing alone. The incontinence episodes are invariably significant, and often the entire bladder volume is drained. Daytime urinary incontinence in conjunction with laughter is also seen in children with OAB and is more common than true giggle incontinence. It is a diagnosis of exclusion and is usually established on history and is supplemented by the absence of other voiding symptoms and normal investigations. Currently, available treatment strategies include biofeedback or methylphenidate.

2. **d. Vaginal reflux.** Vaginal reflux (vaginal entrapment, vaginal voiding) is characterized by incontinence following normal voiding in the absence of other lower urinary tract (LUT) symptoms. It is commonly seen in prepubertal girls, and the typical history is that of wetting of undergarments approximately 10 to 15 minutes following a normal void. It can often be associated with labial adhesions because of chronic irritation and inflammation from skin exposure to relatively caustic urine. Reassurance and postural modification to ensure complete vaginal emptying is the only treatment that is required.

3. **e. The child does not wake to void.** Pollakiuria is a disorder characterized by a very high daytime frequency of micturition (sometimes as high as 50 times per day). A key aspect of this syndrome, which differentiates it from OAB and can often clinch the diagnosis, is that the symptoms are limited to the daytime. It is seen in early childhood (4 to 6 years of age) in both genders and associated with a history of recent death or life-threatening event in the family. Usually, it runs a benign, self-limited course during a period of approximately 6 months.

4. **e. All of the above.** There are long-standing, clear associations between lower urinary tract dysfunction and bowel dysfunction, UTIs, VUR and various psychiatric diagnoses. The incomplete bladder emptying that occurs in children with LUT dysfunction can lead to urinary stasis, with subsequent UTIs causing inflammatory changes in the bladder wall that stimulate hypertrophy and overactivity. It has been theorized that detrusor hypertrophy can alter the closure mechanism at the ureterovesical junction (UVJ), leading to reflux. It has also been shown that ongoing issues with bowel-bladder dysfunction can have a negative effect on VUR resolution rates, and that that addressing bowel dysfunction alone can positively influence LUT function. Finally, clinicians should be cognizant of the association between neuropsychiatric diagnoses and daytime wetting, as the former is likely to interfere with treatment success of the latter.

5. **c. Paralysis of striated muscle of the external sphincter.** Botulinum-A toxin acts by inhibiting acetylcholine (ACh) release at the presynaptic neuromuscular junction. Inhibited ACh release results in regionally decreased muscle contractility and atrophy at the injection site, which in the case of dysfunctional voiding would be the striated muscle of the external urinary sphincter. The chemical denervation that ensues is a reversible process, and eventually the toxin is inactivated and removed. Clinical effects begin within 5 to 7 days of injection, with maximal effects reached within 4 to 6 weeks. The duration of induced paralysis varies depending on the type of muscle treated, with duration of treatment effect lasting between 3 and 12 months.

6. **e.** Voiding diary. Perhaps one of the most helpful diagnostic tools in the armamentarium of providers who care for children with LUT dysfunction is the voiding diary. Its usefulness stems from the fact that this log is an objective record of the child's bowel habits and urinary voiding pattern. The diagnostic information gathered will be the basis for tailoring a treatment regimen and can often be used to demonstrate the child's improvement over time.

7. **d. All of the above.** The three organ systems implicated in the pathogenesis of enuresis include the bladder (reduced nocturnal bladder capacity), the kidney (nocturnal polyuria), and the brain (e.g., a disorder affecting arousal from sleep). Enuresis is logically thought to result from a disruption or maturational lag in one or more of these critical domains.

8. **d. Nocturnal polyuria.** The enuresis alarm and desmopressin are both valid treatment options. There exist patient, caregiver, and disease-related parameters that may aid in offering prognostic information in terms of which therapeutic modality should be first entertained. The enuresis alarm seems best fit for motivated families and for children without polyuria but with low voided volume. Desmopressin seems best suited for children with nocturnal polyuria and normal bladder reservoir function, for those with infrequent wet episodes, and for families in whom alarm treatment has failed or who have refused alarm treatment.

CHAPTER REVIEW

1. In infants and young children, the bladder is an abdominal organ and can readily be palpated when full.

2. Immature detrusor sphincter coordination manifested as detrusor hypercontractility and interrupted voiding commonly occurs in the first 2 years of life and results in functional bladder outflow obstruction.

3. Even in newborns, micturition does not occur during sleep, suggesting modulation of micturition by higher centers.

4. The association of constipation with urologic pathology is referred to as the *dysfunctional elimination syndrome*. Abnormalities of bowel function are commonly present in young children with voiding dysfunction.

5. Giggle incontinence often results in complete emptying of the bladder.

6. In patients who develop acquired bladder sphincter dysfunction, a significant proportion also have bowel dysfunction.

7. There is a significant association of bladder dysfunction with nonresolution of high-grade vesicle ureteral reflux.

8. In children there is a poor correlation between maximal flow rate and outflow resistance. It is better to study the pattern of the flow curve.

9. In any evaluation of voiding dysfunction, abnormalities of the lower spine should be sought.

10. Nocturnal urine output in many enuretic children is in excess of bladder reservoir capacity during sleep.

11. Many enuretic children have a marked reduction in functional bladder capacity when compared with age-matched controls and may have detrusor instability as well.

12. Overactive bladder is the most common lower urinary tract disorder in children, with a peak incidence between 5 and 7 years.

13. Behavioral and emotional disorders occur in 20% to 30% of children with lower urinary tract disorders.

14. Vaginal reflux (vaginal entrapment, vaginal voiding) is characterized by incontinence following normal voiding in the absence of other LUT symptoms. It is commonly seen in prepubertal girls, and the typical history is that of wetting of undergarments about 10 to 15 minutes following a normal void. It can often be associated with labial adhesions.

15. Pollakiuria is a disorder characterized by a very high daytime frequency of micturition (sometimes as high as 50 times per day). A key aspect of this syndrome, which differentiates it from OAB and can often clinch the diagnosis, is that the symptoms are limited to the daytime. It is seen in early childhood (4 to 6 years of age) in both genders and is associated with a history of recent death or life-threatening event in the family. Usually, it runs a benign, self-limited course over a period of approximately 6 months.

16. A voiding diary is perhaps one of the most helpful diagnostic tools in that it is an objective record of the child's bowel habits and urinary voiding pattern.

17. The use of an alarm in the treatment of enuresis seems best fit for motivated families and for children without polyuria but with low voided volume. Desmopressin seems best suited for children with nocturnal polyuria and normal bladder reservoir function, for those with infrequent wet episodes, and for families for whom alarm treatment has failed or who have refused alarm treatment.

144 Management of Defecation Disorders

Martin Allan Koyle and Armando J. Lorenzo

QUESTIONS

1. The Rome III criteria evaluate the following aspects of bowel function EXCEPT:
   a. pain with bowel movements.
   b. production of large stools that can block the toilet.
   c. number of bowel movements per week.
   d. duration of symptoms.
   e. all of the above.

2. A 4-year-old girl presents with a 6-month history of urinary frequency and urgency. Parents report daily small bowel movements, which they attribute to poor diet ("picky eater"). Her physical exam is normal. There is no history of urinary tract infections. Which of the following interventions can lead to paradoxical worsening of her symptoms?
   a. Increase in fluid intake
   b. Polyethylene glycol (PEG)
   c. Oxybutynin
   d. Trimethoprim prophylaxis
   e. Biofeedback

3. Which one of the following aspects of a patient's history and physical examination should raise suspicion for an underlying organic pathology causing constipation?
   a. Early age of onset (before toilet training)
   b. Presence of a palpable mass in the left lower quadrant
   c. Onset after diet change
   d. Poor dietary habits ("picky eater")
   e. All of the above

4. Which part of the physical exam can be safely omitted during initial evaluation of a child with suspected functional constipation?
   a. Height and weight
   b. Inspection of the lower back
   c. Lower extremity muscle tone and reflexes
   d. Digital rectal exam
   e. Visual inspection of the perineum

5. Which of the following metabolic/endocrinologic pathologies is unlikely to cause constipation?
   a. Hypercalcemia
   b. Hypokalemia
   c. Hypothyroidism
   d. Diabetes insipidus
   e. Precocious puberty

6. Regarding the surgical management of refractory constipation, which one of the following statements is CORRECT?
   a. Access for antegrade irrigations should be limited to the cecum.
   b. Open surgical intervention carries a higher success rate than laparoscopic or percutaneous procedures.
   c. Malone antegrade continence enema (MACE) channels and C-tubes provide better procedural independence than retrograde enemas for patients with neuropathic bowel dysfunction.
   d. Similar success rates can be expected irrespective of the underlying pathology.
   e. All of the above.

7. The main principle behind daily antegrade enemas for continence is:
   a. washout with regular evacuation of the entire colon.
   b. direct softening of stools to facilitate passage during the day.
   c. improve hydration.
   d. decrease colon motility.
   e. decrease sphincter tone.

8. Initial workup of a child with constipation is most likely to benefit from including:
   a. abdominal radiograph.
   b. anal manometry
   c. colonic transit time studies
   d. magnetic resonance imaging (MRI) of lumbosacral spine
   e. contrast enema study

9. Which of the following statements regarding creation of a MACE channel is TRUE?
   a. Previous surgical interventions are a contraindication for a laparoscopic approach.
   b. An aggressive bowel washout and mechanical preparation is always warranted before surgery.
   c. Presence of a ventriculoperitoneal shunt is a contraindication for laparoscopic approach.
   d. The appendix may be of sufficient length to be split in order to create a MACE and Mitrofanoff channel for neuropathic bowel and bladder management.
   e. An antireflux mechanism (cecal wrap) is always required in order to prevent stool leakage.

10. Which of the following statements regarding cecostomy tubes is most accurate?
    a. It is a good alternative for patients who have previously undergone an appendectomy.
    b. It avoids the need for regular instrumentation.
    c. It is difficult to remove or convert to a MACE channel.
    d. The most common problem is stenosis and difficulty accessing for fluid instillation.
    e. It is a great alternative for families who have problems with compliance.

11. Recommendations for antegrade enema regimens should include which of the following?
    a. Sterile saline is preferred versus tap water or "home-made" saline solution.
    b. Daily enemas are universally required to achieve continence.
    c. Early morning irrigations are preferable as it allows the patients to enjoy better daytime continence.
    d. Trial and error for more than 6 months may be warranted to reach a reliable enema routine.
    e. All of the above.

12. What is the proposed mechanism of action of prucalopride?
    a. Stool softener
    b. Antispasmodic
    c. Bulking agent
    d. Prokinetic
    e. None of the above

13. Which of the following agents is preferred (first-line) medication for maintenance management of constipation?
    a. Milk of magnesia
    b. Mineral oil
    c. PEG
    d. Prucalopride
    e. Psyllium husk
14. Features of functional constipation include:
    a. recurrence despite recommendations consistent with optimal medical management.
    b. alternating constipation and diarrhea.
    c. episodes of bowel obstruction.
    d. bilious vomiting.
    e. ribbon-like stools.
15. Which one of the following stool characteristics is NOT included in the Bristol scale?
    a. Consistency
    b. Shape
    c. Difficulty having bowel movements
    d. Odor
    e. None of the above
16. Of the following, which one is the best diagnostic test to confirm Hirschsprung disease?
    a. Barium enema
    b. Computed tomography (CT) scan with oral and intravenous contrast
    c. Rectal biopsy
    d. Colonoscopy
    e. Lumbosacral spine MRI
17. New onset of abdominal pain and distention after antegrade instillation of fluid in a child with a cecostomy tube in place for more than 6 months should alert the physician about:
    a. spontaneous cecal perforation.
    b. use of hypotonic fluid for irrigations.
    c. presence of a large fecal load in the rectum and descending colon.
    d. an incompetent ileocecal valve with retrograde irrigation into the terminal ileum.
    e. irritable bowel syndrome.

18. Which of the following statements regarding abdominal plain film during initial assessment of a child with functional constipation is FALSE?
    a. Amount and distribution of fecal material can predict likelihood of response and recurrence with medical therapy.
    b. Helps assess for fecal impaction
    c. Helps assess response to bowel wash out
    d. Aids in demonstrating parents or caretakers the presence of constipation
    e. Detects bony abnormalities that may be associated with neuropathic bowel dysfunction
19. Which statement regarding diagnosis and management of functional constipation is TRUE?
    a. Assessment during evaluation of a child with recurrent urinary tract infections is warranted.
    b. It is an integral part of a program dealing with dysfunctional voiding.
    c. It should be addressed before proceeding with surgical interventions for vesicoureteral reflux.
    d. It can be managed by pediatric urologists and urology nurse practitioners.
    e. All of the above.

Imaging

1. The abdominal radiograph and pelvic ultrasound shown in Figure 144-1 were obtained on a 5-year-old girl with recurrent abdominal pain and distention for the past year. She has a palpable soft, nontender mass in the left lower quadrant. Which one of the following interventions is LEAST likely to help with initial management?
    a. Digital disimpaction under sedation
    b. Enemas
    c. "High-dose" polyethylene glycol
    d. Supplement fiber intake
    e. Increase fluid intake

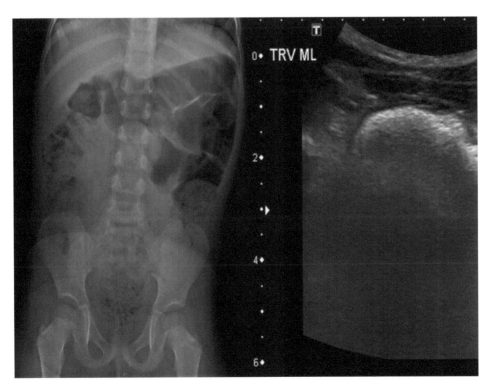

Figure 144-1.

ANSWERS

1. **e. All of the above.** The Rome III criteria requires symptoms to be present for at least 1 or 2 months, and takes into account developmental age and absence of an underlying organic pathology. Pain with defecation, history of large-diameter stools that may obstruct the toilet, and infrequent bowel movements (≤2 defecations per week) are all included in the diagnosis of functional constipation.

2. **c. Oxybutynin.** Constipation is a common side effect of medications used to deal with lower urinary tract symptoms (particularly anticholinergics). Because of this common association, during the past few decades, pediatric urologists have become comfortable with assessing and managing bowel problems. Development or worsening of constipation will sometimes coincide or worsen with precipitating factors, such as change in diet (for example, transitioning out of breastfeeding) and introduction of new medications (such as oxybutynin for management of urinary frequency). Increase in fecal load in the rectum, coupled with toilet avoidance due to lower abdominal pain and discomfort with defecation, may lead to paradoxical worsening of lower urinary tract symptoms. Increase in fluid intake and use of PEG is unlikely to worsen lower urinary tract symptoms and is part of initial recommendations for bowel retraining. Similarly, biofeedback may have a neutral or beneficial effect. Antibiotic prophylaxis, in the absence of recurrent infections, is not expected to influence symptomatology.

3. **a. Early age of onset (before toilet training).** The age of onset of symptoms is one of the easiest and most important pieces of information to obtain, as it can be an important indicator for underlying pathology, particularly if symptoms have been present since early in life (infancy). Other critical information to be actively gathered includes failure to toilet train within an age-appropriate and developmental timeframe, pain with defecation, bleeding per rectum, associated abdominal pain, fecal incontinence, holding behaviors, nausea or vomiting, weight loss, growth pattern (including height and weight), developmental delay, and failure to thrive. Patients with functional constipation often present or worsen after dietary changes. Not uncommonly, otherwise healthy children are described by parents as very selective (or "picky"). In the setting of significant fecal load or impaction in a child with constipation, a palpable mass in the left lower quadrant ("fecaloma") may be detected during examination.

4. **d. Digital rectal exam.** Physical exam should routinely include weight and height, and inspection of the perineum and genital and perianal regions (including anal position, stool present around the anus or on the underwear, signs of trauma, anal fissures, sensation). Although potentially considered to be an integral part of a complete physical exam, digital rectal examination should not routinely conducted in children. It is reserved for difficult-to-treat cases and must be performed by health care professionals comfortable with interpreting features of anorectal anatomical abnormalities, to specifically evaluate for anal stenosis, a large fecal mass, or an empty rectum.

5. **e. Precocious puberty.** Endocrine disorders associated with chronic dehydration (such as diabetes insipidus), electrolyte disorders (most notably hypercalcemia and hypokalemia), hypothyroidism, and hypervitaminosis D are important potential organic etiologies. Precocious puberty presents with development of secondary sexual characteristics at an age before the expected onset during normal development. Constipation is not a presenting or common isolated feature of this condition.

6. **c. Malone antegrade continence enema (MACE) channels and C-tubes provide better procedural independence than retrograde enemas for patients with neuropathic bowel dysfunction.** In cases with severe constipation and a redundant colon, some have advocated the placement of conduits in the left colon rather than the cecum. By doing so, the length of bowel that has to be washed through is reduced and theoretically, so is the time taken for successful enema completion.

Results with this approach have been encouraging. Both open and laparoscopic procedures are associated with similar success rates. Both C-tubes and MACE-type channels provide independence and allow patients greater ability to perform irrigations without assistance in comparison to self-administered retrograde enemas. The underlying diagnosis influences the success rate. Patients with a neuropathic bowel and anorectal malformations seem to fare better than those with chronic idiopathic constipation. Age at operation is also important, with failures more commonly seen in younger patients irrespective of the diagnosis.

7. **a. Washout with regular evacuation of the entire colon.** The success of antegrade enema regimens is based on two important principles: (1) complete colonic emptying can achieve bowel continence, and (2) antegrade colonic emptying is feasible. Regular complete emptying of the colon is the main mechanism associated with fecal continence.

8. **a. Abdominal radiograph.** Although of modest clinical value, abdominal radiographs are commonly used in the diagnosis and management of constipation. Proponents in favor of routine use argue that the study can clearly demonstrate the amount of fecal loading and delineate stool distribution throughout the colon and rectum, as well as help ascertain for the presence of fecal impaction. In addition, it may also reveal associated pathologies, such as bony abnormalities indicative of occult spinal dysraphism or sacral agenesis, and help provide a visual aid for family and patient recognition of stool retention despite a history of regular defecation. Colonic transit time studies are not recommended for routine diagnosis of functional constipation, being reserved for difficult-to-treat or unresponsive cases. Similarly, contrast enema series can be of value in selected cases, such as the evaluation of children with characteristics suggestive of Hirschsprung disease and repaired congenital anatomic abnormalities (i.e., anorectal malformation). Concern for a neuropathic process and/or lower spine stigmata should be evaluated with a spine ultrasound (if detected before calcification of the vertebral bodies in the first 3 to 6 months of life, or a lumbosacral MRI in older children. Anorectal manometry is useful only in very selected cases, such as suspected Hirschsprung disease and internal sphincter achalasia. In these conditions, the rectoanal relaxation reflex is absent. Nevertheless, in patients suspected of having functional constipation, manometry adds little to the diagnosis or therapeutic strategy.

9. **d. The appendix may be of sufficient length to be split to create a MACE and Mitrofanoff channel for neuropathic bowel and bladder management.** In children who require synchronous bladder reconstruction, a simultaneous MACE and Mitrofanoff urinary diversion offers the opportunity for dual fecal and urinary continence. If both a MACE and appendicovesicostomy are considered—and if the appendix is long enough with suitable, robust vascular anatomy—it is possible to split it. Previous surgical interventions are not an absolute contraindication for a laparoscopic approach, although the situation does demand for great care when entering the peritoneal cavity to avoid injuries related to adhesions or fibrosis. Although preoperative bowel preparation may facilitate the initiation of postoperative enemas, an aggressive cleanout is not necessary for the purpose of performing the procedure. Many patients with neuropathic bladder and bowel dysfunction have ventriculoperitoneal shunts. Although it is critical that appropriate use of prophylactic antibiotics and measures to minimize spillage be set in place, the presence of a shunt is not a contraindication for open or laparoscopic reconstruction involving bowel segments. Many descriptions of the MACE procedure propose an "antireflux" valve mechanism to prevent leakage of bowel contents via the cutaneous stoma. This is often achieved by wrapping the appendix with the cecal wall. However, recent reports have suggested that it is not always necessary to construct an antireflux mechanism. Thus far, data appear to support no increase in stomal bowel

incontinence, based on retrospective reviews comparing MACE with and without cecal wrap.

10. **a. It is a good alternative for patients who have previously undergone an appendectomy.** Cecostomy tubes are favored when the appendix is known to be absent (i.e., postappendectomy), when the patient refuses to perform intermittent bowel catheterization, for patients who develop stomal complications such as stenosis (as an alternative to revision of the MACE channel), as a temporary therapeutic challenge to determine response to antegrade enemas, to determine if ideal placement of a permanent MACE should be in the right or left colon, and as a permanent option in cases in which a nonoperative access is favored. The main drawback is that the tube entry site can become unsightly, with granulation tissue and occasional fecal leakage. Stenosis is very rare, in contrast to issues related to MACE channels. In addition, regular instrumentation is needed in order to change the tube on a scheduled basis (i.e., every 6 to 12 months), or sooner if it dislodges or breaks. Patients may opt for subsequent formal conversion to a bowel-based MACE, which can be done either laparoscopically or open. Compliance with antegrade enema regimens is crucial for success, irrespective of how the bowel access has been achieved (C-tube or MACE).

11. **d. Trial and error for more than 6 months may be warranted to reach a reliable enema routine.** One of the most important points, especially in the early weeks and months after surgery, is to advise patients not to expect immediate success with the enema regimen, as early disappointment can lead to frustration and failure. In fact many children may not achieve a steady state or a reliable enema routine for a period of as long as 6 months. Enema protocols differ among centers, and patients and families will frequently modify them to suit their own particular needs. Initially, daily washouts with 20 mL/kg of solution are encouraged, but once the patient is comfortable with the process and a routine has been established, they may attempt to decrease frequency to alternate days. The time of day that the enema is administered is patient dependent, although most families prefer to give the enema during the early evening hours, after dinner. Purges can be done with large-volume tap or salt water, with the judicious mix of additives such as glycerin. The fluid does not have to be sterile.

12. **d. Prokinetic.** Prucalopride is a new oral, selective, high-affinity 5HT$_4$ receptor antagonist with gastrointestinal prokinetic activities, which shows particular promise for management of difficult-to-treat constipation and may eventually represent a reasonable choice for children who fail to respond to more conservative measures. Its main mechanism of action does not influence stool consistency or bulk. As a prokinetic drug, it is likely to stimulate bowel smooth muscle contractions and not provide an antispasmodic effect.

13. **c. PEG.** With the introduction of PEG into routine clinical practice, tolerance of medical management has improved, and it is currently the preferred agent in many centers. PEG is better tolerated and easier to administer than alternative medications such as lactulose, mineral oil, and milk of magnesia (magnesium hydroxide). It is virtually tasteless and dissolves easily within seconds.

14. **a. Recurrence despite recommendations consistent with optimal medical management.** Functional constipation can be difficult to treat and a long-lasting problem for some children. Nevertheless, with adequate management close to 50% of patients monitored for 6 to 12 months can recover and successfully discontinue medications, whereas as many as 80% can be adequately controlled with routine interventions. Unfortunately, subsequent recurrences are fairly common, with as many as 50% of children experiencing one in the first 5 years after successful treatment. All the other listed factors (alternating constipation and diarrhea, episodes of bowel obstruction, bilious vomiting, and ribbon-like stools) are "warning signs and symptoms" that should raise suspicion for alternative diagnosis and an underlying process (i.e., not functional constipation).

15. **d. Odor.** Stool characteristics should be recorded with a validated scale. The most commonly used (Bristol scale) takes into account consistency and stool shape, capturing also the degree of difficulty passing the bowel movement. Smell (odor) is not part of the scale.

16. **c. Rectal biopsy.** If Hirschsprung disease or colon aganglionosis is suspected, a deep suction rectal biopsy (including submucosal) should be obtained, favoring a transanal approach and aiming at a location 2 to 3 cm from the dentate line. Diagnosis is supported by absence of ganglion cells, hypertrophied nerve fibers, and increase in acetylcholinesterase activity in the lamina propria and muscularis mucosa.

17. **c. Presence of a large fecal load in the rectum and descending colon.** Several difficulties can be experienced during enema infusion. The most common problem is pain or discomfort during instillation. In the majority of patients, this is a transient phenomenon that subsides during the first 3 months. It is always important to ensure that the pain is not due to distal fecal impaction, which can occur despite regular washouts. The presence of a large amount of fecal material in the distal colon and rectum can certainly lead to impaction in patients doing infrequent antegrade enemas through a cecostomy access or MACE channel. Attempts at clearing this fecal load with antegrade flushes can lead to abdominal pain, lack of tolerance, and poor response. Spontaneous colon perforation with antegrade enema regimens is exceedingly rare. The use of hypotonic fluids (such as tap water) is commonplace in many centers. Retrograde flow of fluid into the distal ileum is not a common cause of pain with antegrade enemas and is unlikely to develop suddenly in a patient who has been doing enemas for a period of 6 months.

18. **a. Amount and distribution of fecal material can predict likelihood of response and recurrence with medical therapy.** As discussed in question 8, there are some potential benefits to obtaining an abdominal radiograph during the evaluation of children with constipation. These include assessment for fecal impaction, to determine response to a bowel washout, to provide evidence for parents and caretakers, and to detect bony abnormalities suggestive of a possible neuropathic process. The distribution and amount of fecal material on one film has not been described to have any predictive value in terms of response to medical therapy or recurrence.

19. **e. All of the above.** Constipation is common and should be suspected in any patient who presents with lower urinary tract symptoms. Programs dealing with incontinence and dysfunctional voiding have successfully included this aspect of care into their protocols. Dysfunctional voiding and constipation should be addressed before proceeding with surgical correction and can be done by a pediatric urologist or urology nurse practitioner, assisted by the child's primary care physician.

Imaging

1. **d. Supplement fiber intake.** The physical examination and imaging studies are suggestive of severe constipation and stool impaction. Decreasing fecal load in the colon and rectum is the first step towards establishing an optimal medical regimen. Impaction should be suspected when a mass is felt in the lower abdomen and/or left lower quadrant, or a dilated rectum filled with a large amount of stool is seen on pelvic ultrasound or abdominal radiography (as shown in the figure). Approximately 30% of children with functional constipation present with fecal impaction. Disimpaction and bowel washout address the problem in a relatively short period of time, often with enemas or suppositories, in contrast to maintenance therapy. Popular regimens also include "high dose" polyethylene glycol with or without sodium chloride, sodium phosphate or mineral oil enemas. In some circumstances clearance can only be achieved with digital disimpaction under sedation or anesthesia. The addition of fiber to the diet is bound to worsen the problem by increasing fecal load and is generally avoided during the initial management of fecal impaction.

CHAPTER REVIEW

1. Constipation may cause significant voiding dysfunction.
2. Functional constipation is a diagnosis of exclusion.
3. Three stools per day to three stools per week without straining or withholding is considered normal.
4. Organic conditions associated with elimination problems include cystic fibrosis, hypothyroidism, celiac disease, dietary allergies, Hirschsprung disease, anal stenosis, and trisomy 21. In the older child, mental health issues, eating disorders, sexual abuse, and irritable bowel syndrome should also be considered.
5. Initial medical management includes behavioral modification (regular defecation and nonsedentary activity), dietary changes (fluid and fiber intake), stool softeners and laxatives, and judicious use of enemas.
6. Antegrade continence enemas may be given through the cecum or left colon. It often requires that the child sit on the toilet for up to an hour before emptying is complete. The procedure is best employed in children 5 to 12 years of age who are motivated and is more successful in patients with neuropathic bowel or anorectal malformations.
7. Impaction should be suspected when a mass is felt in the lower abdomen and/or left lower quadrant, or a dilated rectum filled with a large amount of stool is seen on pelvic ultrasound or abdominal radiography.
8. In patients with fecal impaction, the addition of fiber to the diet is bound to worsen the problem by increasing fecal load and is generally avoided during the initial management.
9. The age of onset of symptoms is one of the easiest and most important pieces of information to obtain because it can be an important indicator for underlying pathology, particularly if it has been present since early in life (infancy).
10. Endocrine disorders associated with chronic dehydration (such as diabetes insipidus), electrolyte disorders (most notably hypercalcemia and hypokalemia), hypothyroidism, and hypervitaminosis D are important potential organic etiologies.
11. Although of modest clinical value, abdominal radiographs are commonly employed in the diagnosis and management of constipation. Proponents of routine use argue that the study can clearly demonstrate the amount of fecal loading and delineate stool distribution throughout the colon and rectum, as well as help ascertain the presence of fecal impaction. In addition, it may also reveal associated pathologies, such as bony abnormalities indicative of occult spinal dysraphism or sacral agenesis.
12. PEG is better tolerated and easier to administer than alternative medications such as lactulose, mineral oil, and milk of magnesia.
13. The most common problem with antegrade continence enemas is pain or discomfort during instillation. In the majority of patients, this is a transient phenomenon that subsides during the first 3 months. It is always important to ensure that the pain is not due to distal fecal impaction.

145 Lower Urinary Tract Reconstruction in Children

Mark C. Adams, David B. Joseph, and John C. Thomas

QUESTIONS

1. Children with significant bladder or sphincter dysfunction requiring reconstructive surgery most likely have:
   a. bladder exstrophy or epispadias.
   b. posterior urethral valves.
   c. cloacal anomalies.
   d. prune-belly syndrome.
   e. spinal dysraphism.

2. The most important contribution to the field of pediatric reconstructive surgery has been:
   a. Mitrofanoff's description of a continent abdominal wall stoma using appendix.
   b. Lapides' introduction of clean intermittent catheterization (CIC).
   c. Goodwin's description of ileal reconfiguration.
   d. development of several effective means to increase bladder outlet resistance.
   e. recognition that a dilated ureter could be used for bladder augmentation.

3. Normal bladder compliance is based on:
   a. ample collagen type II.
   b. inverse relationship of bladder volume and bladder pressure.
   c. bladder unfolding, elasticity, and viscoelasticity.
   d. subepithelial matrix bridges associated with collagen.
   e. hypertrophic bladder bundles interspersed with collagen.

4. Chronically elevated bladder filling pressures may cause hydronephrosis, vesicoureteral reflux, and impaired renal function. The lowest pressure threshold most often reported to cause problems is:
   a. 20 cm H_2O.
   b. 30 cm H_2O.
   c. 40 cm H_2O.
   d. 50 cm H_2O.
   e. 60 cm H_2O.

5. Upper urinary tract changes associated with a poorly compliant, hyperreflexic bladder are initially treated by:
   a. autoaugmentation.
   b. pharmacologic management and intermittent catheterization.
   c. ileal augmentation.
   d. sigmoid augmentation.
   e. gastric augmentation.

6. Preoperative bladder capacity and compliance are best determined by urodynamics using:
   a. carbon dioxide as an irrigant at a slow fill rate (10% of capacity per minute).
   b. room-temperature saline at a slow fill rate (10% of capacity per minute).
   c. body-temperature saline at a fast fill rate (30% of capacity per minute).
   d. cooled saline at a slow fill rate (10% of capacity per minute).
   e. cooled saline at a fast fill rate (30% of capacity per minute).

7. Urinary tract reconstruction for urinary continence requires:
   a. confirmation of a normal upper urinary tract.
   b. identification of a highly compliant bladder.
   c. documentation of the presence or absence of vesicoureteral reflux.
   d. acceptance of and compliance with intermittent catheterization.
   e. documentation of a serum creatinine value less than 1.4 mg/dL.

8. Mechanical bowel preparation is performed in patients undergoing:
   a. ileocystoplasty.
   b. sigmoid cystoplasty.
   c. gastrocystoplasty.
   d. ureterocystoplasty.
   e. all of the above.

9. A urinary stricture after transureteroureterostomy is most likely due to:
   a. mobilization of the crossing ureter with periureteral tissue.
   b. mobilization of the crossing ureter without angulation beneath the inferior mesenteric artery.
   c. mobilization of the recipient ureter to meet the crossing one.
   d. wide anastomosis of the crossing ureter to the posteromedial aspect of the recipient.
   e. watertight anastomosis.

10. Creating an antireflux mechanism is most difficult with anastomosis to the:
    a. stomach.
    b. ileum.
    c. cecum.
    d. transverse colon.
    e. sigmoid colon.

11. The Young-Dees-Leadbetter bladder neck repair in children with neurogenic sphincter deficiency:
    a. results in limited success because of a lack of muscle tone and activity of the native bladder neck.
    b. can achieve successful continence results similar to those noted in children with bladder exstrophy.
    c. does not often require bladder augmentation or intermittent catheterization.
    d. is best performed in association with a Silastic sling.
    e. limits the necessity for intermittent catheterization in children who could empty by a Valsalva maneuver preoperatively.

12. An ambulatory 15-year-old girl with lumbosacral myelomeningocele voids to completion with a low-pressure detrusor contraction and the Valsalva maneuver. She remains incontinent because of bladder neck and intrinsic sphincter deficiency that is refractory to pharmacologic management. To limit the risk of intermittent catheterization, the next step is:
    a. Young-Dees-Leadbetter bladder neck repair.
    b. artificial urinary sphincter placement.
    c. fascial bladder neck sling placement.
    d. Kropp bladder neck repair.
    e. Pippi-Salle bladder neck repair.

13. One side effect associated with bladder neck repair that can be decreased with good preoperative evaluation is:
    a. recurrent urolithiasis.
    b. recurrent cystitis.
    c. inability to spontaneously void.
    d. associated need for augmentation cystoplasty.
    e. unmasking of detrusor hostility, resulting in upper urinary tract changes.

14. Fascial slings used for increasing outlet resistance in children with neurogenic sphincteric incompetence:
    a. are more effective in girls than in boys.
    b. are dependent on the type of fascial or cadaveric tissue used.
    c. are dependent on the configuration of the sling and wrap used.
    d. rarely result in the need for bladder augmentation and intermittent catheterization.
    e. frequently result in urethral erosion.

15. The least favorable indication for an artificial urinary sphincter is:
    a. neurogenic bladder dysfunction.
    b. bladder exstrophy or epispadias.
    c. inability to empty the bladder by spontaneous voiding.
    d. associated need for bladder augmentation.
    e. prepubertal age.

16. The most common limitation of a Kropp urethral lengthening for continence is:
    a. fistula from the urethra to the bladder, resulting in incontinence.
    b. inability to spontaneously void, resulting in urinary retention.
    c. difficulty with intermittent catheterization, particularly in boys.
    d. new vesicoureteral reflux.
    e. distal ureteral obstruction.

17. Urinary continence is most definitively achieved after:
    a. Young-Dees-Leadbetter bladder repair.
    b. placement of an artificial urinary sphincter.
    c. placement of a circumferential fascial wrap.
    d. urethral lengthening and reimplantation.
    e. bladder neck division.

18. To avoid uninhibited pressure contractions during an enterocystoplasty:
    a. large bowel should be used.
    b. the intestinal segment should be reconfigured.
    c. the majority of the diseased bladder should be excised.

d. a stellate incision into the bladder should be created to increase the circumference of the bowel anastomosis.
    e. small mesenteric windows are created in the bowel segment.

19. Potential ways to prevent reflux when using ileum for continent diversion include all of the following except:
    a. intussuscepted nipple valve.
    b. split nipple cuff of ureter.
    c. placement of the spatulated ureter into an incised mucosal trough.
    d. flap valve created beneath a taenia.
    e. placement of the ureter within a serosa-lined tunnel between two limbs of ileum.

20. The gastrointestinal segment that most often causes permanent gastrointestinal side effects when used in children with a neurogenic bladder is the:
    a. stomach.
    b. jejunum.
    c. ileum.
    d. ileocecal segment.
    e. sigmoid colon.

21. The most likely problem after gastrointestinal bladder augmentation is:
    a. early satiety.
    b. hyperchloremic metabolic acidosis.
    c. small bowel obstruction.
    d. chronic diarrhea.
    e. vitamin B_{12} deficiency with megaloblastic anemia.

22. The gastrointestinal segment resulting in the best long-term capacity and compliance after augmentation cystoplasty is the:
    a. gastric body.
    b. gastric antrum.
    c. ileum.
    d. cecum.
    e. sigmoid colon.

23. The risk of failure to achieve appropriate capacity and compliance after augmentation cystoplasty is:
    a. less than 5%.
    b. 5% to 10%.
    c. 11% to 15%.
    d. 16% to 20%.
    e. more than 20%.

24. The serum metabolic pattern that occurs most often after an ileocystoplasty or colocystoplasty is:
    a. hypochloremic metabolic acidosis.
    b. hyperchloremic metabolic acidosis.
    c. hypochloremic metabolic alkalosis.
    d. hyperchloremic metabolic alkalosis.
    e. hyponatremic metabolic acidosis.

25. The serum metabolic pattern that occurs most often after gastrocystoplasty is:
    a. hypochloremic metabolic acidosis.
    b. hyperchloremic metabolic acidosis.
    c. hypochloremic metabolic alkalosis.
    d. hyperchloremic metabolic alkalosis.
    e. hyponatremic metabolic acidosis.

26. The risk of intermittent hematuria and dysuria after gastrocystoplasty is most influenced by:
    a. the gastric segment used.
    b. persistent urinary incontinence.
    c. decreased renal function.
    d. diagnosis of bladder exstrophy.
    e. neurogenic bladder dysfunction.

27. Bacteriuria should be treated after bladder augmentation when:
    a. associated with CIC.
    b. urinalysis demonstrates microscopic hematuria.
    c. there is increased mucus production.
    d. etiology is posterior urethral valves.
    e. urine culture reveals growth of a urea-splitting organism.

28. The gastrointestinal segment associated with the lowest incidence of stone formation is:
    a. stomach.
    b. jejunum.
    c. ileum.
    d. cecum.
    e. sigmoid colon.

29. Adenocarcinoma of the bladder after augmentation cystoplasty can occur after:
    a. 2 years.
    b. 4 years.
    c. 8 years.
    d. 16 years.
    e. 26 years.

30. The risk of perforation after bladder augmentation includes all but:
    a. high outflow resistance.
    b. persistent hyperreflexia or uninhibited bladder contractions.
    c. use of sigmoid colon.
    d. bladder exstrophy.
    e. neurogenic bladder dysfunction.

31. The initial management of a spontaneous perforation of an augmented bladder in a child with a neurogenic bladder is:
    a. placement of a large-bore urethral catheter for drainage.
    b. placement of a large-bore suprapubic cystotomy tube for drainage.
    c. immediate surgical exploration and repair.
    d. serial abdominal examinations.
    e. urine culture.

32. Pregnancy associated with urinary reconstruction:
    a. is reasonable after urinary diversion but is contraindicated after augmentation cystoplasty.
    b. results in the mesenteric pedicle positioned directly anterior to the uterus.
    c. results in the mesenteric pedicle deflected laterally without vascular compromise to the augmented segment.
    d. is avoided due to mechanical compression of the pedicle and ischemia with loss of the augmented segment.
    e. is contraindicated because of increased risk of systemic sepsis complicating the hydronephrosis.

33. Ureterocystoplasty is limited because:
    a. it requires an intraperitoneal approach.
    b. complete mobilization of the ureter may result in vascular compromise.
    c. a dilated ureter is not as compliant as a similar-sized bowel segment.
    d. a dilated ureter is not available in many patients.
    e. ureterocystoplasty precludes spontaneous voiding.

34. Autoaugmentation is contraindicated with:
    a. serum creatinine value greater than 1.4 ng/dL.
    b. CIC.
    c. vesicoureteral reflux.
    d. uninhibited bladder contractions.
    e. small bladder capacity.

35. A ureterosigmoidostomy should not be undertaken in a patient with a history of:
    a. dilated ureters.
    b. anteriorly placed rectum associated with bladder exstrophy.
    c. recurrent pyelonephritis.
    d. fecal incontinence.
    e. constipation.

36. The use of efferent nipple valves for continence in children:
    a. has not approached the results achieved in adults.
    b. has a higher complication and reoperation rate than a flap valve.
    c. is equivalent to any other continence mechanism.
    d. is often associated with difficulty in catheterization.
    e. often results in stomal stenosis.

37. The least important factor when creating an appendicovesicostomy is:
    a. taking a wide cecal cuff to decrease the risk of stomal stenosis.
    b. creating a tunnel of 4 cm, at least greater than a 5:1 ratio of tunnel length to diameter, to achieve continence.
    c. a small, uniform lumen allowing for easy catheterization.
    d. mobilizing the right colon to adequately free the appendix.
    e. tubularizing a small portion of the cecum in continuity with the appendix to increase length.

38. A frequent occurrence after an appendicovesicostomy is:
    a. urinary incontinence due to inadequate length of the flap valve mechanism.
    b. urinary incontinence due to persistently elevated reservoir pressure.
    c. appendiceal perforation that often occurs due to catheterization.
    d. appendiceal stricture or necrosis.
    e. stomal stenosis.

39. A 12-year-old obese girl with spina bifida undergoes appendico-cecostomy, bladder neck sling, bladder augmentation, and continent catheterizable bladder channel. The upper urinary tract is normal. The best source of tissue for the bladder channel is:
    a. distal right ureter after right-to-left transureteroureterostomy.
    b. tapered segment of small bowel of adequate length.
    c. right fallopian tube.
    d. gastric tube.
    e. tubularized bladder flap.

40. In complex pediatric urinary undiversion procedures it is most difficult to:

    a. provide adequate outflow resistance.

    b. create a compliant urinary reservoir.

    c. achieve an effective antireflux mechanism without upper tract obstruction.

    d. provide a reliable access for intermittent catheterization.

    e. achieve urinary and fecal continence.

ANSWERS

1. **e. Spinal dysraphism.** Most pediatric reconstructive procedures are undertaken to correct a problem of the native urinary tract causing progressive hydronephrosis, urinary incontinence unresponsive to medical management, or temporary diversion. Children with bladder and sphincteric dysfunction are the most complex reconstructive cases seen in pediatric urology; children with the diagnoses of exstrophy, persistent cloaca and urogenital sinus, posterior urethral valves, bilateral single ectopic ureters, and prune-belly syndrome may be involved. However, children with a neurogenic bladder due to a myelomeningocele make up the vast majority of patients requiring this type of surgical intervention.

2. **b. Lapides' introduction of clean intermittent catheterization (CIC).** One of the most important contributions in the care of children with bladder dysfunction came with the acceptance of CIC described by Lapides and colleagues in 1972 and 1976, based on the work of Guttmann and Frankel. The effective use of CIC has allowed the application of augmentation and lower tract reconstruction to groups of patients who had not previously been candidates. The principle of intermittent catheterization allows the reconstructive surgeon to aggressively correct storage problems by providing an adequate reservoir and good outflow resistance. Spontaneous voiding, although a goal, is not imperative because catheterization can be used for emptying.

3. **c. Bladder unfolding, elasticity, and viscoelasticity.** Multiple factors contribute to the property of compliance. Initially the bladder is in a collapsed state, which allows for the storage of urine at low pressure by simply unfolding. While it expands, detrusor properties of elasticity and viscoelasticity take effect. Elasticity allows the detrusor muscle to stretch without an increase in tension until it reaches a critical volume. When filling is slow, as in a natural state, or stops, there is a rapid decay in this pressure known as stress relaxation. Normally, stress relaxation is in balance with the filling rate and prevents an increase in detrusor pressure.

4. **c. 40 cm H$_2$O.** Elevated passive filling pressure becomes clinically pathogenic when a pressure greater than 40 cm H$_2$O is chronically reached. Pressure at this level sustained during a prolonged period of time impairs ureteral drainage and can result in acquired vesicoureteral reflux, pyelocaliceal changes, hydroureteronephrosis, and decreased glomerular filtration rate.

5. **b. Pharmacologic management and intermittent catheterization.** Pharmacologic management can play a role in decreasing filling pressure, particularly when hyperreflexic detrusor contractions are present. A combination of medications and intermittent catheterization has a positive impact, particularly in children with neurogenic dysfunction.

6. **b. Room-temperature saline at a slow fill rate (10% of capacity per minute).** The testing medium and infusion rate can influence the results. Carbon dioxide is not as reliable as fluid infusion, particularly when evaluating bladder compliance and capacity. The most common fluids used for testing are saline and iodinated contrast material; both provide reproducible results. Use of testing media at body temperature is also appropriate, but room temperature has also been shown to be acceptable. End filling pressure and bladder compliance can be dramatically affected by simply changing the filling rate. The cystometrogram should be performed at a fill rate of 10% per minute of the predicted bladder capacity for age.

7. **d. Acceptance of and compliance with intermittent catheterization.** No test ensures that a patient will be able to void spontaneously and empty well after bladder augmentation or other reconstruction. Therefore, all patients must be prepared to perform CIC postoperatively. The native urethra should be examined for the ease of catheterization. Ideally, the patient should learn CIC and practice it preoperatively until the patient, family, and surgeon are comfortable that catheterization can and will be performed reliably. In spite of a technically perfect operation, failure to catheterize and empty the bladder after reconstruction can result in upper tract deterioration, urinary tract infection, or bladder perforation.

8. **e. All of the above.** Each patient undergoes preoperative bowel preparation to minimize the potential risk of surgery if the use of any bowel is contemplated. Even when ureterocystoplasty or other alternatives are planned, intraoperative findings may dictate the need for use of a bowel segment.

9. **c. Mobilization of the recipient ureter to meet the crossing one.** If the native urinary bladder is small and adequate for only a single ureteral tunnel, transureteroureterostomy and a single reimplant may be helpful. Typically, the better ureter should be implanted into the bladder. The contralateral ureter drains into the reimplanted ureter via a transureteroureterostomy. The crossing ureter should follow a smooth path and remain tension free. It should be carefully mobilized with all of its adventitia and as much periureteral tissue as possible to preserve blood supply. Care must be taken not to angulate the crossing ureter beneath the inferior mesenteric artery. The crossing ureter should be widely anastomosed to the posteromedial aspect of the recipient ureter. The recipient ureter should not be mobilized or brought medially to meet the contralateral ureter to minimize devascularization.

10. **b. Ileum.** The necessity of ureteral reimplantation into an intestinal segment may occasionally determine the segment to be used for bladder augmentation or replacement. Long-term experience with ureterosigmoidostomy and colon conduit diversion has established an effective means of creating a nonrefluxing ureteral implant. If a gastric segment is used for bladder augmentation or replacement, the ureters may be implanted into the stomach in a manner remarkably similar to that used in the native bladder. Creating an effective antireflux mechanism into an ileal segment is more difficult. The split nipple technique described by Griffith may prevent reflux at least at low reservoir pressure.

11. **a. Results in limited success because of a lack of muscle tone and activity of the native bladder neck.** Reports of success with the Young-Dees-Leadbetter bladder neck reconstruction in children with neurogenic sphincter dysfunction are limited, not only in the number of series but also in overall improvement of incontinence. Independent reviews of long-term results of this repair show minimal success in individuals with neurogenic dysfunction. These authors speculate that the lack of success was due to a lack of muscle tone and activity in the wrapped muscle related to the neurogenic problem.

12. **b. Artificial urinary sphincter placement.** The artificial urinary sphincter has been recognized as the only procedure that can result in prompt continence in selected children while preserving their ability to void spontaneously.

13. **e. Unmasking of detrusor hostility, resulting in upper urinary tract changes.** It is now recognized that occlusion of the bladder neck in children with neurogenic sphincter incompetence can result in the unmasking or development of detrusor hostility manifest by a decrease in bladder compliance or increase in detrusor hyperreflexia. Careful preoperative urodynamic assessment helps to identify some of the children who are at risk.

14. **a. Are more effective in girls than in boys.** Fascial slings have been used more extensively and with better results in girls with neurogenic sphincter incompetence, although recently some success has been reported in boys. Overall long-term success

with fascial slings in the neurogenic population has varied greatly from 40% to 100%.

15. **c. Inability to empty the bladder by spontaneous voiding.** The ultimate benefits of the artificial urinary sphincter include its ability to achieve a high rate of continence while maintaining the potential for spontaneous voiding. For practical purposes, when intermittent catheterization is required along with augmentation cystoplasty, using native tissue for continence eliminates the long-term concern for infection/erosion and the risk of mechanical failure.

16. **c. Difficulty with intermittent catheterization, particularly in boys.** One study examined the results in 23 children, 22 of whom had neurogenic sphincter incompetence, and noted continence in more than 90% of the children. The most common complication was difficult catheterization, particularly in boys. Fewer than half of the boys in this series were catheterized through the native urethra; the majority were catheterized via an abdominal wall stoma.

17. **e. Bladder neck division.** The ultimate procedure to increase bladder outlet resistance is to divide the bladder neck so that it is no longer in continuity with the urethra. This must be accompanied by creation of a continent abdominal wall stoma and should be performed only in patients who will reliably be able to perform catheterization.

18. **b. The intestinal segment should be reconfigured.** Two studies demonstrated the advantages of opening a bowel segment on its antimesenteric border, which allows detubularization and reconfiguration of that intestinal segment. Reconfiguration into a spherical shape provides multiple advantages, including maximization of the volume achieved for any given surface area, blunting of bowel contractions, and improvement of overall capacity and compliance.

19. **d. Flap valve created beneath a taenia.** Small bowel does not have a taenia; this method is appropriate for large bowel. The split nipple technique described by Griffith may prevent reflux at least at low reservoir pressure. LeDuc and colleagues in 1987 described a technique in which the ureter is brought through a hiatus in the ileal wall. From that hiatus the ileal mucosa is incised and the edges are mobilized so as to create a trough for the ureter. It may also be possible to create antireflux mechanism using a serosal-lined tunnel created between two limbs of ileum as described by Abol-Enein and Ghoneim in 1999. Reinforced nipple valves of ileum have been used extensively to prevent reflux with the Kock pouch. Good long-term results have been achieved by Skinner after several modifications.

20. **d. Ileocecal segment.** Chronic diarrhea after bladder augmentation alone is rare. Diarrhea can occur after removal of large segments of ileum from the gastrointestinal tract, although the length of the segments typically used for augmentation is rarely problematic unless other problems coexist. Removal of the ileum and ileocecal valve from the gastrointestinal tract may cause diarrhea. One study noted that 10% of patients with neurogenic dysfunction have significant diarrhea after such displacement.

21. **b. Hyperchloremic metabolic acidosis.** Postoperative bowel obstruction is uncommon after augmentation cystoplasty, occurring in approximately 3% of patients after augmentation. The rate of obstruction is equivalent to that noted after conduit diversion or continent urinary diversion. Removal of the distal ileum from the gastrointestinal tract may result in vitamin B_{12} deficiency and megaloblastic anemia. The terminal 15 to 20 cm of ileum should not be used for augmentation, although problems may arise even if that segment is preserved. Early satiety may occur after gastrocystoplasty but usually resolves with time. Disorders of gastric emptying should be extremely rare, particularly when using the body of the stomach.

22. **c. Ileum.** Ileal reservoirs have been noted to have lower basal pressures and less motor activity when created for continent urinary diversion. Problems with pressure after augmentation cystoplasty usually occur from uninhibited contractions caused by the bowel segment. It is extremely rare not to achieve an adequate capacity or flat tonus limb unless a technical error has occurred with use of the bowel segment. Rhythmic contractions have been noted postoperatively with all bowel segments, particularly the stomach, although ileum is the least likely to demonstrate a remarkable urodynamic abnormality.

23. **b. 5% to 10%.** Hollensbe and associates at Indiana University reported on one of the largest experiences with pediatric bladder augmentation and found that approximately 5% of patients had significant uninhibited contractions causing clinical problems. Another study found that 6% required secondary augmentation of a previously augmented bladder for similar problems in long-term follow-up.

24. **b. Hyperchloremic metabolic acidosis.** The first recognized metabolic complication related to storage of urine within intestinal segments was the occasional development of hyperchloremic metabolic acidosis after ureterosigmoidostomy. Another study demonstrated the mechanisms by which acid is absorbed from urine in contact with intestinal mucosa. A later report noted that essentially every patient after augmentation with an intestinal segment had an increase in serum chloride and a decrease in serum bicarbonate levels, although clinically significant acidosis was rare if renal function was normal.

25. **c. Hypochloremic metabolic alkalosis.** Gastric mucosa is a barrier to chloride and acid resorption and, in fact, secretes hydrochloric acid. The secretory nature of gastric mucosa may at times be detrimental to the patient and can result in two unique complications of gastrocystoplasty. Severe episodes of hypokalemic hypochloremic metabolic alkalosis after acute gastrointestinal illnesses have been noted after gastrocystoplasty.

26. **e. Neurogenic bladder dysfunction.** Virtually all patients with normal sensation have occasional hematuria or dysuria with voiding or catheterization after gastrocystoplasty beyond that which is expected with other intestinal segments. All patients should be warned of this potential problem, although in most patients these symptoms are intermittent and mild and do not require treatment. The dysuria is less problematic in patients with limited sensation due to neurogenic dysfunction. Patients who are incontinent or have decreased renal function may be at increased risk. These problems occur less frequently after antral gastric cystoplasty in which there is a smaller load of parietal cells.

27. **e. Urine culture reveals growth of a urea-splitting organism.** It appears that the use of CIC is a prominent factor in the development of bacteriuria in patients after augmentation cystoplasty. Every episode of asymptomatic bacteriuria does not require treatment in patients performing CIC. Bacteriuria should be treated when significant symptoms occur such as fever, suprapubic pain, incontinence, and gross hematuria. Bacteriuria should also be treated when the urine culture demonstrates growth of a urea-splitting organism that may lead to stone formation.

28. **a. Stomach.** Most bladder stones in the augmented child are of a struvite composition. Bacteriuria has been thought to be an important risk factor. Stones have been noted after the use of all intestinal segments with no significant difference appreciated between small and large intestine. Struvite stones are less likely after gastrocystoplasty.

29. **b. 4 years.** Patients undergoing augmentation cystoplasty should be made aware of a potential increased risk of tumor development. Yearly surveillance of the augmented bladder with endoscopy should eventually be performed; the latency period until such procedures are necessary is not well defined. The earliest reported tumor after augmentation was found only 4 years after cystoplasty.

30. **d. Bladder exstrophy.** The cause of delayed perforations after bladder augmentation is unknown. Perforations may occur in bladders with significant uninhibited contractions after augmentation. High outflow resistance may maintain bladder pressure rather than allowing urinary leakage and venting of the pressure, potentially increasing ischemia. The majority of patients suffering

perforations after augmentation cystoplasty have a neurogenic etiology. At Indiana University, perforations were noted in 32 of 330 patients undergoing cystoplasty an average of 4.3 years after augmentation. Analysis of this experience suggested that the use of sigmoid colon was the only significant increased risk.

31. **c. Immediate surgical exploration and repair.** The standard treatment of spontaneous perforation of the augmented bladder is surgical repair, as it is for intraperitoneal rupture of the bladder after trauma. The majority of patients with perforations have myelodysplasia and present late in the course of the disease because of impaired sensation. Increasing sepsis and death of the patient may result from a delay in diagnosis or treatment.

32. **c. Results in the mesenteric pedicle deflected laterally without vascular compromise to the augmented segment.** Experience is limited regarding what is known about the changes to the pedicle of a bladder augmentation during pregnancy. It has been reported that the mesenteric pedicle to bladder augmentations is not stretched over the uterus at the time of cesarean section. The pedicle has been found to be deflected laterally. Urinary tract infections may be problematic in women who have undergone urinary reconstruction, including bladder augmentation. Ureteral dilatation, increased residual urine, and diminished tone to the upper tract may all be important risk factors.

33. **d. A dilated ureter is not available in many patients.** Several series have reported good results after ureteral augmentation with a follow-up as long as 8 years. The upper urinary tract has remained stable or improved in virtually all patients. Complications are uncommon. The main disadvantage to ureterocystoplasty is the limited patient population with a poorly functioning kidney drained by a megaureter.

34. **e. Small bladder capacity.** Although autoaugmentation can improve compliance, an increase in volume is "modest at best." In a report of 12 children who had undergone a detrusorotomy, 5 were considered to have excellent results, 2 had acceptable results, and 1 was lost to follow-up. The main disadvantage of autoaugmentation is a limited increase in bladder capacity such that adequate preoperative volume may be the most important predictor of success.

35. **d. Fecal incontinence.** Before ureterosigmoidostomy is considered, anal sphincter competence must be ensured. Tests used to assess sphincter integrity include manometry, electromyography, and practical evaluation of the ability to retain an oatmeal enema in the upright position for a time period without soilage. Incontinence of a mixture of stool and urine results in foul soilage and must be avoided.

36. **b. Has a higher complication and reoperation rate than a flap valve.** The greatest experience with nipple valves for achieving urinary continence has been with the Kock pouch. Skinner and associates made a series of modifications to aid in maintenance of the efferent nipple. Even with experience and these modifications, a failure rate of 15% or higher can be expected. Equivalent results with the nipple valve and a Kock pouch have been achieved in children.

37. **b. Creating a tunnel of 4 cm, at least greater than a 5:1 ratio of tunnel length to diameter, to achieve continence.** The appendix is an ideal natural tubular structure that can be safely removed from the gastrointestinal tract without significant morbidity. The small caliber of the appendix facilitates creation of a short functional tunnel with the bladder wall. Experience has shown that continence can be achieved with only a 2-cm appendiceal tunnel.

38. **e. Stomal stenosis.** Incontinence is rare with the Mitrofanoff procedure and may result from inadequate length of the flap valve mechanism or persistently elevated reservoir pressure. The most common complication has been stomal stenosis and occurs in 10% to 20% of patients. Stenosis resulting in difficult catheterization may occur early in the postoperative course and requires formal revision.

39. **b. Tapered segment of small bowel of adequate length.** When the appendix is unavailable for use, other tubular structures can provide a similar mechanism for catheterization and continence. Mitrofanoff, in 1980, described a similar technique using ureter. Woodhouse and MacNeily, in 1994, as well as others, have used the fallopian tube, which can accommodate catheterization. Monti and Yang have been credited with a novel modification of the tapered intestinal segment, which can be reimplanted according to the Mitrofanoff principle.

40. **c. Achieve an effective antireflux mechanism without upper tract obstruction.** The key to urinary undiversion is understanding the original pathologic condition that led to diversion. One report described a 26-year experience with urinary undiversion in 216 patients. In that series, management of the bladder was relatively straightforward and effective with bladder augmentation as necessary. Inadequate outflow resistance was usually treated with Young-Dees-Ledbetter bladder neck repair. Most complications were related to the ureters; 23 patients required reoperation for persistent reflux, whereas 10 did so for partial obstruction of the ureter. Those reoperation rates are indicative of the difficulty one faces in dealing with short, dilated, and scarred ureters, which may be present after urinary diversion.

CHAPTER REVIEW

1. Bladder volume in children is equal to 30 × (age in years + 2).
2. Intermittent catheterization must be taught and accepted by the patient and caregiver before any urinary reconstruction is performed.
3. There is no test that ensures the patient will be able to void spontaneously and empty well after bladder augmentation or reconstruction.
4. Most patients prefer to catheterize an abdominal wall stoma rather than the native urethra.
5. Bladder neck bulking agents are not particularly effective in children.
6. When placing the artificial sphincter it should be placed at the bladder neck in females and in prepubertal boys.
7. One third of patients will require further surgery after augmentation cystoplasty because of various problems.
8. Bacteriuria is common after intestinal cystoplasty. After intestinal cystoplasty, routine bladder irrigation should be performed to evacuate inspissated mucus.
9. Stomach should be reserved for patients who have short gut syndrome or who have received heavy pelvic irradiation.
10. Delayed spontaneous perforation of the bowel segment after intestinal cystoplasty occurs in approximately 5% of patients.
11. Most secondary reflux will resolve after successful bladder reconstruction.
12. Nonfunctional bladders may need to be cycled to determine their true capacity.
13. Removing the ileal-cecal valve from the gastrointestinal tract in patients with neurogenic bladder and bowel dysfunction may result in intractable diarrhea.
14. It has been noted that there appears to be an increased incidence of malignant tumors in the gastric segment of patients who have had a gastrocystoplasty.
15. When the appendix is used to create a flap valve, the distance to the skin should be as short as possible to facilitate ease of catheterization.
16. The Young-Dees-Leadbetter bladder neck reconstruction in children with neurogenic sphincter dysfunction has had limited success.

17. Occlusion of the bladder neck in children with neurogenic sphincter incompetence can result in the unmasking or development of detrusor hostility manifest by a decrease in bladder compliance or increase in detrusor hyperreflexia.

18. Ileal reservoirs have been noted to have lower basal pressures and less motor activity when created for continent urinary diversion.

19. Essentially every patient after augmentation with an ileal or colonic intestinal segment has an increase in serum chloride and a decrease in serum bicarbonate levels, although severe acidosis is rare if renal function is normal.

20. Severe episodes of hypokalemic hypochloremic metabolic alkalosis after acute gastrointestinal illnesses have been noted after gastrocystoplasty.

21. The majority of patients suffering bladder perforations after augmentation cystoplasty have a neurogenic etiology.

146 Management of Abnormalities of the External Genitalia in Boys

Lane S. Palmer and Jeffrey S. Palmer

QUESTIONS

1. In the male, which of the following stimulates the development of the external genitalia?
   a. Testosterone
   b. Human chorionic gonadotropin
   c. Dihydrotestosterone
   d. Luteinizing hormone and follicle-stimulating hormone
   e. Maternal progesterone
2. What percentage of uncircumcised boys will have persistent phimosis by 17 years of age?
   a. Less than 1%
   b. 5%
   c. 10%
   d. 15%
   e. 20%
3. Circumcision should not be performed in neonates with which condition of the genitalia?
   a. Phimosis
   b. Undescended testis
   c. Inguinal hernia
   d. Penile curvature
   e. Testicular atrophy
4. What is the most common complication associated with circumcision?
   a. Trauma to the glans
   b. Bleeding
   c. Meatal stenosis
   d. Skin bridges
   e. Balanitis xerotica obliterans (BXO)
5. A 4-year-old boy presents with phimosis and BXO of the prepuce. What is the preferred treatment?
   a. Observation
   b. Topical corticosteroids
   c. Excision of BXO skin without circumcision
   d. Warm baths
   e. Circumcision
6. Penile agenesis is associated with all of the following malformations EXCEPT:
   a. cryptorchidism.
   b. vesicoureteral reflux.
   c. horseshoe kidney.
   d. ureteropelvic junction obstruction.
   e. renal agenesis.
7. The etiology of the buried penis includes all of the following EXCEPT:
   a. suprapubic fat pad.
   b. small penis.
   c. poor penopubic fixation of the penis.
   d. obesity.
   e. cicatricial scarring after surgery.
8. A 9-month-old boy who was previously circumcised presents with a buried penis resulting from cicatricial scarring. What is the most appropriate initial treatment?
   a. Topical betamethasone and manual retraction
   b. Revision of circumcision

   c. Penopubic fixation of the penis
   d. Liposuction of the suprapubic fat pad
   e. Observation
9. What is the minimal normal stretched penile length of a full-term neonate?
   a. 1.2 cm
   b. 1.9 cm
   c. 2.5 cm
   d. 3.2 cm
   e. 4.5 cm
10. Which of the following statements is TRUE regarding a micropenis in a term male neonate?
    a. The testes are usually normal in size and not cryptorchid.
    b. It is best managed by gender reassignment.
    c. It has an abnormal ratio of the length of the penile shaft to circumference.
    d. It is unlikely to respond to testosterone stimulation until puberty.
    e. It is less than 1.9 cm in stretched length.
11. What is the most common cause of micropenis?
    a. Hypergonadotropic hypogonadism
    b. Hypogonadotropic hypogonadism
    c. Idiopathic
    d. Growth hormone deficiency
    e. Androgen insensitivity syndrome
12. Which of the following statements regarding penile masses is FALSE?
    a. The treatment of parameatal urethral cysts is complete excision of the cyst.
    b. The most common acquired cystic lesion of the penis is smegma under the unretractable prepuce.
    c. Congenital penile nevi tend to be malignant.
    d. The initial management of juvenile xanthogranulomas is expectant monitoring.
    e. Epidermal inclusion cysts may form after penile surgery.
13. A 13-year-old African-American boy with sickle cell disease has a 6-hour painful erection. The initial management should include all of the following EXCEPT:
    a. alkalization.
    b. hydration.
    c. intracavernous injections of β-adrenergic sympathomimetic agents.
    d. analgesia.
    e. transfusion to reduce hemoglobin S concentration.
14. Which of the following statements is TRUE regarding high-flow priapism?
    a. It is usually a drug-induced etiology.
    b. The aspirated blood is similar to venous blood on blood gas analysis.
    c. Color Doppler ultrasonography commonly demonstrates the fistula.
    d. Surgical intervention is the initial management.
    e. Sickle cell disease is the most common cause

15. Penoscrotal transposition is associated with all of the following anomalies EXCEPT:
    a. sex chromosome abnormalities.
    b. distal shaft hypospadias with chordee.
    c. autosomal chromosome abnormalities.
    d. Aarskog syndrome.
    e. caudal regression.
16. All of the following are associated with patency of the processus vaginalis EXCEPT:
    a. Transverse testicular ectopia
    b. Epididymal anomalies
    c. Cryptorchidism
    d. Spermatic cord torsion
    e. Polyorchidism
17. Abdominoscrotal hydrocele is reported to be associated with all of the following features EXCEPT:
    a. a closed processus vaginalis.
    b. epididymal anomalies.
    c. testicular dysmorphism.
    d. hydronephrosis.
    e. increased pressure within the tunica vaginalis.
18. Irreversible ischemic injury of the testicular parenchyma may begin as early as how many hours after torsion of the spermatic cord?
    a. 1
    b. 2
    c. 4
    d. 6
    e. 8
19. Which of the following is most specific in diagnosing spermatic cord torsion?
    a. High-riding testis
    b. Absence of the cremasteric reflex
    c. Transverse lie of the testis
    d. Spermatic cord twist on high-resolution Doppler ultrasonography
    e. Acute severe pain
20. After manual detorsion of the spermatic chord, which of the following is appropriate management?
    a. Color Doppler ultrasonography
    b. Radionuclide scan
    c. Doppler examination of the testis and spermatic cord
    d. Discharge from the hospital and arrangement for an office reevaluation in 1 week
    e. Immediate scrotal exploration
21. An adolescent is evaluated for a history of self-limited, intermittent episodes of severe unilateral scrotal pain. Physical examination findings are normal. What is the most appropriate course of action?
    a. Color Doppler ultrasonography
    b. Reassessment in 6 months
    c. Elective scrotal exploration
    d. Radionuclide scrotal imaging
    e. Immediate scrotal exploration
22. When the diagnosis of torsion of the appendix epididymis is made, which of the following is optimal management?
    a. Observation
    b. Color Doppler ultrasonography
    c. Radionuclide scrotal imaging
    d. Immediate scrotal exploration
    e. Cord block and manual detorsion
23. Which of the following is the most likely diagnosis in an infant with sterile urine and epididymitis?
    a. Unilateral renal agenesis
    b. Large prostatic utricle
    c. Urethral stricture disease
    d. Persistent vasoureteral fusion
    e. Radiographically normal urinary tract
24. What is the most appropriate course of action in an otherwise healthy neonate with perinatal testicular torsion?
    a. Surgical exploration of the affected testis
    b. Surgical exploration of the affected testis with contralateral scrotal orchidopexy

c. Color Doppler ultrasonography of the scrotum
d. Radionuclide testicular scan
e. Observation
25. Most adolescent varicoceles evaluated by urologists are:
    a. painful.
    b. of cosmetic concern.
    c. asymptomatic.
    d. associated with an ipsilateral hydrocele.
    e. bilateral.
26. Significant testicular volume differential in cases of varicocele is defined as greater than:
    a. 5%.
    b. 5% to 10%.
    c. 10% to 15%.
    d. 15% to 20%.
    e. 25%.
27. Hydrocele formation after varicocele ligation is least likely to occur after which of the following procedures?
    a. Retroperitoneal ligation
    b. Subinguinal ligation
    c. Laparoscopic ligation
    d. Microscopic inguinal ligation
    e. Transvenous embolization
28. Which of the following is NOT a relative indication for elective varicocele repair?
    a. Pain
    b. Oligospermia
    c. Small testes
    d. Continuous spermatic venous reflux
    e. Testicular size discrepancy of greater than 20%

ANSWERS

1. **c. Dihydrotestosterone.** Influence of dihydrotestosterone on the androgen receptors results in the differentiation of the genital tubercle, genital (labioscrotal) folds, and genital swelling at between 9 and 13 weeks of gestation into the male structures of the glans penis, penile shaft, and scrotum, respectively.
2. **a. Less than 1%.** Preputial retractability increases with age with 90% of uncircumcised boys 3 years of age with completely retractable prepuces; less than 1% by 17 years of age have phimosis. Therefore, primary phimosis is almost always resolvable during childhood without intervention.
3. **d. Penile curvature.** Circumcision should not be performed in neonates with other penile conditions that require surgical correction. These conditions include hypospadias, penile curvature, dorsal hood deformity, buried penis, and webbed penis.
4. **b. Bleeding.** The risk of complications after circumcision is 0.2% to 5%. The most common complication is bleeding, which occurs in 0.1% and is more common in older children.
5. **e. Circumcision.** Treatment of BXO includes medical and surgical management. The use of topical corticosteroids has had limited benefit to treat mild BXO of the prepuce with minimal scar formation. Circumcision is the preferred treatment.
6. **d. Ureteropelvic junction obstruction.** Penile agenesis (aphallia) results from failure of development of the genital tubercle. The disorder is rare and has an estimated incidence of 1 in 10 to 30 million births. The karyotype almost always is 46,XY, and the usual appearance is that of a well-developed scrotum with descended testes and an absent penile shaft. The anus is usually displaced anteriorly. Associated malformations are common and include cryptorchidism, vesicoureteral reflux, horseshoe kidney, renal agenesis, imperforate anus, and musculoskeletal and cardiopulmonary abnormalities.
7. **b. Small penis.** A buried penis can be classified into three categories based on etiology for the concealment: (1) poor penopubic fixation of the skin at the base of the penis; (2) obesity; and (3) a trapped penis from cicatricial scarring after penile surgery, typically a circumcision.

8. **a. Topical betamethasone and manual retraction.** Young children with secondary cicatricial scarring after penile surgery can undergo forceful dilation of the cicatrix with a fine hemostat in the office after the application or injection of analgesia. Another option is the combination of topical betamethasone and manual retraction.

9. **b. 1.9 cm.** Stretched penile length is determined by measuring the penis from its attachment to the pubic symphysis to the tip of the glans. One must be careful to depress the suprapubic fat pad completely to obtain an accurate measurement, especially in an obese infant or child. In general, the penis of a full-term neonate should be at least 1.9 cm long.

10. **e. It is less than 1.9 cm in stretched length.** Micropenis is a normally formed penis that is at least 2.5 SD below the mean size in stretched length for age. The ratio of the length of the penile shaft to its circumference is usually normal, but occasionally the corpora cavernosa are severely hypoplastic. The testes are usually small and frequently cryptorchid, whereas the scrotum is usually fused and often diminutive. A stretched penile length less than 1.9 cm long is consistent with a micropenis.

11. **b. Hypogonadotropic hypogonadism.** The most common cause of micropenis is hypogonadotropic hypogonadism, which is the failure of the hypothalamus to produce an adequate amount of gonadotropin-releasing hormone (GnRH). This condition may result from hypothalamic dysfunction, which can occur in Prader-Willi syndrome, Kallmann syndrome (genital-olfactory dysplasia), Laurence-Moon-Biedl syndrome, and the CHARGE association.

12. **c. Congenital penile nevi tend to be malignant.** Congenital penile nevi tend to be superficial and benign. Congenital penile nevi are pigmented lesions that can form on the glans and penile shaft. They tend to be superficial and benign and should be excised.

13. **c. Intracavernous injections of β-adrenergic sympathomimetic agents.** The initial treatment of low-flow priapism resulting from sickle cell disease is conservative with hydration, oxygenation, alkalization, analgesia, and transfusion with the goal of reducing hemoglobin S concentration. Evacuation of blood and irrigation of the corpora cavernosa along with intracavernous injections of α-adrenergic sympathomimetic agents, such as phenylephrine or epinephrine solution, can be a concurrent therapy. Surgical intervention to allow corporeal drainage by shunt procedures is indicated if there is a lack of response to medical therapy.

14. **c. Color Doppler ultrasonography commonly demonstrates the fistula.** High-flow priapism is usually due to perineal trauma, such as a straddle injury. Corporeal irrigation is diagnostic and therapeutic. Typically, the aspirated blood is bright red and the aspirate is similar to arterial blood on blood gas analysis. Color Doppler ultrasonography often will demonstrate the fistula. The initial management is observation because spontaneous resolution may occur. Superselective embolization of cavernous and penile arteries is the next line of therapy. If not, angiographic embolization is indicated.

15. **b. Distal shaft hypospadias with chordee.** Frequently, penoscrotal transposition occurs in conjunction with perineal, scrotal, or penoscrotal hypospadias with chordee. Penoscrotal transposition has also been associated with caudal regression, sex chromosome abnormalities, and Aarskog syndrome. As many as 75% of patients with complete penoscrotal transposition and a normal scrotum have a significant urinary tract abnormality, including renal agenesis and dysplasia, and other nongenitourinary anomalies.

16. **d. Spermatic cord torsion.** Risk of torsion is associated with abnormal development of the tunica vaginalis but not patency of the processus vaginalis.

17. **b. Epididymal anomalies.** The processus vaginalis is closed in cases of abdominoscrotal hydrocele; and an elongated dysmorphic testis, increased pressure within the tunica vaginalis, and hydronephrosis have all been reported.

18. **c. 4.** Irreversible ischemic injury to the testicular parenchyma may begin as soon as 4 hours after occlusion of the cord.

19. **d. Spermatic cord twist on high-resolution Doppler ultrasonography.** Spermatic cord twist on high-resolution Doppler imaging is the most specific finding, that is, the least likely to be false positive, in spermatic cord torsion.

20. **e. Immediate scrotal exploration.** It should be remembered that manual detorsion may not totally correct the rotation that has occurred and that prompt exploration is still indicated.

21. **c. Elective scrotal exploration.** If the suspicion is strong that episodes of intermittent torsion and spontaneous detorsion have occurred, the author's experience has been that the finding of a bell-clapper deformity at exploration can be expected. Elective scrotal exploration should be performed, with scrotal fixation of both testes.

22. **a. Observation.** When the diagnosis of a torsed appendage is confirmed clinically or by imaging, nonoperative management will allow most cases to resolve spontaneously.

23. **e. Radiographically normal urinary tract.** The majority of infants with epididymitis have sterile urine and apparently radiographically normal urinary tracts.

24. **b. Surgical exploration of the affected testis with contralateral scrotal orchidopexy.** Clearly, if the cause of scrotal swelling appears to be related to an acute postnatal event, all efforts should be made to pursue prompt surgical intervention. If torsion is confirmed, contralateral scrotal exploration with testicular fixation should be performed.

25. **c. Asymptomatic.** Most adolescent varicoceles are asymptomatic.

26. **d. 15% to 20%.** In adults and adolescents, testicular size (volume) should be approximately equal bilaterally, with the normal differential not being more than 15% to 20% volume.

27. **e. Transvenous embolization.** Hydrocele formation is related to failure to preserve lymphatic vessels associated with the spermatic cord and its vessels. Hydrocele formation seems most common after retroperitoneal ligation, especially when a mass ligation technique is used, and is least likely to occur after transvenous embolization.

28. **d. Continuous spermatic venous reflux.** Significant pain associated with varicocele, bilateral small testes, and oligospermia are reasonable indications to proceed with repair in an adolescent male. The standard indication is ipsilateral testicular volume loss, or hypotrophy, of at least 15% to 20%, although this should be documented on serial yearly testicular examinations, because variable growth of the testes may occur during puberty. Continuous reflux may be documented on color Doppler imaging but is not a specific indication for surgery.

CHAPTER REVIEW

1. The normal penile size of a neonate is 3.5 ± 0.7 cm in stretched length. It should be at least 1.9 cm. If it is below 1.9 cm, it is classified as a micropenis.
2. The potential benefits of circumcision include prevention of penile cancer; urinary tract infections; sexually transmitted diseases, including human immunodeficiency virus infection; and phimosis.
3. Glanular adhesions and skin bridges are not uncommon complications of circumcision.
4. Meatal stenosis is a condition that occurs almost exclusively in children after infant circumcision.
5. If a meatotomy is performed, suturing the urethral mucosa to the glans with fine, resorbable sutures reduces the risk of recurrence.

6. The causes of micropenis include (a) hypogonadotropic hypogonadism, (b) hypergonadotropic hypogonadism (primary testicular failure), and (c) idiopathic causes.
7. Most men born with micropenis have male gender identity and satisfactory sexual function.
8. Priapism can be ischemic (veno-occlusive, low flow), nonischemic (arterial, high flow), and stuttering (intermittent).
9. In the female and the male with abnormal testosterone and/or dihydrotestosterone production, 5α-reductase deficiency or androgen receptor dysfunction, the genital tubercle, genital folds and genital swelling becomes the clitoris, labia minora and labia majora, respectively.
10. True micropenis is often due to a deficiency of gonadotropins.
11. In penile torsion, the glans may be rotated but the corpora cavernosa and corpora spongiosum at the base of the penis are normal.
12. Urethral duplication usually occurs in the sagittal plane.
13. Inguinal hernias are more common in premature infants.
14. There is a familial predisposition to intravaginal testicular torsion.
15. An absent cremasteric reflex is associated with testicular torsion.
16. There is no convincing evidence that testicular torsion results in antisperm antibodies.
17. The influence of dihydrotestosterone on the androgen receptors during development results in the differentiation of the genital tubercle, genital (labioscrotal) folds, and genital swelling into the male structures of the glans penis, penile shaft, and scrotum, respectively.
18. Circumcision should not be performed in neonates with other penile conditions that require surgical correction. These conditions include hypospadias, penile curvature, dorsal hood deformity, buried penis, and webbed penis.
19. A buried penis has three etiologies: (1) poor penopubic fixation of the skin at the base of the penis; (2) obesity; and (3) a trapped penis from cicatricial scarring after penile surgery, typically a circumcision.
20. High-flow priapism is usually due to perineal trauma, such as a straddle injury. Corporeal irrigation is diagnostic and therapeutic.
21. In testicular torsion, irreversible ischemic injury to the testicular parenchyma may begin as soon as 4 hours after occlusion of the cord.
22. Significant pain associated with varicocele, bilateral small testes, and oligospermia are reasonable indications to proceed with repair in an adolescent male.

147 Hypospadias

Warren T. Snodgrass and Nicol Corbin Bush

QUESTIONS

1. A 6-month-old male presents for evaluation of subcoronal hypospadias. During physical examination, the left testicle is palpated in the groin but cannot be manipulated into the scrotum. The next step is to:
   a. re-examine in 6 months to allow for testicular descent.
   b. perform ultrasonography to rule out testicular retraction.
   c. obtain a karyotype.
   d. schedule hypospadias repair now, and orchiopexy in 6 months.
   e. schedule orchiopexy now, with hypospadias repair in 6 months.

2. During a proximal penile shaft hypospadias repair, a catheter cannot be passed into the bladder. The most likely cause is:
   a. a false passage in the urethra.
   b. an enlarged utricle.
   c. partial urethral duplication ending in a blind pouch.
   d. an elevated bladder neck.
   e. proximal urethral stricture.

3. A 6-month-old infant without other known medical problems is referred for scrotal hypospadias. He is also found to have ventral penile curvature, a deep scrotal cleft, and penoscrotal transposition, but both testes are in the scrotum. The next step is:
   a. proceed with surgery.
   b. obtain a karyotype
   c. order a voiding cystourethrogram (VCUG) to visualize the utricle.
   d. obtain renal sonography.
   e. schedule testicular ultrasonography.

4. A patient with penoscrotal hypospadias has ventral curvature of nearly 90 degrees preoperatively. After the penis is degloved and dartos tissues released, artificial erection shows the curvature has diminished to less than 30 degrees. The best next step is:
   a. transect the urethral plate.
   b. perform dermal grafting of the corpora cavernosa at the point of greatest bending.
   c. proceed with urethroplasty.
   d. perform a midline dorsal plication.
   e. perform midline dorsal plication and ventral dermal corporal grafting.

5. A 6-month-old male is referred for hypospadias. On examination he is found to have a dorsally hooded prepuce, ventral penile curvature, a glanular meatus, and a normal scrotum. The parents should be informed that straightening the penile curvature most likely will require:
   a. only skin degloving and ventral dartos dissection.
   b. multiple dorsal midline plications.
   c. ventral corporal grafting.
   d. transection of the urethra.
   e. single dorsal plication and ventral corporal graft.

6. A 6-week-old infant is evaluated after newborn circumcision. The primary care physician expresses concern for a "bad circ." On examination the meatus is coronal and the glans wings are separated. There is no redundant shaft skin following the circumcision except in the ventral midline near the meatus. The family should be informed that:
   a. these findings indicate urethral injury during circumcision.
   b. urethroplasty will best be performed using a ventral preputial skin flap.
   c. circumcision most likely has affected vascularity to the redundant ventral skin, and so urethroplasty will best be done using the skin as a graft.
   d. following circumcision, urethroplasty will require buccal graft from the lower lip.
   e. their infant has a hypospadias variant.

7. The parents of a 6-month-old male with subcoronal hypospadias request foreskin reconstruction rather than circumcision. The parents should be informed that:
   a. preoperative testosterone therapy to enlarge the foreskin is recommended.
   b. complication rates are significantly greater with prepucioplasty.
   c. they should not retract the foreskin in the first 6 weeks after surgery.
   d. a gentle compression dressing should be used to minimize preputial edema after surgery.
   e. the foreskin most likely will be needed for urethroplasty and so circumcision will likely be necessary.

8. Each of the following is thought to reduce the likelihood for fistula development after hypospadias surgery EXCEPT:
   a. subepithelial suturing of the neourethra.
   b. 2-layer closure of the neourethra.
   c. monofilament sutures.
   d. approximation of the corpus spongiosum over the neourethra.
   e. placement of a dartos flap over the neourethra.

9. A mother reports her 7-year-old child who had a penoscrotal tubularized incised plate (TIP) hypospadias repair took longer to void than a playmate during a sleepover. He does not strain to urinate and has had no urinary tract infections (UTIs). Uroflowmetry shows a peak flow rate of 8 mL/sec with a plateau-shaped curve. The next step is to:
   a. reassure that the flow rate is within the normal range.
   b. recommend VCUG to rule out stricture.
   c. perform urethral dilation.
   d. schedule for flap reoperative urethroplasty.
   e. advise buccal inlay reoperative urethroplasty.

10. An 8-year-old had distal hypospadias repair as an infant. Initially after surgery he was thought to have a normal urinary stream, although the parents only rarely observed urination because he used diapers. During the past year the parents think his stream has slowed and notice he seems to have to "push" to empty his bladder. Examination reveals a faint white discoloration around the meatus. Best management includes:
    a. intraoperative biopsy with frozen section.
    b. meatotomy for meatal stenosis.
    c. flip-flap reoperative urethroplasty.
    d. topical steroids for 6 weeks.
    e. excision of the distal urethra with two-stage buccal graft urethroplasty.

11. A 1-year-old boy had a subcoronal hypospadias repair 6 months ago but has a 2-mm fistula at the site of the original meatus. Distance from the fistula to the neomeatus is approximately 4 mm, and the glans wings still appear approximated. The best treatment of the fistula is:
    a. midline incision through the neomeatus to the fistula with reoperative distal urethroplasty.
    b. rotational skin flap fistula closure.
    c. fistula closure covered with a ventral dartos barrier flap.
    d. inlay buccal graft urethroplasty.
    e. dilation of the meatus for stenosis.

12. A 10-year-old boy presents with midshaft hypospadias persistent after seven operations on his penis. He appears to have ventral curvature greater than 30 degrees and has been circumcised. There is visible scarring between the meatus and the glans, and the scrotum is riding high on the penile shaft to near the meatus. The best procedure is:
    a. TIP reoperation.
    b. flip-flap reoperative urethroplasty.
    c. onlay flap reoperative urethroplasty.
    d. inlay buccal graft urethroplasty.
    e. two-stage buccal graft urethroplasty.

13. A 6-year-old boy who had a tubularized preputial flap hypospadias repair as an infant presents with a slow urinary stream and stranguria worsening over the past year. Physical examination is unremarkable, but the peak flow is 3 mL/sec with a postvoid residual of 75 mL. At surgery cystoscopy shows a 5-mm stricture near the original meatus. This stricture is best corrected by:
    a. urethral dilation.
    b. direct vision internal urethrotomy (DIVU).
    c. DIVU with urethral dilations for 3 months.
    d. inlay buccal urethroplasty.
    e. staged buccal graft reoperation.

14. A 9-year-old prepubertal boy has failed multiple operations for penoscrotal hypospadias. Examination shows a distal shaft meatus, persistent ventral curvature, and a flat ventral glans. During planned two-stage buccal graft reoperation, it becomes apparent the entire neourethra will have to be excised back to the penoscrotal junction. The best plan for first-stage grafting is to:
    a. use cheek tissue on the penile shaft and maintain the remnant prepuce in the glans.
    b. use cheek tissue to graft the entire defect.
    c. use lower lip tissue for the entire graft.
    d. use lip tissue on the penile shaft and cheek tissue within the glans.
    e. use ventral penile shaft skin to graft the entire defect.

15. An infant with distal shaft hypospadias has a narrow, flat appearance to the urethral plate. Artificial erection after degloving shows the penis to be straight. The best option for urethroplasty is:
    a. meatoplasty and glansplasty (MAGPI).
    b. TIP.
    c. flip-flap with V incision meatoplasty.
    d. to incise the urethra to the midshaft and perform onlay preputial flap repair.
    e. to inlay buccal graft from the lip and then tubularize the urethral plate.

16. Parents report that their 1-year-old boy seems to be having difficulty urinating 3 months after TIP repair for coronal hypospadias. They have observed the stream once or twice and thought it looked thin. On examination the glans looks entirely normal, except the meatus appears small. You attempt to calibrate the meatus, and an 8-Fr sound will not pass. The most likely cause for this complication is:
    a. Balanitis xerotica obliterans (BXO).
    b. ischemia of the neomeatus.
    c. postoperative edema of the meatus.
    d. suturing the urethral plate too far distally.
    e. compression from the glans wings closure.

17. Parents report that their 1-year-old boy seems to be voiding without any problems 6 months after TIP repair for coronal hypospadias, although they have not seen the actual urinary stream because he is still in diapers. On examination you observe that the meatus appears small. The next step is:
    a. calibrate the meatus.
    b. obtain VCUG.
    c. schedule examination under anesthesia and meatotomy
    d. recommend reoperative urethroplasty, using either a ventral flip-flap if possible, or inlay buccal grafting from the lip.
    e. begin daily urethral dilations for 6 weeks.

18. A surgeon chooses Koyanagi flap repair for a child with scrotal hypospadias and ventral curvature who also needs rotational flap scrotoplasty for penoscrotal transposition. The surgeon should:
    a. delay scrotoplasty for 6 months to protect skin flap vascularity.
    b. perform urethroplasty and scrotoplasty in a single operation.
    c. straighten ventral curvature and perform scrotoplasty in the first operation and delay urethroplasty for 6 months.
    d. straighten ventral curvature and perform urethroplasty and scrotoplasty at a second procedure in 6 months.
    e. correct ventral curvature and perform scrotoplasty simultaneously, and stage the urethroplasty.

19. A 19-month-old male presents for evaluation of scrotal hypospadias. The mother has noted that his pupils seem enlarged, and she is concerned he might have developmental delay. He is crying during examination, hindering inspection of his eyes. He has scrotal hypospadias with a deep scrotal cleft, but both testes are in the scrotum. His evaluation before surgery should include:
    a. renal sonogram.
    b. testicular sonogram.
    c. VCUG.
    d. testosterone/dihydrotestosterone ratio.
    e. measurement of Müllerian inhibition hormone.

20. A 10-year-old boy had hypospadias reoperation 1 year ago that included a tunica vaginalis barrier flap over the neourethra harvested from the right testicle. He reports no problems voiding, but with erection the penis is pulled to the right side. The next step is to:
    a. reassure him the tension on his penis will resolve at puberty.
    b. make a small scrotal incision and transect the tunica vaginalis flap.
    c. make a midline penile incision and excise the tunica vaginalis flap.
    d. create a tunica vaginalis flap from the left testis to evenly distribute the tension on the penis during erection.
    e. instruct the patient to pull the penis toward the left during erection to relax contracted tissues.

21. A 14-year-old undergoes a first-stage buccal graft reoperation that involves grafting along the entire penile shaft. The next morning he is found to have visible hematoma under the shaft skin. The next step is:
    a. return immediately to the operating room to evacuate the hematoma.
    b. apply a compression dressing over the penis and scrotum.
    c. check coagulation profiles for bleeding diathesis.
    d. observe with continued bed rest.
    e. evacuate the hematoma and regraft the penile shaft.

22. The mother of a patient with coronal hypospadias is pregnant again. She asks, if the child is a male, is he likely to also have hypospadias? She should be told that:
    a. only hypospadias associated with malformation syndromes has familial recurrence.
    b. this would occur only if she was taking birth control pills containing progesterone shortly before she conceived.
    c. this would occur only if her husband also has hypospadias.
    d. it will occur, because hypospadias is a Y-linked disorder.
    e. the odds are greatest that another son would not have hypospadias.

ANSWERS

1. **c. Obtain a karyotype.** The combination of a penile anomaly with undescended testis may indicate a disorder of sex development. Although this is more commonly found with proximal hypospadias and a nonpalpable gonad, it is still advised to obtain a karyotype in any child with hypospadias and cryptorchidism.

2. **b. An enlarged utricle.** The most common reason for difficulty with catheter placement during hypospadias repair is an enlarged utricle, most commonly encountered in boys with proximal hypospadias.

3. **a. Proceed with surgery.** Neither karyotyping nor urinary tract imaging is indicated for isolated hypospadias, even in patients with proximal defects.

4. **d. Perform a midline dorsal plication.** Curvature less than 30 degrees can be straightened by a single dorsal plication without clinically apparent shortening of the penis. Transection of the urethral plate and/or ventral corporal grafting are reserved for cases with curvature greater than 30 degrees after degloving and dartos dissection.

5. **a. Only skin degloving and ventral dartos dissection.** Most often penile curvature noted in so-called chordee without hypospadias is due to shortened ventral skin and dartos and so corrects as the penis is degloved and ventral dartos dissected. Multiple plications should be avoided, ventral corporal grafting is reserved for curvature greater than 30 degrees after degloving and ventral dartos dissection, and urethral transection for a shortened urethra is only rarely indicated in this condition.

6. **e. Their infant has a hypospadias variant.** The patient has megameatus intact prepuce hypospadias variant, and urethroplasty is done without flaps or grafts by tubularizing the urethral plate.

7. **c. They should not retract the foreskin in the first 6 weeks after surgery.** Disruption of the reconstructed prepuce may result from attempts to retract the foreskin early after surgery, before edema subsides and the wound heals. Otherwise complication rates are similar between patients with distal hypospadias undergoing foreskin reconstruction versus circumcision. Dressings do not significantly affect postoperative edema. The foreskin is nearly always adequate for reconstruction in boys with distal hypospadias, with no reports suggesting need for preoperative testosterone therapy. Urethral plate tubularization removes need to use foreskin for urethroplasty.

8. **c. Monofilament sutures.** No study demonstrates outcomes are influenced by suture type.

9. **a. Reassure that the flow rate is within the normal range.** Urethral strictures after hypospadias repair have been reported in patients with peak flow less than 2 standard deviations (SD) from normal, usually less than 5 mL/sec, whereas this child has a peak flow within the normal range for age. Therefore, the likelihood this patient has a stricture is small. Furthermore, TIP repair is uncommonly complicated by stricture.

10. **e. Excision of the distal urethra with two-stage buccal graft urethroplasty.** The history and physical findings suggest BXO. Biopsy with frozen section usually is impractical in children, meaning therapy is directed by clinical suspicion. Meatotomy or skin flap repair of meatal stenosis most often fails in the presence of BXO, whereas excision of all tissues affected by BXO with staged buccal grafting is considered most likely to succeed without recurrent stenosis. Topical steroids may be initially effective, but stenosis recurs when therapy ends, and BXO may extend proximally along the urethra to a level not reached by topical applications.

11. **c. Fistula closure covered with a ventral dartos barrier flap.** A fistula with good glans approximation usually can be primarily corrected with fistula closure covered by a barrier flap. In contrast, only when a thin skin strip holds the glans wings together between the neomeatus and fistula is reoperative distal urethroplasty/glansplasty needed. A rotational skin flap is not a good option in this case because it is necessary to dissect under the corona to completely free the fistula tract and advance a barrier flap. Although meatal stenosis has to be considered in any case with a fistula, appropriate therapy when it is present is reoperation, not dilations.

12. **e. Two-stage buccal graft urethroplasty.** Visible scarring is a relative contraindication to TIP or inlay reoperations, whereas skin flaps are more difficult to raise with adequate vascularity after multiple failed operations. The best plan is to excise scarred tissues and perform staged buccal graft urethroplasty.

13. **d. Inlay buccal urethroplasty.** DIVU has a long-term success less than 10% after tubularized preputial flap repairs. The best treatment in this case is inlay grafting into the stricture.

14. **c. Use lower lip tissue for the entire graft.** It is best to use lip tissue within the glans, because it is thinner than cheek and so facilitates glansplasty. For a long graft covering the entire penile shaft, a combination of cheek tissue on the shaft and lip within the glans is recommended. Given the narrow and flat appearance of the glans and a history of multiple failed repairs, the skin with the glans is best excised to restore a deep groove that ultimately will result in a vertical meatus at the second stage. After multiple failed operations, redundant shaft skin sufficient for grafting and subsequent urethroplasty is not available.

15. **b. TIP.** TIP results for distal hypospadias are not dependent on "characteristics" of the urethral plate. MAGPI is limited to glanular hypospadias. Attempts to create a vertical meatus in conjunction with skin flap repairs usually fail or give suboptimal appearance when the urethral plate is flat. There is no need to convert a distal shaft to more proximal hypospadias to perform onlay preputial flap repair, which has higher complications than does TIP in this situation. It is not necessary to graft the incised plate, and if that were nevertheless considered in a primary operation, preputial graft rather than buccal mucosa would be preferred because it is thinner and more readily accessible.

16. **d. Suturing the urethral plate too far distally.** The most common cause of meatal stenosis after TIP is suturing the urethral plate too far distally. BXO is unlikely early after surgery and often presents with white discoloration at the meatus. Ischemia is possible but unlikely, given the reliable vascularity of the urethral plate and glans tissues. Edema after surgery may slow the urinary stream, but at 3 months it does not prevent passage of a sound. Glans closure does not create urethral obstruction.

17. **a. Calibrate the meatus.** The meatus may appear small after TIP without indicating meatal stenosis. Passage of an 8- or 10-Fr sound would suffice to determine if the meatus is stenotic or not. Meatal stenosis occurs in less than 5% of patients after TIP, and so a small-appearing meatus in an asymptomatic patient should not prompt immediate concern that examination under anesthesia or reoperation is needed.

18. **b. Perform urethroplasty and scrotoplasty in a single operation.** The scrotum and penis develop from different anlage with separate blood supplies, making simultaneous urethroplasty and scrotoplasty possible.

19. **a. Renal sonogram.** The history suggests WAGR (Wilms tumor, Aniridia, Genital abnormalities, mental Retardation) syndrome, and so renal sonography is recommended because of the association with Wilms tumor.

20. **b. Make a small scrotal incision and transect the tunica vaginalis flap.** Failure to dissect the tunica vaginalis flap to the external ring can result in traction on the penis during erection, deviating it toward the base of the flap. The best therapy is to make a small scrotal incision over the flap and transect it.

21. **d. Observe with continued bed rest.** Graft quilting and the tie-over dressing prevent blood from accumulating under the graft. Hematoma under adjacent penile skin and within the scrotum as described here will resolve. It is unlikely that a boy requiring a staged buccal graft repair has an undiagnosed coagulopathy following prior penile operations.

22. **e. The odds are greatest that another son would not have hypospadias.** Sporadic and syndromic hypospadias can have familial recurrence. Although the likelihood a sibling will have hypospadias is increased, the overall risk remains small.

CHAPTER REVIEW

1. Dihydrotestosterone at the 8- to 12-week gestational phase is a key mediator in the proper development of the penis.

2. There is an increased risk of hypospadias in births resulting from assisted reproduction.

3. Physical examination in a patient with hypospadias may reveal a ventral deficient prepuce, downward glans tilt, deviation of the median penile raphe, ventral curvature, scrotal encroachment onto the penile shaft, scrotal cleft, and penile scrotal transposition.

4. Following hypospadias repair, the meatus should calibrate to 8 to 10 Fr.

5. Eighty percent of urethroplasty complications occur within 1 year after surgery.

6. Risk factors for complications following urethroplasty include proximal meatus, reoperation, glans width less than 14 mm, and lack of a barrier flap over the neourethra.

7. Long-term follow-up of patients who have had a hypospadias repair indicates that they are more likely to have ejaculatory problems, are less satisfied with sexual function, and are more likely to be dissatisfied with the appearance of their penis than controls.

8. The combination of a penile anomaly with undescended testis may indicate a disorder of sex development. Although more commonly found with proximal hypospadias and a nonpalpable gonad, it is still advised to obtain a karyotype in any child with hypospadias and cryptorchidism.

9. Curvature less than 30 degrees can be straightened by a single dorsal plication without clinically apparent shortening of the penis. Transection of the urethral plate and/or ventral corporal grafting are reserved for cases with curvature greater than 30 degrees after degloving and dartos dissection.

10. Urethral plate tubularization removes the need to use foreskin for urethroplasty.

11. Meatotomy or skin flap repair of meatal stenosis most often fail in the presence of BXO, whereas excision of all tissues affected by BXO with staged buccal grafting is considered most likely to succeed without recurrent stenosis.

12. It is best to use lip tissue within the glans, because it is thinner than cheek tissue.

148 Etiology, Diagnosis, and Management of Undescended Testis

Julia Spencer Barthold and Jennifer A. Hagerty

QUESTIONS

1. What is the master gene responsible for male sexual differentiation?
   a. *RSPO1*
   b. *SOX9*
   c. *WT1*
   d. *SRY*
   e. *WNT4*

2. During male reproductive tract development, androgens mediate the differentiation of all of the following structures EXCEPT:
   a. seminal vesicles.
   b. ureter.
   c. epididymis.
   d. vas deferens.
   e. ejaculatory ducts.

3. Which of the following does NOT play a direct role in testicular descent?
   a. Testis
   b. Epididymis
   c. Genitofemoral nerve
   d. Gubernaculum
   e. Processus vaginalis

4. Peak levels of testosterone and insulin-like 3 (INSL 3) occur in the male fetus at approximately what gestational week?
   a. 5
   b. 8
   c. 10
   d. 15
   e. 20

5. Cryptorchidism increases the risk of all of the following EXCEPT:
   a. spermatic cord torsion.
   b. clinical hernia.
   c. reactive hydrocele.
   d. infertility.
   e. testicular malignancy.

6. The risk of cryptorchidism is higher in all of the following syndromes EXCEPT:
   a. cerebral palsy.
   b. cystic fibrosis.
   c. arthrogryposis.
   d. prune-belly syndrome.
   e. posterior urethral valves.

7. Abdominal cryptorchidism is associated with all of the following anomalies EXCEPT:
   a. transverse testicular ectopia.
   b. epididymal anomalies.
   c. inguinal hernia.
   d. vanishing testis syndrome.
   e. polyorchidism.

8. Histologic findings in cryptorchid testes may include all of the following EXCEPT:
   a. intratubular germ cell neoplasia, unclassified.
   b. absence of Ad spermatogonia.
   c. early disappearance of gonocytes.
   d. failure of Sertoli cell maturation.
   e. reduced germ cell counts.

9. What percentage of undescended testes are nonpalpable at presentation?
   a. 1%
   b. 3%
   c. 10%
   d. 20%
   e. 30%

10. During laparoscopy, spermatic cord structures exiting an open internal ring ipsilateral to a nonpalpable testis implies:
    a. vanishing testis, inguinal exploration unnecessary.
    b. vanishing testis, inguinal exploration necessary.
    c. intracanalicular atrophic testis, inguinal exploration unnecessary.
    d. intracanalicular testis, inguinal exploration necessary.
    e. further exploration unnecessary if contralateral testicular hypertrophy is present.

11. Advantages of laparoscopic management of an intra-abdominal testis include all of the following EXCEPT:
    a. it more accurately assesses the presence or absence, viability, and anatomy of the testis compared with radiographic imaging.
    b. it allows for laparoscopic repair of the ipsilateral inguinal hernia when present.
    c. it enhances surgical exposure, lighting, and magnification.
    d. it allows a greater degree of proximal dissection of the spermatic vessels.
    e. it allows diagnosis of associated Müllerian ductal abnormalities if present.

12. Which statement is FALSE regarding Fowler-Stephens orchidopexy?
    a. It is less commonly associated with testicular atrophy than laparoscopic orchidopexy.
    b. It has a lower success rate in patients who have undergone previous inguinal surgery.
    c. Blood supply is based on the deferential artery and collateral peritoneal vessels.
    d. It should be performed at a similar age as a standard inguinal orchidopexy.
    e. It should be considered if the testis is not near the internal ring.

13. Which of the following is least consistent with a diagnosis of vanishing testis?
    a. Patent processus vaginalis
    b. Contralateral testicular hypertrophy
    c. Palpable nubbin in scrotum
    d. Increased serum follicle-stimulating hormone (FSH)
    e. Micropenis

14. Lower than expected testicular volume has been associated with all of the following EXCEPT:
    a. cryptorchid testes that have descended spontaneously.
    b. solitary testes in boys with a vanishing testis.
    c. Fowler-Stephens orchidopexy.
    d. increased serum FSH.
    e. surgery for congenital cryptorchidism at 3 years compared with 9 months of age.

15. Regarding epididymal anatomy, which of the following is the most common finding in boys undergoing orchidopexy for acquired cryptorchidism?
    a. Detachment of the cauda epididymis
    b. Detachment of the caput epididymis
    c. Looped epididymis
    d. Long looping epididymis/vas
    e. Normal anatomy

16. All of the following factors may influence the reliability of studies of the efficacy of hormone therapy for cryptorchidism EXCEPT:
    a. treatment of boys with retractile testes.
    b. initial position of the testis.
    c. vanishing testis syndrome.
    d. randomization protocol.
    e. all of the above.

17. A newborn boy presents with a bilateral nonpalpable testes. Next steps in management should be:
    a. karyotype analysis.
    b. hormonal studies.
    c. circumcision.
    d. a and b.
    e. a, b and c.

18. Of the following, which is the least reliable test in confirming the diagnosis of bilateral anorchia?
    a. No change in serum testosterone following human chorionic gonadotropin (hCG) stimulation
    b. FSH level greater than 2 IU/L at 1 year of age
    c. Laparoscopy
    d. Undetectable serum inhibin B
    e. Undetectable serum antimüllerian hormone (AMH)

19. Which of the following is least useful to the provider in determining the diagnosis of retractile versus undescended testes?
    a. Observation of testicular position with abduction of the patient's legs.
    b. History of prior testicular position provided by the patient's family.
    c. Failure of the testis to remain stable in the scrotum with sustained traction on the cord.
    d. Warm room and hands.
    e. Small ipsilateral testis.

20. Which of the following is TRUE regarding spontaneous descent of cryptorchid testes?
    a. Spontaneous descent is independent of testicular position.
    b. Reascent occurs in 40% of patients.
    c. Early descent is more likely in premature boys.
    d. Spontaneous descent is unlikely if the scrotum is small.
    e. The majority of testes that descend spontaneously do so in the first few months of life.

21. The risk of developing testicular germ cell tumor (TGCT) in males with a history of cryptorchidism is:
    a. 2 to 5 times the risk in normal boys.
    b. minimal in boys who undergo orchidopexy in infancy.
    c. determined by placental alkaline phosphatase (PLAP) staining in prepubertal testes.
    d. similar in the contralateral descended testis.
    e. increasing geographically with time.

22. All of the following is more common in association with cryptorchid testes, EXCEPT:
    a. atrophy.
    b. microlithiasis.
    c. mature teratoma.
    d. ectasia of the rete testis.
    e. intratesticular varicocele.

23. The following are possible locations of an ectopic testis, EXCEPT:
    a. peripenile.
    b. perirenal.
    c. perivesical.
    d. perianal.
    e. femoral.

24. Levels of all the following hormones peak after birth and fall to lower levels during childhood EXCEPT:
    a. luteinizing hormone (LH).
    b. FSH.
    c. AMH.
    d. inhibin B.
    e. testosterone.

25. When in fetal development does the testicle pass into the inguinal canal?
    a. 5 to 7 weeks' gestation.
    b. 10 to 14 weeks' gestation.
    c. 20 to 28 weeks' gestation.
    d. 30 to 34 weeks' gestation.
    e. None of the above.

26. How commonly does cryptorchidism occur in full-term males?
    a. Less than 1%
    b. 1% to 4%
    c. 5% to 10%
    d. 15%
    e. None of the above

27. A 6-month-old full-term male presents with a unilateral nonpalpable testis. The next step after a confirmatory exam is:
    a. ultrasound to identify the position of the testis.
    b. hormonal therapy.
    c. surgical intervention.
    d. observation for spontaneous descent until 1 year of age.
    e. a and d.

ANSWERS

1. **d. *SRY*.** The SRY gene appears to be primarily responsible for male sexual differentiation through complex interactions involving both activation and repression of other male-specific genes.

2. **b. Ureter.** Androgens (testosterone, dihydrotestosterone) mediate the differentiation of the paired wolffian ducts into the seminal vesicles, epididymis, vas deferens, and ejaculatory ducts.

3. **b. Epididymis.** Changes in the gubernaculum and processus vaginalis and their innervation by the genitofemoral nerve, as well as hormone secretion by the testis, are all important in the process of testicular descent.

4. **d. 15.** Testosterone production peaks at 14 to 16 weeks and INSL3 peaks at 15-17 weeks.

5. **c. Reactive hydrocele.** All of the others are possible complications of cryptorchidism.

6. **b. Cystic fibrosis.** All the other syndromes are associated with a higher risk of cryptorchidism; mutations of the cystic fibrosis gene are associated with congenital absence of the vas deferens.

7. **d. Vanishing testis syndrome.** All the other entities are more frequently associated with cryptorchid testes located in the abdomen.

8. **c. Early disappearance of gonocytes.** Histological abnormalities that may be present in cryptorchid testes include delayed disappearance of gonocytes, reduced numbers of adult dark (Ad) spermatogonia, reduced number of germ cells per testicular tubule, and carcinoma in situ (CIS).

9. **d. 20%.** Approximately 20% of undescended testes are nonpalpable at presentation.

10. **d. Intracanalicular testis, inguinal exploration necessary.** Although atretic spermatic vessels seen exiting the internal ring may be associated with a distal vanishing testis, the appearance of the spermatic vessels during laparoscopy is subjective, and therefore exploration (inguinal or laparoscopic) is needed to rule out an intracanalicular viable or atrophic testis. Further exploration is unnecessary if blind-ending intra-abdominal spermatic vessels are found. Hypertrophy of a normally descended contralateral testis is suggestive of monorchism.

11. **b. It allows for laparoscopic repair of the ipsilateral inguinal hernia when present.** An inguinal hernia or patent processus vaginalis does not require formal repair at the time of laparoscopic orchidopexy.

12. **a. It is less commonly associated with testicular atrophy than laparoscopic orchidopexy.** Fowler-Stephens orchidopexy, either 1- or 2-stage, has a higher reported testicular atrophy rate compared with laparoscopic orchidopexy. The other statements are true.

13. **a. Patent processus vaginalis.** Contralateral testicular hypertrophy and a palpable scrotal nubbin may present in boys with unilateral vanishing testis and increase serum FSH and micropenis may be seen in boys with bilateral vanishing testes. The processus vaginalis is closed in most cases of vanishing testis.

14. **b. Solitary testes in boys with a vanishing testis.** In vanishing testis syndrome, the contralateral testis may be larger than expected for age.

15. **e. Normal anatomy.** An abnormal epididymis was reported ipsilateral to 11% to 31% of acquired undescended testes at surgery.

16. **e. All of the above.** All are confounding factors that may affect the reliability of studies of the efficacy of hormone therapy for cryptorchidism.

17. **c. a and b.** Circumcision should be avoided in the initial management of phenotypic boys with bilateral nonpalpable testes, pending an evaluation for congenital adrenal hyperplasia.

18. **a. No change in serum testosterone following human chorionic gonadotropin (hCG) stimulation.** Serum testosterone may not increase significantly in response to hCG stimulation in individuals with abnormal testes.

19. **b. History of prior testicular position provided by the patient's family.** Testicular position can change with time and/or be difficult to ascertain in boys with retractile testes; therefore, a careful examination is necessary to differentiate between retractile and undescended testes.

20. **e. The majority of testes that descend spontaneously do so in the first few months of life.** For full-term boys of normal weight, spontaneous testicular descent typically occurs in the first months after birth and is rare after 6 months of age.

21. **a. 2 to 5 times the risk in normal boys.** Surgery may reduce but does not eliminate the risk of TGCT in boys with cryptorchidism, and the risk also exists in the contralateral testis, albeit lower. PLAP+ germ cells can be found in normal testes after birth.

22. **c. Mature teratoma.** The risk of benign testicular tumors is not increased in cryptorchidism.

23. **d. Perianal.** All the other answers reflect possible positions for ectopic testes that are possible although rare.

24. **c. AMH.** AMH levels remain high during childhood and are downregulated at puberty.

25. **a. 20 to 28 weeks' gestation.** The testis passes into the inguinal canal at 20 to 28 weeks' gestation during the fifth phase of testicular descent.

26. **b. 1% to 4%.** Cryptorchidism is one of the most common congenital anomalies, occurring in 1% to 4% of full-term male infants.

27. **c. Surgical intervention.** If descent has not occurred by 6 months of age, surgical treatment should be performed. Diagnostic imaging has not been shown to change the need for surgery. Hormonal therapy is no longer supported, given the lack of evidence to support its use.

CHAPTER REVIEW

1. The Leydig cell hormones insulin-like 3 and testosterone are required for testicular descent.
2. Three fourths of undescended testes are palpable; two thirds are unilateral.
3. The etiology of vanishing testis is most likely due to either in utero torsion or a vascular accident.
4. Confirming that the patient has an absent testis requires identifying a blind-ending spermatic artery.
5. The use of human chorionic gonadotropin for the diagnosis and treatment of undescended testis is not recommended.
6. Laparoscopic identification and mobilization of an abdominal testis is preferred. If the testis can be brought to the opposite internal ring, it can usually be placed in the ipsilateral scrotum.
7. Oligospermia or azoospermia occurs in approximately 75% of patients with bilateral cryptorchidism and in 40% of patients with unilateral cryptorchidism. Paternity in patients with unilateral cryptorchidism is similar to the general population despite the semen abnormalities.
8. Patients with nonsyndromic cryptorchidism have a high incidence of epididymal abnormalities and accompanying inguinal hernias.
9. During fetal development, swelling of the gubernaculum is important to allow for enlargement of the inguinal canal to facilitate testicular passage.
10. Prematurity and low birth weight are risk factors for cryptorchidism; other risk factors include maternal smoking, family history, and maternal exposure to diethylstilbestrol.
11. A karyotype should be obtained if neither gonad is palpable or if there is an undescended testis associated with hypospadias.
12. A two-stage Fowler-Stephens repair is successful approximately 60% of the time.
13. There is a twofold to fivefold increase in the risk of testicular cancer in a cryptorchid testis.
14. Histologic abnormalities that may be present in cryptorchid testes include delayed disappearance of gonocytes, reduced numbers of adult dark (Ad) spermatogonia, reduced number of germ cells per testicular tubule, and carcinoma in situ (CIS).
15. If testicular descent has not occurred by 6 months of age, surgical treatment should be performed.

149 Management of Abnormalities of the Genitalia in Girls

Martin Kaefer

QUESTIONS

1. Which of the following statements is TRUE regarding Mayer-Rokitansky-Küster-Hauser syndrome?
   a. Patients present most commonly with infertility.
   b. It is a homogeneous disorder entailing congenital absence of the uterus and vagina.
   c. It is associated with a spectrum of ovarian abnormalities.
   d. It has associated upper urinary tract anomalies, primarily with the atypical disorder.
   e. It is associated with persistent wolffian duct structures.

2. What is the crucial period in embryogenesis for the formation of the terminal bowel, kidney, paramesonephric ductal system, and lumbosacral spine?
   a. 4 to 6 weeks
   b. 8 to 10 weeks
   c. 10 to 14 weeks
   d. 14 to 18 weeks
   e. After 18 weeks

3. Which of the following is NOT true regarding vaginal agenesis (müllerian aplasia)?
   a. It occurs in approximately 1 in 5000 live female births.
   b. Serum follicle-stimulating hormone and luteinizing hormone levels can be expected to be abnormally high.
   c. Embryologically, it results from a failure of the sinovaginal bulbs to develop and form the vaginal plate.
   d. It is a condition associated with renal abnormalities.
   e. It is a condition associated with skeletal abnormalities.

4. Skeletal anomalies are found in what percentage of patients with Meyer-Rokitansky-Küster-Hauser syndrome?
   a. 10% to 20%
   b. 25% to 35%
   c. 40% to 60%
   d. 70% to 90%
   e. 0% (they are not seen in association with the syndrome)

5. What is the most common cause of primary amenorrhea?
   a. Testicular feminization
   b. Vaginal agenesis
   c. Mixed gonadal dysgenesis
   d. Imperforate hymen
   e. Transverse vaginal septum

6. Which of the following statement is NOT true regarding the genitalia of women with Meyer-Rokitansky-Küster-Hauser syndrome?
   a. In approximately 10% of patients, a normal but obstructed uterus or rudimentary uterus with functional endometrium is present.
   b. Normal fallopian tubes are seen in approximately 35% of patients.
   c. The ovaries are not functional in the majority of patients.
   d. The hymenal fringe is usually present, along with a small vaginal pouch.
   e. The labia majora are typically normal in appearance.

7. Uterus didelphys with unilateral imperforate vagina most commonly present with which condition?
   a. Primary amenorrhea
   b. Cyclical abdominal pain associated with normal cyclical menstruation.
   c. Renal anomalies contralateral to the side of the obstruction
   d. Anomalies of the axial skeleton
   e. Constipation

8. Urethral prolapse is most commonly seen in young females of which ethnic background?
   a. African American
   b. White
   c. Asian
   d. Hispanic
   e. American Indian

9. In most cases of labial adhesions, which of the following is true?
   a. They are believed to occur because of a relative state of hyperestrogenism.
   b. They should be treated with surgical lysis.
   c. They require no treatment.
   d. They occur secondary to sexual abuse.
   e. They have associated renal anomalies.

10. What is the mean age of a child with vaginal rhabdomyosarcoma?
    a. Younger than 2 years
    b. 2 to 4 years
    c. 4 to 8 years
    d. 8 to 12 years
    e. Older than 12 years

11. All of the following statements are true of anogenital condyloma acuminatum EXCEPT:
    a. human papillomavirus is the etiologic agent.
    b. sexual abuse is the only means by which an infant can contract the disease.
    c. many cases in children resolve spontaneously.
    d. pediatric immunization should dramatically reduce the incidence of this disorder.
    e. none of the above.

ANSWERS

1. **d. It has associated upper urinary tract anomalies, primarily with the atypical disorder.** Urinary tract anomalies occur more commonly in patients with the atypical form of the disorder than in patients with the typical syndrome.

2. **a. 4 to 6 weeks.** Laboratory data with teratogens support the concept of a key event occurring between the fourth and fifth weeks of gestation that results in an error in the simultaneous development of the terminal bowel, kidney, bladder, paramesonephric ductal system, and lumbosacral spine.

3. **b. Serum follicle-stimulating hormone and luteinizing hormone levels can be expected to be abnormally high.** Vaginal agenesis, which occurs in approximately 1 in 5000 live female births, is the congenital absence of the proximal portion of the vagina in an otherwise phenotypically (i.e., normal secondary sexual characteristics), chromosomally (i.e., 46,XX), and hormonally (i.e., normal luteinizing hormone and follicle-stimulating hormone levels) intact female. It results from a failure of the sinovaginal bulbs to develop and form the vaginal plate. Hauser brought further attention to the frequent association of renal and skeletal anomalies in these patients and stressed the differences between patients with these findings and those with testicular feminization.

4. **a. 10% to 20%.** Associated congenital abnormalities of the skeletal system have been described in 10% to 20% of cases.

5. **c. Mixed gonadal dysgenesis.** Meyer-Rokitansky-Küster-Hauser syndrome is in fact secondary only to gonadal dysgenesis as a cause of primary amenorrhea.

6. **c. The ovaries are not functional in the majority of patients.** Although occasionally cystic, the ovaries are almost always present and functional.

7. **b. Cyclical abdominal pain associated with normal cyclical menstruation.** As with other obstructive disorders, the patient may present with cyclical or chronic abdominal pain. However, unlike other obstructive processes, duplication anomalies with unilateral obstruction are not associated with primary amenorrhea.

8. **a. African American.** This entity, which was first described by Solinger in 1732, occurs most often in prepubertal black girls and postmenopausal white women.

9. **c. They require no treatment.** Most children do not require treatment unless one of the aforementioned symptoms (urine pooling within the vagina, which may lead to postvoid dribbling; perineal irritation; physical findings of sexual abuse) occurs.

10. **a. Younger than 2 years.** The mean age of patients with primary vaginal tumors is younger than 2 years.

11. **b. Sexual abuse is the only means by which an infant can contract the disease.** Although a very high suspicion for sexual abuse is warranted, it should be kept in mind that perinatal transmission is also a possible mechanism.

CHAPTER REVIEW

1. Remnants of the prostatic ducts give rise to the Skene glands; remnants of the Wolffian ducts give rise to the Gartner ducts.
2. The Bartholin glands are homologues of the bulbourethral glands in the male.
3. The proximal portion of the vagina forms from the fused paired müllerian ducts; the distal portion forms from the sinovaginal bulbs, which later canalize.
4. Clitoral hypertrophy in the newborn should suggest congenital adrenal hyperplasia; other etiologies include neurofibromatosis and an androgen-producing tumor in the mother.
5. A small clitoris may be seen in androgen insensitivity syndrome.
6. In planning treatment for a transverse vaginal septum, it is of critical importance to determine whether there is a cervix and, if present, its exact location relative to the septum.
7. Vaginal atresia differs from vaginal agenesis and testicular feminization in that the müllerian structures are not affected. As a result, the uterus, cervix, and upper portion of the vagina are normal. In vaginal agenesis the uterus is generally absent or rudimentary; there are often associated renal and skeletal abnormalities.
8. A complication of the use of skin grafts to create a neovagina is the increased incidence of vaginal stenosis and the requirement for repeated vaginal dilatation.
9. Most anomalies of lateral fusion have no functional significance.
10. When an intralabial mass appears to be associated with the urethra, workup should always include renal pelvic ultrasonography.
11. Urethral prolapse appears as a doughnut-shaped mass with the urethral orifice in the center; a mass lateral to the orifice may be a periurethral cyst, a prolapsed ureterocele, a urethral polyp, or an ectopic ureter.
12. An imperforate hymen at birth appears as a bulge in the perineum; it may present at puberty as cyclic abdominal pain and amenorrhea.

150 Disorders of Sexual Development: Etiology, Evaluation, and Medical Management

David Andrew Diamond and Richard Nithiphaisal Yu

QUESTIONS

1. Which of the following statements is TRUE about *SRY* (sex-determining region of the Y-chromosome gene)?
   a. It is synonymous with the H-Y antigen.
   b. The expressed SRY protein has a characteristic high-mobility group (HMG), DNA-binding domain.
   c. It is regulated by SOX9 expression.
   d. It was genetically mapped by the study of patients with Klinefelter and Turner syndromes.
   e. It is synonymous with *Zfy* in humans.

2. Which of the following statements is TRUE regarding müllerian-inhibiting substance (MIS)?
   a. It acts systemically to produce müllerian regression.
   b. It is secreted by the fetal Leydig cells.
   c. It functions normally in patients with hernia uteri inguinale.
   d. It is secreted at 7 to 8 weeks of gestation, representing the initial endocrine function of the fetal testis.
   e. It is secreted by the fetal testis at 10 weeks of gestation, after testosterone production has begun.

3. Which description of *WT1* is correct?
   a. Mutations in *WT1* can result in either Denys-Drash or Frasier syndrome.
   b. Mutations in *WT1* are associated with adrenocortical carcinoma.
   c. Loss of *WT1* function has not been associated with genitourinary anomalies.
   d. Duplication of *WT1* has been associated with dosage-sensitive sex reversal.
   e. The gene was originally isolated in cloning experiments and localized to the X chromosome.

4. Which of the following statements is TRUE regarding fetal testosterone?
   a. It results in regression of the müllerian ducts.
   b. It is produced primarily by the adrenal gland.
   c. It acts locally to virilize the urogenital sinus and genital tubercle.
   d. It acts locally to virilize the internal wolffian duct structures.
   e. It enters target tissue by active diffusion.

5. Which of the following statements is TRUE regarding dihydrotestosterone (DHT)?
   a. It produces virilization of wolffian duct structures.
   b. It is converted by 5α-reductase to testosterone in target tissues.
   c. It produces virilization of the urogenital sinus.
   d. It acts locally to produce regression of müllerian structures.
   e. It is secreted in large quantities by the fetal testis.

6. Which of the following statements is TRUE regarding patients with Klinefelter syndrome?
   a. They have at least one X and two Y chromosomes.
   b. They are at increased risk for development of adenocarcinoma of the breast.
   c. They undergo replacement of Leydig cells with hyaline.
   d. They are characteristically fertile.
   e. They bear little resemblance to XX males.

7. The streak gonad of Turner syndrome:
   a. can descend to the scrotum.
   b. has a reduced number of oocytes.
   c. in the presence of a Y chromosome results in increased risk for development of seminoma.
   d. is located in the round ligament.
   e. in the presence of a Y chromosome results in risk for development of gonadoblastoma.

8. Which of the following statements is TRUE regarding patients with "pure" gonadal dysgenesis?
   a. They frequently have chromosomal anomalies.
   b. They are at lesser risk for gonadal tumors than are patients with Turner syndrome.
   c. They lack the somatic defects associated with Turner syndrome.
   d. They have gonadal histology different from that of patients with Turner syndrome.
   e. They derive similar benefit from synthetic growth hormone as do patients with Turner syndrome.

9. What is the common denominator in all cases of Denys-Drash syndrome?
   a. Gonadoblastoma
   b. Nephropathy with early-onset proteinuria
   c. Wilms tumor
   d. Calyceal blunting
   e. Progressive renal failure

10. Which of the following statements is TRUE regarding patients with embryonic testicular regression or bilateral vanishing testes syndromes?
    a. They have normal testosterone and elevated estradiol levels.
    b. They have normal testosterone but decreased DHT levels.
    c. They have castrate testosterone and elevated gonadotropin levels.
    d. They have castrate testosterone and normal gonadotropin levels.
    e. They have normal follicle-stimulating hormone but decreased luteinizing hormone levels.

11. Which of the following statements is TRUE regarding the ovotestis in ovotesticular disorders of sexual development (DSDs)?
    a. It cannot descend from the retroperitoneum.
    b. It is found in the minority of patients.
    c. It can be unilateral or bilateral.
    d. It has testicular and ovarian elements randomly distributed.
    e. It is impossible to cleave surgically.

12. An important consideration for gender assignment in the ovotesticular DSD patient is:
    a. the potential for fertility.
    b. the impossibility of precisely dividing an ovotestis surgically.
    c. that malignant degeneration of gonads does not occur.
    d. the familial pattern of inheritance of the disorder.
    e. the unresponsiveness of the external genitalia to testosterone.

13. Which of the following statements is TRUE regarding the 21-hydroxylase deficiency in congenital adrenal hyperplasia (CAH)?
    a. It accounts for 99% of CAH cases.
    b. It occurs as a result of *CYP21A* gene inactivation in the majority of cases.
    c. It occurs with simple virilization in 75% of cases and salt wasting in 25% of cases.
    d. It occurs with a predictable phenotype.
    e. It is transmitted in an autosomal dominant pattern.

14. Prenatal treatment of patients with CAH with dexamethasone:
    a. is appropriate therapy in seven of eight at-risk fetuses.
    b. is initiated after a diagnosis of CAH is confirmed.
    c. is of no risk to the fetus.
    d. is demonstrated to be effective.
    e. acts by suppressing maternal corticotropin.

15. Which of the following statements is TRUE regarding enzymatic disorders of testosterone biosynthesis?
    a. They are transmitted in an autosomal dominant pattern.
    b. They are associated with persistent müllerian structures.
    c. They appear clinically with a predictable phenotype.
    d. They may involve impaired glucocorticoid and mineralocorticoid synthesis.
    e. They may be associated with fertility.

16. Which of the following statements is TRUE regarding patients with complete androgen insensitivity?
    a. They are appropriately raised as female.
    b. They have normal wolffian duct structures.
    c. They have persistent müllerian duct structures.
    d. They should undergo orchiectomy as early as possible.
    e. They have a 2% incidence of inguinal hernia.

17. What is Reifenstein syndrome?
    a. The group of defects in testosterone biosynthesis that results in male pseudohermaphroditism
    b. A form of 5α-reductase deficiency
    c. Defects of MIS elaboration in utero
    d. A disorder of androgen receptor quantity or function
    e. An autosomal recessively transmitted disorder

18. Which of the following statements is TRUE regarding patients with 5α-reductase deficiency?
    a. Fertility is an important issue in gender assignment.
    b. Isoenzymes 1 and 2 are abnormal.
    c. Serum testosterone levels are normal, but there is a decreased testosterone/DHT ratio.
    d. Masculinization occurs at puberty.
    e. Prostatic enlargement occurs at puberty.

19. Which of the following statements is TRUE regarding patients with persistent müllerian duct syndrome?
    a. They have absent wolffian duct structures.
    b. They represent a homogeneous disorder of involving the MIS receptor.
    c. They should undergo routine removal of müllerian structures.
    d. They experience a high incidence of transverse testicular ectopia.
    e. They are uniformly infertile.

20. Which of the following statements is TRUE regarding Mayer-Rokitansky-Küster-Hauser syndrome?
    a. It presents most commonly as infertility.
    b. It is a homogeneous disorder entailing congenital absence of the uterus and vagina.
    c. It is associated with a spectrum of ovarian abnormalities.
    d. It has associated upper urinary tract anomalies, primarily with the atypical disorder.
    e. It is associated with persistent wolffian duct structures.

21. In an unambiguous neonate with hypospadias and a unilateral cryptorchid testis:
    a. midshaft location of the urethral meatus is an important risk factor for disorder of sexual differentiation.
    b. impalpability of the cryptorchid testis carries a 50% risk of a disorder of sexual differentiation.
    c. palpability of the cryptorchid testis effectively rules out disorder of sexual differentiation.
    d. perineal hypospadias is not a risk factor for a disorder of sexual differentiation.
    e. difference in tissue texture of the poles of the cryptorchid gonad is suggestive of tumor.

22. Gender identity:
    a. is synonymous with gender role.
    b. is primarily determined by prenatal exposure to androgens.
    c. is primarily determined by postnatal environmental influences.
    d. is defined as the identification of self as either male or female.
    e. does not play a role in gender dysphoria.

ANSWERS

1. **b. The expressed SRY protein has a characteristic high-mobility group (HMG), DNA-binding domain.** This domain can induce significant DNA binding when bound to the regulatory regions of target genes. The SRY gene is located on the short arm of the Y chromosome adjacent to the pseudoautosomal boundary. Deletion maps based on the genomes of these individuals were constructed by a number of laboratories, and SRY was mapped to the most distal aspect of the Y-unique region of the short arm of the Y chromosome, adjacent to the pseudoautosomal boundary. SRY expression leads to induction of SOX9 during gonadal differentiation.

2. **d. It is secreted at 7 to 8 weeks of gestation, representing the initial endocrine function of the fetal testis.** The initial endocrine function of the fetal testes is the secretion of MIS by the Sertoli cells at 7 to 8 weeks of gestation.

3. **a. Mutations in WT1 can result in either Denys-Drash or Frasier syndrome.** Denys-Drash syndrome is characterized by a triad of Wilms tumor, congenital nephropathy, and disorder of sexual development (DSD), whereas Frasier syndrome is associated with gonadal dysgenesis, gonadoblastoma, and congenital nephropathy. WT1 is located on chromosome 11 and is not associated with dosage-sensitive sex reversal.

4. **d. It acts locally to virilize the internal wolffian duct structures.** It was clearly demonstrated that androgen is essential for virilization of wolffian duct structures, the urogenital sinus, and genital tubercle. Testosterone, the major androgen secreted by the testes, enters target tissues by passive diffusion. The local source of androgen is important for wolffian duct development, which does not occur if testosterone is supplied only via the peripheral circulation.

5. **c. It produces virilization of the urogenital sinus.** In some cells, such as those in the urogenital sinus, testosterone is converted to DHT by intracellular 5α-reductase. Testosterone or DHT then binds to a high-affinity intracellular receptor protein, and this complex enters the nucleus, where it binds to acceptor sites on DNA, resulting in target gene activation and protein synthesis. Therefore, in tissues equipped with 5α-reductase at the time of sexual differentiation, such as prostate, urogenital sinus, and external genitalia, DHT is the active androgen.

6. **b. They are at increased risk for development of adenocarcinoma of the breast.** Gynecomastia, which can be quite marked, is a common pubertal development in patients with Klinefelter syndrome. As a result, these patients are at eight times the risk for developing breast carcinoma relative to normal males. Males with Klinefelter syndrome have one Y chromosome and at least two X chromosomes. Seminiferous tubular cells undergo replacement with hyaline after pubertal development.

7. **e. In the presence of a Y chromosome results in risk for development of gonadoblastoma.** In patients with occult Y chromosomal material, the risk of gonadoblastoma, an in situ germ cell cancer, is approximately 30%. The streak gonad is usually abdominal in location, is hypoplastic, and predominantly consists of fibrous tissue.

8. **c. They lack the somatic defects associated with Turner syndrome** (e.g., broad chest, neck webbing, cardiac and renal anomalies, and short stature). However, patients with 46,XX "pure" gonadal dysgenesis are closely related to those with Turner syndrome. Because these patients exhibit none of the somatic stigmata associated with Turner syndrome, and their condition entails gonadal dysgenesis only, this type has been regarded by some authors as pure.

9. **b. Nephropathy with early-onset proteinuria.** The full triad of the syndrome includes nephropathy, characterized by the early onset of proteinuria, and hypertension and progressive renal failure in the majority. Because incomplete forms of the syndrome may occur, the nephropathy has become regarded as the common denominator of the syndrome.

10. **c. They have castrate testosterone and elevated gonadotropin levels.** The diagnosis can be made on the basis of a 46,XY karyotype and castrate levels of testosterone, despite persistently elevated serum luteinizing hormone and follicle-stimulating hormone levels. Serum MIS is a useful marker for the presence of testicular tissue and is undetectable in these males.

11. **c. It can be unilateral or bilateral.** Ovotesticular DSD patients are individuals having both testicular tissue with well-developed seminiferous tubules and ovarian tissue with primordial follicles, which may take the form of one ovary and one testis or, more commonly, one or two ovotestes. Histopathology of the ovotestis will typically demonstrate well-developed ovarian tissue and a dysgenetic testicular component.

12. **a. The potential for fertility.** The most important aspect of management in ovotesticular DSD is gender assignment.

13. b. It occurs as a result of gene inactivation in the majority of cases. Mutations leading to gene conversion of the active *CYP21A* gene into the inactive gene occur in 65% to 90% of cases of the classic disorder (salt wasting and simple virilizing) and all cases of nonclassic 21-hydroxylase deficiency. 21-Hydroxylase deficiency accounts for 95% of CAH cases, with 75% of patients presenting with salt wasting and 25% with simple virilization.

14. **d. Is demonstrated to be effective.** Treatment should be initiated before 9 weeks after the last menstrual period, once pregnancy is confirmed. A number of series have established the effectiveness of prenatal treatment of CAH with dexamethasone, which suppresses fetal secretion of adrenocorticotropic hormone. However, a diagnosis of CAH cannot be confirmed before therapy is initiated because the diagnosis is usually made by chorionic villus sampling or amniocentesis. Therefore, if treatment is initiated for all at-risk fetuses, seven of eight may be treated unnecessarily before confirmatory diagnosis.

15. **d. They may involve impaired glucocorticoid and mineralocorticoid synthesis.** A defect in any of the five enzymes required for the conversion of cholesterol to testosterone can cause incomplete (or absent) virilization of the male fetus during embryogenesis. The first three enzymes (cholesterol side chain cleavage enzyme, 3β-hydroxysteroid dehydrogenase, and 17α-hydroxylase) are present in both the adrenals and the testes. Therefore their deficiency results in impaired synthesis of glucocorticoids and mineralocorticoids in addition to testosterone.

16. **a. They are appropriately raised as female.** It is of great interest that, currently, all studies of patients with complete androgen insensitivity support an unequivocal female gender identity, consistent with androgen resistance of brain tissue as well. To date there has been no report of a patient raised as a female who needed gender reassignment to male. Development of wolffian duct structures is androgen dependent. Sertoli cells are present and produce MIS, which results in the regression of müllerian duct structures.

17. **d. A disorder of androgen receptor quantity or function.** Androgen receptor studies in cultured fibroblasts have demonstrated two forms of receptor defect in the partial androgen insensitivity syndrome. These include a reduced number of normally functioning androgen receptors and normal receptor number but decreased binding affinity.

18. **d. Masculinization occurs at puberty.** At puberty, partial masculinization occurs with an increase in muscle mass, development of male body habitus, increase in phallic size, and onset of erections. The type 2 isoenzyme is affected in patients with 5α-reductase deficiency, resulting in an increased testosterone/DHT ratio owing to a reduced testosterone-to-DHT conversion rate.

19. **d. They experience a high incidence of transverse testicular ectopia.** Persistent müllerian duct syndrome is thought to be etiologically important in transverse testicular ectopia, occurring in 30% to 50% of cases. Aberrant MIS function may be secondary to defects in the gene for MIS or in the gene for the MIS receptor.

20. **d. It has associated upper urinary tract anomalies, primarily with the atypical disorder.** Urinary tract anomalies occur more commonly in patients with the atypical form of the disorder than in patients with the typical syndrome. Patients with Mayer-Rokitansky-Küster-Hauser syndrome typically present with primary amenorrhea.

21. **b. Impalpability of the cryptorchid testis carries a 50% risk of a disorder of sexual differentiation.** With a unilateral cryptorchid testis, the incidence of a disorder of sexual differentiation was 30% overall, 15% if the undescended testis was palpable, and 50% if it was impalpable.

22. **d. Is defined as the identification of self as either male or female.** Gender role refers to aspects of behavior that distinguish males and females. The development of gender identity is poorly understood, but is influenced by prenatal and postnatal factors. Individual conflicts with gender identity are central to the concept of gender dysphoria.

CHAPTER REVIEW

1. *SRY* initiates testicular organogenesis. The *SRY* gene is located on the short arm of the Y chromosome.
2. The prostate, urogenital sinus, and external genitalia are all sensitive to dihydrotestosterone.
3. Estrogens are not required for normal female differentiation.
4. Patients with Klinefelter syndrome have eunuchoidism, gynecomastia, azoospermia, and small testes and are tall for their age. Muscle development is poor.
5. Patients with Turner syndrome (XO) have sexual infantilism, web neck, and cubitus valgus; are of the female phenotype; are short in stature; and lack secondary sexual characteristics.
6. In patients with Turner syndrome, any Y-chromosome material increases the risk for the streak gonad developing a gonadoblastoma; these patients also have increased incidence of abnormalities of the kidney, including horseshoe kidney.
7. The diagnosis CAH of the salt-wasting variety is made by obtaining a serum 17-hydroxyprogesterone value 3 to 4 days after birth. If it is elevated, the patient has CAH.
8. In patients who have severe forms of CAH difficult to control medically, bilateral adrenalectomy may be the most effective approach.
9. A distinctly palpable gonad along the pathway of descent is highly suggestive of a testis or rarely of an ovotestis.
10. Patients with bilateral impalpable testes or a unilateral impalpable testis and hypospadias should be regarded as having a disorder of sexual development until proven otherwise whether or not the genitalia appear ambiguous. They should have a karyotype.
11. For normal ovarian development there must be two X chromosomes.
12. In the developing embryo, MIS and testosterone act locally and unilaterally.
13. Mixed gonadal dysgenesis is the second most common cause of DSD after CAH, and it is characterized by a unilateral testis, a contralateral streak gonad, and persistent müllerian structures with varying degrees of inadequate masculinization.

14. The syndrome of complete androgen insensitivity is characterized by 46,XY karyotype, bilateral testes, female-appearing external genitalia, and absence of müllerian structures; the testes are prone to tumors, which usually occur after puberty in 1% to 2% of affected individuals.

15. Persistent müllerian duct syndrome is due to absence of MIS in patients with 46,XY karyotype who have normal male external genitalia and internal müllerian duct structures (fallopian tubes, uterus and upper vagina).

16. The finding of a palpable gonad in a newborn with ambiguous genitalia effectively rules out overt masculinization of the female (congenital adrenal hyperplasia).

17. Patients with Klinefelter syndrome are at 8 times the risk for breast carcinoma relative to normal males.

18. Serum MIS is a useful marker for the presence of testicular tissue in the newborn period.

19. Histopathology of the ovotestis will typically demonstrate well-developed ovarian tissue and a dysgenetic testicular component.

20. Patients with complete androgen insensitivity support an unequivocal female gender identity,

151   Surgical Management of Disorders of Sexual Development and Cloacal and Anorectal Malformations

Richard C. Rink

QUESTIONS

1. Which of the following statements is FALSE regarding the construction of a vagina-utilizing bowel?
   a. Failure to develop an adequate space between the rectum and bladder can result in compromised blood flow to the segment used for vaginal construction.
   b. In general, colon is preferred versus ileum because of its lower incidence of associated postoperative stenosis.
   c. When compared with the McIndoe procedure, the bowel vagina suffers from a higher incidence of postoperative stenosis.
   d. An advantage of a bowel vagina versus the McIndoe procedure includes the lubricating properties of mucus (which may help to facilitate intercourse).
   e. One specific indication for the use of ileum is a previous history of pelvic radiation.
2. Urogenital sinus anomalies in disorders of sexual development states are most commonly seen in association with:
   a. congenital adrenal hyperplasia.
   b. mixed gonadal dysgenesis.
   c. true hermaphroditism.
   d. cloacal anomalies.
   e. gonadal dysgenesis.
3. The most common finding in cloacal anomalies that have been diagnosed by antenatal ultrasonography is:
   a. ascites.
   b. distended rectum.
   c. distended bladder.
   d. distended vagina.
   e. distended bladder and rectum.
4. What is the most common vaginal anatomy in cloacal malformation?
   a. Single vagina, single uterus
   b. Single vagina, double uterus
   c. Two vaginas, two uteri
   d. Two vaginas, one uterus
   e. Single vagina, no uterus
5. Neonatal vaginoplasty combined with clitoroplasty and labioplasty has all of the following advantages EXCEPT:
   a. it allows phallic skin for vaginal reconstruction.
   b. maternal estrogens increase vaginal thickness and vascularity.
   c. tissues are less scarred.
   d. vaginal stenosis is clearly less.
6. The cut-back vaginoplasty is appropriate for:
   a. labial fusion.
   b. low vaginal confluence.
   c. high vaginal confluence.
   d. vaginal atresia.
   e. vaginal agenesis.
7. Surgical management of cloacal malformations involves all of the following steps EXCEPT:
   a. decompression of the gastrointestinal tract.
   b. decompression of the genitourinary tract.

c. vaginostomy.
   d. definitive repair of the cloaca.
   e. correction of nephron destructive anomalies.
8. Fecal continence after cloacal reconstruction is most closely related to:
   a. the level of rectal confluence.
   b. associated urinary anomalies.
   c. neurologic status.
   d. the type of repair.
   e. the timing of the repair.

ANSWERS

1. **c. When compared with the McIndoe procedure, the bowel vagina suffers from a higher incidence of postoperative stenosis.** A high incidence of postoperative vaginal stenosis necessitates postoperative vaginal dilatation in the McIndoe procedure.
2. **a. Congenital adrenal hyperplasia.** Urogenital sinus abnormalities are most often seen in disorders of sexual differentiation states, most commonly in association with congenital adrenal hyperplasia, which has been noted to have an incidence as frequent as 1 in 500 in the nonclassic mild forms.
3. **d. Distended vagina.** The common finding in all reports has been a cystic pelvic mass between the bladder and rectum, representing a distended vagina.
4. **c. Two vaginas, two uteri.** In Hendren's report on 154 patients with cloacal anomalies, 66 patients had one vagina, 68 had two vaginas, and the vagina was absent in 20 (Hendren, 1998). The incidence of vaginal duplication is even higher in the author's own patient population. The uterus anomaly generally is similar to the vaginal anomaly, that is, two vaginas with two uteri.
5. **d. Vaginal stenosis is clearly less.** Other investigators, including the author's group, have thought that vaginoplasty, regardless of the vaginal location, is best combined with clitoroplasty in a single stage. This allows the redundant phallic skin to be used in the reconstruction, adding flexibility for the surgeon, which is compromised when the skin has been previously mobilized. Furthermore, the authors and others have noted that maternal estrogen stimulation of the child's genitalia results in thicker vaginal tissue, which is better vascularized, making vaginal mobilization more easily performed.
6. **a. Labial fusion.** The cut-back vaginoplasty is rarely used and is appropriate only for simple labial fusion.
7. **c. Vaginostomy.** Surgical management now involves four basic steps: decompression of the gastrointestinal tract, decompression of the genitourinary tract, correction of nephron-destructive or potentially lethal urinary anomalies, and definitive repair of the cloaca.
8. **c. Neurologic status.** Fecal continence is directly related to neurologic status.

CHAPTER REVIEW

1. The communication of the vagina with the urinary tract usually occurs in the mid to distal urethra.
2. In patients with congenital adrenal hyperplasia, the location of the confluence of the vagina and the urethra is the critical determinant in the surgical management.
3. Hydrometrocolpos is frequently the initial sign of a urogenital sinus abnormality. It is caused by urine draining into the vagina with poor vaginal drainage.
4. Persistent clitoral hypertrophy may occur in premature infants without DSDs.
5. A cervical impression in the dome of the vagina seen on genitography denotes normal female internal organs.
6. When gonads in the neonatal period require biopsy, a deep biopsy is appropriate because the ovarian component of an ovotestis may cover the testicular component.
7. Renal anomalies commonly occur in patients with a persistent cloaca.
8. Women with CAH are less satisfied as adults with their genitalia than controls.
9. Genital reconstruction must address clitoroplasty, labioplasty, and vaginoplasty.
10. When clitoroplasty is performed, the glans, tunics, and neurovascular bundles should be preserved. The neurovascular bundles should not be mobilized.
11. The timing of surgery for genital reconstruction is controversial: vaginoplasty is best combined with clitoroplasty and labioplasty as a single procedure.
12. Vaginoplasty may be performed with a posterior-based perineal flap for low vaginal confluence, a pull-through vaginoplasty for a high confluence, and vaginal replacement for an absent or rudimentary vagina.
13. The flap in a flap vaginoplasty must reach the normal caliber of the vagina; that is, it must be placed cephalad to the narrowed area of the distal vagina.
14. A vaginoplasty performed in the neonatal period will usually require a secondary procedure after puberty.
15. In cloacal malformations surgical management initially involves decompression of the gastrointestinal tract, generally with a colostomy, and decompression of the genitourinary tract. This is followed by correction of urinary collecting-system abnormalities that impair urine flow. A single stage repair of rectal, vaginal, and urethral abnormalities is performed at a later date when the child is stable.
16. Intermittent catheterization of the vagina may successfully decompress the genitourinary tract in cloacal malformations.
17. Spinal cord abnormalities are frequently found in patients with persistent cloaca.
18. In patients who have had corrective surgery for cloacal abnormalities, a high percentage have a neuropathic component to both urinary and fecal incontinence.
19. In planning treatment for a transverse vaginal septum, it is critical to determine whether there is a cervix and, if present, its exact location relative to the septum.
20. Vaginal atresia differs from vaginal agenesis and testicular feminization in that the Müllerian structures are not affected. As a result, the uterus, cervix, and upper portion of the vagina are normal.

152 Adolescent and Transitional Urology

Christopher R.J. Woodhouse

QUESTIONS

1. Adolescent urology is defined as the care of patients:
   a. from 10 to 19 years old.
   b. from puberty until death.
   c. from 14 to 25 years old for males and from 12 to 21 years old for females.
   d. from puberty to 25 years old.
   e. from puberty until maturity as a young adult.
2. Effective transition requires:
   a. establishment of a care plan for the patient in late childhood.
   b. identification of a destination adolescent clinic.
   c. four or five consults in a transition clinic.
   d. management decisions by an adolescent urology team toward the end of transition.
   e. all of the above.
3. Adolescent urology training requires:
   a. board certification (or equivalent) in urology.
   b. board certification (or equivalent) in pediatric urology.
   c. board certification (or equivalent) in adolescent medicine.
   d. 1 year of training in psychology.
   e. all of the above.
4. In adolescents with congenital abnormalities of the kidneys and urinary tract (CAKUT):
   a. end-stage renal failure within 16 years is unlikely with a glomerular filtration rate (GFR) of 40 mL/min/1.75 m^2.
   b. end-stage renal failure can be prevented with early prescription of angiotensin-converting enzyme inhibitors.
   c. once renal functional deterioration begins, it will usually progress at more than 3 mL/min/yr.
   d. ablation of posterior urethral valves in the first week of life prevents end-stage renal failure in adulthood.
   e. if proteinuria exceeds 50 mg/mmol creatinine (0.5 g/d), renal functional deterioration is inevitable.
5. In which of the following situations should elective cesarean section be performed for urological indications.
   a. Women with spina bifida
   b. Women with intestinal neobladders
   c. Women with a GFR below 40 mL/min/m^2
   d. Women with exstrophy
   e. Women with simple (nonsalt-wasting) congenital adrenal hyperplasia
6. What percentage of adults of working age, born with one of the major congenital urological anomalies (including spina bifida), are likely to be engaged in a profession or administrative occupation
   a. 10% to 19%
   b. 20% to 29%
   c. 30% to 39%
   d. 40% to 49%
   e. 50% to 59%

ANSWERS

1. **b. From puberty until death.** Clearly, the conventional definition of "adolescent" would be the period of growing from childhood to adulthood. That would probably mean from puberty until approximately 20 or 21 years old. When referring to the long-term care of children with congenital genitourinary (GU) anomalies, the term "adolescent urology" has been accepted, for want of a better name. There are no subspecialists of urology to which the children could be sent. Whichever physician them on at puberty is responsbile for their care forever.
2. **e. All of the above.** This answer is really self-explanatory. Parents get very anxious about long-term care for their children while the end of childhood (approximately 9 years old) approaches. They need to be involved in a comprehensive plan that will take them through the several steps to adolescent (adult) urology. This takes time.
3. **a. Board certification (or equivalent) in urology.** In practice, an adolescent urologist will require the skills that are taught in a urology program and will, therefore, be board certified in that specialty. Some training in pediatric urology is needed to understand the nature of the conditions with which the children were born, but not to board level. Adolescent medicine and psychology are required but could be learned through specific courses or online teaching modules.
4. **e. If proteinuria exceeds 50 mg/mmol creatinine (0.5 g/d), renal functional deterioration is inevitable.** A patient who enters in adolescence with a GFR of 40 is likely to go into end-stage renal failure within 16 years. Progression to end-stage renal disease is much slower than in patients with medical renal disease such as glomerular nephritis. Because much of the renal damage occurs before birth in babies with posterior urethral valves (and other conditions), ablating the valve stops further obstruction and allows improvement in GFR, but it does not alter the long-term outcome in most cases. Proteinuria is an ominous sign in all patients with renal disease and, in those with CAKUT, heralds the onset of the final stage.
5. **b. Women with intestinal neobladders.** A reconstructed bladder lies immediately in front of the lower segment of the uterus and is very easy to damage in pelvic surgery. The greatest disasters occur if a cesarean section has to be performed as an emergency. It can take an hour or more to find the uterus. Although many women with reconstructed bladders can and do deliver vaginally, the safe advice is to do an elective cesarean section with an adolescent urologist present to expose the uterus and repair any "urological" damage. In the other conditions, the decision on the mode of delivery should be made jointly by the obstetrician and the adolescent urologist. If there is any doubt, do an elective cesarean section, not a trial of labor.
6. **d. 40% to 49%.** A most important concept of adolescent urology is that successful surgery is not an end in itself. The greater objective is to prepare patients for a normal adult life.

CHAPTER REVIEW

1. The majority of patients in a transitional care clinic will have a diagnosis of either posterior urethral valves or spina bifida.
2. Patients with disorders of sexual development should be seen in a separate clinic.
3. Patients who have had successful hypospadias repairs not infrequently have quality-of-life issues.
4. Ketamine abuse may result in papillary necrosis, retroperitoneal fibrosis, and a shrunken, painful bladder.
5. Adolescents with a GFR greater than 60 mL/min are unlikely to develop end-stage renal disease.
6. Patients who have been reconstructed for significant abnormalities of their bladder or kidneys should be followed up for proteinuria, which is a harbinger of end-stage renal disease.
7. The urine of patients with intestinal diversions may be positive for human chorionic gonadotropin pregnancy test, giving a false-positive result.
8. A reconstructed bladder lies immediately in front of the lower segment of the uterus and is very easy to damage in pelvic surgery. In the pregnant patient, a cesarean section can be difficult, especially if it must be performed as an emergency. It can take an hour or more to find the uterus. Although many women with reconstructed bladders can and do deliver vaginally, the safe advice is to do an elective cesarean section with a urologist knowledgeable about the anatomy.

153 Urologic Considerations in Pediatric Renal Transplantation

Craig A. Peters

QUESTIONS

1. Indications for urodynamic evaluation of a child being prepared for renal transplant include:
   a. poststreptococcal glomerulonephritis-induced renal failure.
   b. end-stage renal disease (ESRD) in a child with wetting but no urinary tract infections (UTIs).
   c. ESRD in a child with nocturnal enuresis.
   d. prolonged anuria after focal segmental glomerulosclerosis (FSGS) renal failure.
   e. ongoing grade III vesicoureteral reflux.

2. Renal transplantation into a child with an augmented bladder is associated with:
   a. cyclosporine toxicity.
   b. hyperchloremic metabolic alkalosis.
   c. refractory rejection.
   d. recurrent infection and risk of sepsis.
   e. no significant change in graft survival.

3. In a 10-year-old boy with a 50-mL capacity bladder, a history of posterior urethral valves, ESRD, and anuria, optimal initial bladder management in preparation for renal transplantation is:
   a. anticholinergic medications and proceeding with transplantation.
   b. bladder cycling by intermittent catheterization.
   c. ileocystoplasty at time of renal transplantation.
   d. gastrocystoplasty and continent catheterizable stoma.
   e. transplant into transverse colon loop and delayed augmentation.

4. Indications for pretransplant native nephrectomy include all of the following EXCEPT:
   a. refractory two-drug hypertension.
   b. multicystic dysplastic kidney (MCDK).
   c. persisting grade III vesicoureteral reflux (VUR) in a 4-year-old.
   d. age under 12 months.
   e. ESRD associated with Denys-Drash syndrome.

5. An antirefluxing transplant ureteroneocystostomy should be performed:
   a. in infants only.
   b. in any child undergoing renal transplantation.
   c. only in children on intermittent catheterization.
   d. in children at risk for UTI or bladder dysfunction.
   e. only in children with neurogenic bladder dysfunction.

6. Following a cadaveric renal transplant for FSGS, a 10-year-old boy is found to have distal ureteral obstruction from a 4-cm stricture that fails balloon dilation and stenting. The best option for management is:
   a. ileal interposition.
   b. Boari flap to graft pelvis.
   c. transplant nephrectomy.
   d. psoas hitch transplant ureteroneocystostomy.
   e. transplant ureter to native ureteroureterostomy.

7. Six months following an uncomplicated living related donor renal transplant, a 7-year-old girl develops acute pyelonephritis of the graft with a rise in creatinine. There is no hydronephrosis on ultrasound. A voiding cystourethrogram (VCUG) demonstrates grade III reflux into the graft, but none in the native ureters. She has normal voiding patterns. The best option for management is:
   a. continuous antibiotic prophylaxis and repeat studies in 18 months, anticipating spontaneous resolution.
   b. open redo transplant ureteroneocystostomy.
   c. transplant ureter to native ureteroureterostomy.
   d. endoscopic injection of subureteral bulking agents.
   e. 6 months of antibiotic prophylaxis and observation.

8. 18 months following an uncomplicated living related renal transplant, a 5-year-old boy with a history of posterior urethral valves develops a rising creatinine, graft hydronephrosis, and two febrile UTIs. VCUG shows grade III reflux into the graft and moderate bladder trabeculation similar to his pretransplant pattern. The best next step in his care is:
   a. psoas hitch ureteral reimplantation.
   b. nontunneled ureteroneocystostomy.
   c. ileocystoplasty and appendicovesicostomy.
   d. transplant ureter to native ureteroureterostomy.
   e. urodynamic evaluation and, likely, anticholinergics and intermittent catheterization.

ANSWERS

1. **b. End-stage renal disease (ESRD) in a child with wetting but no urinary tract infections (UTIs).** The child with ongoing wetting is the most likely to have treatable voiding dysfunction that may put the renal graft at risk. Simple bladder defunctionalization with no history of underlying bladder dysfunction is unlikely to need urodynamic evaluation and often may not need bladder cycling. Reflux alone without recurrent UTI, wetting, or a neurogenic cause is not likely to benefit from urodynamics. Nocturnal enuresis is not an indication for invasive evaluation of bladder function.

2. **e. No significant change in graft survival.** Although early reports implied a high risk due to bladder augmentation in children undergoing renal transplant, modern series have demonstrated the safety, and indeed the benefits, of providing a low-pressure urinary reservoir on graft function. The incidence of positive urine cultures can be increased, but clinically significant infections are not markedly increased.

3. **b. Bladder cycling by intermittent catheterization.** In the child with anuria, bladder function cannot be easily assessed until the bladder has been cycled. Although this child may require augmentation, that cannot be determined until after a trial of cycling is attempted. Transplanting into a diversion is not an acceptable alternative in a child who has the potential for adequate bladder function with medical management and intermittent catheterization.

4. **b. Multicystic dysplastic kidney (MCDK).** All of these clinical situations can justify native nephrectomy except for the presence of an MCDK. There is minimal to no risk in leaving the dysplastic kidney in place. Persisting reflux may be a relative indication, and some practitioners may chose to reimplant the native ureter or simply leave it alone if there is no significant history of infection. Children under 12 months in some centers do not routinely have native nephrectomy, although there is a slightly higher risk of graft loss without this.

5. **d. In children at risk for UTI or bladder dysfunction.** Any child with a risk for UTI or who has bladder dysfunction and may therefore develop a UTI, particularly if immunosuppressed, should have a nonrefluxing ureteroneocystostomy. Some centers perform a nonrefluxing ureteral implantation in all children, although this is probably not essential. Older children and those with no history of bladder dysfunction, recurrent infections, or a structural abnormality can be effectively transplanted with a refluxing ureteroneocystostomy.

6. **b. Boari flap to graft pelvis.** Several options are available for salvage of the graft in this situation, but the most effective is a psoas hitch when there is still some graft ureter available. A transplant to native ureteroureterostomy is effective, but it requires nephrectomy in most cases. Boari flaps may be useful for cases in which the entire ureter is lost or if there is no native ureter remaining. Even with loss of the entire ureter, a renal pelvis–to–native ureter anastomosis is effective. Ileal interposition and graft nephrectomy are not viable options.

7. **b. Open redo transplant ureteroneocystostomy.** The best option in this situation is to redo open reimplantation to create an effective antireflux tunnel. This can be done intravesically or extravesically, or occasionally by using both exposures because of scarring and fibrosis. Spontaneous resolution is highly unlikely, and simply waiting for another episode of pyelonephritis risks graft injury. Transplant to native ureteroureterostomy is an option but requires nephrectomy. Endoscopic injection has a limited success rate in published series, and the durability is undefined. In the setting where another episode of pyelonephritis is associated with significant risk to the graft, such an approach does not seem prudent.

8. **e. Urodynamic evaluation and likely anticholinergics and intermittent catheterization.** This boy is best served by a formal assessment of his bladder function with likely use of anticholinergics to improve capacity and compliance and intermittent catheterization to provide for emptying. One can start this therapy empirically, but having a baseline permits assessment of the treatment effect. Moving directly to augmentation without knowing if medical management can be effective is not appropriate. Simply reimplanting the ureter or performing a ureteroureterostomy without treating the likely bladder dysfunction is also not appropriate.

CHAPTER REVIEW

1. Children who present for renal transplantation often have a congenital obstruction, vesicoureteral reflux, or a neuropathic bladder as the etiology of their renal failure.

2. Indications for urodynamics include neuropathic bladder, posterior urethral valves, voiding dysfunction, hydronephrosis, or recurrent UTIs.

3. The bladder may be refunctionalized with bladder cycling; however, it may take considerable time to reach maximal functional capacity. The goal for refunctionalization should be to achieve 75% of capacity for the expected age and to maintain resting pressures less than 30 cm H_2O for 3 hours. This may require an augmentation cystoplasty.

4. Any major urologic reconstruction should be undertaken well before anticipated transplantation, ideally allowing 3 months for healing to occur before the transplant.

5. Native nephrectomy is indicted in patients with malignant hypertension, profound protein loss due to nephrotic syndrome, recurrent upper tract infections, and massive reflux.

6. For patients on peritoneal dialysis, intraperitoneal surgery will require temporary transition to hemodialysis.

7. An extravesical ureteroneocystostomy is generally preferred for the ureteral vesicle anastomosis for the transplant. There are no data to support routine stenting of the transplanted ureter.

8. In the setting of a rising creatinine level and hydronephrosis, obstruction and rejection may be intermingled.

9. Gastric segments for augmentation are used less often than previously because of the complications, which include acid secretion in a defunctionalized bladder resulting in mucosal erosion, bladder perforation, the hematuria-dysuria syndrome, and the development of malignancy in the segment.

10. Pretransplant psoas hitch and transureteroureterostomy are to be avoided in the pretransplant child, as they may interfere with graft placement.

11. It is important to remember that in the transplanted kidney, obstruction may not be associated with hydronephrosis.

12. Children under 12 months in some centers do not routinely have native nephrectomy, although there is a slightly higher risk of graft loss without this.

154 Pediatric Genitourinary Trauma

Douglas A. Husmann

1. Which of the following signs or symptoms noted after a traumatic insult is suggestive of a preexisting renal abnormality?
   a. Microscopic hematuria with shock
   b. Gross hematuria with shock
   c. Gross hematuria with clot formation
   d. Hematuria disproportionate to severity of trauma
   e. Hematuria in the absence of coexisting injuries to the thorax, spine, pelvis/femur or intra-abdominal organs
2. The radiographic study that is the most sensitive for the presence of a renal injury is:
   a. intravenous pyelogram (IVP).
   b. magnetic resonance imaging (MRI) of abdomen.
   c. focused assessment with sonography for trauma (FAST) ultrasound.
   d. triphasic abdominal computed tomography (CT).
   e. monophasic abdominal CT.
3. Following a traumatic injury, a CT of the abdomen reveals a renal laceration that extends into the collecting system with urinary extravasation. The injury is associated with a devitalized fragment. The grade of renal injury is:
   a. 1.
   b. 2.
   c. 3.
   d. 4.
   e. 5.
4. An 11-year-old boy sustained a renal laceration that extended into the collecting system 2 weeks previously. He has been at home for the past week with grossly clear urine. He presents to the emergency room with the sudden onset of gross hematuria with clots. His blood pressure is normal and his vital signs in the emergency room are stable. The best next step is:
   a. continued observation.
   b. abdominal ultrasound.
   c. a single-phase CT scan.
   d. cystoscopy and stent placement.
   e. angiography.
5. A 9-year-old boy sustained a renal laceration associated with a functional renal fragment that was completely dissociated from the kidney. He has a persistent symptomatic urinary fistula despite combined treatment with a nephrostomy tube, double J stent, and urethral catheter. The best next step is:
   a. angiographic embolization of functional renal fragment.
   b. radio frequency ablation (RFA) of functional renal fragment.
   c. cryotherapy of functional renal fragment.
   d. laparoscopic partial nephrectomy.
   e. open partial nephrectomy.
6. An 8-year-old boy on IV prophylaxis with cefazolin undergoes angiographic embolization of a traumatic arteriovenous fistula (AV) fistula associated with a grade 4 traumatic renal injury. His urine is clear, but on postembolization day 2 he is having febrile temperature spikes to 40°C; blood pressure is stable. Acetaminophen is given for fever and blood and urine cultures are obtained. The best next step in management is:
   a. continued observation.
   b. change in antibiotic coverage to piperacillin.
   c. addition of metronidazole.
   d. CT of abdomen and aspiration of perinephric hematoma/urinoma.
   e. percutaneous nephrostomy drainage of urinoma.
7. A 2-year-old boy sustains a major renal laceration with a tear into his collecting system secondary to child abuse. He has persistent gross hematuria with clots and ileus 5 days following his injury. CT scan reveals a clot filling his renal pelvis, and there is a significant perinephric urinoma. However, good flow of contrast is seen into the patient's ipsilateral distal ureter, findings essentially unchanged from a CT scan done 48 hours earlier. Vital signs and hemoglobin are normal and stable. The best next step is:
   a. continued observation.
   b. angiography.
   c. percutaneous nephrostomy.
   d. cystoscopy, retrograde pyelogram, and stent placement.
   e. surgical exploration and renorrhaphy.
8. Follow-up CT imaging for a grade 2 renal injury should be performed:
   a. only if a patient develops systemic of localized signs or symptoms.
   b. 2 to 3 days after traumatic injury.
   c. 3 to 4 weeks after traumatic injury.
   d. 3 months after traumatic injury
   e. 1 year after traumatic injury.

ANSWERS

1. **d. Hematuria disproportionate to severity of trauma.** The classic patient history that should make the physician think of a preexisting renal anomaly is that the degree of hematuria present is disproportionate to the severity of trauma. None of the other options have been found to be associated with the presence of a preexisting renal abnormality during the evaluation of trauma.
2. **d. Triphasic abdominal computed tomography (CT).** A triphasic CT study (precontrast study, followed by a study immediately following injection and then a 15- to 20-minute delayed study) is the most sensitive method for diagnosis and classification of renal trauma. A single-phase CT study is beneficial in determining renal perfusion and major renal fractures, but may on occasion miss the presence of urinary extravasation and will miss the vast majority of ureteral injuries. FAST sonographic evaluations are operator and experience dependent. It is noteworthy, however, that a normal FAST sonographic evaluation coupled with a serial normal physical examinations during 24 hours will reliably detect all clinically significant genitourinary (GU) injuries.
3. **d. 4.**

GRADE OF RENAL INJURY	DESCRIPTION
1	Renal contusion or subcapsular hematoma
2	Less than 1-cm parenchymal laceration, all renal fragments viable, no urinary extravasations
3	Greater than 1-cm parenchymal laceration, includes renal segmental injuries resulting in devitalized fragments, no urinary extravasation
4	Laceration extending into the collecting system, includes renal segmental injuries resulting in devitalized fragments, urinary extravasation is present. Grade 4 includes shattered kidney, renal pelvic lacerations, and complete ureteropelvic junction disruption.

GRADE OF RENAL INJURY	DESCRIPTION
5	Injury to the main renal vasculature: major renal vessel laceration or avulsion resulting in uncontrollable hemorrhage or renal thrombosis of the major renal vessels

4. **e. Angiography.** Approximately 25% of patients with a grade 3- or 4 renal trauma managed in a nonoperative fashion will have persistent or delayed hemorrhage. Classically, delayed hemorrhage will present 10 to 14 days postinjury, but it may occur as long as 1 month after the insult. Delayed hemorrhage arises from the development of AV fistulas, will not spontaneously resolve, and may be associated with life-threatening hemorrhage. The patient may have had a significant blood loss despite normal vital signs. Shock in a child may be one of the later signs of severe bleeding. IV access should be obtained in the emergency room, and the patient should immediately be transported to the angiography suite for evaluation and embolization of the bleeding site.

5. **a. Angiographic embolization of functional renal fragment.** Persistent urinary fistulae associated with a viable renal fragment that is separate from the remaining portions of traumatically injured kidney are initially managed with percutaneous nephrostomy tube drainage and double J stent placement. If persistent fistula drainage continues, it may be managed by angiographic infarction of the isolated functional segment which may prevent the need for open surgical excision of the functional segment.

6. **a. Continued observation.** Postembolization syndrome is well recognized and self-limiting. It is manifested by pyrexia as high as 40°C, flank pain, and adynamic ileus. Symptoms should resolve within 96 hours after the embolization. When pyrexia develops, blood and urine cultures to rule out bacterial seeding of the necrotic tissue are necessary. Consideration for a repeat CT scan with possible aspiration, culture, and drainage of a perinephric hematoma/urinoma should be given if febrile response persists for longer than 96 hours or if the patient's clinical course should rapidly worsen.

7. **c. Percutaneous nephrostomy.** Most posttraumatic urinomas are asymptomatic and have a spontaneous resolution rate approaching 85%. They will occasionally persist and be associated with continued flank pain, adynamic ileus, and/or low-grade temperature. Frequently these patients are managed via endoscopic intervention, with cystoscopy, retrograde pyelography, and placement of a ureteral stent. It should be noted that both percutaneous nephrostomy drainage and internal stenting are equally efficacious. The advantage of an internal stent is that it prevents possible dislodgment of the draining tube and the need for external drainage devices. The two major disadvantages of internal drainage are that both stent placement and removal, in the pediatric patient population, require general anesthesia. In addition, the small ureteral stents (4 to 5 Fr) placed in young children may become blocked with blood clots from the dissolving hematoma, resulting in persistence of the urinoma. In this young child with large perinephric clots, the best way to manage the problem is with percutaneous nephrostomy. This will allow the physician to externally irrigate the system if the tube becomes blocked with clots.

8. **a. Only if a patient develops systemic of localized signs or symptoms.** Follow-up renal imaging is not recommended for grade 1 or 2 renal injuries or for grade 3 lacerations where all fragments are viable. In patients with grade 3 renal lacerations associated with devitalized fragments, and those with grade 4 or salvaged grade 5 renal injuries, a repeat CT scan with delayed images should be obtained 3 months following the injury. This latter study is obtained to verify resolution of any perinephric urinoma and to define the anatomic configuration and determine the extent of the residual functioning renal parenchyma.

CHAPTER REVIEW

1. Preexisting renal anomalies are commonly found in children who present with traumatic injuries of the kidney.
2. In children, there is a poor correlation between the presence of hematuria and a renal injury.
3. A single-shot IVP intraoperatively is only useful in determining the presence of a contralateral kidney when an ipsilateral nephrectomy is anticipated.
4. The vast majority of AV fistulas that occur after trauma will not spontaneously resolve, unlike AV fistulas following a renal biopsy, where spontaneous resolution is the rule.
5. Most posttraumatic urinomas are asymptomatic and will resolve spontaneously.
6. When there is a coexistence of an intra-abdominal injury adjacent to the urinary tract injury, the two should be separated by interposing tissue such as omentum.
7. Posttraumatic hypertension in children is usually due to a small, poorly functioning kidney; it is renin mediated and nephrectomy is generally the best option.
8. CT findings associated with ureteropelvic junction disruption include medial extravasation, absence of parenchyma lacerations, and no visualization of the distal ureter. Immediate surgical repair is preferred.
9. Traumatic bladder lacerations in children are likely to extend through the bladder neck and require surgical exploration and repair.
10. When a urethral injury is found with a pelvic fracture, a concurrent rectal injury is present in 15%; in females, urethral injuries associated with pelvic fractures are associated 75% of the time with vaginal lacerations and 30% of the time with rectal injury.
11. A diverting colostomy is appropriate in traumatic injuries of the urethra associated with rectal injuries.
12. Penile strangulation caused by hair should be suspected when circumferential edema and/or necrosis is noted from a circumferential point distally.
13. The CT findings following trauma that indicate a need for interventional therapy are: (1) medial extravasation of contrast suggesting a renal pedicle injury, (2) lateral extravasation of contrast with no visualization of the ureter suggesting a ureteral injury, and (3) a large perinephric hematoma that may require angiographic embolization.
14. Radiographic assessment for a genitourinary injury is indicated if the patient has any one of the following: (1) deceleration or high-velocity injury, (2) significant fractures, (3) gross hematuria, and (4) microscopic hematuria with a systolic pressure less than 90 mm Hg.
15. Major renal artery injuries are rarely salvageable.
16. Intraperitoneal bladder injuries require open repair.
17. A triphasic CT study (precontrast study, followed by a study immediately following injection and then a 15- to 20-minute delayed study) is the most sensitive method for diagnosis and classification of renal trauma.
18. Shock in a child may be one of the later signs of severe bleeding.
19. Follow-up renal imaging is not recommended for grade 1 or 2 renal injuries or for grade 3 lacerations where all fragments are viable. In patients with grade 3 renal lacerations associated with devitalized fragments and those with grade 4 or salvaged grade 5 renal injuries, a repeat CT scan with delayed images should be obtained 3 months following the injury.

155 Pediatric Urologic Oncology: Renal and Adrenal

Michael L. Ritchey and Robert C. Shamberger

QUESTIONS

1. A chromosomal abnormality associated with an adverse prognosis in neuroblastoma is:
   a. mutation of chromosome 11p15.
   b. absence of the *MDR* gene.
   c. mutation of the *TP53* gene.
   d. deletion of the short arm of chromosome 1.
   e. loss of heterozygosity (LOH) for chromosome 11p13.

2. In situ neuroblastoma:
   a. invariably progresses to clinical neuroblastoma.
   b. usually regresses spontaneously.
   c. is associated with deletion of chromosome 11.
   d. is usually detected on newborn screening.
   e. is frequently associated with amplification of the *N-MYC* oncogene.

3. Ganglioneuroma is:
   a. a stroma-rich tumor by the Shimada classification.
   b. most commonly located in the adrenal gland.
   c. often found secondary to symptoms from metastatic disease.
   d. associated with acute myoclonic encephalopathy.
   e. associated with an unfavorable prognosis.

4. Screening for neuroblastoma:
   a. has improved survival in patients with neuroblastoma.
   b. has decreased the number of children older than 1 year with advanced staged disease.
   c. has identified more tumors with amplified *N-MYC* oncogene expression.
   d. discovers tumors with an improved prognosis.
   e. is widely performed in the United States.

5. A clinical feature associated with a favorable prognosis in neuroblastoma is:
   a. age older than 2 years.
   b. thoracic location of the primary tumor.
   c. *N-MYC* amplification.
   d. chromosome 1p deletion.
   e. stroma-poor histology.

6. A 1-month-old girl is found to have a right suprarenal mass on abdominal ultrasound. The mass measures 4 cm in diameter. Imaging evaluation detects liver metastases. A skeletal survey is normal. Physical examination reveals multiple subcutaneous skin nodules. The mass is removed and confirmed to be neuroblastoma. Analysis of the tumor reveals no *N-MYC* amplification. The best next step is:
   a. observation.
   b. irradiation to the tumor bed.
   c. vincristine, cyclophosphamide, and doxorubicin.
   d. vincristine, cyclophosphamide, and irradiation to the tumor bed.
   e. autologous bone marrow transplantation after chemotherapy and total-body irradiation.

7. The Wilms tumor, Aniridia, Genital abnormalities, mental Retardation (WAGR) syndrome is most frequently associated with:
   a. deletion of chromosome 15.
   b. advanced-stage Wilms tumor.
   c. neonatal presentation of Wilms tumor.
   d. renal insufficiency.
   e. familial predisposition to Wilms tumor.

8. A 3-year-old boy had undergone treatment for hypospadias and undescended testis as an infant. He develops renal insufficiency. Renal biopsy is consistent with a membranoproliferative glomerulonephritis. Appropriate management before renal transplantation is:
   a. voiding cystourethrogram.
   b. gonadal biopsy.
   c. observation.
   d. bilateral nephrectomy.
   e. serial renal ultrasounds.

9. A 2-year-old boy has a palpable right-sided abdominal mass. Computed tomography (CT) shows this to be a solid lesion. On physical examination, the patient's right arm and leg are noted to be slightly longer in length. His diagnosis is most probably:
   a. Wilms tumor.
   b. neuroblastoma.
   c. angiomyolipoma.
   d. nephroblastomatosis.
   e. renal call carcinoma.

10. A newborn is identified with Beckwith-Wiedemann syndrome. A renal ultrasound is obtained. The clinical finding that best predicts the risk of subsequent Wilms tumor development is:
    a. hepatomegaly.
    b. hemihypertrophy.
    c. nephromegaly.
    d. mutation at chromosome 1p.
    e. family history of Wilms tumor.

11. A 6-month-old girl is diagnosed with aniridia. Ultrasounds are done every 3 months. This will result in:
    a. increased survival.
    b. detection of lower-stage renal tumor.
    c. decreased incidence of bilateral tumors.
    d. decreased surgical morbidity.
    e. detection of tumors smaller than 3 cm in diameter.

12. A deletion of chromosome 11 has been found most frequently in Wilms tumor patients with:
    a. aniridia.
    b. bilateral tumors.
    c. hemihypertrophy.
    d. Denys-Drash syndrome.
    e. Beckwith-Wiedemann syndrome.

13. A 5-year-old boy undergoes nephrectomy for a solid renal mass. Pathology reveals stage 1 favorable-histology Wilms tumor. An increased risk for tumor relapse is associated with:
    a. tumor aneuploidy on flow cytometry.
    b. deletion of chromosome 11p13.
    c. duplication of chromosome 1.
    d. LOH for chromosome 16q.
    e. elevated serum ferritin level.

14. A 2-year-old girl undergoes left nephrectomy for Wilms tumor. A solitary left pulmonary lesion is noted on chest CT. The pathology shows favorable histology but with capsular penetration. The most important prognostic feature is:
    a. capsular penetration.
    b. histologic subtype.
    c. absence of lymph node involvement.

d. age at presentation.

e. presence of pulmonary metastasis.

15. The feature associated with the worse survival in children with Wilms tumor is:

a. diffuse anaplasia.

b. diffuse tumor spill.

c. incomplete tumor resection.

d. tumor spread to periaortic lymph nodes.

e. lung metastasis.

16. An increased risk for metachronous Wilms tumor is associated with:

a. anaplastic histology.

b. clear cell sarcoma.

c. blastemal predominant pattern.

d. renal sinus invasion.

e. nephrogenic rests.

17. A 1-year-old boy undergoes nephrectomy for Wilms tumor. The finding that has the most adverse impact on survival is:

a. hilar lymph node involvement.

b. renal sinus invasion.

c. capsular penetration.

d. ureteral extension of tumor.

e. renal vein thrombus.

18. The factor associated with the lowest risk of local tumor relapse in children with Wilms tumor is:

a. local tumor spill.

b. unfavorable histology.

c. incomplete tumor removal.

d. absence of lymph node sampling.

e. capsular penetration.

19. A 4-year-old girl undergoes removal of a Wilms tumor of favorable histology. Imaging evaluation reveals multiple pulmonary metastases. Treatment should include vincristine, dactinomycin, and:

a. observation.

b. resection of the pulmonary lesions.

c. doxorubicin and chest irradiation.

d. doxorubicin, cyclophosphamide, and irradiation.

e. doxorubicin and etoposide.

20. A 3-month-old boy undergoes removal of a 300-g Wilms tumor of the right kidney. The pathology shows diffuse anaplasia and tumor confined to the kidney. Lymph nodes were negative. The next step is:

a. observation.

b. vincristine and dactinomycin.

c. vincristine, dactinomycin, and irradiation of the tumor bed.

d. doxorubicin, vincristine, dactinomycin, and irradiation of the tumor bed.

e. ifosfamide, etoposide, and doxorubicin.

21. A 5-year-old girl presents with hematuria. CT reveals a right abdominal mass with extension of tumor thrombus into the suprahepatic vena cava. The best next step is:

a. chemotherapy.

b. irradiation.

c. open biopsy followed by chemotherapy.

d. preoperative chemotherapy and radiation therapy.

e. primary surgical removal of the kidney and tumor thrombus.

22. A 2-year-old boy is found to have bilateral Wilms tumor. There is a tumor occupying more than 50% of the left kidney and a 4.0-cm tumor in the upper pole of the right kidney. The best next step is:

a. left nephrectomy and right renal biopsy.

b. bilateral partial nephrectomy.

c. right partial nephrectomy and left renal biopsy.

d. bilateral nephrectomies.

e. chemotherapy.

23. A 1-year-old girl has a stage III Wilms tumor. During the course of chemotherapy she develops an enlarged heart and evidence of congestive heart failure. The drug responsible for these findings is most likely:

a. dactinomycin.

b. etoposide.

c. vincristine.

d. cyclophosphamide.

e. doxorubicin.

24. A 1-year-old boy undergoes left radical nephrectomy for a large renal mass. The pathologic features associated with the worst prognosis are:

a. diffuse anaplasia stage I.

b. focal anaplasia stage III.

c. rhabdoid tumor of the kidney stage III.

d. clear cell sarcoma of the kidney stage III.

e. favorable histology stage IV.

25. A newborn boy was noted to have a left renal mass on prenatal ultrasound. Postnatal evaluation confirms a 5-cm solid mass in the lower pole of the left kidney. The right kidney is normal. Chest radiography and CT of the chest are negative for metastatic disease. The mass was completely removed by a radical nephrectomy. The tumor was confined to the kidney and weighed 300 g. The next step in treatment is:

a. 1200-cGy abdominal irradiation to the left flank.

b. observation only.

c. dactinomycin and vincristine for 10 weeks.

d. dactinomycin and vincristine for 18 weeks.

e. 2000-cGy abdominal irradiation plus dactinomycin and vincristine for 18 weeks.

26. The tuberous sclerosis complex is associated with the development of angiomyolipoma and cystic renal disease. These patients have been found to have an abnormality of chromosome:

a. 1.

b. 7.

c. 9.

d. 12.

e. 14.

Pathology

1. A 4-year-old boy had a right radical nephrectomy for a renal mass. The histology is depicted in Figure 155–1 and is reported as a Wilms tumor with negative margins. Additional information from the pathologist should include a statement as to:

a. differentiation of the blastema.

b. differentiation of the stroma.

c. differentiation of the epithelial component.

d. the presence of an anaplastic variant.

e. the presence of clear cell cancer.

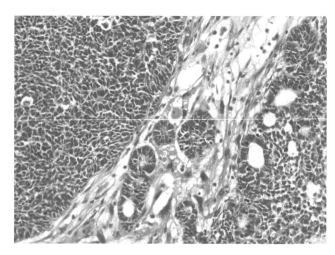

Figure 155–1. (From Bostwick DG, Cheng L. Urologic surgical pathology. 3rd ed. St. Louis: Elsevier; 2014.)

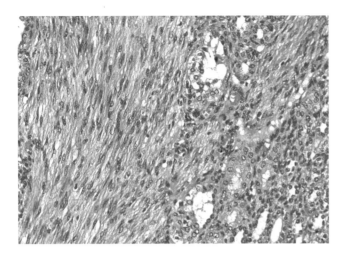

Figure 155–2. (From Bostwick DG, Cheng L. Urologic surgical pathology. 3rd ed. St. Louis: Elsevier; 2014.)

2. A 3-month-old male infant is noted to have a large solid right renal mass. A nephrectomy is performed. The histology is depicted in Figure 155–2 and is reported as a spindle cell tumor. The pathologist should be queried as to:
   a. whether this is a fibrosarcoma.
   b. the degree of anaplasia.
   c. whether this could be a congenital mesoblastic nephroma.
   d. whether there is lymphovascular invasion.
   e. whether there are prominent mitoses.

ANSWERS

1. **d. Deletion of the short arm of chromosome 1.** Deletion of the short arm of chromosome 1 is found in 25% to 35% of neuroblastomas and is an adverse prognostic marker. The deletions are of different size, but in a series of eight cases, a consensus deletion included the segment 1p36.1-2, suggesting that genetic information related to neuroblastoma tumorigenesis is located in this segment.

2. **b. Usually regresses spontaneously.** In 1963, Beckwith and Perrin coined the term in situ neuroblastoma for small nodules of neuroblastoma cells found incidentally within the adrenal gland, which are histologically indistinguishable from neuroblastoma. In infants younger than 3 months of age undergoing postmortem examination, neuroblastoma in situ was found in 1 of 224 infants. This represents an incidence of in situ neuroblastoma 40 to 45 times greater than the incidence of clinical tumors, suggesting that these small tumors regress spontaneously in most cases. However, more recent studies have shown that these neuroblastic nodules are found in all fetuses studied and generally regress.

3. **a. A stroma-rich tumor by the Shimada classification.** The Shimada classification is an age-linked histopathologic classification. One of the important aspects of the Shimada classification is determining whether the tumor is stroma poor or stroma rich. Patients with stroma-poor tumors with unfavorable histopathologic features have a very poor prognosis (less than 10% survival). Stroma-rich tumors can be separated into three subgroups: nodular, intermixed, and well differentiated. Tumors in the last two categories more closely resemble ganglioneuroblastoma or immature ganglioneuroma and have a higher rate of survival.

4. **d. Discovers tumors with an improved prognosis.** The goal of screening programs is to detect disease at an earlier stage and decrease the number of older children with advanced-stage disease and thus improve survival. An increased number of infants younger than 1 year of age have been diagnosed with the mass screening program, and most of these patients have lower-stage

tumors. Regrettably, the number of children older than 1 year of age with advanced-stage disease has not decreased.

5. **b. Thoracic location of the primary tumor.** The site of origin is of significance, with a better survival rate noted for nonadrenal primary tumors. Most children with thoracic neuroblastoma present at a younger age with localized disease and have improved survival even when corrected for age and stage.

6. **a. Observation.** The generally favorable behavior of stage IV-S disease has been explained with the development of biologic markers. The vast majority of these infants have tumors with entirely favorable markers, explaining their nonmalignant behavior. A small percentage, however, have adverse markers, and it is these children who have progressive disease to which they often succumb. Resection of the primary tumor is not mandatory. Although excellent survival has been reported after surgery, information regarding histologic prognostic factors was not available for all of these patients. A more recent review was performed of a large cohort of 110 infants with stage IV-S disease. The entire cohort of infants had an estimated 3-year survival rate of 85%±4%. This survival rate was significantly decreased, however, to 68%±12% for infants who were diploid, 44%±33% for those who were N-MYC amplified, and 33%± 19% for those with unfavorable histology tumors. Of note, there was no statistical difference in survival rate for infants who underwent complete resection of their primary tumor compared with those with partial resection or only biopsy. Patients with extensive metastatic disease who are N-MYC-positive represent a high-risk group. These patients should be considered for a more aggressive treatment with multimodal therapy as per the risk group classification.

7. **d. Renal insufficiency.** Patients with the WAGR syndrome have a germline deletion at 11p13. WT1 mutations and deletions predispose patients to renal insufficiency. Both the Denys-Drash and WAGR syndrome are associated with an increased risk of renal failure. This occurs later in the WAGR syndrome, often in the second decade of life after treatment of the Wilms tumor.

8. **d. Bilateral nephrectomy.** One specific association of male pseudohermaphroditism, renal mesangial sclerosis, and nephroblastoma is the Denys-Drash syndrome. The majority of these patients progress to end-stage renal disease. A specific mutation of the 11p13 Wilms tumor gene has been identified in these children. Although XY individuals have been reported most often, the syndrome has been reported in genotypic/phenotypic females. One should have a high index of suspicion for the development of renal failure and Wilms tumor in patients with male pseudohermaphroditism.

9. **a. Wilms tumor.** Beckwith-Wiedemann syndrome (BWS) is characterized by excess growth at the cellular, organ (macroglossia, nephromegaly, hepatomegaly), or body segment (hemihypertrophy) levels. Most cases of BWS are sporadic, but as many as 15% exhibit heritable characteristics with apparent autosomal dominant inheritance. The risk of nephroblastoma in children with BWS and hemihypertrophy is 4% to 10%.

10. **c. Nephromegaly.** Children with BWS found to have nephromegaly (kidneys at or above the 95th percentile for age-adjusted renal length) are at the greatest risk for the development of Wilms tumor.

11. **b. Detection of lower-stage renal tumor.** Screening with serial renal ultrasonographic scans has been recommended in children with aniridia, hemihypertrophy, and BWS. Review of most studies suggests that 3 to 4 months is the appropriate screening interval. Tumors detected by screening will generally be at a lower stage.

12. **a. Aniridia.** Approximately 50% of patients with WAGR syndrome and a constitutional deletion on chromosome 11 will develop Wilms tumor.

13. **d. LOH for chromosome 16q.** LOH for a portion of chromosome 16q has been noted in 20% of Wilms tumors. A study of 232 patients registered on the National Wilms Tumor Study Group (NWTSG) found LOH for 16q in 17% of the tumors. Patients with tumor-specific LOH for chromosome 16q had

a statistically significantly poorer 2-year relapse-free and overall survival rate than did those patients without LOH for chromosome 16q.

14. **b. Histologic subtype.** Markers associated with unfavorable outcome include nuclear atypia (anaplasia), focal or diffuse, and sarcomatous tumors (rhabdoid and clear cell type). The latter two tumor types, however, are tumor categories distinct from Wilms tumor. These unfavorable features occurred in approximately 10% of patients but accounted for almost half of the tumor deaths in early NWTSG studies.

15. **a. Diffuse anaplasia.** Anaplasia is associated with resistance to chemotherapy. This is evidenced by the similar incidence of anaplasia (5%) in the NWTSG and International Society of Paediatric Oncology studies. Although the presence of anaplasia has clearly been demonstrated to carry a poor prognosis, patients with stage I anaplastic Wilms tumor as well as those with higher stages and focal rather than diffuse anaplasia seem to have a more favorable outcome. This confirms the observation that anaplasia is more a marker of chemoresistance than of inherent aggressiveness of the tumor.

16. **e. Nephrogenic rests.** NWTSG investigators demonstrated the clinical importance of nephrogenic rests. Multiple rests in one kidney usually imply that nephrogenic rests are present in the other kidney. Children younger than 12 months diagnosed with Wilms tumor who also have nephrogenic rests, in particular perilobar nephrogenic rests, have a markedly increased risk of developing contralateral disease and require frequent and regular surveillance for several years.

17. **a. Hilar lymph node involvement.** The most important determinants of outcome in children with Wilms tumor are histopathology and tumor stage. Accurate staging of Wilms tumor allows treatment results to be evaluated and enables universal comparisons of outcomes. The staging system used by the NWTSG is based primarily on the surgical and histopathologic findings. Examination for extension through the capsule, residual disease, vascular involvement, and lymph node involvement is essential to properly assess the extent of the tumor.

18. **e. Capsular penetration.** One study identified risk factors for local tumor recurrence as tumor spillage, unfavorable histology, incomplete tumor removal, and absence of any lymph node sampling. The 2-year survival rate after abdominal recurrence was 43%, emphasizing the importance of the surgeon in performing careful and complete tumor resection.

19. **c. Doxorubicin and chest irradiation.** Patients with stage III favorable histologic type tumors and stage II-III focal anaplasia are treated with dactinomycin, vincristine, and doxorubicin and 10.8-Gy abdominal irradiation. Patients with stage IV favorable histologic type tumors receive abdominal irradiation based on the local tumor stage and 12 Gy to both lungs.

20. **d. Doxorubicin, vincristine, dactinomycin, and irradiation to the tumor bed.** Anaplasia tumors are resistant to chemotherapy. However, if the tumor is confined to the kidney and completely resected the prognosis is good. They do require more intense treatment than children with stage I, favorable histology tumors.

21. **c. Open biopsy followed by chemotherapy.** The current recommendations from the NWTSG are that preoperative chemotherapy is of benefit in patients with bilateral involvement, inoperable at surgical exploration, and inferior vena cava extension above the hepatic veins. All other patients should undergo primary nephrectomy.

22. **e. Chemotherapy.** Patients with bilateral Wilms tumor have an increased risk for renal failure. These patients should receive preoperative chemotherapy without attempts at initial surgery. Repeat imaging after 6 weeks of chemotherapy can assess response to treatment.

23. **e. Doxorubicin.** In recent years, there has been increasing concern regarding the risk of congestive heart failure in children who receive treatment with anthracyclines such as doxorubicin. In addition to the acute cardiotoxicity, cardiac failure can develop many years after treatment.

24. **c. Rhabdoid tumor of the kidney stage III.** Typical clinical features include early age at diagnosis (median age of younger than 16 months), resistance to chemotherapy, and high mortality rate. Unlike Wilms tumor, which typically metastasizes to the lungs, abdomen/flank, and liver, rhabdoid tumor of the kidney, which also metastasizes to these sites, is distinguished by its propensity to metastasize to the brain.

25. **b. Observation only.** The most common renal tumor in a newborn is congenital mesoblastic nephroma. The important aspect of the recognition of these tumors as a separate entity is the usually excellent outcome with radical surgery only. Wilms tumors do occur rarely in neonates, but these patients are eligible for observation only on current protocols.

26. **c. 9.** Two genes have been identified in the tuberous sclerosis complex on chromosome 9 (TSC1) and chromosome 16 (TSC2). It has been postulated that these genes act as tumor suppressor genes and that the LOH of TSC1 or TSC2 may explain the progressive growth pattern of renal lesions seen in these patients.

Pathology

1. **d. The presence of an anaplastic variant.** Wilms tumors have three components as illustrated in the figure: blastema, epithelium forming tubules, and stroma. They are primitive components and are not differentiated. Of critical importance is the presence of an unfavorable histologic type: the anaplastic variant, which profoundly affects treatment and outcome. Clear cell variant is not considered to be a Wilms tumor and is a separate entity.

2. **c. Whether this could be a congenital mesoblastic nephroma.** The figure illustrates a congenital mesoblastic nephroma of the classic type. It is composed of spindle cells that lack cytologic atypia or mitotic activity. This is a classic presentation with a classic histology, and the pathologist should be asked to give a specific diagnosis—"spindle cell tumor" is merely a histologic description.

CHAPTER REVIEW

1. Neuroblastoma is the most common extracranial solid tumor of childhood; 75% arise in the retroperitoneum, 50% in the adrenal, and 25% in the paravertebral ganglia.

2. N-MYC oncogene occurs in 20% of primary neuroblastoma tumors and is an adverse prognostic indicator. Deletion of the short arm of chromosome 1 is found in 25% to 35% of neuroblastomas and is an adverse prognostic marker.

3. Neuroblastoma, ganglioneuroblastoma, and ganglioneuroma form a histologic spectrum of differentiation from malignant to benign.

4. Symptoms of neuroblastoma include those due to catecholamine release, those due to vasoactive intestinal peptide (watery diarrhea), and myoclonic encephalopathy.

5. The finding of intratumor fine stippled calcifications with vascular encasement distinguishes neuroblastoma from Wilms tumor on imaging.

6. Stage IV-S (S meaning special) refers to a small primary tumor with metastases to the liver, skin, and/or bone marrow without radiographic evidence of bone metastases. These patients generally demonstrate a favorable response to treatment, which has been explained by the fact that the vast majority of these infants have tumors with entirely favorable markers explaining their relatively nonmalignant behavior.

7. Complete surgical resection is curative for low-staged neuroblastoma.

8. Familial neuroblastoma has an autosomal dominant pattern of inheritance.

9. Imaging for proper staging of neuroblastoma should include an abdominal CT scan (or MRI), bone scan, and metaiodobenzylguanidine scan.

10. Children who have neuroblastoma and are younger than 1 year have a better prognosis. A better survival rate is also noted for nonadrenal primary tumors.

11. Patients with multiple nephrogenic rests (nephroblastomatosis) are prone to develop Wilms tumors that may be bilateral.

12. In Wilms tumor, loss of heterozygosity at 1p and 16q is associated with an increased risk of tumor relapse and death.

13. There is an association between Wilms tumor and horseshoe kidney.

14. There are three histologic components of Wilms tumor: blastemal, epithelial, and stromal. Tumors with a predominant epithelial component are less aggressive.

15. The anaplastic variant of Wilms tumor is associated with resistance to chemotherapy.

16. Clear cell sarcoma and rhabdoid tumors are not Wilms variants but, rather, distinct histologic types of renal malignancies. They have a high mortality rate and may be associated with brain metastases.

17. There is an increased incidence of second malignant neoplasms in children treated for Wilms tumors.

18. Intraoperative lymph node sampling is mandatory when surgically removing a Wilms tumor.

19. The lung is the most frequent site of distant metastases from a Wilms tumor.

20. Renal cell carcinoma is the most common renal malignancy in the second decade of life; the papillary variant is more common in children.

21. Congenital mesoblastic nephroma is the most common tumor of infants with a peak age of presentation of 3 months; there are three histologic subtypes: classic, cellular, and mixed. Nephrectomy is usually curative; however, the cellular subtype has been associated with recurrence.

22. The Denys-Drash syndrome is characterized by male pseudohermaphroditism, renal mesangial sclerosis, and nephroblastoma.

23. Screening with serial renal ultrasounds has been recommended in children with aniridia, hemihypertrophy, and BWS.

24. The staging system used by the NWTSG is based primarily on the surgical and histopathologic findings. Examination for extension through the capsule, residual disease, vascular involvement, and lymph node involvement is essential to properly assess the extent of the tumor.

25. Preoperative chemotherapy for patients with Wilms tumors is of benefit in patients with bilateral involvement, those inoperable at surgical exploration, and IVC extension above the hepatic veins. All other patients should undergo primary nephrectomy.

26. There is a risk of developing congestive heart failure in children who have received treatment with anthracyclines such as doxorubicin.

156 Pediatric Urologic Oncology: Bladder and Testis

Fernando Ferrer

QUESTIONS

1. A 3-year-old girl has vaginal rhabdomyosarcoma. Her mother has a history of breast cancer. This patient most likely has:
   a. Beckwith-Wiedemann syndrome (BWS).
   b. Li-Fraumeni syndrome.
   c. Perlman syndrome.
   d. fragile X syndrome.
   e. Sotos syndrome.

2. A 3-year-old boy has rhabdomyosarcoma of the prostate. An unfavorable prognostic feature of this tumor is:
   a. alveolar histologic type.
   b. embryonal histology.
   c. loss of heterozygosity (LOH) for chromosome 11p15.
   d. botryoid pattern.
   e. spindle cell variant.

3. A 1-year-old girl previously had a partial cystectomy for rhabdomyosarcoma of the bladder. After completion of vincristine, dactinomycin, and cyclophosphamide (VAC) chemotherapy, biopsy of the bladder reveals rhabdomyoblasts. Abdominal and chest computed tomography (CT) are negative. The next step is:
   a. radiation therapy.
   b. continue chemotherapy.
   c. cystectomy with diversion.
   d. observation.
   e. a change in chemotherapy regimen.

4. A 4-year-old boy has paratesticular rhabdomyosarcoma noted on biopsy of the spermatic cord lesion. The next step is radical orchiectomy and:
   a. vincristine, dactinomycin, and cyclophosphamide.
   b. retroperitoneal lymph node dissection.
   c. retroperitoneal lymph node sampling.
   d. radiation therapy to the retroperitoneum.
   e. cisplatin, etoposide, and vincristine.

5. A 2-year-old boy undergoes left orchiectomy. Pathology reveals a yolk sac tumor confined to the testis. CT findings of the chest and abdomen are negative. No preoperative tumor markers were obtained. At 4 weeks after surgery, tumor markers are negative. The next step is:
   a. lymph node dissection.
   b. observation.
   c. chemotherapy.
   d. staining of the tumor for α-fetoprotein.
   e. retroperitoneal lymph node sampling.

6. A 6-year-old, phenotypic boy with hypospadias and bilateral cryptorchidism has a 3-cm lower abdominal mass. His karyotype is XO/XY. At abdominal exploration, a tumor is found in the right gonad. Right orchiectomy is performed. Frozen section reveals gonadoblastoma. The best next step is:
   a. left orchiopexy.
   b. retroperitoneal lymphadenectomy node sampling.
   c. left orchiectomy.
   d. chemotherapy.
   e. observation.

7. A 2-year-old boy has a left upper pole testicular mass that is cystic on ultrasonography. Excision of the lesion is performed by an inguinal approach leaving the lower half of the testis. Frozen section demonstrates clear margins. Final pathology reveals teratoma, and the margins are negative for tumor. Serum α-fetoprotein and β-human chorionic gonadotropin (hCG) are negative. Chest and abdominal CT are negative. The next step is:
   a. radical orchiectomy and modified retroperitoneal lymph node dissection.
   b. observation.
   c. radical orchiectomy and combination chemotherapy.
   d. radical orchiectomy.
   e. radical orchiectomy and abdominal irradiation.

8. A 3-month-old boy undergoes removal of a solid yolk sac tumor. The margins of resection are negative for tumor. Chest and abdominal CT results show no signs of metastatic disease. Two weeks postoperatively, the serum α-fetoprotein value is 35 ng/dL. The next step is:
   a. chemotherapy.
   b. retroperitoneal lymph node dissection.
   c. observation.
   d. retroperitoneal lymph node sampling.
   e. abdominal irradiation.

9. A 10-year-old boy presents with one episode of gross hematuria. Ultrasound of the bladder demonstrates a small (less than 1-cm) lesion at the bladder base, and cystoscopy reveals a small papillary lesion that is completely resected. Pathology reveals superficial low grade transitional cell carcinoma (TCC). Appropriate next steps include:
   a. a course of bacille Calmette-Guérin (BCG) therapy in an attempt to prevent recurrence.
   b. routine cystoscopic surveillance for 5 years.
   c. no further treatment and surveillance consisting of bladder sonography.
   d. mitomycin C bladder instillations.
   e. staging abdominal-pelvic CT scan and lung radiograph.

10. A 5-year-old male who presents with hematuria is discovered to have a 5-cm mass, which is biopsied and found to be consistent with embryonal rhabdomyosarcoma (RMS). The patient undergoes therapy according to Cooperative Oncology Group intermediate risk protocols (chemotherapy and radiation). At the completion of treatment, the child has a residual 0.5-cm mass, which is biopsied and confirmed to consist of mature rhabdomyoblasts. Future treatment should consist of:
    a. cystoprostatectomy with assessment of margins to determine future treatment.
    b. salvage chemotherapy.
    c. observation only.
    d. cystoprostatectomy followed by adjuvant chemotherapy.
    e. implantation of radiotherapy beads.

11. An 11-year-old male presents with a right paratesticular mass. A inguinal orchiectomy is performed. The pathologic diagnosis is RMS completely excised (clinical group 1). A consulting physician orders a CT scan of the retroperitoneum, which is negative. The next step should be:
    a. observation only.
    b. right staging ipsilateral retroperitoneal lymph node dissection (RPLND).
    c. right staging ipsilateral RPLND plus inguinal lymph node dissection.
    d. right inguinal lymph node dissection.
    e. chemotherapy.

12. A 4-month-old male is noted to have a right testicular mass. Ultrasound reveals a well-circumscribed, heterogenous, cystic mass with calcifications. Serum hCG is within normal limits.

The serum α-fetoprotein is elevated at 90 ng/mL. The most likely appropriate treatment is:
a. radical inguinal orchiectomy.
b. transscrotal exploration and biopsy.
c. inguinal exploration, cord control, biopsy, and partial orchiectomy.
d. transscrotal partial orchiectomy.
e. staging CT scan.

13. A 5-year-old male presents with difficulty voiding and gross hematuria as well as right flank discomfort. Ultrasound demonstrates a 5-cm mass at the level of the trigone with moderate-to-severe right-sided hydronephrosis. A pelvic CT scan confirms these findings and does not suggest the presence of pelvic adenopathy. The next appropriate steps would be:
a. open resection and right ureteral reimplantation.
b. endoscopic biopsy followed by right internal stent placement if possible.
c. attempt a complete endoscopic resection.
d. percutaneous nephrostomy tube placement followed by open biopsy.
e. transrectal sonography-guided needle biopsy.

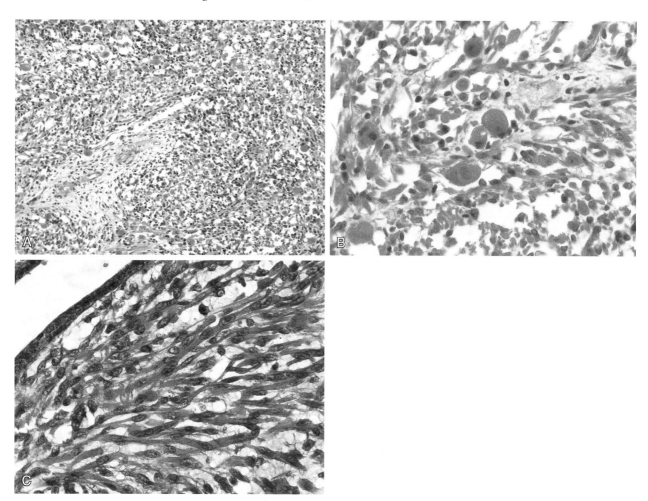

Figure 156-1. From Bostwick DG, Cheng L. Urologic surgical pathology. 3rd ed. Edinburgh: Mosby; 2014.

Pathology

1. A 4-year-old boy presents with urinary retention. He has had constipation and progressively increased stranguria of 2 months' duration. Cystoscopy reveals a polypoid mass arising from the prostate extending into the bladder. The biopsy is depicted in Figure 156-1A, B, and C, which is reported as rhabdomyosarcoma. Note the intensely eosinophilic-stained cytoplasm of the rhabdomyoblasts (Fig. 156-1B). Before treatment is begun, the pathologist should be queried as to:
a. the depth of invasion.
b. the histologic type.
c. the degree of differentiation.
d. the dominant pattern.
e. the percent of rhabdomyoblasts in the tumor.

ANSWERS

1. **b. Li-Fraumeni syndrome.** Subgroups of children with a genetic predisposition to the development of rhabdomyosarcoma have been identified. The Li-Fraumeni syndrome associates childhood sarcomas with mothers who have an excess of premenopausal breast cancer and with siblings who have an increased risk of cancer. A mutation of the *TP53* tumor suppressor gene was found in the tumors in all patients with this syndrome.

2. **a. Alveolar histologic type.** The second most common form is alveolar, which occurs more commonly in the trunk and extremities than in genitourinary sites and has a worse prognosis. Alveolar rhabdomyosarcoma also has a higher rate of local recurrence and spread to regional lymph nodes, bone marrow, and distant sites.

3. **d. Observation.** If tumor is shrinking during chemotherapy, and another biopsy after completing radiotherapy shows maturing rhabdomyoblasts without frank tumor cells, total cystectomy can be postponed or avoided altogether.

4. **a. Vincristine, dactinomycin, and cyclophosphamide.** Before effective chemotherapy, surgery alone produced a 50% 2-year relapse-free survival rate. With current multimodal treatment, survival rates of 90% are expected. Currently, the Intergroup Rhabdomyosarcoma Study Group recommends that children

10 years and older undergo ipsilateral retroperitoneal lymph node dissection before chemotherapy.

5. **b. Observation.** It is important to note that an elevated α-fetoprotein level after orchiectomy for yolk sac tumor in an infant does not always represent persistent disease. Normal adult reference laboratory values for α-fetoprotein cannot be used in young children, because α-fetoprotein synthesis continues after birth. Normal adult levels (less than 10 mg/mL) are not reached until 8 months of age.

6. **c. Left orchiectomy.** Early gonadectomy is advocated, because tumors have been reported in children younger than 5 years. In patients with mixed gonadal dysgenesis who are reared as males, all streak gonads and undescended testes should be removed. Scrotal testes can be preserved, because they are less prone to tumor development.

7. **b. Observation.** Prepubertal mature teratomas have a benign clinical course, which contrasts with the clinical behavior of teratomas in adults, which have the propensity to metastasize. This benign behavior has led to the consideration of testicular-sparing procedures rather than radical orchiectomy.

8. **c. Observation.** The initial treatment for yolk sac tumor is radical inguinal orchiectomy. This treatment is curative in most children. Routine retroperitoneal lymph node dissection and adjuvant chemotherapy are not indicated.

9. **c. No further treatment and surveillance consisting of bladder sonography.** TCC in children is uncommon and the lesions are unifocal, typically low grade and not prone to recurrence; therefore treatment consisting of resection only is adequate. Ultrasound is remarkably accurate and is an adequate surveillance strategy.

10. **c. Observation only.** Mature rhabdomyoblasts found after treatment for RMS do not require further treatment if confirmed by an experienced pathologist. Furthermore, prior studies have demonstrated that some residual mass does not necessarily mean active residual disease exists. In the case presented, further aggressive therapy is not warranted, but serial radiographic evaluation is indicated

11. **b. Right staging ipsilateral retroperitoneal lymph node dissection (RPLND).** Prior studies have shown that children older than age 10 should always undergo siRPLND and not observation because of a high occurrence of retroperitoneal failure. Paratesticular RMS rarely involves the inguinal nodes

12. **e. Inguinal exploration, cord control, biopsy, and partial orchiectomy.** Teratomas are common benign prepubertal tumors that can be treated by partial orchiectomy. Although not always accurate, the ultrasound features of this tumor are suggestive of teratoma. α-Fetoprotein levels do not reach normal adult levels until close to 1 year of life; therefore this elevation is not necessarily reflective of a yolk sac tumor. In fact, yolk sac tumors typically have α-fetoprotein elevations higher than 100 ng/mL. The likelihood of a benign etiology warrants attempt at partial orchiectomy

13. **b. Endoscopic biopsy followed by right internal stent placement if possible.** This presentation is concerning for bladder RMS. In this case organ preservation strategies should be pursued, and endoscopic biopsy is the correct answer. Chemotherapy for RMS can be deleterious to renal function, so stenting to prevent any renal deterioration during treatment should be performed. Internal stent placement is typically more confortable than percutaneous nephrostomy.

Pathology

1. **b. The histologic type.** Rhabdomyosarcomas have three histologic types: embryonal, alveolar, and undifferentiated. The most common type in the genitourinary tract is embryonal and has a better prognosis than the other two. Therapy is determined by stratification as to risk, and histology is one of the parameters used to stratify patients.

CHAPTER REVIEW

1. Of rhabdomyosarcomas, 15% to 20% occur in the genitourinary system. RMS is the most common soft tissue sarcoma in children.
2. Rhabdomyosarcoma has three histologic types: embryonal, alveolar, and undifferentiated.
3. In the genitourinary tract, embryonal histology is by far the most common.
4. Alveolar rhabdomyosarcoma has a higher rate of local recurrence and spread to regional lymph nodes, bone marrow, and distant sites when compared to embryonal.
5. There are two variants of embryonal histology: botryoid (bunch of grapes), which occur in the bladder, and spindle cell, which are common in the paratesticular region.
6. For patients with rhabdomyosarcoma, generally, chemotherapy and radiation precede surgical resection unless the tumor is amenable to a partial cystectomy. Organ preservation is the goal of treatment.
7. Mature rhabdomyoblasts found after treatment do not require further treatment.
8. Radiation therapy for patients with bladder or prostate rhabdomyosarcoma results in a markedly reduced functional bladder capacity and abnormal voiding patterns. Only 40% of patients treated will have normal bladder function—usually these are patients who have not received radiation therapy.
9. Patients with rhabdomyosarcoma of the bladder or prostate typically present with symptoms of outlet obstruction and hematuria. A urethral catheter for the lower tract and an internal stent for the upper tracts are the preferred methods of decompression.
10. In paratesticular rhabdomyosarcoma, children who are 10 years and older should have an ipsilateral retroperitoneal lymph node dissection. Those less than 10 years of age do not require an RPLND.
11. Favorable sites of origin for rhabdomyosarcoma include paratesticular, vulvar-vaginal, and uterine. In the female, the vagina is the most common site. Bladder and prostate are unfavorable sites.
12. Only one third of patients are fertile following treatment for rhabdomyosarcoma.
13. Treated patients are at risk for secondary malignancies, which include osteosarcoma, Ewing sarcoma, lymphoma, cancer of the colon, and cervical cancer.
14. The Li-Fraumeni syndrome associates childhood sarcomas with mothers who have an excess of premenopausal breast cancer and with siblings who have an increased risk of cancer. A mutation of the *TP53* tumor suppressor gene is found in the tumors of these patients.
15. TCC of the bladder in children is uncommon and the lesions are unifocal, often located on the trigone, typically low grade, and not prone to recurrence; therefore, treatment consisting of resection only is adequate. Ultrasound is remarkably accurate and is an adequate surveillance strategy. Cyclophosphamide and dantrolene exposure in selected cases may be etiologic.
16. Patients with a history of smoking, those with end-stage renal disease, and those with transplants who are immunosuppressed and have bladder intestinal augments are at greatest risk for cancer in the augment.